COMMUNITY HEALTH NURSING

Process and Practice for Promoting Health

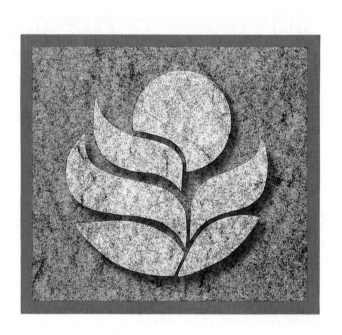

COMMUNITY HEALTH NURSING

Process and Practice for Promoting Health

MARCIA STANHOPE, RN, DSN, FAAN

Professor and Director,
Division of Community Health Nursing and Administration,
College of Nursing, University of Kentucky,
Lexington, Kentucky

JEANETTE LANCASTER, RN, PhD, FAAN

Dean and Sadie Heath Cabaniss Professor
School of Nursing
University of Virginia
Charlottesville, Virginia

with 239 illustrations

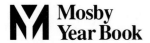
Mosby
Year Book

St. Louis Baltimore Boston Chicago London Philadelphia Sydney Toronto

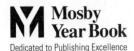
Mosby
Year Book
Dedicated to Publishing Excellence

Executive Editor: Darlene Como
Developmental Editors: Laurie Sparks, Susan R. Epstein, Linda McKinley
Project Manager: Mark Spann
Production Editor: Daniel J. Johnson
Designer: Jeanne Wolfgeher

THIRD EDITION

Printed in the United States of America

Mosby-Year Book, Inc.
11830 Westline Industrial Drive
St. Louis, MO 63146

Library of Congress Cataloging-in-Publication Data

Community health nursing : process and practice for promoting health /
   [edited by] Marcia Stanhope, Jeanette Lancaster. — 3rd ed.
      p.   cm.
   Includes bibliographical references and index.
   ISBN 0-8016-4774-6
   1. Community health nursing. I. Stanhope, Marcia.
   II. Lancaster, Jeanette.
   [DNLM: 1. Community Health Nursing—United States. WY 106 C7356]
  RT98.C6562 1992
  362.1′73—dc20
  DNLM/DLC
  for Library of Congress   91-29999
                                             CIP

GW/VH/VH

CONTRIBUTORS

Mary N. Albrecht, RN, PhD
Post-Doctoral Fellow
Community Health Nursing
University of Michigan
School of Nursing
Ann Arbor, Michigan

Associate Professor
Elmhurst College
Elmhurst, Illinois

Rena Alford, BSN, MN, PNP
State Director of Public Health Nursing
South Carolina Department of Health and Environment Control
Columbia, South Carolina

Sandra Anderson, RN, PhD
Nurse Scientist
World Health Organization Global Programme on AIDS
Geneva, Switzerland

Julia W. Balzer, RN, MN
Staff Educator
Baptist Medical Center
Jacksonville, Florida

Eleanor Bauwens, RN, PhD, FAAN
Professor
University of Arizona
College of Nursing
Tucson, Arizona

Marjorie Glaser Bindner, RN, MA
Continuing Education Consultant and Artist
Kentucky Nurses' Association
Louisville, Kentucky

Kathleen Beckman Blomquist, RN, PhD
Post-Doctoral Scholar
Sanders Brown Center on Aging
University of Kentucky
Lexington, Kentucky

Diane E. Boyer, BSN, RN, MSN, CS
Clinician 2
Neonatal Intensive Care Unit,
University of Virginia Health Sciences Center
Charlottesville, Virginia

Jacquelyn Campbell, RN, PhD, FAAN
Associate Professor
College of Nursing
Wayne State University
Detroit, Michigan

Ann Cary, BSN, PhD, MPH
Professor and Associate Dean for Student and Alumni Affairs
Louisiana State University
Medical Center
School of Nursing
New Orleans, Louisiana

Carol J. Loveland-Cherry, RN, PhD
Assistant Professor
Community Health Nursing
The University of Michigan
School of Nursing
Ann Arbor, Michigan

Marcia Cowan, RN, C, MSN, PNP
Clinical Nurse Specialist
Vanderbilt University Medical Center
Nashville, Tennessee

Beverly C. Flynn, RN, PhD, FAAN
Professor, Community Health Nursing
Indiana University
School of Nursing
Director
Institute of Action Research for Community Health
Head, World Health Organization Collaborating Center on
    Healthy Cities
Director, Healthy Cities Indiana
Indianapolis, Indiana

Sara T. Fry, RN, PhD, FAAN
Associate Professor
School of Nursing
University of Maryland at Baltimore
Baltimore, Maryland

Jean Goeppinger, RN, MS, PhD
Professor
University of Michigan
School of Nursing
Ann Arbor, Michigan

Phyllis Graves, RN, MPH, DSN
Professor (Retired)
College of Nursing
Northwestern State University
Shreveport, Louisiana

Patty J. Hale, RN, MSN
Assistant Professor
School of Nursing
University of Virginia
Charlottesville, Virginia

Nancy Dickenson-Hazard, RN, CPNP, MSN
Executive Director
The National Certification Board of Pediatric Nurse Practitioners
    and Nurses
Rockville, Maryland

Irma Heppner, RN, MS, CS
Director of Emergency Services
Region 10 Community Services Board
Charlottesville, Virgina

Judith B. Igoe, MS, RN, FAAN
Associate Professor
Director, School Health Programs
University of Colorado
School of Nursing
Denver, Colorado

Rosemary Johnson, RN, MPH
Professor Emeritus
College of Nursing
Arizona State University
Tempe, Arizona

Karen T. Labuhn, RN, PhD
Senior Research Associate
Kaiser Permanente Center for Health Research
Portland, Oregon

Jeanette Lancaster, RN, PhD, FAAN
Sadie Heath Cabaniss Professor of Nursing
Dean, School of Nursing
University of Virginia
Charlottesville, Virginia

Wade Lancaster, PhD
Marketing Analyst
University of Virginia
Health Sciences Center
Charlottesville, Virginia

Peggye Guess Lassiter, RN, BSN, MSN
Assistant Professor
Howard University
College of Nursing
Washington, DC

Gwendolen Lee, RN, EdD
Associate Professor and Director
Division of Parent-Child Nursing
College of Nursing
University of Kentucky
Lexington, KY

Roberta K. Lee, RN, DrPH
Associate Professor
University of Texas Medical Branch at Galveston
College of Nursing
Galveston, Texas

Myra Lovvorn, RN, MSN
Clinic Coordinator
The 1917 Clinic (AIDS Outpatient Care)
University of Alabama at Birmingham
Birmingham, Alabama

Lois W. Lowry, RN, DNSc
Assistant Professor
College of Nursing
University of South Florida
Health Sciences Center
Tampa, Florida

Karen S. Martin, RN, MSN, FAAN
Director of Research
Visiting Nurses Association of Omaha
Omaha, Nebraska

Mary Lynn Mathre, RN, MSN, CARN
Clinician 4
Addiction Treatment Program
University of Virginia Health Sciences Center
Blue Ridge Hospital
Charlottesville, Virginia

Beverly McElmurry, RN, EdD, FAAN
Professor and Program Director
Primary Health Care in Urban Communities
Associate Dean
Office for International Studies
Director of Women's Studies
University of Illinois at Chicago
College of Nursing
Chicago, Illinois

Geneva W. Morris, RN, PhD
Assistant Professor
University of Texas
Health Science Center at Houston
School of Nursing
Houston, Texas

Cynthia E. Northrop, RN, MS, JD
Nurse Attorney
Member of Maryland Bar
New York, NY
(deceased)

Charlene C. Ossler, PhD, COHN
Executive Director
American Board for Occupational Health Nurses, Inc.
Mequon, Wisconsin

Juliann G. Sebastian, RN, MSN
Associate Professor
College of Nursing
University of Kentucky
Lexington, Kentucky

Nancy J. Scheet, RN, MSN
Director of Hospice
Visiting Nurses Association of Omaha
Omaha, Nebraska

Cynthia S. Selleck, RN, C, DSN, FNP
Assistant Professor
Chair, Family Health Nursing
College of Nursing
University of South Florida
Tampa, Florida

Linda Shortridge, RN, PhD
Assistant Professor
College of Nursing and Health
University of Cincinnati
Cincinnati, Ohio

George F. Shuster, III, RN, DNSc
Assistant Professor
College of Nursing
University of New Mexico
Albuquerque, New Mexico

Ann T. Sirles, RN, DSN, CFNP
Professor
Community Health Nursing
School of Nursing
University of Alabama at Birmingham
Birmingham, Alabama

Delois H. Skipwith, RN, DSN
Professor
School of Nursing
University of Alabama at Birmingham
Birmingham, Alabama

Rebecca H. Sloan, RN, MSN, CRNP
Family Nurse Practitioner
Geriatric Resource Center
Carraway Methodist Medical Center
Birmingham, Alabama

Sudie Elizabeth Speer, RN, BS, MS
Level III Staff Nurse, Home Care
The Children's Hospital
Denver, Colorado

Patricia L. Starck, RN, DSN
Dean and Professor
School of Nursing
University of Texas Health Science Center at Houston
Houston, Texas

Marcia Stanhope, RN, DSN, FAAN
Professor and Director
Community Health Nursing and Administration Division
College of Nursing
University of Kentucky
Lexington, Kentucky

Susan M. Swider, RN, PhD
Clinical Assistant Professor
University of Illinois at Chicago
Project Co-Director
Primary Health Care in Urban Communities
College of Nursing
Chicago, Illinois

Joan G. Turner, RN, DSN
Associate Professor
School of Nursing
University of Alabama at Birmingham
Birmingham, Alabama

Barbara Valanis, RN, DrPH
Senior Investigator
Kaiser Permanente Center for Health Research
Portland, Oregon

Prapin Watanakij, RN, MEd
Research Assistant
Primary Health Care in Urban Communities Project
University of Illinois at Chicago
College of Nursing
Chicago, Illinois

Deputy Director, Nursing Division
Ministry of Public Health
Bangkok, Thailand

Carolyn A. Williams, PhD, RN, FAAN
Dean and Professor
College of Nursing
University of Kentucky
Lexington, Kentucky

CONSULTANTS

Barbara K. Andersen, RN, EdD
Associate Professor
University of Tennessee at Chattanooga
Chattanooga, Tennessee

Arlene Gray Blix, RN, DrPh, CHES
Associate Professor
Department of Nursing
California State University, Fullerton
Fullerton, California

Mary Woods Byrne, RN, PhD
Associate Professor and Chairperson
Undergraduate Nursing Program
College of Mount Saint Vincent
Riverdale, New York

Patricia F. Conley, RN, MS
Assistant Professor of Nursing
University of Wisconsin at Oshkosh
College of Nursing
Oshkosh, Wisconsin

Barbara Crosson, RN, MSN
Case Manager
SPRANS (Special Project of Regional and National
    Significance) Case Managerment Project
Children's Medical Services
District 8-1
Valdosa, Georgia

Elizabeth L. Foster, RN, MS
Assistant Professor of Nursing
Community Health Nursing
Husson College
Eastern Maine Medical Center Baccalaureate Nursing Program
Bangor, Maine

Nancy Bernice Jones, MSN, RN
Assistant Professor, Nursing in the Community
Kent State University
Henderson Hall, School of Nursing
Kent, Ohio

Shirley Stevenson, RN, PhD, CS
Professor of Nursing
Pittsburg State University
Pittsburg, Kansas

Patricia Torsella, RN, MSN, CS
Assistant Professor, Community Health Nursing Coordinator
Department of Nursing
Bloomsburg University
Bloomsburg, Pennsylvania

It is not often that one attains a measure of success in a career without the support and mentoring of others. I am fortunate to have been the recipient of such relationships. They are truly gifts that require special interest, time, and energy, and an understanding of when and how to help, when to push, and when to quit. This edition of the text is dedicated to those who helped shape my career and who were instrumental in my choice of community health nursing as my specialty area. It was the public health nurse who visited my home when I was a child who piqued my curiosity about the specialty, and my high school principal, Clyde T. Lassiter, who paved the road for my entrance into my first nursing program. Beyond that I have enjoyed the colleagueship of many but it is that special few who are foremost in my thoughts: Paulina Sloan, Charlotte Denny, Mary Hall, Carolyn Williams, Norma Mobley, and Jeanette Lancaster. Each has contributed in her own way to my career development. I owe each a special thanks.

Marcia Stanhope

It is always hard to know where to start when I write a dedication to the people who were so supportive and who helped in so many ways to make this monumental project possible. Certainly, I will always be grateful to my parents, Howard and Glada Miller, who never thought anything was impossible for me to accomplish and who were so proud of the achievements I have had. My husband, Wade, and daughters, Melinda and Jennifer, have missed meals, talked to me when all I could think of were deadlines, and been supportive when my writing upset their plans and desires. In this edition I have been privileged to have a wonderful secretary, Agnes Toms, who has worked to help me meet deadlines and prepare materials. Marcia and I have been privileged to work with a great group of contributors who made considerable sacrifices of their time and energy to meet deadlines and to keep revising until we finally got this edition "right." With my dear friend, Marcia, I have enjoyed a special closeness that comes from trust, respect, caring, and 13 years of working together to meet a goal that we both cherish.

Jeanette Lancaster

A Tribute To Cynthia Ellen Northrop
1950-1989

Cynthia Northrop was an author that every editor dreamed of working with; she was consistent in the high quality of her work; efficient in meeting deadlines; and always professional in working to meet mutually agreed upon goals. When Cynthia died in 1989 at the age of 39, nursing lost a fine nursing law practitioner and a leader in both community health nursing and law.

Among the many roles in which she achieved success were nurse educator in community health nursing, practicing nurse attorney, author, and speaker. She acted upon the strength of her convictions and was a leader in many areas, including the founding in 1982 of the American Association of Nurse Attorneys. She subsequently served as president and board member of this organization whose members now number more than 600.

Cynthia will be remembered for her many contributions to nursing, particularly nursing law. Perhaps she will be more vividly remembered as a friend, colleague, member of a loving family, and person who had the courage to live each day to the fullest even though she knew for the last several months of her life that she would not be allowed the long life she so deserved.

We all miss Cynthia, friend and colleague to so many.

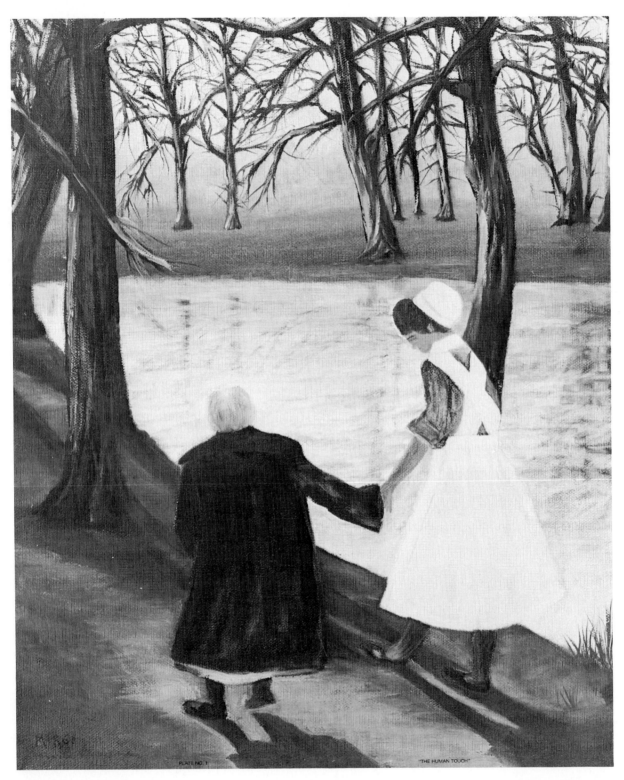

The Human Touch by Marjorie Glaser Bindner
Copyright 1980

Limited Edition
Full-color print

FOREWORD

The challenge of today's nursing educator is the preparation of the practitioners and leaders of the future. Rather than focus on giving lectures and providing "content," the model of the effective educator is increasingly being conceptualized as that of a "coach" whose expertise is directed to assessing the needs of students and identifying resources and opportunities that they can use in addressing their learning needs. Although a wide range of materials and experiences may be useful in assisting students to meet their goals, the need for a progressive, authoritative, and readable textbook persists. Stanhope and Lancaster's third edition of *Community Health Nursing: Process and Practice for Promoting Health* remains a compelling choice.

This latest edition of what has become a classic resource in the field of community health nursing maintains strengths of the two previous editions and incorporates new material to deal with current health problems and management strategies. In one single volume the user has access to guidance from acknowledged experts and leaders in community health nursing, who consider a wide range of topics from the history of the field and conceptual foundations to models for program planning and evaluation. In addition, contemporary epidemics and concerns such as AIDS, adolescent pregnancy, substance abuse, and homelessness are addressed as are the latest approaches to nursing diagnosis and case management in community-based services.

The provision of high quality, direct care nursing service to individuals is the heart of nursing, but for a profession that aspires to make a difference, a focus that is limited to direct care clinical concerns at the individual level is not a sufficient response to the present and future health care needs of the nation. If nursing is to have a positive and significant impact, its practitioners must become seriously involved in structuring the political agenda and adopting strategies to deal with promoting health and providing health care services at the community level. With the aging of the population and the growing recognition that the ever increasing cost of medical care must be slowed, it has never been more important to focus attention on community-based, population-focused approaches to health promotion and disease prevention. And, with the recognition that current knowledge is sufficient to prevent many of the major health problems of these times and significantly reduce the negative sequelae of others, it has never been more timely to do so. For those who seek to understand the elements and strategies inherent in such practice, which is the essence of community health nursing, and for those who seek to prepare for the challenges and rewards that go with it, Stanhope and Lancaster's third edition is the resource of choice.

Carolyn A. Williams, RN, PhD, FAAN
Dean and Professor
College of Nursing
University of Kentucky
Lexington, Kentucky

PREFACE

The current critical state of the health care system is reflected in triple digit inflation, questionable quality of care, and inaccessible care for 27% of the population who are underinsured or uninsured. Though the health of the average American is said to be better today than ever before in the history of the nation, medical practices have not markedly influenced the overall decline in mortality in the United States since the early 1900s. In fact, despite the vast sums of money spent on health care and the increasing number of health providers, the United States still lags behind several industrialized nations when one compares mortality and morbidity statistics.

The improved health of the population and the slight decline in mortality related to the leading causes of death are primarily attributed to the many advances in public health across the decades, advances such as improved sanitation, food pasteurization, refrigeration, immunization, and emphasis on personal lifestyle and environmental changes.

Recent estimates indicate that 50% of disease, disability, and death is due to lifestyle influences and is preventable. Control or risk factors such as diet, exercise, use of tobacco, drugs and alcohol, sexual promiscuity, and seatbelt use could prevent between 40% to 70% of all premature death, 33% of all disability, and 66% of all chronic disability. Yet most health care dollars are spent to treat the ten percent of the population who may be ill at any one time.

These factors have led to the formation of a resolution to focus attention on the development of a healthy public policy for the nation. This policy is reflected in the Year 2000 National Health Objectives designed to reduce the overall need for institutional care for both acute and chronic illness and reduce the need for use of technologies while increasing the health of individuals.

Disease prevention and health promotion activities designed to change personal lifestyle are to be planned through the establishment of partnerships between government, business, voluntary organizations, consumers, and health providers. The purposes to be accomplished through these partnerships are to reduce health disparities among Americans by targeting care to children, minorities, elderly, and the uninsured; to increase the healthy lifespan of Americans and to achieve access to preventive services for all Americans. The overall goal is to develop healthy communities.

To develop healthy communities, commitment from the individual, family, community, and society is essential. People must understand the need for changes in personal health-related practices. Society, and especially health care providers, must provide support including education, alterations in health policy priorities, changes in financing, and research to demonstrate the benefits of health promotion.

What does this mean for nurses? Nursing as a caring and helping profession exists because people are not always healthy and self-sufficient. Nursing's challenge is to become the central catalyst for change. Community health nursing is a practice that is continuous and comprehensive, is directed toward all age groups, takes place in a wide variety of settings, and includes health education, maintenance, coordination, and evaluation of care for individuals, families, groups, and communities.

To meet the demands of a constantly changing health care environment, nursing must become increasingly futuristic in developing roles and practice areas. To do this the nurse must know the importance of several key factors, including a knowledge of public health tradition and principles, the current and evolving characteristics of the health care system, a heightened awareness of the role and responsibilities of nurses, the importance of a health promotion orientation, and the necessity for consumer responsibility for health.

This text was written to provide nursing students and practitioners with a comprehensive source book that offers a foundation for designing community health nursing strategies for individuals, families, groups, and communities. The unifying *theme* for the book is the integration of health promotion concepts into the multifaceted role of the community health nurse. Such a preventive focus emphasizes traditional public health practice with increased attention to the effects of the internal and external environment and lifestyle on health.

To achieve this goal, the text is divided into seven sections: (1) introduction to the contemporary health care delivery system that describes the historical and current status of the health care system, including factors that influence community health nursing services; (2) discussion of the conceptual foundations for community health practice, including selected models from nursing and related sciences; (3) focus on the community as client, which describes the aggregate concept, the influence of groups in communities, and the extent to which environment affects the health of the community; (4) a review of common community health problems that affect the quality of life in society; (5) a developmental approach to describe risk factors and health problems of individuals and families; (6) health promotion strategies; and (7) a look at the diversity in the role of community health nurses that describes the changing roles, functions, and practice settings.

We wish to take this opportunity to express sincere appreciation to our families and friends who supported and encouraged us through this herculean task and to the administration and staff of the University of Kentucky College of Nursing and to the staff at the University of Virginia who generously contributed their time, effort, and support to this endeavor. In addition, we wish to thank Darlene Como, Laurie Sparks, Susan R. Epstein, and Linda McKinley, of Mosby-Year Book, Inc., and the reviewers for their time and effort in assisting with the refinement of this text. The cooperation and commitment to quality by those who worked with us on this project are greatly appreciated.

A special thanks to past contributors to the first and second editions of this text. Their expertise and commitment to quality continue to be reflected in this edition of the text. Much appreciation to Nannette Worel, Vivienne Brown, David Kerschner, Denise Geolot, Doris Wagner Ferguson, Margaret Millsap, Cora Withrow, Sharon Sheahan, Ellen Kent Bailey, Eileen Wiles, Paula Pointer, Marjorie Keller, and Jacquelyne Logue.

Marcia Stanhope

Jeanette Lancaster

CONTENTS

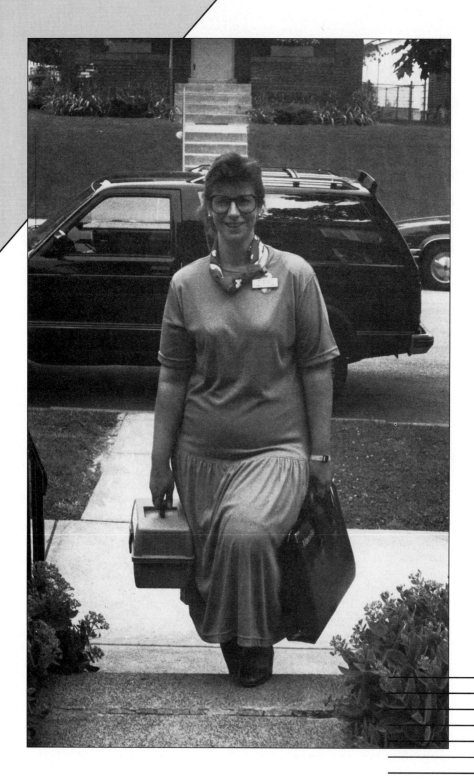

PART ONE

Contemporary Health Care Delivery and Community Health Nursing

Since the late 1800s, community health nurses have been leaders in improving the quality of health care for individuals, families, and communities. The importance of legal, economic, ethical, social, cultural, and political forces has been recognized. It has also become clear that community health nursing throughout the world has more similarities than differences from one country to another.

In recent years the U.S. health care system has been under attack because of rapidly rising health care costs, inconsistency in the level of services provided from one area to another, and a general inconsistency in the quality and accessibility of health services. With 37 million Americans uninsured and 18 million underinsured, it has been recognized that access to health care services is not a right for all. The public health system has eroded as a major force for promoting the health of all people. It is unable to protect and improve the health of the most needy individuals and families.

In September 1990 Secretary of Health and Human Services Louis Sullivan called together in Washington over 1500 leaders of 300 national organizations and governmental agencies to announce the Health Objectives for the Nation for the Year 2000. Based upon the success in achieving the 1990 objectives, there is every reason to believe that these latest objectives will improve the overall health of the nation.

If community health nurses are to be effective forces for promoting the health of Americans, it is necessary to understand the history of community health nursing and the current status of the public health system. The challenges currently facing community health nurses are similar to those facing nurses in earlier times. The approaches that have proved successful in the past often can be modified and implemented to deal with contemporary challenges. We can learn not only from the past but also from others. This edition includes content related to health care delivery in Canada because many people believe that Americans could learn how to improve services from the Canadian model of health care delivery.

Part One presents information about significant factors affecting health in the United States. Some contrasts and comparisons, especially in primary health care, are made with Canada and Thailand. The amount of money spent on health services is tremendous. An understanding of the political, legal, ethical, and cultural factors that affect decisions about health care priorities is imperative. It is said that "knowledge is power." To influence the national health care agenda and be instrumental in changing the level and quality of services and the priorities for funding, requires informed, courageous, and committed nurses. The chapters in Part One are designed to provide crucial information so that community health nurses can make a difference in health care.

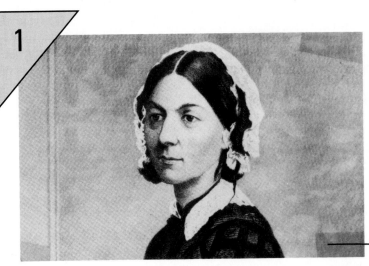

1

History of Community Health and Community Health Nursing

Jeanette Lancaster

OBJECTIVES

After reading this chapter, the student should be able to:

Trace current community health practices from the pre-Christian era and compare the past activities with those occurring at the present time.

Describe two leaders in nursing who made a profound difference in community health nursing practice.

Summarize two famous health care reports of the early twentieth century that led to lasting changes in medical education and public health.

Discuss the importance of voluntary health organizations and use one major organization as an example.

Discuss the development of two major nursing organizations and assess their effect on public health nursing.

Summarize the history of home health care and compare its significance today with that of the early Sisters of Charity.

Briefly describe the development of community health nursing in Canada.

Compare community health nursing from its inception until the present time in the United States and in Canada.

KEY TERMS

American Nurses' Association	Frontier Nursing Service	public health settlement houses
American Public Health Association	home health care instructive district nursing	Shattuck Report The Report of the
American Red Cross	Lillian Wald	Committee for Study of Nursing Education
Mary Breckenridge	National League for	voluntary agencies
district nursing	Nursing	

The roles of the community health nurse are varied, complex, and challenging. Many of the current roles can be traced to the early nineteenth century when public health efforts focused on environmental conditions such as sanitation, control of communicable diseases, education in personal hygiene, disease prevention, and care of the sick in their homes. Over the years health threats from the environment, communicable diseases, and general wearing out of the body have changed. Many diseases such as diphtheria, cholera, and typhoid fever have been eradicated in developed countries only to be replaced by hepatitis, AIDS, and a resurgence of such diseases such as measles and tuberculosis, which were considered eradicated in North America during the current century.

Similarly the environment in industrialized countries is no longer polluted with garbage in the streets but now is threatened by overcrowded garbage dumps, the seepage of garbage into the waters that feed crops, and toxins in the air, water, and soil. The body is being worn out not by physical toll but rather by the debilitating diseases of the current era, which are often stress related.

Throughout history the roles of the community health nurse have changed to respond effectively to the prevailing public health problems. The roles have been dynamic and multifaceted and have relied heavily on the science of public health. Part of the excitement of community health nursing is due to the autonomy of the practice and use of problem-solving and astute decision making skills in the role.

To understand the current scope of community health nursing it is necessary to briefly trace the history of health care from the pre-Christian era to the present. The early role of the public health nurse in the United States was patterned after the European model of nursing, therefore the history of public health nursing in North America can be understood by looking first at forerunners in Western Europe. Though the majority of the chapter focuses on the United States, attention is also paid to the development of community health nursing in Canada. The development of community health nursing in Canada parallels that of the United States.

EARLY HEALTH PRACTICES

A review of the dominant cultural ideas of each era is useful in understanding the antecedents of the current community health system. The patterns of health care in previous eras reflect the prevalent patterns of medical and nursing practice.

Pre-Christian Era

People have always been concerned with the events surrounding birth, death, and illness. With few exceptions primitive tribes had a certain amount of group spirit and a sense of hygiene. In their struggles to exist, early people tried to understand disease so they could cope with disease-producing agents. However, their success was limited because their health practices were largely based on magic and superstition rather than on facts about the causes and effects of actions and the subsequent health consequences. Shamans, or medicine men, cared for both health and religious needs and were highly esteemed.

Rudiments of community health can be traced to the earliest recorded civilizations. Excavations from the Middle Kingdom (2100-1700 BC) reflect community health practices in ancient Egypt. Two thousand years before the Christian era, securing an adequate supply of drinking water was a major concern. In Babylonia the "notion persisted that illness was caused by sin and displeasures of the gods; that disease was inflicted as a punishment for sinning" (Dolan, 1978, p. 10). Sick people were seen as unclean and in need of purification, and temples became the seat of medical care. Sick people were often taken to a busy market where passersby could offer suggestions for treatment. In spite of their primitive practices, both the Babylonians and Egyptians emphasized hygiene and possessed some medical skills.

The Egyptians of about 1000 BC, the healthiest of all early civilizations, used principles based on observations and empirical knowledge rather than on magic. They also developed a variety of pharmaceutical preparations and constructed earth closets and public drainage systems.

The Mosaic health code of the Hebrews is clearly reflected in the Old Testament. This code discussed many aspects of individual, family, and community hygiene and provided a sound basis for practices to maintain health and prolong life. Also, Hebrew nurses participated in carefully planned programs of visiting the sick in their homes and caring for them by bringing physical and spiritual refreshment for the sick person and the family.

Greek Era

The early Greeks viewed people as part of nature and believed health resulted from a harmonious relationship with nature. The Greeks saw health care delivery as a responsibility of civilized man, and the medical ethics established in Greece guided contemporary medical practice. The Greeks also paid attention to personal cleanliness, exercise, diet, and sanitation. Despite their many farsighted practices, the Greeks ignored or destroyed the weak, sick, and crippled.

The first notation of women being associated with healing is found in connection with the Greek mythological character of Aesculapius, who eventually became deified as the god of healing. One of his five children, Hygeia, became the goddess of health and another, Panacea, the restorer of health. In later Greek civilizations, healing largely occurred in shrines where patients congregated and were looked after by attendants called "basket healers" (Deloughery, 1977).

The first clear-cut evidence of acute communicable disease is recorded in classical Greek literature. There are numerous references to severe sore throats that often ended in death. The Greek work *Kynanche* mentioned acute inflammatory processes of the throat and larynx and probably referred to what is now known as diphtheria. In ancient Greece, medicine was an itinerant vocation, with practitioners going from town to town, knocking on doors and offering their services. Larger cities appointed physicians and paid for their services from public funds; these probably were the earliest community physicians.

Roman Empire

The Roman view of health shared many concepts with the Greeks yet focused much more on pragmatic application of ideas rather than on astute observation and a continual search for new knowledge. The Roman Empire is remembered for its administrative and engineering efforts. According to Pellegrino (1963), Romans viewed medicine from a community health and social medicine perspective. They emphasized regulation of medical practice, punishment for negligence, drainage of swamps, provision of pure water, establishment of sewage systems, and supervision of street cleaning and public food preparation.

Appius Claudius Crassus Caecus, who built the first great Roman road, the Appian Way, was responsible for bringing a supply of water to Rome by means of an aqueduct (Rosen, 1958, p. 39). To monitor the purity of water, settling basins were established at points along the aqueduct to allow sediment to deposit. When the water reached Rome, it was received in large reservoirs from which emerged smaller reservoirs so that water could be segregated according to its purpose. The Romans not only valued pure water but also had sewage systems in major cities. The Romans developed community health services with an effective and systematic organization, which continued to function as the Empire disintegrated. Additionally, at the peak of the Roman Empire women visited and cared for the sick. Special hospitals were established when it became impractical to shelter patients in the bishops' houses, which had previously been their practice.

Middle Ages

The decline of the Greco-Roman era led to both a decay of urban culture and a disintegration of community health organization and practice (Rosen, 1958, p. 50). The period between 500 and 1500 AD was a heterogeneous phase in history during which superstitions dominated thinking yet advances such as the development of health care facilities originated. As cities grew, they built great walls to protect their inhabitants against invasions by hostile groups. These encircling walls, though necessary for safety and protection, also led to considerable crowding and poor sanitary and hygienic conditions. Clean water supplies and elimination of refuse in the streets were difficult to ensure.

With the dawn of the Christian era, a new conceptualization of man influenced health practices. The early Christian church believed that the Roman and Grecian ways pampered the body at the expense of the soul. Disease was seen as punishment for sin.

During this era thinking reverted to mysticism and superstition, and there was religious persecution of those who tried to introduce new ideas. Progress in medicine came to a halt. People considered it immoral to look at their own bodies. People seldom bathed and often wore dirty clothes. Sanitation was not important, and refuse and body wastes were allowed to accumulate near dwellings. However, despite this reversal in thinking about health, hospitals for the poor and neglected were developed.

The rise of monasteries and convents as places for caring for the sick led to the early development of nursing activities. Between 1091 and 1291, early male and female nurses joined military orders during the Crusades. As the early Christian church developed, those who had devoted their lives to Christian service cared for the poor, fatherless, and sick. Initially they cared for all three groups under the same roof. However, the knowledge the Crusaders gained from the Arabs led to the establishment of hospitals. Early hospitals were known as a Hotel Dieu, with the best known located in Paris. During this era several orders of nuns provided simple nursing care directed primarily toward meeting the patient's physiological needs (Griffin and Griffin, 1973). Health education and personal hygiene knowledge also increased during the Middle Ages. Books were written that talked about healthful living and encouraged moderate eating to ensure health.

Renaissance

The great epidemics of the Middle Ages led to attitudes of fatalism and a general depressed orientation toward health. However, during the Renaissance people started opening their minds to new ideas, and between 1500 and 1700 medicine began to advance. In general, the Renaissance was characterized by achievement in the arts and scholarly efforts and by a rise in commerce and industry. A belief in humanism developed. Human dignity and worth began to influence health practices.

The Renaissance ushered in a new period of history during which community health as currently known was begun (Rosen, 1958). The many technological advances designed to cure the epidemics of the Middle Ages provided the impetus and resources necessary for the changes that took place in the Renaissance. These changes, though not directly influencing community health, supplemented the foundation of modern community health.

A matter of serious debate during the Renaissance was whether diseases prominent at the time—including scarlet fever, rickets, scurvy, syphilis, smallpox, and malaria—were caused by contagion or constitution. The invention of the microscope by Anton van Leeuwenhoek in the late seventeenth century supported the contagion view by permitting the observation of microorganisms in soil and water.

Although establishment of a systematic national health policy in Europe failed, health problems began to be analyzed and proposals for national action were set forth (Rosen, 1958). William Perry contributed significantly with his belief that communicable disease control would save the lives of infants and improve the lot of the people. Although this idea made sense, there was no way of enforcing it because local authorities had no jurisdiction outside their boundaries and ships frequently brought contagious diseases into the ports.

During the time residents supposedly kept the streets clean. They had no sewage disposal system, and private enterprises supplied water. Towns provided assistance for the sick and lame. Hospitals during this period became places not only to care for the sick but also to study and teach medicine. These advances were forerunners of later scientific discoveries and gains.

EARLY COMMUNITY HEALTH NURSING

Community health nursing has evolved dramatically since the first visiting nurses were sponsored by St. Vincent de Paul in Paris in 1669. Table 1-1 chronicles the milestones in early community health nursing.

TABLE 1-1

Milestones in the history of community health and community health nursing: 1600-1866

1601	Elizabethan Poor Law written
1617	Sisterhood of the Dames de Charite organized in France by St. Vincent de Paul
1789	Marine Hospital Service and Baltimore Health Department established
1812	Sisters of Mercy established in Dublin where nuns visited the poor
1813	Ladies' Benevolent Society of Charleston, South Carolina founded
1834	Poor Law Amendment in England sets up a Commission of Inquiry on the Poor Laws administered by Edwin Chadwick
1836	Modern order of Lutheran Deaconesses created by Pastor Fliedner at Kaiserwerth
1850	Shattuck Report prepared on the status of medical education
1851	Florence Nightingale goes to Kaiserwerth; first International Sanitary Conference in Paris
1855	Quarantine Board established in New Orleans; beginning of tuberculosis campaign in the United States
1859	District nursing established in Liverpool by William Rathbone
1860	Florence Nightingale Training School for Nurses established at St. Thomas Hospital in London; nursing program started at New England Hospital
1864	Factory Act of 1864 passed to control treatment of children in industries; Treaty of Geneva; inauguration of Red Cross
1866	New York Metropolitan Board of Health established

St. Francis De Sales (1567-1662) developed a voluntary association of friendly visitors to go to the homes of the poor and care for the sick. The ensuing organization, cofounded and directed by Madame de Chantal, and supported with time and money by influential women, was an early form of visiting nursing. She and the members of her group visited the sick in their homes, cleaned and dressed their wounds, made their beds, and gave them clothes (Dolan, 1978).

St. Vincent De Paul (1576-1669) was another prominent figure in the history of nursing and social welfare. In 1617 in Paris, he organized the Sisterhood of the Dames de Charite, which systematically introduced the modern principles of visiting nursing and social welfare. His aim was to help people learn to help themselves. The Sisterhood comprised a group of women who went from cottage to cottage, much like the plan used by de Sales, to provide home care. As their numbers increased and the demands for their services grew, Mademoiselle Le Gras was appointed as supervisor. The work of the sisterhood conveyed the beliefs that home nursing should be carried out if based on sound principles rather than on just kindness and intuition and that nurses' activities should be supervised. They based their work on a belief in teaching nurses and the people they visited (Maynard, 1939).

Industrial Revolution

The Industrial Revolution, with its emphasis on power and profits, reversed many of the gains of the Renaissance. Also, as urban populations grew because of the emphasis on industry and production, the number of people needing health care outpaced the voluntary and often piecemeal efforts to provide services. The 80 years between 1750 and 1830 influenced the future design of community health because of the upheaval and change prevalent at that time.

Major problems of this time included a high infant mortality rate, neglect and often murder of illegitimate infants, poor working conditions, diseases of certain occupations, and the growing incidence of mental illness. During the eighteenth century people with mental illness were locked in jails, workhouses, or madhouses. An early defender of the mentally ill, Vincenzo Chiarugi, brought about major reforms at St. Bonifacio in Florence, Italy, where in 1788 he established a system in which properly trained nurses cared for mentally ill people under the direct supervision of a physician. Other such asylums followed suit, providing patients with kindness, physical exercise, good food, and fresh air. In 1770 Eastern State Hospital, known as the "Lunnatick Hospital," was established in Williamsburg, Virginia. This was one of the first American state hospitals for the mentally ill.

The growth of hospitals paralleled the development of asylums. In 1731 Blockley Hospital, later known as Philadelphia General, was established to receive the sick, poor, insane, prisoners, and orphans. In 1737 Charity Hospital was established in New Orleans. In 1751 Pennsylvania Hospital was founded in Philadelphia to admit acutely ill or injured people (Dolan, 1978). Most early U.S. hospitals were begun on the Northeast coast, following the pattern of settlement in the United States. Community-minded citizens established New York Hospital in 1771, and the Philadelphia Dispensary opened in 1786, thanks to the work of Quakers (Dolan, 1978, p. 111).

The Industrial Revolution witnessed tremendous advances in transportation, communication, and other forms of technology. Modern public health efforts began in England, the first modern industrial nation. The prevailing social problem of that time was caring for the poor, and the Elizabethan Poor Law of 1601 guaranteed medical and nursing care for the poor, blind and lame. A Commission of Inquiry on the Poor Laws was established and administered by Edwin Chadwick, who subsequently devoted his entire career to helping the poor. Chadwick campaigned vigorously to get bills passed in Parliament that would not only help poor people but would eliminate some of the unsanitary environmental conditions of that time.

Early forerunners of community health nursing are found in the work of the first two nursing orders in the British Isles. Mary Aikenhead (Sister Mary Augustine) started the Irish Sisters of Charity in Dublin in 1812, and the nuns visited among the poor. The Sisters of Mercy founded a home for destitute girls and visited the sick in their homes.

Toward the end of the Industrial Revolution, women performing nursing functions changed from a caring group of women largely supported by a religious order to a group often referred to as the "dregs of the community: dirty, drunken, and dishonest" (Swinson, 1965, p. 22). Charles Dickens' *Martin Chuzzlewit,* first published in 1843, provided a lasting impression of nursing in the eighteenth century with his description of Sairy Gamp, a drunk, untrained servant who reportedly provided a semblance of nursing care. However, not all nurses were Sairy Gamps; by far, the majority provided safe and humane care.

Colonial Period

During the Industrial Revolution in Europe, events occurred that influenced the course of community health in what would later be the United States. Epidemics, especially smallpox, occurred in the early years of North American settlement. It is possible that the colonists were able to settle in North America because the diseases they brought with them were fatal to natives who lacked immunity to them.

Early Colonial community health efforts included the collection of vital statistics, improved sanitation, and the avoidance of exotic diseases brought in from trade routes. However, they lacked a continuing and organized mechanism for ensuring that community health efforts would be supported and enforced (Rosen, 1958).

Because of the pressure to establish a federation of states, community health received little attention before the American Revolution. Following the American Revolution, the threat of a variety of diseases, especially yellow fever, influenced the establishment of official boards of health. By the end of the eighteenth century, New York City, with a population of 75,000, had established a public health committee for monitoring water quality, sewer construction, drainage of marshes, planting of trees and vegetables, construction of a masonry wall along the waterfront, and interment of the dead (Rosen, 1958).

THE NINETEENTH CENTURY

Although the United States grew tremendously between 1800 and 1850, community health efforts by no means kept pace. During this period threats to health escalated as epidemics of smallpox, yellow fever, cholera, typhoid, and typhus entered the country along with the influx of migrants from many parts of the world. By 1850 the living conditions and the average life span in the older American settlements were worse than in London, which at that time was well-known for its deprived living conditions.

The quality of medical care reflected the inadequacies of this period. At this time medical education followed the pattern originally established by law schools of having lectures and no clinical work in the curriculum. Any applicant who could pay was accepted, and an apprenticeship followed the lecture series (Schudson, 1974).

At the same time hospitals were generally unsanitary places staffed by poorly trained workers; hospitals were a place where people, especially the poor, could go to die. In the early hospitals, many people developed infections and died following surgery.

Just as American cities began establishing community health efforts an influx of immigrants poured in from Europe. These immigrants taxed the stability of cities, especially those on the East Coast. Housing and sanitation became major problems. As urban communities grew and their sanitary conditions worsened, conflict arose between those wanting health reforms and those wishing to maintain the status quo. A number of voluntary health associations developed to mobilize forces for protecting the community.

The earliest local health departments were established in Baltimore (1798), Charleston, S.C. (1815), Philadelphia (1818), Providence, R.I. (1832), Cambridge, Mass. (1846), and New York City (1866). These early health departments focused on eliminating environmental hazards associated with poor living conditions, crowding, and the proximity of slaughterhouses to homes. Local health departments subsequently developed in rural areas and other cities.

From the 1840s on, attention focused on attacking community health problems and improving urban living conditions. The National Institute, a distinguished scientific body, was formed in Washington, D.C., in 1845. Founded in 1847, the American Medical Association (AMA) responded to pressure to form a hygiene committee in 1848 to carry out sanitary surveys and develop a system for collecting vital statistics.

Concurrently, efforts were being carried out in Massachusetts, which produced the famous Shattuck Report. This report was published in 1850 by the Massachusetts Sanitary Commission. Major recommendations called for the establishment of a state health department and local health boards in every town; sanitary surveys; varying kinds of vital statistics; environmental sanitation, food, drug, and communicable disease control; well-child care, including immunizations and health education; and proposals on smoke and alcohol control, town planning, and the teaching of preventive medicine in medical schools. Although the Shattuck Report now receives credit as a noteworthy and farsighted document, it was virtually ignored in its own time. Implementation of the actions recommended by the report came 19 years after its publication.

Some claim that Louisiana's quarantine board, established in 1855 to deal with yellow fever and other epidemics, was the first state health department. However, Massachusetts established the first operational state board of health in 1869. The power of this first official state board of health was limited to investigation and advice. The board began with a budget of $5000, no trained staff, and no predecessors from which to learn. The second state health department was established in California in 1870. By the end of the nineteenth century there were 38 state health departments in the United States (Pickett and Hanlon, 1990).

In July 1798 Congress created a Marine Service Hospital to provide care for sick and disabled seamen. This service was significant for at least three reasons: (1) it served as the stimulus for what later became the United States Public Health Service; (2) it supplied an organized effort to bring about national quarantine efforts and prevented dreaded diseases from entering the United States at its seaports; and (3) it was one of the first recorded examples of prepaid medical insurance, because for 20¢ monthly, merchant seamen were guaranteed medical and hospital care. During that same year, the first local health department was established in the United States in Baltimore, Maryland.

The most significant national public health agency is the Public Health Service, officially established in 1879 with the appointment of the first medical director. However, as previously mentioned, the Marine Hospital Service, which began in 1798, was the forerunner of the Public Health Service. The development of a national public health agency paralleled the development of the United States. The country was just being settled and relied heavily on its expanding maritime activities. Ships from around the world were landing on the East Coast. Merchant seamen on U.S. ships often had no permanent homes, yet they were American citizens. The introduction of epidemics into the country via the ports led, in 1878, to the passage of the first port quarantine act. To illustrate the magnitude of these epidemics, between the time of the Louisiana Purchase in 1803 and the beginning of the twentieth century, New Orleans witnessed 37 severe yellow fever epidemics.

In 1890 Congress authorized the Marine Hospital Service to inspect all immigrants. Because the incidence of contagious diseases was the greatest at ports, Marine Hospital Service physicians had the greatest skill in preventing epidemics. Initially, this authority was intended to bar "lunatics and others unable to care for themselves." The following year, authority was extended to include "persons suffering from loathsome and contagious diseases" (Pickett and Hanlon, 1990, p. 35).

Because of the severity of these epidemics a series of national quarantine conferences resulting from the efforts of Wilson Jewell, a health officer in Philadelphia, began with a 3-day meeting in Philadelphia in 1859. The 54 attendees discussed subjects of common interest, including prevention of epidemic diseases such as cholera, typhus, and yellow fever and the role of stagnant water, filthy bedding, and baggage and clothing of immigrant passengers in the spread of disease. This convention recommended that immigrants not previously protected from smallpox be vaccinated. The second convention was held in 1858 in Baltimore. Major outcomes of the second conference were proposals for a system of quarantine laws and the organization of a Committee on Internal Hygiene or the Sanitary Arrangement of Cities. Two additional conferences were held in New York and Boston before the Civil War broke out and interrupted public health efforts.

However, the work of the conventions seemed to plant the seed that led to the establishment of the American Public Health Association (Pickett and Hanlon, 1990). This influential organization, now with over 150,000 members, began in 1872. There are 23 sections in the APHA that represent member interests and include groups such as public health nursing, epidemiology, health administration, environmental health, and social work. The association meets annually, publishes a well-respected journal *(The American Journal of Public Health)* and a variety of monographs, books, and a monthly newsletter for members, lobbies for improved public health, and issues thoughtful position papers on public health issues.

The Beginnings of Home Health Care

The next significant era for community health nursing began with William Rathbone in Liverpool, England, in 1859. Because of the outstanding care provided to his dying wife, Rathbone promoted the establishment of a district nursing service. Based on his experience, Rathbone concluded that many people with long-term illnesses could be better cared for in their own homes than in a hospital. He urged his wife's nurse, Mary Robinson, to begin a program of home nursing care for poor people. Subsequently, at Rathbone's urging, the Liverpool Relief Society divided the city into nursing districts and assigned a committee of "Friendly Visitors" to each district to provide health care to needy people (Kalisch and Kalisch, 1977).

Based on the Liverpool experience, Rathbone wrote a book entitled *Social Organization of Effort in Works of Benevolence and Public Charity by a Man of Business,* in which he outlined a philosophy for home health care. Rathbone's work spurred Florence Nightingale to publish a pamphlet on nursing entitled *Suggestions for Improving Nursing Service,* which recommended steps for nursing care in the home. Rathbone ultimately founded the Metropolitan Nursing Association to provide home health nursing (Bullough and Bullough, 1964). During this time the largest religious organization in London, the Bible and Domestic Mission, sent women into the slums to read the Bible. In 1868 they added nursing care to their program (Dolan, 1978).

In nineteenth century America, the first visiting nurse society began in Philadelphia in 1886 to provide home health care to the sick. Earlier efforts had been noted in New Amsterdam (New York) in the works of the *Krankenbezoekers* (visitors of the sick) and *Ziekentroosters* (one who gives comfort to the sick). Following the War of 1812, a Ladies Benevolent Society was organized to aid sick and impoverished people. In 1877 the Women's Board of the New York Mission hired Frances Root, a graduate of Bellevue Hospital's first nursing class, to visit the sick poor and provide nursing care and religious instruction (Bullough and Bullough, 1964).

Nurses at the first visiting nursing society in Philadelphia strictly followed physician's orders, gave selected treatments, and kept temperature and pulse records. Because their visits were brief, the nurse soon recognized the need to teach family members basic elements of care. Thus from the very beginning, community health nursing included teaching and prevention.

In 1886 two women in Boston approached the Women's Education Association to seek support for district nursing. They used the term *instructive district nursing* to emphasize the relationship to education and to increase their likelihood of receiving support from this group. They then met with representatives of the Boston Dispensary, which was providing free medical care to the poor according to the dispensary district in which they lived. In February 1886 the first district nurse was hired in Boston. As the number of district nurses increased, they worked closely with physicians to carry out medical orders. Patients paid no fees, and initially two lay managers of the association supervised the nurses. In 1888 the Instructive District Nursing Association became incorporated as an independent voluntary agency to provide care to the sick poor under the direction of a trained physician. These nurses also taught families to take better care of themselves and their neighbors by living a wholesome life (Brainard, 1922).

Early Settlement Houses

During this era wealthy people became interested in charitable activities and began to fund settlement houses in the poorer sections of many larger cities. These settlement houses offered a variety of services for members of the community. For example, in 1893 Lillian Wald and her friend Mary Brewster, both trained nurses and wealthy women, organized a visiting nursing service for the poor of New York (see box below.)

In 1909, along with Lee Fraskel, Lillian Wald established the first community health nursing program for workers at the Metropolitan Life Insurance Company. Believing that keeping workers healthier would increase their productivity, she urged that nurses at agencies such as Henry Street Settlement provide skilled nursing care. Wald convinced the company that it would be more economical to use the services of community health nurses than to employ their own nurses. She also convinced them that services could be available to anyone desiring them, with fees graduated according to the ability to pay. This nursing service designed by Wald continued for 44 years and contributed several significant accomplishments to community health nursing, including the following:

1. Availability of home nursing care on a fee-for-service basis
2. Establishment of an effective cost-accounting system for visiting nurses
3. Use of advertisements in newspapers and on radio to recruit nurses
4. Reduction of mortality rates from infectious diseases

Lillian Wald also believed that the nursing efforts at Henry Street Settlement should be aligned with an official health agency, and she arranged for nurses to wear an insignia that signified that they served under the auspices of the Board of Health. Also, she established rural health nursing services through the American Red Cross. Her other accomplishments included helping to establish the Children's Bureau, fighting in New York City for better tenement living conditions, city recreation centers, parks, pure food laws, graded classes for mentally handicapped children, and assistance to immigrants (Figure 1-1).

About this same time a group of women in Los Angeles established the College Settlement. They requested that the City Council give them a monthly allowance so a district nurse could visit the sick poor. In 1898 public funds paid the first nurse to provide nursing care in the home.

THE TWENTIETH CENTURY

In 1912 Congress broadened the Marine Hospital Service, and it became the United States Public Health Service (USPHS). The chief officer of the USPHS became the Surgeon General. The Public Health Service is directed by the Assistant Secretary for Health. It is organized into six functional units: (1) the Centers for Disease Control, (2) the Food and Drug Administration, (3) the Health Resources and Services Administration, (4) the National Institutes of Health, (5) the Alcohol, Drug Abuse, and Mental Health Administration, and (6) the Agency for Toxic Substances and Disease Registry. The functioning of the USPHS is discussed in greater detail in Chapter 4.

By 1920 all states and most large cities had established health departments. Nurses comprised the majority of their staff. The development of the public health nursing role is described later in the chapter.

During the next several decades substantial changes took place at the federal level, affecting the structure of community health resources. The Federal Social Security Act of 1935 was the first of these changes. Title VI of the act affected the scope of community health through its original mission to assist states and their subdivisions in the establishment and maintenance of adequate community health services. These services included the training of personnel for both state and local health activities.

As the Social Security Act of 1935 attempted to overcome the national setbacks of the Great Depression, it expanded community health nursing. Title VI stipulated protection and health promotion for all people. Two major provisions of Title VI included (1) the appropriation of $8 million to help states, counties, and medical districts establish and maintain adequate health services and train public health

---

LILLIAN WALD: FIRST PUBLIC HEALTH NURSE IN THE UNITED STATES

Public health nursing evolved in the United States in the late nineteenth and early twentieth centuries, largely due to the pioneering work of Lillian Wald. Born on March 10, 1867, Lillian Wald decided to become a nurse after Vassar College refused to admit her at age 16. She graduated in 1891 from the New York Hospital Training School for Nurses and spent the next year working at the New York Juvenile Asylum. To supplement what she thought had been inadequate training in the sciences, she enrolled in the Woman's Medical College in New York (Frachel, 1988).

Having grown up in a warm, nurturing family in Rochester, New York, Wald found her work in New York City introduced her to an entirely different side of life. In 1883 while conducting a class in home nursing for immigrant families on the Lower East Side of New York, a small child asked Wald to visit her sick mother. Wald found the mother in bed, having hemorrhaged for two days. This home visit confirmed for Wald all of the injustices in society and the differences in health care for the poor and those able to pay.

She simply could not tolerate seeing poor people with no access to health care. With her friend Mary Brewster and the financial support of two wealthy lay people, Mrs. Soloman Loeb and Joseph H. Schiff, she moved to the East Side and occupied the top floor of a tenement house on Jefferson Street. This move eventually led to the establishment of the now famous Henry Street Settlement. In the beginning she and Brewster helped individual families. Wald believed that the nurse's visit "should be like that of a very interested friend rather than that of an impersonal, paid visitor" (Dolan, 1978, p. 227).

Ever discontent to deal only with the present and convinced that environmental conditions and social conditions were the causes of ill health and poverty, Wald became actively involved in using epidemiological methods to campaign for health-promoting social policies. She not only wrote *The House on Henry Street* to describe her own public health nursing work but also led the development of payment by insurance companies for nursing services.

workers and (2) the allocation of $2 million for research and the investigation of disease and sanitation. This act also provided funds for the education and employment of public health nurses.

Finally, in 1939 the Public Health Service relocated from the Treasury Department to the newly created Federal Security Agency. The Division of Environmental Health Sciences was established within the Public Health Service in 1966. When the Environmental Protection Agency opened in 1970, most of the environmental health activities of the Public Health Service were transferred to it. Additionally, for more effective service to states, the Public Health Service developed 10 regional offices located in Boston, New York, Philadelphia, Atlanta, Chicago, Kansas City, Dallas, Denver, San Francisco, and Seattle.

Although the government retains a major responsibility for the health and welfare of its citizens, voluntary organizations play key roles in community health. Health-related voluntary agencies, many of which are supported by citizen contributions and donations, fall into several categories.

1. Those dealing with specific diseases such as cancer or diabetes. Examples include the American Cancer Society, the Cystic Fibrosis Foundation, and the American Diabetes Association.
2. Those involved with certain organs of the body, for example, the American Lung Association or the American Heart Association.
3. Those involved with the health and welfare of special groups such as the aged or children and including groups such as the National Council on Aging or the National Society for Crippled Children.
4. Those dealing with health problems that affect the community as a whole, such as the National Safety Council and the Planned Parenthood Federation of America.

A second group of organizations engaged in health activities are those established by private philanthropy, such as the Rockefeller Foundation, the WK Kellogg Foundation, the Carnegie Foundation, the Milbank Memorial Fund, and the Pew Charitable Trust. The third influential group of voluntary health agencies is made up of professional associations such as the American Public Health Association, the ANA, the NLN, and their state and local affiliates. These groups not only meet the needs of their professional members for meetings and dissemination of information but they also establish and improve standards for practice and education, encourage research, further health education, and promote educational programs for professionals and consumers (Figure 1-2).

Nurses play a significant role in voluntary efforts to promote health. Nurses often serve on local, state, and national boards of voluntary organizations, work as employees, serve as volunteers in carrying out the mission of the agency, and develop many of the health-related materials, literature,

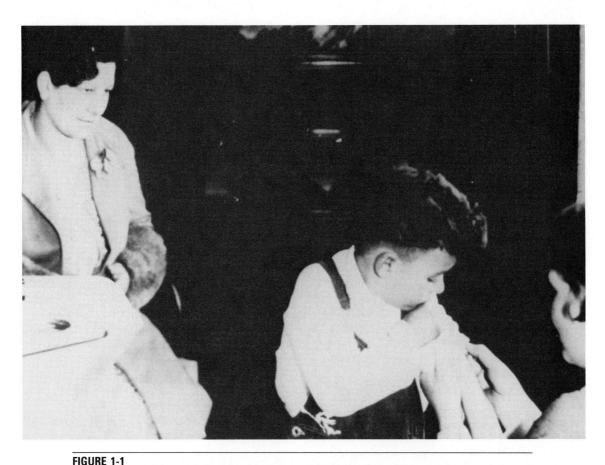

FIGURE 1-1

Clinic visit for immunization. (Donated by the Jefferson County Department of Health, Birmingham, Ala., Myra Downs, Director, Bureau of Public Health Nursing.)

and teaching aids provided by the agency. Nurses are also the recipients of grants to improve health care from both voluntary agencies and foundations.

Nursing Organizations and Nursing Education

Beginning in the late nineteenth century and continuing until the present, nursing organizations and specialized education in public health have been evolving. The early organizations, just as today's groups are, were instrumental in recommending how curricula should be shaped to effectively include public health content.

Nursing Organizations in the United States

Concurrently, nurses were organizing into national groups. In 1893 Isabel Hampton Robb led the effort to establish the Society of Superintendents of Training Schools of Nurses in the United States and Canada. The society, which later became the National League for Nursing (NLN), established training standards, and promoted colleagueship among nurses. Two years later the Nurses' Associated Alumnae of the United States and Canada, which later became the American Nurses Association (ANA), was organized to strengthen the union of nursing organizations, improve nursing education, and promote ethical standards.

In 1911 a joint committee composed of representatives of the ANA and the American Society of Superintendents of Training Schools was appointed to standardize nurses' services outside the hospital. Lillian Wald chaired and Mary Gardner served as secretary of the committee that recommended that a new organization be formed to meet the needs of community health nurses. They subsequently invited 800 agencies known to be involved in community health nursing activities to send delegates to an organizational meeting in Chicago in June 1912. A heated debate commenced concerning the name and purpose of this organization; however, at noon on June 7, 1912, the delegates unanimously voted the National Organization for Public Health Nursing (NOPHN) into existence, with Lillian Wald as its first president.

The new organization sought "to standardize public health nursing activities on a high level and coordinate all efforts in the field" (Deloughery, 1977, p. 116). Although it was primarily a nursing organization, anyone interested in community health nursing could participate. Because of its willingness to cooperate with other groups with similar interests, the organization grew rapidly and remained in existence until the American Public Health Association (APHA) came into being.

Community Health Nursing Education

Initially, community health nursing required special education. Debate ensued as to whether community health

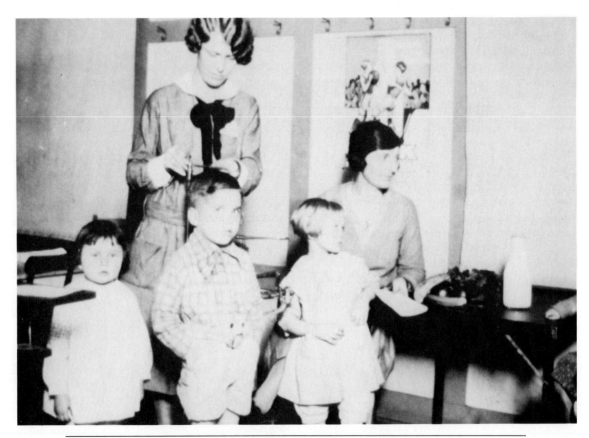

FIGURE 1-2

Instruction of dietetics in school in early 1900. (Donated by the Jefferson County Department of Health, Birmingham, Ala., Myra Downs, Director, Bureau of Public Health Nursing.)

nurses needed a basic nursing education or just special training in home care. Nursing leaders decided that all nurses needed some community health content; hence, basic undergraduate courses began to include the topic of community health, with Boston leading the way with the first undergraduate community health course.

As community health nursing grew as a specialized and respected area of nursing, it became apparent that the inclusion of this content in basic curricula was insufficient. In 1914 Mary Adelaide Nutting offered the first postgraduate nursing course in community health at Teachers College, in affiliation with the Henry Street Settlement (Deloughery, 1977). When this turned out to be successful, Boston began a special training program for community health nurses, which developed into an 8-month course affiliated with Simmons College.

During World War I the Vassar Camp School for nurses started in 1918 as a unique and patriotic aspect of nursing education. The American Red Cross and the Council of National Defense jointly supported this novel program, which proposed that nursing education could be shortened from 3 years to 2 years for college graduates. The Vassar Camp School, modeled after the Plattsburg Military Camp in New York, gave intensive training to college graduates so they could become army reserve officers and meet urgent wartime needs. A total of 435 graduates of this program represented many colleges across the country. The program ended when peace was declared.

Nursing education profited from the landmark study published in 1923 as *The Report of the Committee for Study of Nursing Education*. This study, directed by Josephine Goldmark, led to the Rockefeller Foundation's endowment of the School of Nursing at Yale University. During this same time, Frances Payne Bolton, a wealthy Cleveland citizen, contributed financial support to establish the School of Nursing at Western Reserve University. She had become interested in nursing education on reading the Goldmark report and subsequently contributed significantly to nursing education.

Schools of nursing proliferated during the 1920s amid turmoil and change. In 1925 the three major nursing organizations (NLN, ANA, and NOPHN) authorized a program for grading schools, and in 1926 the Committee on the Grading of Nursing Schools began with 21 members. The committee had three major goals: to study the supply and demand for nursing service, to complete a job analysis of nurses, and to grade nursing schools. Grading began in 1929 and was repeated again in 1932, leading to the closing of several hundred weak schools.

Collegiate programs increasingly included content in community health nursing. The first basic program in nursing was accredited in 1944 and included sufficient community health content so that graduates did not need additional training courses to practice community health nursing (National Organization for Public Health Nursing, 1944, p. 371).

Training for Nurses for National Defense, the GI Bill, the Nurse Training Act of 1943, and Public Health and Professional Nurse Traineeships provided additional educational funds (McNeil, 1967).

In 1946 a committee of representatives for agencies interested in community health met to establish guidelines for this area of nursing (Public Health Nursing 1946, p. 387). These guidelines became necessary because community health nursing evolved in an unplanned fashion with sponsorship by many voluntary agencies, thereby leading to a great deal of overlap. The guidelines took into account this history of community health nursing and proposed that a population of 50,000 be required to support a community health program and that there should be one nurse for each 2200 people. Other principles addressed were that (1) the function of community health nursing includes health teaching, disease control, and care of the sick and (2) the community should adopt one of the following three organizational patterns (Public Health Nursing, 1946):

1. All community health nurse services will be administered by the local health department.
2. Preventive health care will be provided by health departments and home health care will be by a cooperating voluntary agency.
3. A combination service will be jointly administered and financed by official and voluntary agencies, with all services provided by one group of community health nurses.

By the early 1960s community health nursing began to assume a more active role in society. Practice in community health nursing became a requirement of all baccalaureate programs in nursing. In 1964 the ANA defined a community health nurse as a graduate from a baccalaureate program in nursing accredited by the NLN.

Over the next 30 years several major changes in nursing education occurred, including the development and rapid expansion of practical nursing programs and the establishment of associate degree nursing programs in 1953, with Mildred Montag's doctoral dissertation at Teachers College in New York City. Moreover, starting in 1963 the NLN required baccalaureate programs to include public health nursing in order to be eligible for accreditation. Additionally, a major conceptual change in nursing resulted from the 1965 ANA's position paper on nursing practice, which proposed that the education of nurses should take place in institutions of higher learning. In 1966 the APHA and NLN jointly developed a program for accrediting community health nursing services. This was the first effort to accredit the delivery of nursing services and continues today as a vital and sought after program.

In recent decades, nursing has advanced as a scholarly profession characterized by increased research among practitioners and the development of a conceptual basis for practice.

Health Departments and Community Health Nursing

Advances in community health nursing paralleled those in both nursing and community health (Table 1-2). During the 1920s community health nursing recognized the relationship between health and economic security and began to assume responsibility for community health. By 1920 all states and most large cities had health departments, with the majority of the staff being community health nurses. During this period community health nursing assumed a leadership role in establishing standards for nursing practice. As mentioned earlier, community health nurses received advanced preparation, and the major community health nursing organization provided for collaboration among citizens, nurses, and other health providers. All who desired community health nursing care received it, regardless of their ability to pay. During the early decades of the twentieth century the scope of community health nursing included disease pre-

vention, health promotion, and family-oriented services (Figure 1-3). This type of nursing care serves as a prototype of contemporary community health nursing.

World Wars I and II and Community Health Nursing

The onset of World War I in 1915 threatened the role of community health nurses. The large numbers of nurses involved in the war left very few to practice in the community

TABLE 1-2
Milestones in the history of community health and community health nursing: 1866-1946

1872	American Public Health Association established
1873	Training schools established at Bellevue Hospital, New Haven Hospital, and Massachusetts General Hospital; Linda Richards becomes first nurse to graduate in the United States
1877	Women's Board of the New York Mission hires Frances Root to visit the sick poor
1878	National Quarantine Act passed by Congress
1879	New York Ethical Society places trained nurses in dispensaries
1880	Division of Child Hygiene established in New York Health Department
1885	District Nursing Association in Buffalo established
1886	First visiting nurse society in Philadelphia provides home health care; instructive district nursing begins in Boston
1889	Chicago Visiting Nursing Association established
1893	Visiting nursing service for the poor in New York organized by Lillian Wald and Mary Brewster; American Society of Superintendents of Training Schools for Nurses organized (became National League for Nursing Education in 1912)
1895	Industrial nursing program initiated at Vermont Marble Works
1896	Nurses' Associated Alumnae of United States and Canada organized (became ANA in 1911)
1898	Public health nurses hired by Los Angeles Health Department; Detroit Visiting Nurse Association formed
1899	International Council of Nurses organized; university education for nurses introduced at Teachers College, New York
1900	American Journal of Nursing begins publication
1902	School nursing started in New York (Lina Rogers)
1903	First nurse practice acts; tuberculosis nursing in Baltimore
1905	200 organizations providing public health nursing (about 440 nurses)
1906	First post graduate course in district nursing offered by the Instructive District Nursing Association (Boston)
1907	Alabama law permitting employment of public health nurses passed
1908	Detroit Health Department hires public health nurses
1909	The Visiting Nurse Quarterly first published in Cleveland (in 1918 became a monthly, The Public Health Nurse, and in 1931 name changed to Public Health Nursing); Metropolitan Life Insurance initiates offer of home nursing to its industrial policy holders
1910	Public health nursing program instituted at Teachers College, New York
1911	First state public health nursing laws passed
1912	National Organization for Public Health Nursing formed with Lillian Wald as first president; Rural Nursing Service of American Red Cross established; National League for Nursing Education started
1913	Division of Public Health Nursing, New York State Department of Public Health organized
1914	First undergraduate nursing education course in public health offered by Adelaide Nutting at Teachers College
1916	1922 organizations providing 5152 public health nurses
1917	Publication of the Standard Curriculum for Nursing Schools
1918	Vassar Camp School for Nurses organized; USPHS establishes division of public health nursing to work in extracantonment zones
1919	Public Health Nursing written by Mary S. Gardner
1920	NOPHN approves university programs in public health nursing; passage of Sheppard-Towner Act
1922	4040 public health agencies providing 11,548 nurses
1923	Report issued by Committee for Study of Nursing Education (Goldmark Report)
1924	U.S. Indian Bureau Nursing Service established
1925	Frontier Nursing Service using nurse-midwives organized (Mary Breckenridge); first NOPHN statement of qualifications for public health nurses; John Hancock Mutual Life Insurance Company starts Visiting Nurse Service
1926	Committee on Grading of Nursing Schools begins studies
1931	4255 public health organizations providing 15,865 nurses
1933	Pearl McIver becomes first nurse employed by USPHS
1934	Survey of Public Health Nursing published by NOPHN
1935	Facts about Nursing first published by ANA: Passage of Social Security Act
1942	American Association of Industrial Nurses established
1943	Bolton-Bailey Act for nursing education and Cadet Nurse Program passed; Division of Nursing Education started by USPHS (Lucille Petry appointed chief of Cadet Nurse Corps)
1944	First basic program in nursing accredited as including sufficient public health content

setting. However, the American Red Cross helped to sustain community health nursing by establishing a roster of nurses who could be enlisted to supply health care.

During the war the NOPHN loaned a nurse to the U.S. Public Health Service to establish a community health nursing program for military outposts, which led to the first community health nursing program sponsored by the federal government (Gardner, 1919, p. 44).

After World War I, many changes occurred that subsequently affected community health nursing. Despite the economic constraints of the depression, this era witnessed many advancements in community health nursing. Because of limited local and national resources many people volunteered to assist others, and these volunteers rapidly learned the value of community health nursing. Also, many federally funded relief projects utilized nurses, which led to the need for these federally employed nurses to provide consultation to the states. In 1933 Pearl McIver became the first nurse employed by the U.S. Public Health Service to provide consultation services to state health departments. Before 1936 only a few states had budgeted community health nursing positions; by 1936 all states included some type of community health nursing consultation services in their budgets.

The onset of World War II in 1941 accelerated the need for nurses. Many nurses joined the Army and Navy Nurse Corps, and substantial funding was provided by the Bolton Act of 1943 to establish the Cadet Nurses Corps. The National Nursing Council, comprising six national nursing organizations and assisted by the U.S. Department of Education, received a million dollars to expand facilities for nursing education. The U.S. Public Health Service managed these nursing education funds. During this time community health nursing expanded its scope of practice. Community health nurses moved into rural area, and many official agencies began to provide bedside nursing care.

Frontier Nursing Service

The Frontier Nursing Service (FNS), characterized by a unique pioneering spirit, was influential in the development of community health programs. Its historical development is detailed here because of the contributions of FNS nurses in improving the health care of a rural and often inaccessible population. The FNS developed as the result of nurse Mary Breckenridge's commitment to provide care to isolated and needy people in Appalachian sections of Kentucky. Mary Breckenridge is described in the box on p. 14.

Having volunteered after World War I with the American Committee for Devastated France, she had considerable experience in public health nursing services for the sick of all ages. When she returned to the United States she used money her grandmother had left her to start the forerunner

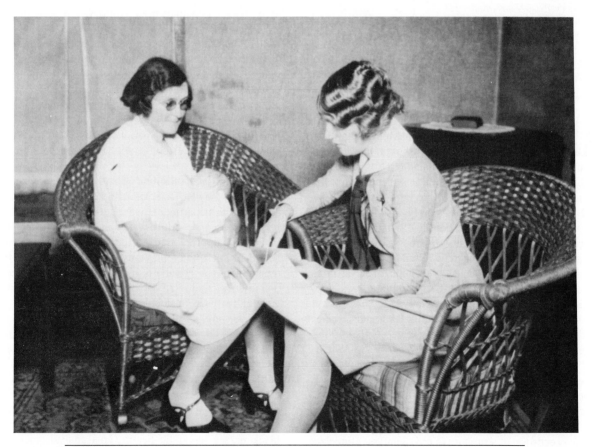

FIGURE 1-3

Early public health nurse making home visits to mother and newborn. (Donated by the Jefferson County Department of Health, Birmingham, Ala., Myra Downs, Director, Bureau of Public Health Nursing.)

MARY BRECKENRIDGE

Born in 1881 into the fifth generation of a Kentucky family, Mary Breckenridge devoted her life to the establishment of the Frontier Nursing Service. Learning from her grandmother, who used a large part of her fortune to improve the education of Southern children, she later used money left to her by her grandmother to start the FNS.

She was tutored in childhood and later attended private schools, but she did not consider becoming a nurse until her husband died. In 1907 she began studying nursing at St. Luke's Hospital School of Nursing in New York. She later married for a second time and had two children. Her son died at the age of four and her daughter died at birth. From the time of her son's death in 1918, she devoted her considerable energy to promoting the health care of disadvantaged women and children (Browne, 1966).

After World War I and her work in postwar France, Breckenridge returned to the United States, passionate about helping the neglected children of rural America. To prepare herself for what would become her life's work, she studied for a year at Teacher's College, Columbia University, to learn more about public health nursing.

Early in 1925, she returned to Kentucky. She decided that the mountains of Kentucky were an excellent place to demonstrate the value of public health nursing to remote, disadvantaged families. She thought that if she could establish a nursing center in rural Kentucky, this effort could then be duplicated anywhere.

Like her nurses, Mary Breckenridge traveled many miles through the mountains of Kentucky on her horse, Babette, providing food, supplies, and health care to mountain families. A hard worker, she had little patience with laggards (Browne, 1966).

of the FNS, the Kentucky Committee for Mothers and Babies. The first health center was established in a five room cabin in Hyden, Kentucky. Establishing the center took more than nursing skills; the construction of the center and later the hospital and other buildings required extensive knowledge about securing a water supply, disposing of sewage, getting electric power, and building in a mountain area in which landslides could occur (Browne, 1966).

Despite many obstacles inherent in building in the mountains, six outpost nursing centers were built between 1927 and 1930. The FNS hospital in Hyden, Kentucky, was completed in 1928, and physicians began entering service. Payment of fees ranged from giving in return labor and supplies to funds raised through annual family dues, philanthropy, and the fund-raising efforts of Mary Breckenridge (Holloway, 1975). During the early years, the Frontier Nursing Service established medical, surgical, and dental clinics; provided nursing and midwifery services 24 hours a day; and served nearly 10,000 people spread out over 700 square miles.

At the suggestion of a supportive physician, baseline data were obtained on infant and maternal mortality rates before beginning services. The reduced mortality rates following the inception of the FNS are especially remarkable considering the environmental conditions in which these rural Kentuckians lived. Many homes had no heat, electricity, or running water; often physicians were located over 40 miles from their patients (Tirpak, 1975). During the 1930s nurses lived and saw patients from one of the six outposts and often had to make their visits on horseback (Figure 1-4).

Medicaid and Medicare made available to the FNS a more predictable source of revenue than they had been assured through gifts and contributions. In 1939 Mary Breckenridge established the FNS School of Midwifery. Over the years, deliveries increasingly took place in hospitals, thereby reducing the need for midwifery and accelerating the demand for family nursing. By 1975, with only 7% of nursing time devoted to midwifery, the 41 FNS nurses devoted their attention to meeting the primary care needs of the residents of Leslie County, Kentucky (Frontier Nursing Service, 1978). Once admitted to a nurse's district, clients are seen at least once a year until they die or move.

Over the years several hundred nurses have worked at the FNS. Despite the fact that Mary Breckenridge died in 1965, the FNS has continued to grow and provide needed services to people in the mountains of Kentucky. This service continues today as a vital and creative way to deliver public health services to rural families. The role of nurses in the FNS has always been similar to that of family nurse practitioners and nurse midwives.

The Years Following World War II

Many societal changes after World War II subsequently affected community health nursing (Table 1-3). These included a more prosperous economy and increasing use of the automobile. Where community health nurses had previously made visits on foot, in horse-drawn buggies, or on bicycles, automobiles made it possible to see far more people. Additionally, wartime service called national attention to the poor health of young and middle-age males. Approximately 29% of all men called up for military service were rejected because of poor and often preventable health conditions.

Due to the level of military health care, veterans returning home from the war expected a higher quality of health care. Local health departments were soon faced with a group of patients who expected services and with a sudden increase in emotional problems, accidents, alcoholism, and other health problems not previously considered to be in their treatment domain (Roberts and Heinrich, 1985). Funds were increased and targeted to specific health problems such as venereal disease, cancer, tuberculosis and mental illness. Likewise, funding through the GI bill was available to send veterans to school, and many chose to study public health.

Local health departments increased dramatically; by 1955, 72% of all counties in the continental United States had full-time local health services. Public health nurses comprised a large proportion of the staff in these health departments. During the 1950s there was considerable interest in nurse-midwifery, equality and advancement of black nurses in public health, cost analysis methods and studies, inclusion of nursing services in health insurance programs, and better coordination of organized nursing (Roberts and Heinrich, 1985). One considerable setback in this decade was the dilution of public health content in nursing curricula. Students received limited information on groups and the community as a unit of service. Instead, as nursing education focused heavily on the care of individuals, new graduates were not adequately prepared to work in public health without considerable agency orientation and teaching.

The 1960s witnessed a revolution in health care that affected public health and public health nursing. In 1964 the passage of the Economic Opportunity Act provided funds for neighborhood health centers, Head Start, and many other community action programs. Funding was also increased for maternal and child health, mental health and mental retardation, and public health training. In 1965, Congress amended the Social Security Act to include health insurance benfits for the elderly (Medicare) and increased care for the poor (Medicaid). Unfortunately, the revised Act did not include coverage for preventive services, and home health care was reimbursed only when ordered by the physician. However, this latter coverage prompted the rapid proliferation of home health care agencies. Many local and state health departments rapidly changed their policies to allow them to provide reimbursable home care. This often led to the decline of their health promotion and disease prevention activities. From 1960 to 1968 the number of official agencies that provided home care services grew from 250 to 1328. Many for-profit agencies began during this era also.

Two additional major factors influenced public health nursing during the 1960s: the development of the nurse practitioner movement and the call for the evaluation of the

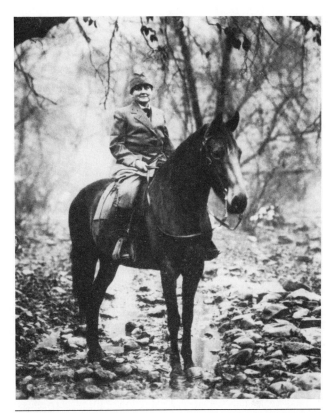

FIGURE 1-4

Mary Breckenridge, founder of the Frontier Nursing Service.

TABLE 1-3	
Milestones in the history of community health and community health nursing: 1946-1990	

1946	Nurses classified as professionals by U.S. Civil Service Commission; Hill-Burton Act approved; passage of National Mental Health Act
1948	NLN established accrediting service
1949	National Federation of Licensed Practical Nurses organized
1950	25,091 nurses employed in public health field
1951	NLN recommends collegiate basic nursing education include content in public health nursing; National Association of Colored Graduate Nurses merges with ANA
1952	Six nursing organizations merge into two: ANA and NLN; associate degree nursing started; Boston University begins program in general nursing approved for preparation of public health nurses
1953	*Nursing Outlook* published
1955	27,112 nurses employed in public health field
1959	NLN votes that no new specialized baccalaureate program be accredited (move toward general education in nursing); after 1963 only baccalaureate programs including public health nursing to be eligible for accreditation
1960	NLN establishes criteria for evaluation of educational programs in nursing that lead to baccalaureate and master's degrees
1964	Nurse Training Act passed
1965	Position paper of ANA proposes that education for nurses take place in institutions of higher learning
1970	National Commission on Nursing and Nursing Education offers Abstract for Action
1977	Passage of Rural Health Clinic Services Act, which provides indirect reimbursement for nurse practitioners in rural health clinics
1978	President Carter vetoes Nurse Training Act
1978	Establishment of Association of Graduate Faculty in Community Health Nursing/Public Health Nursing (later became Association of Community Health Nursing Educators)
1980	Medicaid amendment to the Social Security Act for direct reimbursement for nurse practitioners in rural health clinics
1980	Both ANA and APHA developed statements on the role and conceptual foundations of community health nursing.
1983	Advent of prospective payment for the Medicare program, that is, diagnostic-related groups (DRGs)
1985	Establishment of Center for Nursing Research
1990	Association of Community Health Nursing Educators publishes *Essentials of Baccalaureate Nursing Education*

effectiveness of public health programs. The nurse practitioner movement began in 1965 at the University of Colorado and opened a new era for nursing involvement in primary health care. Initially, the nurse practitioner was a public health nurse with additional skills in the diagnosis and treatment of common illnesses. Although many nurse practitioners remained in public health, others migrated to a variety of clinical areas. In public health, they have made sustained contributions in providing primary health care to people in rural areas and the inner cities and in other medically underserved areas (Roberts and Heinrich, 1985).

Historically, public health nursing relied on case studies and numerical reports of services provided to evaluate their programs. By 1965 federal regulations were developed that required states to submit plans for how they would reduce major health problems. These new regulations required considerable work and a major refocusing of how evaluation was done.

The enthusiasm of the 1960s continued into the 1970s, and several new developments occurred that influenced public health nursing. Prevention regained prominence at the federal level, and the question of "What is public health nursing?" reemerged. The individual orientation of health care in the 1960s gave way in the 1970s to a review of what broader views needed to be considered to provide comprehensive health care services. Evaluation of the effectiveness of care continued, and nursing was increasingly viewed as a powerful force in improving the health care of communities. Nurse practitioners became increasingly accepted as cost effective providers of primary health care services, and educational programs to prepare nurse practitioners grew.

Public health nursing and nursing in general were on the move. Nurses made significant contributions to the hospice movement, the development of birthing centers, day care for the elderly and disabled, drug abuse programs, and rehabilitation services in long-term care (Roberts and Heinrich, 1985).

The 1980s witnessed an unheralded concern in the United States with cost effectiveness in health care. Health promotion and disease prevention programs received less priority as funding was shifted to meet the escalating costs of hospital care and medical procedures. The use of ambulatory services, including health maintenance organizations, was encouraged; home health care and services of nurse practitioners grew. People were encouraged to assume more responsibility for their own health status. Health education, always a part of public health nursing, became popular and people seemed to think this was something new. Consumer groups urged laws to prohibit unhealthy practices such as smoking in public areas and driving under the influence of alcohol. As funds grew scarce the presence of nurses in official agencies diminished. Public health nurses, steadfast in their determination to improve the health care of Americans, have pressed for greater involvement in official and private agencies.

The 1980s saw an increase in the presence of public health nurses in many states. The establishment in 1985 of the National Center for Nursing Research within the National Institutes of Health in Washington, D.C., will be a major tool in promoting the work of nurses. Through research nurses can document the quality of care they give by looking at the cost-effectiveness of their actions and also the outcomes of nursing intervention.

COMMUNITY HEALTH NURSING IN CANADA

There are many similarities in the history and beliefs of community health nurses in the United States and in Canada. The roots of community health nursing in both Canada and in the United States can be traced to St. Vincent de Paul of France, who campaigned for helping the poor become more skilled and useful and, if this was not possible, to at least visit the poor in the homes and provide the needed care and support (Allemang, 1985). The actual beginning of community nursing in New France (Canada) is attributed to the Duchesse d'Aiguillon, who sent nurses to the New World to begin a hospital, and Mademoiselle Jeanne Mance, who founded the Hotel Dieu. The Hotel Dieu provided care for the sick and people in need of shelter and attention. Unconditional care was given to new settlers waiting to build homes, seamen, soldiers, and Indians.

The regionalism that was characteristic of the nineteenth century in Canada began in 1763 when New France was ceded to Great Britian. As Allemang (1985, p. 4) says, during this time "human life was threatened by wars, the hazards of immigration, the dangers of pioneer life, epidemics of infectious diseases, and the scarcity of health care and services." The regions of the land that later became Canada were very different in geography, environmental conditions, and stages of development.

Wars brought sickness, casualities, and the disruption of families. The arrival of poor, malnourished immigrants brought typhus fever, cholera, and other infectious diseases. Clearing the land to build homes and towns caused injuries and death, and for women, childbirth remained dangerous. Missionaries cared for the sick; hospitals were established and medical education began in 1824 with the establishment of the first school in Montreal (Allemang, 1985). The work of the Grey Nuns in the remote areas of Canada is similar to that of the Frontier Nursing Service in the United States.

The establishment of training schools for nurses greatly influenced the development of community health nursing in Canada. As in the United States, nursing and nursing education in Canada was greatly influenced by the work of Florence Nightingale and took into account the role of the environment on health status. The first training school was established in 1874 in St. Catharines, Ontario. Graduate nurses joined the existing group of medical missionaries who were providing care to people in remote areas.

The first Board of Health was established in Ontario, Canada, in 1882, and legislation establishing health boards in all provinces except New Brunswick and Prince Edward Island was soon passed.

The First Visiting Nurses in Canada

The first visiting nurses in Canada were the Grey Nuns, established in Montreal in 1747 by Marguerite D'Youville, a wealthy widow (Pringle, 1988). In addition to providing good nursing care in hospitals, these nuns visited the sick in their homes. Despite their effectiveness, home health care did not actually develop for 150 more years.

Following the model of William Rathbone in England as previously discussed, the Victorian Order of Nurses was established in 1897 with branches in Halifax, Montreal, Ottawa, and Toronto. In her travels across the country, Lady Aberdeen, the wife of the Governor General of Canada from 1894 to 1898 and President of the National Council of Women, became increasingly alarmed at the lack of health services for women. She suggested that an order, similar to the "Queen's Nurses" in the United Kingdom, be established to provide visiting nurses and cottage hospitals to small communities (Allemang, 1985). Despite opposition from the medical community, which feared that standards of care would be lowered, the Victorian Order of Nurses for Canada (VON) was established in 1897 with Charlotte Macleod as the first superintendent. Nurses working at the VON were required to be graduates of a training school for nurses and have six additional months of training in district nursing at a VON center.

In each community the VON established a "house which served as office, residence for the nurses, and training school in district nursing" (Pringle, 1988, p. 124). In the early years, the VON was involved in a range of public health activities in addition to its initial purpose of providing home care. By the 1950s and 1960s public health units had developed and assumed many of the general functions of the VON, thereby freeing up the VON to devote 98% of its time to care of the ill either following hospitalization or as a result of a chronic illness.

Currently, VON is a voluntary nonprofit organization with responsibility for identifying unmet needs in the community and developing services to meet them. This organization has been remarkably successful in weathering the storms of change as Canada has implemented a national health plan and in remaining viable by virtue of being creative and identifying new health care needs as times and conditions change. At present, health promotion and disease prevention programs are emerging as significant VON services.

The Twentieth Century

The early twentieth century witnessed a rapidly growing population, a national optimism, and a belief in the ability of individuals to master and control circumstances (Allemang, 1985). The decades of optimism and prosperity had a dark side: tuberculosis was a leading cause of death; cities became crowded; reservation Indians were victims of epidemics of typhoid fever, measles, smallpox, tuberculosis; and war resulted in broken families and disabled veterans.

Small and large hospitals grew after World War I, and groups such as the VON, Canadian Red Cross Society, religious sisterhoods, and mission boards extended services out of the hospitals into the homes. Health promotion became popular, and industries, insurance companies, and department stores developed health services to keep their employees well.

Nurses became an integral part of the public health system in Canada. In addition to schools of nursing, hospitals, and visiting nursing services that relied on nurses, Divisions of Public Health Nursing were formed in provincial and municipal health departments. The role of the public health nurse became one of health teaching, case finding, and preventive care in a variety of settings. As in the United States, the debate began in Canada about whether public health nurses needed specialty training or if their basic educational programs prepared them for this work. The first 5-year nursing program was begun in 1919 at the University of British Columbia. The 5-year program offered liberal and scientific education, then an opportunity for students to choose public health nursing or the teaching of nursing. Critics said that too much of the educational program resided under the control of the hospital. In 1933 a new type of 3-year program was established that taught students how to practice in both the hospital and the community. In 1942 this program was replaced with a 4-year program leading to the Bachelor of Science in Nursing degree.

Origins of Government Health Insurance

The origins of government health insurance in Canada can be traced to 1665 when a Montreal physician offered a form of prepaid coverage to 26 families in his city. Saskatchewan, with its 1916 Union Hospital Act, launched the modern era of prepaid insurance. The financial ravages of the Depression of the 1930s increased awareness of the need for a better way to finance health care. In 1935, the same year that the Social Security Act was passed in the United States, the federal government attempted to implement the Employment and Social Insurance Act, but the provinces challenged such legislation. By 1957 the federal government had succeeded in convincing five provinces to provide a hospital insurance program. By 1961 all Canadian provinces, together with the Northwest and Yukon Territories, were participating in a federal health program to provide hospital insurance to 99% of all Canadian residents.

The initiation of medical insurance was more provocative than had been the hospital insurance. The Medical Care Act was implemented in 1968. In 1984 financial arrangements for health care in Canada were incorporated into the Canada Health Act. The most controversial part of the bill was the banning of extra billing by physicians and hospitals. In recent years, Canada like the United States has been fighting the high costs of health care and must consider such unpopular options as rationing services and deinsuring services (Baumgart, 1988).

Goal of "Health for All"

Canada subscribes to the World Health Organization's goal of "Health for All." In 1978 the World Health Organization (WHO) adopted as a goal "the attainment by all peoples of the world by the year 2000 of a level of health that will permit them to lead a socially and economically productive life. Primary health care is the key to attaining this target" (WHO, 1978, p. 1). This goal, now known as the Declaration of Alma Ata, has been endorsed by many nations. For many years Canada has placed a high value upon primary health care and has financed initiatives to implement a philosophy that supports health promotion and disease prevention.

SUMMARY

The history of community health nursing can be traced to the earliest record of civilization. Throughout history, periods of progress have been overshadowed by setbacks as health has been alternatively given high priority and then ignored. Many of the advances in community health arose out of necessity. Wars, massive immigration, epidemics, and other devastating health conditions demanded immediate resolutions.

Major social, economic, and political developments have influenced community health programs in the United States, with many advances made as a result of congressional action. Community health nursing has been at the forefront in developing and encouraging other groups to institute healthier living conditions and care for all people.

The history of the early Christian church is replete with

examples of home health care. St. Vincent de Paul influenced home care in both the United States and Canada, as did the work of Florence Nightingale, who influenced all future nursing practices. Lillian Wald organized visiting nursing in New York, established the unique program at the Henry Street Settlement, and was responsible for many improvements in living conditions in New York City. She also established the first program of nursing services provided by an insurance company. Over the years, community health nursing in both the United States and Canada has evolved from a home care service delivered by caring women who ministered to both the health and spiritual needs of individuals and families to a broadly based, population-focused discipline that considers individuals, families, groups, and communities as the scope of practice.

KEY CONCEPTS

An understanding of the dominant cultural ideas of each era since early recorded history is useful in understanding the antecedents of the current community health care system.

Rudiments of community health can be traced to the earliest civilizations.

With the dawn of the Christian era, a new conceptualization of man influenced health practices. The early Church believed that the Roman and Grecian ways pampered the body at the expense of the soul. Disease was viewed as a punishment for sin.

The Renaissance ushered in a new period of history during which community health as currently known was begun.

The history of the early Christian Church is replete with examples of home health care. Of considerable importance was the work of St. Vincent de Paul and Mademoiselle Le Gras, who established what was probably the first actual community health nursing program.

The Industrial Revolution witnessed tremendous advances in transportation, communication, and other forms of technology. Modern public health efforts began in England, the first modern industrial nation.

The Poor Law Amendment Act of 1834 ushered in a new era of social welfare and community health in England.

Lillian Wald organized visiting nursing in New York in the nineteenth century, established the unique program at the Henry Street Settlement, and was responsible for many improvements in living conditions in New York City.

The first visiting nurse society in America began in Philadelphia in 1886 to provide home health care to the sick.

The early twentieth century witnessed multiple improvements that both directly and indirectly affected health status.

Several significant events influenced the further development of community health efforts in the first half of the twentieth century, including two major wars and an economic depression.

As the Social Security Act of 1935 attempted to overcome the national setbacks of the depression, it expanded community health nursing.

The Frontier Nursing Service (FNS) was influential in the development of community health programs and was characterized by a unique pioneering spirit.

Although the government retains a major responsibility for the health and welfare of its citizens, voluntary organizations play key roles in community health.

Over the years, community health nursing has evolved from a home care service characterized as being delivered by caring women who ministered to both the health and spiritual needs of individuals and families to a broadly based, population-focused discipline that considers individuals, families, groups, and communities as the scope of practice.

The development of community health nursing in the United States and Canada have many common characteristics.

LEARNING ACTIVITIES

1. Write a summary of what you believe were Lillian Wald's greatest contributions to community health nursing.

2. If you were Lillian Wald and chose to devote your energy to critical forces affecting the health of Americans, what would be your three highest priority efforts?

3. Of the three efforts, take one and develop a realistic plan for (a) implementation and (b) evaluation.

4. Telephone or visit one voluntary agency in your community and describe its purpose, source of funding, major programs or services, and eligibility of recipients of services.

5. Interview three nurses employed in community health nursing to determine how they currently define their role.

6. Describe what you see as (a) the three primary *similarities* between community health nursing in Canada and in the United States and (b) the two major *differences*.

BIBLIOGRAPHY

Allemang MM: Development of community health nursing in Canada. In Stewart M, Innes J, Searl S, and Smillie C: Community health nursing in Canada. Toronto, 1985, Gage Educational Publishing Co.

Baumgart AJ, and Larsen J (editor): Canadian nursing faces the future, St. Louis, 1988, The CV Mosby Co.

Baumgart AJ, and Larsen J: Overview: nursing practice in Canada. In Baumgart AJ, and Larsen J: Canadian nursing faces the future, St. Louis, 1988, The CV Mosby Co.

Brainard AM: Evolution of public nursing, Philadelphia, 1922, WB Saunders Co.

Brown EL: Nursing for the future, New York, 1948, Russell Sage Foundation.

Browne H: A tribute to Mary Breckenridge, Nurs Outlook 14:54-55, May 1966.

Buhler-Wilkerson J: Public health nursing: then and now, Am J Public Health 75:1155-1161, 1985.

Bullough V, and Bullough B: The emergence of modern nursing, New York, 1964, Macmillan Publishing Co.

Cohen IB: Florence Nightingale, Sci Am 250(3):128-137, 1984.

Deloughery GL: History and trends of professional nursing, ed, 8, St. Louis, 1977, The CV Mosby Co.

Desirable organization for public health nursing for family service, Public Health Nurs 38:387-389, Aug. 1946.

Dickens, C: Martin Chuzzlewit, New York, 1975, Penguin Books (Edited by PN Furbank).

Dock L, and Steward I: A short history of nursing, ed. 4, New York, 1983, GP Putnam's Sons.

Dolan J: History of nursing, ed. 14, Philadelphia, 1978, WB Saunders Co.

Frachel RR: A new profession: the evolution of public health nursing, Public Health Nurs 5(2):86-90, 1988.

Frontier Nursing Service: FNS Q Bull 540(2):3-6, 1978.

Gardner MS: Public health nursing, ed. 3, New York, 1919, MacMillan Publishing Company.

Griffin GJ, and Griffin JK: History and trends of professional nursing, ed. 7, St. Louis, 1973, The CV Mosby Co.

Holloway JB: Frontier Nursing Service 1925-1975, J Ky, Med. Assoc. 13:491-492, Sept. 1975.

Kalisch P, and Kalisch BJ: Nursing involvement in the health planning process, DHEW pub. no HRA 78-25, Hyattsville, Md, 1977, U.S. Department of Health, Education and Welfare.

Kalisch P, and Kalisch BJ: The advance of American nursing, ed. 2, Boston, 1986, Little, Brown & Co.

Maynard T: The apostle of charity: the life of St. Vincent de Paul, New York, 1939, Dial Press.

McNeil EE: Transition in public health nursing, John Sundwall Lecture, University of Michigan, February 27, 1967.

National Organization for Public Health Nursing: approval of Skidmore College of Nursing as preparing students for public health nursing, Public Health Nurs. 36:371, July 1944.

Pellegrino ED: Medicine, history, and the idea of man, Ann Am Acad Pol Soc Sci 346:9-20, March 1963.

Pickett G, and Hanlon JJ: Public health administration and practice, ed. 9, St. Louis, 1990, Times Mirror/Mosby College Publishing.

Pringle DM: Nursing practice in the home: the role of the Victorian Order of Nurses. In Baumgart AJ and Larsen J (editor). Canadian nursing faces the future, St. Louis, 1988, The CV Mosby Co.

Roberts DE, and Heinrich J: Public health nursing comes of age, American Journal of Public Health. 75(10):1162-1172, 1985.

Rosen G: A history of public health, New York, 1958, MD Publications.

Schudson M: The Flexner Report and the Reed Report on the history of professional education in the United States, Soc Sci Q 55:347-361, Sept. 1974.

Shyrock H: The history of nursing, Philadelphia, 1959, WB Saunders Co.

Swinson A: The history of public health, Exeter, England, 1965, A. Wheaton & Co.

Tirpak H: The Frontier Nursing Service—fifty years in the mountains, Nurs. Outlook 33:308-310, May, 1975.

Wilner DM, Walkey RP, and O'Neill EJ: Introduction to public health, ed. 7, New York, 1978, Macmillan Publishing Co.

World Health Organization: Primary health care: report of the international conference on primary health care, Alma Ata, Ussr 6-12 September 1978, Geneva, Switzerland, World Health Organization.

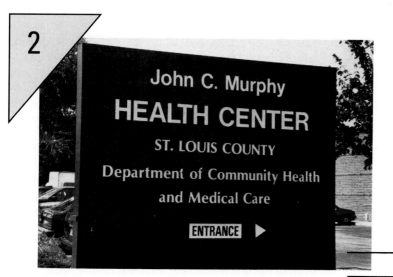

2

Current Status of the Health Care System

Jeanette Lancaster

Wade Lancaster

OBJECTIVES

After reading this chapter, the student should be able to:

Define health, health care, and public health.
Differentiate between health promotion and disease prevention.
Describe the current public health system in the United States.
Identify three factors that people identify as flaws in the US health care system.
Describe three trends in the United States that are affecting health care.
Compare the US health care system with the Canadian system.
Discuss current community health nursing in both the United States and Canada.

KEY TERMS

alternate delivery
  system
ambulatory care center
community health
  nursing
consumerism
demographic trends
dependent practitioner
disease prevention
health promotion

Health Maintenance
  Organization (HMO)
home health agency
hospice
independent
  practitioner
Preferred Provider
  Organization (PPO)
prevention
primary care
primary prevention

public health
Public Health Service
public health agency:
  federal, state, and
  local
public health nursing
secondary care
secondary prevention
tertiary care
tertiary prevention

The American health care system has done a remarkable job in many ways in providing health care to the American people. New technologies have been developed, and skilled providers have been trained. Today's health care facilities would defy the imagination of our predecessors. Public and private health insurance programs protect most Americans from the financial ravages of illnesses. However, the system is not without serious liabilities. Major concerns include cost, accessibility, and quality of care.

The cost of health care in the United States has increased dramatically in the last decade. The American public has become increasingly skeptical of physicians and hospitals because of the high costs associated with their services.

Americans spent $550 billion or more than 11.5% of the gross national product on health care in 1990. This is more than any other country in the world spent on health care. The cost containment efforts that have been instituted since 1983 have curbed the growth of *costs*, but they have not solved this tremendous problem. Chapter 4 describes in detail the economics of health care.

Increasing costs have been accompanied by another significant problem: poor *access* to health care. The American health care system is described as a two class system: private and public. People with insurance or those who can personally pay for health care are viewed as receiving superior care compared to people whose only source of care depends upon public funds. People who are uninsured or underinsured tend to seek health care only when they are very sick. This places a considerable burden on the health care system.

The gradual erosion of public health services has added to the access problems. Clinics in rural and heavily populated urban areas are not funded as well as they have been in the past. This forces many people to seek emergency rather than preventive care.

Quality of health care is the third major concern in the United States. Recent studies document that in both the tertiary and public health system, there are considerable variations in quality from one part of the country to another (Institute of Medicine, 1988; Lee and Estes, 1990).

In the landmark document, *The Future of Public Health*, published by the Institute of Medicine in 1988, the state of public health was found to be in disarray. Chapter one of this book stated that many of the improvements in the health of Americans have been accomplished through public health efforts. These improvements include control of epidemic diseases, provision of safe water, food, and environment, and advances in maternal and child health. Now that many of the earlier problems in these areas have been solved, public health has been taken for granted and funding to support preventive health programs has diminished.

This chapter will discuss briefly the current health care system in the United States. Attention will be paid to the development and organization of the public health system and the role of public health nursing in the United States. Also, the public health system in Canada and the role of its public health nurses will be discussed.

HEALTH, HEALTH CARE, AND PUBLIC HEALTH

The term *health* is defined in many different ways. The World Health Organization (1986, p. 1) describes health as "a state of complete physical, mental and social well-being and not merely the absence of disease or infirmity." Pickett and Hanlon (1990, p. 5) describe health as being on a continuum and representing the absence of disability. They go on to say that "a disease or injury is any phenomenon that may lead to an impairment." The definition of *public health* has changed over time. Early definitions discussed the use of sanitary measures against nuisances and health hazards. A recent definition of public health describes it as "organized community efforts aimed at the prevention of disease and promotion of health." It links many disciplines and rests upon the scientific core of epidemiology (Institute of Medicine, 1988, p. 41).

The concepts of health promotion and disease prevention are important in understanding public health. They are defined in the box below.

The levels of prevention parallel the delivery of health care. *Primary care*, typically the entry point into the health care system, focuses on promotion of health, prevention of disease, the management of commonly occurring diseases, and the maintenance of people with chronic diseases. *Secondary care* responds to more severe illnesses or chronic illnesses that erupt periodically into acute phases. Tertiary care deals with serious and often life-threatening illnesses.

Public health emphasizes health promotion and disease prevention. The box offers several additional definitions relevant to the health care system.

TRENDS AFFECTING THE HEALTH CARE SYSTEM

The American health care system is undergoing a revolution. Disgusted with years of escalating costs, big purchasers of health care services—governments, corporations, and unions—are demanding changes in the ways physicians, hospitals, and other providers are used and paid (Califano,

HEALTH PROMOTION AND DISEASE PREVENTION TERMS

Health promotion	Activities aimed at increasing the well-being of individuals, families, and communities.
Prevention	Behaviors designed to avoid disease.
Primary prevention	Actions designed to prevent a disease from occurring; reduces the probability of a specific illness occurring and includes active protection against unnecessary stressors or threats.
Secondary prevention	Early diagnosis and prompt treatment; includes activities such as screening for diseases, e.d., hypertension, breast cancer, cancer of the cervix, blindness, and deafness.
Tertiary prevention	Treatment, care, and rehabilitation of people to prevent further progression of the disease (Pender, 1987).

1986). Most people agree that change is needed. They disagree, however, about what will solve the problems of cost, access, and quality. Several trends, demographic, social, economic, political, and technical, are affecting the health care system.

Demographic Trends

The world's population is growing fast and is expected to double in the next 30 years. Population growth is a function of three factors: fertility, mortality, and immigration into the country. Today, the most explosive growth is occurring in Third World countries. In contrast, in the United States growth has slowed dramatically. Two factors must be considered: the size of the population and the characteristics of its members.

Size of the Population

The Census Bureau reports that the US population increased by 19.2 million between 1980 and 1989. It predicts that the population will continue to grow until 2038, hitting a record high of 302 million before declining in the latter part of the next century (Bureau of the Census, 1989). Interestingly, much of this future growth is expected to be the result of immigration of people from other countries into the United States.

The US birth rate has fluctuated greatly in the last 50 years. From 1946 to 1964, Americans witnessed a "baby boom." This was followed by the "baby bust" of the 1970s, in which the population reached its low point in 1976. In the late 1970s the birth rate began rising again. This increase resulted from the fact that the "baby boom" women had begun having children of their own. A continuation of this trend is not expected, because the "baby boom" women will no longer be of childbearing age (US Bureau of the Census, 1989).

Characteristics of the Population

There will be major changes in American society due to the continuing rise in the average age (Bureau of the Census, 1989). In the last decade, mortality rates for both sexes in all age groups have declined (Exter, 1990). A more significant reason for the changing age distribution is that the baby boom produced about 20% of the present population (US Bureau of the Census, 1990).

The US population is aging. Demographers predict a 74% increase in the number of people aged 50 or older by the year 2020, while the number of people under 50 will only grow approximately 1% (Exter, 1990). The elderly population will increase slowly during the next 20 years, and then rapidly for the following 20 years. From 2010 to 2030, the number of people 65 and older will increase substantially, because the first "baby boomer" will turn 65 in the year 2011. The number of people over 85 is growing so rapidly that by 2050 this group will comprise approximately 24% of the elderly population.

The middle-aged population will also continue to increase since nearly one-third of Americans were born between 1945 and 1960. The entire "baby boom" generation will be over the age of 35 by the turn of the century.

As a result of medical progress, the leading causes of death have changed from infectious diseases to chronic and degenerative diseases. Substantial gains against infectious diseases resulted in steady declines of mortality among children. The mortality rates for older Americans also declined, especially during the 1970s and 1980s. However, people aged 50 and older have higher rates of chronic illness, and they consume a larger portion of health care services than other age groups.

These changing demographic trends will affect the health care system dramatically. It is expected that the nature of hospital admissions will change, with more admissions dealing with acute, intensive, and complicated illnesses. Community care will increase as consumers seek more cost-effective health care than that provided in hospitals. It is also anticipated that the aging population will require more home health care and nursing-home services than previous generations because of their increasing longevity and the chronic nature of their illnesses. Chapter 4 discusses the economic impact of these demographic trends.

Social Trends

In addition to the size and changing age distribution of the population, other factors also affect the health care system. Several social trends that influence health care include changing lifestyles, a growing appreciation of the quality of life, changing composition of families and living patterns, rising household incomes, and a revised definition of quality health care.

Historically, US citizens have been driven by the "American dream." This dream emphasized hard work, getting a good education, and achieving a better life than the previous generation. However, the drive to achieve these goals has diminished. There have been major shifts in American values and lifestyles. Replacing the work ethic is an increasing emphasis on an improved quality of life and the fulfillment of personal goals. This shift in values is reordering the relative importance of economic success. It can be seen in a variety of behaviors, such as increased attention to leisure pursuits, self-help, fitness, and nutrition.

The self-help movement, for example, has emphasized

SELECTED HEALTH CARE DEFINITIONS

Health care system: The organization and distribution of all the resources a society allocates for the delivery of health services.

Health services: Individual and institutional public service activities that have as their goal maintaining or restoring health.

Medical care: The delivery of personal or individually oriented health services.

Health care: The output of health services.

Health promotion: Activities that have as their goal developing human resources and behaviors that maintain or enhance well-being.

Disease prevention: Activities that have as their goal protecting people from the ill-effects of actual or potential health threats.

the belief that people are responsible for their own health. Increasingly, people are learning that health is a valuable asset and efforts should be taken to improve it. Centers for promoting all aspects of health are developing in response to this movement.

The composition of households in the United States is also changing. The Census Bureau categorizes households as being either *family* or *nonfamily*. Families are further classified as *married couple*, *female householder*, or *male householder*. The nature, mix, and size of these households has changed considerably. Over the last two decades the percentage of family households has declined from 81% to 72%. Similar declines are reported for married couple families. People are marrying at a later age, delaying child bearing, and having fewer children. Couples with no children under 18 now account for almost half of all families. People are not staying together as long as they did in the past. About 4 of 10 marriages end in divorce. Also, more people are marrying at a later age, and there is an increasing number of divorced and never-married people. More adults are, therefore, living alone. In fact, about 20% of all households are single adult households (Bureau of the Census, 1989; Exter, 1990).

There is a growing number of both single and married women in the work force. Since 1950, the number of married women in the work force increased from less than 25% to more than 50%. It is projected that more than 80% of new entrants into the work force in the next decade will be women, minorities, and immigrants (Schwartz, 1989).

Economic Trends

Sixty years ago income was distributed in such a way that a relatively small proportion of households earned high incomes; a somewhat larger proportion of families were in the middle-income range; and the largest proportion of households were at the low end of the income scale. By the 1970s, household income had risen and income was more evenly distributed. This meant that more families had choices about how to spend their money.

Although the distribution of income has dramatically changed over time, it is important to remember that more than 12 million families—about 20% of households—receive only 5% of the total income. Two-thirds of this group are below the poverty level. This means that a sizable proportion of low-income Americans will continue to rely on public support to maintain a minimum standard of living.

The emphasis on quality health care is diminishing as costs escalate. According to Stevens (1985, p. 27), "Until recently, people sought to preserve life at all costs. But today, society twists and turns on subtle issues of life's quality." The funds available for health care influence the range of services from health promotion to rehabilitation that will be available in any community. Chapter 4 provides a detailed discussion of the economics of health care and how financial constraints influence decisions about public health services.

Health Workforce Trends

Throughout the 1980s the health care industry accounted for 7% to 8% of civilian employment in the United States.

8.8 million people were employed in the health care industry in 1988. About half of them worked in hospitals, 17% worked in nursing and personal care facilities, and 11% worked in physicians' offices. Total employment in the health care field is expected to increase to about 10.3 million by 1995 (US Bureau of the Census, 1990). It is projected that 700,000 physicians will be practicing in the United States by the year 2000, reflecting a 54% increase from 1980 and a surplus of physicians in selected specialties and areas of the country.

Historically, nursing care has been provided in a variety of settings, with the hospital being the dominant setting. Currently, two thirds of all registered nurses are employed in hospitals. It is predicted that as alternative health settings gain popularity, a redistribution of the nurse work force will follow. There will be an increasing need for nurses in non-hospital settings, such as outpatient clinics, health maintenance organizations, home health care, nursing homes, and group and solo medical practice arrangements. It is estimated that by 2000, the need for nursing personnel will be about 1.8 million, a 65% increase from 1980. Between 1987 and 1988 first-year enrollment in nursing schools rose by 4% to 95,000, reversing the 27% decline observed over the previous 3 years (US Bureau of the Census, 1990). Enrollment increased by 5.9% in 1989-1990 and by more than 10.9% in 1990-1991 (AACN, 1991). These gains in enrollment will help to offset the previous substantial declines in nursing school enrollment, but still will not produce sufficient nurses to meet the increasing demand.

Political Trends

The federal government plays a major role in the US health care system by establishing a national health care policy. Currently, three interrelated trends are changing the nature of the system and the roles of the various participants.

The first trend is the pro-competition environment advocated by former President Reagan and other supporters of supply-side economics. Proponents of this theory argue that if prices are not regulated there will be more competition in the marketplace, and price will greatly influence what products and services are purchased. A goal of the pro-competitive environment and one emphasized by the second trend is to reduce total health care expenditures by reducing the amount of money spent by the federal government, primarily through Medicare and Medicaid programs (Weil, 1985). The Prospective Payment System (PPS) was devised in 1983 as a new way to pay hospitals for the services they provide to Medicare patients (Fagin, 1986). From 1981 through 1986, Medicare spending dropped $22 billion and federal Medicaid expenditures fell by $3.8 billion. The goal of this federal policy is to shift the burden of health care costs from the government to other groups including patients, hospitals, and health care providers who are encouraged to work more efficiently and charge less for their services (Weil, 1985).

The third trend is to shift to the states the responsibility of providing appropriate incentives when regulatory policies are enacted. This will slow down the rising rate of health care costs, especially until the pro-competition/supply-side economic policies are well in place (Weil, 1985).

Technological Trends

Improved technology is rapidly changing the health care system. Changes in technology include advances in computer hardware and software, new instruments and drugs, as well as new ways of thinking about and performing diagnostic techniques and surgical procedures (Andreoli and Musser, 1985; Stevens, 1985).

Technology has had both positive and negative effects on the health care system. On the positive side, technological advances promise improved health care services and reduced costs. Recent biomedical developments have reduced the length of hospital stays, cut labor costs, and intervened in what were previously fatal conditions. Technology has increased the number of procedures and techniques that can be performed by home health nurses and family members. Some of the high-technology services that can be delivered in nonhospital settings include chemotherapy, kidney dialysis, intravenous (hydration) therapies and feeding, insulin therapy, antibiotic therapy, apnea monitoring, parenteral and enteral nutritional support services, and biotelemetry (ANA, 1985).

Cost is the most significant negative aspect of advanced health care technology. High-technology equipment is expensive, quickly becomes outdated when newer developments occur, and often requires highly trained personnel.

Unquestionably, advances in medical technology will continue. However, it is anticipated that the emphasis will shift away from expensive diagnostic and therapeutic technologies. Efforts will focus on devising simpler, more mobile, cheaper tests and procedures that are less oriented to tertiary care and can be used in nonhospital settings.

ORGANIZATION OF THE HEALTH CARE SYSTEM

For the last decade, health care in the United States has been a growing enterprise. Since World War II the health care system has grown from one consisting of a general medical practitioner who sent patients to a community hospital to a vast, complex, and often seemingly overwhelming network of providers and institutions. The most elementary model of health care, that of consumers and providers, is shown in Figure 2-1. An enormous number and range of facilities and providers make up the health care system. These include physicians' and dentists' offices, hospitals, health maintenance organizations, nursing homes and other related inpatient facilities, mental health centers, ambulatory care centers, rehabilitation centers, and local, state and federal official and voluntary agencies. See Figure 2-2 for a depiction of the health care system.

Hospitals

Hospitals are the most conspicuous component of the health care system. Generally, hospitals attempt to carry out four major services: patient care, education of health care providers, research, and community service. There are three predominant forms of ownership: government (federal, state, or local); private not-for-profit (voluntary); and private-for-profit (proprietary). The most common type of hospital in the United States is the community hospital, a nonfederal short-term general or specialized hospital.

Before the late 1970s the corporate structure in hospitals

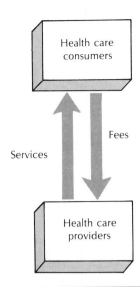

FIGURE 2-1

Elementary model of the health care delivery system.

was reasonably simple, and most were privately owned, not-for-profit institutions. As hospitals felt the effect of prospective payment they began to look at ways to cut costs, and adopting a new corporate structure arose as one alternative. Multihospital systems offered a way to cut overheads in administration and to share services and make purchases in bulk.

Alternative Delivery Systems

The type of organizations grouped under the umbrella of alternative delivery systems (ADSs) include health maintenance organizations (HMOs) and preferred provider organizations (PPOs). "Alternative delivery systems are no longer alternative; they are fast becoming the mainstream" (Ellwood, 1985, p. 1). Health maintenance organizations have been in existence for over 30 years. They are an organized system of health care that, for a fixed fee, provide physician services, emergency and preventive treatment, and hospital care to people who have agreed to obtain their medical care from the HMO for an extended period of time. The HMO is owned by a specific group, and services are provided in one facility or in a group of facilities in close proximity to one another.

The chief advantage of HMOs lies in the economic incentive to keep costs under control. Prevention is emphasized to reduce the need for costly services. The greatest potential for savings from HMOs, which is reduction of the costs of unnecessary hospitalization, also accounts for the greatest fear: that providers will underuse necessary services to save money. Additional details about HMOs are found in Chapter 4.

A PPO is defined as an organization of providers that contracts on a fee-for-service basis with third-party payers to provide comprehensive medical services to subscribers. The agreement between the PPO and the third-party payer allows subscribers to receive medical services at lower-than-usual rates (Roble, Knowlton, and Rosenberg, 1984).

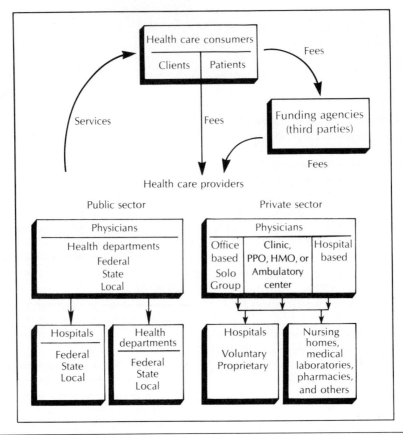

FIGURE 2-2

Health care delivery model: public and private sectors.

The PPO concept appears to have a number of advantages over the traditional delivery system. However, current experience with them is too limited to make a full evaluation. PPOs have several obvious disadvantages. First, measuring the cost effectiveness of PPOs is difficult. This problem is complicated by the fact that consumers are permitted to use both PPO and non-PPO services concurrently. Second, the third-party payer assumes a volume risk because there is no way to control subscriber use. Third, there is no way of evaluating whether a PPO physician's discounted fees are actually lower than those of non-PPO providers (NAQ Forum, 1985).

Other Health Care Delivery Organizations

As shown in the health care delivery models, a number of additional facilities and organizations make up the contemporary US health care system. The importance of many of these has grown as hospital use patterns have changed in recent years.

For example, *home health services* have grown considerably. Home care programs are provided by a variety of organizations such as hospitals, health departments, visiting nurse associations, and independent agencies. Home health care is covered in detail in Chapter 42; however, it is important to recognize the significant growth and shift in market share by these organizations. The significance of this growth is that for years visiting nurse associations (VNAs) and public health departments provided high-quality, low-

cost services, and commerical organizations were relatively unsuccessful in this field. All that has changed. Proprietary home health organizations have successfully penetrated the market in the past few years and taken over half the market away from VNAs and public health departments (Fagin, 1986).

Originating in nineteenth-century England, *hospice care* refers to " . . . caring for people near the end of their journey through life . . . " (Vines and Hartzell, 1981, p. 3). Hospice care offers the terminally ill person an alternative: to spend the end of life at home rather than in a hospital. A team of professionals bring the needed care to the home and teach family members how to participate in the care of their dying loved one. Palliative rather than curative care is the objective. Patients are enrolled in hospice programs only after they have been diagnosed as being terminally ill and are in the last few months of their life.

Another group of health care facilities, collectively known as *ambulatory centers*, provide a wide range of services. These facilities are either hospital based or community based. Hospital-based services are provided in either ambulatory care units or clinics. Community-based settings include neighborhood health centers, ambulatory health centers, and mental health centers. Neighborhood health centers provide a comprehensive array of health services to the population within a defined geographical area. Their major focus is on health promotion and disease prevention. Ambulatory centers, also known as surgicenters, emergicenters, and medical care walk-in centers are being established in many middle-class urban and suburban neighborhoods to provide services similar to those provided by physicians' offices and hospital-based programs (Fagin, 1986). One advantage of these centers is that they are open for many hours per day, and many are open 7 days a week.

Community mental health centers provide comprehensive mental health services to defined geographic areas. The types of services available are often based on community needs. Chapter 21 provides an in-depth discussion of the services of community mental health centers.

As the population ages, the need for *long-term care facilities* also grows. One type of organization dedicated to serving this need is the nursing home. These long-term care facilities can be classified according to the level of health care services they provide, ranging from minimal to continuous professional nursing services.

Long-term care in nursing homes is expensive. The average cost in 1985 per year for each resident was $23,600 (Schneider and Guralnik, 1990). About half of the country's total nursing home bill is paid by residents and their families, and coverage is limited under both Medicare and Medicaid (Coile, 1990). Another alternative to nursing home care includes board and care homes or personal care homes, (DHEW Pub No 81-1232, 1980). It is estimated that at present there are over 200,000 state-certified beds in such homes. Other options for providing long-term care include home health care, chronic disease hospitals, mental institutions, and community-based day care centers (DHEW Pub No 82-1232, 1981).

ORGANIZATION OF THE PUBLIC HEALTH SYSTEM

In general, public health is concerned with four broad areas: (1) lifestyle and behavior, (2) the environment, (3) human biology and (4) the organization of health programs and systems (Pickett and Hanlon, 1990, p. 8). Public health is both a concept and an agency for providing services. As a concept, public health represents a defined body of information that guides the organization and delivery of preventive care to individuals, families, and communities. Federal, state, and local governments are responsible for ensuring that an agreed upon set of services is provided in every community; in this it functions as an agency. How this is done varies from one community to another (Pickett and Hanlon, 1990). A local health department or a part of the state health department ensures that all agreed-upon services are provided and that the standards that have been set are actually met.

Local Health Agencies

All local governmental units are created by the state. In 1987, there were 83,166 units of local government in the United States. Most local health departments are part of county or municipal units of government. Cities have more autonomy because they have charters that allow them to do almost anything that is not prohibited by state law. Counties are limited in that they can only do those things that are permitted by the state. Other than in Connecticut and Rhode Island, counties are the universal form of government in the United States.

There are 3,232 local health departments in the 3,024 counties in the United States. More than half are single-county units (Pickett and Hanlon, 1990). The size and scope of services that can be offered by a local health department vary in proportion to the size of the local unit of government. In rural and small urban areas, the local board of health is given legal responsibility for the health of people within its jurisdiction. The members of the board of health are appointed by local elected officials such as the mayor or a county board of supervisors. The board of health typically employs a county health officer who then appoints other personnel as need demands and budget allows. The type of workers that would be added include public health nurses, environmental health workers, office personnel, nutritionists, and dentists. Typically, about half of the funds and positions are allocated to public health nursing. Larger agencies are able to add people to manage statistics, records, laboratory, and epidemiologic services, and health educators. Maternal and child health constitutes a large part of the work of public health agencies. Mental health is usually provided for by a separate agency.

State Health Agencies

The variation in state health agencies is almost as remarkable as it is with local agencies. Interestingly, most of the major federal health initiatives had their origins in a specific state program. Examples of state initiatives that led to federal programs include: occupational health, maternal and child health, and compulsory immunization of school children. Currently, the bulk of public health policy is being formed at the state level. Each of the 50 states has devised a unique structure to meet its needs; some are highly centralized, others quite decentralized. State boards of health play a minor role in forming public health policy.

FEDERAL PUBLIC HEALTH ORGANIZATIONS

Federal agencies responsible for public health fall into four categories: those with broad health interests (Public Health Service); those that deal with the interests of special populations (Administration on Aging, Veteran's Administration); those that deal with special problems or programs (Social Security Administration); those concerned with international health (Agency for International Development of the Department of State).

Perhaps the two agencies most important for public health are the Public Health Service and the Department of Health and Human Services. These organizations are fully described in Chapter 7. The Public Health Service, directed by the Assistant Secretary for Health, is organized into eight functional units: (1) the Centers for Disease Control (CDC), (2) the Food and Drug Administration (FDA), (3) the Health Resources and Services Administration (HRSA), (4) the National Institutes of Health (NIH), (5) the Alcohol, Drug Abuse, and Mental Health Administration, (6) the Agency for Toxic Substances and Disease Registry, (7) the Indian Health Service, and (8) the Agency for Health Care Policy and Research.

Figure 7-3 in Chapter 7 shows the organizational chart of the US Department of Health and Human Services, Public

Health Service (PHS). There is considerable variation in how the units of the PHS operate. The NIH and CDC carry out extensive research both within their agencies and by means of grants and contracts to other agencies, including universities in the United States and other parts of the world. The CDC serves as the nation's epidemiologic surveillance and emergency unit and the NIH has responsibility for a variety of federal centers including the National Library of Medicine.

Health Work Force

Health care providers have typically been divided into three separate groups: independent practitioners, dependent practitioners, and support staff. Independent practitioners are legally permitted to provide a specific range of services without relying on supervision from any other provider. The most commonly known independent practitioners are physicians, both medical and osteopathic, dentists, chiropractors, optometrists, podiatrists, and chiropodists.

Dependent practitioners are allowed by law to deliver a specified range of services that must be performed under the supervision and authorization of independent practitioners. Dependent practitioners have included nurses, psychologists, social workers, pharmacists, physicians' assistants, dental hygienists, and various others such as occupational, physical, and speech therapists. The line separating dependent and independent practitioners has become blurred as many groups, including nurses, have been approved for more autonomous forms of practice. For example, in many states, nurse practitioners can prescribe a certain type of drug. Other professionals, including physical, occupational, and speech therapists, are increasingly becoming more independent in their practices.

The federal government is actively trying to improve access to health care in physician-shortage areas by supporting the education and employment of health care providers who are not physicians. Two types making major contributions in primary care are *nurse practitioners* (NPs) and *physician assistants* (PAs). The primary distinction between these groups is that besides their nursing duties, NPs perform functions that were previously within the domain of physicians. In contrast, PAs assist or substitute for the physician in the performance of specific medical tasks. The best use of both NPs and PAs is not as a substitute for the physician but rather as members of a collaborative health care team. PAs and NPs perform the following basic functions (DHHS Pub No 81, 1232, 1980, p. 83):

1. Take medical histories and do physical examinations to define health and medical problems
2. Institute therapeutic regiments within established protocols and recognize when to refer the patient to a physician or other health care provider
3. Provide counseling to individuals, families, and groups in the area of health promotion and maintenance

Like NPs and PAs, nurse-midwives emphasize the care of well rather than ill persons. The American College of Nurse Midwives (ACNM) defines nurse-midwifery as "the independent management and care of essentially normal newborns and women antepartally, intrapartally, postpartally, and gynecologically, occurring within a health care system that provides for medical consultation, collaborative management, or referral . . . " (DHEW Pub No 80-1232, 1979, p. 50). The mother is the primary focus of care for nurse-midwives, who spend the majority of their time on prenatal care, labor, delivery, and postpartum care, as well as family planning services.

Research findings have indicated that NPs, PAs, and nurse-midwives have a definite place in the health care delivery system. These providers have been judged capable of carrying out a substantial number of tasks previously reserved for physicians, without compromising the quality of care. In general, services can be provided at considerable savings to consumers while quality and a high level of consumer acceptance and satisfaction is maintained. In recent years, these groups have received considerable pressure to limit their practice so as to avoid infringing on what physicians perceive as their role. Nurse practitioners, nurse midwives, and physician assistants have been effectively used in the Public Health Service as well as in other federal, state, and community health care practices.

Supporting staff members carry out work tasks authorized and often delegated by either independent or dependent practitioners. The work of members of this group is not always regulated by laws directly pertaining to them, in which case they work under the legal sanctions provided by their supervisors. Members of the supporting staff group include research assistants, various types of technicians, and clerical, maintenance, housekeeping, and food processing workers.

CURRENT STATUS OF COMMUNITY HEALTH NURSING IN THE UNITED STATES

Community health nursing focuses on care of individuals, families, groups, and communities. Although nurses in other speciality areas work in the community, the focus and orientation that they bring to the community setting may not include the concept of public health. Community health nursing is a specific and specialized orientation to care that embodies principles of public health as guiding concepts. The key difference between community health nursing and other areas of nursing practice is the emphasis on the personal and environmental health of the total population, not just the health of selected individuals.

The terms *community health nursing* and *public health nursing* have different meanings. In this book, the term *community health nursing* is used to include the body of public health knowledge that is associated with the term *public health nursing*. Many people believe there is a significant difference in the scope of practice of community health vs. public health nurses; i.e., community health nurses "provide direct primary care in settings outside of health care institutions," for example, in the home, workplace, clinic, school, and/or recreational setting" (Rothman, 1990, p. 481). In contrast, public health nurses "function in a community-based setting established to address the health problems of specific identified populations" (Rothman, 1990, p. 481). The public health nurse engages in identifying high-risk populations and instituting programs to prevent health disruption, or, if health has already been affected, to intervene as quickly as possible to reduce further illness or disability. The primary difference is that the scope of practice has shifted from the individual to the community.

Several chapters describe in detail aspects of the current status of community health nursing. For example, Chapter 8 compares the ANA and the APHA conceptual frameworks for community health nursing. Primary health care, a key component of community health nursing, is described in Chapter 3. Community health (or public health) nursing focuses on the physical, biological, social, psychological, and environmental health of a population group, whereas primary care is a "coordinated system of personal health care, emphasizing first-contact care and continuity" (Ruth and Partridge, 1978, p. 625). Primary care generally focuses on the individual whereas community health nursing emphasizes individuals as clients within the context of the community.

Chapter 15, *Population-Focused Practice*, helps to clarify the scope of community health nursing by emphasizing the focus on aggregates or population groups. Aggregates may be defined at many levels: age, risk for certain health problems, race, sex, and so on. A major characteristic of community health nursing is its focus on promoting health-related behaviors as well as providing personal health services to members of populations or communities. Rather than serving only the subgroups who need care, community health nurses anticipate, estimate, and design measures to interrupt the onset of personal health problems.

CANADIAN SYSTEM OF HEALTH CARE

Chapter 1 described selected historical events that led to the current system of health care in Canada. Many would say that Canada has been able to deal with two of the chief complaints of the American health care system, cost and access, more effectively than the United States. Comprehensive, government-administered health insurance plans were established in all provinces of Canada in the late 1960s. The impetus for comprehensive coverage arose as scientific medicine began to extend its boundaries to offer a diverse and expensive array of services. The poor were eligible for public services and the rich could pay; the middle-class soon began to feel excluded from access to quality health care.

By the mid-1950s public pressure for a national plan to provide health care was growing. In 1956, the federal government proposed a cost-sharing hospital insurance program as a combined federal and provincial venture (Baumgart, 1988). Legislation to provide such coverage was passed in 1957 with the Hospital and Diagnostic Services Act. By 1961, all provinces including the Northwest and Yukon Territories were participating.

Services varied somewhat from province to province but all provided standard benefits that included the basic cost of acute treatment and convalescent and chronic care in approved facilities; laboratory, radiological, and other diagnostic procedures; and a range of emergency and outpatient services. The organization and administration of hospital services were left in the hands of local authorities, and as a result, most Canadian hospitals are owned and governed by local voluntary boards (Baumgart, 1988).

The second phase in the establishment of a national health care plan, the development of insurance for medical care, was more controversial than had been the hospital component of the plan. The 1984 Canada Health Act consolidated the former Hospital Insurance and Diagnostic Services and Medical Care Acts and asserted federal power over such previous features as extra physician billing. Currently, all provinces have outlawed extra billing over and above what the government health plan will cover.

The Canadian health care system allows each province/ territory freedom to determine how it will allocate costs between hospitals and medical care; medical care is provided by subsidizing private medical providers rather than via public clinics; to be eligible for cost-sharing under the Medical Care Act, provinces must meet four criteria, called the "Four Points": comprehensive, universally available (accessible), portable (beneficiaries can use it in more than one province) and publicly administered.

The Department of National Health and Welfare, the major official agency responsible for health, is primarily accountable for:

◇ Enforcing federal laws regarding harmful foods and drugs
◇ Providing health services for certain categories of people
◇ The promotion of fitness and amateur sports
◇ Administration of various social welfare programs
◇ Financial and technical assistance to provincially operated health care programs

Public Health in Canada

In Canada, the public and private health care systems are operated under the same federal financial umbrella. However, the curative services (i.e., hospitals) and preventive and public health services are maintained as separate operations. Like the United States, public health departments and community health agencies in Canada administer services that deal with public health problems such as communicable diseases, environmental health, maternal and child health, nutrition, and health promotion. In Canada, school health services are provided through the public health system whereas in some areas of the United States they are provided through the local department of education. In Canada, the regulation of occupational health is generally accomplished through one of several provincial governmental departments such as Labour, Worker's Compensation, Health, and Mines and Industry. Some provinces have established divisions of Occupational Safety and Health (Storch, 1985).

Role of Voluntary Agencies

Voluntary agencies play a significant role in Canada's health care system. Often, they pioneer new services and promote public awareness and action in regard to specific health problems. Like in the United States, citizen-organized and nongovernmental agencies provide resources and services for specific health problems or diseases. Increasingly, voluntary organizations such as the Victorian Order of Nurses, the Canadian Mental Health Association, or the Red Cross have received government grants or contracts to provide designated services for the government (Storch, 1985).

Other voluntary organizations such as the Heart Foundation and the Cancer Society raise their own funds to promote research and education related to a specific disease.

Criticism of the System

Critics of the Canadian health care system focus on its high cost, although health care costs in Canada are lower than in the United States. In 1990, health care in the United States accounted for 11.5% of the gross national product compared with 9% in Canada. After adjusting for population size and the overall purchasing power of the dollar in Canada, Americans spend 72% more than Canadians on physicians' services and 34% more on hospital care (Healthline, 1990, p. 4). Critics also complain about having to wait for some surgeries because of the substantial back log of people waiting and the focus on cure rather than on prevention. There is also concern about the current discussion about whether to "de-insure" some categories of health, such as those that are wanted by the client but are not essential to life and health. There is also some suggestion that perhaps the private sector would be more efficient than the public sector (Baumgart, 1988).

Public Health Nursing in Canada

Approximately 10% of all Canadian nurses practice outside the hospital (Jones and Craig, 1988) in physicians' offices and community health, school health, occupational health, visiting nursing, and community health services. Current nursing practice in the community focuses on health promotion and disease prevention for individuals, families, and groups. Strategies for aggregates (groups) are usually undertaken by multidisciplinary teams. Community health nursing is a vital part of the Canadian health care system. Because the government pays for health care, it is advantageous to spend money to keep people healthy and to prevent costly hospitalizations. Community health nurses also follow up hospital stays with home care so that early discharge can be more effective.

Community health nursing has input into the national structure through the Health Services and Promotion Branch of the Department of National Health and Welfare. The Principal Nursing Officer has direct access to the Deputy Minister of the Department on matters of health and nursing (Clarke-Slater and Walsh, 1985).

As described in Chapter 1, the Victorian Order of Nurses for Canada (VON) continues to provide community services through 69 branches across nine of the provinces and the Northwest Territories. The major part of their service time is spent in providing nursing care to individuals in their homes, community projects such as health counseling programs for senior citizens, and activities such as running adult day care centers or providing transportation with their vans (Clarke-Slater and Walsh, 1985).

At the present time, public health nurses in Canada are university educated and play diverse roles within a rapidly changing health care delivery system. They are a vital part of the interdisciplinary health care team. They visit individuals, families, and groups across the life span. Public health nurses provide health-promotion and disease-prevention services including health education and screening, life-style and nutrition teaching, counseling, and referrals (Matuk and Hornsburgh, 1989).

The issues facing public health nurses in Canada are much the same as those facing their counterparts in the United States:

◇ To clarify their role
◇ To heighten government and public recognition of the importance of preventive health services
◇ To gain recognition for being a unique subspecialty of nursing
◇ To increase their political involvement
◇ To develop an adequate supply of well-prepared nurse administrators

CONSUMERISM

Consumerism is not a new concept. Early consumer participation can be traced to medieval times (400 to 1400 AD) when guilds of workers in Europe joined together to protect their common interests. These guilds developed "sick chests" to provide funds to pay for medical care needed for sickness or disability resulting from accidents. This early evidence of health insurance was devised by consumers. Similarly in seventeenth-century England, societies such as the Oddfellows and the Ancient Order of Foresters extended the "sick chest" idea to include people outside their guilds. The friendly society concept also developed in the American colonies, and by 1867 more than 24,000 benevolent societies operated in the United States (Hamilton, 1982). Over the years the consumer movement has taken many forms, with its guiding aim being to secure health care that is accessible, effective, and reasonable in cost. This movement is based on the belief that people have both a right and a responsibility to be knowledgeable about and involved in the choices made about their health and illness care.

Passive Consumers

Consumerism is "an organized movement of citizens and government to improve the rights and power of buyers in relation to sellers" (Kotler and Armstrong, 1989, p. 605). This movement, which began in the 1960s with Ralph Nader, assumes that consumers will take time to acquaint themselves with selected health-related information and that health care professionals will provide health information in easily understood forms.

In the past, health care consumers have been different from consumers of many other products and services. Health care consumers too often invest complete, unquestioning trust in health care providers, especially physicians. Few consumers devote as much time to researching the relative merits of a proposed medical treatment as they devote to choosing an automobile. Health care consumers are often hesitant to raise questions about costs or to do any comparative shopping. This is changing. Today's consumers are becoming more cost-conscious and many are choosing HMOs so their costs will be predictable (Coile, 1986). The reasons for the lack of informed health consumers care are discussed in this section.

A major hurdle for consumers to overcome is their perceived or actual lack of power. According to Hamilton (1982, p. 14), "Power, or the lack of it, is at the root of all consumer issues."

Consumer Sovereignty

Consumerism in health care discounts the basic notions held by economists about the role and influence of consumers. According to classic economic theory, consumers create mandates for producers, who then concede to consumer demands.

For consumers to have the sovereignty or power to influence the behavior of providers of services or producers of products, the following four conditions must exist (Hamilton, 1982, p. 15):

1. Consumer demand must determine production of goods and provision of services.
2. Consumers must have the information necessary to judge the quality, utility, and safety of products and services.
3. Consumers must choose products and services that give the greatest utility for the lowest prices.
4. Both consumers and providers must have free access to the marketplace.

These conditions do not presently exist in health care. First, demand is not determined by consumers; it is determined by providers, who decide what services and products are needed. One reason providers have so much control is that consumers have not had sufficient information to make informed choices; this is the second condition for consumer sovereignty. Only recently have unbiased sources of information become available to consumers. In recent years the US Food and Drug Administration (FDA) has taken an active role in informing consumers about the hazards of health care. Consumers now serve on FDA advisory panels and participate in the review of drugs, diagnostic and treatment devices, and radiological equipment (Hamilton, 1982).

In most other consumer-provider interactions advertising plays a much greater role than it does in health care. Although in many instances advertising is biased in favor of the product being discussed, it does inform consumers about prices, the relative merits of products, and where they can be purchased. Traditionally, health care providers have looked down on advertising as being inappropriate for their services. However, the use of advertising has increased in recent years because of the increasingly competitive nature of health care and the decline and restrictions on third-party reimbursement.

The third condition of consumer sovereignty, that consumers try to obtain the greatest utility at the lowest price, does not always hold true in health care. Because of the fear of illness and disability, people do not consistently seek second opinions, negotiate prices, or question the treatment proposed by the provider. Consumers erroneously equate quality with high prices. This tendency has, however, been changing recently as both consumers and their insurers have become more cost conscious.

The last condition of consumer sovereignty says that consumers and providers have free access to the marketplace. In the present health care system, access is largely influenced by physicians and third-party payers. Physicians prescribe and order services, many of which would be otherwise unavailable. In many instances, consumer participation in hospital-sponsored health education provided by nurses must also be prescribed by physicians. Further, insurance carriers and Medicare and Medicaid influence which services will be reimbursed and at what rate.

Promoting Consumerism

What can and should be done to alter the power ratio in health care? Should consumers become more involved in their care and, if so, how should they begin? The place to begin is with a recognition of consumer rights. There have been several attempts on the part of providers to draft documents setting forth patient rights. However, consumers themselves must assume responsibility for their rights. They have the most to gain if their rights are acknowledged and respected, and the most to lose if their rights are ignored or violated. Consumers are entitled to privacy, confidentiality, and self-determination of care, yet these rights are only realized when providers are sincerely committed to client-centered care.

The tendency to passively rely on health care providers to repair one's physical and emotional maladies has changed considerably in recent years. People increasingly recognize their personal responsibility for health and realize that many health problems can be avoided by proper care, including preventive maintenance such as health promotion. People are encouraged to scrutinize both the products and services they purchase by reading about them, asking carefully formulated questions, and thinking critically about what is best for them.

To become participants in the health care system, consumers must become better informed and also gain more power. Consumers, individually and collectively, need to know what choices are available and the potential consequences of selecting one rather than another. Nurses can play a key role in advancing the cause of consumerism by informing clients of their choices, encouraging them to seek additional information, and motivating them to become involved in consumer issues beyond those that affect them at the present time. Consumers can organize groups to promote health care by approaching various power groups in the community and enlisting their support.

CLINICAL APPLICATION

The goal of community health nursing is to promote and preserve the health of the population. The practice is general and comprehensive and is not limited to a particular age group. As a community health nurse it is important to guide and direct clients so they can seek the health care services that best meet their needs and resources.

During a well-child clinic visit, Jenna Wells, RN, met Sandra Farr and her 24-month-old daughter, Jessica. The Farrs had recently moved to the community. Mrs. Farr states that she knew Jessica needed the last in a series of immunizations and because they did not have health insurance, she brought her daughter to the public health clinic. Upon initial assessment, Mrs. Farr tells Nurse Wells that her husband is newly employed and will not have any health care coverage for 30 days. The Farrs also need to decide which health care package they want. Mr. Farr's company offers a major medical plan and an HMO plan to all employees. Neither Mr. or Mrs. Farr have ever used an HMO, and they are not sure what services it provides. Almost under her breath, Mrs. Farr admits that she does not even know what an HMO is.

Recognizing that Mrs. Farr is sensitive about her lack of information about health care coverage but wants to make an informed decision, Nurse Wells continues with her initial assessment of the Farrs, completes the well-child assessment, and gives Jessica her immunizations. As Mrs. Farr dresses Jessica, Nurse Wells collects several pamphlets and handouts on insurance and the type of health coverage each plan provides.

Upon returning to Mrs. Farr and Jessica, the nurse asks Mrs. Farr if she would like to look at some of the material on health insurance. Together, they review the information. Initially, Mrs. Farr looks confused and asks which choice the nurse would make. Nurse Wells says that she cannot really say which would work best for the Farrs, but she recommends that Mrs. Farr talk about the options with her husband. The nurse asks if she can call Mrs. Farr in 2 days to see if she has any questions about the insurance. Mrs. Farr looks pleased by this offer and comments that she will probably adjust better to the community once she chooses an insurance plan and finishes getting the immunizations for Jessica.

The next day, the nurse telephones Mrs. Farr and learns that after carefully reviewing the information, the Farrs decided on the HMO. Both Mrs. and Mr. Farr believe that health promotion is important, and this service is provided by the HMO. They also thought that since they did not know any of the local physicians or dentists, the HMO would give them enough choices to meet their needs.

Mrs. Farr reports that Jessica slept well on the night following the immunization and that there is no irritation around the site of the immunization nor any generalized discomfort. Before ending the conversation, the nurse asks Mrs. Farr if she would like the community welcome wagon to visit her. Following Mrs. Farr's enthusiastic response, the nurse contacts the local community service group that manages the welcome wagon and asks them to visit the Farrs.

SUMMARY

The health care system in the United States continues to be criticized for its high cost, its lack of access to consumers, and the lack of availability of services in all parts of the country. In many sections of the country, health personnel and resources are poorly distributed. Some urban areas have an abundance of providers and facilities whereas people in many rural and some inner-city areas have virtually no services available within a reasonable commuting distance.

As discussed in Chapter 1, community health providers have consistently advocated that it is less costly to prevent illness than to provide adequate treatment once disruption has occurred. However, the study of the cost of preventive measures has been neglected in the past, therefore there are few statistics that support cost effectiveness of prevention. Nurses who work in preventive care are in a key position to contribute to research efforts in this much-needed area.

Additionally, changes in the health care system need to recognize that the community itself is a major determinant of the health of its residents. Clean water, adequate sewage disposal, food, heat, and proper personal health practices are major factors in determining the health of the residents. Nursing has a major role to play in the ultimate restructuring of the health care system by continuing to urge communities and other health care providers to focus on health, personal responsibility for health, and a view that takes into account the needs, sources of support, and resources in a given community.

KEY CONCEPTS

Health is a concern of all Americans; it is inextricably linked with all aspects of daily living and is a prerequisite for living a healthy and productive life.

Public health refers to organized community efforts designed to prevent disease and promote health.

Health promotion focuses on maintaining or enhancing well-being; disease prevention focuses on protection from health threats.

Several important trends affecting the health care system are demographic, social, economic, political, and technological trends.

The federal government plays a major role in our health care system by establishing a national health care policy.

Among the major issues related to the health care system are recent challenges to the notion that health care should be available to all regardless of their ability to pay, the rapid growth of health care systems and providers, and competition among for-profit health care providers.

The health care system is composed of consumers, providers, and mechanisms for delivery of health care services. However, the consumer of health care services is a client, not a customer.

Consumerism is a major movement affecting the health care industry.

Canada established a national plan for health care in 1957 when it passed the Hospital and Diagnostic Services Act.

The issues facing public health nurses in Canada, like those faculty U.S. nurses deal with role clarity, the need for more preventive services, the need for stronger political impact, and the need for educating more nurse managers.

LEARNING ACTIVITIES

1. Describe three health promotion activities that community health nurses should be able to implement.

2. If you were asked to plan a program designed for disease prevention in your community, what would you do? Describe the plan you would implement.

3. If there is an HMO in your community, interview three providers and three consumers to determine what each sees as the advantages and disadvantages of this type of care delivery system.

4. Debate whether consumerism should exist in health care as it exists in the distribution of other products and/or services.

5. Debate the following: The major problem with the health care system is (choose one of the following topics):

   Escalating costs
   Fragmentation
   Inaccessibility
   Quality of care

BIBLIOGRAPHY

American Association of Colleges of Nursing: News: reduced resources prompt nursing schools to turn away qualified students, AACN survey shows. Washington, DC, January 13, 1991.

American Nurses' Association: Environmental assessment: factors affecting long-range planning for nursing and health care, Kansas City, Mo, 1985, American Nurses' Association.

Andreoli KG and Musser LA: Trends that may affect nursing's future, Nurs Health Care 6(1):47-51, 1985.

Baumgart AJ: Evolution of the Canadian health care system. In Baumgart AJ and Larsen J, editors: Canadian nursing faces the future, St Louis, 1988, The CV Mosby Co, 19-38.

Bureau of the Census, Current Population Reports: Population Profile of the United States, 1989, Special Studies Series P-23, No 159, Washington, DC, 1989, US Department of Commerce.

Califano JA: America's health care revolution, New York, 1986, Random House Inc.

Canadian physicians provide more services for lower fees, Healthline, 9(12):4, Dec 1990.

Clarke-Slater M and Walsh E: Official and voluntary agencies—a generalist role. In Stewart M et al, editors: Community health nursing in Canada, Toronto, 1985, Gage Educational Publishing Co. 147-177.

Coile RC Jr: The new hospital: future strategies for a changing industry, Rockville Md, 1986, Aspen Publishers Inc.

Coile RC Jr: The new medicine: reshaping medical practice and health care management, Rockville, Md, 1990, Aspen Publishers, Inc.

Ellwood PN: Alternative delivery systems: health care on the move, J Ambulatory Care Management 8(4):1-2, 1985.

Exter T: Demographic forecasts, American Demographics 12(2):55, 1990.

Fagin CM: Opening the door on nursing's cost advantage, Nursing and Health Care 7(7):352-357, 1986.

Guralnik JM and Schneider EL: The compression of morbidity: a dream which may come true someday! In Lee PR and Estes CL (editors): The nation's health, ed 3, Boston, 1990, Jones and Bartlett Publishers.

Hamilton PA: Health care consumerism, St Louis, 1982, The CV Mosby Co.

Health: United States, 1979, DHEW Pub No (PHS) 80-1232, Washington, DC, Dec 1979, Department of Health, Education and Welfare.

Health: United States, 1980, DHHS Pub No (PHS) 81-1232, Washington, DC, Dec 1980, Department of Health and Human Services.

Health: United States, 1981, DHHS Pub No (PHS) 82-1232, Washington, DC, Dec 1981, Department of Health and Human Services.

Institute of Medicine: The future of public health, Washington, DC, 1988, National Academy Press.

Jones PE and Craig DM: Nursing practice in the community: primary health care. In Baumgart AJ and Larsen J, editors: Canadian nursing faces the future, St. Louis, 1988, The CV Mosby Co.

Kotler P and Armstrong G: Principles of marketing, ed 4, Englewood Cliffs, 1989, Prentice Hall.

Matuk LC and Horsburg MEC: Rebuilding public health nursing practice: a Canadian perspective, Publ Health Nurs 6(4):169-173, 1989.

NAQ Forum, Trandel-Korenchuk K, and Trandel-Korenchuk L: Alternative delivery systems, Nurs Admin Q 10(1):61-64, 1985.

Pender NJ: Health promotion in nursing practice, ed 2, Norwalk, Ct, 1987, Appleton & Lange.

Pickett G and Hanlon JJ: Public health administration and practice, St Louis, 1990, Times Mirror/Mosby College Publishing.

Roble DT, Knowlton WA, and Rosenberg GA: Hospital-sponsored preferred provider organizations, Law, Medicine Health Care 12(5):204-209, 1984.

Rothman NL: Toward description: public health nursing and community health nursing are different, Nurs Health Care 11(9):481-483, 1990.

Ruth MV and Partridge KB: Differences in perception of education and practice, Nurs Outlook 26:622-629, Oct 1978.

Schwartz JN: Management women and the new facts of life, Harvard Business Review 89(1):65-76, 1989.

Stevens BJ: Tackling a changing society head on, Nurs Health Care 6(1):27-30, 1985.

Storch JL: The Canadian health care delivery system: policies, programs, services. In Stewart M et al, editors: Community health nursing in Canada, Toronto, 1985, Gage Educational Publishing Co, 33-47.

US Bureau of the Census: Statistical abstract of the United States, 1990. Washington, DC, 1990, US Department of Commerce.

Vines E and Hartzell DH: The hospice movement in the United States, National Health Standards and Quality Information Clearinghouse Bulletin, Baltimore, March, 1981.

Weil RP: Procompetition or more regulation? Health Care Manage Rev 10(3):27-35, 1985.

World Health Organization: Basic documents, ed 36, Geneva, 1986, WHO.

3

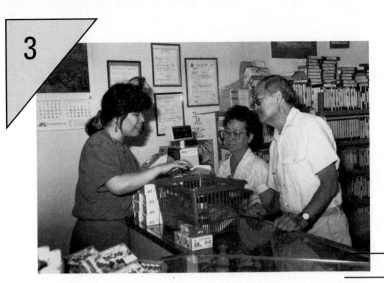

Primary Health Care

Beverly J. McElmurry

Susan M. Swider

Prapin Watanakij

Historical Overview

The Concept of Primary
Health Care

Application of Primary
Health Care
  Primary Health Care in Canada
  Primary Health Care in Thailand
  Primary Health Care in the United
    States

Primary Health Care and
Community Health Nursing

Clinical Application: PHC Nursing
Demonstration Project

Summary

OBJECTIVES

After reading this chapter, the student should be able to:

Describe the relationship of primary health care (PHC) to community health nursing.

Discuss key components of the PHC approach: equity, social participation, essential health care, and health as integrally related to social/economic development.

Differentiate between PHC and primary care.

Explain the value of PHC as a strategy for dealing with the interaction between health and socioeconomic conditions.

Explain the difference between an international nursing perspective and the global strategy of PHC.

Define nursing roles in a PHC team.

Suggest at least two methods to change nursing roles in relation to PHC.

Compare the US health system to the idea of PHC as a national health care approach.

KEY TERMS

community
  involvement
community
  participation
decentralization
empowerment

environmental
  conditions
Health for All by the
  Year 2000
right to health care

self-care
self-determination
self-reliance
socioeconomic status

P rimary health care (PHC) is a strategy that may be used to guarantee a minimum level of basic health care for all people. PHC emphasizes the development of universally acceptable, affordable, and accessible essential health care services that are community based and emphasize health promotion and maintenance, self-reliance, and community participation in decision making about health. The United States has not adopted PHC as a national strategy nor any alternative strategy that guarantees everyone a minimum level of health care. However, changes in health policy often occur when members of the community become aware of what needs to change and how others have brought about change. The community health nurse has an important role in helping people learn to care for themselves and to work with other community residents to develop the capacity or infrastructure needed to ensure essential health care for everyone.

This chapter provides a historical perspective on the development of the primary health care approach, identifies some of the key ideas inherent in PHC, emphasizes PHC as an important community health nursing approach, and shows how PHC has been applied in several countries. By the conclusion of this chapter, the community health nurse should be able to identify ways to incorporate some of the important ideas from PHC in his or her practice.

HISTORICAL OVERVIEW

The PHC movement officially began in 1977 when the 30th World Health Organization (WHO) Health Assembly adopted a resolution accepting the goal of attaining a level of health that permitted all citizens of the world to live socially and economically productive lives. At the International Conference in 1978 in Alma Ata, USSR, it was determined that this goal was to be met through PHC. This resolution became known by the slogan "Health for All (HFA) by the Year 2000" and captured the official health target for all of the member-nations of the WHO.

In 1981, after identifying the goal of HFA and the PHC strategy for realizing that goal, the WHO established global indicators for monitoring and evaluating the achievement of HFA. In the *World Health Statistics Annual* (1986) these indicators are grouped into four categories: health policies; social and economic development; provision of health care; and health status. An important part of understanding such global indicators is the stress on health as an objective or part of socioeconomic development (Mahler, 1981). In this context, health improvements are a result of efforts in many areas (multisectoral) in addition to the health field, including agriculture, industry, education, housing, and communications.

Although the original definition of PHC has at times been misunderstood, it is important to understand the Alma Ata declaration as the basis for PHC and the global evolvement of this strategy over the past 10 to 15 years. For this reason, the complete declaration is presented in the box on p. 36 (WHO, 1978, p. 226):

A key nurse leader in launching PHC nursing efforts was Dr. Amelia Mengay Maglacas. In 1986 she proposed a network of WHO Collaborating Centres in Nursing. She believed that organizing at a global level could speed the mobilization of the nursing profession to reorient nursing education, practice, and research to the goal of health for all through primary health care. In her official capacity at the WHO, she was able to facilitate and coordinate the establishment of this network. Each nursing collaborating center was encouraged to identify a plan for national nursing development. In addition, the centers of the network were encouraged to support each other through the transfer and exchange of ideas and technologies and by cooperating on specific projects and research. The importance of identifying nursing leaders and centers in each country was to ensure the stimulation of activities and changes that would be required in nursing service, education, and research to advance PHC (Maglacas, 1986).

When the global network was proposed in 1986, two types of collaborating centers were evolving. Some centers existed to carry out a regional plan for advancing health care through nursing activity. Others were designated as global collaborating centers willing to carry out nursing activities in support of the WHO's program for health. The centers that became members of the network were designated by the WHO as centers with global significance. However, outside of the assistance or facilitation of the WHO in organizing the network, the global network was an independent organization. Thus, when representatives from the collaborating centers met in Bangkok, Thailand in 1987 to form the network, they also established a constitution and bylaws to govern their work. The network is a worldwide concerted action for nursing development toward the attainment of health for all through PHC. It is interesting that only 2 years later, in 1989, the National League for Nursing (NLN) members of the Council of Baccalaureate and Higher Degree Programs (CBHDP) adopted the following resolution: "Thus the NLN promotes the practice of primary health care by nurses within its educational and lobbying activities" (NLN, June 1989).

The HFA/2000 goal was renewed in 1988 when a WHO Technical Session was held in Riga, USSR. The action agenda recommended by participants at this conference emphasized the following: empowering people to participate in health decisions and the implementation of those decisions; the delivery of PHC in decentralized health care systems; the preparation and support of health professional participants in PHC; the application of advances in science and technology to developing new approaches to persistent problems, and accepting that assisting least developed countries was an international priority. Thus, for well over a decade the leadership of the WHO has continued to reaffirm HFA. In May 1990, Dr. Hiroshi Nakajima, the Director General of the WHO, reaffirmed HFA as a health and social justice challenge for the 1990s (WHO Press, WHA/4).

It is important to distinguish the focus on PHC as a global strategy to implement "at home" from the usual use of the term *international nursing*. Those who work in international nursing offer their knowledge and expertise to the advancement of nursing research, education, or practice in another country. An example of international nursing is when a nurse provides consultation to colleagues in another country or goes to live and work in another country for a period of time. The primary organization for the advancement of international nursing is the International Council of Nurses (ICN). The actual members of the ICN are national nursing associations, and a primary goal of the ICN is to work toward enhancing the work of nurses in those associations. Therefore, while one can consider PHC as being of global significance, it is important to understand it as a strategy applicable for improving the health of people in any community.

THE CONCEPT OF PRIMARY HEALTH CARE

Primary health care is essential health care made universally accessible to individuals and families in the community. Health care is made available to them through their full participation, and is provided at a cost that the community and country can afford. The focus of primary health care is broad and encompasses all aspects of the community and its health needs. The community as a whole, rather than the individual, is considered the client. The word *primary* refers to the most important and central concept of the health care system. Primary health care occurs at a transdisciplinary level. The setting for primary health care is within all communities of a country, and permeates all aspects of society. It is important to note that the concept of PHC differs from the concept of primary care, which originated within the medical profession. Primary care refers to the delivery of health care that may be directed by medicine, nursing, or other specialized branches of the health care system. Primary care is one part of the traditional health model that divides health care into primary, secondary, and tertiary levels of care. The focus of primary care is usually on the individual or an individual family. In this sense, the word 'primary' refers to the first contact an individual has with the health care system. See Smith, Forchuck, and Martin

---

DECLARATION OF ALMA-ATA

The International Conference on primary health care, meeting in Alma-Ata this twelfth day of September in the year nineteen hundred and seventy-eight, expressing the need for urgent action of all governments, all health and development workers, and the world community to protect and promote the health of all the people of the world, hereby makes the following Declaration:

I

The Conference strongly reaffirms that health, which is a state of complete physical, mental, and social well being, and not merely the absence of disease or infirmity, is a fundamental human right and that the attainment of the highest possible level of health is a most important world-wide social goal, whose realization requires the action of many other social and economic sectors in addition to the health sector.

II

The existing gross inequality in the health status of the people particularly between developed and developing countries as well as within countries is politically, socially, and economically unacceptable and is, therefore, of common concern to all countries.

III

Economic and social development, based on a new international economic order, is of basic importance to the fullest attainment of health for all and to the reduction of the gap between the health status of the developing and developed countries. The promotion and protection of the health of the people is essential to sustained economic and social development and contributes to a better quality of life and to world peace.

IV

The people have the right and duty to participate individually and collectively in the planning and implementation of their health care.

V

Governments have a responsibility for the health of their people which can be fulfilled only by the provision of adequate health and social measures. A main social target of governments, international organizations, and the whole world community in the coming decades should be the attainment by all peoples of the world by the year 2000 of a level of health that will permit them to lead a socially and economically productive life. Primary health care is the key to attaining this target as part of development in the spirit of social justice.

VI

Primary health care is essential health care based on practical, scientifically sound, and socially acceptable methods and technology made universally accessible to individuals and families in the community through their full participation and at a cost that the community and country can afford to maintain at every stage of their development in the spirit of self-reliance and self-determination. It forms an integral part both of the country's health system, of which it is the central function and main focus, and of the overall social and economic development of the community. It is the first level of contact for individuals, the family, and the community with the national health system, bringing health care as close as possible to where people live and work, and it constitutes the first element of a continuing health care process.

VII

Primary health care:
1. reflects and evolves from the economic conditions and sociocultural and political characteristics of the country and its communities and is based on the application of the relevant results of social, biomedical and health services research and public health experience;
2. addresses the main health problems in the community, providing promotive, preventive, curative, and rehabilitative services accordingly;
3. includes at least: education concerning prevailing health problems and the methods of preventing and controlling them; promotion of food supply and proper nutrition; an adequate supply of safe water and basic sanitation; maternal and child health care, including family planning; immunization against the major infectious diseases; prevention and control of locally endemic diseases; appropriate treatment of common diseases and injuries; and provision of essential drugs;

Continued.

DECLARATION OF ALMA-ATA—cont'd

4. involves, in addition to the health sector, all related sectors and aspects of national and community development, in particular agriculture, animal husbandry, food, industry, education, housing, public works, communication, and other sectors; and demands the coordinated efforts of all those sectors;

5. requires and promotes maximum community and individual self-reliance and participation in the planning, organization, operation, and control of primary health care, making fullest use of local, national and other available resources; and to this end, develops through appropriate education the ability of communities to participate;

6. should be sustained by integrated, functional and mutually supportive referral systems, leading to the progressive improvement of comprehensive health care for all, giving priority to those most in need;

7. relies, at local and referral levels, on health workers, including physicians, nurses, midwives, auxiliaries, and community workers, as applicable, as well as on traditional practitioners as needed, suitably trained socially and technically to work as a health team and to respond to the expressed health needs of the community.

VIII

All governments should formulate national policies, strategies, and plans of action to launch and sustain primary health care as part of a comprehensive national health system and

in coordination with other sectors. To this end, it will be necessary to exercise political will, to mobilize the country's resources, and to use available external resources rationally.

IX

All countries should cooperate in a spirit of partnership and service to ensure primary health care for all people because the attainment of health by people in any one country directly concerns and benefits every other country. In this context the joint WHO UNICEF report* on primary health care constitutes a solid basis for the further development and operation of Primary Health Care through the world.

X

An acceptable level of health for all the people of the world by the year 2000 can be attained through a fuller and better use of the world's resources, a considerable part of which is now spent on armaments and military conflicts. A genuine policy of independence, peace, detente, and disarmament could and should release additional resources that could well be devoted to peaceful aims and in particular to the acceleration of social and economic development of which Primary Health Care, as an essential part, should be allotted its proper share.

*World Health Organization: Primary health care: report of the International Conference on Primary Health Care, Alma-Ata, USSR, Sept 6-12, 1978, Geneva, 1978, The Organization.

(1985) and Egwu (1984) for further discussions of the importance of understanding the differences between PHC and primary care.

PHC is a pattern of health care delivery in which the consumers of health care are partners with professionals and participate in achieving the common goal of improved health. The PHC strategy encourages self-care and self-management in health and social welfare aspects of daily life. People are educated and empowered to use their knowledge, attitudes, and skills in activities that improve health for themselves, their families, and their neighbors. The desired outcome from the PHC strategy is individual, family, and community self-reliance and competence.

The key to a PHC program is not the government or local health personnel but the people in a community. The total population is the major target of PHC. It can be said that this strategy of health care delivery is "by the people, of the people, and for the people." Governmental officials and health personnel support technologies and facilities that are of most benefit to the population.

Primary health care thus requires the development, adaptation, and application of appropriate health technology that the people can use and afford. Such health care includes an adequate supply of low-cost, good-quality essential drugs, vaccines, biologicals, and other supplies and equipment, as well as counseling and advisory services to help people review their health practices and make healthy choices. PHC includes functionally efficient supportive

health care facilities such as health centers and hospitals. Drawing from the WHO definitions of essential elements in health services, there are at least eight essential health elements in the provision of PHC:

1. Education concerning prevailing health problems and the methods of preventing and controlling them
2. Promotion of food supply and proper nutrition
3. Maternal and child health care, including family planning
4. Adequate, safe water supply and basic sanitation
5. Immunization against major infectious diseases
6. Prevention and control of local endemic diseases
7. Appropriate treatment of common diseases and injuries
8. Provision of essential basic household drugs for the community

The PHC approach includes dimensions of social and economic development. The services are determined by social goals, such as the improvement of the *quality of life* (QOL) and maximum health benefits for the greatest numbers. Society benefits from healthier people who are more likely to be able to contribute to social and economic development.

Improved QOL is a goal of PHC. QOL relates to internal phenomena that determine health matters or external phenomena such as social conditions and environmental influences on human life. A high quality of life is evident when community members have the prerequisites for good health and happiness in their daily lives (Watanakij, 1990).

The preceding material on PHC illustrates two things. First, that PHC is a global strategy that has been with us for some time, and second, that we have yet to fully discern the significance of this movement for realizing changes in US health care. The following sections discuss the application of PHC to health care in Canada, Thailand, and the United States. The Canadian example emphasizes extending an existing health care system to the poor or underserved population. Thailand is an example of a national political strategy to improve health care. The third example, a demonstration project in the United States, illustrates an effort to enhance local community development in order to improve the health of the residents in that community.

APPLICATION OF PRIMARY HEALTH CARE
Primary Health Care in Canada

The status of PHC in Canada is emerging as an issue of concern to nurses who understand the potential benefits of the PHC strategy. Indeed, Chamberlain and Beckingham (1987) make the point that Canada must distinguish between declarations of support for PHC, such as found in the Ottawa Charter for Health Prevention, and a serious financial commitment to establish PHC as a unifying health strategy.

It is important to recognize the value of PHC as a strategy for dealing with the problems facing poor and underserved communities. However, overemphasis on PHC as a strategy for delivery of health services to low-income or uninsured populations perpetuates the view held by the general public that community health strategies do not apply to all socioeconomic groups. Further, Mardiros (1987) cites the native populations in Canada as an example of a situation in which considerable professional energy and governmental funding have not achieved the desired health changes because the local communities and their ideologies have been omitted from the decision process.

A joint demonstration project under way in Canada and Denmark is the PHC nursing model coordinated by Dorothy C. Hall. In the initial descriptions of the Canadian aspects of this project (Hall, 1990), it is noted that Canada has not yet implemented the PHC strategy, and this will be the first attempt to launch a comprehensive PHC program consistent with the WHO declaration at Alma Ata. The demonstration in the province of Newfoundland has the endorsement of various nursing organizations in Canada and Denmark, as well as of governmental entities, and is coordinated by a person with extensive experience in international nursing and PHC. When the results of this project are available in the mid-1990s the project is expected to serve as an example of the changes in health care that nurses can initiate.

Primary Health Care in Thailand

The health care system in Thailand has changed dramatically in the past 25 years. From a focus that emphasized primary, secondary, and tertiary care for the sick, Thailand has adopted the 1978 WHO policy and integrated PHC as a national strategy to achieve the goals of HFA/2000.

In the development of a national PHC program, the government officials sponsored several pilot projects between 1965 and 1981 to identify effective strategies for delivering health care services to the population. The goal of these projects was to ensure health care for all people, particularly the rural majority of the Thai population (80%). Special attention was paid in the pilot projects to finding ways to improve health planning, intersectoral collaboration, decentralized management, and local leadership development. When completed, the pilot projects had helped Thailand establish health planning and health management activities at the grass roots level that were linked to the national level of health care delivery. The specific foci of the early studies were:

◊ The use of village health volunteers (VHVs) and village health communicators (VHCs);
◊ The provision of maternal and child health, family planning, and nutrition services to the majority of the population in a defined area;
◊ Achieving an intersectoral and integrated rural health and development model;
◊ An understanding of the role of community leadership in PHC development and;
◊ The achievement of village funds through cooperative means to ensure availability of essential drugs to the village residents (Royal Thai Government, 1988).

At this point, Thailand has realized the goal of promoting health and prevention of disease through the designation of community people as VHVs and VHCs to work with the health personnel at the local level. This strategy results in community involvement, using available and appropriate local resources, government support, grassroots health reports, local records, and intersectoral and interdisciplinary cooperation for health care services. The desired outcomes of the PHC program in Thailand include:

1. Individual health behaviors consistent with self-reliance and self-care.
2. Health outcomes for women, infants, and children that ensure:
   ◊ Infants of normal birth weight and growth rate who are fully immunized, well nourished, and free from chronic illness and endemic diseases.
   ◊ Children with normal physical and mental growth who are well nourished, maintain immunization schedules, use practices to prevent endemic and epidemic diseases, and attend school regularly.
   ◊ Women with normal pregnancies and deliveries who are free of child-bearing complications.
3. Family size that is compatible with the cultural and socioeconomic conditions of family life in a literate, interdependent society.
4. Sanitary and environmental conditions that ensure well-maintained homes, uncontaminated water, sewage, garbage disposal, emergency services, toilets, and clean air.
5. A national system for maintaining and responding to mortality and morbidity rates.
6. Community reliance and social conditions that foster village resident participation in primary health care matters and local community management.
7. Recognition of the interrelationships between socioeconomic development and health.

8. The identification of appropriate strategies to achieve intersectoral and interdisciplinary cooperation in health care delivery including rights of the people to voice their ideas, opinions, and knowledge and to suggest to the various governmental and private sectors ways to improve or solve daily health problems.

9. Eradication of endemic and epidemic diseases—PHC begins at the village level.

These responsibilities are assigned to a PHC team that includes health educators, dietitians, pharmacists, nurses, physicians, sanitarians, junior health workers, midwives, and volunteers from the local communities.

Nurses provide the liaison between the community volunteers and other health professionals. Most professionals on the PHC team visit the community only periodically to work with the local people on a particular aspect of PHC. The nursing team is responsible for collecting the health and social data, maintaining records, and working closely with the volunteers from the community.

The PHC activities of the nurse combine health promotion, disease prevention, and curative and rehabilitative dimensions. Nurses strive to empower the volunteers and their neighbors to understand and work with the nursing team for each PHC element. Nurses must be careful not to assume responsibilities that are appropriate for community residents to assume. The following PHC concerns illustrate the nurse's role:

1. Nutritious food: in communities without dietitians or nutritionists, nurses are responsible for teaching community members to cook the supplementary food for the malnourished children as well as for teaching people about meal preparation, balance, and how to select food in sufficient quality and quantity. In addition, they provide information on the five food groups and how to preserve food. Basic sanitary conditions are fostered by teaching people to clean their hands before cooking or handling food, and to wash dishes and appliances so as to prevent endemic and epidemic diseases.

2. Maternal and child health, including family planning: nurses are assigned to carry out this element of PHC, which includes prenatal, perinatal, and postnatal care to ensure the normal growth and development of all infants. Pregnant women are a special target population of PHC along with newborns and school-age children.

3. Water supply and sanitation: sanitarians and junior health workers are responsible for safe and clean running and drinking water, hygienic latrines, and sewage and garbage disposal. Nurses coordinate and cooperate with sanitarians to inform people about germ theory, hygienic personal health habits, causes of unclean environments, and the advantages of regulations in sanitation. Nurses also supervise and monitor volunteers in dealing with sanitary and hygienic problems.

4. Immunization to prevent endemic and epidemic diseases: nurses and the nursing team plan immunization programs for adults and children, particularly infants and pregnant women. Encouragement and persuasion are strategies used in monitoring and scheduling immunization. Volunteers are assigned to visit and remind the target population to obtain immunizations from the nearby community health centers.

5. Disease control and prevention: nurses and the nursing team collect and record data about communicable diseases, provide care for the ill, offer health education, visit and follow up cases, and provide surveillance over the target population to ensure that communicable diseases are eradicated.

6. Treatment of diseases and injuries: in Thailand, nurses are educated to treat patients under a physician's standing order. The emergency treatment and infirmary care provided by nurses helps to lower mortality rates. Because there are not enough physicians to have one in each local community, physicians are available or scheduled to treat the sick in the rural community twice a week, and nurses are expected to provide such care at all other times.

These PHC activities in Thailand are undertaken with the involvement of the local community residents and supported by government technologies, human resources, and advisory information. Implementing PHC has made health delivery in Thailand more effective and progressive. More health problems are resolved and the prevalence of endemic and epidemic diseases has declined. The successful PHC community is characterized by cooperation and involvement of people in the management of safety, security, health and social education, socioeconomic development, social welfare, and social awareness.

Primary Health Care in the United States
Essential Health Care

As indicated in the earlier discussion, PHC is as much a political statement as a methodology or system of care. As a political statement agreed on by the UN member countries, it needs to be interpreted by each country in the context of its culture, health needs, resources, and system of government.

As a WHO member nation, the United States has endorsed PHC as a strategy for achieving the goal of Health For All by the year 2000. However, PHC is not the primary US strategy for improving the health of the American people. The Pan American Health Organization (PAHO) description of a local health system (1988) is a PHC model that has been submitted to the WHO and may eventually be found useful in the United States. To date, health care in the United States has developed as a system dominated by hospital-based medical care for disease-specific treatment. This system exists in a country with fairly high overall levels of social and economic development, a high national life expectancy, and low national disease rates as compared to other countries. Thus, the national health plan for the United States focuses on disease prevention and health promotion in the areas of most concern in the nation.

This focus is exemplified by the health objectives for the nation, *Promoting Health/Preventing Disease: Year 2000 Objectives for the Nation* (PHS, 1991, p. 43). These objectives were published by the Public Health Service, Department of Health and Human Services, following a process of gathering data from health professionals and organizations throughout the country. The final document was made available for public comment and revision so as to gain as much support as possible for the goals described therein.

The objectives focus on three overarching goals: increase the lifespan of healthy Americans; reduce health disparities among Americans and provide all Americans with access to preventive services; and decrease the race-based disparity in life expectancy.

Specific areas of concern for each of these goals include:

Health promotion: nutrition, physical activity and fitness, consumption of tobacco, alcohol, and other drugs, family planning, violent and abusive behavior, mental health, and educational and community-based programs.

Health protection: environmental health, occupational safety and health, accidental unintentional injuries, food and drug safety, and oral health.

Preventive services priorities: maternal and infant health, immunizations and infectious diseases, HIV infection, sexually transmitted diseases, heart disease and stroke, cancer, diabetes, other chronic disabling conditions; and clinical preventive services for these. Also, chronic disorders, and mental and behavioral disorders; and

System improvement priorities: health education and preventive services, and surveillance and data systems. (PHS, 1991).

This particular set of objectives has only recently been published, and it is too soon to judge national success in meeting the goals and objectives. There is considerable overlap between the essential elements of PHC and the areas of concern stated in the objectives. In Table 3-1 the eight essential elements of PHC are related to the US priority areas, as defined by the Public Health Service.

Health and Social/Economic Development

PHC is an approach to health care that can be adapted to varying cultures and health needs. Thus, the objectives to be achieved by the year 2000 have much in common with the eight essential elements of PHC. However, several other aspects of the PHC approach are not included in the Year 2000 objectives for the United States. The following comparisons of the Year 2000 objectives with the PHC approach will illustrate continuing concerns in moving toward a national health plan for the United States.

As stated earlier, health care in the United States is directed at disease-specific treatment and prevention. This emphasis has been successful, and the United States is known throughout the world as the center of medical technology and treatment. The pluralistic American health care system is issue driven, responsive to dramatic cases or illnesses, scientific or technological research, and supported by a combination of govenment and private sector funds (Institute of Medicine, 1988).

However, as dramatic and impressive as the American system may be, the more common causes of death and disability are related to socioeconomic conditions and personal behavior (McKinlay, 1979; McKeown, 1976; McKinlay and McKinlay, 1977). Because such causes of illness are not addressed by sophisticated scientific and technological research, the US health care system fares less well in these areas. In the US health care system at present, costs of care are such that only minimal benefits to health will be realized from large treatment expenditures (WHO, 1986; Anderson and Mullner, 1990). A good example of this is infant mortality. The United States has poor infant mortality rates as compared to other developed countries, despite enormous expenditures on neonatal intensive care units and high-technology medical care. Such medical measures did have success in decreasing infant mortality rates for a time (PHS, 1991); however, they have reached the limits of their effectiveness, and early infant death could now be better prevented by low-cost public health measures such as improved access to prenatal care, improved nutrition and overall standard of living of young mothers, and a decrease in substance abuse by pregnant women. These measures require that the social, economic, and behavioral concerns of reproduction be attended to.

Another example of the relationship between social and economic conditions and health is the health status indicators for poor and minority populations in the United States. In the objectives for the year 1990, even among those that were achieved, morbidity and mortality rates were appreciably higher in the poor and minority groups. These class and

---

TABLE 3-1
Year 2000 objectives and PHC

Eight essential elements (PHC)	USA year 2000 priority areas
Health education	Physical activity and fitness; tobacco, alcohol and other drugs; mental health; surveillance and data systems; violence and abusive behavior
Proper nutrition	Nutrition;
Maternal and child health care; family planning	Maternal and infant health; family planning
Safe water and basic sanitation	Environmental health
Immunization	Immunization and infectious diseases
Prevention and control of locally endemic diseases	HIV infection; chronic disorders; cancer; heart disease and stroke; sexually transmitted diseases; immunization and infectious diseases; clinical preventive services
Treatment of common diseases and injuries	Unintentional injuries; occupational safety and health
Provision of essential drugs	

race differences reflect living conditions in the United States and illustrate a lack of equity and access to care in a developed country. The Year 2000 objectives addressed this issue by identifying a reduction in racial disparity in life expectancy as one of the three national health goals.

The issue of health and its relation to social and economic conditions is addressed in the PHC approach to improving health. However, consistent with the PHC approach, the specifics of implementation are unique to each country. The PHC approach includes a focus on equity whereby all populations receive a comparable level of services. This requires social programs to decrease poverty via eliminating joblessness and homelessness, educate the population to lead productive lives, and provide safe shelter and adequate nutrition for all. Other factors such as education, housing, and agriculture must be improved if opportunities for healthy and productive lives are to be maximized. Health professionals must recognize that housing and education experts are part of the multisectoral effort required to improve health, which can be done primarily in the community where people live and work.

Community Participation

Another key component of PHC is community participation in defining health problems and developing approaches to address the problems. The premise here is that lasting changes in community health occur if the community agrees that addressing a given problem is a priority. In addition, community residents have a unique perspective on their own health issues; their perspective must be integrated into the effort to improve health if health planning is to be effective. An effective PHC approach involves the community in definition of health concerns, identification and implementation of possible solutions, and evaluation of results.

The development of the Year 2000 objectives were based on the experience of implementing and evaluating the 1990 objectives and input from the health provider community. Specific objectives for each general area were developed by agencies within the Public Health Service and reviewed by health providers in the individual states where much of the implementation is expected to take place. This approach was valuable in obtaining input from health providers and resulted in notable improvements in the Year 2000 objectives as compared to the 1990 objectives. Many of the 1990 objectives were not stated in measurable terms, nor were goals and baseline data provided for comparison (Anderson and Mullner, 1990). The Year 2000 objectives addressed this problem by providing baseline data and more specific measurable objectives, thus increasing the ability to evaluate national progress towards meeting the objectives.

The Year 2000 objectives pay little attention to the role of personal behavior in health and the motivation of individuals to change unhealthy behaviors. In 1985 in written reports to the WHO regarding PHC in the United States, the Department of Health and Human Services mentioned the importance of personal behavior and lifestyle in improving health status. Further, this report related the needed behavior change with the need for greater public involvement in public health planning and implementation. How-

ever, the emphasis of the reports to the WHO was on individual responsibility for health rather than on the country's responsibility to foster conditions and to provide lifestyle choices that enhance health.

The PHC approach stresses that community involvement is necessary to realize behavioral change. If the residents of a community understand health issues, it is more likely that they will endeavor to participate in health programs. In addition, as Beauchamp argued in 1976, society has some responsibility for providing people with healthy environments and choices, in addition to encouraging increased personal responsibility for health. PHC stresses increasing self-reliance in health matters, and this includes helping communities attain the skills and knowledge needed for increased self-reliance. One of the key aspects of PHC is collaboration between health professionals and community residents to define and address health concerns. The Year 2000 objectives were developed in collaboration with the health community, with some input from ordinary citizens. Such involvement is key to achieving public support for and making efforts towards improving health.

There remain larger issues of concern regarding the US public health system. The mission of public health is to ensure societal conditions in which people can be healthy (IOM, 1988). Clearly, such a mission must address the social, environmental, and economic factors associated with health and emphasize that health is not an isolated commodity. The development of a national will to improve health requires leadership in raising public health questions for debate in the public arena. Important questions to discuss include: what does the United States owe its citizens and vice versa? How should national resources be distributed to achieve national goals and commitments? A national debate about health would foster a national strategy for improving health that could be implemented locally. Involving citizens in the clarification of health issues and priorities will motivate behavioral change and promote changes in social, economic, and environmental conditions that would be conducive to good health. Such efforts are consistent with the PHC approach.

Developing a national will to realize the goal of PHC requires involvement of the formal health sector and the educational, economic, and social sectors for a coordinated strategy to improve the quality of life for all American citizens. Quality of life includes attention to health, work opportunities, positive social and environmental conditions, and other factors that allow people to participate fully in society. The responsibility for improving our nation's health is shared by all sectors of society.

The Year 2000 objectives demonstrate considerable national effort towards improving the health of the nation. Because the objectives were developed nationally, considerable effort is needed to disseminate this plan to state and local areas, and to elicit community participation in achieving its objectives. The Department of Health and Human Services (1988) has recognized this and has plans for disseminating the objectives at a local level, with guidelines for implementation, in an effort to obtain local involvement. This is a beginning in making health a priority for policy and community/individual action.

PRIMARY HEALTH CARE AND COMMUNITY HEALTH NURSING

To implement the PHC concept, nurses must focus on the prevention of disease and the promotion of health, as well as on care of the acutely ill and those in need of rehabilitation. These dimensions of nursing care delivery offer an integrated nursing service in community health nursing and apply to rural and urban communities as well as community and hospital settings.

The management processes in community health nursing are applicable to PHC nursing, and include community diagnosis based on assessing and prioritizing community problems and planning nursing interventions. The evaluation of interventions is followed by reassessment of the situation in order to improve and adapt the PHC nursing interventions. In this process people from the community are involved in working with nurses at every step.

Moreover, strong nursing leadership and management roles are necessary in PHC and nurses are encouraged to become leaders of the health team. In preparing for leadership roles, nurses need to develop skills in human and public relations, management, administrative psychology, scientific problem-solving, and the sociology of groups and communities. Most importantly, nurses must help the health care team learn to work *with* communities, thus sharing that knowledge and decision-making authority with the public. This often requires a rethinking of the role of health professionals and a willingness to collaborate with the public to improve health.

In recruiting nurses to primary health care delivery, it is important that the methods of teaching and learning focus on problem-based learning both in theory and in experiential community-based situations. In practice areas, in community and hospital settings (including rural and urban areas), nurses must demonstrate the PHC emphasis on working with and educating people about health. Nurses need to learn to assess the potential opportunities to participate in working situations focused on competency-based and community-oriented PHC.

The concepts and practices of PHC can and should be implemented and developed in today's practice settings. PHC encourages a focus on health as interrelated with social and economic development; a concern with equity between races, classes, and genders; community participation in setting national goals and developing local strategies for improving health; and implementation at the local level. Within the strategy of PHC, health is a political and social right, measured in terms of both health effectiveness and social impact (Morley, Rhode, and Williams, 1983). "Health for All" means

> that people will use much better approaches than they do now for preventing disease and alleviating unavoidable illness and disability, and that there will be better ways of growing up, growing old, and dying gracefully. And it means that health begins at home and at the workplace, because it is there, where people live and work, that health is made or broken. And it means that essential health care will be accessible to all individuals and families in an acceptable and affordable way, and with their full participation (Mahler, 1982).

It will never be easy to realize the goal of PHC, but it is an important ideal. In its best form, the PHC system allows both professionals and community residents an opportunity to share their expertise and to negotiate a mutually acceptable decision about the health priorities for their community. The task before us is a creative opportunity to learn how to share power or authority and how to use limited resources wisely in advancing the health of a community.

CLINICAL APPLICATION: PHC NURSING DEMONSTRATION PROJECT

A group of nurses from the College of Nursing, University of Illinois at Chicago, have been involved in a project implementing the PHC approach in two Chicago neighborhoods. The project involves the selection of a small group of community residents, primarily women, for training as community health advocates. The training program has been designed to include didactic and experiential learning activities basic to promoting and maintaining health. After training, the *community health workers* (CHW) work with a public health nurse to assess the health status and resources of their community; provide information and referral to care for residents; provide health education for the residents based on their needs and interests; and organize groups of community residents to take action to improve the health and social and economic conditions of their neighborhood.

This project implements the essence of PHC: community involvement in defining and addressing health problems; the integral relationship between social, economic, and health status; a commitment to essential health services; and collaboration between community residents and health professionals. The project is involved in the social and economic development of several low-income, inner-city neighborhoods and serves as an example of the leadership of public/community health nurses in implementing PHC. Other such efforts at local and national levels will help to demonstrate the need to make the PHC approach the focus of US health policy and planning (McElmurry et al, 1986; McElmurry et al, 1990; Swider and McElmurry, 1990).

SUMMARY

This chapter describes PHC as an essential goal for communities throughout the world. Primary health care, which emphasizes the availability of affordable, accessible community-based services to individuals, families, and communities as a whole is different from primary care which typically is directed toward individuals or an individual family. The total population is the target for PHC.

This chapter examines and compares the use of PHC in the United States, Canada, and Thailand. The use of PHC is more fully developed in Thailand than in the United States or Canada. To be successful, PHC should involve more than just health care providers and consumers. The social and economic structures of the community must also support the concept of PHC and cooperate in the management of safety, security, health and social education, socioeconomic development, social welfare, and social awareness.

KEY CONCEPTS

PHC is a strategy for delivering essential health care to the community.

The health personnel in a PHC system are partners in their activities with community members.

PHC emphasizes affordable, accessible, available, and acceptable health services.

Community assessment, establishing health priorities, implementing activities, and conducting evaluations are aspects of community health nursing used in PHC.

Encouraging people from the community to help themselves provides them with the opportunity to perform self-care activities in health and social matters.

Educating people about health and social development helps them to achieve self-care, self-determination, and self-reliance.

The target of PHC is the community as a whole, rather than individuals.

PHC differs from primary care. Primary care is a component of PHC.

Community health workers participate in the implementation of PHC.

A PHC team includes nurses, physicians, dentists, pharmacists, health educators, sanitarians, and dietitians.

Effective nurses in a PHC system work closely with the people, the community, and its resources as well as other professionals in that community.

The nurse in a PHC team requires leadership and management skills.

LEARNING ACTIVITIES

1. From what you know about your community, select one population group and identify whether it has access to primary health care.

2. If it does, describe the care in terms of how it is accessible, affordable, and supportive of self-management.

3. If it does not, what would need to happen in that community to make such care available?

4. Using the WHO definitions of essential elements in health services, describe how you would apply a PHC approach to one part of your community.

5. If improved quality of life is a goal of PHC, what steps should a university take to ensure it?

6. Name three approaches to PHC that are operational in Thailand and that would have real value for the United States.

7. Describe three factors that discourage a true approach to PHC in the United States.

BIBLIOGRAPHY

American Public Health Association, Public Health Nursing Section: Definitions and role of public health nursing in the delivery of health care, Washington, DC, 1980.

Andersen R and Mullner R: Assessing the health objectives of the nation, Health Aff 9(2):152-162, 1990.

Beauchamp D: Public health as social justice, Inquiry 13:3-14, March 1976.

Chamberlain M and Beckingham A: Primary health care in Canada: in praise of the nurse, Int Nurs Rev 34(6):158-160, 1987.

Council for Community-based Development: Expanding horizons: foundations grant support of community-based development, New York, 1989.

Department of Health and Human Services: Monitoring the strategies for health for all by the year 2000, United States of America Report to the World Health Organization, 1988.

Durning AB: Worldwatch Paper 88: Action at the grassroots: fighting poverty and environmental decline, Washington, DC, 1989, Worldwatch Institute.

Egwu IN: Update: primary care is not the same as primary health care, or is it? Family and Community Health, 7(3):83-88, 1984.

Hall DC: Primary health care: a nursing model: a Danish-Newfoundland (Canada) project, St. John's Newfoundland, Canada, 1989, Association of Registered Nurses of Newfoundland.

Health Planning Division: The sixth five-year national health development, 1987-1991, Bangkok, Thailand, Ministry of Public Health.

Institute of Medicine: The future of public health, Washington, DC, 1988.

Magleas AM: Proposal for networking of WHO collaborating centers in nursing. In Leadership in nursing for health for all: echoing in the area of the Americas, Chicago, 1986, The University of Illinois at Chicago.

Mahler H: The meaning of "Health for All by the Year 2000," World Health Forum 2(1):5-22, 1981.

Mahler H: Essential drugs for all. Address given by the Director-Genral of the WHO to the eleventh assembly of the International Federation of Pharmaceutical Manufacturers Associations, Washington, DC, 1982.

Mardiros M: PHC: Primary health care and Canada's indigenous people, The Canadian Nurse 88(6):20-24, 1987.

McElmurry BJ, Swider SM, Bless C, Murphy D, et al: Community health advocacy: primary health care nurse-advocate teams in urban communities, In NLN Perspectives in Nursing, 1989-91, New York 1990, NLN.

McElmurry BJ, Swider SM, Grimes MJ, Dan AJ, et al: Health advocacy for young, low-income, inner-city women, Adv Nurs Sciences 9(4):62-75, 1986.

McKeown T: The role of medicine: dream, mirage or nemesis, London; 1976, Nuffield Provincial Hospitals Trust.

McKinlay JB and McKinlay SM: The questionable contribution of medical measures to the decline of mortality in the United States in the twentieth century, Milbank Q 53(3):405-428, 1977.

McKinlay JB: Epidemiological and political determinants of social policies regarding the public health, Sci Med 13A:541-558, 1979.

Ministry of Public Health: Health and social development in Thailand, Bangkok, Thailand, 1988, Royal Thai Government, World Health Organization, and the government of the Netherlands.

Morley R, Rhode JE, and Williams G, editors: Practicing health for all, Oxford, UK, 1983, Oxford University Press.

National League of Nursing: The Council of Baccalaureate and Higher Degree Program (CBHDP), The biennial conference in Seattle, Wash, June 1989.

Nondasuta A, editor: The realization of primary health care in Thailand, Bangkok, 1988, Amarin Printing Group Co, Ltd.

Pan American Health Association: Development and strengthening of local health systems in the transforming of national health system, Washington, DC, 1988, The Association.

Public Health Service, US Department of Health and Human Services: 1991. Healthy people 2000: national health program and disease prevention, Washington, DC, US Government Printing Office.

Royal Thai Government: Health and social development in Thailand, Bangkok, 1988, Ministry of Public Health.

Smith RH, Forchuck C, and Martin M: Primary what? Int Nurs Rev 32(6):174-176, 180, 1985.

Swider SM and McElmurry BJ: A women's health perspective in primary health care: a nursing and community health worker demonstration project in urban America, J Fam Comm Health 13(3):1-17, 1990.

Watanakij P: Quality of life: goal of health for all by the year 2000, unpublished paper, College of Nursing, University of Illinois at Chicago, 1990.

World Health Organization: Health for all, Series #1, Geneva, 1978, The Organization.

World Health Organization: Primary health care: Alma-Ata Conference, Geneva, 1978, The Organization.

World Health Organization: Leadership for health for all: the challenge to nursing, Geneva, 1986, The Organization.

World Health Organization: The community health workers, Geneva, 1987, The Organization.

World Health Organization: World Health Technical Report: A meeting of a technical group at Riga, USSR, 22-28. Geneva, 1988, The Organization.

World Health Organization: Strengthening the performance of community health workers in primary health care, (technical report services), Geneva, 1989, The Organization.

World Health Organization: Health and social justice: challenge for the 1990s. In World Health Organization Press: Release WHA/4, Geneva, 1990, The Organization.

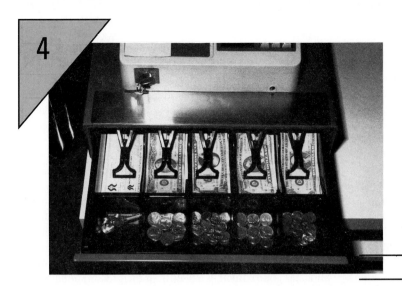

4

Economics of Health Care Delivery

Marcia Stanhope

OBJECTIVES

After reading this chapter, the student should be able to:

Define health economics.
Identify levels of economic theories.
Trace the evolution of the components of health care services.
Identify the factors influencing health care economics.
Trace the involvement of government and other third-party payers in health care financing.
Discuss national health care financing and direct service delivery plans.
Discuss proposed health care financing for the future.
Analyze the impact of a primary prevention goal on health care economics.
Discuss health care rationing.
Describe the relationship between poverty and health care financing.

KEY TERMS

benefit schedule	gross domestic product (GDP)	medically indigent
capitation	gross national product (GNP)	Medicare Program
cost-plus reimbursement		population demography
diagnosis-related groups	health economics	price inflation
	health care rationing	prospective cost reimbursement
economics	Health Maintenance Organization Act	prospective payment system
efficacy	managed care	retrospective cost reimbursement
enabling legislation	Medicaid Program	
fee-screen system	medical technology	third-party payments

T he health care delivery system of the 1960s and 1970s experienced vast expansions, unlimited financial resources, an open job market, and a nursing discipline that was expanding and broadening its responsibilities and influence. In contrast, the present health care delivery system is characterized by limited resources, regulatory restrictions, increased technological advances, increased competition, a nursing shortage, and more emphasis on health care delivery in the community.

Because of these, the concerns of the 1990s and the twenty-first century will focus on examining the economics of health care delivery, limiting the continuous growth of the largest employing industry in the United States, and organizing and assigning priorities to use the available resources at the least cost. Nursing will be concerned with establishing its contribution to the health of the nation and ensuring its economic viability in the market structure as a major contributor in health care delivery.

With the current emphasis on cost consciousness in health care delivery, nurses are being challenged to implement changes in practice and participate in research and policy activities designed to reduce health care costs. These activities will require a basic understanding of economics and the economics of the delivery system (IOM, 1983).

This chapter provides an overview of the economic issues of the health care delivery system. Discussion focuses on factors influencing health care, schema for financing health care, economics of primary prevention, methods for evaluating health and nursing costs, and the value of human life in health care spending. A brief view of health care financing and the impact of the issues of accessibility, acceptability, affordability, and organization of the industry is also included.

DEFINITIONS

To grasp the importance of the economics of health care and its significance to nursing, a basic understanding of key economic terms is essential.

Economics is the social science concerned with the problems of using or administering scarce resources in the most efficient way to attain maximum fulfillment of society's unlimited wants (Heider-Dorneich, 1978). *Health economics* is concerned with the problems of producing and distributing the health care resources.

The goal of health economics is not unlike the goal of public health—to provide the most good for the most people, given available knowledge and resources.

The goal of health economics is to provide the best quality health care to the largest number of people, given available financial resources. The provision of health goods (services) requires money. Spending money on health goods limits the amount of money available for other goods, such as food, clothing, shelter, transportation, education, and recreation.

Society must begin to make tough decisions about the allocation of available resources. Today the United States allocates approximately a twelfth of the gross national product (GNP) for health goods. This represented $500 billion spent in 1987. Health care expenditures are projected to reach 15% of the gross national product by the year 2000 (Table 4-1).

The *gross national product (GNP)* is defined as the total value of all goods and services produced in the economy in 1 year (Health: United States, 1988). The GNP is the most comprehensive measure of a nation's total output of goods and services. For example, all cars, food, clothes, and houses that are made and sold are a part of the **goods** that help to describe the GNP. It is useful for comparing how much is spent in a year and tells people where society's values are. The value, or price, of a **service** is determined by using the consumer price index. The *consumer price index* is a shopping basket approach that compares prices of all consumed goods and services purchased by urban wage earners and clerical workers and their families on a monthly or quarterly basis. The medical care component of the consumer price index compares selected prices of hospital, medical, dental, and pharmaceutical products and services (Health: United States, 1988).

The *gross domestic product (GDP)* is a statistical measure that is used to compare health care spending between countries. The GDP defines the total value of all goods

---

TABLE 4-1

Gross national product and national health expenditures in United States for selected years from 1929 to 1987*

| | | National Health Expenditures | | |
| | Gross national | Amount | Percent of | |
Year	product in billions	in billions	gross national product	Amount per capita
1929	$ 103.9	$3.6	3.5	$29
1940	100.4	4.0	4.0	29
1950	288.3	12.7	4.4	80
1960	515.3	26.9	5.2	142
1970	1015.5	75.0	7.4	349
1980	2731.9	248.1	9.1	1055
1987	4526.7	500.3	11.1	1987

From Office of National Cost Estimates, Office of the Actuary: National health expenditures, 1987, Health Care Financing Review, vol. 10, no 2. FCFA Pub. No. 03276, Health Care Financing Administration, Washington, D.C., 1989, U.S. Government Printing Office, 1989.
*Note: These data reflect Bureau of Economic Analysis, Department of Commerce, revisions to the gross national product as of December 1988 and Social Security Administration revisions to the population as of April 1988.

and services produced in the United States plus the value of services performed in the United States by foreign subjects minus the value of services performed in other countries by U.S. citizens (Health: United States, 1988). Whereas the GNP is used in the United States to compare costs of health care to other costs, such as defense, the GDP helps in comparing costs of health and nursing care in the United States to other countries such as Canada because it is a more exact measure of international comparisons than the GNP.

ECONOMIC THEORIES

Two basic theories are applicable to the study and understanding of economics: microeconomic theory and macroeconomic theory.

Microeconomic theory is concerned with the study of allocation and distribution of income. What should be produced and in what quantity? How should income be distributed among the members of society? The basic principles applied to microeconomic theory are those of supply and demand. When the supply of a product or service increases, the demand decreases. This results in lower prices. Conversely, when demand goes up and supply goes down, the price goes up.

The primary objective of this level of theory is to explain the factors that determine prices, which affect resource allocation and result in income being distributed. This theory focuses on factors, including behaviors, related to individuals, agencies and corporations (Landreth, 1976).

Macroeconomic theory concerns itself with the study of stability and growth of the total economy, the factors which determine levels of income and employment, general price levels, and the rate of economic growth. This theory is concerned with aggregate (group) variables that affect the total economy.

An outgrowth of microeconomic theory was a branch called welfare theory, which was policy oriented and proposed to establish criteria for making objective judgements about welfare. This theory assumed that permitting citizens to follow their own self-interests would promote the social good, and that a governmental policy that did not interfere with their activities would lead to maximum national welfare. This theory further assumes that a competitive market would result in maximum resource allocation and a maximum economic welfare (Landreth, 1976).

Each of these theories is applicable to the following discussion in which global factors (macroeconomics) are examined that affect the health state. Aggregate and organizational factors are examined in considering health care financing or a national health insurance, rationing, the new concept of managed care, and the poverty of health care.

An interesting point to remember is that to date the laws of supply and demand (microeconomic theory) have not worked in the health care industry because it is a monopoly with a captive consumer market instead of a competitive market. Regardless of supply and demand, prices continue to go up. It remains to be seen whether the new spirit of competitiveness will have a positive effect on health care costs and if supply and demand will eventually work to control prices.

HEALTH SERVICES COMPONENTS: SYSTEM EVOLUTION

From the 1800s through the late 1900s, the U.S. health care delivery system experienced four developmental stages with differing emphasis on health care economics. The health services component framework is used to describe the evolution of the organization of health care delivery.

Four basic components provide the framework for health services delivery: *labor* (work force), *facilities, technology,* and *service intensity.* Historically, changes in these components have occurred as macro level changes have occurred in morbidity, mortality, national health policy, and economic and social forces.

The *first developmental stage* of the health care delivery system occurred during the period 1800 to 1900. As mentioned in Chapter 1, the period was characterized by epidemics of infectious diseases, such as plague, cholera, typhoid, smallpox, influenza, malaria, yellow fever, and gastric disorders. The health problems of the period were related to contaminated food and water supplies, inadequate sewage disposal, and poor housing conditions (Banta, 1990; Pickett and Hanlon, 1990).

Minimal technology was available to aid in disease control. The doctor's black bag contained the few medicines and tools available for health care in the era, and hospitals were characterized by overcrowding, disease, and lack of cleanliness. Because the sick, if cared for in a hospital, usually died because of hospital conditions, most people were cared for at home by family and friends (Rushmer, 1984).

During this period the labor force was composed of poorly trained physicians who attained their skills through apprenticeships with practicing physicians who were trained the same way. Nurses were typically volunteers recruited from the lower social strata or from religious orders. Their primary focus was to assist the clients with activities of daily living. In 1867 the first nurse training school was established at the New England Hospital for Women and Children to provide formal preparation for nursing in the United States; by 1877, organized district nursing (home nursing) had been established (Gardner, 1936; Kalish, 1986). In this first developmental phase the methods of financing were private pay for those who could afford health care, bartering with the physicians, or charitable contributions from individuals and organizations.

The *second developmental phase* of the health care delivery system, dating from 1900 to 1945, was marked by the control of acute infectious diseases. Environmental conditions began to improve, with major advances in water purification, sanitary sewage disposal, milk and water quality, and urban housing quality. The health problems of the era changed from mass epidemics to individual acute infections or traumatic episodes (Pickett and Hanlon, 1990; Rushmer, 1984).

The workers of the period were better educated. Physician education evolved from apprenticeships to scientifically based college education; the change occurred after the publication of the Flexner Report of 1910. Clinical medicine was in its "golden age" because of major advances in surgery and childbirth, identification of the cause of pernicious anemia, and such technological discoveries as insulin in 1922 for control of diabetes, sulfa drugs in 1932 for treatment of infectious diseases, and antibiotics such as penicillin in the 1940s (Rice, 1990; Rushmer, 1984).

Nurses of the era were trained primarily in hospital schools of nursing, whose goal was to educate nurses in the dependent function of following physicians' orders. Hospitals and health departments were growing in numbers and strength. The public health departments' major emphasis was on quarantine and case finding. These tasks were delegated to the public health nurse. Also, 225 visiting nurse organizations were offering skilled attendance and were focusing on the teaching of cleanliness and the proper care of the sick in the home. Thus health education was identified as a nursing function early in the development of the health care delivery system (Lee, 1981; Rushmer, 1984).

In addition to private and charitable financing of health care, city, county, and state governments were beginning to contribute through the provision of hospitals and clinics for the poor, state mental institutions, and other specialized hospitals, such as tuberculosis hospitals.

The *third developmental stage*, from 1945 to 1984, showed a shift away from acute infectious health problems toward chronic health problems such as heart disease, cancer, and stroke. Major technological advances of the era included the development of chemotherapeutic agents, immunological prophylaxis, advances in anesthesia, advances in electrolyte and cardiopulmonary physiology, expansion of diagnostic laboratories and complex equipment such as the CT scanner, organ and tissue transplants, radiation therapy, and specialty units for critical care, coronary care, and intensive care.

The numbers and kinds of health service facilities increased; health care providers constituted more than 5% of the total U.S. work force. The three largest employers were hospitals, convalescent institutions, and physician's offices. Between 1970 and 1984 alone the number of persons employed in the health care industry grew by 90%. The numbers of personnel employed in "other sites," such as the community, also increased.

During this third developmental stage the system appeared to have unlimited resources for growth and expansion. The period was marked by the introduction of the health insurance industry and substantial growth of the federal government's role in financing health care.

Current problems and realities in the health care delivery system are reflected in a *fourth developmental stage,* one of increasingly limited resources, restricted growth, and a reorganization of methods of financing and care delivery. Health care providers are being forced to be more introspective, to look at alternatives and options to the unlimited resources, growth, and services of previous decades. With substantial federal health policy changes, emphasis is slowly moving toward increased health care delivery in the community and increased emphasis on preventive care.

Unfortunately, a shift backward toward increases in communicable, infectious, and environmental illnesses is now occurring. Table 4-2 provides a comparison of the leading causes of mortality from 1900 to 1987. Infant mortality is increasing whereas life expectancy is increasing. Chronic illnesses resulting from environmental and lifestyle influences are increasing and, with the resurgence of commu-

TABLE 4-2
Leading causes of death in the United States, 1900 and 1987

Cause	Death rate per 100,000 population
1900	
Influenza and pneumonia	202.2
Tuberculosis	194.4
Diarrhea and enteritis	139.9
Heart disease	137.4
Cerebral hemorrhage	106.9
Nephritis	88.7
Accidents	72.3
Cancer	64.0
Diseases of early infancy	62.6
Diphtheria	40.3
Simple meningitis	33.8
Typhoid and paratyphoid	31.3
All causes	1719.1
1987	
Heart diseases	312.4
Malignant neoplasms	195.9
Cerebrovascular accidents	61.6
Accidents	39.0
Chronic obstructive pulmonary disease	32.2
Influenza and pneumonia	28.4
Diabetes mellitus	15.8
Suicide	12.7
Liver cirrhosis	10.8
Homicide	8.7
AIDS (#15)	5.5
All causes	872.4

nicable and infectious diseases, promise to be the major health threats of the twenty-first century.

Health Care Providers

The types of health care providers and the number of practitioners of each type also influence the economics of health care. Before 1940 there were fewer than 40 types of health care providers; in 1990 the number, as reported by the U.S. Department of Labor, had risen to more than 200. The increase in specialization led to changes in certification, qualifications, education, and standards of care in each professional area. The combination of these factors contributed to the increased number and kinds of providers to meet the demands of the health care system. As of 1988, there were approximately 560,000 physicians and 1.6 million nurses in the United States providing health care services to a population of 245 million. Of the practicing nurses, approximately 21% were employed in areas of community health. The above total represents approximately 223 physicians per 100,000 population and 668 registered nurses per 100,000 population. Since 1970 the physician population has grown by 71% and the nurse population by 126%. Table 4-3 shows the increase in the number of people employed in the health industry from 1970 through 1988.

During the fourth developmental period the supply of physicians has continued to increase whereas the demand has declined. This will lead to more competition, different practice arrangements, and different payment mechanisms. Conversely, the demand for nurses has increased faster than the supply. The primary reason for this increase is the change in the health care market philosophy from that of unlimited spending and care at any cost to one of a competitive and cost-driven market. Therefore the federal government and other payers are supporting the use of nurses and other health care workers to provide care previously given by the more expensive physician. Nurse-managed clinics, more emphasis on home care, community care, and preventive programs are being supported as less costly methods to provide quality care (micro level theory).

As *economic philosophy* has changed, other changes have included prospective payment, managed care (providing a given set of coordinated services to a client group at the best price), industry self-insurance, decline in insurance benefits, nonphysician provider reimbursement, community based services, a shift away from for-profit back to nonprofit health care, and an emphasis on evaluating the effectiveness of interventions and technologies.

Health Care Changes

This era will be noted as an era of vast changes in all sectors of health care delivery. Technological advances of the era continue to focus on development of new biogenetic and drug therapies for problems such as AIDS, cancer, Alzheimer's and Parkinson's Diseases and fertility problems. Alternative health care delivery units are increasing and are community-based. The electronic fetal monitor and magnetic resonance imaging (MRI) are a few of the latest advances in technical equipment, whereas intrauterine fetal surgery exemplifies the latest surgical techniques. Meanwhile, however, the country faces its first major epidemic in decades.

FACTORS INFLUENCING THE ECONOMICS OF HEALTH CARE

Four major factors are instrumental in influencing the economic growth of the health care system: price inflation, technology, intensity, and changes in population demography.

Price Inflation

Price inflation was the major economic problem between 1950 and 1980. General inflation affected the prices of all goods and services in the United States, including health care costs, which increased approximately 12% faster than the consumer price index. By 1990 health care costs outdistanced general inflation by 10%.

Table 4-4 shows the changes in money spent for health care from 1950 to 1987. Note that this table shows a rise in health care expenditures from $12.7 billion in 1950 to $500.3 billion in 1987. Whereas the population had increased by 62% over this 37 year period, all health care costs had increased by 4000%. Thus, the amount spent per person increased by approximately 2000%, or from less than $100 per person in 1950 to $2000 per person in 1990. Health services and supplies accounted for 92% to 97% of the total money spent, whereas research and construction costs decreased from 7.6% to 3%.

▼	**TABLE 4-3**

Persons employed in selected health service sites, according to place of employment in United States from 1970 to 1988

Site	1970*	1980	1988
Number of persons in thousands All employed civilians	76,805	99,303	114,968
All health service sites	4246	7339	8781
Offices of physicians	477	777	985
Offices of dentists	222	415	521
Offices of chiropractors†	19	40	77
Hospitals	2690	4036	4520
Nursing and personal care facilities	509	1199	1467
Other health service sites	330	872	1211

From U.S. Bureau of the Census: 1970 Census of population: occupation by industry, Subject Reports, Final Report PC(2)-7C. Washington, D.C., 1972, U.S. Government Printing Office, U.S. Bureau of Labor Statistics: Labor force statistics derived from: Current population survey: a databook, vol. 1. Washington, D.C., 1982 U.S. Government Printing Office; Employment and Earnings, January 1983-89, vol. 30, no. 1, vol. 31, no. 1, vol. 32, no. 1, vol. 33, no. 1, vol. 34, no. 1, vol. 35, no. 1, and vol. 36, no. 1, Washington, D.C., 1983-1989 U.S. Government Printing Office; American Chiropractic Association: Unpublished data.
*April 1, derived from decennial census; all other data years are annual averages from the Current Population Survey.
†Data for 1980 are from the American Chiropractic Association; data for all other years are from the U.S. Bureau of Labor Statistics.
NOTES: Totals exclude persons in health-related occupations who are working in nonhealth industries, as classified by the U.S. Bureau of the Census, such as pharmacists employed in drugstores, school nurses, and nurses working in private households. Totals include federal, state, and county health workers. In the period 1970 to 1982, employed persons were classified according to the industry groups used in the 1970 Census of Population. Beginning in 1983, persons were classified according to the system used in the 1980 Census of Population.

In the early 1980s inflation began to decline. In 1984 with the decline in prices for other goods and services came the lowest annual increase in health care prices since 1960. Nevertheless, hospital services continued to increase at twice the overall inflation rate. During these years hospitals and physicians were the two major recipients of health care expenditures, whereas government-sponsored public health care programs received less than 3% of the total health care dollars.

Inflation in health care delivery remains the dominant factor in health economic issues today. By 1987 dental services and physician services were increasing more rapidly than hospital services. Whereas the slowdown in price increases, especially in hospital care, may be attributed to the new *prospective payment system* (see page 55), a number of assumptions have been made regarding reasons for price inflation in health care delivery:

1. As earnings increase and more people acquire health insurance, use of the system and the demand for services also increases.
2. Expenditures are rising in response to increased hospital wages, whereas lagging employee productivity requires more personnel.

3. Increases in supply, equipment, and salary expenditures result from the growth and the number of insurance plans.

4. New and costlier methods of care force prices up.

5. Prices rise because of the building of costly, expensive-to-maintain hospital facilities that already exist in sufficient supply.

6. Changes in consumer lifestyles and environmental hazards have created a new set of health problems that require services.

7. New kinds of health insurance coverage encourage increased use of services such as dental care and organ transplantation.

8. Increased community-based care services add to the overall costs.

9. Discontinuation of the federal Economic Stabilization Program, which controlled prices of health care, resulted in increases in costs and services offered (Health: United States, 1985; Joel, 1985).

Although all factors mentioned have contributed to inflation in health care costs, some have had more effect than others. The availability of insurance to cover health care costs and the development of new and costlier methods of health care technology appear to be the major contributors to increased costs. Increased wages for the new categories of health care personnel, such as nurse practitioners, physician's assistants, and dental technicians, have also contributed to increased costs. The increased numbers of health care facilities and the vast duplication of services offered have contributed to the need for more employees, supplies, and equipment, and thus to increased costs through the 37-year period.

However, some change is occurring. For example, although hospitals have traditionally been the single largest employer of health personnel in the United States, the number of community-based employees increased in 1987. Health care reimbursement schemes have changed and will cover the cost of more community based care, such as home care, well child screening, and prenatal care.

Technology and Intensity

Medical technology has been defined by the Congressional Office of Technology Assessment as "the set of techniques, drugs, equipment, and procedures used by health care professionals in delivering medical care to individuals and the system within which such care is delivered" (Banta, 1990). Included in any discussion of costs of technology is the cost of use of technology.

Intensity refers to the use of technologies, supplies, and health care services by or on behalf of the client. Intensity includes and is a partial measure of the use of technologies.

Health care professionals, such as physicians, have become dependent on technology for diagnosis and treatment. They have become the principal purchasing agents of technology for the client. Nurses, too, have become dependent upon technologies to monitor client progress and make decisions about client care. The population, with an increasing sophistication about health and health care needs, demands the use of laboratory, radiological, diagnostic, palliative, and therapeutic services for treatment.

TABLE 4-4
National health expenditures and percent distribution according to type of expenditure in United States for selected years from 1950 to 1987

Type of expenditure	1950	1960	1970	1980	1987
			Amount in billions		
Total	$ 12.7	$ 26.9	$ 75.0	$248.1	$500.3
			Percent distribution		
All expenditures	100	100	100	100	100
Health service and supplies	92	94	93	95	97
Personal health care	86	88	87	89	88
Hospital care	30	34	37	41	39
Physician services	22	21	19	19	21
Dentist services	8	7	6	6	7
Nursing home care	2	2	6	8	8
Other professional services	3	3	2	2	3
Drugs and medical sundries	14	14	11	8	7
Eyeglasses and appliances	4	3	3	2	2
Other health services	4	4	3	2	2
Program administration and net cost of health insurance	4	4	4	4	5
Government public health activities	3	2	2	3	3
Research and construction	8	6	7	5	3
Noncommercial research	1	3	3	2	2
Construction	7	4	5	3	2

From Office of National Cost Estimates, Office of the Actuary: National health expenditures, 1987, Health Care Financing Review, vol. 10, no. 2, HCFA Pub. No. 03276. Health Care Financing Administration, Washington, D.C., 1989, U.S. Government Printing Office.
NOTE: Some numbers in this table have been revised and differ from previous editions of Health, United States.

As new and more complex technology is introduced into the system, the trend toward increasing use and cost is evident. For example, between 1979 and 1988 there was a 400% increase in CT scans performed on hospital inpatients; meanwhile ultrasound diagnostic procedures and angiocardiography tripled (Health: United States, 1988).

One of the most significant examples of a technology contributing to increasing costs is that of renal dialysis. After a 1972 congressional amendment to the Social Security Act extended Medicare coverage to pay for renal dialysis, approximately 16,000 people received care under this program at a cost of $250 million. By 1979 costs had risen to $1 billion for 51,000 clients. Costs were projected to reach $2.8 billion by 1986. In 1987, 130,939 persons served by Medicare received renal dialysis, a 156% increase in 8 years.

Renal dialysis programs and other new technologies demand personnel and investments in equipment and facilities. They also add to administrative costs, especially when the federal government is involved in the financing and regulating of the technology. All clients who qualify for health care financing through one of the federally funded programs qualifies for the use of these and other technologies.

An example of a health care problem that has contributed to the cost of health care through research and development of new technologies is the recent AIDS epidemic. This is the first problem to reach epidemic proportions in recent memory. It is a prime example of a problem that while affecting a growing number of people who will require a wide array of services (intensity), expensive treatments (technologies), and care, will also exacerbate already existing concerns about health care financing. Expenditures by the federal government alone for the AIDS epidemic increased from $6 million to $1.5 billion between 1982 and 1988. Projections indicate a rise in cost to $8.5 billion in 1991 to care for the 1 million people who are currently HIV sero positive on testing. In 1982 there were only 9000 cases.

The technologies and service intensity included in these figures are: research, education and prevention, veterans and Department of Defense medical care, Medicaid and Medicare funded medical care, and cash assistance. One medication alone was estimated to cost $6400 per year in 1989. The cost per individual case was approximately $147,000 (Green, 1989; Health: United States: 1988; Lyon, 1988; Scitovsky, 1987; Wagner, M., 1989). The box lists a few federal regulatory mechanisms that have contributed to the control and cost of technology.

Changes in Population Demography

The fourth major contributor to rising health care costs is the changing *population demography*. As discussed in chapter 2, the population of the United States is aging. It is projected that by the year 2000, 35% of the total population will be over 65 years of age, with the 85-years-old and older group growing at a rapid rate (JAH, 1987; Korn, 1989; Rubin et al., 1989; Theilheimer, 1989). These population changes are summarized in Table 4-5.

This is expected to lead to pressure to spend more money, especially for long-term care, research, and prevention of chronic disease in this population group. Data indicate that the major increases in health care expenditures have already

---

EXAMPLES OF FEDERAL REGULATORY MECHANISMS CONTRIBUTING TO TECHNOLOGY COSTS/CONTROL

1906 Prescription drug regulation passes—Food, Drug, and Cosmetic Act

1938 Manufacturers required to prove drug safety—Food, Drug, and Cosmetic Act

1952 Hill-Burton Act provides construction monies and requires a specified volume of "free care" in exchange

1962 Manufacturers required to prove drug efficacy—Food, Drug, and Cosmetic Act

1965 Amendments to Social Security Act providing Medicare and Medicaid result in increased use of technologies

1972 Social Security Act amendments extending coverage for end-stage renal disease provide payment for use of treatment technologies

1972 Social Security Act amendments provide for Professional Standards Review Organizations to review appropriateness of hospital care for Medicare and Medicaid recipients

1974 Health Planning and Resources Development Act introduces certificate-of-need authority to limit major capital expenditures at local and state levels

1976 Medical Devices Amendments regulates safety and effectiveness of medical equipment, such as pacemakers

1978 Medicare End-Stage Renal Disease Amendment provides for home dialysis and for kidney transplantation

1978 Health Services Research, Health Statistics, and Health Care Technology Act establishes a national council on health care technology to develop standards, criteria, and norms for the use of particular medical technologies

1982 Tax Equity and Fiscal Responsibilities Act establishes prospective payment system providing lump sum payment for hospitalized medicare patients by DRG category

1985 Gramm-Rudman-Hollings Balanced Budget and Emergency Deficit Control Act resulted in reduced funding to Medicare and Medicaid programs

1986 Omnibus Reconciliation Act (OBRA) directed the development of a model PPS for outpatient hospital services

1989 Medicare regulations introduced eight payment groups for ambulatory surgery centers and a flat payment amount for intraocular lens insertions. A precursor to prospective payment for ambulatory care

1989 OBRA created a physician resource-based fee schedule to be implemented by 1992, with more emphasis on family practice and less emphasis on the "high tech" specialties of surgery

1989 OBRA created the Agency for Health Care Policy and Research to perform research on effectiveness of medical services, interventions, and technologies, including nursing

---

been for the elderly population, whereas the least expenditures have been for people under 19 years of age.

Since the Social Security Amendments of 1965, the increase in Medicare expenditures for health care for the elderly has been greater than the rate of increased expenditures for the remainder of the population. Reasons for the increased rate of expenditures are the rapid growth of the

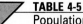

TABLE 4-5
Population data, in millions, for selected age groups from 1950 to 1987

Age (years)	1950	1970	1987
Under 15	40.4	57.9	52.4
15-24	22.0	35.4	38.2
25-44	45.2	47.9	77.6
45-64	30.8	41.9	45.2
65 and over	11.1	20.0	29.8

numbers of elderly in the United States, the increased number of elderly women who are heavier users of health services than men, the decline in family social support requiring the elderly to seek care and assistance outside the family structure, the greater use of more complex medical and surgical services, and the increased ability of the elderly to pay for services received.

Table 4-6 depicts the distribution of the four factors affecting increased costs of health care delivery from 1967 to 1987. Clearly, population has been a significant contributor after inflation and technology. In 1967 prices and intensity had similar effects. In 1977 inflation began to outdistance all other factors influencing health care expenditures. In 1987 prices contributed 53% to the growth of all health care expenditures. From 1977 to 1987 intensity increased in contribution to overall costs while prices were declining.

FINANCING OF HEALTH CARE: PRIVATE AND PUBLIC

Health care financing has evolved through the twentieth century from a system financed primarily by the consumer to a system financed primarily by third-party payers, i.e., private insurance companies and governments. This section will discuss changes in government, private insurance, consumer, and public health funding of care.

Table 4-7 shows changes in the percentages of financing from various sources. From 1950 to 1987 direct consumer payment decreased, philanthropic payments decreased, and third-party governmental and private insurance payments increased dramatically. The combined state and federal governments' contributions as third-party payers are currently

higher than those of private payers. In 1987, third-party payers contributed 71% toward the total costs of health care for the consumer, leaving only 29% to be covered by out-of-pocket money.

Third-Party Payments

Medical insurance in the private sector was first offered in 1847 by a commercial insurance company. The purpose of the insurance was to defray financial losses from disability attributable to accidents and later to defray income losses caused by specific sicknesses attributable to catastrophic communicable diseases, such as smallpox and scarlet fever.

A comprehensive study in the 1920s by the Committee on the Costs of Medical Care showed that a small portion of the population was paying most of the costs of medical care for the majority of the people. The Depression, rising medical costs, and the need to spread financial risk across communities spurred the development of the *third-party payment* system.

The system began as a major industry in the 1930s with the Blue Cross system, which initially provided prepayment for hospital care. It was modeled on the Baylor University prepayment plan established in 1929 to provide teachers with hospital coverage. In 1939 Blue Shield created plans to provide physician payment. The Blue Cross plans began as taxfree, nonprofit organizations established under special *enabling legislation* in various states.

In the 1940s and 1950s hospital and medical-surgical coverage increased substantially. Employee group coverage appeared and profit-making commercial insurance underwriters began offering health insurance packages with competitive premiums. The commercial insurance companies could offer lower premium rates becaue of the methods used to set rates. Blue Cross used a *community rate*, establishing a similar premium rate for all subscribers regardless of illness risk. In contrast, the commercial companies used an *experience rate* in which the premium was based on an estimate of the risk or the number of claims by the subscriber.

The premium competition, the popularity of health insurance packages as a fringe benefit, and the use of health insurance as a negotiable collective bargaining item led to increased numbers of covered benefits, payment of higher

TABLE 4-6
Average annual percent change in personal health care expenditures and percent distribution of factors affecting growth in United States

Period	Average annual percent change	Percent distribution of factors affecting growth			
		All factors	Prices	Population	Intensity*
1966-67	12.2	100	55	9	36
1976-77	12.3	100	64	7	29
1986-87	10.2	100	53	9	38

From Office of National Cost Estimates, Office of the Actuary: National health expenditures, 1987, Health Care Financing Review, vol. 10, no. 2. HCFA Pub. No. 03276, Health Care Financing Administration, Washington, D.C., U.S. Government Printing Office.
*Represents changes in use and/or kinds of services and supplies.
NOTE: Some numbers in this table have been revised and differ from previous editions of Health, United States.

TABLE 4-7
Personal health care expenditures and percent distribution, according to source of payment in United States for selected years, from 1929 to 1987

Year	Total in billions*	Per capita	All sources	Direct payment	Private health insurance	Philanthropy and industry	Government Total	Government Federal	Government State and local
1929	$ 3.2	$ 26	100.0	88.4†	‡	2.6	9.0	2.7	6.3
1940	$ 3.5	$ 26	100.0	81.3†	‡	2.6	16.1	4.1	12.0
1950	10.9	70	100.0	65.5	9.1	2.9	22.4	10.4	12.0
1960	23.7	129	100.0	54.9	21.1	2.3	21.8	9.3	12.5
1970	65.4	305	100.0	40.5	23.4	1.7	34.3	22.2	12.1
1980	219.7	934	100.0	28.7	30.7	1.2	39.4	28.4	10.9
1987	442.6	1758	100.0	27.8	31.4	1.2	39.6	29.6	10.0

From Office of National Cost Estimates, Office of the Actuary: National health expenditures, 1987, Health Care Financing Review, vol. 10, no. 2, HCFA Pub. No. 03276, Health Care Financing Administration, Washington, D.C., 1989, U.S. Government Printing Office.
*Includes all expenditures for health services and supplies other than expenses for prepayment and administration and government public health activities.
†Includes any insurance benefits and expenses for prepayment (insurance premiums less insurance benefits).
‡Figures are not separable from direct payment.
NOTE: Some numbers in this table have been revised and differ from previous editions of Health, United States.

portions of medical care expenses, and increased employer-paid premiums. These factors led to higher premium costs, higher health care costs, and plans that could economically cover high-risk segments of the population, such as the aged, poor, and disabled. The average monthly cost for private health insurance increased 70% from 1988 to 1990, bringing the average employees' share of family health care insurance premiums to more than $100 per month. It is projected that continued health care inflation could increase the bill to $5000 per year for middle income workers in 5 years (Tokarski, 1990).

The needs of high-risk populations led to passage of Medicare and Medicaid legislation. These and other national health programs were authorized to provide health care coverage for specific population segments. These new programs, federal regulations, and insurance company reimbursement methods contributed to increased technological costs. Because money was available to be paid, physicians, hospital managers, and clients used more medical technology, and service intensity increased.

Three reimbursement methods have been or are currently used to pay agencies for health goods and services:

1. *Cost-plus reimbursement*. An agency may be reimbursed for the actual costs of treatment and care plus added allowable costs. These added costs include depreciation of costs of a building and equipment and administrative costs (e.g., administrative salaries, utilities, and office supplies).
2. *Retrospective cost reimbursement*. An agency may be reimbursed per unit of service, according to an agreed-on price usually predetermined by the state insurance departments or departments of health. In home health the unit of service is the home visit and the agreed upon price is a set amount of money paid for a home visit in the region of the country in which the home care agency is located.

3. *Prospective cost reimbursement*. Based on previous experience and current rates for care, agencies and insurance companies attempt to predict an agency's costs for the year. The agency plans an annual budget with projected goals for services. The insurance company reimburses the agency based on predicted costs for services. For example, a home care agency may receive a check for 6 months to cover home care visits they predict they will make.

Positive and negative incentives were built into these reimbursement schemes. The cost-plus reimbursement scheme encouraged agencies to add depreciation and administrative costs that inflated actual treatment and care costs. The retrospective cost reimbursement method encouraged agencies to pad unit cost prices to cover unexpected cost increases, like increased postal service. The prospective cost reimbursement scheme encouraged agencies to stay within budget limits and added an incentive for providing less service to contain or reduce costs.

Along with agency reimbursement, physician reimbursement is a key factor in the use and cost of technology and service intensity. The two primary methods for physician reimbursement have been:

1. *Benefit schedule*—a list of specific physician services that identifies the amount third parties must pay for them.
2. *Fee screen system*—a method that determines the usual, customary, and reasonable charge (UCR) for specific services, based on a regional evaluation of physician charges in all specialties. A maximum reimbursement limit by third parties is determined by the UCR for a specific service.

These fee-for-service reimbursement schemes were shown to be inflationary. Physicians controlled the numbers and kinds of services provided a client. As third-party reimbursement increased, physicians' fees increased. The consumer was responsible for the costs over and above the third-party coverage. Negative experience with fee-for-service physician reimbursement and the inflationary nature of the system has impeded progress toward third-party reimbursement for other health care providers, such as nurses.

The third-party pay system is often blamed for rising health care costs. Factors that support this belief include the following:

1. The cost-plus reimbursement scheme previously used to pay hospital care for Medicaid-Medicare and Blue Cross clients provided little incentive to control costs.
2. The third-party payers provided better coverage for the more expensive hospital services than for ambulatory care, home health care, or nursing home care. This encouraged consumer use of hospitals because more of the clients' bill was paid by the insurer. If there was a choice between hospital and home care, hospital care was chosen.
3. Consumer demand for services increased and provider incentives to use less costly services were lacking because government or private insurers paid most hospital and physician bills. The providers did not develop more ambulatory services because of the need for the consumer to pay out-of-pocket.
4. The UCR charge pay system encouraged physicians to charge maximum fees so they could boost the UCR charge schedule.
5. Third-party reimbursement for surgery, diagnostic procedures, and other technological interventions encouraged the provision of these services, regardless of their necessity.

Generally, health care costs have risen faster than the cost of all goods and services.

Consumer Payments

Before 1930 and the beginning of Blue Cross, the consumer had more influence over health care costs because nearly all health care costs were paid out-of-pocket. However, the health care system has always been a sellers' market. Once the buyer (the client) makes the decision to enter the health care market, all goods and services are provided and controlled by the seller (the physician).

When the health care system was economically controlled by the consumer market, entrance into the system was restricted to those who could afford to pay or to those few who could find care financed by charitable and philanthropic organizations.

Today the consumer pays directly approximately 26% of all physician fees and 20% of all hospital bills. However, these figures do not reflect the amount of money the consumer pays in taxes to finance government-supported programs such as Medicare and Medicaid, the insurance premiums averaging $1200 per year that come from wages and therefore decrease the size of paychecks, or the direct insurance premiums paid for supplemental insurance to plug the gaps in the primary health insurance policy and Medicare.

It is estimated that the elderly pay approximately 60% of all health care costs directly (Grau, 1988). This is due to limits in coverage in Medicare and Medicaid programs,

payment of premiums for Medicare, and the need to have additional insurance to cover these gaps. It is also due to the limited number of physicians, hospitals, and other agencies who accept Medicare and Medicaid payment. The aged then are left to cover the difference between Medicare and Medicaid services and additional costs. In reality, the working consumer pays all health care costs directly or indirectly and should be more concerned about health care costs.

Until the mid 1980s, consumer demands increased and strengthened the benefits of private health insurance packages, the numbers of government programs available to the aged and poor, and the availability and accessibility of health care services. These consumer demands contributed to health care inflation and caused a financial drain on the economic potential of the individual and the government. Beginning in the 1980s health insurance benefits were cut back. Medicare and Medicaid program benefits were reduced, prospective payment to hospitals was introduced, and more emphasis was placed on care in the home and community. To attempt to control physician costs, a new Medicare fee schedule, called a relative value scale, was adopted in 1991. This scale replaces the previously described methods of physician payment, placing more emphasis on payment of care received through primary care physicians in the community. It also places more value on prevention, health promotion, and evaluation with less value for surgery and the use of high technologies. This is an attempt to reduce inappropriate and unnecessary care (Lee, 1990).

Government Payments

The federal government became involved in health care financing for population segments early in U.S. history. As mentioned in Chapter 1, in 1798 the federal government created the Marine Hospital Service to provide medical service for sick and disabled sailors and to protect the nation's borders against importation of disease through seaports. The Marine Hospital Service is considered the first national health insurance plan in the United States. The original plan cost each sailor 20 cents per month in a payroll deduction for illness care.

The National Health Board was established in 1879. The board was later renamed the United States Public Health Service (USPHS). Within the USPHS, the federal government developed a public health liaison with state and local health departments for the purpose of controlling communicable diseases and improving sanitation. Additional health programs were also developed to meet obligations to federal beneficiaries, including American Indians (Indian Health Service), the armed forces (Department of Defense), and veterans of wars (Veterans Administration).

Today, the federal government is involved in health care research, training, financing, and delivery and provides money for four aspects of public health: (1) broad national health interests, such as AIDS research; (2) special groups, such as mothers, infants, and the aged through WIC, Medicare, and Medicaid funds; (3) special problems or programs, such as food and drugs through FDA requirements, food inspection; and (4) international health through its affiliation with World Health Organization.

Appendix G contains an overview of the major historical events depicting the federal government's increasing involvement in financing health care research, training, and delivery.

Public Health Care Funding

Most public governmental agencies operate on an annual budget and plan for costs by estimating salaries, expenses, and costs of services for a budgetary period. Public health agencies, such as the health departments and WIC programs, receive primary funding from tax revenues, with additional reimbursement for select goods and services through private third-party payers. Selected public health programs receive reimbursement for services as follows: through block grants given by the federal government to states for prenatal and child health; through Medicare and Medicaid for home health, nursing home, WIC programs, early periodic screening and childhood development programs (EPSDT); and through collection of fees on a sliding scale for select client services through health departments, such as immunizations.

Although only 3% of all federal funds expended are for government public health programs, such as mental health and WIC, as opposed to 97% for illness care in hospitals, public health expenditures by states and territorial health agencies have increased at a rate of 11% per year between 1977 and 1987. Table 4-8 indicates the amount, source of funds, and program areas supported since 1976. Note a declining emphasis on personal health programs and an increasing emphasis on the supplemental food program for women and children (WIC). The effect of the fee-for-service issue is not as great in public health care as in private health care because most providers are salaried. However, the increasing costs of health care goods and increasing salaries of providers has contributed to the rising costs of public health care as well.

National Health Care Plans

The *Medicare Program,* Title XVIII of the Social Security Act of 1965, provides hospital insurance, Part A, and medical insurance, Part B, to the elderly, the permanently and totally disabled, and people with end-stage renal disease (Health: United States, 1988).

The hospital insurance package, Part A, is available without cost to all elderly individuals who have paid Social Security taxes. Estimates indicate that 98% of the elderly population are covered by Part A. Part A provides payment for hospital services, home health services, and extended care facilities. This includes an annual deductible based on a rate equal to a 1-day stay in the hospital. That deductible has increased over the years as daily hospital costs have increased; in 1991 it was $628.

The medical insurance package, Part B, is available to all people who wish to pay a monthly premium for the coverage. Approximately 96% of the elderly population is covered. The premium cost was $29.90 per month in 1991. Part B of Medicare provides coverage for services other than hospitalization, such as physician services, outpatient hospital care, outpatient physical therapy and speech therapy, home health care, laboratory services, ambulance

TABLE 4-8
Public health expenditures by State and territorial health agencies, according to source of funds and program area: United States, selected fiscal years 1976-87

Funds and program area	1976	1980	1987
	Amount in millions		
Total	$2539.8	$4450.8	$8127.6
Source of funds			
Federal grants and contracts	796.9	1573.1	2821.7
Department of Agriculture	153.7	678.4	1651.6
Other	643.2	894.7	1170.1
State	1485.7	2513.3	4562.1
Local	96.1	114.0	139.7
Fees, reimbursements, and other	161.2	250.3	604.1
Program area			
WIC*	137.7	660.7	1622.1
Noninstitutional personal health other than WIC†	1079.0	1698.2	3129.5
State health agency-operated institutions	531.1	819.3	1226.7
Environmental health	199.2	298.0	528.2
Health resources	208.2	356.5	709.4
Laboratory	104.1	161.1	264.7
Other‡	280.6	457.0	646.9

From Public Health Foundation: Public health agencies 1987: expenditures and sources of funds, Washington, D.C., 1987, Unpublished data.
*Supplemental Food Program for Women, Infants, and Children.
†Includes funds for maternal and child health services other than WIC, handicapped children's services, communicable disease control, dental health, chronic disease control, mental health, alcohol and drug abuse, and supporting personal health programs.
‡Funds for general administration and funds to local health departments not allocated to program areas.
NOTE: Data are reported for 55 health agencies in 50 states, the District of Columbia, and 4 territories (Puerto Rico, American Samoa, Guam, and the Virgin Islands).

transportation, prostheses, equipment, and some supplies. After a $100 deductible, up to 80% of reasonable charges are paid for these services. Part B resembles the major medical insurance coverage of private insurance carriers. Table 4-9 shows the increasing cost of the Medicare program from 1967 to 1987.

Since the passage of the Medicare amendments to the Social Security Act in 1965, the cost of Medicare has increased dramatically. Hospital care continues to be the major factor contributing to Medicare costs.

As a result of the increasing costs, Congress passed a law in 1983 that radically changed Medicare's method of payment for hospital services. The Social Security amendments of 1983 (PL 98-21) mandated an end to cost-plus reimbursement by Medicare and instituted a 3-year transition to a *prospective payment system (PPS)* for inpatient hospital services. The purpose of the new hospital payment scheme was to shift the financial incentives away from the provision of more care, the use of more technology, and the

TABLE 4-9
Medicare expenditures and percent distribution, according to type of service, in United States for selected years, from 1967 to 1987*

Type of service	1967	1970	1980	1987
AMOUNT IN BILLIONS				
All expenditures	$4.5	$7.1	$35.7	$88.5
PERCENT DISTRIBUTION				
All services	100.0	100.0	100.0	100.0
Hospital care	69.1	71.5	72.6	67.3
Physician services	24.7	22.8	22.1	27.4
Nursing home care	4.6	3.7	1.1	0.8
Home health service	2.1	2.4	3.9	4.5

*Data compiled by the Health Care Financing Administration.

TABLE 4-10
Medicaid expenditures and percent distribution, according to type of service, in United States for selected years from 1967 to 1987

Type of service	1967	1970	1980	1987
AMOUNT IN BILLIONS				
All expenditures	$2.9	$5.2	$25.2	$45.1
PERCENT DISTRIBUTION				
All services	100.0	100.0	100.0	100.0
Hospital care	42.3	42.9	38.1	29.8
Physician services	10.9	13.3	9.7	6.1
Dentist services	4.4	3.2	2.0	1.2
Other professional services	0.9	1.4	2.2	0.6
Drugs and drug sundries	7.2	7.9	5.5	6.8
Nursing home care	31.7	27.2	38.1	41.7
Home health service	—	0.4	1.4	4.1
Other*	2.6	4.1	3.7	8.7

From Health Care Financing Administration.
*Other services include laboratory and radiological services, family planning services, EPSDT, clinics, and pro rated care.

use of more hospital care. Reimbursement is based on a fixed price per case for clients in 468 *diagnosis-related group (DRGs)*. The objective of this system was to reduce hospital costs while maintaining an acceptable level of quality health care and access. Although this type of reimbursement was mandated for hospitals only, prospective payment for physicians, home health, long-term care, and ambulatory care is slowly being introduced.

The *Medicaid program,* Title XIX of the Social Security Act of 1965, provides financial assistance to states and counties to pay for medical services for the aged poor, the blind, the disabled, and families with dependent children. The Medicaid program is jointly sponsored and financed with matching funds from the federal and state governments. Currently, 22 million people are enrolled in Medicaid.

Full payment for four types of service was provided originally: (1) inpatient and outpatient hospital care; (2) laboratory and radiological services; (3) physician services; and (4) skilled nursing care, at home or in a nursing home, for people over 21. The 1972 Social Security Amendments added family planning to the list of full-pay services. Prescriptions, dental services, eyeglasses, intermediate facilities care, and coverage for the *medically indigent* are allowable program options. By law, the medically indigent are required to pay a monthly premium.

Any state participating in the Medicaid program is required to provide the five basic services to participants who are below state poverty income levels. The optional programs are provided at the discretion of each state.

In 1989 changes in Medicaid required states to provide care for children under age 6 and to pregnant women under 133% of the poverty level. These changes also provided for pediatric and family nurse practitioner reimbursement.

Federal government reorganization of the Medicaid program in the 1990s may include a requirement for states to begin prospective payment systems to reduce costs. Table 4-10 indicates the increased cost of the Medicaid program from 1967 to 1987.

In contrast to Medicare, the major contributor to costs in the Medicaid program has been nursing home care. When combined with hospital care, it accounts for 76% of all costs

to the program. See Table 4-11 for a comparison of Medicare and Medicaid programs.

With Medicare and Medicaid, the federal government purchases goods and services for population segments through independent health care systems. In contrast, the *military medical care system* is a federal program that provides health care and insurance to military personnel and their dependents at no direct cost to the recipient.

The military medical system comprises 168 hospitals and clinics, which provide military personnel with health care wherever they are located. This health care system has several important characteristics: (1) the system is all-inclusive and ever-present; (2) coverage is effective at all times; (3) prevention, early case-finding, and health promotion are emphasized; and (4) dependents and families are served by a subsystem that combines military and civilian health services (Sharfstein, 1990). This system also places the federal government in the direct health service business.

The *Civilian Health and Medical Program of the Uniformed Services* (CHAMPUS) allows families and dependents to obtain private sector care if service is unavailable in the military system. The program is provided, financed, and supervised by the military system. In 1981 the CHAMPUS Program began direct, independent reimbursement of nurse practitioners and physician assistants for services to military dependents.

As with all other programs, military medical care systems' costs have increased. From 1981 to 1989, costs increased by 148% to $13 billion, whereas the CHAMPUS program costs climbed 200% to $2.4 billion (Tokarski, 1989).

The *Veterans Administration health care system,* linked to the military health care system, operates within the United States for retired, disabled, and other specified categories of military service veterans. The system, comprising 172 hospitals and more than 200 outpatient departments, is one

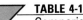

TABLE 4-11
Comparison of Medicare and Medicaid programs

Feature	Medicare	Medicaid
Obtain information	Social Security Office	Welfare Office
Recipients	Persons aged 65 +; disabled under 65 eligible after 2 years	Needy and low income, persons aged 65 +, blind, disabled, families with dependent children, some other children
Type of program	Insurance	Assistance
Government affiliation	Federal	Federal/state partnership
Availability	All states	All states
Hospital insurance	Financed by working persons' payroll contributions	Financed by federal and state government
Medical insurance	Monthly premiums paid by recipients (25%) and federal government (75%)	Federal and state government
Types of coverage	Inpatient and outpatient hospital care	Inpatient and outpatient hospital care
	Posthospital skilled nursing facility	Skilled nursing facilities
	Home health care	Home health care
	Physician services	Physician services
	Medical services and supplies	Other laboratory and x-ray services
	Hospice care	Screening, diagnosis, and treatment of children under 21
		Family planning
		Rural health clinic services
		Supplements Medicare payments

Modified from Medicaid/Medicare: which is which? USDHHS pub. no. 02129, Washington, D.C., 1984, National Health Care Financing Administration.

part of a benefit package received by veterans. Eligibility for health care is often tied to other financial benefits within the system structure. Current cost of this program is $11 billion per year.

The Indian Health Service provides direct care to Native Americans living on reservations. This agency operates approximately 50 hospitals and 340 clinics to serve over 1 million Native Americans. This service was established in 1911 through the Bureau of Indian Affairs in the Department of the Interior. This service, like the military service provides a combination of public and private health care. Legislation passed in 1976 provides opportunity for tribes to assume responsibility of operating their own facilities. This service cost the Public Health Service $41 billion in 1988.

POVERTY AND HEALTH CARE FINANCING

In 1987, 64% of the United States population had health insurance provided through their employers. Another 10.2% purchased private coverage directly from insurance companies or through groups, such as unions, bringing the total population to 74.5% insured. An additional 10% received insurance through public programs leaving 15.5% uninsured (36.9 million people). Of the 74.5% *insured*, 30 million, or 12.6% of the total population, were *underinsured*. These figures indicate that one in four citizens are not prepared for a health care crisis. This number includes 34 million Americans living in poverty (Grace, 1990; Nemes, 1989).

The typical uninsured person is a member of a family, child or adult, whose adults do not work and, therefore, do not have access to insurance as an employment benefit. Others who are typically uninsured are young adults, minorities, and/or unmarried persons. These people may be in minimum wage jobs and their employers may not offer health insurance as a benefit. Their salary levels are such that they cannot afford to purchase it on their own, or because of their age, they may not see the need for it. For these people, a major illness can result in debt and/or disability that will keep them or place them at poverty level. This may ultimately deny them access to health care. For those who are underinsured, poverty, homelessness, continuing ill health, disability, and loss of employment are but a few of the effects of a catastrophic illness.

The elderly, in spite of Medicare and sometimes private insurance supplements, pay a large portion of their health care bill out-of-pocket. Long-term care is the most common cause of catastrophic health care bills for this group. The cost of a year in a nursing home averaged $20,000 to $30,000 in 1989 (Korn, 1989). To receive Medicaid and certain Medicare benefits, elderly persons must "spend down" their life savings, including selling their homes, until they have only $1500 to $2000 left. It should be noted that long-term care is not used solely for the elderly. In 1985, 12% of those in nursing homes were under age 65, whereas 10% of all disabled persons were under 65. Therefore this issue is a concern to all ages. Although the majority of the elderly today are economically, physically, and socially sound, 13% live in poverty. The majority of these are women (Grau, 1988). Those in poverty are more likely to experience ill health, whereas others may experience age related situational factors that put them at risk for poverty.

Poverty and health care funding are directly and indirectly related in three ways: (1) when an individual is impoverished and unable to qualify for public supported programs, health care access may be denied to him; (2) when a person is underinsured, a catastrophic illness may lead to poverty; (3) when a person is elderly and in poverty, illness is more likely to occur.

HEALTH CARE TRENDS

The economic viability of the health care delivery system is affected by a number of factors. Trends explored in this section include managed care, health care rationing, health care financing schemes, and payments for nursing services.

Managed Care

To spur the development of a comprehensive health care system for the entire U.S. population, the *Health Maintenance Organization Act* became law in 1972. As discussed in Chapter 2, health maintenance organizations (HMOs) are prepaid systems that provide comprehensive health care services to participants for a basic monthly premium or a *capitation fee:* one fee covering all services. Prepaid group practice plans existing in the United States since the 1940s served as models for the HMO Act. The intent of HMOs was to prevent costly hospitalization by educating consumers in illness prevention and health maintenance. A degree of success has been realized, as shown by up to 40% reduction in hospital use for HMO clients (Knichman, 1990).

HMO plans usually provide more coverage to an enrollee without copayment or deductible than is typical of other health insurance schemes. Federal and state governments continue to encourage the development of HMOs by providing grants and loans for planning and operation. Some states require employers to offer HMOs as health insurance options in benefit packages. There are more than 604 HMOs in the United States with 32 million enrollees, including 385 independent practice associations (IPAs), thereby offering a competitive system to other health insurance schemes (Kenkel, 1989).

Though an HMO may be a freestanding health care agency providing its own staff, the IPA is a type of HMO whereby a third-party payer contracts with a range of independent providers to give service to the HMO enrollees. Preferred Provider Organizations (PPOs) are arrangements using multiple physicians who agree to offer services to clients of a third-party payer at a discount rate. In 1987 there were 17.5 million people enrolled in PPOs (Lee, 1990).

All of these schemes are called managed care programs, or services which organize and provide the type of care needed by the client. Some believe that this is not managed care but "utilization review" (See chapter 13) or care based on selecting services at a price (Modern Health Care, 1989). Managed care currently involves second surgical opinions, preauthorization of selected hospital admissions, concurrent review of care, outpatient surgery, and testing requirements to attempt to alleviate use of "inappropriate care" (Thorpe, 1990).

Health Care Rationing

The crisis in health care financing has spurred a renewed effort to ration health care. With unsuccessful attempts at cost containment and cost reduction, new plans are being introduced to control use of services and technologies.

Rationing is not new to health care delivery. For decades the uninsured and those who do not qualify for governmental programs have been denied services or have been eligible for restricted services only. The absence of a universal health plan and the existence of federal program eligibility criteria are other examples of health care rationing.

With the introduction of new and limited technologies, "death committees" were formed and criteria established to determine who would benefit from the technology and who would be allowed to advance to terminal stages and death. Examples included committees, and in some instances one physician, who made decisions about dialysis and/or organ transplantation.

In the mid 1970s, discussions were held about future policies to limit intensity of services and technologies, such as surgery for those who became ill because of personal lifestyles, i.e., smokers and lung cancer treatment, alcoholics and treatment for cirrhosis, the obese and treatment for cardiovascular disease. In fact, involvement in lifestyle risks today such as lack of seat belt use, drinking, and smoking habits often lead to increased insurance premiums. This concept of rationing is termed "blaming the victim" (Banta, 1990).

By 1990, the Oregon State Health Plan had been passed to ensure basic health care to all state citizens. This plan, recognized as a model health plan, required the use of managed care and ranking health services according to their effectiveness and benefit. The most effective and beneficial services were to be prioritized and paid for to the extent that the state legislature had the money to pay. These services were to be available to the poor and uninsured who were also ranked from those with the greatest need to those with the least need. Services that exceeded the state budget limit would not be included in the benefits, thus rationing of services.

Other plans that preceded the Oregon Plan were Arizona's Medicaid plan to provide managed care to qualified recipients (1982) and Massachusetts Universal Health Plan (1988). Some plans have been successful in reducing overall costs and others have not.

Several issues emerge as one considers the concept of rationing. Rationing implies limiting care that may be beneficial to the client's well being. When resources become scarce, policy makers determine what will be rationed. Individual characteristics and effectiveness of technologies are most likely to affect a rationing decision. The elderly, whose life value may not be considered important may be affected the most by such plans. Others who may be affected include women, minorities, and children in poverty. Children comprise 40% of those living in poverty. The quality of care under rationing may be inferior to care received in a totally competitive market because of the restricted services offered.

Rationing of health care in any form implies reduced access to care and a potential decrease in acceptability, as well as quality, of services offered. There is the potential for more appropriate care through managed care and care that is better organized to meet the basic health care needs of the total population. Plans must include a mechanism for informed choice (Enthoven, 1989; Grace, 1990; Larkin, 1988; Levine, 1989; Popp, 1988; Rooks, 1990; Williams, 1988).

One could argue that rationing restricts the individual's right of choice and thereby restricts total society's freedom. This is the opposite response suggested by welfare economic theory. However, to allow continuing skyrocketing prices in health care restricts the monies available to spend on education, transportation, housing. The answer is not simple. The Rand Corporation studies have shown that clients and providers will make choices based on who pays. The ability and willingness to pay through a fee-for-service system, or any cost sharing, such as an insurance deductible, decreases contact with the health care system (client self-rationing). "Free-care" results in quicker decisions by clients to seek health care. Conversely when the client is paying, quicker decisions are made by the provider to offer more complex care. Such provider decisions are often delayed in the managed care system, with set capitation payments, or in a free service, market-controlled rationing (Newhouse, 1988).

Health Care Financing

Though the government and third-party payers continue to be the major source of funding, new trends in health care financing have emerged. Although prospective payment was introduced in 1983 to control government health care costs, private insurance has followed suit by requiring precontract arrangements and approval before the client can receive certain services, i.e., hospital admission. Also, reimbursement for selected services has been omitted, curtailed, or payment rates are set, i.e., routine chest x-rays, surgical procedures, and number of hospital days.

A growth in competitive bidding for health care services, designed to create incentives for providers to compete on price, has also occurred. This concept was introduced in states to provide Medicaid services to eligible recipients. In this scheme hospitals and others who do not receive a bid are not eligible to receive Medicaid payments. The California program is highlighted as the greatest success in reducing overall program costs (Thorpe, 1990).

The reform of physician reimbursement, the first modern attempt to regulate and change physician fee structure, was introduced in 1990 in the Omnibus Reconciliation Act. After a study by the Physician Payment Review Commission established by Congress, the *resource-based relative value scale* was established, which is designed to shift physician fees toward increased reimbursement for such services as physical examinations, diagnostic services, teaching, and counseling, and decreased reimbursement for use of surgical procedures and technologies. This is an attempt to place more emphasis on prevention and promotion and lessen incentive to place clients in sick roles and to use unnecessary technologies (Knickman, 1990; Thorpe, 1990).

Though PPS was intended to reduce health care costs, costs were again on the increase after a reduction the first year. "Unbundling" of hospital services and an emphasis on community services shifted the costs from hospital to other services rather than reducing them. (For example, to "unbundle" services, hospitals separated laboratory, radiology, and outpatient surgery to cost units outside the hospitals.) Home health care, adult day care, ambulatory clinics, emergi-centers, nursing home care and, in some instances, payment of a family member to care for the sick in the home were services on the increase.

In addition to the comprehensive health care organizations, other alternative health care delivery services were emerging or expanding, as discussed in chapter 2. These services represented a major change in the structure and pattern for delivering health care and reflected the increasing emphasis on direct out-of-pocket payment for health care services. Although the development of such health care alternatives provided ready access to a number of services to those who could pay, it encouraged fragmentation of care.

Insurance companies were beginning to reduce benefits while premiums and deductibles rose. Private insurers were moving more toward establishing experience rate premiums, placing further burden on employers and employees.

While the federal government imposed taxes on a certain portion of insurance premiums paid by employers and employees, omitting the "free benefits" received as a result of employment, Medicare and Medicaid eligibility became more restrictive. These factors resulted in increased out-of-pocket expenses for all persons, regardless of age, if they chose hospitals or providers who were nonparticipants in Medicare, Medicaid, or private insurance programs. A nonparticipating provider or agency will not accept the usual, customary, and reasonable fees for services established by third-party payers, therefore the consumer must make up the difference. In some instances, nonparticipants will not accept Medicaid clients because of the fee structures of the governmental programs, thereby limiting access.

A major change that has had a positive impact for nurses is the growth in the number of self-insured or self-funded health plans. These funds are primarily found in major industries. When an industry or group of corporations band together to self-insure, emphasis switches from sick care to prevention and health promotion. The purpose of the switch is to reduce sick care costs, to increase productivity, reduce absenteeism, and enhance employee morale.

These programs use nurses to provide wellness programs, health assessment, and screening and monitoring of employees and their families. This change in health care provider emphasis results in a savings to the company and has benefitted industry by reducing overall sick care costs (Christenson, 1989; Gillis, 1988; Knickman, 1990; Walker, 1989).

The reported health care crisis of the 1980s and 1990s has led to increased emphasis on managed care and health care rationing. New health care financing plans are reflecting these changes.

Health Care Financing Plans

Although there is no definitive answer to the questions of cost containment and cost reduction, it has been suggested that the only way to provide health care for all is to implement a three-tiered health care system (Reinhardt, 1986; Thurow, 1985).

The first tier would provide a publicly financed health

care program, funded primarily by a competitively bid, pre-paid *capitation* plan with rationing of health care services. Social Security taxes, individual taxation, or taxation of employer health insurance contributions, and individual health insurance benefits may be used to finance this health care program. The government would pay health care providers a fixed fee to provide a minimal level of health care to the uninsured, poor, and elderly.

The second tier would be established by private industry and would depend on the level of health care they are willing to provide their employees. Corporations would likely establish a self-insurance program and purchase a package of services through HMOs, PPOs, or IPAs. The traditional private insurance fee-for-service system would continue to be an option.

The third tier would be a free market system in which individual health care could be purchased in excess of that provided by employers or government. Care would be limited only by the amount of money a person is willing to pay.

Examples of a three-tiered system already exist. Home care waivers through Medicaid are an example of the first tier. Wellness programs, industry self-insurance plans, and managed care programs are part of the second tier. Private physicians and hospitals are examples of the third tier.

The implications of the three-tiered system are many. The quality of care is of major concern. Quality of care in the first tier would depend largely on the ethics and expertise of the health care providers. If providers who are motivated by the need to help others are employed in the first tier, the quality of care may be higher than that currently offered to these population groups. If, on the other hand, first tier providers are primarily those who cannot find positions in the second and third tiers, quality may become an issue.

Access to care would become more equitable across population groups by such a system. Costs and use would be controlled by the buyers of service—the government and corporations in the first and second levels, and the consumer in the third.

As changes in health care financing occur, nurses must plan for the future. They must be aware of the cost of nursing services and become more knowledgeable about economics and finance. They need to develop new interventions or methods of care that provide efficient quality care, take advantage of opportunities to play a leading role in the new alternative delivery systems, and assume a greater role in decision making and evaluating client care and nurse performance.

Cost Applied to Nursing Care Delivery

Excessive and inefficient use of goods and services in health care delivery have been viewed by many as the major causes of rising costs in health care delivery. For this reason, in 1978 Congress established the Center for National Health Care Technology and mandated the center to define the safety, efficiency, and cost effectiveness of medical procedures. Nursing is one service in the health care system, and recent studies released by the center present a strong argument for the cost-effectiveness of nurse practitioners (LeRoy and Solkowitz, 1981; Nurse practitioners, 1986).

Many studies appear in the literature about the cost effectiveness of nurse practitioners and cost benefit, efficiency, efficacy, and effectiveness of medical procedures and programs; however, data are becoming more available about the cost benefit, efficiency, and effectiveness of nurses generally (OTA, 1990; Stanhope, 1990).

A recent statement issued by the American Nurses' Association indicated that nurses should receive third-party reimbursement. The ANA recommended that nursing care should become a separate budget item in all organizations so that cost studies can show the efficiency and effectiveness of the nursing profession. At present, hospitals include nursing care costs in daily patient room charges. Other agencies, such as home health care agencies, include nursing care costs with administrative costs, supplies, and equipment costs. Major efforts are underway that can be used by nurses to show actual costs of nursing care and their contributions to the system (Grimaldi et al, 1982; McKibbin et al, 1985; Reitz, 1985; Thompson, 1984; Stanhope, 1990).

At present, a movement exists in the United States to provide third-party reimbursement for nurses. Medicare and Medicaid have provided *indirect nurse reimbursement* to agencies offering home health care services for a number of years. The Rural Health Clinic Services Act of 1977 provided for indirect reimbursement for the services of nurse practitioners in rural health clinics, with payment going to the clinics for nurses salaries. In 1978 Maryland was the first state to provide direct reimbursement for nurse practitioners and nurse-midwives; Maryland extended the legislation in 1979 to provide direct reimbursement for "any duly licensed health care providers" for services within their lawful scope of practice. Currently, more than 50% of the states provide direct reimbursement for nurse practitioner or nurse-midwifery services and many others are pursuing reimbursement legislation.

The 1980 and 1989 Medicaid amendments to the Social Security Act provided for *direct reimbursement* of nurse-midwives, pediatric nurse practitioners, and family nurse practitioners. The 1989 amendments allow these nurses to provide services without physician supervision. A bill is now being considered in Congress to establish community nursing centers to provide direct reimbursement for ambulatory nursing and related care to defined community populations. Today, there are already over 100 nurse-managed clinics providing care to select client groups such as the elderly, homeless, and school children. Data show that nurses can care for 70% to 80% of all needs of these groups independently (Stanhope, 1990). Beginning in 1990, under Medicare changes, nurse practitioners were allowed indirect reimbursement when, in collaboration with a physician, they provided services to nursing home residents.

In the 1990 Omnibus Budget Reconciliation Act, Medicare amendments included a provision for direct reimbursement of nurse practitioners and clinical nurse specialists, working in collaboration with a physician, for services provided in a rural area. Direct reimbursement may also be obtained under the Federal Employee Health Benefit Plan without physician supervision. All of these changes are moving toward more autonomous practice and are showing recognition of nurses' contributions to health care delivery.

COST EFFECTIVENESS OF PRIMARY PREVENTION

An area in the health care delivery system that is beginning to show cost effectiveness is primary prevention. Primary prevention has three major aspects: personal health services, such as immunization against infectious diseases; environmental services, such as adequate water and sewage treatment to prevent parasitic diseases or water fluoridation to prevent dental caries; and health behavior practices, such as nonsmoking programs to prevent lung cancer, the use of seatbelts to prevent accident fatalities, and good nutrition to prevent obesity and ensuing complications.

Benefits

Estimates indicate that 97% of the health care dollars are spent on secondary and tertiary prevention. A growing body of evidence links personal health behaviors to leading causes of illness and death in the United States. For example, smoking results in one out of every six deaths from cancer, coronary artery disease, cerebrovascular disease, and chronic obstructive pulmonary disease. Failure to wear safety belts and driving while intoxicated result in injuries from motor vehicle accidents. Physical inactivity and poor diet are related to atherosclerosis, cancer, diabetes, osteoporosis. Unsafe sexual practices cause unwanted pregnancy, sexually transmitted diseases, and AIDS.

The principal reasons given for lack of emphasis on prevention in clinical practice and on spending less money for prevention include lack of third-party reimbursement, insufficient time to deal with client behaviors, and skepticism about clinical effectiveness of prevention techniques (e.g., relaxation, exercise, and diet (Fischer, 1989). Preventive services produce dramatic reductions in morbidity and mortality. The major causes of mortality in our adult population have shown major decline since 1970. Several assumptions are made about the causes of the decline in mortality in the past two decades. These were discussed in the previous section.

Reimbursement

Primary prevention measures could reduce the risk of early death, disease, disability, discomfort from disease, and reduce care costs. Why then have the federal and third-party payers not provided coverage for such measures? The answer is in the following discussion. In addition to the benefit of improved health status of the population, a focus on prevention could mean a reduction in the need for and use of medical, dental, hospital, and health provider services. This would mean that the health care system, the largest employer in the United States, would be reduced in size and become more controlled by the client than by the seller of these services. However, with the increasing costs of health care, consumer demand, and changes in financing mechanisms, there is a new trend toward financing more preventive care services. Today, the third-party payers are beginning to cover preventive services, recognizing that the growth of the health care system can no longer be supported.

Preventive Services

The *goal* of public health is to provide activities to improve and protect the well-being and health of the nation. Preventive community health services include health planning, disease prevention and control, consumer safety, and occupational safety and health. National health priorities are set by the federal government, and financial support through block grants is provided to the 55 state and territorial health agencies and to the over 3000 local health departments. These health departments use funds to provide direct community services, such as public health nursing, home health care, immunizations, venereal disease control, chronic disease screening, and consumer protection.

The possible increases in communicable diseases and increased awareness of measures to prevent chronic diseases, mental illnesses, suicide, accidents, substance abuse, homicide, and sexually transmitted diseases may influence the resources allocated to public health activities (Freeland and Schendler, 1984).

Federal Recommendations

In 1979, the Surgeon General of the United States published a report entitled *Healthy People*. The report called for a renewed preventive health care commitment through the identification of priorities and specific goals. The central theme of the report was that the health of the nation could be significantly improved through actions taken by individuals and by policy makers to promote a safer, healthier environment for all at home, at work, and at play.

The report suggested that most people could improve their personal health by observing the following practices:
◇ Elimination of cigarette smoking
◇ Reduction of alcohol abuse
◇ Moderate dietary changes to reduce intake of excess calories, fat, salt, and sugar
◇ Moderate exercise
◇ Periodic screening for major causes of morbidity and mortality, such as blood pressure and cancer
◇ Adherence to speed laws and usage of seat belts.

The report also emphasized the link between physical and mental health and the need to maintain strong family ties, the assistance of supportive friends, and the use of community support systems.

For the policy makers, the report suggested a need to recognize the relationship between health and the physical environment, which could lead to the reduction of morbidity and mortality caused by air, water and food contamination, accidents, radiation exposure, excessive noise, occupational hazard, dangerous consumer products, and unsafe highway design.

Subsequently, in 1980 the Secretary of DHHS presented a report, *Promoting Health/Preventing Disease—Objectives for the Nation*, that outlined the national health status and objectives to be attained by the health care system by 1990. The following target areas were identified in the report: control of high blood pressure; pregnancy and infant health; immunization; sexually transmitted diseases; toxic agents; occupational health; fluoridation and dental health; surveillance of infectious disease; smoking; misuse of alcohol and drugs; nutrition; physical fitness and exercise; and stress. The objectives of the report were aimed at reducing death rates and related measures of poor health, reducing measurable risks, increasing public and professional awareness of risk and reduction possibilities, and improving services (*Health: United States,* 1980). Preliminary data indicate progress toward achieving the national goal of reduction of mortality at every life stage (Prevention, 89/90).

In 1990 the Office of Disease Prevention and Health Promotion released the report *Healthy People 2000.* The new national health objectives are designed to build on the 1990 objectives, setting targets to improve health status, reduce risk, and improve services. The priorities of the year 2000 objectives appear in the box. Three overall goals are to be met by the year 2000: (1) Increased span of healthy life for Americans, (2) Reduce health disparities among Americans, and (3) Achieve access to preventive services for all Americans. (see Appendix M.)

Reducing the burden of avoidable illness and disability will reduce the human and economic costs imposed on the U.S. population. To accomplish the goals of prevention, changes will have to occur in environmental protection, lifestyles, and orientation of health providers and institutions toward health promotion. Support is being gained from employers, schools, product designers and manufacturers, food distributors, and the insurance industry for preventing injury and promoting healthier life-styles, thereby reducing the overall economic burden of health care delivery in the United States.

The Value of Human Life

The concept of *human capital* has evolved in economics as a way of measuring the value society places on the worth of the individual. The value is quantified and expressed in dollar amounts, and it constitutes a real limit on how much money either people or society will pay for personal health care.

A major goal of the health care delivery system today is to preserve and maximize human capital by offering health-preserving and social practices that result in avoidance of disease (primary prevention) and by offering diagnosis, treatment, and rehabilitation services for existing diseases (secondary and tertiary prevention). The past goal of the health care delivery system has been to emphasize the "sickness system." DHHS health goals suggest that a higher value should be placed on primary prevention. Table 4-12 shows the potential life lost for those who died prematurely from the leading causes of death. Though over 12 million years of potential life were lost, the years lost were twice as great for the black population than for the white.

An example of the costs of life-style–related illness to the health care system can be found by looking at the cost of alcohol abuse. In 1983 the cost to the nation was $117 billion, whereas nonalcoholic drug abuse cost $60 billion. Costs of alcohol abuse were expected to exceed $130 billion by 1990.

The outcome of health care goals should be the provision of a quality of life that will promote happiness, productivity, efficiency, and the capacity to engage in and enjoy life activities. Quantifying life is meaningless to the person unless the quality of life can be maximized and unless functional days become more valuable than dollars spent. An emphasis on primary prevention may hold the key to reducing dollars spent while increasing the quality of life.

Healthy People 2000 is a national public-private initiative led by the U.S. Public Health Service (PHS) to reduce preventable death, disease, and disability by the year 2000. The cornerstone of this initiative, the National Health Promotion and Disease Prevention Objectives, was developed through a three-year, broad-based effort involving groups and individuals in the health care system, business and industry, voluntary organizations, communities, and federal, state, and local agencies.

The new health objectives, which build on the 1990 objectives established in 1980, set targets to improve Americans' health status, reduce risks, and improve services. Many will challenge the Nation to confront such issues as quality of life and health disparities among our citizens. Priorities are emerging in the areas of health promotion, health protection, and preventive services. Special sections also summarize needs related to specific age groups and data collection systems.

PRIORITIES

Health Promotion	**Preventive Services**
Physical activity and fitness	Maternal and infant health
Nutrition	Heart disease and stroke
Tobacco	Cancer
Alcohol and other drugs	Other chronic and disabling conditions
Family planning	HIV infection
Mental health	Sexually transmitted diseases
Violent and abusive behavior	Immunizations and infectious diseases
Educational and community-based programs	Clinical preventive services
Health Protection	**Age-Related**
Unintentional injuries	Healthy babies
Occupational safety and health	Healthy children
Environmental health	Healthy adolescents and youth
Food and drug safety	Healthy older people
Oral health	

Surveillance and Data Systems

CLINICAL APPLICATION

The goal of health economics is to provide maximum benefit to the clients of health care services. Thus the goal of a community health nursing service should be to provide a program that will provide quality of care and meet the needs of the clients served. The amount of money the client and the community spend and the agency spends in offering a service is beneficial if the client is satisfied and if there are enough clients in the community to justify the employment of nurses to provide the service.

Connie, a community health nursing student, has identified a case load of five families in a home health nursing program, offered by the local health department. She is interested in *assessing* the costs of care to her clients and to the agency. Connie approaches the appropriate administrator or director of nurses and asks the following questions: how is the agency reimbursed for home care visits

TABLE 4-12
Years of potential life lost before aged 65 for selected causes of death: United States, 1980 and 1987. (Data are based on the National Vital Statistics System.)

Cause of death	Years lost in thousands		Years lost per 1000 population under 65 years of age	
	1980	1987	1980	1987
All causes	12,896	12,074	64.2	56.5
Diseases of the heart	1691	1520	8.4	7.1
Cerebrovascular diseases	283	248	1.4	1.2
Malignant neoplasms	1824	1817	9.1	8.5
Chronic obstructive pulmonary diseases	115	132	0.6	0.6
Pneumonia and influenza	196	172	1.0	0.8
Chronic liver disease and cirrhosis	292	235	1.5	1.1
Diabetes mellitus	113	123	0.6	0.6
Accidents and adverse effects	2760	2306	13.7	10.8
Motor vehicle accidents	1690	1442	8.4	6.8
Suicide	621	671	3.1	3.1
Homicide and legal intervention	751	656	3.7	3.1
Human immunodeficiency virus infection	—	363	—	1.7

From National Center for Health Statistics: Vital statistics of the United States, vol II, mortality, part A, for data years 1980-1987, Public Health Service, Washington, D.C., U.S. Government Printing Office; Data computed by the Division of Analysis from data compiled by the Division of Vital Statistics and from Table 1.
NOTE: For data years shown, the code numbers for cause of death are based on the International Classification of Diseases, Ninth Revision, described in Appendix II, Table V.

and how much does each visit cost? Who pays? Also, she asks if nursing care costs are known. When she finds that the agency is primarily a Medicare financed agency and that the cost of a home visit is determined by a regional standard of the Health Care Financing Administration, she knows that her families must be eligible for Medicare, unless they have private insurance that will cover home visits or Medicaid eligibility for their children. (Few clients are able to quality for services with private insurance and Medicaid.)

When she finds that nursing costs are known, she asks why the visit costs are so high. The administrator shares with Connie that lights, water, nurse supplies, buying cars for the nurses to drive and secretarial and administrative salaries are a part of the per visit costs. Although Connie's work occurs in the client's home, support services through a central office must be available to help Connie with her work, accounting for the cost of the visit.

Connie then asks about the criteria clients must meet to be able to use the service. She wants to determine for herself

if the service is rationed. Connie learns that Medicare, Medicaid, and private insurance limit the services her clients are able to receive. When they reach the limits of the criteria they must seek care through private payments, hospital, nursing home, or family support.

The stated goal for offering a service is to provide nursing care in the home to reduce the need for clients to be hospitalized. Unless clients have someone at home to care for them between nurse visits, they may need to go to the hospital or nursing home.

Connie inquires at the local hospital about the room cost per client day. She divides the number of nursing visits by the home health program into the total cost of visits the client received for the year. She then recognizes the differences between the costs of staying at home and staying the same number of days in the hospital. This sample formula provides Connie with some data to compare cost of care per day in the hospital to the cost of care per visit in the home.

In one of her families, the Smiths, the husband has died and the wife can no longer be cared for at home. Connie is informed that the client will need to be admitted to a nursing home for a period of time. In *planning* for the transition from home care to nursing home, Connie contacts social services to consult with the client about the "spend down" process, so the client may be eligible for Medicare and Medicaid coverage of nursing home costs.

As Connie *implements* her nursing care plan for her families, she knows, for the three families covered by Medicare within the limited criteria, all costs of care are paid, except for certain medicines, homemaker services, and some supplies and equipment. For the client going to the nursing home, Connie recognizes that this move will deplete most of her financial assets. Connie talks with the director of nurses about implementing a homemaker/aide service which can be covered by third-party payers to reduce the possibility that others may need nursing home placement.

Connie discharged the fifth family, after the number of visits covered by private insurance was depleted, and upon *evaluation* it was determined that Mr. Jones could be assisted by his wife until he returned to work. She recognized that a safety program in the factory in which Mr. Jones worked could have prevented the back injury he received from a fall. This fall required nursing care and physical therapy as follow-up to hospitalization.

Connie then asked her clients for permission to perform a client or family satisfaction survey. An example of the satisfaction survey Connie used appears in Appendix A1. Connie performed the client satisfaction survey and tallied her results as an *evaluation* of the care she had given them. The clients were satisfied with the home health service, and the cost of visits to the clients was lower than that of a hospital day. Connie considered the service appropriate.

Note: In this example it is assumed that one home visit will equal one hospital day, that hospital nursing care costs are included in the room charge, and that the home nursing visit cost includes other agency charges, such as administrative overhead.

SUMMARY

Economics is concerned with the most efficient use of resources to fulfill society's unlimited wants. Health economics is concerned with the distribution of health care resources to provide maximum benefit to the most people.

As the cost of health care services increases, the consumer has less money to spend for other needs and wants. Economic indicators show that the health care costs continue to increase per year and have risen to a cost of $500 billion, or over $1987 per person per year.

The major factors influencing the costs of health care delivery are inflation, technology, intensity and population changes. The availability of insurance and government funds to cover health care costs, the method of reimbursement, and the development of new and costlier methods of health care technology appear to be the major contributors to rising health care costs. The rising numbers of elderly in the population, the increasing proportion of women, and the decline in family support systems are viewed as the major population changes contributing to increased demand for services and increased costs of services.

The new financing mechanisms, competition, and alternative health care delivery methods appear to be contributing to a three-tiered health care system that provides care for all people.

Another problem in health care delivery is establishing the value of primary preventive care. Studies show the savings society could have with a preventive emphasis in its health care delivery system. The large amount of money society spends annually on health care indicates that society values human life. However, the focus of this society's future investment should be to provide more than longevity. The goal of health economics should be to provide a quality of life that offers happiness, productivity, and the capacity to engage in life activities, through the provision of reasonably priced quality services focused on illness prevention, health promotion, and health protection. Nursing has a major role to play in meeting this goal.

KEY CONCEPTS

From 1800 to the 1980s the U.S. health care delivery system experienced three developmental stages, with different emphasis on health care economics. Since 1985, the health care delivery system appears to have entered a fourth developmental stage.

Four basic components provide the framework for health care delivery: Labor (work force), facilities, technology, and intensity.

Four major factors have been instrumental in influencing the growth of the health care delivery system: price inflation, technology, intensity and changes in population demographics.

Health care financing has evolved through the twentieth century from a system financed primarily by the consumer to a system financed primarily by third-party payers.

To solve the problems of rising health care costs, a number of plans for future payments of health care are being considered, including rationing.

Excessive and inefficient use of goods and services in health care delivery have been viewed as the major causes of rising health care costs.

The concept of human capital has evolved in economics as a way of measuring the value society places on the worth of an individual.

The goal of health economics is maximum benefits from services of health providers, leading to health and wellness of the population

LEARNING ACTIVITIES

1. Define in your own words the following terms: economics, health economics, gross national product, consumer price index, human capital.

2. State the goal of health economics and compare to the goal of public health.

3. Review Chapter 5, Ethics in Community Health Nursing Practice. Debate in class the ethical implications of the goal of rationing. Focus your debate on the implications for community health nursing practice.

4. Invite a community health nurse administrator to meet with your class or clinical conference group. Ask how inflation, changes in population, and technology have changed the community health care delivery system and community health nursing.

BIBLIOGRAPHY

Ancona-Berk V and Chalmers T: An analysis of ambulatory and inpatient care, Am J Pub Health 76:1102, 1986.

Arno P et al: Economic and policy implications of early intervention in HIV diseases, JAMA 262(11):1493, 1989.

Banta HD: Technology assessment in health care. In Kovner A: Health care delivery in the United States, New York, 1990, Springer Publishing Co, Inc.

Banta HD: What is health care? In Kovner A: Health care delivery in the United States, New York, 1990, Springer Publishing Co, Inc.

Becker E et al: Refinement and expansion of the Harvard resource-based relative value scale: the second phase, Am J Pub Health 80(7):799, 1990.

Beyers M: Perspectives on prospective payment: challenges and opportunities for nurses, Rockville, Md, 1985, Aspen Systems Corp.

Bloch H and Pupp R: Supply, demand, and rising health care costs, Nurs Econ 3(2):119, 1985.

Brecher C: The government's role in health care. In Kovner A: Health care delivery in the United States, New York, 1990, Springer Publishing Co, Inc.

Blendon R and Donelan K: The public and emerging debate over national health insurance, New Engl J Med 323(3):208, 1990.

Bocchino C: An interview with Bruce Vladeck: perspectives on prospective payment and medical gridlock, Nurs Econ 7(2):71, 1989.

Brandon D and Huber C: Evaluating cost-effectiveness of preevaluation client contacts, Nurs Econ 5(2):65, 1987.

Bullough B: The Gramm-Rudman-Hollings budget deficit control act, J Prof Nurs 207, 1986.

Burda D: Changing ownership: not-for-profit hospitals become major players in hospital takeovers, Modern Health Care 24, 1988.

Burke T: The economic impact of alcohol abuse and alcoholism, Public Health Reports 103 (6):564, 1988.

Carney K et al: Hospice costs and medicare reimbursement: an application of break-even analysis, Nurs Econ 7(1):41, 1989.

Caplan R: The commodification of American health care, Soc Sci Med 28(11):1139, 1989.

Christenson G and Kiefhaber A: Highlights from the national survey of worksite health promotion activities, Health Values 12(2):29, 1988.

Cook A: Comparable worth: an economic issue, Nursing Management 21(2):28, 1990.

Cournoyer P: The veterans administration's resource allocation system, Nurs Clin North Am 23(3):531, 1988.

Cummings S et al: The cost effectiveness of counseling smokers to quit, JAMA 261(1):75, 1989.

Curtin L: Economics and nursing care: nursing practice in the 21st century, Kansas City, Mo, 1988, American Nurses' Foundation, Inc.

Dornbusch R and Fischer S: Macroeconomics, ed 2, New York, 1981, McGraw-Hill Book Co.

Enthoven A and Kronick R: A consumer choice health plan for the 1990s, New Engl J Med 320(1):30.

Fagin C: Opening the door on nursing's cost advantage, Nursing and Health Care 7(7):352, 1986.

Fischer M, editor: Guide to clinical preventive services: an assessment of effectiveness of 169 interventions, Report of the United States preventive services task force, Baltimore, 1989, Williams & Wilkins.

Frank K: Rationally rationing health care: effectiveness research by another name? Nurs Econ 7(6):289, 1989.

Freeland M and Schendler C: Health spending in the 1980s: integration of clinical practice patterns with management, Health Care Fin Rev 8(3):1, 1984.

Fuchs V: The economics of health in a postindustrial society, Pub Interest 56:3-20, 1979.

Gabel J and Ermann D: Preferred provider organizations: performance, problems, and promise, Health Affairs 4(1):25, 1985.

Gardner M: Public Health Nursing, New York, 1936, MacMillan.

Gillis D: Employers ally with nursing in the war on health care costs, Nursing and Health Care 9(4):173, 1988.

Ginzberg E: Health care reform — why so slow? New Engl J Med 322(20):1464, 1990.

Goldsmith J: National health insurance catches corporate attention, Modern Healthcare 89:33, 1989.

Grace H: Can health care costs be contained? Nursing and Health Care 11(3):125, 1990.

Grau L: Illness-engendered poverty among the elderly, Women's Health 12(3/4):103, 1987.

Green J and Arno P: AIDS: the cost and financing of care, Caring 15, 1989.

Greenwald H: HMO membership, copayment, and initiation of care for cancer: a study of working adults, Am J Pub Health 77(4):461, 1987.

Grimaldi P et al: RIMs and the cost of nursing care, Nursing Management 13, 1982.

Grimaldi P: New Medicare rates for ambulatory surgery, Nursing Management 21(4):20, 1990.

Grimaldi P: Final 1987 PPS regulations issued, Nursing Management 16(12):20, 1986.

Haddon R: An economic agenda for health care, Nursing and Health Care 11(1):21, 1990.

Haddon R: The final frontier: nursing in the emerging health-care environment, Nurs Econ 7(3):155, 1989.

Hamm-Vida D: Cost of nonnursing tasks, Nursing Management 21(4):46, 1990.

Harrington C and Culbertson R: Nurses left out of health care reimbursement reform, Nurs Outlook 38(4):156, 1990.

Harris M: The changing scene in community health nursing, Nurs Clin North Am 23(3):559, 1988.

Hawken P and Hillestad A: Promoting nursing's health care agenda through collaboration, Nursing and Health Care 11(1):17, 1990.

Havas S et al: Report of the New England Task Force on reducing heart disease and stroke risk, Public Health Reports 104(2):134, 1989.

Health care financing administration statistics, 1989, Bureau of Data Management and Strategy, Washington, DC.

Health care in rural America, Congress of the United States, Office of Technology Assessment, 1990, US Government Printing Office, Washington, DC.

Health: United States, 1989 and Prevention Profile, USDHHS Pub No (PHS) 90-1232, Hyattsville, Md, 1990, Department of Health and Human Services.

Health: United States, 1988, DHHS Pub No (PHS) 89-1232, Washington, DC, 1989, Department of Health and Human Services.

Health: United States, 1985, DHEW Pub No (PHS) 86-1232, Washington, DC, 1985, Department of Health and Human Services.

Healthy People: the Surgeon General's report on health promotion and disease prevention, DHEW Pub No (PHS) 79-55071, Washington, DC, 1979, Department of Health, Education, and Welfare.

Heider-Dorneich P: Social control in health economics, Rev Soc Economy 36(1):1-18, 1978.

Hicks L: Using benefit-cost and cost-effectiveness analysis in health care resource allocation, Nurs Econ 3(2):78, 1985.

Higgins C: The economics of health promotion, Health Values 12(2):38, 1988.

Hoyer R: Private insurance where does long-term care fit in? Caring 12, 1989.

Huey F: To the president and Congress: nurses know that US citizens can get better access to better health care at affordable costs: are you ready to change the system? Am J Nurs 1483, 1988.

Institute of Medicine: Nursing and nursing education: public policies and private actions, Bethesda, Md, 1983.

Ives J and Kerfoot K: Pitfalls and promises of diversification, Nurs Econ 7(4):200, 1989.

Joel L: DRGs and RIMs: implications for nursing. In Beyes M, editor: Perspectives on prospective payment: challenges and opportunities for nurses, Rockville, Md, 1985, Aspen Publishers, Inc.

Jones K: Evolution of the prospective payment system: implications for nursing, Nurs Econ 7(6):299, 1989.

Jonas S: Health manpower: with an emphasis on physicians. In Kovner A: Health care delivery in the United States, New York, 1990, Springer Publishing Co, Inc.

Kalish P and Kalish B: The advance of american nursing, Boston, 1986, Little, Brown, & Co.

Kass D: Economics of scale and scope in the provision of home health services, J Health Econ 6:129, 1987.

Kelley M: The omnibus budget reconciliation act of 1987, Nurs Clin North Am 24(3):791, 1989.

Kelly L: Nursing's velvet revolution, Nurs Outlook 38(1):15, 1990.

Kenkel P and Morrissey J: Managing to survive: it may come down to size or entrenchment, Modern Healthcare: 21, 1989.

Kenkel P and Morrissey J: Enthoven's proposal: managed-care solution to plight of uninsured, Modern Healthcare: 28, 1989.

Kenkel P: HMO profit outlook begins to brighten, Modern Healthcare: 28, 1989.

Knickman J, and Thorpe K: Financing for health care. In Kovner A: Health care delivery in the United States, New York, 1990, Springer Publishing Co, Inc.

Kilner J: Selecting patients when resources are limited: a study of US medical directors of kidney dialysis and transplantation facilities, AJPH 78(2):144, 1988.

Kinzer D: Why the conservatives gave us universal health care: a parable, Health Services Administration 34(3):299, 1989.

Korn K et al: The need to reform the long-term care system, Caring 42, 1989.

Kovner A: Health care delivery in the United States, New York, 1990, Springer Publishing Co, Inc.

Lamm R: Rationing of health care: the inevitable meets the unthinkable, Nurse Pract 11(5):57, 1986.

Landfeld J and Seskin E: The economic value of life: linking theory to practice, Am J Public Health 72(6):555, 1982.

Landreth H: History of economic theory: scope, method, and content, Boston, 1976, Houghton Mifflin Co.

Larkin H: Will the public support health care rationing? Hospitals 79, 1988.

LaRochelle D: The moral dilemma of rationing nursing resources, J Prof Nurs 5(4):173, 1989.

Lauver E: Where will the money go? Economic forecasting and nursing's future, Nurs Health Care, 1985.

Lawrence R and Jonas S: Ambulatory care. In Kovner A: Health care delivery in the United States, New York, 1990, Springer Publishing Co, Inc.

Lee PR: Technology and the cost of medical care. In Lee P, Brown N, and Red I, editors: The nation's health, San Francisco, 1981, Boyd & Fraser Publishing Co.

Lee P, Brown N, and Red I: Health costs: what limit? The nation's health, San Francisco, 1981, Boyd & Fraser Publishing Co.

Lee P and Estes C: The nation's health, ed 3, Boston, 1990, Jones & Bartlett.

Leigh J: Gender, firm size, industry, and estimates of the value of life, J Health Econ 6:255, 1987.

Leroy L and Solkowitz S: The implications of cost-effectiveness analysis of medical technology, Congress of the United States, Office of Technology Assessment, case study no 16, Washington DC, 1981, US Government Printing Office.

Levine M: Ration or rescue: the elderly patient in critical care, Critical Care Nursing Quarterly 12(1):82, 1989.

Loucine D and Huckabay R: Identification of issues in determining the cost of nursing services, Nursing Administration Quarterly 13(1):72, 1988.

Lyons J: AIDS: what are the costs? Who will pay? Nurs Econ 6(5):241, 1988.

Mahoney M et al: Years of potential life lost among a native American population, Public Health Reports 104(3):279, 1989.

Mansfield D: Study guide for principles of microeconomics, ed 5 New York, 1986, WW Norton & Co.

Maraldo P: An interview with Claire Fagin: perspectives on nursing in today's health care environment, Nurs Econ 7(4):186, 1989.

Markus G: Considered approaches to physician payment in the '90s. Nurs Econ 6(2):63, 1988.

McCombie S: Politics of immunization in public health, Soc Sci Med 28(8):843, 1989.

McGivern D: Teaching nurses the language of the marketplace, Nursing and Health Care 9(3):127, 1988.

McKeown T: Determinants of health. In Lee P, Brown N, and Red I, editors: The nation's health, San Francisco, 1981, Boyd & Fraser Publishing Co.

McKibbin R, et al: DRGs and nursing care, HCFA Grant # 15-C-98421/7-02 Kansas City, Mo, June 1985, Center for Research, American Nurses' Association.

McKinlay JB and McKinlay SM: The questionable contribution of medical measures to the decline of mortality in the United States in the twentieth century, Milbank Mem Fund Q 55(3):405-H428, 1977.

McMahon L: A critique of the Harvard resource-based relative value scale, AJPH 80(7):793, 1990.

Medicare's prospective payment system: strategies for evaluating cost, quality, and medical technology, Congress of the United States, Office of Technology Assessment, OTA-H-263, Washington, DC, 1985, U.S. Government Printing Office.

Melnick G and Mann J: Are Medicaid patients more expensive? A review and analysis, Medical Care Review 46(3):229, 1989.

Mitchell K: Lean, mean, and fiscally fit, Nurs Econ 3(3):134, 1985.

National Center for Health Services Research: National health care expenditures study: changes in health insurance status full-year and part-year coverage, Data preview 21, USDHHS Pub No (PHS) 85-3377, Washington DC, 1985, Department of Health and Human Services.

National Center for Health Services Research: National health care expenditures study: private insurance and public programs: coverage of health services, Data preview 20, USDHHS Pub No (PHS) 85-3374, Washington, DC, March 1985, Department of Health and Human Services.

National Center for Health Services Research: Research summary series: morbidity costs: national estimates and economic determinants, USDHHS Pub No (PHS) 86-3393, Washington DC, 1985, Department of Health and Human Services.

National Center for Health Statistics: Provisional data from health promotion and disease prevention supplement to the national health interview survey: United States, January-March, 1985, USDHHS, vol 113, 1985, Department of Health and Human Services.

National Center for Health Statistics: Advance data: provisional data from health promotion and disease prevention supplement to the national health interview survey: United States, January-March, 1985, USDHHS Pub No (PHS) 86-1250, vol 113, 1985, Department of Health and Human Services.

National Center for Health Services Research: Employers and Medicare as partners in financing health care for the elderly, Pub No (NCHSR) 88-1, USDHHS, 1987, Rockville, Md.

National Center for Health Services Research: Health insurance coverage of retired persons: research findings 2, Pub No (PHS) 89-3444, USDHHS, 1989, Rockville, Md.

National Center for Health Services Research: A profile of uninsured Americans: research findings 1, Pub No (PHS) 89-3443, USDHHS, 1989, Rockville, Md.

Navarro V: Why some countries have national health insurance, others have national health services, and the United States has neither, Soc Sci Med 28(9):887, 1989.

Nemes J: Health care stocking up on ESOPS, Modern Healthcare 89:24, 1989.

Newhouse J et al: Are fee-for-service costs increasing faster than HMO costs? Medical Care 23(8):960, 1985.

Newswatch: Catastrophic legislation provides new dose of SNF, home health, and spouse benefits, Geriatr Nurs 260, 1988.

Nurse practitioners, physician assistants, and certified nurse midwives: quality, access, cost and payment issues, Congress of the United States, Office of Technology Assessment, Health Program, Unpublished report, 1986.

Ostrander V: Consumers look to nurses, Nursing and Health Care 7(7):368, 1986.

Pallarito K: Managed care reaches for access to capital, Modern Healthcare 89:68, 1989.

Parkin D: Aggregate health care expenditures and national income: is health care a luxury good? J Health Econ 6:209, 1987.

Pepper C: Long-term care insurance, Caring 4, 1989.

Pfaff M: Differences in health care spending across countries: statistical evidence, J Health Polit Policy Law 15(1):1, 1990.

Phillips B: Epidemiological issues in health promotion and cost containment, Health Values 12(2):31, 1988.

Phillips C: Reimbursement for nursing services revisited, Econ 5(5):220, 1987.

Phillips E et al: DRG ripple and the shifting burden of care to home health, Nursing and Health Care 10(6):324, 1989.

Pickett G and Hanlon J: Public health administration and practice, St. Louis, 1990, Times Mirror/Mosby College Publishing.

Pillar B et al: Technology, its assessment, and nursing, Nurs Outlook 38(1):16, 1990.

Polich C: Financing long-term care: the role of the federal govenment, Caring:16, 1989.

Popp R: Health care for the poor: where has all the money gone? J Nurs Adm 18(1):8, 1988.

Prevention 89/90 federal programs and progress, Washington, DC, 1990, Department of Health and Human Services, US Government Printing Office.

Pruitt R: Economics of health promotion, Nurs Econ 5(3):118, 1987.

Redman B et al: Policy perspectives on economic investment in professional nursing education, Nurs Econ 8(1):27, 1990.

Reinhardt U: Rationing the health care surplus: an American tragedy, Nurs Econ 4(3):101, 1986.

Relman A: Economic incentives in clinical investigation, New Engl J Med 320(14):933, 1989.

Rice D: The medical care system: past trends and future projections. In Lee P, editor: The nation's health, 1990, Jones & Bartlett.

Richardson H: Long-term care. In Kovner A: Health care delivery in the United States, New York, 1990, Springer Publishing Co, Inc.

Rodwin V: Comparative health systems. In Kovner A: Health care delivery in the United States, New York, 1990, Springer Publishing Co, Inc.

Rooks J: Let's admit we ration health care—then set priorities, Am J Nurs 90(6):39, 1990.

Rubin R, et al: Private long-term care insurance; simulations of a potential market, Medical Care Review 27(14):182, 1989.

Rushmer R: Technological resources for health. In Williams S and Torrens P, editors: Introduction to health services, New York, 1984, John Wiley & Sons, Inc.

Schell E: Lessons from the Canadian health care system, Nurs Econ 7(6):306, 1989.

Scitovsky A and Rice D: Estimates of the direct and indirect costs of acquired immunodeficiency syndrome in the United States, 1985, 1986, and 1991, Public Health Reports 102(1):5, 1987.

Sofaer S and Kenney E: The effect of changes in the financing and organization of health services on health promotion and disease prevention, Medical Care Review 46(3):313, 1989.

Smith D: Health promotion for older adults, Health Values 12(2):46, 1988.

Stevens J: Access to health care and the future of nursing, Journal of Community Health Nursing 4(2):65, 1987.

Theilheimer L: Aging and long-term care: a consumers' view, Caring 25, 1989.

Thompson J: The measurement of nursing intensity. In USDHHS health care financing review: 1984 annual supplement, Baltimore, 1984, Health Care Financing Administration.

Thorpe K: Health care cost containment. In Kovner A: Health care delivery in the United States, New York, 1990, Springer Publishing Co, Inc.

Thurow L: Medicine vs. economics, N Engl J Med 313(10):611, 1985.

Traska M: HMO uses quality measures to pay its physicians, Hospitals 34, 1988.

Tokarski C: Medicare payments to hospitals targeted, Modern Healthcare 88:4, 1988.

Tokarski C: Employees' insurance costs jump 70%, Modern Healthcare 89:20, 1989.

Tokarski C: Vet group wants health systems of the VA and defense to boost sharing efforts, Modern Healthcare 89:19, 1989.

Tokarski C: Health care costs mount an assault on defense department, Modern Healthcare, 89:28, 1989.

Ulin P: Global collaboration in primary health care, Nurs Outlook, 37(3):134, 1989.

USDHHS: Nursing—sixth report to the president and Congress on the status of health personnel in the United States, Accession No HRP 0907204, Springfield, Va, 1988, National Technical Information Service.

Wagner L: Rules on home-care training rapped as vague, expensive, Modern Healthcare 89:4, 1989.

Wagner L: HCFA revises rules on home-care claims, Modern Healthcare 89:4, 1989.

Wagner L: Shift in mortality seen as evidence of PPS efficiency, Modern Healthcare 89:4, 1989.

Wagner L: AIDS forecast update, Modern Healthcare 89:4, 1989.

Walker V: Ready, set, go: wellness movement focuses business efforts on improved worker fitness, health, Occupational Health and Safety 12(3):13, 1987.

Warner S: Third-party payments for nurses: untangling the web, Nursing and Health Care 9(4):181, 1988.

Washington focus: Political trends and health care reform, Nursing and Health Care 10(4):178, 1989.

Wedig G: Health status and demand for health, J Health Econ 6:151, 1988.

Williams A: Priority setting in public and private health care, J Health Econ 6:173, 1988.

Wright J: Changes in federal funding for health services: effect on nursing, Nursing Management 68, 1987.

5

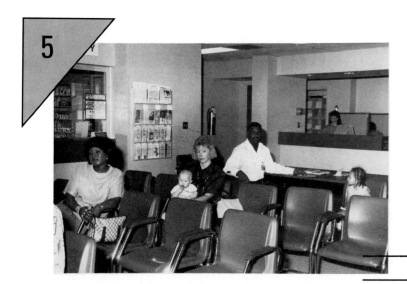

Ethics in Community Health Nursing Practice

Sara T. Fry

OBJECTIVES

After reading this chapter, the student should be able to:

Describe the meaning of accountability in community health nursing.

Identify the relationship of ethical rules, principles, and theories in community health nursing decisions.

Discuss the application of ethical principles, including their potential conflicts, in community health nursing practice.

Given an appropriate case example of community health nursing practice, identify the following:
1. The basis for clients' rights claims
2. Specific professional responsibilities in response to clients' rights
3. Limitations of clients' rights in today's health care delivery system

Given a hypothetical community health need requiring the fair and just distribution of community health nursing resources to a specific aggregate group, formulate a plan of nursing care delivery using the following:
1. A theory of distributive justice
2. Ethical principles and their priority or influence
3. Evaluation of the potential benefits and harms of the plan
4. Evaluation of the extent to which moral requirements of community health nursing practice are met by the plan

KEY TERMS

advocacy	egalitarian theory	public health ethic
autonomy	entitlement theory	right to health
beneficence	ethical decision	right to health care
caring	making	rules
Code for Nurses	informed consent	rule of utility
codes of ethics	justice	theories
coercive health	maximin theory	utilitarian theory
measures	moral accountability	veracity
confidentiality	Patient's Bill of Rights	
clients' rights	principles	

Community health nurses experience many ethical conflicts in today's health care delivery system. The nursing profession has traditionally upheld the rights and needs of the individual client. Yet today this focus is difficult to maintain when nurses have the additional goal of maximizing the health of populations at risk. The traditional focus is also difficult to maintain when nursing resources are influenced by legislation and funding for specific population groups. One result of this latter difficulty is that other populations identified as being at risk are not adequately served by community health nursing efforts because of the lack of funds. Nurses who experience this conflict between the individualistic focus of the professional ethic and the aggregate focus of community health recognize the dilemma of professional nursing in community health settings.

The purpose of this chapter is to analyze traditional ethics of professional nursing and apply these principles to the practice of community health nursing. Since the client is the focus of all nursing actions, clients' rights are discussed first.

Not all nursing actions are simply correlative to clients' rights. General ethical principles, moral rules, and the various theories of social justice also influence health care delivery and nursing services. These principles, their definitions, and applications in community health nursing are presented, and their priority in community health nursing is discussed. Accountability—being answerable to someone for what has been done in the nursing role—is a strong value in nursing, directing the nurse to practice professional skills and expertise in a certain way. Thus the development of methods to measure accountability is also a high priority in community health nursing. It is a priority in that community health nursing must not only demonstrate the cost-effectiveness of its services in promoting health and preventing illness but must also show how it meets normal requirements for professional practice. If community health nursing can demonstrate its ability to increase the community's health while meeting requirements for accountability to clients, then great gains will be made in the name of community health nursing services.

CLIENTS' RIGHTS AND PROFESSIONAL RESPONSIBILITIES IN COMMUNITY HEALTH CARE
Clients' Rights

One of the earliest recognitions of *clients' rights* concerning health was made by the National Convention of the French Revolution in 1793. Underscoring the theme of basic human rights, the leaders of the revolution declared that there should only be one patient to a bed in hospitals and that hospital beds were to be placed at least three feet apart (Annas, 1978). This kind of direction by a government or legislating body in the recognition and assertion of clients' rights has continued to be prominent in considerations of the right to health and the right to health care as extensions of basic human rights. However, the recognition of other clients' rights—such as rights to informed consent, to refusal of treatment, or to privacy—have apparently been aided by consumer groups and health care providers such as the American Hospital Association (Annas, 1978).

Right to Health

A right to health has been historically recognized as one of the basic human rights of all persons. When introducing the Public Health Act of 1875 to the British Parliament, Prime Minister Disraeli noted that "the health of the people is really the foundation upon which all their happiness and all their powers of state depend" (Brockington, 1956, p. 47). In modern times, the right to health has been considered comparable to the rights of life and to liberty, which obligates "the State to prevent individuals from depriving each other of their health" (Szasz, 1976, p. 478).

In the United States, early nineteenth-century public health measures such as sanitation and water supply regulations to control the spread of disease demonstrate early protective laws in matters of human health and hygiene. However, most of these measures protected a negative right to health—the right to not have one's health endangered by the actions of others. The state or government recognized its obligation to enact those measures that prevent the actions of others from adversely affecting the health of an individual.

It is important to note that positive obligations to provide services may seemingly "flow from negative rights" (Beauchamp and Faden, 1979, p. 124). In other words, the negative right to be free to enjoy good health may lead to the positive right to obtain certain services or community health safeguards. For example, the negative right to not have one's health endangered by others led to the provision of public health measures concerning sewage disposal, water supplies, and the regulation of prostitution (Brockington, 1956). It has even led to regulations concerning housing and measures to protect the health of children. More recently it has encouraged some community health advocates to propose broad, federally supported programs and services to protect citizens against preventable diseases and disability (in particular, alcoholism and smoking-related illness) caused, in part, by social conditions (Beauchamp, 1976, 1980, 1985).

Thus advocacy—in the guise of protecting a negative right to health—has helped open the door to consideration of the right to health as a positive right. It has been aided by documents such as the Universal Declaration of Human Rights of the United Nations Assembly. Noting the right of all persons to a standard of living adequate to provide for health and well-being and the right "to food, clothing, housing, and medical care" (UNESCO, 1949), this document suggests that persons not only have a strong negative right to health but a strong positive right to health care as well. It suggests that persons are entitled to certain services, programs, and goods in order to maintain or achieve health as a basic human right.

Right to Health Care

Even though it is sometimes claimed that the "right to health" is an elliptical term for the expression "the right to health care" (Daniels, 1979), the two terms denote different kinds of rights and should be kept separate. The right to health is a negative right to a natural human good, which can be of various degrees. It is a right to not have one's health interfered with by others. However, the *right to health care* is a positive right to goods and services in order to maintain and improve whatever state of health exists. It is a rights claim against the state or its agencies to provide specific health care services that one requests or is entitled to receive. For example, immunization programs, kidney dialysis services, home health services for Medicare and Medicaid recipients, and federally funded prenatal and family planning services all recognize the positive right to specific health care services.

The distinction between the two terms is often blurred for two reasons. First, the World Health Organization defines *health* as "a state of complete physical, mental, and social well-being and not merely the absence of disease or infirmity" (World Health Organization, 1958). The emphasis on complete physical, mental, and social well-being in this definition tends to suggest that one is unhealthy without complete well-being. Since persons experience, as a result of the natural lottery, various degrees of health (but are not necessarily "unhealthy"), this would mean that services must be provided to bring about physical, mental, and social well-being for one to possess complete health. Thus, in recognizing a right to health, the right to health care services to achieve complete health would also have to be recognized.

This is obviously a mistake. The World Health Organization's definition of health should merely be considered as an ideal state of health—one which very few persons actually possess or maintain over a long period of time. As a definition of an ideal state of health, it has no bearing on the provision of health care services as a right of all persons and should not be construed as a state that must, in fact, exist.

A second reason why the distinction between the two terms has become blurred stems from the recent advancements of modern medicine and the willingness of government to subsidize medical treatment for specific disorders such as renal disease (Public Law 92-603, 1972) and some genetic disorders (Public Law 92-278, 1976). This tendency has created an escalation of expectations in terms of services to achieve optimal health. It seems as if government, in recognizing a right of citizens to be as healthy as possible, must necessarily recognize a right of citizens to those services to achieve optimal health. Therefore by subsidizing treatment of some diseases and genetic disorders, government has created the idea that the right to health means a right to good health, a state that can only be achieved through the provision of specific health care services.

Yet this is clearly wrong. In an analysis of Szasz's position (1976), Bell points out that "the right to health does not entail a right to health care because it does not entail a right to good health (only a right to good health if I already have it)" (1979, p. 162). Recognition of the right to health simply does not mean that the state is obligated to initiate health services to maintain health or improve it. Although there may be other reasons why the difference between the right to health and the right to health care are not very clear, these two reasons are certainly pertinent.

Other Rights

The rights to health and health care are not the only rights of clients recognized by the health care delivery system. Other basic human rights are recognized as well.

In 1972 the American Hospital Association issued its study entitled *"The Patient's Bill of Rights."* Soon health care facilities began to use this document as a means for health care providers to communicate rights to their clients. The bill affirmed the basic human rights of all clients who seek health care services (American Hospital Association, 1973). It included the rights to (1) receive considerate and respectful care, (2) obtain complete medical information, (3) receive information necessary for giving informed consent, (4) refuse treatment, (5) request services, (6) refuse participation in research projects, (7) expect reasonable continuity of care, and (8) be informed of institutional regulations. It also included as clients' rights (1) considerations of privacy, (2) confidential treatment of personal information and medical records, (3) provision of information on other institutions and individuals related to care and treatment, and (4) the ability to examine and obtain explanations of financial charges.

Societal Obligations

The issue of client rights is a problem in health care delivery because society does not articulate its obligations to citizens regarding health. As a result, health care providers fail to recognize and protect basic rights of clients. To correct this problem, health professionals need to ask: What are societal obligations to citizens regarding health? What kind of responsibilities do health care providers have in response to client rights?

In a lengthy document entitled *Securing Access to Health Care* (1983), the President's Commission for the Study of Ethical Problems in Medicine and Biomedical and Behavioral Research reported the differences in the availability of health services according to an individual's income or residence. The commission reached several conclusions concerning current patterns of access to health care and made significant recommendations for changes.

The cornerstone of their conclusions is the assertion that "society has an ethical obligation to ensure equitable access to health care for all" (President's Commission, 1983, p. 4). It noted that this obligation "rests on the special importance of health care and is derived from its role in relieving suffering, preventing premature death, (and) restoring functioning, . . ." (p. 29). Considering these obligations, the commission recommended that costs for health care for those unable to pay ought to be spread equitably at the national level and that costs should not be "allowed to fall more heavily on the shoulders of residents at different localities" (p. 30). The commission further recommended that the federal government assume ultimate responsibility for ensuring that equitable access to health care for all is achieved "through a combination of public and private sector arrangements" (p. 29). These conclusions and recommendations are summarized in the box on p. 72.

Professional Responsibilities

In response to clients' rights, health care professionals have particular duties or responsibilities as illustrated in Figure 5-1. Some of these duties are supported by professional codes of ethics and are correlative to basic liberty rights of the client.

ETHICAL FRAMEWORK OF THE PRESIDENT'S COMMISSION

The Commission concludes that:

Society has an ethical obligation to ensure equitable access to health care for all.

The societal obligation is balanced by individual obligations.

Equitable access to health care requires that all citizens be able to secure an adequate level of care without excessive burdens.

When equity occurs through the operation of private forces, there is no need for government involvement, but the ultimate responsibility for ensuring that society's obligation is met, through a combination of public and private sector arrangements, rests with the federal government.

The cost of achieving equitable access to health care ought to be shared fairly.

Efforts to contain rising health care costs are important but should not focus on limiting the attainment of equitable access for the least well served portion of the public.

From President's Commission for the Study of Ethical Problems in Medicine and Biomedical and Behavioral Research: Securing access to health care. vol. 1, Washington, DC, 1983, U.S. Government Printing Office.

Code Duties

Professional *codes of ethics* are statements encompassing rules that apply to persons in professional roles. Two questions generally arise concerning the importance of these codes in health care delivery. (1) What is their relation to universal moral principles? and (2) What is their relation to legal requirements for professional practice? (Beauchamp and Walters, 1978).

In answering the first question, we should consider the rules contained in professional codes of ethics for nurses to be specific applications of more universal moral principles. While some professional codes of ethics are merely statements about professional etiquette or conduct between professional groups and have no relation to external principles, this is not the case in nursing. The professional code of ethics for nurses prescribes moral behavior and actions based on moral principles (Fry, 1982). Thus the professional nurse has a moral obligation to follow the rules in a code of ethics such as the *Code for Nurses with Interpretive Statements* of the American Nurses' Association (1985).*

In answering the second question, we should consider many of the rules in the **Code for Nurses** to be morally obligatory and legally required. Some of the rules may even have legal ties to licensure requirements concerning professional acts. For example, the rules of respecting client confidentiality and accountability are mentioned in the *Code for Nurses* as both morally obligatory and legally required.

Codes of ethics also prescribe duties that are required of the professional in response to rights of the client. The duties

of veracity and advocacy are specifically mentioned in the *Code for Nurses* as being correlative to clients' rights.

Veracity

Truthfulness has long been regarded as fundamental to the existence of trust among human beings. Persons have a duty of **veracity**—a duty to tell the truth and not lie or deceive others. In health care relationships several arguments are usually given in support of a duty to tell the truth (Beauchamp and Childress, 1989).

One argument claims that telling the truth and forbearing from lying or deceiving is part of the respect we owe other persons. We respect persons because they are self-determining, or autonomous, individuals with all the rights and privileges of autonomous persons, including the right to be told the truth and not be lied to or deceived. Because we respect persons and their autonomy, we have a duty of veracity. An example is being truthful to clients regarding the nature of the care they are receiving.

A second argument claims that the duty of veracity is derived from, or is a way of expressing, the duty of keeping promises (Ross, 1930). Communicating with the client creates an implicit contract to tell the truth and not lie or deceive. The contract between client and community health nurse creates the expectation that nurses will, in interacting with the client, speak truthfully.

A third argument claims that relationships of trust are necessary for cooperation between clients and health care professionals. After all, to not tell the truth or to deceive clients will, in the long run, undermine relationships and cause undesirable consequences for future relationships with clients. Thus the community health nurse has a responsibility to maintain truthful relationships with clients in order to protect and strengthen other health care relationships in general.

Yet community health nurses often have difficulty heeding or observing a duty of veracity. The truth is sometimes withheld or filtered because a nurse may think certain information will cause a client anxiety. This tendency is illustrated in a 1975 survey in which over 15,000 nurses were asked how knowledge of the client's condition should be handled by the nurse. The question was asked, "When a patient who has a terminal illness bluntly asks you if he is dying and his physician does not want him to know, what do you usually do?" Of those surveyed, 1% said that they would tell him; 1% would avoid the question or try to distract him; 1% would reassure him that he was just ill, not dying; 2% would lie, saying they did not know; 14% would tell him that only the physician could answer the question; and the majority (81%) would ask why he brought up the question or would try to get him to talk about his feelings (Popoff, 1975, p. 24).

Nurses also withhold information because they think that clients, particularly if very sick or dying, do not really want to know the truth about their conditions. But this belief is not substantiated by surveys of the sick and dying. In a survey of 100 cancer patients, 89% preferred knowing their condition; in a survey of 100 non-cancer patients, 82% said they preferred knowing; in a survey of 740 patients being diagnosed in a cancer detection center, 98.5% said they

*Hereafter referred to as *Code for Nurses*.

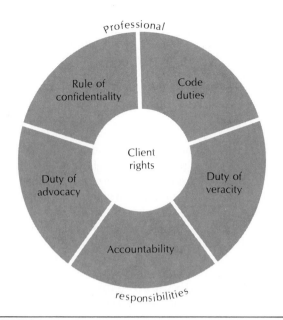

FIGURE 5-1

Client rights and professional responsibilities.

wanted to know their condition (Veatch, 1978).

Regardless of the reasons for not telling the truth to clients or withholding information, it is clear that community health professionals have a duty of veracity. As the *Code for Nurses**notes, "clients have the moral right . . . to be given accurate information, and all the information necessary for making informed judgments . . ." (American Nurses' Association, 1985, p. 2). In fact, the duty to not lie or deceive is a stronger moral duty than the duty to disclose information.† The duty of veracity correlates with the patient's right to know and includes a strong moral obligation not to lie or deceive.

Confidentiality

In general social interaction, certain information is regarded as confidential. Regarding information as confidential enables us to control the disclosure of personal information and to limit the access of others to sensitive information (Fry, 1984).

In community health care relationships, **confidentiality** of information is maintained for several reasons. First, if health care professionals did not follow a rule of confidentiality, clients might not seek help when they needed it. They would reveal necessary information relating to their illnesses that would facilitate treatment. For example, family

---

*Quotations from *Code for Nurses* reprinted with permission of ANA.
†The duty to disclose information evolves from special relationships between agents. In such relationships, one agent can claim a right to information that the other agent would not be obligated to provide to a stranger. The duty to not lie, however, does not depend on special relationships. Lying threatens any relationship because, as Beauchamp and Childress point out, lying is "telling another person what one believes to be false in order to deceive that person" (1989, p. 309).

planning clients might not reveal information relating to their reproductive history that would facilitate appropriate and safe nursing care and follow-up treatment. In short, maintaining confidentiality helps protect the functioning of nurse-client relationships.

A second reason for maintaining confidentiality is that privacy is recognized as a basic human right. Because persons are self-determining moral agents, they have a right to determine how personal information, especially health information, is communicated. As the *Code for Nurses* points out, "The nurse safeguards the client's right to privacy by judiciously protecting information of a confidential nature" (American Nurses' Association, 1985, p. 4). Because of respect for persons, nurses respect clients' rights to privacy by maintaining the moral rule of confidentiality.

In health care relationships, however, the duty to observe the rule of confidentiality is not always absolute. It is merely a *prima facie* duty, meaning that it may be overridden when in conflict with other duties that are morally stronger. The duty to observe confidentiality may be overridden for several reasons:

1. *When in conflict with other duties toward the client.* For example, the duty to preserve life may outweigh the duty to respect confidential information concerning self-destructive wishes of the client.

2. *When in conflict with duties toward identified others.* For example, if a mental health client tells the nurse of intent to harm or kill another member of the community, the nurse's duty to protect others by warning the intended victim will override the duty of confidentiality. This action may even be required by law (Tarasoff, 1976).

3. *When in conflict with duties toward nonidentified others or the rights and interests of society in general.* For example, communicable diseases such as tuberculosis or venereal disease are required by law to be reported regardless of the confidential nature of that information. Another example occurs when health records are used for epidemiological research without the client's knowledge. There are, of course, stringent constraints placed on the use of this information by epidemiologists in health research (Gordis and Gold, 1980; Kelsey, 1981). But in general, the duty to increase or protect the health of the community through research outweighs the duty to respect the confidentiality of health records.

Advocacy

The nursing profession recognizes a strong duty of **advocacy** where the care or safety of clients is concerned. As the *Code of Nurses* states, " . . . the nurse must be alert to and take appropriate action regarding any instances of incompetent, unethical, or illegal practice by any member of the health care team or the health care system, or any action on the part of others that places the rights or best interests of the client in jeopardy" (American Nurses' Association, 1976, 1985, p. 6). In the role of advocate, the nurse speaks for or in support of the best interests of the individual client or vulnerable client populations.

The role of advocate can be difficult for the community health nurse. First, it must be recognized that clients should always determine what is in their best interests. Acting on the basis of what the nurse thinks is in the best interests of clients can lead to paternalism when the wishes of clients are never ascertained.

Second, the duty of advocacy extends to populations at risk, which may bring the community health nurse into conflict with health policy or established professional practices within a community or institution. Nurse advocates who have experienced this kind of conflict have sometimes found their jobs and other professional relationships in jeopardy (Smith, 1980). Needless to say, positions of advocacy can be difficult to maintain when they conflict with accepted professional practices.

Third, it has been questioned whether the duty of advocacy requires the community health nurse to put one's own job, health, or professional standing at risk on behalf of advocacy for the client. According to Beauchamp and Childress, this is not a moral requirement of the principle of beneficence (1989). What is required is that the nurse fulfill the primary commitment to client care and safety by protecting the client from harm. While the implicit contract of the nurse-client relationship does, in general, require positive acts of benefiting from care rendered, this does not extend to the role of advocate. Thus the community health nurse is only required, in the role of advocate, to protect, speak for, and support the interests of the client to *not* be harmed in the provision of health care services.

Caring

The value of **caring** is widely recognized as important to the nurse-client relationship (Fry, 1988). Caring behavior is expected of the nurse and is generally considered fundamental to the nursing role. Leininger (1984a), for example, argues that caring has a direct relationship to human health. Her research demonstrates that all cultures and communities practice caring behaviors which serve to reduce intercultural stresses and conflicts. Such behaviors also protect human survival.

Recent feminist interpretations of the phenomenon of human caring relate caring to ethical behaviors and choices. Noddings (1984) states that " . . . to care may mean to be charged with the protection, welfare, or maintenance of something or someone" (p. 9). This means that nurse caring is specifically directed toward the protection of the health and welfare of clients in the community. When caring is valued as important to the nursing role, it indicates a commitment toward the protection of human dignity and the preservation of human health as well.

Pellegrino (1985) also characterizes caring as a moral obligation or duty among health professionals. He believes that one is obligated to promote the good of another person with whom a special relationship exists. Since nurses have special relationships with their clients, they are called upon and expected to provide caring behaviors to those who have health needs. Caring is a form of involvement with others that is directly related to concern about how other individuals experience their world (Benner and Wrubel, 1989). Caring is therefore always practiced within some context, and its significance is interpreted in terms of the special duties or obligations between individuals within that context.

Accountability

The need within the nursing practice for **moral accountability** in response to basic human rights has long been recognized. Even Florence Nightingale reputedly made strong objections to the overriding of a person's will for the benefit of others in the performance of nursing care (Palmer, 1977).

Modern leaders in nursing have also noted that means must be sought to promote progress in health care delivery while simultaneously protecting the rights of the individual (Gortner, 1974). In the *Code for Nurses*, accountability is defined as "being answerable to someone for something one has done" (American Nurses' Association, 1985, p. 8). It includes providing an explanation to one's self, to the client, to the employing agency, and to the nursing profession for what one has done in the role of nurse. It is an obligation that has both moral and legal components and implies a contractual agreement between two parties. This means that when a community health nurse enters into a contractual agreement to perform a service for a client, the nurse will be held answerable for performing this service according to agreed-upon terms, within an established time period, and with stipulated use of resources and performance standards. The nurse as contractor is responsible for the quality of the services rendered and is accountable to the individual client, the health service agency, the nursing profession, and even his or her own conscience for what has been done (Fry, 1983a).

Referring to accountability in nursing as a moral obligation means that being answerable for one's services is correlative to a client's right to an accepted level of competent nursing care and the right to self-determination in health care. As a moral obligation, accountability directs the professional to act in a particular way according to moral norms (Fry, 1981, 1986b).

In nursing, and especially in community health nursing, accountability appears to be the quality that defines the kinds of relationships among client, nurse, other professionals, and the public at large that form the moral foundations of the professional ethic. Furthermore, since accountability correlates to clients' rights to competent levels of nursing care, it is responsive to the humanistic traditions that permeate nursing's history. Viewed in this manner, accountability enables the nurse to achieve the protection of the client's human dignity and right to self-determination in matters of health.

ETHICAL PRINCIPLES IN COMMUNITY HEALTH
Relationship of Ethical Rules, Principles, and Theories

In making moral decisions we usually appeal to various rules, principles, or theories (Figure 5-2). *Rules* state that certain actions should (or should not) be performed because they are right (or wrong). An example would be that "nurses ought to always tell the truth to clients." *Principles* are more abstract than rules and serve as the foundation of rules. For example, the ethical principle of autonomy is the foundation for such rules as "Always support the right to informed consent," "Tell the truth," and "Protect the privacy of the client." Likewise, the principle of justice serves as the foundation of rules such as "treat equals equally" and "divide

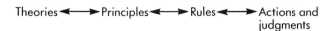

FIGURE 5-2

The relationship of ethical theories, principles, and rules.

your time on the basis of needs." ***Theories***, however, are collections of principles and rules. They provide theoretical foundations for deciding what to do when principles or rules conflict. Examples of a few major theories are *utilitarianism, deontologism,* and *natural law* (see Glossary for exact definitions).

Within theories, the various moral rules and principles are arranged according to their importance or justifiability. For example, in utilitarianism the principle of beneficence often carries more weight than the ethical principles of autonomy or justice.

However, ethical principles are not absolute. Each ethical principle is always morally significant but may not always prevail when in conflict with other principles. Ethical theories simply suggest which ethical principles will more likely prevail when moral decisions have to be made.

But what makes some judgments moral and others non-moral? Moral judgments are evaluations of what is good or bad, right or wrong, having certain characteristics that separate them from non-moral evaluations such as personal preferences, beliefs, or matters of taste. The difference between the evaluations lies in the reasons for or the characteristics of the judgments themselves (Frankena, 1973).

Moral judgments are generally made concerning human actions, institutions, or character traits. What makes them moral (instead of non-moral) is that they (1) are ultimate or preemptive, meaning that older values or human ends cannot, as a rule, override them (Fried, 1978); (2) have universality, meaning that they apply to everyone under relevantly similar circumstances (Baier, 1958); and (3) have an other-regarding focus, meaning that they treat the good of everyone alike and do not give a special value to one's own welfare (Beauchamp and Childress, 1989).

Community health nurses frequently make moral judgments. When the nurse decides to arrange a home visiting schedule on the basis of need or seriousness of illness, a moral judgment is made. When the nurse decides to refer a client to a physician for further evaluation based on the expressed wishes of the client and his condition, a moral judgment is made. When in response to a request for an abortion a nurse decides, regardless of personal beliefs, to inform the client of all the options available, a moral judgment is made. When a nurse, resisting pressure from other individuals, decides not to participate in political activities that might lessen health care coverage for vulnerable populations, a moral judgment is made.

Principle of Beneficence
Definition

The principle of ***beneficence*** states that "we ought to do good and prevent or avoid doing harm" (Frankena, 1973, p. 45). Beneficence is a duty to help others gain what is of

benefit to them but does not carry the obligation to risk one's own welfare or interests in helping others. In fact, some theorists maintain that beneficence does not morally require us to always benefit others even when we can do so. Rather, we are only morally required to prevent harm to people. This may be true in general social interactions among persons. But the implicit contract underlying the nature of the nurse-client relationship seems to indicate that positive benefiting or acts of beneficence should take place.

The need for health care forms the basis of the relationship between community health nurse and client and imposes a moral duty on the nurse to benefit the client through nursing actions. However, there may be limits on the amount of beneficial nursing care a client should expect. Certainly nurses should not be expected to provide nursing care to individual clients or client populations if they are putting themselves at risk; nor should it be expected if clients' needs infringe either on their personal lives or on their responsibilities to other clients, themselves, or their own families. While the duty to prevent harm to clients is a stringent one, the claim to positive benefiting is limited.

Applications in Community Health

In community health nursing, the principle of beneficence can be applied in (1) balancing harms and benefits to client populations and (2) in the use of cost benefit analyses in decisions affecting client populations.

BALANCING HARMS AND BENEFITS. Service that brings about the greatest balance of good over evil, or benefit over harm, is in accordance with a ***rule of utility***. This rule is derived from the principle of beneficence and includes a moral duty to weigh and balance benefits against harms to increase benefits and reduce the occurrence of harms (Beauchamp and Childress, 1989).

In community health a rule of utility may be the basis for deciding whether to fund certain health programs more than others, whether to conduct screening programs for communicable diseases, or whether to conduct research projects where individual rights to privacy may be concerned. In each example, the decision is made by balancing the possible harms and benefits of several alternative courses of action. The community health nurse should accurately assess the known benefits and harms to clients from the point of view of nursing care and should present them with other relevant facts that might enter into the decision-making process.

COST-BENEFIT ANALYSIS. Cost-benefit analysis is a specific application of the principle of beneficence. It is a device for measuring the harms and benefits of providing various health programs or methods of care while also figuring the costs of the potential relative trade-offs in selecting certain courses of actions. All of the units taken into consideration, such as lives saved, costs averted, taxes saved, and illness prevented, are eventually converted into one common unit—usually money—to measure the benefits and costs of alternative approaches to a problem or to decide how to distribute health program funds.

Problems and Conflicts

Decision-making in community health settings on the basis of a principle of beneficence and the weighing of harms and benefits raises moral questions concerning (1) paternalism in health care decisions and (2) the extent of the rule of utility in decision making.

PATERNALISM. Paternalism is a liberty-limiting principle that is frequently invoked to override people's actions or expressed wishes for their own good or best interests. Parents may override a child's desire to play with the interesting knobs on a stove because they do not want the child to get burned. Community health nurses may override clients' expressed wishes "not to hear any bad news" by telling them the results of laboratory testing so that their health status can be treated and improved. Nurses do this because they feel it is in clients' best interests in the long run to know the status of their health.

In general, it is morally justified to restrict a person's liberty when not doing so could cause physical harm, possibly life-threatening. However, it is more difficult to justify paternalistic actions for perceived psychological harms. For example, it might seem morally justified to override a teen-ager's desire to participate in a research project that poses a potential health risk but not to withhold information of a defective fetus from a woman who is six months pregnant because it might cause her psychological harm and grief during the remaining months of pregnancy.

It is also difficult to justify paternalistic actions for the purpose of benefiting the person whose liberty is restricted. For example, it is hard to morally justify remaining and forcibly giving medication to a mental health client who has refused chemotherapy simply because the medication will benefit him by reducing his paranoia or irrational fears. Yet we recognize that health care practitioners often carry out paternalistic actions. If this is the case, are there some acts of paternalism which are morally justified and if so, what are the criteria for justified paternalism in community health decisions?

Since paternalism always violates the moral principle of autonomy and the moral rule to treat persons as self-determining moral agents, justified paternalism is a very limited area. According to Gert and Culver (1979), paternalism is justified only if (1) the evils that would be prevented are much greater than the evils, if any, that would be caused by the violation of the moral rule and (2) we would be willing to universally allow the violation of the moral rule in these same circumstances and be able to publicly advocate this kind of violation. Thus acts involving justified paternalism seem to be limited to those acts that prevent a person from committing some grave bodily harm to himself—self-mutilating or self-destructing behaviors and acts committed out of ignorance, such as unknowingly ingesting harmful substances. Beyond these and similar acts, it is hard to justify paternalism in community health. Few situations meet the criteria for justified paternalism.

EXTENT OF THE RULE OF UTILITY. Attempting to bring about the greatest possible balance of benefit over harm in community health may lead to two problems. The first is the potential overriding of individual liberties and values for the common good (Fry, 1985). For example, in calculating the benefits of a health policy to citizens in terms of tax savings and other economic benefits, the health needs of individual citizens may be overlooked or simply not deemed as important. Human needs and wants that cannot be easily or accurately converted into monetary units may simply be left out in deciding for the greatest amount of overall benefit. As pointed out by MacIntyre, the methodology of cost-benefit analysis in particular cannot truly represent the value choices of individuals (1979). Incommensurable value choices pertaining to health and life are distorted or ignored in figuring perceived harms and benefits into the calculations of the analysis. Thus policy decisions based on the rule of utility as expressed in cost-benefit analysis may be inaccurate and irrelevant to the health needs of individuals.

A second problem arises when the rule of utility is applied in health policy decisions having long-term effects. For example, it is often unclear how short-term harms and benefits ought to be weighed against long-term consequences in cost-benefit analysis. If the benefits and harms to individual health or economic savings in the future are judged more important than present savings or health conditions, then individual and collective interests in health may be sacrificed for future benefits.

Principle of Autonomy
Definition

Autonomy refers to freedom of action as chosen by an individual. Persons who are autonomous are capable of choosing and acting on plans they themselves have selected.

To respect persons as autonomous individuals is to acknowledge their personal rights to make choices and act accordingly. They are respected as self-determining moral agents or persons. Thus when nurses respect persons as moral agents, they are acting in accordance with the requirements of the moral principle of autonomy.

Applications in Community Health

The principle of autonomy is applied in community health through considerations of (1) respect for persons, (2) the protection of privacy, (3) the provision of informed consent, (4) freedom of choice, including treatment refusal, and (5) the protection of diminished autonomy.

RESPECT FOR PERSONS. In community health, clients are respected because they are persons and have the right to determine their own plan of life. Community health nurses acknowledge respect by seriously considering the opinions and choices of clients and not obstructing their actions unless they are harmful to themselves or others. Denying clients freedom to act on their own judgments or withholding information necessary to make judgments demonstrates a lack of respect for clients.

Elderly clients provide an example. Community health nurses often find it easier and quicker to communicate with family members than with the clients themselves. They may simply tell the client what treatment has to be performed, not giving them choices or even involving them in deciding on the treatment plan. Age, however, does not render a client less worthy of our respect (Figure 5-3). The elderly have the right to determine their life and health plans insofar as they have the capacity to do so. To deny them the opportunity to choose according to their capacities demonstrates a lack of respect for persons and is an infringement of the principle of autonomy.

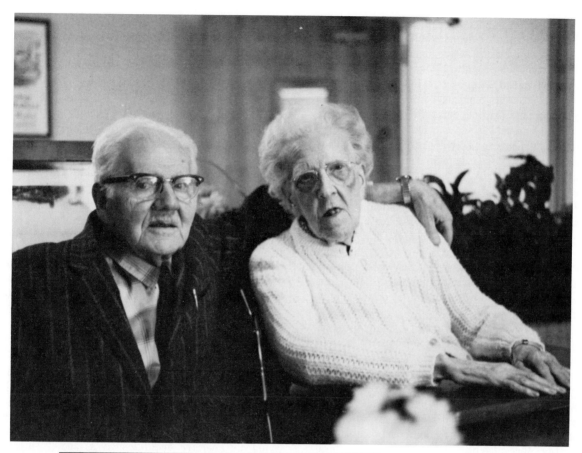

FIGURE 5-3

Age does not render clients less worthy of our respect.

PROTECTION OF PRIVACY. The nature of community health nursing care involves close observation of clients, physical touching, and access to personal health and economic information about clients and their families. All of these aspects of nursing care may invade the privacy of clients or threaten their right to control personal information.

Since the relationship between nurse and client is built on trust, the nurse has a responsibility to protect the privacy of clients and their families insofar as their health is concerned. This means that personal information gathered in the home assessment of clients must be recorded in a manner that acknowledges respect for clients' privacy and is communicated only to those directly concerned with client care.

When personal economic information must be shared with third parties for payment of nursing care, clients have the right to authorize or withhold disclosure of information. Even though the information may be essential for continuity of nursing care services, the client retains control of all information.

When clients' records are examined for quality assurance purposes, or when notes about home or clinic visits are included in research studies, the protection of privacy may be a genuine problem. Utilization of health records in determining funding levels for community health nursing services does not justify the use of nurse-generated information about the client without the client's knowledge and per-

mission. Health record information can only be used for quality assurance purposes or research studies and can be shared with others only under clearly defined policies and written guidelines protecting client privacy. In addition, community health nursing services are responsible for making sure that policies and guidelines appropriately protect client privacy and that clients are informed of this protection *before* their personal information is released to any source. Only when measures to protect the privacy of clients are fully carried out can it be said that community health nursing meets the requirements of the ethical principle of autonomy.

PROVISION OF INFORMED CONSENT. The principle of autonomy requires that clients be given "the opportunity to choose what shall or shall not happen to them" (National Commission, 1978, p. 10). Clients are provided this opportunity when adequate disclosure standards for ***informed consent*** are included in the contract for community health nursing services. Three elements are essential for adequate informed consent: information, comprehension, and voluntariness.

1. *Information.* The nurse must disclose information pertaining to treatment procedures, their purposes, any discomforts and anticipated benefits, alternative procedures for therapy, and options for questioning procedures or ending the contract at any time. Clients should also be adequately informed as to how confidentiality of their health records will be maintained.

2. *Comprehension*. The manner and context in which information is conveyed to clients is also important for informed consent requirements. Clients must be allowed time to consider information provided by the community health nurse, as well as time to ask questions. If the client is unable to comprehend because of a language barrier the nurse must provide an intepreter. This, of course, implies that the client is competent to understand and can make decisions rationally. Competent clients are those able to understand a treatment procedure or proposed care plan, weigh its discomforts and benefits, and then make decisions about undertaking the procedure or plan.

3. *Voluntariness*. Any contract or agreement with the client constitutes valid consent only if it is given voluntarily and is free of coercion or undue influences. Voluntariness includes the ability to choose one's own health goals and the ability to choose among several goals when offered a choice of options (Beauchamp and Childress, 1983). Again, the principle of autonomy is the main ethical principle guiding this provision.

These three elements—information, comprehension, and voluntariness—constitute informed consent in community health nursing practice. Informed consent is not valid without all elements, and no contract between client and nurse is ethically acceptable without valid informed consent.

INDIVIDUAL FREEDOM OF CHOICE. Respecting the client's right to self-determination includes respecting a decision to refuse treatment. The client's personal freedom, the potential harm to the client or other citizens, the cost of treatment refusal, and the values of society are all factors that enter into the nurse's acceptance of treatment refusal (Capron, 1978). But as long as a client is judged competent to make this kind of decision, it is difficult to infringe on autonomy by not allowing treatment refusal.

Some of the most interesting and difficult legal cases involving treatment refusal have involved the exercise of religious beliefs (*In re estate of Brooks*, 1965). Others have involved the autonomy of the teenage minor to refuse life saving treatment such as kidney dialysis (Veatch, 1976). More recent cases affecting the values of entire communities have involved the right of parents to refuse lifesaving treatment for their defective newborns (Lyons, 1985; Will, 1982) and the right of the terminally ill to refuse life-sustaining food and water (Annas, 1985; Fry, 1986b; Lynn and Childress, 1983).

In community health nursing, respect for the client's or guardian's right to refuse treatment may hinge on the nurse's judgment of the competency of the client to make such choices. The physical competency of the elderly or severely ill client, the psychological competency of former mental patients, and the maturity or legal competency of minors may, in part, rely on the assessment of client abilities by the community health nurse.

In situations of questionable competency, decisions have generally opted for the preservation of life (Beauchamp and Childress, 1989). In situations where competency to make decisions has been established, other factors such as obligations to others (such as dependent children) may determine whether autonomy of choice will be respected. No hard or fast rule on treatment refusal can be made. Yet

community health nurses should recognize that respect for persons may involve allowing clients and their legal guardians to make decisions concerning their lives and health that may be very difficult for the nurses to accept.

PROTECTING DIMINISHED AUTONOMY. The principle of autonomy is generally applied only to persons capable of autonomous choice. Persons who have diminished autonomy, whether from immaturity or physical or psychological incapacities, are not considered fully autonomous persons. Thus it is thought justifiable to interfere with the actions of those not fully autonomous to protect them from harmful results of their choices and actions. This interference, however, requires appeals to other principles, such as beneficence.

The community health nurse may have difficulty recognizing when diminished capacities render clients incapable of self-determination. The capacity for self-determination is relative to maturity, chronological age, the presence or absence of illness, mental disability, or social factors. Yet respect for the principle of autonomy requires that practitioners recognize when persons lack the capacity to act autonomously and therefore are entitled to protection in health care delivery (Figure 5-4).

Problems and Conflicts

Respecting the ethical principle of autonomy can be difficult in community health nursing practice. Those areas creating the most conflict for nurses have included (1) carrying out *coercive health measures* and (2) invasions of privacy for health reasons.

COERCIVE HEALTH MEASURES. Clients consulting a community health agency may have a communicable disease that not only is harmful to themselves if untreated but also may affect the health of family members, neighbors, or co-workers. The client may not want to receive treatment and may even refuse to take medications or attend follow-up care recommended for the illness. For example, many areas of the United States still require clients diagnosed with active tuberculosis to be confined until their disease process is no longer considered active or communicable to others. Clients have no choice in the matter. They must be admitted and must take treatment, regardless of their own wishes, choices, or life plans.

The community health nurse may be the one to enforce these regulations or be the agent to override a client's expressed wishes in this matter. Thus nurses may find the conflict between individual rights to self-determination in health matters and the protection of the community's health to be especially difficult when they are the agents carrying out this kind of coercive health measure.

INVASIONS OF PRIVACY. In protecting the health of vulnerable populations the community health nurse may infringe on rights to privacy by actively gathering information of a private nature. For example, a sharp rise in the incidence of venereal disease among a high school population may require interviewing teenagers diagnosed with the disease and accurately following up with all named contacts. This action may lead to invasions of individual privacy through discussion of sexual habits and preferences and potential disclosures to adults, including parents.

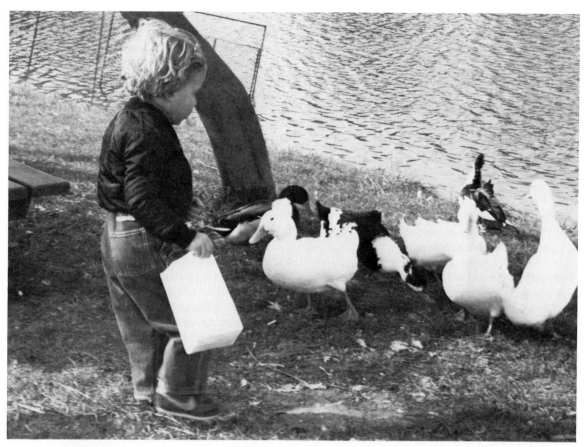

FIGURE 5-4

Children have diminished autonomy and are entitled to protection in health care delivery.

All of these actions are infringements of self-determining behavior but are considered justifiable on the basis of potential harm to others. Nonetheless, it is the nurse's responsibility to inform those whose privacy is invaded that information will be recorded and communicated in a way that does not infringe on their future privacy.

Privacy may also be invaded by the assessment and recording of personal client information. For example, the community health nurse may record information about the social habits and life-styles of pregnant women, and that information may subsequently be used in research studies correlating neonatal mortality and morbidity with social habits during pregnancy. This type of personal information is often freely communicated on the basis of the trust relationship between nurse and client. It may also be recorded in the client's record without full understanding of the potential impact of this information if, in fact, a child is born with anomalies related to social habits or life-styles during pregnancy. The presence of this information in prenatal records means that it might eventually be shared with other health professionals and members of the client's family, constituting further invasions of the client's right to privacy of personal information.

In community health these invasions of privacy may be justified on the basis of preventing harm to innocent third parties. However, communicating this information while remaining sensitive to the client's right to privacy may create conflicts of interest for the nurse.

Principle of Justice
Definition

The formal principle of *justice* claims that equals should be treated equally and that those who are unequal should be treated differently according to their differences (Beauchamp and Childress, 1989). In considerations of a community's health we appeal to a principle of justice in determining the manner in which social burdens and benefits, including health goods, ought to be distributed among all individuals in the community.

Applications in Community Health

Different theories of justice may be considered in deciding how to distribute health care resources. These theories include (1) the entitlement theory, (2) the utilitarian theory, (3) the maximum theory, and (4) the egalitarian theory. Each theory has its advantages and disadvantages in terms of the distribution of health goods in the community.

ENTITLEMENT THEORY. The *entitlement theory* claims that everyone is entitled to whatever they get in the natural lottery at birth and there is no responsibility for government or its agencies to improve the lot of those less fortunate than others. If people are healthy and rich, and have been able to acquire possessions by purchase, gift, or legitimate exchange, they are entitled to what they have. They may also increase their possessions in any way possible as long as they do not cheat others (Nozick, 1974).

It is, of course, considered unfortunate that some people are mentally or physically handicapped in society; yet others have no obligation to give money to the handicapped to make their lives more comfortable. Aiding the unfortunate is simply an act of charity on the part of members in the community.

In this theory, inequalities between individuals in matters of health, position, and wealth are tolerated. Only aggressions or harms against others and the unjust acquisitions of goods are prohibited. Thus the actual distribution of goods seems more in line with a principle of autonomy or the exercise of the right to liberty than a principle of justice (Veatch, 1981).

UTILITARIAN THEORY. The *utilitarian theory* of justice claims that the best way to distribute resources among the citizenry is to decide how expenditures or the use of resources will achieve the greatest net total of good and serve the largest number of people (Mill, 1957). In times of limited resources, when all that is needed or wanted cannot be provided in the community, this method of distribution is appealing. While it does tend to overlook the needs and wants of individuals, it manages to maximize net benefits over costs and serves the greatest number of people.

In this theory the needs and wants of some individuals will not be satisfied, and they may, indeed, be harmed in the process. This would be considered unfortunate, but in distributing limited resources so that "the greatest good for the greatest number" is achieved, government and its agencies would have fulfilled their obligations to citizenry. It is easy to see that the principle of beneficence dominates other considerations in utilitarianism. Justice is served by benefiting the greatest number at the least cost.

MAXIMIN THEORY. The *maximin* theory* of justice first identifies the least advantaged members of the community (for example, the economically poor, the elderly, the mentally retarded, and children under one year of age) and decides how they might be benefited rather than deciding on greatest net aggregate benefit. It then permits free exercise of liberty on the part of all citizens and allows social and economic inequalities to evolve in such a manner that these inequalities are of benefit to the least advantaged or least well-off members in society (Rawls, 1971). Many kinds of inequalities in terms of health, health care resources, and possession of economic benefits will be tolerated and considered, just as long as the position of the least advantaged is improved or benefited. For example, health professionals can charge high fees or receive substantial salaries as long as they also serve the interests of the disadvantaged. In a similar manner costly health care resources such as kidney dialysis, CT scans, and artificial hearts can be developed and purchased by those who can afford them, as long as the lot of the least advantaged is also improved in the process.

Obviously, distributing health goods according to this theory will create problems in times of limited resources. Providing benefit first to the least advantaged is a constraint on the expansion of health care resources and technological advancement. Thus it is possible that technological advancement and the development of more sophisticated health care goods cannot be made widely available to the public in times of limited economic resources. The result is that interests and needs in matters of health may not be satisfied within this system of justice.

EGALITARIAN THEORY. The *egalitarian theory* of justice claims that justice requires the "equality of net welfare for individuals" (Veatch, 1981, p. 265). In this theory the distribution of goods in the community takes the needs of all citizens into account equally. Thus everyone would have a claim to an equal amount of all goods and resources, including health care.

Clearly, this is a goal that cannot be achieved. It would be virtually impossible for any system of justice to guarantee equality of goods and resources for everyone, let alone equal health care. At least with respect to health care, the egalitarian theory must be amended. Instead of health care being a good that everyone should have in equal amounts, basic health care should be viewed as a good to which all should have equal access. In short, everyone should have equal access to those basic health goods and resources to improve their health according to the need (Green, 1976; Veatch, 1981).

This is a system that respects the autonomy of individuals to seek the health services they need or want and gives equal consideration to the positive benefiting of individuals in terms of improved health. Most important, it is just in that it follows the dictates of a principle of justice while, at the same time, not limiting the liberty of anyone in terms of basic health needs. It treats equals equally and unequals unequally and provides a just manner for the distribution of health resources in the community.

Problems and Conflicts

The application of a principle of justice in community health nursing creates conflicts in two areas: (1) establishing priorities for the distribution of basic goods and health services in the community and (2) determining which population or individuals shall obtain available health goods and nursing services.

DISTRIBUTING BASIC GOODS AND SERVICES. In deciding how to distribute basic health care assets or resources within a community, the first decision is to set the priorities for distribution. Should the protection and promotion of health be the main consideration? Or should a major portion of resources be set aside for other social goods, such as housing or education? If community leaders agree that everyone has a right to equal access to basic health care according to need and that this right must be satisfied for justice to be served, then enough community assets and financial resources will be allotted to meet the requirements of this basic right (Milio, 1975).

A second decision concerns the most effective and efficient methods of meeting this basic right while preventing catastrophic events needing immediate and more concen-

---

*Maximin is a short term for maximizing the minimum position in society.

trated attention, which may lead to death or disability. Should the emphasis be placed on direct health care services to care for illness (such as clinics and programs) or should indirect services to prevent illness or promote health (such as health education and transportation services) receive equal emphasis?

Third, decisions will have to be made for the appropriate relationship between rescue services and preventive services (Beauchamp and Childress, 1989). In other words, is it more effective to concentrate on kidney dialysis and terminal cancer services, or should concentrated effort and economic resources be devoted to prevention of disease and disabilty through, for example, hypertension and diabetes screening?

Fourth, decisions will need to be made as to whether certain diseases or categories of illness receive more emphasis than others. For example, should the prevention and treatment of coronary heart disease take precedence over the prevention and treatment of venereal disease? Decisions in this area may result in allocating money and services to certain socioeconomic groups or racial groups and will require careful consideration to avoid conflicts of interest.

Fifth, in establishing certain priorities, it is necessary to ascertain whether these priorities will compromise important values or principles. For example, preventive strategies aimed at discouraging alcohol consumption or smoking may involve emphasis on behavioral change or the altering of life-styles by members of the community. The nurse might question whether priority setting in terms of these preventive strategies would have a substantial impact on the autonomy of community members, particularly regarding their choice to engage in health risking behaviors.

Clearly, the prioritizing of health interests and the various ways to carry out these priorities may create conflicts of interest among health care providers, with subsequent influence on the actual delivery of needed nursing care. These conflicts of interest continue into the next area of decision making.

DISTRIBUTING NURSING RESOURCES. Once the priorities for health are designated, community health nursing services need to decide who will receive services and what criteria can be used to determine services equally in accordance with client needs.

One strategy may be to focus services on those who have the most reasonable chance of benefiting from services; examples are children and childbearing families (Beauchamp and Childress, 1989). This is a utilitarian approach to distributing services aimed at providing the greatest overall benefit. It is questionable whether this strategy meets the moral requirements of a principle of justice, which holds that everyone has a claim of equal access to basic health care services according to need. Certainly a strategy that focuses on one age group in the community will overlook many individual needs in terms of health care services and cannot be considered just.

A second strategy is to provide basic services in all categories in limited amounts and accommodate requests for nursing care services on a first-come, first-served basis. This approach may certainly cost more in terms of services provided. It may even overlap with similar services provided in the community through health maintenance organizations

or group practices of private family physicians. It does meet the basic requirement of providing the opportunity for everyone to have equal access to services, even though they may have to wait a long time to be served. Yet it may not be the most efficient means of disbursing nursing resources according to the needs of clients.

A third strategy is to focus nursing services on those who are most able to pay for services, an approach that is all too frequently used in today's health care delivery system. This approach has been fostered by legislation and funding by government and its agencies. Unfortunately, this approach may have limited relevance to the needs of a particular community. For example, focusing the majority of nursing resources on a home health care program because of Medicare reimbursements would be unjust with respect to the other community health needs if the community had only a small elderly population.

A fourth approach is to categorize those in the community according to health needs and decide who should receive first priority. Those who cannot survive without nursing resources (those receiving kidney dialysis or respiratory therapy at home) would have first priority. Those who can be assisted to prevent long-term disability (populations at high risk; the preeclamptic client; children with minor cardiac anomalies) would come next. Those who do not have an acute disabling illness or are not at risk of long-term disability (school-aged children, the elderly, or some persons with chronic diseases) would come last. Other groups whose health needs can be easily met and who can benefit the health of others (women with uncomplicated pregnancy, mothers with children under 2 years of age) may also be accorded a high priority in this system.

This approach has a decidedly utilitarian twist, and it limits the access of some groups to nursing services according to their priority (Figure 5-5). While it does distribute nursing resources according to who can benefit the most, some clients (such as dying cancer clients) would have no access to the system at all. This can hardly be considered just if we adopt the principle of justice (rather than a utilitarian principle of beneficence) as the guiding principle for distributing health goods.

As can be demonstrated by all of these various approaches to distributing nursing care resources, the moral requirements of justice create numerous conflicts of interest for health practitioners when they face specific choices.

APPLICATION OF ETHICS TO COMMUNITY HEALTH NURSING PRACTICE
The Priority of Ethical Principles

In community health nursing, ethical principles direct and guide nursing actions with individuals and aggregate groups. The professional ethic, in general, places a greater emphasis in most nursing actions on the observance of the principles of autonomy and beneficence than on the principle of justice (Fry, 1982). For example, in the *Code for Nurses*, respect for the principle of autonomy is emphasized by such statements as "the nurse provides services with respect for human dignity and the uniqueness of the client;" that "clients have the moral right to determine what will be done with their own person;" and that "the nurse's respect for the worth

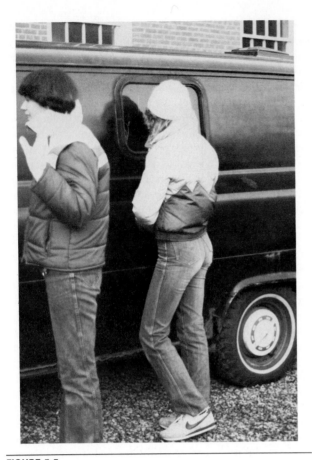

FIGURE 5-5

Teenage populations have a low priority in the allocation of health and nursing resources.

and dignity of the individual human being applies irrespective of the nature of the health problem" (American Nurses' Association, 1985, pp. 2, 3). All of these statements indicate a high respect for client autonomy or claim that the nurse has a strong, primary duty to respect the client's right to self-determination.

The ethical principle of beneficence is given slightly less emphasis in the *Code for Nurses*. For example, the code claims that "the nurse's primary commitment is to the health, welfare, and safety of the client;" that "the nurse safeguards the client's right to privacy by judiciously protecting information of a confidential nature;" and that "nurses are responsible for advising clients against the use of products that endanger the client's safety and welfare . . . The nurse may use knowledge of specific services or products in advising an individual client, since this may contribute to the client's health and well-being" (American Nurses' Association, 1985, pp. 4, 6, 15). Acts of beneficence may even include overriding the autonomy of individuals in the interests of other clients. The *Code for Nurses* describes the occurrence of this nursing action when "the nurse recognizes those situations in which individual rights to autonomy in health care may temporarily be overridden to preserve the life of the human community . . ." (American Nurses' Association, 1985, pp. 2, 3).

However, the principle of justice is not strongly empha-

sized in the professional code of ethics. It is noted in passing that nursing practice is not influenced by age, sex, race, color, personality, or other personal attributes or individual differences in customs, beliefs, or attitudes. The code states that "nursing care is delivered without prejudicial behavior;" that "the nurse adheres to the principle of nondiscriminatory, nonprejudicial care in every situation and endeavors to promote its acceptance by others;" and that "the setting shall not determine the nurse's readiness to respect clients and to render or obtain needed services" (American Nurses' Association, 1985, pp. 3, 4). Clearly, these statements related to the moral requirements of the principle of justice are not as strong as those related to the moral requirements of the principles of autonomy and beneficence.

In community health nursing, nursing actions are guided not only by the professional ethic and its priority of ethical principles, but also by the **public health ethic,** which has a different priority of principles. This ethic is strongly modeled on the priority of the principle of beneficence and follows the rule of utility in disease detection and prevention and in health maintenance (Beauchamp, 1976; Shindell, 1980). This emphasis certainly influences the practice of community health nursing, as is evidenced by the statement of the definition and role of public health nursing from the Public Health Nursing Section, American Public Health Association (1980). It describes public health nursing accomplishing its goal of improving the health of the community by identifying aggregates and by moving "away from solely meeting the needs of consumers as individually presented and toward practicing public health nursing for the 'sum' of individuals or families within the program" (American Public Health Association, 1980, p. 9).

This statement indicates an orientation in community health nursing toward following a rule of utility in matters of health pertaining to clients. The needs of aggregates or groups of individuals is determined for the purpose of providing population groups with net benefit over possible health harms (Fry, 1985). This emphasis on the moral requirements of the principle of beneficence does not align with the highly individualistic approach for the *Code for Nurses*, with its emphasis on respect for client autonomy.

Accountability in Community Health Nursing

Moral accountability in nursing practice means that nurses are answerable for how they promote, protect, and meet the health needs of clients while respecting individual rights to self-determination in health care. In community health nursing, where the greater emphasis is on aggregates rather than individual clients, moral accountability means being answerable for how the health of aggregate groups has been promoted, protected, and met (Figure 5-6). Meeting accountability requirements in community health nursing will thus be different from meeting accountability requirements in other spheres of nursing practice.

For example, whereas the professional ethic clearly indicates that nurses are morally accountable for how they respect the client's right to self-determination and provide health services with respect for "the uniqueness of the client," the application of this ethic in community health nursing indicates that community nurses are morally ac-

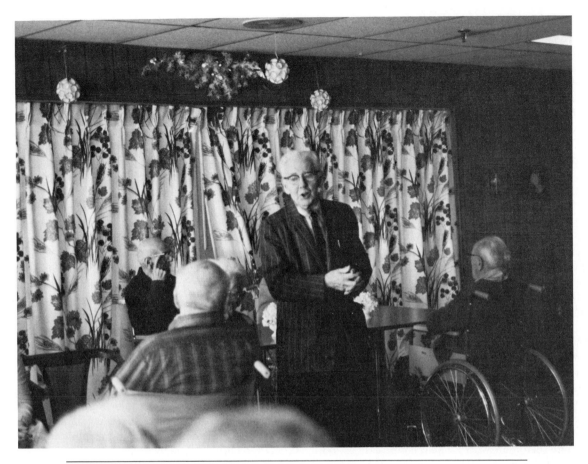

FIGURE 5-6

Community health nurses are accountable for the health of aggregate groups, such as the elderly in a nursing home.

countable for how they provide health services so as to maximize total net health in population groups. It further indicates that they are accountable for demonstrating the increased health of aggregate groups through various research methods and studies while containing costs (Schlotfeldt, 1976). This is the meaning of accountability in community health nursing. Rather than being primarily accountable for how the moral requirements of the principle of autonomy are met, the community health nurse is primarily accountable for how the moral requirements of the principle of beneficence are met by nursing services.

The moral requirements of the principles of autonomy and justice are still important in community health nursing, but they are less important than the requirements of the principle of beneficence. In community health nursing, the emphasis of the professional ethic is slanted toward benefit to aggregates, which implies following a rule of utility in planning, implementing, and evaluating community health nursing services.

Future Directions

The emphasis on the moral requirements of a principle of beneficence in community health nursing has two implications. The first implication is heralded by the position paper *The Definition and Role of Public Health Nursing in the Delivery of Health Care*, which defines public health nursing as deriving its theoretical direction from both the public health services and professional nursing theories and has as its goal "improving the health of the entire community" (American Public Health Association, 1980, p. 4). If this is how community health nursing is to be defined, then it is important that the planning, implementation, and evaluation of nursing services in the community be clearly differentiated from the provision of nursing services in other spheres of health care delivery. While community health nursing is a synthesis of the sciences of both public health and nursing (Archer, 1982), there needs to be a clear understanding of how the ethical components of professional practice, including the observance of clients' rights and professional responsibilities, are considered in the provision of nursing services. There is also a need for clarity and agreement on the priority of ethical principles in community health nursing. The goal of improving the health of the entire community by identifying aggregates and directing resources to them indicates an orientation toward meeting health needs according to the rule of utility. Is the ethical principle of beneficence the principle that should primarily guide community health nursing practice? The moral underpinnings of community health nursing clearly need to be given careful consideration in any statement defining the role of the discipline.

The second implication concerns the evaluation of accountability in community health nursing practice. Just as community health nursing has been affected by changes in both the health care delivery system and nursing practice in recent years, accountability requirements have likewise been affected by changes in public and professional expectations and the scope of nursing practice (Cushing, 1983; Warren, 1983). For example, the expanded role of the nurse has increased the legal accountability of the nurse practitioner who is certified to function as an independent care giver. Thus there is a current and future need for periodic assessment of the moral and legal requirements of accountability in community nursing services.

There is also the need to determine how accountability will be measured in community health nursing and how existing programs and services will be evaluated to determine the effectiveness of various nursing services in meeting accountability requirements. This is a task that has yet to be accomplished by today's community health nursing leaders.

CLINICAL APPLICATIONS

Ethical decision making in the clinical area involves many variables and can be enhanced by an orderly process that considers ethical principles, client values, and professional obligations. The need for this orderly process is demonstrated by the increasing use of ethical decision-making frameworks in nursing practice (Thompson and Thompson, 1985). While such frameworks should not be used as foolproof formulas for ethical decision making, they help individual nurses to explore moral issues and relevant values to arrive at specific decisions (Fry, 1989).

Jameton's Method for Resolving Nursing Ethics Problems is a representative framework that can be used in community health nursing practice (1984). His framework involves six steps.

1. *Identify the problem.* The nurse should clarify what is at issue in the situation in terms of values, conflicts, and matters of conscience.
2. *Gather additional information.* The nurse should decide who is the main decision maker for the situation and what the client or his surrogate decision maker wants.
3. *Identify all the options open to the decision maker.* All possible courses of action and their outcomes should be considered. The likelihood should also be evaluated about whether future decisions might have to be made.
4. *Think the situation through.* Consider the basic values and the professional obligations involved. The ethical principles and relevant rules should also be explored.
5. *Make the decision.* The decision maker should choose the course of action that reflects his or her best judgment.
6. *Act and assess the decision and its outcomes.* The nurse should compare the actual outcomes of the situation with the projected outcomes. Can the process of decision making be improved for future situations having similar characteristics? Can this decision be generalized to other patient care situations?

The use of ethical decision-making frameworks can assist the community health nurse in situations laden with conflicting values. They are not used to "solve" the moral conflict, but they do provide an orderly means for considering the issues involved.

The following are typical case situations encountered in community health nursing practice. Use Jameton's Method for Resolving Nursing Ethics Problems to analyze the issues and clarify the decision-making process. The questions after each case will help you apply the moral concepts and ethical principles in this chapter to the nurse-client relationship in community health nursing practice.

Case 1: What Are Society's Obligations to the Client?

Mr. H is a 48-year-old man referred to the visiting nurse association for evaluation and treatment of stasis ulcers on his legs and for maintenance of a weight-reduction program for both Mr. H and his wife. Mr. H is 6 feet tall and weighs over 380 pounds. The Hs have a 27-year-old mentally retarded son.

When she visited the home, Karla Lowe, the VNA nurse, found large, oozing, sticky areas of raw tissue on Mr. H's legs. Ms. Lowe cleaned and dressed the ulcers and continued visiting the H's every other day for the next 3 months. As the ulcers began to heal, Ms. Lowe attempted to engage the Hs in discussion about nutrition and hygiene and to encourage them to start a weight-reduction program. Mr. and Mrs. H were not interested and chose not to participate in any type of weight-reduction program.

Several months went by and Mr. H's ulcers stopped healing. When they began to deteriorate, he was hospitalized. Within a few weeks, they had healed enough that he could return home. Ms. Lowe visited his home to change dressings as before, but despite her efforts the ulcers deteriorated once again. It was too soon for him to return to the local hospital under his SSI benefits, so it was arranged to have him admitted to the state hospital. Two days later he signed himself out of this hospital. "It was too far away and I didn't know anybody. Besides, they were too rough on me," he stated.

Angered by Mr. H's decision, his physician refused to continue treating him, and Ms. Lowe was left without any current physician orders. This meant that she could no longer give Mr. H physical care or receive reimbursement for her visits. Mr. H's unwillingness to cooperate in the development of "healthy behaviors" made him ineligible for the agency's health maintenance program. When Ms. Lowe explained the situation to her patient, Mr. H said that Mrs. H could wash his legs and apply the medicine that Ms. Lowe had been applying. Besides, he did not think that his physicians had really helped him and he had no intention of ever going to one again. He would miss Ms. Lowe's visits but thought he would manage. Ms. Lowe left the VNA number to call if they ran into any unforeseen problems.

Nearly a year passed. One summer day Mrs. H called Ms. Lowe. She said that Mr. H was "awful sick" and had been in bed for nearly a month. VNA policy allowed a one-time evaluation visit, so Ms. Lowe visited the home. She found Mr. H's legs alive with the larvae of the summer flies attracted to the steamy bedroom. She urged Mr. H to seek hospitalization. He would not be turned away, even if he no longer had a physician. Mr. H agreed, an ambulance was called, and Mr. H was transported to the local hospital. Because of the condition of his legs, a bilateral leg amputation was performed.

When news of Mr. H's general condition got out (he had created quite a sensation in the emergency room of the local hospital) the people of the small town were aghast. How could a man be allowed to rot away? Where were all the services? Who was responsible? The mayor appointed a special task force to investigate the matter. Months (and endless newspaper columns) later "no fault" was found, and it was announced that the town's health services "had sufficient mechanisms to prevent such a thing from ever happening again." Mr. H recovered, obtained prostheses, and moved to another state where he had family to help him.

Yet Ms. Lowe was not satisfied. Didn't the system fail patients like Mr. H? Did patients have an obligation to accept the services offered to them and the recommendations of health workers who took care of them? If they refused to follow recommendations, does it mean that health care services should be totally withdrawn? Couldn't the amputations have been prevented if Ms. Lowe had at least continued her visits and prevented the extreme condition of Mr. H's legs before his last hospitalization?

Discussion Questions

1. What are society's health care obligations to Mr. H?
2. How are professional obligations constrained by society's obligations?
3. Can the conclusions in the report of the President's Commission, *Securing Access to Health Care*, help Ms. Lowe?

Case 2: The Visiting Nurse and the Obstinate Patient: Are Professional Responsibilities Ever Limited?*

Mr. Jeff Williams, team leader in Home Health Care Services at the county health department, was preparing to visit Mr. Rufus Chisholm, a 59-year-old patient recently diagnosed as having emphysema. Well known to the health department, Mr. Chisholm was unemployed as a result of a farming accident several years earlier. Hypertensive and overweight, he was also a heavy long-term cigarette smoker despite his decreased lung function. Mr. William's reason for visiting him was to find out why Mr. Chisholm had missed his latest chest clinic appointment. He also wanted to find out if the patient was continuing his medications as ordered.

As Mr. Williams parked his car in front of his patient's house, he could see Mr. Chisholm sitting on the front porch smoking a cigarette. A flash of anger made him wonder why he continued trying to teach Mr. Chisholm reasons for not smoking and why he took the time from his busy home-care schedule to follow up on Mr. Chisholm's missed clinical appointments. This client certainly did not seem to care enough about his own health to give up smoking.

During the home visit, Mr. Williams determined that Mr. Chisholm had discontinued the use of his prophylactic antibiotic and was not taking his expectorant and bronchodilator medication on a regular basis. Mr. Chisholm's blood pressure was 210/114, and he coughed almost continuously. Although he listened politely to Mr. Williams's concerns about his respiratory function and the continued use of his medications, Mr. Chisholm simply made no effort to take responsibility for his health care. Even so, another clinic appointment was made and Mr. Williams encouraged the client to attend.

As he drove to his next home visit, Mr. Williams wondered to what extent he was obligated as a nurse to spend time on patients who took no personal responsibility for their health. He also wondered if there was a limit to the amount of nursing care a noncooperative client could expect from a community health service.

Discussion Questions

1. What are Mr. Williams's professional responsibilities in response to Mr. Chisholm's rights to health care?
2. *Is* there a limit to the amount of care nurses should be expected to give to clients?
3. What authority defines the moral requirements and moral limits of nursing care to clients?

Case 3: When the Family Asks the Nurse Not to Tell the Truth

Ralph Bradley, a recently widowed man in his mid-sixties, was discharged from the hospital following exploratory surgery that disclosed colon cancer with metastasis to the lymph nodes. His physician referred him to a community health agency for nursing care follow-up. In reading the referral, the nurse learned that Mr. Bradley had been living with a married daughter and her family since his wife's death. An unmarried daughter apparently lived nearby, visiting him regularly and helping with his daily care. The referral did not explain what, if anything, the patient had been told by his physician concerning his condition.

During the first home visit it became apparent that Mr. Bradley did not know that the tumor removed from his body had been diagnosed as cancerous or that it had metastasized to the lymph nodes. He did not realize the seriousness of his condition, but he did express concern about his health. He complained of vague pain in the abdomen, asked for information about the results of the tests performed before discharge from the hospital, and wanted to know how soon he would be able to return to his work as a cabinet maker. When the nurse avoided a direct answer to these questions, Mr. Bradley asked directly, "Is everything all right?" The married daughter, who was present when her father was asking these questions, assured him that everything was all right and that he would soon be up and around.

Walking the nurse to her car when the visit was over, the married daughter confided that it was the family's wish that their father not be told how serious his condition was. She said that her mother's recent death had been very difficult for him to accept. They did not want him to be further burdened with the knowledge of his condition. The nurse listened, acknowledging the difficulties posed by the wife's recent death and the father's serious condition. She told the daughter, however, that it would be very difficult, if not impossible, for anyone from her agency to continue to provide nursing care to Mr. Bradley without his knowledge of his condition.

When she returned to her office, the nurse discussed Mr. Bradley's situation with her supervisor. The nurse did not want to continue visiting the patient, knowing he was being deceived by the physician and family. The supervisor suggested that she consult with the attending physician as soon as possible and explain that Mr. Bradley was asking questions about his condition. Luckily, the nurse was able to reach the physician before it was time to make the next home visit. She asked the physician what the patient had been told about his condition. The physician said that at the family's request Mr. Bradley had not been told that he had cancer. He said he agreed with the family that Mr. Bradley could probably not withstand the anxiety of knowing he had a terminal illness so soon after his wife's death. The physician also expressed concern about Mr. Bradley's daughters who, as he put it, "need a little time to accept the mother's death, as well as accept the impending death of the old man." The physician went on to state that he would consider any act of disclosure on the nurse's part at this time to be inappropriate to her role as a visiting nurse and inconsistent with the well-being of the patient and his family.

Discussion Questions

1. What is the professional duty of veracity?
2. What reasons might the community health nurse give for telling the truth to Mr. Bradley?
3. What reasons might the community health nurse give for *not* telling Mr. Bradley the truth?
4. How does not telling the truth constrain nursing care in the community?

Case 4: The Nurse Who Could Not Protect the Patient's Right to Confidentiality

Jane Sanborn was the occupational health nurse in a federal health agency. Among her responsibilities was the completion of the health status section of a form that included both personal and health history for periodic health examinations of the facility's employees. The physician completed the medical portion of the health report, recorded a decision about the employee's fitness for work, and returned the report to Ms. Sanborn, who maintained a confidential file for employees' health reports and records. Employees were asked to sign a statement on the health report to the effect that information in the report relating to employee fitness for the job could be shared with the employer as necessary.

One day Ms. Sanborn received a memo directing her to send a copy of an employee's health report to Washington, D.C., for filing in a centralized data bank. Ms. Sanborn questioned the request and asked for an explanation of the purpose of the centralized file. No explanation was provided, and the original request was repeated. Ms. Sanborn responded to the request by saying that she would send the health record as soon as she obtained the consent of the employee. The employee's original consent was to share

information only with his immediate employer. Before she could contact the employee, however, Ms. Sanborn was again asked to send the health record immediately; additional consent from the employee was not required. When she discussed the matter with the physician and the administrator of the health facility, Ms. Sanborn was told that she should comply with the request—it was the accepted practice to send any requested employee health records to the centralized file without obtaining consent from employees. Under pressure from both the physician and the administrator, she sent the health record to the centralized data bank.

Discussion Questions

1. Why did Jane Sanborn break confidentiality in this situation?
2. Is there a morally justifiable reason to override the employee's right to confidentiality in this case situation?
3. Why is following the rule of confidentiality important in community health nursing?

Case 5: The Nurse Epidemiologist and Newborn Morbidity Statistics

Ms. Sharon Smith was the community health nurse responsible for interpreting mortality and morbidity statistics for her county health department. Based on a preliminary listing of figures, she initiated a comparative study of newborn morbidity from the death certificates of infants delivered at five county hospitals. The study revealed that one hospital had a high rate of newborn deaths. On closer look, the nurse found that the interns and residents of this hospital were using a particular kind of instrument-assisted delivery. When she presented her findings to the county health officer, he shelved the report. She persisted and eventually went public with her findings. Despite eventual investigation into the matter and a change of the procedures at the hospital in question, Ms. Smith was labeled "a traitor" by officials at her health department, and she lost the support of nurse colleagues employed by the county health agency. After several months of this treatment, she resigned her position.

Discussion Questions

1. What does the duty of advocacy mean in this case situation?
2. What is the appropriate action for the nurse in protecting the health, welfare, and safety of the client?
3. Does the duty of advocacy override personal concerns of the nurse? Why or why not?

Case 6: The Patient Who Did Not Want to be Clean

Marion Downs, a community health nurse, must decide whether or not to refer her patient, 72-year-old Sadie Jenkins, to the community fiduciary for consideration of conservatorship and guardianship. Miss Jenkins has no living relatives and lives alone in a one-room apartment furnished with a bed, refrigerator, table, chair, lamp, and small sink. Since she does not have a stove, two meals per day are supplied by her landlord. With the support of her Social Security check and food stamps, she has adequate money for her needs and has lived for over 10 years in these arrangements. She is also in good physical health.

Marion has made four home visits to Miss Jenkins to check her vital signs and medication routine following recent treatment in the Health Center's Hypertension Clinic. Although Miss Jenkins has made excellent progress and no longer requires visits from the community health nurse, her landlord, the other residents of her small apartment building, and her immediate neighbors are urging the nurse to "do something" about Miss Jenkins. Admittedly, Miss Jenkins' apartment has a strong odor from the long-term accumulation of dust, dirt, and mold. There are visible cockroaches in the apartment, and an unemptied bedpan is often sitting next to Miss Jenkins' bed (it is "too much trouble," Miss Jenkins stated, to walk to the hall bathroom shared by Miss Jenkins and two other tenants). Marion has noticed that Miss Jenkins has worn the same soiled clothes every time she has been to her apartment. It is also obvious that Miss Jenkins has not bathed for a long time, her hair is unwashed, and she apparently does not clean her nails and dentures. In addition, her toenails are so long that they have perforated the canvas of her tennis shoes, apparently the only shoes that she likes to wear.

Yet, Miss Jenkins is comfortable with her life-style and does not want to change her living arrangements. Although Marion has offered to contact agencies to help Miss Jenkins—homemaker service, counseling, and Senior Citizens—Miss Jenkins says that she is comfortable and does not want or need help from anyone.

Discussion Questions

1. Should Marion use her role of community health nurse to create an arrangement by which Miss Jenkins would lose the right to control her person, her financial resources, and her environment?
2. Can an individual in the community be forced to be clean and to live in a clean environment?
3. How far should a nurse go in providing "good" for a patient, and who determines what is "good"?

Case 7: When Aging Parents Can No Longer Live Independently

Joyce Fisher, a home health agency nurse, has just received a telephone call from the daughter of a patient, 82-year-old Mr. Sims, whom she had visited some months before. The daughter was very distraught, telling Joyce that her father had fallen at home but refused to be seen by a physician. Ms. Sims's mother had called her at her place of business and pleaded with her to come to the home and stay with them. The daughter was exasperated by the frequency of these types of phone calls from her parents in recent weeks and was appealing to Joyce for help in making some long-term decisions for the care and safety of her parents.

Joyce clearly remembers the conversations that she had with Mr. and Mrs. Sims and their daughter several months ago after Mr. Sim's last hospitalization. Mr. and Mrs. Sims live alone in a small home and are frequently visited by the daughter, who buys their groceries and takes them to their various health appointments. Mr. Sims has always been the decision maker of the family but allows this amount of assistance from the daughter "for Mama's sake." Another daughter lives in a nearby city but has chronic health problems that prohibit her active involvement in the affairs of her parents. A son lives on the West Coast and travels constantly in his line of business. He supports his parents by sending money for their expenses to his sister (Mr. Sims has refused direct financial aid from any of the children). All three children are concerned about the future welfare of their parents but have been unsuccessful in persuading them to change their mode of living.

The present problem is created by the fact that Mr. and Mrs. Sims are losing their ability to live independently and make their own decisions. Mr. Sim's unexplained falls are also increasing, a continued source of worry for Mrs. Sims and a genuine concern for their daughter. They all look toward Joyce Fisher as the person who can help them make and support a decision that will preserve some autonomy for the aging parents and respect their choices and life-style. Yet Joyce doubts that what is best for all concerned can avoid infringing upon the choices and self-respect of the parents.

Discussion Questions

1. What is the role of the home health nurse in assisting individuals to reach a decision they can live with?
2. What does it mean to respect Mr. and Mrs. Sims as autonomous individuals?
3. Do clients really have the right to refuse services or treatment from the community health nurse? Does such refusal limit future treatment? Why or why not?
4. Is there any happy medium for aging parents when they can no longer live independently?

SUMMARY

The practice of community health nursing is influenced both by traditional ethics of professional nursing and the aggregate focus of community health. In providing nursing care services to individuals and aggregate groups within the community, the nurse must necessarily balance both of these influences. Client's rights to equal access to health care services as well as aggregate groups' needs and interests in matters of health will often compete for the attention and services of the practicing community health nurse. Thus the nurse must become familiar with the moral requirements of nursing practice in general and the community health nursing practice in particular.

Community health nursing practice, as a synthesis of both public health science and nursing science, is theoretically responsive to our prevailing ideas of social justice and the methods of distributing health care resources as chosen by the community. Yet community health nursing practice, as a composite of the individualistic ethic of nursing and the aggregate ethic of public health, is also responsive to the moral requirements of ethical principles as prioritized within these ethics. How the individual community health nurse and community health nursing services view these moral requirements may well determine the future direction and influence of the discipline in meeting the health needs of communities.

KEY CONCEPTS

Because clients have rights, health care professionals have responsibilities to tell the truth, respect confidentiality, function as client advocates, and accept accountability for providing proper health care.

The development of methods to measure accountability is a high priority in community health nursing.

A right to health has been historically recognized as a basic human right.

The negative right to be free to enjoy good health may lead to the positive right to obtain certain services or community health safeguards.

"Right to health" and "right to health care" are different kinds of rights and should be kept separate.

Use of the Patient's Bill of Rights has been the means by which many health care providers communicate rights to their patients. However, the Patient's Bill of Rights has been criticized for several reasons.

According to a recent presidential commission, "society has an ethical obligation to ensure equitable access to health care for all."

The professional code of ethics for nurses prescribes moral behavior and actions based on moral principles.

The need for moral accountability within nursing practice has been recognized ever since Florence Nightingale began her nurse training program.

The ethical principles operable in community health nursing are beneficence, autonomy, and justice.

The four major theories of justice used to decide the allocation of health care resources are the entitlement theory, the utilitarian theory, the maximin theory, and the egalitarian theory. The moral requirements of justice create numerous conflicts of interest for health practitioners when specific choices must be made.

The professional ethic generally places a greater emphasis on observance of the principles of autonomy and beneficence than on the principle of justice in most nursing actions.

In community health nursing, moral accountability means being answerable for how the health of aggregate groups has been promoted, protected, and met.

Clients' rights to equal access to health care and the aggregate's needs and interests in health matters will often compete for the attention and services of the nurse.

LEARNING ACTIVITIES

1. Hold a conference among two or three nursing students and two or three practicing community health nurses. Discuss how community health nurses assume responsibility and accountability for individual nursing judgments and actions in their areas of practice. Be sure to distinguish moral accountability from legal accountability.

2. Suggest three ways by which community health nursing might extend the scope of accountability for nurses in delivering nursing care services to aggregate groups in the community.

3. Select an aggregate group at risk in your community. Formulate a plan of nursing care delivery in response to a health care need using a specific theory of distributive justice.

4. Determine how client's rights to privacy are respected and protected in a community health care agency. To what extent do community health nurses contribute to the protection of client privacy? Are client records used in research studies? If so, how is personal information about the client protected? Suggest two methods by which client privacy could be more adequately protected. What would be the relative costs and benefits of your proposed methods?

BIBLIOGRAPHY

American Hospital Association: Statement on a patient's bill of rights, Hospitals 47:41, 16, 1973.

American Nurses' Association: Code for nurses with interpretive statements, Kansas City, Mo, 1976, 1985, The Association.

American Public Health Association, Public Health Nursing Section: The definition and role of public health nursing practice in the delivery of health care: a statement of the public health nursing section, Washington, DC, 1980, The Association.

Annas GJ: Patients' rights movement. In Reich WT, editor: Encyclopedia of bioethics, vol 3, New York, 1978, The Free Press.

Annas GJ: Fashion and freedom: When artificial feedings should be withdrawn, Am J Pub Health 75:685-688, 1985.

Archer SE: Synthesis of public health science and nursing science, Nurs Outlook 30:442-46, 1982.

Baier K: The moral point of view, Ithaca, NY, 1958, Cornell University Press.

Beauchamp DE: Public health and social justice, Inquiry 13:3-14, 1976.

Beauchamp DE: Public health and individual liberty, Ann Rev Pub Health 1:121-36, 1980.

Beauchamp DE: Community: the neglected tradition of public health, Hastings Center Rep 15:28-36, 1985.

Beauchamp TL and Childress JF: Principles of biomedical ethics, ed 3, New York, 1989, Oxford Press.

Beauchamp TL and Faden RR: The right to health and the right to health care, J Med Philos 4:118-31, 1979.

Beauchamp TL and Walters L: Patients' rights and professional responsibilities. In Beauchamp TL and Walters L, editors: Contemporary issues in bioethics, Belmont, Calif, 1978, Wadsworth Publishing Co.

Bell NK: The scarcity of medical resources: are there rights to health care? J Med Philos 4:158-69, 1979.

Benner P and Wrubel J: The primacy of caring: stress and coping in health and illness, Menlo Park, Calif, 1989, Addison-Wesley Publishing Co.

Brockington C: A short history of public health, London, 1956, Churchill.

Capron AM: Right to refuse medical treatment. In Reich WT, editor: Encyclopedia of bioethics, vol 4, New York, 1978, The Free Press.

Cushing M: Expanding the meaning of accountability, Am J Nurs 83:1202-1203, 1983.

Daniels N: Rights to health care and distributive justice: programmatic worries, J Med Philos 4:174-91, 1979.

Feinberg J: Social philosophy, Englewood Cliffs, NJ, 1973, Prentice-Hall, Inc.

Frankena WK: Ethics, Englewood Cliffs, NJ, 1973, Prentice-Hall, Inc.

Fried C: Right and wrong, Cambridge, Mass, 1978, Harvard University Press.

Fry ST: Accountability in research: the relationship of scientific and humanistic values, Adv Nurs Sci 4:1-13, 1981.

Fry ST: Ethical principles in nursing education and practice: a missing link in the unification issue, Nurs Health Care 3:363-68, Sept 1982.

Fry ST: Dilemma in community health ethics, Nurs Outlook, 31:176-179, 1983a.

Fry ST: Rationing health care: the ethics of cost containment, Nurs Econ 1:165-169, 1983b.

Fry ST: Confidentiality in health care: a decrepit concept? Nurs Economics 2:413-418, 1984.

Fry ST: Individual vs. aggregate good: ethical tension in nursing practice, Int J Nurs Studies 22:303-310, 1985.

Fry ST: Ethical aspects of decision-making in the feeding of cancer patients, Semin Oncol Nurs 2:59-62, Feb 1986a.

Fry ST: Ethical inquiry in nursing: the definition and method of biomedical ethics, Periop Nurs Q 2:1-8, June 1986b.

Fry ST: The ethic of caring: can it survive in nursing? Nurs. Outlook, 36:48, 1988.

Fry ST: Ethical decision making. Part I: selecting a framework, Nurs Outlook 37:248, 1989.

Gert B and Culver CM: The justification of paternalism. In Robinson WL and Pritchard MS, editors: Medical responsibility: paternalism, informed consent, and euthanasia, Clifton, NJ, 1979, Humana Press.

Gordis L and Gold E: Privacy, confidentiality, and the use of medical records in research, Science 207:153-56, 1980.

Gortner SR: Scientific accountability in nursing, Nurs Outlook 22:764-68, 1974.

Green R: Health care and justice in contract theory perspective. In Veatch RM and Branson R, editors: Ethics and health policy, Cambridge, Mass, 1976, Ballinger Publishing Co.

In re estate of Brooks, 32 Ill, 2d 361, 205 N.E. 2d 435, 1965.

Jameton A: Nursing practice: the ethical issues, Englewood Cliffs, NJ, 1984, Prentice-Hall Inc.

Kant L: Groundwork of the metaphysic of morals, New York, 1964, Harper & Row Publishers, Inc. (Translated by H.J. Paton: originally published in 1785.)

Kelsey JL: Privacy and confidentiality in epidemiological research involving patients, IRB 3:1-4, 1981.

Leininger MM: Care: the essence of nursing and health, Detroit, Mich, 1984, Wayne State University Press.

Lynn J and Childress J: Must patients always be given food and water? Hastings Center Rep 13:17-21, 1983.

Lyons J: Playing god in the nursery, New York, 1985, WW Norton Co.

MacIntyre A: Utilitarianism and cost-benefit analysis. In Beauchamp TL and Bowie NE, editors: Ethical theory and business, Englewood Cliffs, NJ, 1979, Prentice-Hall, Inc.

Milio N: The care of health in communities: access for outcasts, New York, 1975, Macmillan Publishing Co, Inc.

Mill JS: Utilitarianism, New York, 1957, The Bobbs-Merrill Co, Inc. (Edited by O. Priest; originally published in 1863.)

National Commission for the Protection of Human Subjects of Biomedical and Behavioral Research: The Belmont report: ethical principles and guidelines for the protection of human subjects of research, DHEW Pub No. (OS) 78-0012, Washington, DC, 1978.

Noddings N: Caring: a feminine approach to ethics and moral education, Berkeley, 1984, University of California Press.

Nozick R: Anarchy, state, and utopia. New York, 1974, Basic Books Inc., Publishers.

Palmer LS: Florence Nightingale: reformer, reactionary, researcher, Nurs Res 26:84-89, 1977.

Pellegrino E: The caring ethic: the relation of physician to patient. In Bishop AH and Scudder JR, editors: Caring, curing, coping: nurse, physician, patient relationships, Birmingham, Ala, 1985, University of Alabama Press.

Popoff D: What are your feelings about death and dying? Part 1, Nursing 5:15-24, 1975.

President's Commission for the Study of Ethical Problems in Medicine and Biomedical and Behavioral Research: Securing access to health care, vol 1. Report on the ethical implications of differences in the availability in health services, Washington, DC, 1983, US Government Printing Office.

Public Law 92-603, Social Security amendments of 1972, 92nd Congress, Oct. 30, 1972.

Public Law 92-278, The national sickle cell anemia, Cooley's anemia, Tay-Sachs and Genetic Disease Act, Title IV, 90 stat, Section 410, 1976.

Rawls J: A theory of justice, Cambridge, Mass, 1971, Harvard University Press.

Rosen G: Preventive medicine in the United States: 1900-1975, New York, 1975, Science History Publishers.

Ross WD: The right and the good, Oxford, 1930, Oxford University Press.

Schlotfeldt RM: Accountability: a critical dimension of health care, Health Care Dimen 3:137-48, 1976.

Shindell S: Legal and ethical aspects of public health. In Last JM, editor: Maxcy-Rosenau public health and preventive medicine, ed 11, New York, Norwalk, Conn, 1980, Appleton-Century-Crofts.

Smith CS: Outrageous or outraged: a nurse advocate story, Nurs Outlook 28:624-25, 1980.

Szasz T: The right to health. In Gorovitz S et al., editors: Moral problems in medicine, Englewood Cliffs, NJ, 1976, Prentice-Hall Inc.

Tarasoff v. Regents of The University of California, 131 Cal Rptr 14, 551 P.2d 334, 1976.

Thompson JB and Thompson HO: Bioethical decision making for nurses, Norwalk, Conn, 1985, Appleton-Century-Crofts.

UNESCO: Human rights, a symposium, New York, 1949, Allan Wingate.

Veatch RM: Death, dying, and the biological revolution, New Haven, Conn, 1976, Yale University Press.

Veatch RM: Truth-telling: attitudes. In Reich WT, editor: Encyclopedia of bioethics, vol 4, New York, 1978, The Free Press.

Veatch RM: A theory of medical ethics, New York, 1981, Basic Books, Inc, Publishers.

Veatch RM and Fry ST: Case studies in nursing ethics, Philadelphia, JB Lippincott, 1987.

Warren JJ: Accountability and nursing diagnosis, Am J Nurs Admin 13:34-37, 1983.

Will GF: The killing will not stop, The Washington Post, April 22, 1982, p A-29.

Williams C: Community health nursing: what is it? Nurs Outlook 25:250-52, 1977.

World Health Organization: The first ten years of the World Health Organization, New York, 1958, WHO.

6

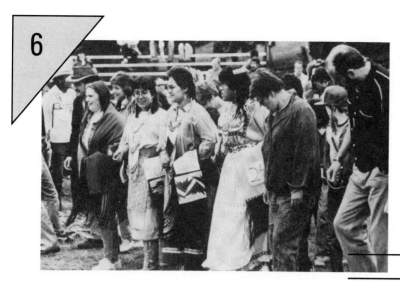

Social and Cultural Influences on Health Care

Eleanor Bauwens

Sandra Anderson

Meaning of Culture

Concepts Relevant to Culture
Holism
Culture Change
Enculturation
Culture-Bound
Ethnocentrism
Stereotypes
Cultural Values

Cultural Differences
Ethnic Collectivity
Cultural Shock
Communication Patterns
Personal Space and Contact
Sociocultural Views of Disease and
Illness

Diverse Cultures of the U.S.
Asian Americans
Black Americans
Mexican Americans
Middle Eastern - Arab Americans
Native Americans
Refugee and Immigrant Populations

Poverty
Absolute and Relative Standards
Culture of Poverty
Poverty and Health

Sociocultural Assessment
Community Sociocultural Factors
Family/Individual Factors

**Guidelines for Culturally
Appropriate Health Care**
Client's Exploratory Model
Client's Perception of Symptoms
Cultural Health Practices

Clinical Application

Summary

OBJECTIVES

After reading this chapter, the student should be able to:

Define culture and how it relates to health and illness behavior.

Identify concepts relevant to culture and health care.

Recognize the variety of influences that cultural differences have on the interpretations of health and illness.

Evaluate the effects of variation between one's own value and belief systems and those of clients from different cultures, particularly regarding implications for nursing care.

List factors that produce diversity in health-seeking behavior between and within ethnic groups.

Describe the nature of poverty and its effect on health status and health behavior.

Assess sociocultural factors and their impact on health care for the individual, family, and community.

Provide culturally appropriate nursing care based on assessment, planning, and evaluation.

KEY TERMS

absolute standard	culture change	minority
beliefs	culture of poverty	poverty
bicultural	enculturation	race
cultural relativism	ethnic collectivity	relative standard
cultural shock	ethnicity	stereotype
cultural values	ethnocentrism	values
culture	holism	yang
culture-bound	iatrogenic	yin

T he premise of this chapter is that health care is based not only on knowledge of the physical causes of disease but also on sociocultural influences. Often nurses must plan and give care to individuals and families whose health beliefs and practices differ from their own. To give effective and appropriate care, nurses must recognize the importance of cultural influences and of specific cultural values.

This chapter will help nurses deliver more personalized, culturally appropriate care to all clients. Ideally it will increase nurses' sensitivity to sociocultural influences on health care and thereby improve their ability to assess, intervene in, and evaluate health problems. The chapter explores the meaning of culture, cultural differences, specific cultural groups in the United States, and poverty. It also provides guidelines for cultural assessment and culture-relevant health care.

MEANING OF CULTURE

Culture enables us to interpret our surroundings and the actions of people around us and to behave appropriately. "Culture consists of standards for deciding what is, what can be, how one feels about it, and how to go about doing it" (Goodenough, 1966, pp. 257-258). Some anthropologists describe culture as a set of rules that provides the individual with a means for behaving and interpreting the behavior of others. This set of rules may be compared with cultural grammar. Harrison and Ritenbaugh (1981) elaborate on the idea that "culture is to behavior" as "language is to speech." This analogy implies that people may not always be consciously aware of the rules, but become uncomfortable if they are broken. For example, if greetings and farewells are not exchanged in an appropriate manner, either party may feel uncomfortable and the relationship may be awkward.

Viewing culture as a set of rules also implies that there are methods of learning explicit and implicit rules. People are consciously aware of explicit cultural rules and do not consciously recognize implicit rules. Explicit rules are more easily learned. Implicit rules can be learned through talking with people and observing their behavior. The rules can be inferred from what people say they should do and from observations and descriptions of what people actually do.

An individual does not need to know all the rules of grammar to communicate through speech; neither does a person need to know all the cultural rules to act appropriately and understand the behavior of others. When enough grammar is known, individuals can create new sentences and make themselves understood in a variety of situations. Understanding cultural rules allows for the interpretation of behavior and helps a person act appropriately.

CONCEPTS RELEVANT TO CULTURE
Holism

Anthropologists believe that culture is a functional, integrated whole with interrelated and interdependent parts. The concept of *holism* requires that human behavior be considered within the context in which it occurs. Similarly, culture is best viewed and analyzed as a whole. The various components of a culture, such as the political, economic, religious, kinship, and health systems, perform separate func-

tions and mesh to form an operating whole. Thus to understand any one system, one must view each in relation to the others and to the entire culture. A culture is often said to be more than the sum of its parts (Benedict, 1934).

Culture Change

Any change in one or more systems affects the whole. Culture is never static but is constantly adding or deleting elements. This process of *culture change* is a result of contact between groups and of forces within a group. Culture change usually creates new challenges and problems. It involves creative adaptation of behavioral precedents that are passed on through language, customs, beliefs, attitudes, values, goals, laws, traditions, and moral codes. At times precedents become outmoded or maladaptive and thus provide a potential source of conflict (Elling, 1977).

The health status of a society is related to its ability to adapt to change. In an increasingly technological society such as the United States, some individuals have become alienated from orthodox medicine. For example, chiropractic medicine has gained status because of political, social, and legal changes.

Enculturation

Cultural behavior, or knowing how to act appropriately, is socially acquired, not inherited. Patterns of cultural behavior are learned through the process of *enculturation,* sometimes called socialization. Enculturation is the process of acquiring knowledge and internalizing values. Through this process people achieve competence in their own culture. Children acquire their culture by watching adults and making inferences about the rules for behavior. Cultural patterns provide explanations for life events such as birth, death, puberty, childbearing, rearing of children, illness, and disease. It is important for the nurse to understand these explanations. As children grow in society, they learn certain beliefs, attitudes, and values about these life events. They retain this knowledge throughout their lives unless necessity or force compels them to learn different ways.

Culture-Bound

Whenever people learn a culture, they are to some extent imprisoned without knowing it. Anthropologists refer to this existence as being *culture-bound;* that is, living within a particular reality that is considered as *the* reality. Everyone has learned ways to interpret the world based on their enculturation. Their interpretations are understandable and persuasive to those who share the same frame of reference but may sometimes make little sense out of context. Nurses are culture-bound within their own culture and profession. Being culture-bound within nursing means that nurses are likely to view the modern scientific approach to health and illness as the only possibility. Clients may view this modern scientific approach differently, judging that in some ways it meets their needs, and in other ways it does not. Dissatisfaction with medical treatment and practitioners, the movement toward self-care, and the striving for freedom of choice and individual responsibility have led to increased interest in alternative health services. Western medicine is often practiced in unscientific ways. Desirable outcomes may occur independently of the physician's intervention, or the physician's intervention may lead to *iatrogenic* (treatment-related) consequences such as adverse drug reactions (Gevitz, 1988; Young, 1978).

Ethnocentrism

Ethnocentrism is the belief that one's own cultural viewpoint is the best. It is important for nurses not to consider their own way the best and other people's ideas as ignorant or inferior. The ideas of lay individuals may be valid and certainly influence their health care behavior. Culturally appropriate health care begins with the awareness that people may live by different rules and priorities from those of the health care provider, and these rules and priorities decisively influence health-related behavior. Health care providers tend to act on the assumption that their world view conforms to the way the world really is or ought to be. When people are judgmental of other cultures, they go beyond healthy cultural identification. The term *cultural relativism* denotes that cultures are neither inferior nor superior to one another. Cultural relativists believe that there is no single scale for measuring the value of a culture; rather, the value of a culture can only be defined by its meaning to its members. The following comment by Jelliffe (1969, p. 61) refers specifically to nutrition, but applies to any aspect of culture:

> . . . all different cultures, whether in a tropical village or in a highly urbanized and technologically sophisticated community, contain some practices and customs which are beneficial to the health and nutrition of the group, and some which are harmful. No culture has a monopoly on wisdom or absurdity.

Health professionals must recognize the role of cultural relativism in regard to modern scientific medicine. Nurses must realize that not even their own beliefs and professional practice are immune to scientifically unsound behavior. Tripp-Reimer (1982) studied ethnocentrism and cultural relativity in an Appalachian population served by both Appalachian and non-Appalachian health professionals. She observed that both the client and the health care provider enter the clinical situation with predetermined values, beliefs, and perceptions. She noted that "the provider's culture biases the interpretation and understanding of client behavior . . . [and] it will diminish the quality of care available for minority clients" (Tripp-Reimer, 1982, p. 188).

Stereotypes

Stereotypes are exaggerated beliefs and images that are popularly depicted in the mass media and folklore. Usually these images are false; they obscure important differences among members of a group and exaggerate those between groups. The perceived, exaggerated differences between two groups are used to justify negative behavior of people in one group toward the other group. Although individuals may be found to fit the stereotypes, most do not. Stereotypes are commonly reflected by false and insensitive statements such as "Indians are drunks," "blacks are lazy," "poor whites are trash," or "nurses are passive." Stereotyping can lead to inaccurate assessments and interventions based on preconceived notions. Health professionals must remain sensitive to individual variation within groups.

Cultural Values

The cultural system is composed of value orientations. A *value* is a type of belief about how one should or should not behave. *Beliefs* are "statements which the subject holds as true, but which may or may not be based on empirical evidence. Thus the strength of a belief does not depend on its degree of correspondence with objective fact. . ." (Horn, 1979, p. 63). All belief systems are culture-bound because they are based on cultural factors and the meaning that individuals ascribe to these factors. Individuals assign meaning to health and illness based on their values and beliefs. Therefore the behavior of clients in regard to health and illness can be more accurately understood by knowing something about their beliefs and values.

Cultural values are the prevailing and persistent guides influencing how people think and act. Beliefs and values influence the kind of health care a person considers acceptable or desirable. Values provide powerful motivation and standards for behavior. For instance, if people value prevention, they will generally have their children immunized against disease. If they do not value prevention, they will likely ignore immunizations even if they are provided free of charge.

There are two types of values: public and personal (Goodenough, 1966). Public values tend to be objectified by policies and laws; personal values are usually unstated and individualized. People may agree on public values but may vary greatly on personal values. Acceptance of rules requires that public values may be reasonably compatible with personal values. When incompatibility exists, the society strives for agreement between public and personal values. An example of this is the conflict over abortion in the United States.

One of the most important elements shared by a culture is its values. Shared values give a culture stability and security, providing a standard for behavior. If two people share a similar culture and their experiences tend to be similar, their values tend to be similar. Although no two people have exactly the same value pattern, they are enough alike to recognize similarities and to identify the other as "one of my kind" (Goodenough, 1966).

The nurse should not expect to understand the value system of a family or cultural group after the first contact. The nurse should realize the importance of gathering data, because different people will view health care as good or bad, adequate or inadequate, depending upon their cultural values (Leininger, 1976). Even in situations where the cultural backgrounds of the client and nurse are assumed to be similar, problems can arise if the nurse fails to recognize the sociocultural aspects influencing health and illness.

Although it is important to understand the client's ideas about disease, it is equally important to understand what the client views as appropriate treatment and acceptable behavior on the part of the health care provider. The degree to which the client's actions to resolve a health problem agree with those of the health care provider is influenced by the similarity in cultural backgrounds of the client and provider. Health care providers need to consider what clients actually believe about their health problems and how they should be treated. Both have their own ways of explaining and treating ill health and specifying how the health care provider and client should interact in the treatment encounter. If health care providers have a working knowledge of the culture, they can more accurately interpret and influence the client's behavior.

CULTURAL DIFFERENCES

All segments of the population in the United States share certain common elements in life patterns and basic beliefs. However, because of different cultural traditions and increasing mobility, a homogeneous culture is seldom found. In a homogeneous culture individuals tend to share the same attitudes, interests, and goals. Generally people are likely to do what is expected or to follow the norms, but discrepancies occur in all cultures. Society prescribes what individuals should ideally do, but their real behavior only approximates the norm, especially if the norm is not highly valued. The actual behaviors tend to cluster toward a trend or mode. Individuals who grow up in the same society acquire certain standardized ways of dealing with objects and people. This means that even among total strangers in a unique situation, general standards guide behavior.

Ethnic Collectivity

An *ethnic collectivity* is a group with common origins, a sense of identity, and shared standards for behavior. Individuals reared within such a group are enculturated by norms that determine their thoughts and behaviors (Harwood, 1981). The effects of this enculturation carry over to health care and become an important influence for activities related to health and illness.

Social scientists speak about American culture as if it included a set of values shared by everyone. However, even within an ethnic collectivity intra-ethnic variations can be expected and are apparent in health behaviors. For example, variations are seen in conceptions of mental illness (Guttmacher and Elinson, 1971), in definitions of health and illness, in skepticism about medical care, in use of health care services (Berkanovic and Reeder, 1973), and in willingness to assume a dependent role when ill (Greenblum, 1974; Suchman, 1964).

The term *bicultural* implies that a person straddles two cultures, life-styles, and sets of values. To understand biculturalism it is necessary to discuss the different meanings of ethnicity, race, and minority. Ethnicity is frequently used to mean race, but it includes more than a biological identification. *Ethnicity* refers to groups whose members share a common social and cultural heritage passed on to each successive generation. Members of an ethnic group feel a sense of identity. *Race* is a biological term. Racial group members share distinguishing physical features such as skin color and bone structure and genetic traits such as blood grouping. Ethnic and racial groups may overlap, in which case the biological and cultural similarities can reinforce one another. A *minority* may consist of a particular racial, religious, or occupational group that constitutes a numerical minority of the population. In this sense all of us belong to various kinds of minorities (Bullough and Bullough, 1982). Bicultural group members may share ethnic and/or social characteristics of the larger group of which they are a part,

but they also share a common culture different from that of the larger group. For example, Mexican Americans share the larger society's perspective of health and illness, but for many Mexican Americans folk medicine is a cultural choice.

Cultural Shock

Cultural shock is one of the effects of working with individuals from different cultural backgrounds. Leininger (1976, p. 7) describes *cultural shock* as "the feelings of helplessness and discomfort and the state of disorientation experienced by an outsider attempting to comprehend or effectively adapt to a different cultural group because of differences in cultural practices, values, and beliefs." Cultural shock sometimes makes health care providers feel uncomfortable or even angry. Kubricht and Clark (1982) surveyed nurses and foreign clients to identify areas in which clients' needs were unmet and nurses encountered problems. The survey revealed that foreign clients experienced boredom, anxiety, and fear; nurses experienced frustration and inadequacy. Communication was either inadequate or nonexistent and the lack of culture-specific information was a significant problem. The resources to overcome these problems were not consistently available.

Nurses can help reduce cultural shock by learning about the different cultural groups they encounter. Methods of learning include transcultural course work and experiences. Even with some knowledge of a variety of cultures, the nurse may regard certain clients as strange and have difficulty communicating with them. Likewise, the client may perceive the health system and health care providers as unusual and incomprehensible. It is important for nurses to develop respect for others who are culturally different while maintaining their own sense of worth. Community health nursing practice requires tolerance of beliefs that may oppose those of the nurse.

Communication Patterns

Obvious barriers are present when two people speak different languages. Familiarity with the language of the client is one of the best ways to gain insight into a culture. Kluckhohn (1972) wrote that every language is also a special way of looking at the world and interpreting experiences. Each language makes a whole set of unconscious assumptions about the world and life. Kluckhohn believed that the grammatical system of a language alerts its speakers to what they see and hear. Cultural differences are reflected in language by the actual terms that are used, the appropriate times for speech, acceptable and taboo topics, and the social situation. For example, Saunders (1954, p. 116) describes how the English speaker's assessment of Spanish-speaking people's worth can be affected by being unable to understand their way of looking at things: ". . . in English a clock runs, while in Spanish, it walks *(el reloj anda)*. Such a simple difference as this has enormous implications for appreciating differences in the behavior of English-speaking persons. If time is moving rapidly, as Anglo usage declares, we must hurry. . . . If time walks, as the Spanish-speaking say, one can take a more leisurely attitude toward it. . . ." An attempt to understand a people's world view through their language can avert some major misunderstandings.

Barriers to communication may exist even when individuals speak the same language. Nurses have difficulty explaining things in simple, jargon-free language that clients can understand. It is important to determine that the message was received and understood as intended. The nurse and client can employ a feedback mechanism to facilitate communication. Much of the information we transmit to each other is conveyed by facial expression, posture, body movement, and voice tone. For example, an Anglo may value straightforward criticism to the person's face, but a Tohono O'odham Indian (formerly the Papago) finds that action impolite. Thus Tohono O'odham clients may be unwilling to criticize health personnel directly even if they are dissatisfied with their health care.

Personal Space and Contact

Personal space is an invisible, flexible boundary. Insel (1978) describes personal space as a "portable bubble" that continuously surrounds the individual. This invisible cushion provides a margin of safety and security. The bubble expands and shrinks, according to the social situation, the physical area, the culture of the individual, and the relation to others present (Meisenhelder, 1982). Body or eye contact accepted or even expected in one culture may be taboo in another. Touching may be considered an intrusion of personal space in some cultures. In others, many forms of traditional healing require touching as a part of the healing process or as a comfort measure.

Hall (1966) observed and interviewed northeastern Americans to learn about their use of personal space. He identified four zones (Figure 6-1):

    Intimate distance: 0 to 18 inches from the individual
    Personal distance: 18 inches to 4 feet
    Social distance: 4 feet to 12 feet
    Public distance: 12 feet or greater

People are usually not aware of the use of personal space according to zones; nevertheless, the use of personal space is certainly influenced by culture.

Watson (1970) studied cultural differences in the use of personal space. He compiled a range of space by nationality and found that Americans, Canadians, and British require the most personal space, whereas Latin Americans and Arabs need the least. He noted that within the same cultural group individuals interacted at a uniform distance according to the situation. Because people do not consciously recognize their own use of personal space, they have difficulty understanding a different cultural pattern. As a result, acts of friendliness may be misinterpreted as threatening behavior if personal space has been invaded.

An understanding of personal space by the community health nurse can facilitate the assessment process and improve nurse-client interaction. Health professionals often feel that they have access to any area of the client's body. The client may develop patterns of avoidance and withdrawal to protect personal space. Close contact is often necessary, such as when the nurse does a physical assessment. The nurse should attempt to reduce anxiety by recognizing the individual's need for personal space and taking the appropriate action to provide privacy. Clients should be allowed to direct the use of their personal space, whether

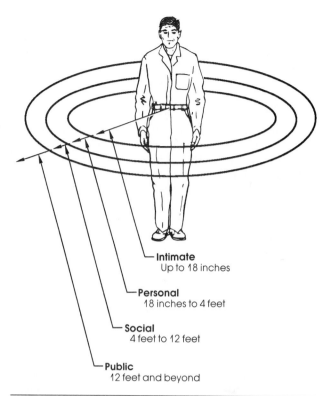

FIGURE 6-1

Proxemics focuses on four zones of space in human interaction. *(From Beck, C.K., Rawlins, R.P., and Williams, S.: Mental health-psychiatric nursing: a holistic life-cycle approach, ed. 2, 1988, The C.V. Mosby Co.)*

they are in their homes or in the hospital, so that individual identity and integrity are preserved.

Sociocultural Views of Disease and Illness

In countries such as the United States there is an extremely complex system of health beliefs and practices. Variations in these beliefs and practices may be found across ethnic and social class boundaries and even within families. Currently the generally accepted approach is the biomedical model, which emphasizes biological concerns. These concerns are often considered more "real," significant, and interesting than psychological and sociocultural issues (Kleinman et al., 1978). Most health professionals in modern Western settings are primarily interested in the treatment of diseases and abnormalities of body systems. Kleinman et al. view the biomedical approach as culture-specific (culture-bound) and value-laden. The biomedical model represents one end of a continuum. At the other end is traditional content, the popular beliefs and practices that usually differ from medical science (Chrisman, 1977). Health beliefs and practices of individuals vary along the continuum.

There is a distinction between illness and disease. The human experience of illness is not necessarily identical to the biomedical interpretation of disease. Illness is the individual's perception of being sick. Disease is only diagnosed when the condition is a deviation from norms established by Western biomedical science (Helman, 1990; Fabrega, 1971). Illness may occur in the absence of disease. "Illness is culturally shaped in the sense that how we per-

Figure labels:

Intimate
Up to 18 inches

Personal
18 inches to 4 feet

Social
4 feet to 12 feet

Public
12 feet and beyond

ceive, experience and cope with disease is based on our explanations of sickness" (Kleinman et al., 1978, p. 252).

Culture influences people's expectations and perceptions of symptoms as well as the way they label sickness. It also affects when, how, and to whom they communicate their health problems and how long they remain under care. Because health and illness are shaped by cultural factors, there is variation in health care behavior, health status, and patterns of sickness and care within and between different cultures. Health care behavior refers to an individual's social and biological activities with respect to maintaining an acceptable health status or altering an unacceptable condition. Health status refers to the success with which a person has adapted to the total environment. Health care behavior and health status are interrelated, and both are affected by sociocultural forces such as economics, politics, environmental influences, and the health system (Elling, 1977).

The model in Figure 6-2 shows the relation of sociocultural patterns to the health care system and many other factors that have a bearing on health. As the model illustrates, sociocultural influences affect not only the individual's health status but also the entire health system. Other factors depicted in the model also produce changes in the health status of a population. Demographic factors including age, gender, marital status, and migration have a strong influence on health status. The arrows indicate a causal direction of influence. Biomedical factors, including race, weight, height, and genetic inheritance are linked to various deviations from the normal, influencing the health status of an individual. Most of the relationships shown in the model are reciprocal. The many interrelations indicate that a change in any one factor affects the others.

Health care providers and clients may define disease and illness differently. If so, they may disagree about the best method of care. Such a disagreement may cause the client to be uncooperative. If the provider and the client share the same beliefs and values, agree on a plan of care, and desire the same outcome, the client is more likely to cooperate. The community health nurse should not attempt to change clients' values but instead should involve the client in making decisions about the plan of care. If the client is involved, cooperation is more likely and the client's health status will be improved.

DIVERSE CULTURES OF THE UNITED STATES

The United States comprises many diverse cultures. Although broad cultural values are shared by most people, a rich diversity of values and beliefs exists, including variation in health and illness beliefs. Nevertheless, nurses tend to practice in an ethnocentric manner. Nursing has generally been taught and practiced as if all clients were members of the dominant American group: white, Christian, and of European ancestry (Ruiz, 1981). Because most people are familiar with this American group, it is not discussed in this chapter. (For information on low-income Anglos see Bauwens [1977], and for middle-income Anglos see Hautman and Harrison [1981]).

Information about the cultural backgrounds of Asian Americans, black Americans, Mexican Americans, Middle Eastern-Arab Americans, and Native Americans is pre-

sented to illustrate how cultural factors can and do influence client behavior and to highlight the importance of using cultural background data in providing nursing care. The purpose of these examples of specific ethnic groups is to emphasize the wide array of factors that influences health and illness beliefs. Factors that produce diversity between and within ethnic groups include historical factors, education, sex, place of birth, geographical location, socioeconomic status, and religious affiliation.

Asian Americans

The likelihood of nurses having contact with Asians (or more specifically, Orientals) in the United States is greater than ever before. Historically, the largest groups have been the Japanese, Chinese, Filipino, and Korean. More recently refugees from Viet Nam, Cambodia, and Laos have increased the Asian population, especially on the West Coast. A wide range of health beliefs and behaviors exists within each group.

The Asian health system is based on the ancient principle of hot and cold forces (yin and yang). Yin, the "female" force, represents negative elements such as darkness, cold, weakness, and death. Yang, the opposite "male" force, represents positive forces such as light, heat, regeneration, and strength. The body contains both elements. An imbalance in these forces may cause discomfort and illness. If one's body is too "cold," one takes "hot" foods and/or herbs to correct the imbalance. Most spices, sweets, eggs, and onions are viewed as "hot" whereas vegetables, fruits, rice, and potatoes are thought to be "cold." Foods such as watermelon soup, beef broth, and vegetables are used to prevent illness (Tien-Hyatt, 1989; Spector, 1985; Oraque, 1983).

Some Asian Americans also believe that illness can be due to supernatural entities such as gods and spirits. Illness may be an individual's punishment for offending a god or spirit. They also believe that some illnesses are due to naturalistic causes. For example, one may become ill from exposure to bad weather and cold draughts.

Health and other aspects of daily life are the responsibility of the family. Therefore in order to assess and intervene appropriately, nurses must be familiar with the prescribed roles in Asian American families. Special care is needed when dealing with individuals' and families' expressions of feelings even though they may be nonverbal (Muecke, 1983; Henderson and Primeaux, 1981). Most Asians strongly emphasize harmony and avoidance of conflict in groups. Direct confrontations are usually avoided. It is important for all to maintain self-esteem and not lose face, and this is sometimes achieved by non-responsiveness.

The community health nurse needs to be aware that although there are many similarities among Asians, variations exist among generations and subgroups. Individual values may contribute to different responses to the health care system. The nurse will need to ask the client and family about their cultural beliefs and health care practices before intervening (Tien-Hyatt, 1987).

Black Americans (African Americans)

In the past, various terms have been used to describe blacks: colored, Negro, Afro-American, and black. Caution is ad-

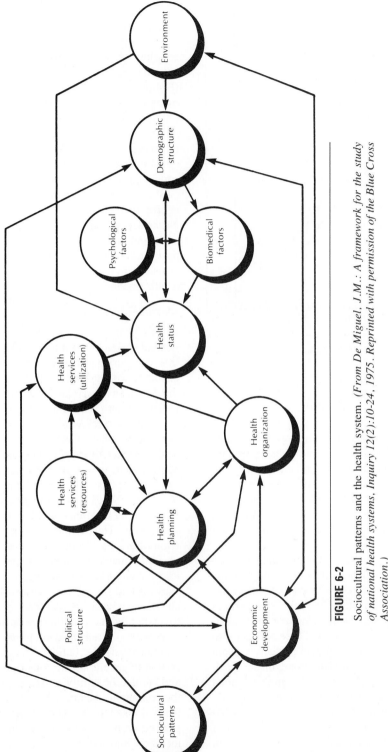

FIGURE 6-2

Sociocultural patterns and the health system. *(From De Miguel, J.M.: A framework for the study of national health systems, Inquiry 12(2):10-24, 1975. Reprinted with permission of the Blue Cross Association.)*

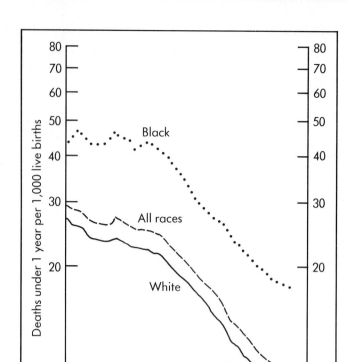

FIGURE 6-3

Infant mortality rates by race: United States, 1950 to 1987. *(From National Center for Health Statistics.)*

vised in labeling because clients of various age groups may prefer different terms. Jackson (1981) notes that blacks constitute a highly heterogeneous group; in other words, no "typical" black individual exists. Because blacks are readily identified by their skin color, many health professionals have a tendency to treat blacks as if they were all alike. However, black Americans display considerable variation in their health attitudes and behaviors.

Some of the differences in health problems are the result of varying genetic pools and hereditary immunity. Some differences are closely associated with poverty, discrimination, and social and psychological barriers. Such barriers tend to keep people from using health care services (Zaida, 1988; Townsend and Davidson, 1982). These barriers also interact and reinforce each other and may partially explain why mortality and morbidity are higher among blacks (Bullough and Bullough, 1982). For example, in the United States proportionately more blacks than whites have hypertension. Evidence indicates that explanations for this discrepancy in morbidity rates should be sought in the area of social pressures arising from enduring racism, not only in dietary or genetic differences (Szathmary and Ferrell, 1990).

Black Americans have a higher infant mortality rate (17.9 per 1000 live births in 1987) than do white Americans (8.6 per 1000 live births in 1987). The downward trend in infant mortality has decreased among both the white and black populations: since the late 1970s it has slowed for white

infants, and it began to decline for black infants in 1981 (Figure 6-3).

The black family is often oriented around women (matrifocal). Within the family the wife and/or mother is often responsible for protecting the health of family members. She is expected to assist them in maintaining good health and in determining treatment for illness.

In general, black Americans have a strong religious orientation. Most belong to Protestant denominations. A common and frequently cited method of treating illness is prayer (Helman, 1990; Spector, 1985). Snow (1977) noted that many of the individuals in her study found it impossible to separate religious beliefs from medical ones. In some instances illnesses may be viewed as punishment for failure to abide by God's rules. Thus spiritual healers, who frequently have their own special curing techniques, are often sought for curing illnesses.

It is important for the community health nurse to recognize that black Americans are a heterogeneous group. Nevertheless, many are still influenced by ethnic group customs and traditions. Nurses have the responsibility to improve accessibility to health care, to provide culturally relevant health care, and to assist blacks to improve their own health status.

Mexican Americans

In this chapter the term *Mexican American* is used as a general designation for individuals of Mexican ancestry who live only in the southwestern states. Given the regional enculturation and socioeconomic variation existing within the Mexican American populations, it is difficult to formulate conclusions about an entire ethnic group with such diversity as rural villagers in New Mexico and Colorado (Saunders, 1954; Weaver, 1970), agricultural laborers in Texas (Rubel, 1966; Trotter and Chavira, 1981; Trotter et al., 1989), low-income residents in Arizona (Kay, 1977), or urban lower socioeconomic class individuals in California (Clark, 1970). Not only do studies represent different populations, but they also differ in their definitions of Mexican Americans. Thus any discussion of Mexican Americans is complicated by the problem of defining this population.

Traditionally the family is important in Mexican American culture and is characterized by a close-knit kin group. Ties beyond the nuclear family link grandparents, uncles, aunts, and cousins. A Mexican American is expected to turn to the family first to fulfill needs; seeking outside help often is done at the expense of pride and dignity of both the individual and the family. Practices are passed from generation to generation. If strong ties exist between the client and family, the family's advice may be followed rather than the community health nurse's. The nurse may suggest that the client solicit the opinions of other family members regarding proposed actions. The nurse should involve family members in planning care. This demonstrates that the nurse understands the family's importance in health matters.

Language may influence health care practices of Mexican Americans. If a language barrier exists, it can be overcome by providing translators or Spanish-speaking health care providers. Mexican American clients may be fairly fluent in English; yet when exposed to treatment plans in technical language, they may not comply with the regimen because of miscommunication or terminology.

Religion is often an important cultural factor affecting health beliefs and practices. Many Mexican Americans are Catholic and turn to religious practices to overcome illness. Folk cures often include prayers before treatment begins (Kay, 1977; Spector, 1985; Kay and Yoder, 1987).

Health is viewed as harmonious relations within the social and spiritual realms. Disrupting social relations or breaking cultural rules is believed to have a negative effect on an individual's mental and physical well-being (Madsen, 1964; Mardiros, 1989). Rubel (1966) and Trotter and Chavira (1981) noted that Mexican Americans structure folk illness concepts into two major categories: (1) *males naturales* (natural illnesses) and (2) *mal puesto* (the supernatural or bewitchment). The first category includes four prominent folk syndromes: *molera caida* (fallen fontanel), *empacho* (indigestion infection), *mal ojo* (evil eye), and *susto* (fright); the second category includes such disorders as *brujeria* (witchcraft). Belief in mal puesto is declining, and it is generally considered only after several other diagnoses have been tried and treatment has been unsuccessful (Kay et al., 1988; Mardiros, 1989; Trotter et al., 1989).

A wide variety of folk practitioners may be used by Mexican Americans including *curanderos* (folk healers), *sobadoras* (masseuses), and *parteras* (lay midwives). An individual is usually referred to these folk practitioners by a family member, relative, or friend (Trotter and Chavira, 1981).

Mexican Americans acknowledge folk concepts of illness and also a number of categories of scientifically recognized diseases. However, recognition does not necessarily imply acceptance of scientific causes of disease. The cause may still be attributed to a lack of harmonious relations (Kay, 1977). Folk or scientific beliefs may be selectively chosen depending on factors such as the nature of the illness or the ability of folk or scientific treatment to produce a satisfactory outcome. Kay indicated that curanderos refer individuals to biomedical practitioners for serious illness, while often encouraging treatment for folk illnesses alternately by traditional or scientific means.

Nurses should elicit the client's view of the illness and recognize that many Mexican Americans have their own culturally derived concepts and interpretations about specific health problems. Denial of folk disorders by health professionals only reinforces the belief that these disorders lie outside scientific medicine's competence. Thus the client is encouraged to continue other forms of treatment. Folk medicine continues to exist because it satisfies health needs of the Mexican American community. One of the reasons for the continued existence of *curanderos* is their use of the family as a support system (Trotter and Chavira, 1981; Kay et al., 1988; Trotter et al., 1989).

Identifying cultural patterns is important in collecting data for planning nursing care. It is essential that the community health nurse be familiar with and understand the various cultural factors that may influence the health beliefs and practices of Mexican Americans and that may determine their acceptance or rejection of health care services.

Middle Eastern–Arab Americans

Only recently have Arabs immigrated to the United States in significant numbers. There are between 2 and 3 million permanent and temporary Arab residents in the United States (Lipson and Meleis, 1985). Arab identity is characterized by the use of the Arabic language and practice of the Islamic religion. They share the values, customs, and beliefs of the Arab culture.

Social properties of the Arab culture that are of interest to health care providers have been described by Meleis (1981), Meleis and Sorrell (1981) and Lipson and Meleis (1985). Affiliation with family enables an Arab American to cope satisfactorily with daily events and/or life crises. Arab Americans usually do not seek advice but feel that help should be offered. Visiting between family members is viewed as a social obligation during illness and other significant life events. The nurse should keep this in mind in regard to hospital visitation.

Western medicine is usually highly valued even though the "will of God," the "evil eye," and hot and cold shifts in temperature may be used to explain certain diseases. An effective cure is expected of the health care system, but Arab Americans prefer to receive personal care from their families. Many believe that the more intrusive the procedure, the better the chance for recovery.

Arab Americans tend to give as little information as possible about themselves and their families to strangers. They may be concerned about the personal nature of questions that might appear routine to others. They may view the nurse's questions about illness as intrusive.

Arab society is oriented to the present, and many believe that planning for the future may defy God's will. Arab American women tend not to plan ahead for labor, delivery, and the new baby. Lack of planning should not be interpreted as maternal disinterest. Their values concerning planning and prevention make it difficult for some Arab Americans to use contraceptives. When birth control is practiced, Arab American women are most likely to prefer intrauterine devices because of the value placed on intrusive treatment.

Arab American women usually dress conservatively. Since they value modesty, it is important to protect them from unnecessary exposure. Topics related to sex and reproduction are discussed with female relatives and friends but not with men or strangers. "Extreme tact needs to be exercised when involving the wife in any discussion without the husband . . . he can be employed to enhance the compliance of the family in all areas of health care including contraception" (Meleis and Sorrell, 1981, p. 176).

Like any profile, this description of Arab Americans does not fit any individual exactly but broadly applies to some degree. Meleis (1981, p. 1183) offers an important caveat: "The line between individualizing care based on cultural diversity and stereotyping is a very fine one."

Native Americans (American Indians)

As defined in the 1980 census, the largest concentrations of Native American populations in the United States were in California (201,489) and Oklahoma (169,450). Two other states, Arizona and New Mexico, had 152,145 and 107,481 Native American residents, respectively. Alaska, North Carolina, South Dakota, New York, Montana, Washington, and Minnesota are other states with large numbers of Native Americans (U.S. Congress, Office of Technology Assessment, 1986).

Providing effective health care to Native Americans is complicated by the fact that each nation or tribe has its own language, religion, and belief system regarding health and illness and its treatment. There are also variations in geography, distribution of wealth, and social organization. What is effective among one group may not be among another group (Vogel, 1970). The community health nurse must fit traditional customs into effective preventive health care. The nurse must be aware that individual Native Americans range from those uneducated in Anglo ways to those well educated in their own and Anglo cultures. The nurse needs to determine the client's level of knowledge.

The Native American family is frequently an extended family that includes several households. In addition, formal religious ceremonies can render other individuals as parental equivalents in the family network. Grandparents are family leaders, and age increases one's status. The family is important during periods of crises, when family members serve as sources of support and security. The family structure has implications for the community health nurse, since family members need to be included in actively caring for the client (Primeaux and Henderson, 1981).

Religion, pervasive in Native American life, is integrated into the lifestyle and interpretation of life. Traditional healing ceremonies are ritualistic ways to handle illness and deaths. Some rituals may be performed by the family; others require the services of a traditional specialist (Primeaux and Henderson, 1981). It is important for the community health nurse to recognize that Native Americans' health beliefs and practices today are a combination of Western medicine and traditional religious practices. Even though Anglo physicians and hospitals have been made available to Native Americans on reservations, traditional methods are still employed to treat illnesses and are sometimes incorporated into the modern referral system. For example, a Navajo nursing student related an incident about her mother-in-law who lives on the Navajo reservation. A physician diagnosed the woman as having breast cancer, based on positive mammography and a biopsy. Surgery was recommended (radical mastectomy), but her mother-in-law refused. Instead she went to a medicine man who "sucked out" the inflicting cause. The mother-in-law still returns to the physician for periodic checks that include mammography. The student stated that her mother-in-law was still well, but the physician remains appalled by this outcome, which included no further problems.

Statistics for 1985 indicated that the infant mortality rate for Native Americans had fallen to 9.3 per 1000 live births. The rate was 7% lower than the United States "All Races" rate for 1985, which was 10.4 (Indian Health Service, 1989). Although the Indian Health Service has been successful in reducing infant mortality in the general Native American population in the United States, those living in urban areas have not been part of the success story. Infant mortality rates for urban Native Americans in Arizona, at 14 deaths per 1000 live births, are 60% higher than the Surgeon General's 1990 objective for the nation, which is 9 deaths per 1000 live births (American Indian Health Care Association, 1989).

Infant mortality is influenced by the use of prenatal care, birth weight of the infant, feeding patterns, nutritional status of the infant and mother, and pregnancy complications. Improvements in the future will probably depend upon better living conditions and improved socioeconomic status rather than improved medical care (Oakland and Kane, 1973).

Knowledge of health beliefs and practices assists the community health nurse in the management of the individual client and in the planning of health care for specific cultural groups. Clients may use a variety of services and simultaneously switch from traditional to Western scientific medicine or other forms of practice. As illustrated in the example about the nursing student's mother-in-law, there is a strong tendency to accept modern medicine, but at the same time there are pragmatic reasons to use traditional practitioners.

Refugee and Immigrant Populations

New immigrants are a growing segment of the American population. These individuals are first-generation immigrants and therefore have not been acculturated to prevailing American norms of health belief or behavior.

Social factors such as settlement patterns, communication networks, social class, and education help immigrants and refugees to maintain their cultural traditions. In addition, most have their own community churches, stores, newspapers, physicians, and folk healers. Settling in an area with others of the same origin assists immigrants in adapting to new demands and assures that they have someone to call on during illness or other crises. An individual's social class, education, and residential background also help to predict health practices. All of these factors tend to discourage immigrants from seeking Western health care. Fear of disease and past illness experience may also inhibit seeking treatment.

Immigrants often initially experience medical culture conflict when their expression and interpretation of discomfort conflicts with that of current Western medical practice. Most health care professionals cannot learn all the folk health care of their client groups. Without a holistic view of the immigrant or refugee culture, health professionals find themselves confronted with what appears to be strange and curious notions held by the clients. They begin to overgeneralize and think that all individuals in this group are alike; for example, "Vietnamese have a present-time orientation." This leads to stereotyping, which can decrease the quality of care. The provider may give the Vietnamese immediate care to treat the illness but may not be inclined to plan for the prevention of future problems.

The community health nurse should evaluate each person to determine the individual needs and the degree to which the client adheres to cultural standards of health behavior. The nurse must recognize that the behavior of all members of a specific ethnic group is not necessarily uniform and may vary according to factors such as income, occupation, education, length of time since immigration, and experiences with health care services.

Southeast Asian Refugees

Since 1975, over half a million persons from Vietnam, Cambodia, and Laos have entered the United States. There is much variation among these individuals based on socio-economic factors such as ethnic group membership, socioeconomic status, geographical residence, gender, and degree of urbanization (Montero, 1978; Lipson and Meleis, 1989).

One ethnic group, the Hmong, are sufficiently similar to the other refugee groups from Southeast Asia to serve as a model for discussion. The Hmong in Southeast Asia are members of a large group found in China, North Vietnam, Thailand, and Laos. Non-refugee Hmong in Southeast Asia have very high birth rates, large extended family households, and relatively low infant and crude mortality rates. The Hmong in the United States have posed special problems because of minimal use of health care services and psychiatric problems associated with refugee migration (Westermeyer et al., 1983). Their low utilization of health services may be caused by difficulties in communicating with American providers. Migration may change family and network structures, and this disruption or loss of social support systems may have adverse effects on health. The Hmong in the United States can be expected to face challenges to their belief that spirits cause illness, since this belief conflicts with modern medical understanding of illness (Kunstadter, 1985). This affects their use of health services and their health.

The community health nurse must communicate a genuine respect for the Hmong cultural heritage and recognize this group's dependence on folk medicine. Often the Hmong do not distinguish between religion and medicine and, although not opposed to Western medicine, they prefer traditional folk medicines. The nurse will need to recognize her own folk beliefs, ethnocentrism, and assumptions about refugees and to be alert to culturally diverse expectations and other significant clues concerning how health care might be better directed.

POVERTY

There is no agreement about how *poverty* should be defined or measured; in fact, no one really knows the extent of poverty in the United States. Any attempt at defining and measuring poverty must consider numerous variables. The federal government's poverty standards are defined and measured strictly in terms of income; that is, an absolute standard is used. Some have agreed that poverty should be defined in relative terms, by accepted standards of what human life requires.

Absolute and Relative Standards

An *absolute standard* attempts to define some basic set of resources necessary for adequate existence. The federal government defines poverty using as the official measure an absolute standard, the Social Security Administration (SSA) standard. This standard varies by place of residence, family size, and gender of the family head. The basis for the standard is the cost of food. Increases in the SSA poverty standard are based on the consumer price index. The consumer price index reflects, among other factors, current market prices for food as determined by the United States Depart-

ment of Agriculture. (See Chapter 4 for a discussion of the Consumer Price Index.)

A *relative standard* attempts to define poverty in terms of the median standard of living in a society. Townsend (1974, p. 15) stated that "Individuals, families and groups . . . can be said to be in poverty when they lack the resources to obtain the type of diets, participate in activities, and have the living conditions and amenities which are customary, or are at least widely encouraged or approved, in the societies to which they belong." If a relative standard were to be used, the poor might be defined as those who earn 50% of the median income for their family size. For example, in 1988 the median income for four-person families was $27,230. Any four-person family with an income less than $13,615 would be considered poor by this standard. This would raise the poverty level for a four-person family to $1,523 over the estimated 1988 SSA standard of $12,092, significantly increasing the poverty count. A major attraction of the relative standard is that it more clearly delineates the overall distribution of wealth in the United States.

Health and welfare programs for the poor are based on absolute standards, which are misleading because they do not consider factors such as access to basic services, regional variations, and assets. As a result, many of the deserving poor do not receive assistance. The working poor have incomes too high to be considered eligible for public assistance programs; yet because of inflation, common needs such as food and health care are inaccessible.

Culture of Poverty

In *The Children of Sanchez* (1961) and *La Vida* (1966), Oscar Lewis formulated the concept "culture of poverty." The main idea of this concept is that poverty is not merely economic deprivation but also entails personality traits, some of which are psychologically compensatory and rewarding. Like other aspects of culture, such elements are passed from generation to generation through enculturation. Many of the poor have beliefs, values, and lifestyles that do not reflect an adjustment to low income but an ingrained way of life that is self-perpetuating and reinforced by each new generation. Lewis (1968) noted that the socioeconomic interests and values of the larger society perpetuate poverty by focusing on changing poor people rather than the society as a whole. He contended that these lifestyles and the ways the poor perceive the world and their place in it must be abolished if poverty is to be eradicated. This has led to solutions which demand no major changes in the structure of inequality or distribution of resources. Reforms necessary to remedy poverty must involve a larger part of society than just the poor alone, and these reforms can be implemented only by forces greater than those available to poor people (Valentine, 1971; Roby, 1974).

Numerous critics have disagreed with Lewis' concept. Valentine disagrees with the causes of behavior, the reasons for the deprivation of the poor, and the direction that social policies should take. He and other critics of the concept (Kahn, 1969; Leacock, 1971; Harrington, 1984) fear that those unsympathetic to the poor will use the concept to withdraw aid or institute programs that will require some type of menial work to receive aid.

There are dangers associated with the culture of poverty concept. For example, if the existence of a distinct and self-perpetuating culture of poverty were widely accepted, public funds might be diverted from programs to create more jobs, more housing, and better schools to those for more social work and re-education of a psychiatric nature. Moreover, the culture of poverty concept serves to sustain the complacency of the more affluent by shifting the blame away from themselves and onto the shoulders of the poor. Another danger associated with the concept is that if the poor can be characterized as disorganized, deviant, or even sick, it would be foolhardy to permit them to share in decisions about the allocation of funds or to give them control over their lives.

However, the culture of poverty may be a valuable concept. For example, the controversy and research about the concept may help define the range of values for the poor, the functions of their specific values, and in what situations they emerge. Attention to lifestyles can reveal how and why certain groups are excluded from the mainstream and are unable to obtain adequate services. The insight gained from this can guide health care planners and others to restructure health care to make it equally available to the poor.

Poverty and Health

There is a direct relation between poverty and health. It has long been recognized that economic deprivation and health status are intertwined. For example, in 1828 Villerme showed that mortality in France was closely linked to the living conditions of different social classes (Rosen, 1963).

In the early twentieth century the health of the poor was deplorable. Campaigns demanded government action to eliminate or ameliorate the consequences of poverty with respect to health.

By the 1960s it was evident that poverty and its attendant ills had not disappeared. With the passage of the Economic Opportunity Act in 1964, the United States declared war on poverty and rediscovered the poor. In 1965 Congress enacted the Medicare and Medicaid programs.

According to most indicators the health status of rural people is poor, particularly when contrasted with the health of the total population. The death rates of infants and mothers are significantly higher in rural areas than in urban areas. Additionally, work-related disability rates are high in rural areas because of accidents resulting from hazardous work environments (Health Status in Rural America, 1977). Most sparsely settled rural areas lack medical personnel and resources as well as strong lobbies in special interest areas. The poor are unlikely to use preventive health care because of more pressing priorities (Koos, 1954; Bauwens, 1977; Orque et al., 1983).

Although the health problems of the general rural populations are severe, they are even more critical for migrant farm workers. Migrant workers suffer a higher rate of acute and chronic illness than the majority of Americans (Barrett et al., 1980; O'Brien, 1982; Johnston, 1985). The accident rate among children of migrants is high because there is little supervision while the parents are working in the fields. Lack of sanitary facilities and overcrowding contribute to the spread of infectious diseases. Housing is frequently improvised and inadequate. The migratory conditions and state of poverty reduce the migrants' ability to seek health care. These conditions account for the greater probability of their acquiring diseases. As a rule, poor people get sick more often and stay sick longer because of inadequate health maintenance, lack of prevention, poor nutrition, and limited access to adequate health services.

Because of this vulnerability, community health programs should ideally focus attention on populations in which there are high incidences of chronic and communicable diseases, high infant death rates, high birth rates, environmental hazards, and multiple social problems. The community health nurse needs to involve the affected individuals in the planning and implementation of such programs. The programs should consider social and cultural factors, community values, and local resources. To meet these needs, health programs may encounter difficulties for at least four reasons:

1. The methods that are used may have to be adapted or specially designed to reach the individuals.
2. The individuals may be geographically remote from health centers, adding the problems of transportation.
3. The individuals may have little political power and therefore little influence on the allocation of resources.
4. The values held by the individuals may be different from those of the program planners and administrators, and setting objectives and appraising results of the programs may have to follow unique criteria.

When working with the poor, nurses need to be able to identify the strengths and weaknesses of poor clients without imposing their own values. Facts regarding poverty lifestyles need to be distinguished from myth and prejudice. The nurse must consider numerous questions. For instance, are the values of the poor client perceived as different from the nurse's? If so, how do the values differ? Does the nurse expect the poor client to conform to his/her values? What does the client expect of the nurse as a health professional? This value clarification enables nurses to examine their own attitudes with respect to poor clients.

SOCIOCULTURAL ASSESSMENT

The material in this section is meant to assist nurses to be aware of and sensitive to sociocultural factors that affect a health care system. The nurse must be aware of sociocultural factors when assessing a community, family, and individual. Sociocultural assessment provides a data base from which the nurse can obtain an idea of the client's attitudes, values, and beliefs about the world. If culture provides standards for behavior, then nurses should assess their own culture of health care, both from the viewpoint of the culture of origin (what they were taught to believe when growing up) and from that of the system into which they have been socialized. Nurses need to explore values, since values form one's basis for behavior. What were the nurse's earliest experiences with deviations from health? Which symptoms were the nurse taught to notice and attend to?

Assessment tools or guides may be geared to a broad area (e.g., mental health) or have a narrow focus specific to particular practices (e.g., nutrition). A number of sociocultural assessment guides for nurses are available.* Brown-lee (1978) has identified several relevant factors to guide the nurse in the assessment of community, family, and/or individual sociocultural factors.

Community Sociocultural Factors

The following is a list of pertinent or sociocultural factors to be assessed in the community:

1. Existing influences that divide people into groups within the community, such as ethnicity, religion, social class, occupation, place of residence, language, education, sex, race, and age
2. Conditions that lead to social conflict and/or social cohesion
3. Attitudes toward minority groups, youth and the elderly, and males and females and age and gender groups
4. Division of the community into neighborhoods or districts and the characteristics of these
5. Formal and informal channels of communication between health programs and the community
6. Barriers that may be the result of differences in cultural beliefs and practices
7. Political orientation in the community (attitudes toward authority and its use in health problems)
8. Patterns of migration either in or out of a community and their effect on health care services
9. Relation of religion and medicine within the community (who and what causes various illnesses and how they can be prevented)
10. Types of diseases or illnesses thought by various members of the community to exist (culture-specific conditions, such as illnesses caused by hot and cold imbalances or diseases of magical origin)

Family and/or Individual Sociocultural Factors

When assessing families or individuals, the community health nurse needs to be aware of the following:

1. Typical family households, roles played by family members and kinship groups, and patterns of residence
2. Events, rituals, and ceremonies considered important within the life cycle, such as birth, baptism, puberty, marriage, and death
3. The health beliefs and values of the family members and the social meaning attached to wellness and illness
   a. Beliefs concerning body organs and/or systems and how they function
   b. Particular methods used to help maintain health, such as hygienic and self-care practices
   c. Attitudes toward immunizations, screening tests, and other preventive health measures
   d. Beliefs and practices surrounding conception, pregnancy, childbirth, lactation, and rearing of children
   e. Attitudes toward mental illness, deformities, and death and dying
4. The person(s) in a family responsible for various health-related decisions, such as what to do when ill, where to go, who to see, and what advice to follow
5. Health topics that may be sensitive or taboo to the client
6. Possible conflicts between family health beliefs and practices and the teachings and practices of an established health program
7. Beliefs, rules, and preferences or prejudices concerning food, such as those believed to cause or cure illness
8. Culturally appropriate ways to enter and leave situations, including greetings, farewells, and convenient hours to make a home visit

Sociocultural assessment of the community, family, or individual includes all the preceding factors. The community health nurse needs to spend time to learn the culture before beginning any efforts at intervention or change. Specific families and individuals do not always reflect the "typical" cultural pattern. The nurse must remain sensitive to individual variations.

The nurse should also assess cultural standards about appropriate roles for participants in a health care system. How does the nurse feel about the use of medical doctors, osteopaths, chiropractors, Christian Science practitioners, psychologists? What about faith healers and folk curers? The client is also expected to cooperate with treatment recommendations. What constitutes "cooperation" is, however, culturally determined. Which aspects of care and treatment are the responsibility of the client? Should the client question health care management or is that disrespectful?

Assessment in the nursing process is done to identify the client's needs. Culture affects the way these needs are perceived, understood, and attended to. Social factors such as age, education, income, religion, generation removed from mother country, and opportunities for obtaining health care all influence health beliefs and practices. Sociocultural assessment leads to relevant nursing diagnoses, planning, and interventions. An intervention may be adapted to meet the client's expectations, or an acceptable compromise for treatment may be necessary. Not every element of culture needs to be included in any one assessment; sociocultural factors will vary in importance based on the particular situation.

GUIDELINES FOR CULTURALLY APPROPRIATE HEALTH CARE

Modern Western medicine considers the biomedical model to be the best, if not the only, view of disease. This cultural conditioning of health professionals leads to depreciation or even denial of the client's view. To compensate for this inherent bias, nurses should elicit clients' interpretations of their health problems.

Client's Explanatory Model

Kleinman (1980) developed the client explanatory model. In this model an individual pulls together various beliefs and applies them to an illness to provide a meaningful explanation of the events surrounding the illness and to choose an

---

*Branch and Paxton, 1976; Leininger, 1976; Kay, 1977; Brownlee, 1978; Block, 1983; Orque, 1983; Tripp-Reimer, et al., 1984; Steiger and Lipson, 1985.

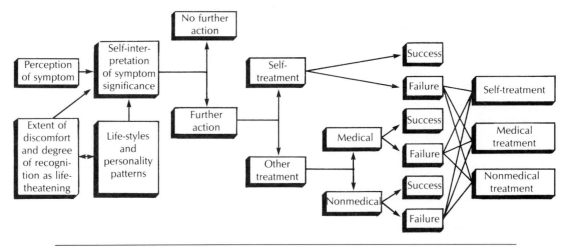

FIGURE 6-4

Process of symptom management. *(From Jackson, J.J.: Urban black Americans. In Harwood, A.I., editor: Ethnicity and medical care, Cambridge, Mass., 1981, Harvard University Press. Reprinted by permission.)*

appropriate course of action. The client's model deals with one or more of the same five questions for illness as used in the medical model: (1) etiology, (2) onset of symptoms, (3) pathophysiology, (4) course of illness, and (5) treatment. Usually the client's model is more concrete, is not completely articulated, and may be inconsistent and based on erroneous evaluation of evidence. "Nonetheless, they [clients' models] are comparable to clinical models . . . as attempts to explain clinical phenomena" (Kleinman et al., 1978, p. 256). The client's model reflects cultural beliefs, social class, education, occupation, religious affiliation, and past experience with illness and health care.

Clients often hesitate to disclose their models to health professionals. Once clients are assured that the health care provider is genuinely interested, their models can usually be elicited by the nurse with a few direct questions. The following set of questions will help elicit the client's explanation of the illness (Kleinman et al., 1978, p. 256):

1. What do you think caused your problem?
2. Why do you think it started when it did?
3. What do you think your sickness does to you? How does it work?
4. How severe is your sickness? Will it have a short or long course?
5. What kind of treatment do you think you should receive?

Client's Perception of Symptoms

A model developed by Jackson (1981) illustrates the process that a client might use from the initial self-perception of illness symptoms to treatment, whether that treatment is self-care, medical, or non-medical (Figure 6-4). The model begins with the perception of a symptom, which implies that the individual has identified that something is wrong. The individual then evaluates the significance of the symptom. Many factors influence the interpretative process, such as cultural beliefs and values, extent of discomfort, and previous experience with illness. Jackson (1981) believes that the level of income, social class, education, and disruption

of activity are major variables determining the client's process of symptom management. Based on the interpretation, the client may or may not initiate further action and may choose self-treatment or treatment by others and either medical or nonmedical treatment. The client then makes a decision about the success or failure of the selected treatment. If the treatment is deemed a failure, the client may vacillate among alternative sources of health care or simultaneously use two or more alternatives.

Cultural Health Practices

Cultural health practices may be considered as efficacious, neutral, or dysfunctional (Pillsbury, 1982). Efficacious practices are recognized by Western medicine as being beneficial to health even though they may be very different from scientific practices. Beneficial practices should be actively encouraged by community health nurses, although they may seem foreign. A treatment strategy that conforms to the client's own beliefs has a better chance of success. For example, cultural beliefs about the efficacy of herbal teas must be considered by the community health nurse, since some are therapeutic (dehydration can be treated with tea). Treatment with tea may be as efficacious as water. Another example is the preference of some cultural groups to kneel during childbirth rather than to lie down. (Cominsky, 1977).

Neutral (harmless) practices are of no significance one way or the other to the health of the individual. They may be considered unimportant by the health professional, but for the individual the health practices may be linked with beliefs that are closely integrated into everyday behavior. Examples of neutral practices include "the ritual disposal of the placenta and cord, avoidance of sexual activity during various stages of pregnancy, culturally prescribed hygiene practices and avoidance of exposure during a lunar eclipse" (Johnston, 1980, p. 13). Even though these practices do not require intervention by the practitioner, the nurses should respect their significance and meaning to the individual.

In all cultures there are practices that are dysfunctional

or harmful from a health point of view. In Western countries the excessive use of sugar and overrefined flour is partially responsible for the high incidence of dental caries and obesity. Health education should be focused on dysfunctional or harmful health practices. Efforts should be made to assist clients to modify harmful practices.

In addition to culturally specific health care practices, individuals may turn to alternative health practitioners for a variety of reasons. Harwood (1981) listed the following general reasons why individuals might use alternative healers: (1) lack of availability and accessibility of mainstream health services, (2) lack of satisfaction with treatment, (3) lack of trust in the ability of Western medical practitioners to effectively treat psychosocial problems, and (4) lack of knowledge on the part of Western medical practitioners in the treatment of culture-bound syndromes.

In many cases alternative healers complement the delivery of mainstream health care services. Often they are more available and accessible than Western health care providers. They are familiar with culture-bound syndromes and cultural traditions. In addition, they often establish warm relations with clients and their families. Based on the discussion of culture and cultural differences, principles for nursing practice can be identified for application in clinical practice (Table 6-1).

CLINICAL APPLICATION

Ella Johnson is a 56-year-old divorced black woman who was recently discharged from the hospital following an acute hypertensive crisis. She has been referred to the community health nurse for health maintenance and prevention of future hypertensive problems. The physician has prescribed an antihypertensive drug and a low sodium diet. Ms. Easton, a student nurse, has been assigned to visit Mrs. Johnson. The nurse prepares for the home visit by reading literature about blacks and their health and illness practices. During the home visit the nurse learns that Mrs. Johnson believes her "high blood" is due to "impurities" that have entered her body. She tells the nurse that avoiding salt and taking medicines will help her get well. She correctly describes how the prescribed drug will help her. She tells the nurse, "Don't overeat, don't drink too much, don't overwork— you must protect your body."

The nurse is surprised that Mrs. Johnson does not "fit" some of the information that she obtained from her readings about the black client in the health care system.

1. Based on the information above, what additional assessment data should be collected by the nurse during the first home visit?
2. What principles for culturally appropriate care must be considered?

TABLE 6-1

Principles for providing culturally appropriate nursing care

Principle	Intervention
Culture affects clients' interpretations of health, illness, and health care.	Ask clients nonjudgmental questions concerning their ideas about health and illness.
Culture may be a source of discrepancy between clients' and health providers' concepts of health or illness.	Clarify with clients their meaning of terms used to label an illness or symptoms.
	Identify discrepancies.
Cultural values affect clients' use of the health care system.	Use culturally preferred treatment interventions when possible.

3. How can the nurse know what care will be perceived to be appropriate?
4. Analyze the assessment data using Kleinman's explanatory model.

SUMMARY

Sociocultural variables related to health care have been discussed. The premise that health care is based not only on knowledge of physical causes but also on sociocultural influences has been introduced. Culture has been defined as a set of rules that help people act appropriately. The following cultural concepts have been discussed: holism, culture change, enculturation, stereotypes, and cultural values.

The mobility of people and their cultural diversity increase the likelihood that nurses will come in contact with a variety of cultural lifestyles and traditions. Often nurses must provide care for individuals from different cultural groups. This chapter has explored cultural aspects in the following areas: ethnic collectivity, cultural shock, communication patterns, personal space and contact, and cultural views of health and illness. Diverse cultures of the United States, namely Asian, African-American, Mexican, Arab and Native American, have been presented as examples to provide cultural background data to assist nurses in providing culturally relevant nursing care. Poverty has been addressed from the economic, psychological, and cultural perspective, and the reciprocal relation between poverty and health has been discussed.

KEY CONCEPTS

Culture enables us to interpret our surroundings and the actions of people around us and to behave in appropriate ways.

Some anthropologists conceive of culture as a set of rules providing the individual with a means for behaving and interpreting the behavior of others.

The concept of holism requires that human behavior not be isolated from the context in which it occurs and that the culture is best viewed and analyzed as a whole.

Culture is never static but is in a constant process of adding or deleting elements.

Enculturation is the process of acquiring knowledge and internalizing values; through this process persons achieve competence in their own culture.

Because we look at the world from our own particular cultural viewpoint, we often believe our way is best; such a viewpoint is called "ethnocentrism." It is important for nurses not to consider their own way as best and other people's ideas as ignorant or inferior.

Stereotypes are exaggerated beliefs and images that are popularly depicted in the mass media and folklore. Usually these images are false; they obscure important differences among members of a group and exaggerate those between groups.

Cultural values are the prevailing and persistent guides influencing thinking and actions of people.

People who have been reared in an "ethnic collectivity" (a shared group with common origins, a sense of identity, and shared standards for behavior) often acquire from that experience cultural norms that determine the thought and behavior of individual members.

"Cultural shock" is one of the effects of working with individuals from different cultural backgrounds. Nurses can reduce cultural shock by knowing about the different cultural groups with whom they are working.

Poverty may be defined in absolute or relative terms. An absolute standard attempts to define some basic set of resources necessary for adequate existence. A relative standard attempts to define poverty in terms of the median standard of living in a society.

There is a direct relationship between poverty and health. It has long been recognized that economic deprivation and health status are intertwined.

The mobility of the population and its cultural diversity increase the likelihood that nurses will come in contact with a variety of cultural life-styles and traditions.

LEARNING ACTIVITIES

1. Define culture and how it relates to health and illness behavior.

2. Identify concepts relevant to culture and health care.

3. Before asking clients questions that have cultural relevance, ask yourself the same question about your own culture.

4. Recognize the variety of influences that cultural differences have on the interpretation of health and illness.

5. Identify factors that produce diversity in health-seeking behavior between and within ethnic groups.

6. Describe the nature of poverty and its effect on health status and health behavior.

7. Assess sociocultural factors and their impact on health care for the individual, family, and community.

BIBLIOGRAPHY

American Indian Health Care Association: Assessment of the health care needs of the urban Indian population in the state of Arizona, A.I.H.C.A., St. Paul, Minnesota, 1989.

Barrett SE, Gillespie J, and Call RL: Migrant health revisited, Am J Public Health 70(10): 1092-1094, 1980.

Bauwens EE: Medical beliefs and practices among lower-income Anglos. In Spicer EH, editor: Ethnic medicine in the Southwest, Tucson, 1977, University of Arizona Press.

Benedict R: Patterns of culture, Boston, 1934, Houghton Mifflin Co.

Berkanovic E and Reeder LG: Ethnic, economic, and social psychological factors in the source of medical care, Soc Prob 21:246-259, 1973.

Block B: Block's assessment guide for ethnic/cultural variations. In Orque MS, Block B, and Monrroy LS, editors: Ethnic nursing care, St. Louis, 1983, The CV Mosby Co.

Branch MF and Paxton PP: Providing safe nursing care for ethnic people of color, New York, 1976, Appleton-Century-Crofts.

Brownlee AT: Community, culture, and care, St. Louis, 1978, The CV Mosby Co.

Bullough VL and Bullough B: Health care for the other Americans, New York, 1982, Appleton-Century-Crofts.

Calhoun MA: Providing health care to Vietnamese in America: what practitioners need to know, Home Healthcare Nurse 4(5):14-22, May 1986.

Chrisman NJ: The health seeking process, Cult Med Psychiatry 1:351-377, 1977.

Chrisman NJ and Kleinman A: Popular health care, social networks, and cultural meanings: the orientation of medical anthropology. In Handbook of Health, Health Care, and the Health Professions, New York, 1983, The Free Press.

Clark M: Health in the Mexican-American culture, Berkeley, 1970, University of California Press.

Cominsky S: Childbirth and midwifery on a Guatemalan finca, Med Anthropol 1:94, 1977.

Currer C and Stacey M, editors: Concepts of health, illness, and disease, Leamington, 1986, Berg Publishers.

DeMigul JM: A framework for the study of national health systems, Inquiry 12(2):10-24, June 1975.

Dohrenwend BP: Sociocultural and social-psychological factors in the genesis of mental disorders. J Health Soc Behav 16:365-392, 1975.

Dohrenwend BP and Dohrenwend BS: Social status and psychological disorder: a causal inquiry, New York, 1969, John Wiley & Sons, Inc.

Dohrenwend BS and Dohrenwend BP: Stressful life events: their nature and effects, New York, 1974, John Wiley & Sons, Inc.

Dunham HW: Community and schizophrenia: an epidemiological analysis, Detroit, 1965, Wayne State University.

Elling RH: Socio-cultural influences on health and health care, New York, 1977, Springer Publishing Co., Inc.

Fabrega H: Medical anthropology. In Siegel BJ, editor: Biennial review of anthropology, Standard, Calif., 1971, Stanford University Press.

Foster GM: Relationships between theoretical and applied anthropology: a public health analysis, Hum Organization 11:5-16, 1952.

Fox R: The Indochinese: strategies for health survival, Intl J Soc Psych 30(4):285-291, 1984.

Geddes W: Migrants of the mountains: the cultural ecology of the Blue Miao (Hmong Njcca) of Thailand, Oxford, 1976, Clarendon Press.

Gevitz N, editor: Other healers, unorthodox medicine in America, Baltimore, 1988, Johns Hopkins Press.

Goodenough WH: Cooperation in change, New York, 1966, Russell Sage Foundation.

Greenblum J: Medical and health orientations of American Jews: a case of diminishing distinctiveness, Soc Sci Med 8:127-134, 1974.

Greene L and Johnston F: Social and biological predictors of nutritional status, growth, and development, New York, 1980, Academic Press, Inc.

Guttmacher S and Elinson J: Ethno-religious variation in perceptions of illness: the use of illness as an explanation for deviant behavior, Soc Sci Med 5:117-125, 1971.

Hall ET: The silent language, New York, 1959, Doubleday & Co., Inc.

Harrington M: The new American poverty, New York, 1984, Holt, Rinehart, and Winston.

Harrison G and Ritenbaugh C: Anthropology and nutrition: a perspective on two scientific subcultures, Fed Proc 4(11):2595-2600, Sept 1981.

Harwood A, editor: Ethnicity and medical care, Cambridge, Mass, 1981, Harvard University Press.

Hautman MA and Harrison JK: Health beliefs and practices in a middle-income Anglo-American neighborhood, Adv Nurs Sci 4(3):49-64, 1982.

Health status in rural America, Rural Health Report no. 1, Washington, DC, 1977, Rural America.

Helman CG: Culture, health, and illness, ed 2, Kent, England, 1990, Wright.

Henderson G and Primeaux M: Transcultural health care, Reading, Mass, 1981, Addison-Wesley Publishing Co, Inc.

Hoang GN and Erickson RV: Guidelines for providing medical care to Southeast Asian refugees, JAMA 248(6):710-714, 1982.

Hollander J: The abolition of poverty, Boston, 1914, Houghton Mifflin Co.

Hollingshead AB and Redlich FC: Social class and medical illness, New York, 1958, John Wiley & Sons, Inc.

Horn BM: Transcultural nursing and child-rearing of the Muckleshoot people. In Leininger M, editor: Transcultural nursing, New York, 1979, Masson International Nursing Publications.

Indian Health Service: Indian Health Service chart series tables, Office of Program Statistics, Rockville, Md, 1986.

Indian Health Service: Trends in Indian health 1989, Dept of Health and Human Services, Public Health Service, 1989.

Insel PM: Too close for comfort, Englewood Cliffs, NJ, 1978, Prentice-Hall, Inc.

Jackson JJ: Urban black Americans. In Harwood A, editor: Ethnicity and medical care, Cambridge, Mass, 1981, Harvard University.

Jelliffe DB: Child nutrition in developing countries, Washington, DC, 1969, U.S. Department of Health, Education and Welfare.

Johnston HL: Health for the nation's harvesters, Farmington Hills, Mich, 1985, National Migrant Workers Council, Inc.

Josephy AM, Jr: The Indian heritage of America, New York, 1969, Alfred A. Knopf, Inc.

Kahn AO: Studies in social policy and planning, New York, 1969, Russell Sage Foundation.

Kay MA: Health in the Mexican-American barrio. In Spicer EH, editor: Ethnic medicine in the southwest, Tucson, 1977, University of Arizona Press.

Kay MA, Tobias C, Ide B, Guernsey J, et al: The health and symptom care of Mexican-American widows, J Cross-Cultural Geron 3:197-208, 1988.

Kay MA and Yoder M: Hot and cold in women's ethnotherapeutics: the American-Mexican West, Soc Sci Med 25(4):347-355, 1987.

Keefe S and Padilla A: Chicano ethnicity, Albuquerque, 1987, University of New Mexico Press.

Kleinman A: Patients and healers in the context of culture, Berkeley, 1980, University of California Press.

Kleinman A, Eisenberg L, and Good B: Culture, illness and care, Ann Intern Med 88:251-258, 1978.

Kluckhohn C: The gifts of tongues. In Samover LA and Porter RE, editors: Intercultural communication: a reader, Belmont, Calif, 1972, Wadsworth, Inc.

Kniep-Hardy M and Burkhardt M: Nursing the Navajo, Am J Nurs 77:95-96, 1977.

Koos E: Health in Regionville, New York, 1954, Columbia University Press.

Kubricht DW and Clark JA: Foreign patients: a system for providing care, Nurs Outlook 30(1):55-57, Jan 1982.

Kunitz IJ and Levy JE: Navajos. In Harwood A, editor: Ethnicity and medical care, Cambridge, Mass, 1981, Harvard University Press.

Kunstadter P: Health of Hmong in Thailand: risk factors, morbidity and mortality in comparison with other ethnic groups, Cult Med Psychiatry 9(4):329-351, Dec 1985.

Laderman C: Commentary on E Szathmary and R Farrell: Glucose level, acculturation, and glycosylated hemoglobin: an example of biocultural interaction, Med Anth Quart 4(3):354-358, Sept 1990.

Leacock E: The culture of poverty: a critique, New York, 1971, Simon & Schuster.

Leininger M: Transcultural health care issues and conditions, Philadelphia, 1976, FA Davis Co.

Lewis O: The children of Sanchez, New York, 1961, Random House, Inc.

Lewis O: La Vida, New York, 1966, Random House, Inc.

Lewis O: A study of slum culture, New York, 1968, Random House, Inc.

Lipson J and Meleis A: Culturally appropriate care: the case of immigrants, Top Clin Nurs 7(3):48-56, 1985.

Lipson J and Meleis A: Methodological issues in research with immigrants. In Morse J, editor: Cross-cultural nursing, New York, 1989, Gordon and Breach Science Publishers, Inc.

Madsen M: The Mexican-Americans of south Texas, New York, 1964, Holt, Rinehart & Winston General Book.

Mardiros M: Conception of childhood disability among Mexican-American parents. In Morse J, editor: Cross-cultural nursing, New York, 1989, Gordon and Breach Science Publishers, Inc.

Markides K and Coreil J: The health of Hispanics in the southwestern United States, Public Health Rep 101(3):253-265, 1986.

Mechanic D: Illness and cure. In Kosa J, Antonovsky A, and Zola I, editors: Poverty and health: a sociological analysis, Cambridge, Mass, 1969, Harvard University Press.

Meisenhelder JB: Boundaries of personal space, Image 14(1):16-19, Feb-March 1982.

Meleis AI: The Arab American in the health care system, Am J Nurs 81:1180-1183, 1981.

Meleis AI and Sorrell L: Arab American women and their birth experiences, Am J Matern Child Nurs 6:171-176, 1981.

Melnyk KA: Barriers: a critical review of recent literature, Nurs Res 37(4):196-201, 1988.

Moccia P and Mason DJ: Poverty trends: implications for nursing, Nurs Outlook 34(1):20-24, Jan/Feb 1986.

Montero D: The Vietnamese refugees in America: patterns of socioeconomic adaptation and assimilation, College Park, MD, 1978, Institute of Urban Studies, University of Maryland.

Muecke M: Caring for Southeastern Asian refugee patients in the USA, Am J Public Health 73:431-437, 1983.

National Center for Health Statistics: Advance report of final mortality statistics, monthly vital statistics report, 38(5), Hyattsville, Md, 1989, Public Health Service.

National Center for Health Statistics: Vital statistics of the United States, 1977, vol II, Mortality, Part A, Hyattsville, MD, 1981, US Government Printing Office.

Nichter M: Anthropology and international health, Norwell, Mass, 1989, Kluwer Academic Publishers.

O'Brien ME: Pragmatic survivalism: behavior patterns affecting low-level wellness among minority group members, Adv Nurs Sc 4(3):13-26, April 1982.

Oakland L and Kane RL: The working mother and child neglect on the Navajo reservation, Pediatrics 51:849-853, 1973.

Orque MS: Orque's ethnic/cultural system: a framework for ethnic nursing care. In Orque, MS, Bloch B, and Monrroy LS, editors: Ethnic nursing care, St. Louis, 1983, The CV Mosby Co.

Pillsbury B: Doing the month: confinement and convalescence of Chinese women after childbirth. In Kay M, editor: Anthropology of human birth, Philadelphia, 1982, FA Davis Co.

Primeaux M and Henderson G: American Indian

patient care. In Henderson S and Primeaux M, editors: Transcultural health care, Philadelphia, 1981, FA Davis Co.

Quesada GM: Mexican Americans: Mexicans or Americans? Lubbock, Tex, 1973, Southwestern Council of Latin-American Studies.

Reinert BR: The health care beliefs and values of Mexican-Americans, Home Healthcare Nurse 4(5):23-31, May 1986.

Rosen G: The evaluation of social medicine. In Freeman HE, Levin S, and Reeder LB, editors: Handbook of medical sociology, Englewood Cliffs, NJ, 1963, Prentice-Hall, Inc.

Rubel A: Across the tracks: Mexican Americans in a Texas city, Austin, 1966, University of Texas Press.

Ruiz MCJ: Open-closed mindedness, intolerance of ambiguity and nursing faculty attitudes toward culturally different patients, Nurs Res 30(3):177-181, 1981.

Ryan W: Blaming the victim, New York, 1971, Pantheon Books.

Samora J: Conceptions of health and disease among Spanish-Americans, Am Cath Sociol Rev 22:314-323, 1961.

Saunders L: Cultural difference and medical care, New York, 1954, Russell Sage Foundation.

Simons R and Hughes C: The culture-bound syndrome, Dordrecht, 1985, D Reidel.

Snow LF: Popular medicine in a black neighborhood. In Spicer EH, editor: Ethnic medicine in the southwest, Tucson, 1977, University of Arizona Press.

Spector RE: Cultural diversity in health and ill-

ness, ed 2, Norwalk, 1985, Appleton-Century-Crofts.

Suchman EA: Sociomedical variations among ethnic groups, Am J Sociol 70:319-331, 1964.

Tien-Hyatt JI: Keying in on the unique care needs of Asian Clients, Nurs and Health Care 8(5):269-271, 1987.

Townsend P: Poverty as relative deprivation: resources and style of living. In Weaderburn D, editor: Poverty inequality and class structure, London, 1974, Cambridge University Press.

Townsend P and Davidson D, editors: Inequalities in health: the black report, Harmondsworth, 1982, Penguin Books, Inc.

Tripp-Reimer T: Barriers to health care: variations in interpretation of Appalachian client behavior by Appalachian and non-Appalachian health professionals, West J Nurs Res 4(2):179-191, 1982.

Tripp-Reimer T and Brink P: Cultural brokerage. In Bulechek GM and McCloskey JC, editors: Nursing interventions, treatments for nursing diagnosis, Philadelphia, 1985, WB Saunders.

Tripp-Reimer T, Brink P, and Saunders J: Cultural assessment: content and process, Nurs Outlook 32(2):78-82, March/April 1984.

Trotter RT and Chavira JA: Curanderismo: Mexican-American folk healing, Athens, 1981, The University of Georgia Press.

Trotter RT, Ortiz de Montellano B, and Logan M: Fallen fontanel in the American Southwest, Med Anthro 10:211-221, 1989.

U.S. Bureau of the Census: Statistical abstracts of the United States, 1989, Washington, DC, 1989, U.S. Government Printing Office.

U.S. Congress, Office of Technology Assessment: Indian health care, OTA-H-290, Washington, DC, 1986, U.S. Government Printing Office.

Valentine CA: Culture and poverty, Chicago, 1968, University of Chicago Press.

Valentine CA: The culture of poverty: its scientific significance and its implications for action. In Leacock EB, editor: The culture of poverty: a critique, New York, 1971, Touchstone-Simon and Schuster.

Vogel VJ: American Indian medicine, Norman, Okla, 1970, University of Oklahoma Press.

Watson OM: Proxemic behavior: a cross-cultural study, The Hague, Netherlands, 1970, Monitor & Co.

Weaver T: Use of hypothetical situations in a study of Spanish-American illness referral systems, Hum Org 29:140, 1970.

Westermeyer J, Vang TF, and Neider J: Migration and mental health among Hmong refugees, J Nerv Ment Disorders 171(2):92-96, 1983.

White EH: Giving health care to minority patients, Nurs Clin North Am 12:27-40, 1977.

Williams C and Jelliffe D: Mother and child health: delivering the services, London, 1972, Oxford University Press.

Young AA: Rethinking the Western health enterprise, Med Anthropol 2(2):1-9, 1978.

Yu E: The low mortality rates of Chinese infants: some plausible explanatory factors, Soc Sci Med 16(3):253-265, 1982.

Zaida SA: Poverty and disease: need for structural change, Soc Sci Med 27:119-127.

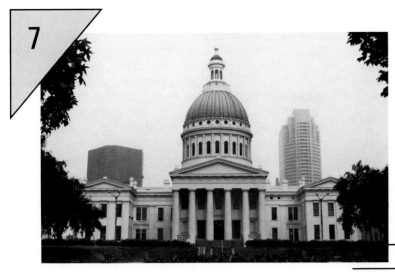

7

Governmental, Political, and Legal Influences on the Practice of Community Health Nursing

Cynthia E. Northrop*

OBJECTIVES

After reading this chapter, the student should be able to:

Describe the trends and roles of several levels of government.
Identify the impact of changing governmental roles and structures on health care.
Describe the major governmental functions in health care.
Discuss community health nursing roles in selected governmental agencies.
Shape health policy by participating in the regulation-making process and the political arena.
Describe selected laws that affect community health nursing practice, both generally and in special areas of practice.
Conduct a brief exercise in legal research as one means of staying informed about current law.

KEY TERMS

constitutional law	legislative process	public sector
Department of Health and Human Services (DHHS)	National Center for Nursing Research	Public Health Service (PHS)
Federal Register	Occupational Safety and Health Act (OSHA)	regulation
Codes of Regulation		scope of practice
judicial and common law	police power	*Scorpio*
legislation	Practice Acts	self regulation
Lexis	private sector	World Health Organization (WHO)
	professional negligence	

*Updated by Marcia Stanhope

C ommunity health nurses are significantly affected by governments and the legal system. This chapter will provide descriptions of these institutions, including organization and primary functions of governments, governmental regulation, and professional self-regulation. The chapter concludes with an overview of laws affecting community health nursing practice.

GOVERNMENTAL ROLE IN HEALTH CARE

The federal and most state governments are comprised of three branches: the executive branch comprises the President (or governor), cabinets, and regulatory units such as the Department of Health and Human Services; the legislative branch comprises two houses of Congress: the Senate and the House of Representatives; and the judicial branch comprised of the Supreme Court. Each of these branches plays a significant role in development and implementation of health policy. The executive branch administers and regulates policy, e.g., the Division of Nursing of the Department of Health and Human Services writes criteria to fund nursing education. The legislative branch passes laws which become policy; e.g., the Medicare Amendments of the 1966 Social Security Act. The judicial branch interprets laws and the meaning of policy, as in its interpretation of states' rights to grant abortions.

One of the first constitutional challenges to congressional legislation in the area of health and welfare came in 1937, when Congress established unemployment compensation and old-age benefits. Although Congress had created other health programs, its legal basis for doing so had never been challenged before. The Supreme Court interpreted the meaning of the Constitution and decided that such federal government action was within congressional powers to promote the general welfare. Most legal bases for congressional action in health care are found in Article I, Section 8 of the U.S. Constitution. They include the following:

1. Provide for the general welfare
2. Regulate commerce among the states
3. Raise funds to support the military
4. Provide spending power

These statements have been interpreted by the Court to include a wide variety of federal powers and activities.

State power concerning health care is mostly **police power.** This means that states may act to protect the health, safety, and welfare of their citizens. Such police power must be reasonably exercised, and the state must demonstrate that it has a compelling interest in taking actions, especially actions that might infringe on individual rights.

Examples of a state exercising its police powers include requiring immunization of children before school admission and requiring casefinding, reporting, follow-up care, and treatment of tuberculosis. These activities protect the health, safety, and welfare of state citizens.

Trends and Shifts in Governmental Roles

Governmental involvement in health care at both the state and federal levels began gradually. Many historical events correspond closely with the role that has developed. Wars, economic instability, depressions, different viewpoints, and political parties have all shaped the governmental role. The New Deal, Roosevelt's post-Depression plans to revive the country, established major precedents for government spending on health care for Americans. In 1930, federal laws were passed to promote the public health of merchant seamen and the Native Americans. The Social Security Act of 1935 was a substantial piece of legislation, which has grown to include not only the aged and unemployed but also survivors' insurance for widows and children, child welfare, health department grants, and maternal and child health projects. In 1934, Senator Wagner of New York initiated the first national health insurance bill. Debate still continues on the extent of governmental responsibilities in health care.

Before the 1930s the only major governmental action relating to health was the creation in 1798 of the Public Health Service. The *Department of Health and Human Services (DHHS),* a regulatory agency known until 1980 as the Department of Health, Education, and Welfare (DHEW), was not created until 1953. It had a small predecessor that had been established in 1939, the Federal Security Agency. In 1946 Congress enacted a mental health bill and the Hospital Survey and Construction Act and created the National Institutes of Health in 1948. These legislative acts created entities that became part of the executive branch, now within the DHHS.

In a democracy the role of government in the area of health care depends on the beliefs of its citizens. Strong beliefs of self-determination and self-sufficiency mixed with beliefs about social responsibilities are hallmarks of a multiple approach to solving societal problems. Political party platforms provide the best example for demonstrating how different beliefs yield different approaches to problems.

Goldsmith (1973) studied twelve health platforms written by the two major parties between 1948 and 1968 and found them to be indicative of subsequent governmental directions in health care. Goldsmith stated that the platforms particularly pointed to areas of future health legislation. He recommended that influential health policy leaders in each party be identified and that health care providers and others examine the party platforms. Nurses are becoming more aware of the influence of political parties on health care delivery.

A major effort of the Reagan administration was to shift federal government activities to the states. In addition, passage in 1985 of the Gramm-Rudman Act, which was designed to decrease the federal budget deficit, not only promoted the continued shift of federal programs to states but also resulted in significant cutbacks in health and social programs.

This discussion has focused primarily on trends and shifts within and among different levels of government. An additional aspect of governmental responsibilities is the relationship between government and individuals. Freedom of individuals must be balanced with government powers. Citizens express their views on the amount of governmental interference that will be tolerated. For example, the issue of sex education in public schools delineates at least two viewpoints on the government-individual relationship:

1. Ever since the legislative branch of government established a system of education, some citizens believe that education should include content on sex.

2. Some citizens believe sex education belongs in the family and should not be interfered with by public schools, which are governmentally established.

These are only two of the views expressed in the literature. There are strong feelings about this issue, and the example shows how opinions about governmental vs. individual responsibilities can be divided.

Governmental Health Care Functions

Federal, state, and local governments all carry out four general categories of health care functions: (1) direct services, (2) financing, (3) information, and (4) policy setting.

Direct Services

Federal, state, and local governments provide direct health services to certain individuals and groups. For example, the federal government provides health care to Native Americans, members and dependents of the military, veterans, and federal prisoners. State and local governments employ community health nurses to deliver services to individuals and families, usually based on financial need. State and local governments also may provide direct specific services to all individuals, such as hypertension or tuberculosis screening and immunizations for children and inmates in local jails or state prisons.

Financing

Governments pay for some health care services, training of personnel, and research. Financial support in these areas has significantly contributed to and affected consumers and health care providers. State and federal governments finance the direct care of clients through the Medicare, Medicaid, and Social Security programs. Many nurses have been educated with government funds; schools of nursing have been built and equipped through federal capitation funds. Other health care providers have also been financially supported by governments. Monies in the form of grants have been given by governments for specific research and demonstration projects. One of the best-known centers of medical research is the federally funded National Institutes of Health.

Information

All branches and levels of government at one time or another have collected, analyzed, and made available data about health care and health status in the United States. An example is the annual report, *Health: United States,* compiled by the DHHS. Collection of vital statistics, including mortality and morbidity data, gathering of census data, and sponsoring health care status surveys are all government activities. Table 7-1 lists examples of available international and federal government data sources on the health status of the total U.S. population. These sources are available in the government documents sections of most large libraries.

Policy Setting

A *policy* is an agreed upon course of action to solve a problem. Policy setting relates to all government functions. Decisions about health care are made by governments at all levels and within all branches. Governments often show

TABLE 7-1	
International and national sources of data on the health status of the U.S. population	
Organization	**Data source**
INTERNATIONAL	
United Nations	Demographic Yearbook
World Health Organization	World Health Statistics Annual
FEDERAL	
Public Health Service	National Vital Statistics System
	National Survey of Family Growth
	National Health Interview Survey
	National Health Examination Survey
	National Health and Nutrition Examination Survey
	National Master Facility Inventory
	National Hospital Discharge Survey
	National Nursing Home Survey
	National Ambulatory Medical Care Survey
	National Morbidity Reporting System
	U.S. Immunization Survey
	Surveys of Mental Health Facilities
	Estimates of National Health Expenditures
	AIDs Surveillance
	Abortion Surveillance
	Nurse Supply Estimates
Department of Commerce	U.S. Census of Population
	Current Population Survey
	Population Estimates and Projections
Department of Labor	Consumer Price Index
	Employment and Earnings

preference between groups when giving financial support. Such decisions affect the health care resources of each group and show the influence of government policy-setting. Health policy decisions, or courses of action, usually have broad implications for economic growth, resource allocation, and development in the health care field. Examples of policy setting include the passage of amendments to the Social Security Act that established Medicare and the Professional Standards Review Organization (PSRO). The law that has had the most significant impact on the development of public health policy, public health nursing, and social welfare policy in the U.S. was the Sheppard-Towner Act of 1921.

In 1912 the Child Health Bureau was established as part of the U.S. Public Health Service (see Chapter 1). In 1917 the Bureau published a report, "Public Protection of Maternity and Infancy," to highlight findings of studies on infant and maternal mortality and consequently on the plight of women and children in the United States. In 1918 the first congresswoman, Jeanette Rankin, introduced a bill that later became the Sheppard-Towner Act. This act made public health nurses available to provide health services for women and children; offered well-child and development services; provided adequate hospital services and facilities for women and children; and provided grants-in-aid for the establishment of maternal and child welfare programs.

The Sheppard-Towner Act helped to establish precedent and set patterns for the growth of modern-day public health policy. It established the federal government's involvement in health care and the system for federal matching grants-in-aid awarded to states. The Act set the role of the federal government in creating standards to be followed by states in conducting categorical programs such as today's Women, Infants, and Children (WIC) and Early Periodic Screening and Developmental Testing programs (EPSDT). Also established were the position of the consumer in influencing, formulating, and conducting public policy; the government's role in research; a system for collecting national health statistics; and the integration of health and social services (Fromer, 1979; Pickett and Hanlon, 1990). This policy established the importance of prenatal care, anticipatory guidance, client education, and nurse-client conferences, all of which are viewed today as essential community health nursing responsibilities.

ORGANIZATION OF GOVERNMENTAL AGENCIES

Community health nurses (CHNs) are actively involved with many levels of international and national government. This section discusses international organizations and roles of community health nurses in different national governmental agencies.

International Organizations

In June of 1945 many national governments joined together to create the United Nations. Aims and goals described in its charter include several dealing with human rights, world peace, security, and promotion of economic and social advancement of all people. The United Nations is headquartered in New York City and is made up of six principal organs. Several other organs and many specialized agencies and autonomous organizations are also within the system. One of the special autonomous organizations is the *World Health Organization (WHO)*.

Established in 1946, WHO relates to the United Nations through the Economic and Social Council to attain its goal of the highest possible level of health for all. Headquartered in Geneva, Switzerland, WHO is composed of three main branches: the Assembly, the Executive Board, and the Secretariat (Figure 7-1). The organization has six regional offices. The office for the Americas is located in Washington, D.C., and is known as the Pan American Health Organization (PAHO). (See Chapter 1.)

The World Health Assembly, to which all United Nations members belong, meets annually and is the policy-making body of WHO. WHO provides worldwide services to promote health, cooperates with member countries in their health efforts, and coordinates biomedical research. Its services, which benefit all countries, include a day-to-day information service on the occurrence of internationally important diseases; publication of the international list of causes of disease, injury, and death; monitoring of adverse reactions to drugs; and establishment of world standards for antibiotics and vaccines. Assistance available to individual countries includes support for national programs to fight disease, train workers, and strengthen health services. An example of biomedical research collaboration is a special program to study six widespread tropical diseases: malaria, leprosy, "snail fever," filariasis, leishmaniasis, and "sleeping sickness."

The number of community health nursing roles in international health is increasing. Besides offering direct health services, nurses serve as consultants, educators, and program planners and evaluators. They focus their work on a variety of community health concepts, including environment, sanitation, communicable disease, wellness, and primary care.

In 1978 the International Conference on Primary Health Care sponsored by WHO, held in Alma-Ata, USSR, declared that the world community's goal should be the attainment of a level of health by the year 2000 that would permit all peoples to live socially and economically productive lives (WHO, 1978). The conference resolved that primary health care was the key to attaining this goal.

At about the same time, the WHO Expert Committee on Community Health Nursing convened and outlined the broad role of community health nurses in primary health care. WHO is encouraging strengthened regulation of nursing education and practice related to primary health care, and it is in support of nurses in their efforts to become forces in attaining the goal of "health for all" (Mahler, 1985; WHO, 1986). This is an example of an international organization and policy that is certain to affect the future of nursing education and community health nursing practice.

Federal Agencies

Many federal agencies are involved in governmental health care functions. Legislation passed by Congress may be delegated to any regulatory agency within the executive branch for implementation, surveillance, regulation, and enforcement. Congress decides which agency will monitor specific laws. For example, most health care legislation is delegated to the Department of Health and Human Services (DHHS); however, legislation concerning the environment or occupational health would probably be monitored by the Environmental Protection Agency or the Labor Department. Examples of those departments most involved with health care will be included in the following discussion.

Department of Health and Human Services (DHHS)

DHHS is the agency most heavily involved with the health and welfare concerns of U.S. citizens. It touches more lives than any other federal agency. As mentioned earlier, the organizational chart of DHHS (Figure 7-2) depicts the office of the Secretary and four principal operating components: the Social Security Administration, the Health Care Financing Administration, the Office of Human Development Services, and the Public Health Service. The Public Health Service is charged with regulating health care and overseeing the health status of Americans.

Public Health Service

The major components of the *Public Health Service (PHS)* are shown in Figure 7-3. The PHS has been a long-standing, significant contributor to the improved health status of Americans. The Health Resources and Services Administration of the PHS contains the Bureau of Health Professions, which includes a Division of Nursing. Medicine, Dentistry, and Allied Health Professions have divisions of their own.

Structure of the Secretariat of the World Health Organization

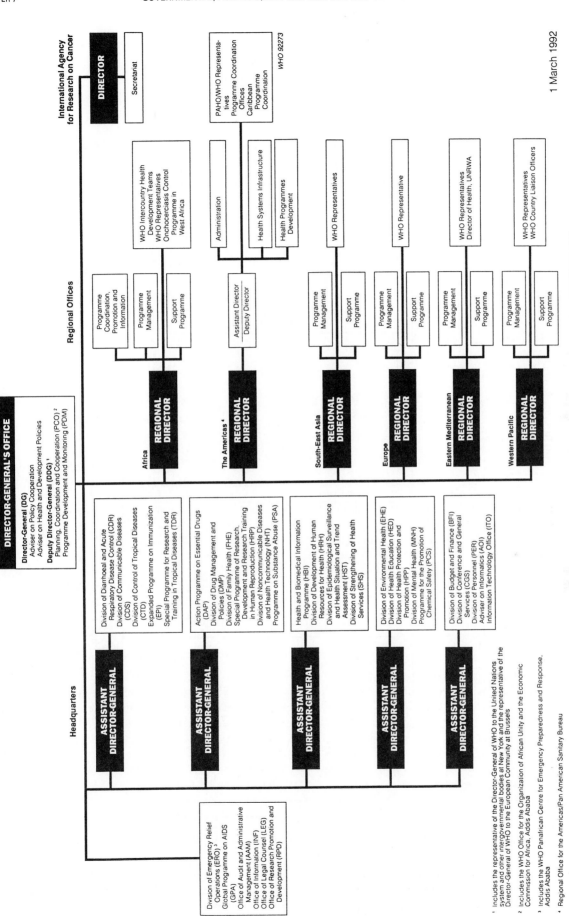

FIGURE 7-1

Structure of the World Health Organization. (Used with permission of the Office of Publication, WHO, Geneva, 1992.)

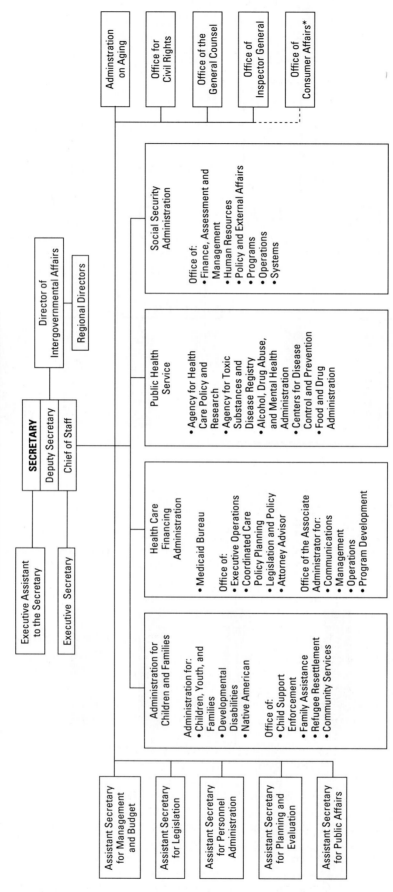

FIGURE 7-2

Organizational chart of the Department of Health and Human Services. (From Office of Federal Register: United States Government Manual, Washington, DC, 1992, US Government Printing Office.)

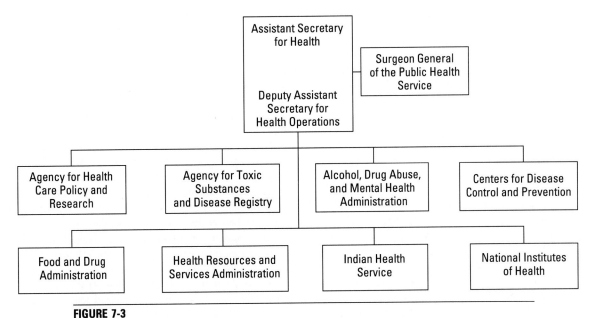

FIGURE 7-3

U.S. Department of Health and Human Services: Public Health Service (Office of Federal Register, 1990.)

The Division of Nursing has these specific goals:

1. To provide the professional nursing expertise and leadership required to coordinate, evaluate, and support development and utilization of the nation's health workforce resources;
2. To support and conduct programs on the development, use, quality, and certification of nursing personnel. This includes registered nurses, practical or vocational nurses, and nursing aides;
3. In cooperation with other organizations, to assist states and regions in planning, developing, and improving nursing services and educational programs;
4. To conduct and support programs related to the provision of nursing care to advance the health status of individuals, families, and communities;
5. To engage with other federal health provider programs in cooperative efforts of research into, and development and demonstration of programs that show the interrelationships between individual members of the health care team, as well as their tasks, education requirements, and related training models;
6. To maintain liaison with health professional groups and others, including consumers, who have a common interest in the nation's capacity to deliver nursing services;
7. To foster, support, and conduct projects to expand the scientific base of nursing practice and role delineation and to develop and incorporate new knowledge into practice and education; and
8. To provide consultation and technical assistance to public and private organizations, agencies, and institutions, including PHS regional offices and other agencies of the federal government, on all aspects of nursing relevant to the division's functions (Division of Nursing, PHS, 1985).

In late 1985 Congress overrode a Presidential veto, al-lowing the creation of the **National Center for Nursing Research,** within the National Institutes of Health. The research and research-related training activities previously supported by the Division of Nursing were transferred to this new Center. The Center is the focal point of the nation's nursing research activities. It promotes the growth and quality of research in nursing and patient care, provides important leadership, expands the pool of experienced nurse researchers, and serves as a point of interaction with other bases of health care research.

A significant addition to the PHS in 1990 was the creation of the Agency for Health Care Policy and Research. This agency is charged with conducting research on effectiveness of medical services, interventions, and technologies, including research related to nursing interventions and outcomes that contribute to the improved health status of the nation.

Other Federal Government Agencies

DHHS has primary responsibility for federal health functions. The cabinet departments of the federal government carry out certain other functions. Those departments include Commerce, Defense, Labor, Agriculture, and Justice.

DEPARTMENT OF COMMERCE. Within the Department of Commerce (DOC) is the Bureau of the Census, which carries out an information function in health care. Established in 1902, this bureau conducts a census of the population every 10 years. The most recent was in 1990. Also a part of the DOC is the National Oceanic and Atmospheric Administration, which provides special services in support of controlling urban air quality, a major factor in community health today.

DEPARTMENT OF DEFENSE. The Department of Defense (DOD) delivers health care to members of the military and their dependents. The Assistant Secretary of Defense for Health Affairs administers the Civilian Health and Medical

Program of the Uniformed Services (CHAMPUS). The departments within Defense (Army, Navy, Air Force, and Marines) each have a surgeon general. Health services, including community health services for members of the military, are delivered by a Health Services Command in each department. In each command, nurses of high military rank, including brigadier general, are part of the administration of health services.

DEPARTMENT OF LABOR. The Department of Labor has two agencies with health functions: the Occupational Safety and Health Administration and the Mine Safety and Health Administration. Both are charged with writing safety and health standards and ensuring compliance in the workplace. This includes conducting inspections, investigating complaints, and issuing citations if necessary. Each agency coordinates its activities with state departments of labor and health.

DEPARTMENT OF AGRICULTURE. The Department of Agriculture is involved in health care primarily through administering the Food and Nutrition Service. Although plant, product, and animal inspection by the Department of Agriculture is also related to health, the Food and Nutrition Service oversees a variety of food assistance activities. This service collaborates with state and local government welfare agencies to provide food stamps to needy persons to increase their food purchasing power. Other programs include school breakfast and lunch programs; the Supplemental Food Program for Women, Infants, and Children (WIC); and grants to states for nutrition education and training.

DEPARTMENT OF JUSTICE. Health services to federal prisoners are administered within the Department of Justice. The Medical and Services Division of the Bureau of Prisons includes medical, psychiatric, dental, and health support services. It also administers environmental health and safety, farm operations, and food service, along with commissary, laundry, and other personal services for inmates.

State and Local Government Departments

Most state and local (county and city) jurisdictions perform governmental activities that affect the health care field. At the state level, three executive branch departments will be described: health, education, and corrections. The organization of a local health department will also be outlined, and community health roles will be discussed.

Selected Health Departments

Selected programs within a typical state health department are as follows:

Legal services
Services to the chronically ill and aging
Juvenile services
Medical assistance: policy, compliance, operations
Mental health and addictions
Mental retardation and developmental disabilities
Environmental programs
Departmental licensing boards
Division of vital records
Health services cost review
Health planning and development
Preventive medicine and medical affairs

In most state health departments, community health nurses serve in many capacities. These capacities are similar to those in international and federal agencies: consultation, direct services, research, teaching, supervision, planning, and evaluation of health programs. Most health departments have a division or department of community health nursing.

Every state has a board of examiners of nurses. The board may be found either in the department of licensing boards of the health department or in an administrative agency of the governor's office. Created by legislation known as a state nurse practice act, the examiner's board is made up of nurses and consumers. A few states have other providers or administrators as members. The functions of this board are described in the practice act of each state and generally include licensing and examination of registered nurses and licensed practical nurses; approval of schools of nursing in the state; revocation, suspension, or denial of licenses; and writing of regulations about nursing practice and education. Nurse practice acts will be discussed later in a section on the scope of nursing practice.

State Education Departments

Some state departments of education coordinate health curricula and services provided within local school systems. Other state legislatures mandate coordination of services solely within the health department or jointly between the health and education departments. Often liaison groups or councils are formed to facilitate joint coordination. These councils develop policy and guidelines for school health services and health education. Community health nurses often represent health and education departments at these councils and help shape health policy. Community health nurses also serve in departments of education in capacities similar to those in health departments.

State Departments of Corrections

Community health nurses work in state departments of corrections as planners and coordinators and sometimes as supervisors of health and nursing services for inmates in state prisons. Community health nurses in such state positions may also coordinate the health service efforts of local jails. Local jails may hire nurses directly or use the services of community health nurses in local health departments.

Local Health Departments

Depending on funding and other resources, programs offered by local health departments vary greatly. A fairly comprehensive list of such programs, taken from an urban-suburban county health department in a mid-Atlantic state, is shown in the box on page 117. At the local level, as at the state level, coordination of health efforts between health departments and other county or city departments is essential. For example, local boards of education and departments of social services are an integral part of activities of local governments. More often than at other levels of government, community health nurses at the local level provide direct services. Some community health nurses deliver special or selected services, such as follow-up of contacts in cases of tuberculosis or venereal disease, or providing child im-

---

**EXAMPLES OF PROGRAMS PROVIDED
BY LOCAL HEALTH DEPARTMENTS**

Addictions and alcoholism clinics
Adult health
Birth and death records
Child day care and development
Child health clinics
Crippled children's services
Dental health clinic
Environmental health
Epidemiology and disease control
Family planning
Geriatric evaluation
Health education
Home health agency
Hospital discharge planning
Hypertension clinics
Immunization clinics
Information services
Maternal health
Medical social work
Mental health
Mental retardation and developmental disabilities
Nursing
Nursing home licensure
Nutrition division
Occupational therapy
Physical therapy
School health
Speech and audiology
Vision and hearing screening

---

munization clinics. Other community health nurses have a more generalized practice, delivering services to families in certain geographical areas. This method of delivery of community health nursing services involves broader needs and a wider variety of nursing interventions.

Social Welfare Programs

In addition to health programs, federal, state, and local governments also provide social welfare programs. Generally these programs provide monetary benefits to the poor, elderly, disabled, and unemployed.

The federal Social Security Act established a number of programs, which include the social insurance programs, Social Security, unemployment insurance, and welfare programs.

The Social Security Administration, which is within the DHHS, administers the following programs:

1. Old Age Survivors and Disability Insurance (OASDI)
2. Aid to Families with Dependent Children (AFDC) and
3. Supplemental Security Income (SSI).

OASDI provides monthly benefits to retired and disabled workers, their spouses and children, and to survivors of insured workers. AFDC, which is a federal and state program, helps needy families with children. AFDC subsidizes

children deprived of the financial support of one of their parents as a result of death, disability, absence from the home, or, in some states, unemployment.

SSI is a federal program for the aged, blind, and disabled that may be supplemented by state support. The funds for these programs are provided by contributions from employees, employers, and self-employed individuals. These contributions are pooled into a special trust fund that is paid to a worker on retirement, death, or disability as partial replacement of the earnings the family has lost.

In 1965, amendments to the Social Security Act created Medicare and Medicaid. These programs are administered by the Health Care Financing Administration (HCFA) within the DHHS; in the case of Medicaid the administration is done in conjunction with state governments. (See Chapter 4 for additional discussion of Medicare and Medicaid programs.)

In addition, there are human development services coordinated by the Office of Human Development Services within DHHS. Programs are focused on the aging, children, youth and families, Native Americans, and the developmentally disabled.

The Older Americans Act is designed to promote the welfare and needs of older people. Through this act the federal government promotes the development of state-administered community-based systems of comprehensive social services for the elderly.

Social programs focused on children and families include programs on adoption opportunities, Head Start services, runaway-youth facilities, child-abuse prevention and treatment, juvenile justice, and delinquency prevention. Other programs promote the social and economic development of Native Americans.

The Administration on Developmental Disabilities assists states in increasing the provision of quality services to persons with developmental disabilities. Grants are administered that support projects aimed at removing physical, mental, social, and environmental barriers for these disabled individuals.

Social welfare policies and programs affect community health nursing practice. Community resources that improve the quality of life for specific populations help nurses to assist clients in attaining optimal health.

Impact of Governmental Health Functions and Structures on Community Health Nursing

The variety and range of functions of government agencies has had a major impact on the practice of community health nursing. Funding in particular has shaped roles and tasks of community health nurses. The designation of money for specific needs has led to special, more narrowly focused community health nursing roles. For example, funds assigned to communicable disease programs or family planning usually will not support home care services. Therefore nurses develop specialty roles related to these funded programs (e.g., immunization nurses, family planning nurses, etc.).

Training grants for nurse practitioners in primary care have provided incentives to individual nurses to attend programs and develop new community health nursing roles within the health care system. Finally, school, adult, and pediatric nurse practitioners emerged primarily because of the funding provided by government agencies.

Other health policy information, funding, and direct services functions of government have influenced community health nursing. Legislatures have identified special needs and programs to meet the needs of special populations such as migrant workers, pregnant women, or at-risk children. Often community health nurses are called upon to implement these programs. Vital statistics and other epidemiological data collected by government agencies have influenced the location, work force, planning, and evaluation of community health nursing services.

According to the evolving policies of the federal government and administrations of the 1980s, federal money given to the states was in the form of block grants. A sum of money with no specific program tags, the block grant had a great impact on community health nursing. Having less money in special programs resulted in a shift of community health nursing roles toward more generalized practice. Whether community health nursing should be a specialty or a generalized practice is an age-old debate. The purpose of mentioning the debate here is to show how government funding has shaped the functions of community health nurses within all levels of government. When governments give money to special programs, community health nursing roles become specialized and take care of needs of certain clients only. When governments give money to states to spend as they wish, community health nursing roles become generalized, and the nurse takes care of all of the client needs.

COMMUNITY HEALTH NURSE'S ROLE IN THE POLITICAL PROCESS

The number and type of laws influencing health care are increasing. Because of this, involvement in the *political process* at all possible points is most important to community health nursing. The community health nurse's basic understanding of this political process should include knowing who the lawmakers are, how bills become law, the regulation-writing process, and methods of influencing the process and shaping health policy.

The federal and state legislatures are composed of two houses: an assembly, or house, and a senate. Representatives and senators are elected by the people within geographic jurisdictions. Each state has two federal senators and one or more representatives, depending on the state's population. Each state has its own rules for deciding on representation within the state for the state legislature.

Although Congress meets throughout the year, state legislatures have sessions of varying lengths. Each legislature has its own leadership, usually dominated by either the Democratic or Republican party. Roles include the presiding officers, party floor leaders, and committee chairpersons.

An important part of this *legislative process* is the work of the staffs of the legislatures. These individuals do the legwork, research, paperwork, and other activities that move ideas into bills and then into law. In addition to the individual legislators' staffs, committee staffs are also im-

portant. Both of these can provide valuable information for constituents, as well as for their legislators. Nurses often serve as staff to legislators.

The legislative process begins with ideas that are developed into bills. After a bill is drafted, it is introduced to the legislature, given a number, read, and assigned to a committee. Hearings, testimony, lobbying, education, research, and informal discussion follow. If the bill is passed from the committee, the entire house hears the bill, amending it as necessary, and votes on it. A majority vote moves the bill to the other house, where it is read, amended, and voted on.

Community health nurses can be involved in this process at any point. Many professional nursing associations have professional lobbyists, legislative committees, and political action committees (PACs) to shape health policy.

Common methods of lobbying include face-to-face encounters, personal letters, mailgrams, telegrams, telephone calls, testimony, petitions, reports, position papers, fact sheets, letters to the editor, news releases, speeches, coalition-building, demonstrations, and litigation. Depending on the issue, each of these can be equally effective.

Behind the scenes of this process lies the political party activity in which community health nurses should be involved. A wide variety of activities are available, including voting, participating in the party organization, registering voters, getting out the vote, fundraising, building networks or communication links, and participating in political action committees.

The passage of the National Health Research Extension Act of 1985 is an example of how nurses can use their influence. This act included the establishment of the National Center for Nursing Research. The Center began as the idea of a small group of nurses who worked to gain the support of colleagues and major national nursing organizations. Individual nurses provided testimony to Congress on the importance of nursing research. Some visited their congressional representatives to lobby for the bill. Many wrote letters and provided position papers and fact sheets to help legislators understand the need for the Center. Although the process took several years, the idea became a reality. Both the nursing profession and the consumer will benefit from the research and the knowledge base developed through the Center.

PRIVATE SECTOR INFLUENCE ON REGULATION AND HEALTH POLICY

In each level of government the executive branch can, and in most cases must, prepare regulations. These regulations are detailed, and they establish, fix, and control standards and criteria for carrying out certain laws. Figure 7-4 shows the steps in the typical regulation-writing process.

When the legislature passes a law and delegates its administration to an agency, it gives that agency the power to make regulations. Because regulations flow from legislation, they have the force of law.

The *private sector,* which includes everyone that is not part of the government or *public sector,* can influence and shape legislation through many means. Through the same means, the private sector also influences the writing of reg-

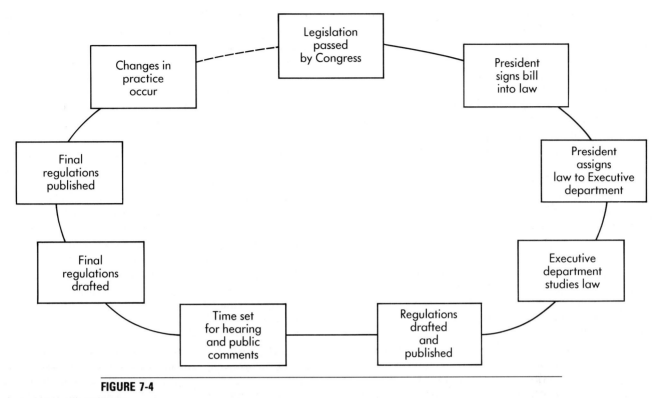

FIGURE 7-4

The regulation-writing process.

ulations. This part of the chapter will describe the process of regulation writing and ways to influence it. Community health nursing students and clinicians are members of the private sector and are influenced by regulations that affect nursing practice.

Process of Regulation

After a law is passed, the appropriate executive department begins the process of regulation by studying the topic or issue. Advisory groups or special task forces, including nondepartmental members, are sometimes formed to provide the content of the regulations. As the work of the groups or individual department members progresses, initial drafts of the proposed regulations are written. Community health nurses, including students, can influence these regulations by writing letters to the regulatory agency in charge or by speaking at public hearings.

After refinement, the proposed regulations are put into final draft form and printed in the legally required publication. At the federal level the legally mandated channel is the *Federal Register.*

Similar registers exist in most states where regulations from state departments, including state health departments, are published. The publication of proposed regulations includes notice about a time period within which public comment will be accepted. Public comment in this situation is usually in written form. The notice may also give a date, time, and place for a hearing that is open to the public. Anyone may attend; if one wishes to speak at the hearing, published rules for that procedure must be followed. This usually involves notifying the agency of one's intent to speak and limiting the length of testimony as specified by the agency.

Revisions made to the proposed regulations are based on public comment and public hearing. Depending on the amount and content of the public reaction, final regulations are prepared or more study of the area and issues is conducted. Final published regulations carry the force of law. The date when regulations become effective is also published. It is at this point that practice is changed to conform to the new regulations.

Close monitoring by, and participation of, the private sector in regulation writing can begin as soon as a law is passed and delegated to an executive branch agency. Government manuals, updated at least yearly, list names and phone numbers of individuals within the executive branch. Early contact and expression of interest in how a particular law gets administered may result in membership on a task force or advisory board. The membership of such groups is public information, and one can contact these members to determine their thoughts on the direction the regulations will take.

Regular surveillance of the *Federal Register* or state registers is essential. Once proposed resolutions are published, members of the private sector may influence regulations by attending the hearings, providing comments, testifying, and engaging in lobbying aimed at individuals involved in the writing. Concrete, written suggestions for revision submitted to these individuals are usually persuasive.

Final regulations, published in a *Code of Regulations* (both federal and state), usually lead to changes in practice. Regulations need to be made available to all individuals whose practice is affected. This dissemination can be effectively helped by private sector involvement. Regulations need to become included in manuals of policies and procedures of the agencies affected by them. For example, Medicare regulations setting standards for nursing homes and home health are incorporated into these agencies' manuals.

LAWS AFFECTING COMMUNITY HEALTH NURSING PRACTICE

Community health nursing combines nursing practice and public health practice. The community health nurse is subject to the laws relating to nursing practice and public health practice.

This part of the chapter will discuss the various types of laws, how they affect community health nurses, and the legal resources available.

Types of Laws

Several definitions of laws are available. However, many of these tend to describe what law is *not* rather than what it is. Definitions of law include the following:
1. A rule established by authority, society, or custom
2. The body of rules governing the affairs of people within a community or among states; social order; the common law
3. A set of rules or customs governing a discrete field or activity; e.g., criminal law, contract law
4. The system of courts, judicial process, and legal officers, or lawyers giving effect to the laws of a society

These definitions reflect the close relationship of law to community and to society's customs and beliefs. Since community health nursing reflects society's beliefs and customs, law has had a major impact on this practice. Although community health nursing practice emerged from individual voluntary activities, society soon recognized the need for it. Through legal mandates, positions and functions for nurses in community settings were created. These functions in many instances carry with them the "force of law." For example, if the community health nurse discovers a person with smallpox, the law directs the nurse and others legally designated in the community to take specific action. This is just one example of how the law has shaped community health nursing practice.

There are three types of laws in the U.S: (1) constitutional law; (2) legislation and regulation; and (3) judicial and common law.

Constitutional Law

Constitutional law emerges from federal and state constitutions. From this type of law community health nurses can get answers to questions in selected practice situations. For example, on what basis can the state require quarantine or isolation of individuals with tuberculosis? The answer to this question can be found in constitutional law.

The U.S. Constitution specifies explicit and limited functions of the federal government. All other powers and functions are left to the individual states. The major power of the states relating to community health nursing practice is the right to intervene in a reasonable manner to protect the health, safety, and welfare of the citizenry. As described earlier in this chapter, the state's "police power" is not without limitation. First, it must be a "reasonable" exercise of power. Second, if the power interferes or infringes on individual rights, the state must demonstrate that there is a "compelling state interest" in exercising its power. Hence, isolating an individual or separating one from a community because he has a communicable disease has been deemed an appropriate exercise of state powers. The state can isolate an individual even though it infringes on individual rights (freedom, autonomy), under the following conditions:
1. If the isolation is done in a reasonable manner
2. If there is a compelling state interest in the prevention of an epidemic
3. If the isolation is necessary to protect the health, safety, and welfare of individuals in the community or the public as a whole

Legislation and Regulation

Legislation is the type of law that comes from the legislative branches of federal, state, or local government. Much legislation has an impact on community health nursing. *Regulations* are very specific statements of law that relate to individual pieces of legislation.

Community health nurses are often employed by the executive branch through the state or local health department. Hence, nursing interventions often implement legislation and regulations. Nurses employed in other community settings—those with no governmental responsibilities or legal mandates—are nevertheless often subject to legislation and regulations. For example, community health nurses employed by private agencies who are rendering home health care must deliver care according to federal Medicare legislation and regulations or state Medicaid legislations and regulations in order for the agency to be reimbursed for those services. Private and public health care services rendered by community health nurses are subject to many government regulations.

Judicial and Common Law

Judicial and *common law* is the last group of laws having an impact on community health nursing. Judicial law is law based on court or jury decisions.

The opinions of the courts are judicial opinion and are referred to as "case law." The court uses other types of laws to make its decision, including previous court decisions or cases. Precedent is one principle of common law. Judges are bound by previous decisions unless they are convinced that the "old law" is no longer relevant or valid. This process is called "distinguishing" and usually involves a demonstration of how the currently disputed situation differs from the previously decided situation. Other principles of common law are part of a court's rationale and the basis of making a particular decision. Such principles include justice, fairness, respect for individuals, autonomy, and self-determination. These play an important role in decisions made by courts.

General Community Health Nursing Practice and the Law

Despite the broad nature and varied roles of community health nursing practice, two legal aspects apply to most practice situations. The first aspect is *professional negligence,* or malpractice; the second is the *scope of practice* defined by custom and state practice acts.

Professional Negligence

Professional negligence or malpractice is defined as an act or failure to act on behalf of a client which leads to injury of that client. To prove that a nurse was negligent, the client must prove *all* of the following:

1. The nurse owed a duty to the client, or was responsible for the client's care.
2. The duty to act as a reasonable, prudent nurse, or as another community health nurse would act under the circumstances, was breached or not fulfilled.
3. The failure to be reasonable under the circumstances led to the alleged injuries.
4. The injuries provide the basis for a monetary claim through the legal system.

Reported cases involving negligence and community health nurses are almost nonexistent. As one example, a case involving an occupational health nurse is discussed. Although occurring some years ago, this example clearly represents the four criteria which must be present to prove negligence. Since nurses still use standing orders, a similar problem could happen to a nurse today.

The California case of *Cooper vs Motor Bearing Co.,* 288P 2d 581, involved an occupational health nurse who negligently implemented standing orders on an injury involving a puncture wound. The nurse, by her own testimony, did not examine or probe the wound, nor did she refer the worker to a physician; she simply swabbed and bandaged it. Only after 10 months, in which time there were many documented visits to the dispensary and the worker complained that the wound was not healing, did the nurse refer him to the company doctor. On referral, basal cell carcinoma was found and surgery followed.

The fact that the nurse was employed by the industry to render first aid established the first element of negligence: a duty was owed the worker. The nurse acknowledged that it was her duty to refer any unfamiliar or questionable condition or injury to the doctor for diagnosis. The standard of good nursing care in the community was to examine the wound for the presence of foreign bodies. The nurse knew the normal healing time was one to two weeks. If a wound persisted and did not heal, proper nursing care would indicate referral to a physician. Testimony was given that the practice of an occupational health nurse in this particular type of industry is to probe wounds for foreign bodies. According to the nurse's education and experience, she should have been aware of the possibility of foreign objects being present in such a wound.

In this case the nurse's failure to detect the foreign body was the proximate cause of the basal cell carcinoma. The pain, suffering, lost time and wages, and bodily disfigurement were all injuries that could be calculated and totaled as a monetary amount. The nurse and the company were found negligent by the California Court.

An integral part of negligence suits is the question of who should be sued. Obviously, those who made the mistakes should be sued, but part of the consideration has to do with who can best compensate for the injuries. When a nurse is employed and functioning within the scope of that employment, the employer is responsible for the nurse's negligent actions. This is referred to as the doctrine of *respondeat superior.* By directing a nurse to carry out a particular function, the employer becomes responsible for negligence, along with the individual nurse. The scope of employment is usually more inclusive than a job description but does not include criminal activities. Because employers are usually better able to compensate for the injuries suffered, they are more often sued than the nurses themselves.

Community health nurses employed by government agencies need to ascertain whether that agency has *sovereign immunity.* Under this doctrine the agency may be exempt from suit for particular kinds of actions such as negligence. However, sovereign immunity will not protect nurses who are acting under the auspices of the government when the negligence occurs. Individual public health nurses may have personal immunity for particular practice areas such as giving immunizations. In some states the legislature has granted personal immunity to community health nurses to cover all aspects of their practice.

Community health nursing students need to be aware that they are governed by the same laws and rules governing the graduate nurse. Students are expected to meet the same standard of care of any licensed nurse practicing under the same or similar circumstances. Lower standards of care by students are not acceptable. Students are expected to be able to perform all tasks and make clinical decisions based on the knowledge they have gained or been offered, according to their progress in their educational programs. If a faculty member gives a student an assignment based on the student's progress in the program, the faculty member is not considered liable for the student's actions.

Scope of Practice

The issue of *scope of practice* involves differentiating between the practices of physicians, nurses, and other health care providers. *Scope of practice* is assessed by (1) examining the usual and customary practice of a profession, and (2) taking into account how legislation defines the practice of a particular profession in a jurisdiction. The issue is especially important to community health nurses who have traditionally practiced in a wide scope.

The usual and customary practice of community health nursing can be determined through a variety of sources, including the following:

1. Contents of community health nursing educational programs, general and special
2. Experience of other practicing nurses (peers)
3. Activities and statements, including standards, of community health nursing professional organizations
4. Policies and procedures of agencies employing nurses
5. Needs and interests of the community
6. Literature, including books, texts, and journals

All these sources can describe and help determine the scope of the usual practice of a community health nurse.

Every community health nurse should know and follow closely the proposed changes in practice acts in nursing, medicine, pharmacy, and other related professions. These pieces of state legislation define the scope of practice for professionals in these areas. The nurse should always examine *all* definitions related to nursing practice. For example, a review of the Pharmacy Act will let the nurse know whether to question the right to "dispense" medications in a methadone clinic in a local health department, when following physician prescription and preparing several identical doses for the client to take between clinic visits. Defining scope forces one to clarify both independent and dependent community health nursing functions. The failure to know one's limitations could lead, for example, to charges of practicing as a pharmacist without a license, with subsequent fines and possible suspension or revocation of license. Just as practice acts vary, so do the issues of scope of practice. It is best to refer directly to practice acts for a particular state code.

Because of the variety of legal aspects, the following section will deal with areas of practice having special focuses.

Special Community Health Nursing Practice and the Law

Legal aspects of community health nursing vary, depending on (1) the setting where care is delivered, (2) the clinical specialty, and (3) the functional role. Four special areas of community health nursing practice and their respective legal aspects will be discussed to illustrate how the law affects specific practice areas. Those four areas are school and family health, occupational health, home care and hospice services, and correctional health. Examples of legislation and judicial opinions affecting community health nurses within these selected areas will be included.

School and Family Health

School and family health nursing may be delivered by community health nurses employed by health departments or boards of education. School health legislation establishes a minimum of services that must be provided to children in public and private schools. For example, most states require that children be immunized against certain communicable diseases before entering school. Children must have had a physical examination by that time, and most states require at least one physical at a later time in their schooling. Legislation also specifies when and what type of health screening will be conducted in schools; examples are vision and hearing testing.

Legislation treating child abuse and neglect makes a large impact on community health nursing practice within schools and families. Most states require nurses to notify police or a social service agency of any situation in which they suspect a child is being abused or neglected. This is one instance in which society permits a professional to breach confidentiality to protect someone who may be in a helpless and vulnerable position. There is civil immunity for such reports, and the nurse may be called as a witness in any subsequent hearing. In fact, the majority of legal cases involving community health nurses concern child abuse.

Other examples of federal legislation affecting community health nursing practice with regard to schools and families are Head Start, early diagnostic screening programs, nutritional programs, services for the handicapped, and special education. Most of this legislation, although written by the U.S. Congress, requires cooperative federal and state funding, planning, and implementation. Each nurse working within a service based on legislation should be oriented to the legislation. It is advisable that the legislation and its regulations be included in the nursing agency's manual of policies and procedures so that the nurse may refer to it.

Occupational Health

Occupational health is another special area of practice that is greatly affected by state and federal laws. The *Occupational Safety and Health Act (OSHA)* imposes many requirements on industries. These requirements shape the functions of community health nurses and the types of services given to workers. OSHA also establishes a reporting system for workers exposed to toxic agents in the workplace. A record-keeping system required by OSHA greatly affects health records in the workplace. Each state has an agency similar to OSHA that also monitors and inspects industries, as well as the health services rendered to them by nurses. Most states have a "worker's right to know" law requiring employers to provide employees with information concerning the nature of toxic substances they may encounter in the workplace during their employment. In addition, all states have workers' compensation statutes that provide a legal opportunity for claims of workers injured on the job. Access to records, confidentiality, and the use of standing orders are legal issues of great significance to nurses employed in industries.

Home Care and Hospice

Home care and hospice services rendered by community health nurses are greatly affected by state laws that require licensing and certification. Compliance with these laws is integrally linked to the method of payment for the services. For example, a service must be licensed and certified to obtain payment for services through Medicare. Federal regulations implementing Medicare have an effect on much of community health nursing practice, including how nurses record details of their visits.

Many states have passed laws requiring nurses to report elder abuse to the proper authorities. Legislation affecting home care and hospice services has related to such issues as the right to death with dignity, rights of residents of long-term facilities, definitions of death, and the use of living wills. The legal and ethical dimensions of community health nursing practice are particularly important in this area of practice. Individual rights, such as the right to refuse treatment, and nursing responsibilities, such as the legal duty to render reasonable and prudent care, may often be in conflict in delivering home and hospice services. Much case discussion, sometimes including outside consultation, is required when rights and responsibilities are in conflict and a decision must be made to resolve that conflict.

Correctional Health

Nursing practice in correctional health systems is controlled by state and federal laws and regulations, as well as by recent Supreme Court decisions. The laws and decisions relate to the type and amount of services that must be provided for incarcerated individuals. For example, physical examinations are required of all prisoners after they are sentenced. Regulations specify basic levels of care that must be provided for prisoners, and care during illness is particularly addressed. Court decisions requiring adequate health services are based on constitutional law. If minimum services are not provided, it is a violation of a prisoner's right to freedom from cruel and unusual punishment. Such decisions provide a framework that strongly influences the setting of nursing priorities. For example, providing sick calls would take priority over nutritional classes.

Each of the preceding areas of special community health nursing practice are significantly shaped by legislation and judicial opinion. Those nurses responsible for setting and implementing program priorities need to identify and monitor laws related to each special area of practice.

Legal Resources

In addition to seeking legal counsel, community health nurses can actively remain current with respect to nursing-related laws and regulations. There are many resources in public libraries and law libraries, including the following:

    State bar association publications
    State code
    State annotated code
    Indexes to codes
    Supplements to codes and indexes
    Federal Register and state registers
    Codes of regulations (federal and state)
    Administrative agency rules and decisions
    Case law
    Opinions of attorney generals
    Legal dictionaries
    Legislative histories
    Legal periodicals

In using these legal resources, begin by reviewing the topical index to each source. As the headings are reviewed, several can be identified as relating to the content areas of practice (such as immunizations or family planning) and the types of clients (e.g., minors, adolescents, and children) served by the community health nurse. Computer search tools are often available. One legal computerized search tool is called *Lexis.* The Library of Congress has a service called *Scorpio.* Both services will search not only books and journals but also recent case laws, bills, amendments, and legislation. One of the best ways to stay informed is to read the area newspaper.

CLINICAL APPLICATION

Larry was in his final rotation in the bachelor of science in nursing program at State University. He was anxious to complete his community health nursing course because upon graduation he would begin a position as a staff nurse specializing in school health at the local health department. His wife was expecting their first child, and she had been receiving prenatal care at the health department.

Larry was aware that a few years ago the federal government had, by law, provided block grants to states for primary care, maternal child health programs, and other health care needs of states. He had read the Federal Register and knew that the regulations for these grants had been written through DHHS departments. He was aware that these regulations did not require states to fund specific programs.

Larry read in the local paper that the health department was closing their prenatal clinic at the end of the month. When this state had received its block grant, they decided to spend their money for programs other than prenatal care.

The next day Larry began the process of *assessing* the situation. He knew that his wife and others like her were in jeopardy of losing their prenatal care, placing them at risk for premature delivery, low birth weight, or other such complications. In the law library, he reviewed the state register to see if regulations for the block grants had been finalized. He also checked state health statistics, which include vital statistics providing the current infant and maternity mortality rates in the state. In addition to comparing these data with national statistics, he reviewed the literature for research that would show the relationship between neonatal care, normal deliveries, and complications of pregnancy and delivery.

To his surprise, Larry found that a three-year study in his own state showed improved pregnancy outcomes as a result of prenatal care. The results were further improved when the care was delivered by community health nurses.

Larry was concerned that, as a student, he would have little influence. However, he decided to call his classmates together to *plan* a course of action. After some discussion, a representative contacted the local nurses' association and found that the association was also extremely concerned about the problem. Together the groups contacted their local senators and representatives and asked for a meeting to discuss the issue. Larry also contacted the legal aid society. He found a lawyer interested in consulting with them in preparing written and oral testimony. The testimony was to be presented to the state health department during the process of preparing the regulations for the block grants.

Since Larry had been the leader in rallying support for the issue, he was asked to present this testimony. To *implement* the planned action, he used the national and state statistics, his literature review, and his own family situation to present his argument for the needed support for prenatal care.

Because his own senators and representatives were sympathetic to the issue, he was able to get their support for his testimony. The regulatory process took approximately 180 days. Larry wanted to *evaluate* the outcome of lack of prenatal care and found that during this time the infant mortality rate in the state was already on the rise. This incident, the support of the nursing organization, and congressional influence led to changes in the state Medicaid law, increasing the number of women in the state who could obtain prenatal care through the health departments.

SUMMARY

This chapter has presented information about governmental and legal influences on the practice of community health nursing. The influence of government and law on community health nursing is significant. However, community health nurses can participate in influencing government through writing regulations and lobbying. Organizations, functions, and structures of government, as well as the process of regulation writing, are all important areas for community health nurses to understand. Legal aspects of the roles and functions of community health nursing, especially scope of practice and negligence, will prove to be useful information for nurses in community health.

Every community health nurse must consider legal implications of practice in each clinical encounter. Because the community health nurse may be the agent of the government when implementing a particular health program, consideration must be given to the power of the state or the relationship of this power to individual rights.

In each clinical encounter, before treating the client, the community health nurse should know what standard of care applies to the situation. Standards of care can be learned from expert nurse witnesses and can be found in agency policies and procedures, nursing, and health care literature, ANA and other professional associations' standards, community health nursing curricula, legislation such as the state nurse practice act, and accreditation and certification criteria. A community health nurse can review nursing documentation to see if an agency's policy requirements were met. Conducting a self-audit ensures that standards of care are met.

KEY CONCEPTS

Many historical events have been significant in developing the role of government in health care.

The legal basis for most congressional action in health care can be found in Article I, Section 8 of the U.S. Constitution.

The four major health care functions of the federal government are direct service, financing, information, and policy setting.

The goal of the World Health Organization is the attainment by all people of the highest possible level of health.

Many federal agencies are involved in government health care functions. The agency most directly involved with the health and welfare of Americans is the Department of Health and Human Services (DHHS).

Most state and local jurisdictions have government activities that affect the health care field.

The variety and range of functions of government agencies have had a major impact on community health nursing. Funding in particular has shaped the role and tasks of community health nurses.

The private sector can influence legislation in many ways, especially through influencing the process of writing regulations. Nurses are a part of the private sector.

The number and types of laws influencing health care are increasing. Because of this, involvement in the political process is most important to community health nurses.

Professional negligence and the scope of practice are two legal aspects particularly relevant to nursing practice.

Community health nurses must consider the legal implications of their own practice in each clinical encounter.

LEARNING ACTIVITIES

1. Conduct an interview with the local health officer. Ask for information from a 10-year period. See if you can see trends in population size and needs and corresponding roles and activities of government that were implemented to meet these changes.

2. Examine a current health department budget and compare it with a budget from previous years. Has there been any impact on health care because of changes in government spending?

3. Select a community health nursing role you would like to examine more closely. Interview a person in that role, asking questions about job function, organizational structure, agency goals, salary, mobility within the agency, and potential contributions of this role to the health of the community.

4. Locate your state register or other documents such as newspapers that publish proposed regulations. Select one set of proposed regulations and critique them. Submit your opinion

in writing as public comment, or attend the hearing and testify on the regulations. Be sure to submit something in writing. Evaluate your participation by stating what you learned and whether the proposed regulations were changed in your favor.

5. Find and review your state nurse practice act and define your scope of practice.

6. Contact your local public health agency to discuss the state's official powers in regulating epidemics such as the recent AIDS outbreak. Explore the state's right to protect the health, safety, and welfare of the citizens. Ask about the conflict between the state's rights and individual rights and how such issues are resolved. Ask about the standards of care that apply to this issue and how it is decided which services offered to clients should be mandatory and which should be voluntary. Explore how the role of public health differs in these epidemics compared with the past epidemics of smallpox and tuberculosis.

BIBLIOGRAPHY

Altman S and Sapolsky H: Federal health programs, Lexington, Mass, 1981, DC Heath & Co.

American Nurses' Association: Guidelines for implementing the code for nurses, Kansas City, Mo, 1980, The Association.

American Nurses' Association: A conceptual model of community health nursing, Kansas City, Mo, 1982, The Association.

American Nurses' Association: Code for nurses, Kansas City, Mo, 1985, The Association.

American Nurses' Association: Standards of community health nursing practice, Kansas City, Mo, 1986, The Association.

American Public Health Association: The definition and role of public health nursing in the delivery of health care, Washington, DC, 1981, The Association.

Aroskar MA: Ethical issues in community health nursing, Nurs Clin North Am 14(1):35-44, 1979.

Bagwell M and Clemens S: A political handbook for health professionals, ed 2, Boston, 1985, Little, Brown, & Co.

Beauchamp T and Childress J: Principles of biomedical ethics, ed 2, New York, 1983, Oxford University Press.

Betz C: Promoting visibility, J Pediatr Nurs 2:1-2, 1987.

Blum H: Planning for health, New York, 1981, Health Sciences Press.

Bullough B: The law and the expanding nursing role, ed 2, New York, 1980, Appleton-Century-Crofts.

Campazzi B: Nurses, nursing, and malpractice litigation, Nurs Adm Q 5(1):1-18, 1981.

Chaney E: Personal and vicarious liability, J Pediatr Nurs 2(2):132, 1987.

Christofel, T: Health and the law: a handbook for health professionals, New York, 1982, MacMillan, Free Press.

Cohen W and Milburn L: Political action, Nursing and Health Care 9(6):294, 1988.

Creighton H: Law every nurse should know, ed 5, Philadelphia, 1986, WB Saunders Co.

Creighton H: Legal implications of home health care, Nurs Mgt 18(2):14, 1987.

Creighton H: Legal implications of policy and procedure manual, part 1, Nurs Mgt 18(5):22, 1987.

Curtin L and Flaherty M: Nursing ethics: theories and pragmatics, Bowie, Md, 1982, Robert J Brady Co.

Cushing M: Million-dollar errors, Am J Nurs 4:435, 1987.

Cushing M: Keeping watch, Am J Nurs 8:1021, 1987.

Cushing M: A strong defense, Am J Nurs 10:1278, 1987.

Cushing M: Perils of home care, Am J Nurs 4:441, 1988.

Dahl R: Democracy in the United States: promise and performance, ed 2, Chicago, 1972, Rand McNally & Co.

Davis A and Aroskar M: Ethical dilemmas and nursing practice, ed 2, New York, 1983, Appleton-Century-Crofts.

Division of Nursing, Bureau of Health Professionals, Health Services and Resources Administration, Public Health Service: The division of nursing, Hyattsville, Md, 1985, The Division.

Feutz S: The expansiveness of liability to third parties, J Nurs Adm (4):9, 1987.

Fiesta J: The nursing shortage: whose liability problem? Part 1, Nurs Mgt 21(1):24, 1990.

Fiesta J: The nursing shortage: whose liability problem? Part 2, Nurs Mgt 21(2):22, 1990.

Fox J: Controversial and legal issues, Family Community Health 2(3):62-68, 1979.

Fromer M: Ethical issues in health care, St. Louis, 1981, The CV Mosby Co.

Halpern S: Government involvement in maternal and child health care: a learning resource for the nurse-midwife, J Nurse Midwifery 32(1):34, 1987.

Health: United States, 1989, DHHS Pub. No. (PHS) 1232, Hyattsville, Md, 1990, Department of Health and Human Services.

Healthy People: The Surgeon General's report on health promotion and disease prevention, DHEW Pub. No. (PHS) 79-55071, Washington, DC, 1979, Department of Health, Education, and Welfare.

Hemelt M and Mackert M: Dynamics of law in nursing and health care, ed 2, Reston, Va, 1982, Reston Publishing Co, Inc.

Hogue E: Nursing and legal liability, a case study approach, Owings Mills, Md, 1985, National Health Publishing.

Kalisch B and Kalisch P: Politics of nursing, Philadelphia, 1982, JB Lippincott Co.

Kapp M: Hospital reimbursement by diagnosis-related groups: legal and ethical implications for nursing homes, J Long-Term Care Adm (3):20, 1986.

Luquire R: Six common causes of nursing liability, Nursing 88(1):61, 1988.

Malher H: Nurses lead the way, WHO features, No. 97, June 1985.

Marks D: Legal implications of increased autonomy, J Gerontol Nurs 13(3):26, 1987.

Martin J et al: Preparing students to shape health policy, Nurs Outlook 37(2):89, 1989.

Northrop C and Kelly M: Legal issues in nursing, St. Louis, 1987, The CV Mosby Co.

Northrop C: Current status of nursing litigation, Nurs Economics 2(6):423-427, 1984.

Northrop C: Filling in charting gaps . . . in court, Nursing 87(9):43, 1987.

Northrop C: Adequate staffing . . . whose problem is it? Nursing 87 (6):43, 1988.

Northrop C: Legal content in the nursing curriculum: what students need and how to provide it, Nurs Outlook 37(4):200, 1989.

Northrop C and Mech A: The nurse as expert witness, Nurs Law Ethics 2(2):1,2,6,8, 1981.

Office of Federal Register: United States government manual, Washington, DC, 1990, US Government Printing Office.

Painter S: Shield yourself from liability, Nursing 87(5):47, 1987.

Parsons M: Five common legal risks: could these stories have happened to you? Nursing Life (6):26, 1986.

Pickett G and Hanlon J: Public health administration and practice, St Louis, 1990, Times Mirror/Mosby College Publishing.

Primary health care needs. Conclusion and recommendations of a WHO study group, Int Nurs Rev 34(2):52, 1987.

Rogge M: Nursing and politics: a forgotten legacy, Nurs Res (1):26, 1987.

Scearse P: Public policy and the conservatives, traditionals, and influentials, J Prof Nurs 3(3):132, 1987.

Scearse P: Disease, debts, and the political process, J Prof Nurs 4(4):239, 1988.

Schanz S: Health care provider liability: traditional principles, Nurs Econ 5(6):311, 1987.

Smith C: Patient teaching: it's the law, Nursing 87(7):67, 1987.

Smith G, Using the public agenda to shape PHN practice, Nurs Outlook 37(2):72, 1989.

Solomon S and Roe S: Integrating public policy into the curriculum, 1986, National League for Nursing.

Solomon S and Roe S: Key concepts in public policy: student workbook, 1986, National League for Nursing.

Szasz A: The labor impacts of policy change in health care: how federal policy transformed home health organizations and their labor practices, J Health Polit Policy Law 15(1):191, 1990.

United Nations: Basic facts about the UN, New York, 1990, The UN.

Weaver J: National health policy and the underserved, St. Louis, 1976, The CV Mosby Co.

Wiley L: Liability for death: nine nurses' legal ordeals, Nursing 2(9):34-43, 1981.

Wing K: The law and the public's health, ed 2, Ann Arbor, Mich, 1985, Health Administration Press.

World Health Organization: The work of WHO, 1988-1990: biennial report of the Director-General, Geneva, 1990, WHO.

World Health Organization: Technical report series, 738, Geneva, 1986.

PART TWO

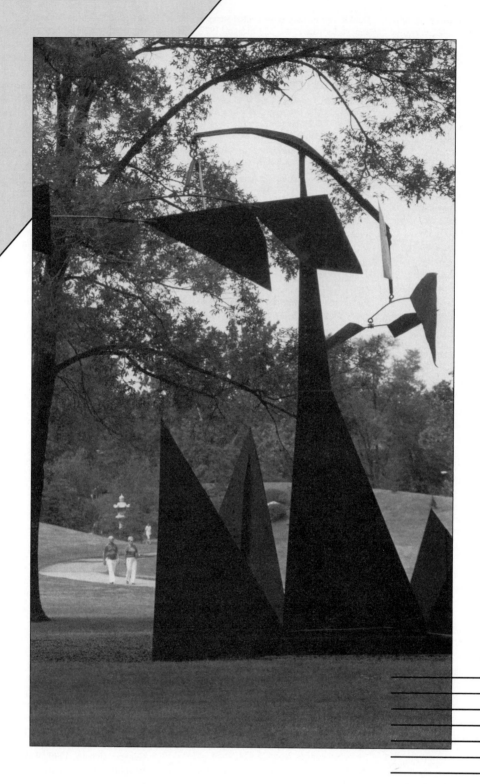

Conceptual Foundations for Community Health Nursing Practice

I n 1988 the National Center for Nursing Research (NCNR) was established under the National Institutes of Health for the purpose of facilitating nursing research. The establishment of the NCNR has been crucial to the profession's movement to build a stronger base for practice. Though no conceptual or theoretical model will meet the needs of all community health nurses, several nursing and public health models serve as frameworks for organizing educational programs and for making practice decisions.

The scientific base provided by public health as a specialty continues to lay a useful foundation for community health nursing. In Part Two, seven chapters provide information about how to use conceptual models, epidemiology, research, nursing diagnoses, principles of education, program planning, and quality assurance to organize community health practice.

Each chapter provides both theory and practical application of the specific topic to the clinical area. The goal of this section is to provide readers with a helpful set of tools that can be used to influence public health and community health nursing practice.

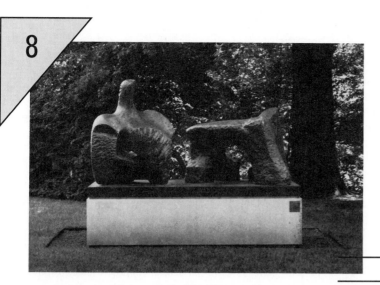

8

Conceptual Models for Community Health Nursing

Jeanette Lancaster

Lois Lowry

Gwendolyn Lee

OBJECTIVES

After reading this chapter, the student should be able to:

Define the terms **theory, model, concept, and conceptual model.**

Differentiate between conceptual model and theory.

Describe key components of current conceptual models in nursing.

Identify at least three uses of conceptual models in nursing.

Differentiate between the ANA and the APHA models of community health nursing.

List the chief characteristics of these interdisciplinary theories: systems, developmental, and interaction.

List the chief characteristics of the following models: Roy, Rogers, Johnson, Orem, Neuman, King.

Apply the Neuman Systems model to community health practice.

KEY TERMS

boundary	Interaction models	openness
concept	Johnson's behavioral	Orem's self-care
conceptual model	systems	model
developmental theory	King's theory	Rogers' science of
entropy	Maslow's hierarchy of	unitary man
equifinality	needs	Roy's adaptation
feedback	model	model
General Systems	negentropy	theory
Theory (GST)	Neuman's systems	wholeness
hypothesis	model	

A s described in Chapter 1, community health nursing has historically demonstrated both the art and science of nursing. In recent years there has been considerable discussion about the extent of a scientific basis for nursing. According to Walker and Avant (1988, p. 3), "As nursing has come of age both as a profession and a scholarly discipline, there has been increasing concern with delineating its theory base." Study of theory calls attention to the relationships that influence nursing. The development of conceptual models has stimulated the refinement of theory utilization in nursing. This chapter will discuss several theories that influence current thinking in nursing.

This chapter also includes a discussion of selected conceptual models that can guide community health practice. Several important terms are defined, and the usefulness of conceptual models for guiding practice is explained. The "Conceptual Model of Community Health Nursing" of the American Nurses' Association (1980) and the "Role and Definition of Public Health Nursing in the Delivery of Health Care" by the American Public Health Association (1981) are summarized and compared. The Neuman model is used to demonstrate the value of theory in guiding community health practice.

DEFINITION OF TERMS

Historically, nursing knowledge developed informally and was characterized as the *art* of nursing. However, during the 1950s, nurse scholars began to formally develop theories that would establish nursing as a profession separate and distinct from medicine (Chinn & Jacobs, 1991).

"A *conceptual model* and synonymous terms, *conceptual framework* and *conceptual system*, refer to global ideas about individuals, groups, situations and events of interest to a discipline" (Fawcett, 1989, p. 2). The box at right defines key terms that are used in explaining the conceptual approach to nursing. Conceptual models provide a frame of reference for members of a discipline to guide their thinking, observations, and interpretations. A model is inductively developed when specific events are seen as examples of more general events (Fawcett, 1989). Thus conceptual models are approximations or simplifications of reality and are based on the concepts the model builder considers relevant. Thus nursing models facilitate communication among nurses and can provide a unified approach to nursing practice, education, administration, and research.

Although the terms model and theory are often used interchangeably, they are different in several ways. One main difference is in the level of abstraction. A conceptual model is a highly abstract system of global concepts and propositional statements. In contrast, a theory focuses on one or more concrete, specific concepts and statements. A second difference involves the ability to test the model or theory. A conceptual model cannot be tested directly because the concepts are not operationally defined, nor are the relationships observable. A theory, on the other hand, is clearly stated and operationally defined, and hypotheses are formulated so they can be tested through research. Conceptual models constitute a key stage in theory development by providing focus, identifying relevant variables and ruling out others as unrelated.

DEFINITIONS OF KEY TERMS

Conceptual model (framework): Provides a frame of reference for members of a discipline to guide their thinking, observations, and interpretations; made up of concepts; propositions of a conceptual model are abstract and general.

Concepts: The building blocks of theory; describe mental images of phenomena, and can be concrete (chair) or abstract (body temperature).

Constructs: Concepts describing phenomena that are not directly observable; e.g., society, intelligence, age.

Propositions: Statements that describe the relationship between concepts; e.g., "persons and their environments are in constant interaction" is a proposition.

Theory: A set of interrelated constructs (concepts), definitions, and propositions that present a systematic view of phenomena by specifying relationships among variables, with the purpose of explaining and predicting phenomena (Kerlinger, 1973, p. 9).

In conceptual models with the greatest application to community health nursing, people are viewed as being in continuous interaction with the environment. The environment is dynamic and can be either positive or negative. The unique feature of community health nursing is the emphasis on assisting individuals, families, groups, and communities to maintain their highest possible levels of health. To accomplish this, the community is viewed from a holistic perspective as a motivator or disrupter of health. The nursing goal is to assess, plan, implement, and evaluate ways to make the community a healthier place to live.

USING CONCEPTUAL MODELS

To some extent everyone has developed a conceptual model, because all people have assumptions and beliefs about how the world operates. Everyone has a unique set of concepts guiding how ideas and information are categorized. In nursing, people view situations differently and respond in their own ways to others. Whether implicit or explicit, a person's conceptual models influence behavior. Conceptual models guide actions either consciously or unconsciously. As will be seen later, a variety of conceptual models are useful in community health.

Many nurses use one particular nursing model to guide practice; others merge more than one model into a unique guide for practice; still others integrate theories borrowed from other disciplines such as psychology, sociology, and the biological sciences. Conceptual models are especially useful in nursing education, research, administration, and practice.

Nursing Education

Conceptual models can provide a general outline for organizing curricular content and for selecting teaching-learning approaches. To guide curriculum, conceptual models must be linked with theories about education and the teaching-learning process and must draw upon substantive theoretical content from nursing and other relevant disciplines.

Nursing Research

Conceptual models cannot be tested directly. However, the propositions linking constructs of the model can be indirectly tested when they are operationally defined. Data are collected using actual instruments or through a variety of experiments. A three-level representation of theory development is evident in research. The conceptual model is the most abstract level that guides the study; the second level includes propositional statements; and the third and most concrete level contains the empirical indicators (Fawcett & Downs, 1987, p. 87).

Conceptual models provide the essential conceptual, instrumental, and methodological rules for guiding nursing research. The model helps define the concepts from which specific variables are derived. It defines research questions and thereby serves as an overall map for the study. Specific research endeavors may focus on one or several aspects of a conceptual model.

Nursing Administration

Conceptual models have been used by nursing service administrators for nearly three decades as guides to determine methods of providing client care. Models serve as paradigms that connect the structural environment to the patterns of relationships within the organization. Administrative models reflect the interrelationship of nursing education, practice, administration, and research within a service setting (Nelson, 1989). Models provide a means for uniting service, education, and research through collaboration toward achieving a unified goal. This results in quality client care based on knowledge as well as professional accountability (Chance, 1982).

Nursing Practice

A model provides practitioners with a general perspective on what is important to observe (Broncatello, 1980). The framework provides categories into which assessment data can be organized, thus reducing the possibility of overlooking critical information. The practitioner can then better plan interventions for client care. Specific theories are employed to describe, explain, and predict client manifestations of actual or potential health problems (Fawcett, 1989, p. 30). Nurses using models in practice are able to identify problems from which hypotheses can be generated. In this way, clinical research becomes an integral part of nursing practice.

THE ANA CONCEPTUAL MODEL OF COMMUNITY HEALTH NURSING PRACTICE

The definition of community health nursing set forth in the ANA Conceptual Model of Community Health Nursing emphasizes health promotion and consumer involvement and considers health as influenced by multiple factors within people and by the environments in which people live. The definition reads as follows (American Nurses' Association, 1980, p. 2):

> Community health nursing is a synthesis of nursing and public health practice applied to promoting and preserving the health of populations. The practice is general and comprehensive. It is not limited to a particular age group or

---

ASSUMPTIONS AND BELIEFS ABOUT COMMUNITY HEALTH NURSING

Assumption 1: The health care system is complex.

Assumption 2: Primary, secondary, and tertiary health care are components of the health care system.

Assumption 3: Nursing, as a subsystem of the health care system, is the product of education and practice based upon research.

Assumption 4: Provision of primary care predominates in community health nursing practice, with lesser involvement in secondary and tertiary health care.

Assumption 5: Community health nursing occurs principally in primary health care settings.

Belief 1: Health care should be available, accessible, and acceptable to all persons.

Belief 2: In making health policy, recipients of health care services should be included.

Belief 3: The nurse as a provider and the client as a consumer of health care services can form a conjoint relationship to advocate and effect change in health policies and services.

Belief 4: The environment affects the health of populations, groups, families, and individuals.

Belief 5: Prevention of illness is essential to promote health.

Belief 6: A health axis intersects with the life span axis.

Belief 7: The client is the only constant member of the health care team.

Belief 8: Individuals within a community are ultimately responsible for their own health and must be encouraged and taught to be active participants in their own health care.

© American Nurses' Association, 1980. Reprinted with permission.

---

diagnosis, and is continuing, not episodic. The dominant responsibility is to the population as a whole; nursing directed to individuals, families, or groups contributes to the health of the total population. Health promotion, health maintenance, health education, and management, coordination, and continuity of care are utilized in a holistic approach to the management of the health care of individuals, families and groups in a community.

This definition encompasses both direct and indirect services to individuals, families, groups, and communities. Its scope is concerned with both wellness and illness in providing, as well as facilitating, the delivery of services. A set of assumptions and beliefs further elaborates on the goal of community health nursing and describes the scope of practice (see box above).

According to the ANA conceptual model, the focus of community health nursing is on the prevention of illness and promotion and maintenance of health. To achieve these goals, nursing activities include client education, counseling, advocacy, and management of care. The major emphasis in community health nursing is on primary care. This begins when clients enter the health care system and continues throughout the duration of the client's care. Secondary and tertiary care are emphasized less. Clients are considered to be active members of the health care team, and the goal of care is to help clients assume self-responsibility for health care.

The specific functions viewed as priorities in the role of the community health nurse are seen in the nine standards identified by the Division on Community Health Nursing Practice and given in Appendix F (American Nurses' Association, 1980).

The major goal of the community health nurse, as pointed out in Chapter 1, is the preservation and improvement of the health of the community. This overall objective is accomplished in two major ways. The first is through direct care to individuals, families, and groups within a designated community. The second is by considering the health of the total population and how community health problems and issues affect individuals, families, and groups. For example, the problem of improper waste disposal or stagnant water near a residential area would be considered a community health nursing problem because it could adversely affect the health of area residents.

Practicing in the first mode, community health nurses work directly with clients to promote optimal health, and where health has been disrupted, to assist in its restoration and stabilization. The pattern of practice takes place through clinics, home health care, and group work with clients having common health needs. Practice is collaborative with other members of the health care team, is holistic in orientation, and emphasizes the evaluation of nursing care to individuals, families, and the community.

In the second mode the focus is on the community as client, and the aim is to assist communities to identify health needs, establish priorities, plan and implement actions, and identify and intervene in factors affecting the health of the community. This mode emphasizes the ongoing interaction between people and their environment. The role of the community health nurse embraces all three levels of prevention—primary, secondary, and tertiary—with emphasis on primary. As will be noted in the following discussion, many similarities exist between the ANA Conceptual Model of Community Health Nursing and the definition and role delineation established by the APHA Public Health Nursing Section.

THE APHA DEFINITION OF PUBLIC HEALTH NURSING AND ITS ROLE IN THE DELIVERY OF HEALTH CARE

Like the ANA, a work group of the APHA Public Health Nursing Section was established as an ad hoc committee to define public health nursing* and delineate its scope of practice. To state a clear and concise position, the following definition of public health nursing was recommended (American Public Health Association, 1981, p. 4):

> Public health nursing synthesizes the body of knowledge from the public health sciences and professional nursing theories for the purpose of improving the health of the entire community. This goal lies at the heart of primary prevention and health promotion and is the foundation for public health nursing practice. To accomplish this goal, public health nurses work with groups, families, and individuals as well

as in multidisciplinary teams and programs. Identifying the subgroups (aggregates) within the population which are at high risk of illness, disability, or premature death and directing resources toward three groups is the most effective approach for accomplishng the goal of public health nursing. Success in reducing the risks and in improving the health of the community depends on the involvement of consumers, especially groups experiencing health risks, and others in the community, in health planning, and in self-help activities.

The position paper of the APHA committee further noted that public health nursing practice is a systematic process in which the following occur (American Public Health Association, 1980, pp. 4-5):

1. The health and health care needs of a population are assessed by nurses or in collaboration with other disciplines in order to identify subpopulations (aggregates), families, and individuals at increased risk of illness, disability, or premature death.
2. A plan for intervention is developed to meet these needs that includes available resources and those activities that contribute to health and its recovery and to the prevention of illness, disability, and premature death.
3. A health care plan is implemented effectively, efficiently, and equitably.
4. An evaluation is made to determine the extent to which these activities have an impact on the health status of the population.

Both the ANA and APHA definitions emphasize the blending of nursing and public health knowledge as a foundation for determining the scope of practice. They both acknowledge that community health nursing efforts are directed toward all people, whether they are cared for as individuals, as part of a family, in a community, or as a community at large. Each definition emphasizes a multidisciplinary role for the successful implementation of public health practice, and they both focus on the increasing priority of health promotion. However, the APHA definition emphasizes primary care more than the ANA definition does. It also clearly points out the need to determine within a community those groups at greatest risk for health disruption, so that nursing intervention can be targeted toward them to prevent the onset of disease.

MODELS APPLICABLE TO NURSING PRACTICE

Conceptual models have proliferated in the physical, biological, and social sciences during the twentieth century, providing a frame of reference for members of a discipline (Lippett, 1973). A model directs the world view: what is considered relevant, what is eliminated, which concepts or constructs are identified, and how they are defined. The world view refers to philosophic assumptions about the nature of person-environment interactions. Not every world view is the same, so one model may be logically incompatible with another (Fawcett, 1989).

In addition to reflecting diverse world views, conceptual models can be classified according to the approach from which they were derived. Systems, developmental models, and interaction models are different classes of approaches to understanding phenomena (Riehl & Roy, 1980). Most

---

*The term *public health nursing* will be used in this section of the discussion instead of *community health nursing* because APHA uses this term to refer to their nursing clinical section.

nursing models fall within these classifications because each suggests a way to interpret personenvironment interactions, perceptions of health/illness, and the role of nursing. Nursing models that reflect more than one approach are classified within the most dominant category.

Systems Models

Systems models focus on the "organization, interaction, interdependency and integration of parts and elements" (Chinn, 1980, p. 24). Systems models are based on general systems theory as postulated by von Bertalanffy (1952, p. 11), who wrote that "every organism represents a system, by which term we mean a complex of elements in mutual interaction." The elements are wholeness, organization, and dynamic order, and von Bertalanffy delineates how these concepts are important phenomena in physics, biology, psychology, and philosophy (1952, pp. 176-204).

Characteristics

Concepts frequently discussed in relation to general systems theory are wholeness, organization, openness, boundary, entropy, negentropy, and equifinality. Wholeness refers to that property of a system in which a collection of parts responds as an integrated single part. The arrangement of the elements and their relationships to each other represent their organization.

Openness of a system refers to the extent to which it exchanges energy with the environment. An open system is affected by the environment (receives input) and in turn affects the environment by its output. In a closed system, no energy is exchanged.

Boundary refers to a line or border that defines what elements comprise the system. In biological terms the cell membrane is a boundary encompassing the contents of a cell. In social systems the boundary is more like an imaginary line that groups certain individuals together.

Entropy is a concept based on a major implication of the second law of thermodynamics, which states that elements in a closed environment will proceed toward greater randomness or less order. Entropy is also described as disordered energy, or energy that is bound and cannot be converted to work. Negentropy is the energy that is "free," can be used for work, and tends toward order. Because living systems are open systems, they do not adhere to the implications of the second law of thermodynamics. *Equifinality* refers to the concept that the end state of the open system is independent of the beginning state.

Feedback is the process whereby the output of the system is redirected as the input to the same system. The body as a physiological system uses feedback to regulate temperature, heart rate, and respiration. Every system contains parameters representing input, thruput, output, and feedback.

Advantages and Disadvantages

Systems theory can be applied across disciplines so that universal laws are identified and can be used with individuals, groups, and communities. It emphasizes how each isolated variable affects the whole and how the whole affects each part. A disadvantage is that it does not explicitly emphasize growth and change toward a higher level of organization.

Application to Community Health Nursing

The community as a whole is a social system made up of interrelated and interdependent subsystems. The subsystems include the economic, educational, religious, health care, political, welfare, law enforcement, energy, and recreational systems. When any one of the subsystems is affected, it affects the community as a whole. One subsystem in which changes immediately and obviously affect the whole is the economic system.

All of the subsystems of the larger social system, the community, are organized and related to each other in a specific way. Specific communication channels exist for the organizations to relate to each other and to the whole.

According to systems theory, the community is an open system that exchanges materials such as energy, goods and services, values, and ideals with the environment outside the community. The community as a system has boundaries, the most obvious being geographical lines. The imaginary boundary is one that encompasses all the subsystems in the community and identifies what is inside and outside the community. Entropy can be compared with landfill garbage dumps or with problems such as crime, violence, and poor health in the community. Negentropy can be compared with the resources, health, wealth, and altruistic values of the people. Equifinality indicates that the community, no matter how poor and unattractive, may attain economic balance and beauty if given the proper resources and energy.

Systems thinking was popular in the 60s and 70s. Four nurse theorists, King, Johnson, Roy, and Neuman, formulated systems models between 1968 and 1972. Each of these models is used today in community health nursing. They are discussed later in the chapter.

Developmental Theory

Developmental theory is a way of thinking about how changes occur based on theories of development of the human organism. Lewis (1982) classifies theories of child development as reactive and structural. Reactive theories emphasize the influence of the environment on the development of the child. These include stimulus-response theory, learning theories, classical conditioning, and operant conditioning. Structural theories emphasize the genetically determined program for development, which is usually described in stages (Lewis, 1982, p. 10). Examples of structural theories include Freud's psychosexual stages, Erikson's psychosocial phases, and Piaget's stages of cognitive development (Lewis, 1982, pp. 12-13). Although Lewis (1982) refers to these as structural theories, they are generally referred to as developmental theories.

Characteristics

Chinn (1980, pp. 30-31), describes the major characteristics of developmental models as direction; stages (also referred to as phases or levels); progression; potentiality; and forces. These characteristics refer to the process of growth or change.

Direction refers to the fact that growth proceeds in a specific direction toward an end state or goal. In development of the individual, a direction of physical growth is toward being taller, and a direction of mental growth is toward complexity in thought and language.

Stages, phases, and levels are synonymous terms used to describe periods when the individual or group is concentrating on a particular task or developmental milestone. Certain facets of growth or behavior are unique to each stage. For example, an infant develops motor capabilities sequentially by crawling, pulling to a standing position, and then walking.

Progression suggests that the way in which change occurs over time has a characteristic form. Chinn (1980, p. 31) describes four types or characteristics of progression: linear, spiral, oscillation, and differentiation. Linear refers to changes, such as aging, that proceed in a unidirectional manner. Spiral refers to the fact that similar behaviors may be repeated, but at a more complex level. For example, thinking and problem solving are behaviors that are repeated but are performed at higher levels as development progresses. Oscillation refers to the individual going back and forth for a time between behaviors of two stages. Differentiation refers to changes in which the functions of the individual become more specialized.

The last characteristic, forces, include genetic and environmental factors. Individuals are genetically programmed for growth and development. The environmental forces can enhance or deter that development. Potentiality refers to the genetic capabilities of the individual given a supporting and nurturing environment. Although it is easier to understand these characteristics in the development of the individual, the reader should remember that the developmental model is also applied to change in groups or social organizations such as health care delivery systems.

Advantages and Disadvantages

Developmental models have two advantages. First, their characteristics are easy to understand. In relation to the human organism, the developmental changes can be observed. Second, growth is emphasized and viewed as a positive event, which may be experienced psychologically even when physical growth has ceased. A disadvantage of developmental models is that major variables such as environment, sociocultural factors, or circumstances may not be considered or may be minimized.

Application to Community Health Nursing

The usefulness of developmental theory in working with infants and children is evidenced by the fact that growth and development is an inherent part of every nursing curriculum. A major part of the nurse's role in working with infants and children is assessing their developmental progress and helping parents promote that progress with a stimulating environment. One of the most widely used screening tools to assess child development is the Denver Developmental Screening Test (DDST). The DDST was developed and tested to yield a developmental profile in the areas of gross motor, language, fine motor-adaptive, and personal-social skills. The developmental approach also has been widely used with families. Duvall (1977, p. 144) described the family life cycle in eight stages: beginning, early childbearing, preschool, school, teenagers, launching center, middle years, retirement, and old age. The nurse can use each of these stages of development and their respective

tasks for each stage in the assessment and the promotion of family development.

The nursing models of Rogers and Orem can be classified as developmental models.

Interaction Models

Interaction models are based on theories that stem from philosophical writings such as those of Cooley (1909) and Mead (1934). Mead was influential in the development of social psychology. He viewed a human being as a reflection of human society, that is, primarily a social and cultural being. Further, he contended that a newborn develops a self as a consequence of relationships with others and the environment. The major concepts used in interaction models are communication, perception, role, and self-concept.

Characteristics

Communication is the act of giving and receiving information and consists of both verbal and nonverbal language. Perception is the way a person perceives a situation or an event. It is influenced by antecedent, cognitive, and emotional factors already present in the person's background. Role refers to the set of prescriptions defining what the behavior of a position member should be. Variations in meanings attached to role are best illustrated by the qualifiers or descriptors attached to role. Multiple roles refer to the fact that one human being has several roles. Each role brings expectations, and sometimes role strain occurs as a result of role conflict. Self-concept refers to the way in which persons visualize and think about themselves. The picture that we have of ourselves influences the way we interact with others.

Advantages and Disadvantages

Interaction theory calls attention to how elements affect each other, especially the individuality of human beings. However, attention can be focused on interaction to the exclusion of other variables.

Application to Community Health Nursing

The phenomenon of family dynamics is frequently addressed in the nursing literature. The interaction model can be useful in analyzing family dynamics. Each of the four concepts of interaction theory has specific application to community health nursing.

COMMUNICATION. When working with families, assessment of communication patterns is an important element of community health nursing. The reason for the family's contact with the nurse may be health related, but the manner in which the family is coping with the health problems may be intricately related to communication patterns. These patterns include who talks to whom about what and in what way. It is also important to know who listens, what is heard by the person listening, if the message sent is the message received, and what kind of feedback the members of the family give to each other.

ROLE. Assessment of the role structure is also important in working with families. Role refers to a set of expected behaviors by virtue of occupying or holding a given position, and every person assumes multiple roles. Problems or illnesses that generally bring the person to the health care system will affect the person's ability to function in many of the roles. The person may worry about the inability to function in all the roles. An obvious and perhaps overused example is the executive who worries that a heart attack will interfere with the role as provider for the family. In the health maintenance function, the nurse uses knowledge about role to identify such things as role conflict or role strains. Role conflict is a situation in which a person is confronted with incompatible expectations. Role strain involves anxiety, work, and stress associated with the role. The nurse will also have contact with first-time parents who are undergoing the role transition from husband and wife to father and mother.

SELF-CONCEPT. Self-concept is an important aspect of health and well-being. It probably influences health-seeking behaviors and adaptation to problems of a health-illness nature. The change from being a well person to someone who requires health care may result in a lower self-concept. Thus it is important that the nurse listen for cues and help the person use self-concept positively.

PERCEPTION. Perception of events and situations (for example, accidents) differs from one person to another. In the same way, people's perceptions of events and situations involving themselves are affected by previous experiences including attitudes, beliefs, and socialization into a particular culture. It is useful to the nurse to recognize the differences in perception. The client's perception of the situation may not be the same as that of the nurse.

NURSING MODELS WITH APPLICATION TO COMMUNITY HEALTH NURSING

Several conceptual models have been developed and described by nurses for use in nursing. Among the models with greatest application to community health nursing are those developed by Roy, Rogers, Johnson, Neuman, Orem, and King. These are described briefly.

King

Imogene King's theory (1968) was first introduced as a "conceptual frame of reference." King refers to her work as a derivation from systems theory, with emphasis on interaction theory.

Nursing intervention is carried out through the process of action, reaction, interaction, and transaction between the client and the nurse. King also described a theory of goal attainment through a goal-oriented nursing record. This consists of five major elements: a data base, a problem list, a goal list, a plan, and progress notes (King, 1981, p. 165). King describes her conceptual framework as a general systems model with three subsystems: personal system, interpersonal system, and social system. The personal system is made up of the concepts of perception, self, growth and development, body image, space, and time. The interpersonal system is made up of the concepts of human interactions, communication, transactions, role, and stress. The social system is made up of the concepts of organization, authority, power, status, and decision making. The three systems are dynamic and interacting (King, 1981).

Application to Community Health Nursing Practice

The goal of nursing is "human beings interacting with their environment leading to a state of health for individuals, which is an ability to function in social roles" (King, 1981, p. 143). Emphasis on client participation in goal setting and goal achievement is a major strength of this model. The theory of goal attainment has been tested and has received support, advancing nursing knowledge. The Goal-Oriented Nursing Record (GONR), derived from the theory of goal attainment, has been implemented in service agencies. King's model is a useful framework for nurses whose social interactions with clients are a key focus of their practice.

Johnson

Dorothy Johnson's Behavioral Systems Model was first presented as an unpublished paper at Vanderbilt University in 1968. It is clearly a systems model with the behavioral system having subsystems. The system and the subsystems are linked to each other and are open. Johnson assumed that the person can be viewed as a behavioral system in the same way that the human body is viewed as a biological system. The behavioral system consists of seven subsystems: achievement, affiliation, aggression, dependency, elimination, ingestion, and sexuality. Each subsystem has four structural elements: drive or goal, set or predisposition to act, choices of action alternatives, and the ultimate action or behavior. The behavioral system as a whole and each of the subsystems have functional requirements: protection, nurturance, and stimulation. The outcome of the behavioral system is a patterned, repetitive, and purposeful way of behaving. If behavior is efficient and effective, it will be orderly, purposeful, and predictable.

Application to Community Health Nursing Practice

"The goal of nursing action in each case is to restore, maintain, or attain behavioral system balance and stability at the highest possible level for the individual" (Johnson, 1980, p. 214). This means that the nurse is concerned with promoting efficient and effective behavior in the client to prevent illness and promote health. Johnson did not identify a specific nursing process but suggested listing all significant behaviors in each of the seven subsystems and identifying them as functional or dysfunctional.

Variables influencing or causing the behaviors are also identified. The nursing problem or diagnosis is made and is placed in one of four diagnostic classifications: (1) insufficiency, which indicates the subsystem is not functioning; (2) discrepancy, which indicates the behavior is not meeting the intended goal; (3) incompatibility, which indicates that goals or behaviors of two subsystems are in conflict; and (4) dominance, which indicates that the behavior in one subsystem is used more than any other. Long- and short-term goals are set before intervention. There are four modes of nursing intervention: (1) restrict or place limits on behavior; (2) defend or protect from negative stressors; (3) inhibit or suppress ineffective responses; and (4) facilitate or give nurturance and stimulation. Following intervention, evaluation is made in terms of long- and short-term goals.

The conceptualization of man as a behavioral system gives an alternative to the medical model as a way of viewing a human. In this way the nursing role can be differentiated from medicine's role. Johnson demonstrated how the model can be used to focus on a person's behavior rather than on the health state or disease condition. Limitations of this model include a nurse-centered focus and incomplete linkages among the four concepts of the paradigm. Johnson had a positive influence on Roy and Neuman in the development of their models.

Roy

The Roy Adaptation Model of Nursing was first presented in the periodical literature (Roy, 1970) and has since been used as a conceptual framework for nursing curricula, nursing practice, and nursing research. Roy (Riehl and Roy, 1980, p. 179) maintains that her model is a systems theory model although it also contains interactionist levels of analysis. A human is viewed as an adaptive system. Changes occur in the system in response to stimuli (input). If the changes promote integrity of the individual (such as growth or self-mastery), the response is adaptive. Otherwise, the response is considered maladaptive. The system has two major mechanisms for adapting or coping: the regulator and cognator. The regulator system is concerned with the neural, endocrine, and perception-psychomotor processes. The cognator mechanism is concerned with the processes of perception, learning, judgment, and emotion (Roy and Roberts, 1981, pp. 60-63). Additionally, four modes for effecting adaptation of the system include physiological needs, self-concept, role function, and interdependence.

The nursing process, according to Roy, consists of a first and second level assessment, problem identification, nursing diagnosis, setting priorities, setting goals, intervention, and evaluation (Roy, 1984, p. 43). In the first level assessment, client behaviors in each of the adaptive modes (physiological, self-concept, role function, and interdependence) are observed and described. In the second level assessment, the nurse identifies the focal, contextual, and residual factors influencing client behavior. The focal stimuli represent the situation, such as stress, injury, or illness, immediately confronting the individual. The contextual stimuli are the other factors present, such as family milieu or environment. The residual stimuli are influencing factors from the client's background: beliefs, attitudes, experiences, and traits. Following the second level assessment, problems are identified, nursing diagnoses are made, priorities are set, and goals are formulated. The next step, intervention, manipulates the stimuli to promote adaptation. Finally, evaluation is used to judge the effectiveness of the nursing approach.

Application to Community Health Nursing Practice

The goal of the nurse is to "maintain and enhance adaptive behavior and to change ineffective behavior to adaptive" (Roy, 1984, p. 59). The nurse achieves this goal by manipulating or changing the stimuli that are causing the stress, thus helping the person cope more effectively. When individuals encounter more than the usual amount of stress, their established coping mechanisms may be ineffective. Thus a nursing intervention is required.

Strengths of the model include the following: (1) most of the terminology is familiar or is clearly described; (2) the nursing process is similar to the standard of assessment, planning, implementation, and evaluation; (3) the focus is on behaviors offering greater individuality in assessment; (4) assessment of psychosocial needs is emphasized; and (5) it has been applied in practice, education, and research (Fawcett, 1989).

Limitations of the model include the following: (1) the adaptive modes overlap, especially in the modes of self-concept, role function, and interdependence, (2) the judgment of behavior as adaptive or maladaptive will be influenced by the value system of the nurse assessing the client, and (3) the term "adaptation" generally does not convey a meaning of growth as intended in the model.

Neuman

Betty Neuman's Health-Care Systems Model was first developed as a total person approach to viewing client problems in response to expressed needs of graduate students in the school of nursing at the University of California at Los Angeles (Neuman & Young, 1972). Neuman claims that the model depicts an open system in which persons and their environments are in dynamic interaction (Neuman, 1989). The client system is composed of five interacting variables: physiological, psychological, sociocultural, developmental, and spiritual. These variables have a basic core structure unique to the individual, but with a range of responses common to all human beings. Client systems may be individuals, families, groups, or communities.

The model is depicted as concentric rings surrounding the core. The inner rings represent lines of resistance against stressors, such as the immune system and defense mechanisms. An outer ring is the normal line of defense representing a clients' normal wellness state. External to the normal line of defense is an accordion-like flexible line of defense that acts as a buffer zone to cushion the client from stressor invasion (Neuman, 1989).

The environment is seen as all factors affecting and affected by the system. Stressors occurring within and outside the client create tension and reactions to the tension. The stressors are defined as interpersonal, intrapersonal, or extrapersonal in nature (Neuman, 1989). Gestalt, stress-adaptation, systems, and wholeness theories have influenced Neuman's thinking. Neuman's model is flexible and applicable to a variety of settings.

Application to Community Health Nursing Practice

The major goal of nursing is "system stability" (Neuman, 1989). Nurses intervene to reduce the client's encounter with stressors. Primary prevention strengthens the flexible line of defense; secondary prevention reduces the degree of reaction to stressors; and tertiary prevention assists reconstitution to attain maximum wellness (Neuman, 1989). Neuman emphasizes assessing both the client's and nurse's perceptions of stressors to determine the existence of any discrepancies.

The nursing process format for the Neuman Systems Model consists of three steps: nursing diagnosis, nursing goals, and nursing outcomes. Nursing goals are mutually determined by the client and nurse according to the three preventive categories and are evaluated as nursing outcomes (Neuman, 1989).

The Neuman Systems Model has been adopted by 14 countries to guide nursing curricula, nursing practice, and administration. Its popularity stems from its basic vocabulary, an open structure that facilitates the use of many supporting theories, an interdisciplinary approach, and emphasis on the three preventions familiar to community health nursing. Its primary limitation is that nursing theory has yet to be derived from this model.

Rogers

Martha Rogers' Science of Unitary Man first appeared in the literature in 1970. It has been used as the conceptual base for nursing curricula, research projects, and to a lesser extent to guide nursing practice. Rogers' model has strong ties to general systems theory, and elements of the developmental model are inherent.

Rogers describes energy fields, universe of open systems, pattern and organization, and four dimensionality as the four building blocks for her conceptual system (Rogers, 1980, p. 330). Energy fields refers to the conceptualization of humans and their environment as matter or energy evidenced by wave patterns. Rogers emphasizes the energy field as part of a person's wholeness: "The human field is more than and different from the sum of its parts" (Rogers, 1980, p. 330). Openness refers to the view of persons as open systems who interact continuously with the environment. Pattern and organization refer to the way the energy fields emerge, and are characterized by wave pattern and organization. Four dimensionality is another characteristic of energy fields. This has been described by Johnson and Fitzpatrick (1982, p. 10) as "transcendence of the time-space interaction." Four dimensionality is easier to understand by thinking of the phenomenon of clairvoyance; a person who is clairvoyant sees the future and transcends time for an instant.

Rogers (1980, p. 333) describes the development of unitary persons by use of three principles of homeodynamics. Helicy refers to life as proceeding in one direction, rhythmically, along a spiral. Resonancy refers to the wave pattern and organization of the energy fields. Complementarity refers to integrality, the simultaneous mutual interaction of the human and environmental fields.

Application to Community Health Nursing Practice

Rogers' background in public health obviously influenced her statement of nursing's goal: "Maintenance and promotion of health, prevention of disease, nursing diagnosis, intervention, and rehabilitation encompass the scope of nursing's goals" (Rogers, 1970, p. 86). She also emphasizes that nursing is for the well and the sick, the rich and the poor, and is practiced in all settings—home, school, work, and play.

Rogers made the goal of nursing clear: individuals should achieve their maximum health potential (1970, p. 86). However, it was others who developed her model into a framework for the nursing process. Therapeutic touch (Krieger, 1981; Heidt, 1981) is an application of the Rogers frame-

work to the nursing process. Whelton (1979, pp. 10-14) illustrates assessment and nursing process in the areas of wholeness, openness, pattern and organization, unidirectionality, and sentience and thought.

Falco and Lobo (1985) illustrated the process of assessment using the principles of homeodynamics: integrality, resonancy, and helicy. Whall (1981, pp. 33-34) operationalized Rogers' theory by illustrating the assessment of families under the categories of (1) individual sub-system; (2) interactional patterns; (3) unique characteristics of the whole; and (4) environmental interface synchrony.

Strengths of this model are (1) emphasis on the total context of the universe; (2) the goal of maximum health potential; and (3) emphasis on the effect of environment on a person's health. Limitations of the model include (1) terminology that is not easily understood; and (2) the need for application to practice to be more clearly operationalized.

Orem

The Orem Self-Care Nursing Model began when Orem (1959, p. 5) described the nurse's role as assisting the person who has inabilities in self-care. It was further developed by the Nursing Model Committee of the School of Nursing Faculty of the Catholic University of America, initiated in 1965 (Nursing Development Conference Group, 1973). The first full description, *Nursing: Concepts of Practice*, was published in 1971 and revised in 1991. Orem's model was categorized by Riehl and Roy (1980) as a systems model; however, Fawcett (1989) more appropriately classifies it as a developmental model.

Orem's model (1985) evolves from the way she conceptualizes nursing, especially from her perspective that nursing is concerned with self-care. Important terms in the model are self-care, self-care agency, therapeutic self-care demand, and self-care deficit. Each of these are addressed from a developmental perspective.

Self-care consists of those activities that an individual does for himself to maintain life, health, and well-being. Self-care agency refers to the person who provides the self-care. Every individual has need of a composite of self-care actions called therapeutic self-care demand. If the therapeutic self-care demand is greater than the self-care agency, a self-care deficit exists. When this occurs nursing intervention is needed.

Application to Community Health Nursing Practice

Orem's goal of nursing is to meet the client's self-care demand until the family is capable of providing it. Orem categorized self-care requirements into three types: (1) universal, self-care to meet physiological and psychosocial needs; (2) developmental, the self-care required when one goes through developmental stages; and (3) health deviation, the self-care required when an individual deviates from health. Using the Orem model, assessment is made of the therapeutic self-care demand, the self-care agency, and the self-care deficits in the areas of knowledge, skills, motivation, and orientation.

Following the nursing assessment, a design is formulated for the nursing system, which is the approach the nurse uses to meet the client's self-care deficit. These are categorized into three systems: (1) wholly compensatory, in which the client has no active role; (2) partly compensatory, in which both the client and the nurse have an actual role; and (3) educative development, in which the client can meet his need for self-care with some assistance from the nurse. To implement the nursing system the nurse does one of the following: (1) acting for, or doing for; (2) guiding; (3) supporting; (4) providing; and (5) teaching.

The model builds on self-care, a function for which nurses have historically assumed responsibility. Orem emphasized the client's role in planning and implementing care according to his or her capability. Structure in the model focuses on the client as a learner and the nurse as a teacher.

Similarities and Differences between Models

One way to examine the similarities and differences of nursing models is to consider how each author defines components of the nursing paradigm: person, environment, health, and nursing (Table 8-1). Similarities in the models include their consideration of the impact of environment on humans and human interaction with the environment. Behavioral patterning, the holistic human, and maximum functioning of the organism are common themes. For the most part, the differences are more in their emphasis, although there are some unique views (e.g., Rogers' emphasis on energy fields and Johnson's conceptualization of a human as a behavioral system). In others, particular attention is focused on themes previously introduced in nursing. Neuman emphasizes primary, secondary, and tertiary prevention; Orem's model is organized around self-care; Roy recognizes the human as a psychosocial human being. King emphasizes transactions in interpersonal contacts.

PSYCHOSOCIAL THEORIES APPLICABLE TO COMMUNITY HEALTH NURSING

Various psychosocial theories are applicable to nursing. Four theories that are particularly relevant to community health nursing are motivation, change, communication, and leadership.

Motivation

The influence of motives on behavior and the influence of motivation on achievement or work productivity have long been recognized. Between 1900 and 1930 classical theory postulated that the basic motive of man was economic gain; the emphasis in organizations was on tasks. However, following the studies at the Hawthorne Plant of the Western Electric Company, the classical theory was abandoned for the human relations theory. The human relations theory advocated the importance of job satisfaction and the feeling of belonging to a group (interpersonal relations). Thus, in the work setting the emphasis in organizations should be on relationships (Hersey and Blanchard, 1977, p. 91).

An early advocate of the human relations movement was Elton Mayo, who noted that the assumptions of many managers about workers was that workers wanted to make as much money as possible for as little work as possible (Hersey and Blanchard, 1977, p. 54). Douglas McGregor developed this thesis further and is now widely known for his list of assumptions about human nature and human moti-

vation, called Theory X and Theory Y. McGregor (1960) drew heavily from Maslow's work on motivation. Although there are other motivation theories, including that of Herzberg (1976), Maslow's are described because his writings have been used most widely in nursing.

Chief Characteristics

Maslow's theory (1970) states that the basic driving force or basic motive of people arises from a hierarchy of needs (Fig. 8-1). When needs of the lower hierarchy are met, the need at the next higher level becomes the basic motivating need. The hierarchy of human needs progresses from lower to higher needs as follows: physiological requirements, safety and security, social affiliation (love and belonging), esteem and self-actualizations. Needs can be met out of order, although they typically follow a pattern similar to Maslow's hierarchy.

Advantages and Disadvantages

Perhaps more than any other single work, Maslow's writings have given nursing the impetus to view clients as human beings with needs beyond physiological ones. It has promoted a movement to look beyond the pathophysiology of disease to the psychosocial needs of clients. However, the broad categories may obscure individuality of clients and their unique reactions to illness.

Application to Community Health Nursing

Many nursing programs have used Maslow's hierarchy of needs as a model for curriculum. An example of how it

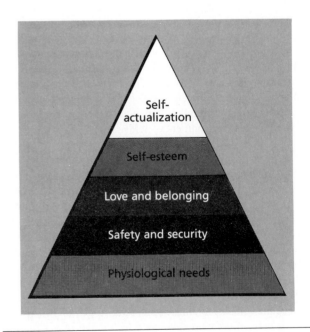

FIGURE 8-1

Maslow's hierarchy of needs.

generally is applied to nursing care planning is as follows: (1) Problem: failure to thrive, (2) Interference with basic human need: social affiliation or love and belonging, (3) Nursing plan and implementation: set goals for mother or mother-surrogate to meet need of social affiliation, and (4) Evaluation: assess alleviation of problem.

As mentioned above, the categories of needs are broad, and how the need is being impeded often must be further delineated before action can be taken.

Change

Change is constant and inevitable: some changes are planned; others are unplanned. Since an objective of most baccalaureate programs is for their graduates to be change agents, planned change is of concern here. "Planned change is a conscious, deliberate, and collaborative effort to improve operations of human systems . . . through the utilization of valid knowledge" (Bennis, Benne, Chin, and Corey, 1976, p. 4). Lewin (1951), the noted psychologist, applied concepts from field theory to the process of change.

Chief Characteristics

According to field theory, change occurs in a three-step process: unfreezing, moving, and refreezing. Unfreezing begins with dissatisfaction with the present system. The dissatisfaction may occur first among or within the group members. The leader must promote the unfreezing process or the willingness of the group members to give up their old ways of doing things and to be willing to consider alternatives. A major part of unfreezing is called force field

TABLE 8-1
Definitions of Person, Environment, Health, and Nursing

Person or Patient/Client	Environment	Health	Nursing
Roy An adaptive system (Roy, 1984, p. 28) can be a person or group.	"All conditions, circumstances, and influences surrounding and affecting the development and behavior of persons or groups" (Roy, 1984, p. 39).	"A state and a process of being and becoming an integrated and whole person. Integrity means soundness or an unimpaired condition that can lead to completeness or unity" (Roy, 1983, p. 269).	The science that observes, classifies, and relates the processes by which persons positively affect their health status, and the practice discipline that uses this particular scientific knowledge in providing a service to people (Roy, 1984, p. 4).
Rogers "Unitary man—a four-dimensional, negentropic energy field identified by pattern and organization and manifesting characteristics and behaviors that are different from those of the parts and which cannot be predicted from knowledge of the parts" (Rogers, 1980, p. 332).	A four dimensional, negentropic energy field identified by pattern and organization and encompassing all that is outside any given human field (Rogers, 1980, p. 332).	Health not specifically defined; but disease and pathology are value terms (Rogers, 1980, p. 336) and since values change, phenomena perceived as disease such as hyperactivity may change over time and not be perceived as disease.	Goal of nursing is that individuals achieve their maximum health potential through maintenance and promotion of health, prevention of disease, nursing diagnosis, intervention, and rehabilitation (Rogers, 1970, p. 86).
Johnson Behavioral system (Johnson, 1980, p. 207).	Malfunctions in behavioral systems are frequently caused by "sudden internal or external environmental change" (Johnson, 1980, p. 212; refers to man's interaction with environment p. 209).	"It seems reasonable to assume that health would be considered behavior that is orderly, purposeful, predictable, and functionally efficient and effective" (Johnson, 1980, p. 209).	Goal of nursing is to "restore, maintain, or attain behavioral system balance and stability at the highest possible level for the individual" (Johnson, 1980, p. 214).
Orem "A receiver of care, someone who is under the care of a health professional at this time, in some place or places" (Orem, 1985, p. 49).	Although not explicitly defined, speaks to the role of the nurse in providing a developmental environment (Orem, 1985, p. 141) may be physical or psychosocial; is the total environment.	"The state of wholeness of developed human structures and of bodily and mental functioning" Orem, 1985, p. 179.	"Deliberate action to bring about humanely desirable conditions in persons and their environments" (Orem, 1985, p. 15).

Continued.

> **TABLE 8-1**
> Definitions of Person, Environment, Health, and Nursing—cont'd

Person or Patient/Client	Environment	Health	Nursing
Neuman "A composite of the interrelationship of the five variables (physiologic, psychologic, sociocultural, developmental and spiritual) that are always present" (Neuman, 1989).	"All internal and external forces that could affect life and development" (Neuman, 1983, p. 246); "consists of the internal and external forces surrounding man at any point in time. Created environment represents an open system exchanging energy with both the internal and external environments (Neuman, 1989, p. 32).	"Health or wellness is the condition in which all parts and subparts (variables) are in harmony with the whole of man." Disharmony "reduces the wellness state." (Neuman, 1983, p. 246). Health is equated with system stability. The wellness-illness continuum implies energy flow is continuous between client system and environment (Neuman, 1989).	"Nursing can use this model to assist individuals, families, and groups to attain, retain and maintain a maximum of total wellness by three modes of prevention as intervention" (Neuman, 1989, p. 35).
King A social, sentient, rational, reacting, perceiving, controlling, purposeful, action-oriented, and time-oriented being (King, 1981, p. 143).	Writes about environment, but does not define it "the internal environment of human beings transforms energy to enable them to adjust to continuous external environmental changes. . . ." (King, 1981, p. 5).	"dynamic life experiences of a human being, which implies continuous adjustment to stressors in the internal and external environment through optimum use of one's resources to achieve maximum potential for daily living" (King, 1981, p. 5).	"Nursing is perceiving, thinking, relating, judging, and acting vis-a-vis the behavior of individuals who come to a nursing situation" (King, 1981, p. 2). "Nursing is a process of human interactions between nurse and client whereby each perceives the other and the situation; and through communication, they set goals, explore means, and agree on means to achieve goals."

analysis. This involves identifying forces that support the change (driving forces) and those that fail to support or are against the change (restraining forces) (Bernhard and Walsh, 1981, p. 143).

The second step in the change process, moving, involves implementing the change. Three change strategies are: empirical-rational, normative-reeducative, and power-coercive (Chin and Benne, 1976, p. 23). The empirical-rational strategy provides knowledge that the change will improve the situation. For example, chlorine added to the water supply makes it safe for drinking. The normative-reeducative strategy goes beyond an increase in knowledge to include change in values and attitudes. For example, a change in the format of a nursing procedure would require that the nurse value the change. The power-coercive strategy implements change by the use of power. An administrator may make a change without any input from the staff members, using her power base to effect the change.

The final stage in the change process is called refreezing. In refreezing, the newly acquired behavior has been practiced and is stable.

Advantages and Disadvantages

The model of change as related to field theory enables change agents to recognize the elements in a situation that must be assessed and known and to develop a way to proceed. A change agent who has taken into consideration all of the elements involved in the change process is much more likely to achieve an accepted and lasting change.

Application to Community Health Nursing

Suppose a community health nurse in a middle management position has just attended a conference on problem-oriented records and thinks such a system would be an improvement over the system currently being used. According to the first stage in change theory, unfreezing, the manager would need to determine if any of the staff were dissatisfied with their own method. If dissatisfactions about the current method exist, the unfreezing process has begun. The nurse then needs to ask the staff to discuss their views on the process currently used. In this way the nurse can identify the driving and restraining forces in the staff and move toward presenting the proposed change to administration to see if they support the change. If there is enough support for the next stage, then it is time for the moving stage. This stage may mean sending others to a conference on problem-oriented medical records or inviting someone to come in and present a conference. This would be the normative-reeducative strategy. Then the change would be implemented and the refreezing phase would begin.

Communication

Communication, or the act of giving or exchanging information, can be described by the use of two simple models. The first model (Figure 8-2) is linear and consists of a sender, a message, and a receiver. The second, seen in Figure 8-3, is circular and includes a sender, a message receiver, and feedback.

More elaborate models exist in the literature and Lancaster (1982, pp. 111-112) has described four models of communication theory:

1. The systems approach, which consists of input, processing, output, and feedback.
2. The questioning approach, which consists of asking the questions, who?, what?, how?, to whom?, and to what effect? (is a way to obtain feedback).
3. The human relations model, described as generation of idea, encoding, transmission, receipt of message, decoding, and action.
4. A composite model, which consists of generation of idea, encoding transmission, receipt of message, decoding, action, and feedback to encoding.

Chief Characteristics

Communication is the expression of a mesage in at least four forms: artistic, written, verbal, and non-verbal. Music, art, poetry, and literature are all forms of expression and communication. The written word, in the forms of books, articles, and letters, is another way of communicating. Verbal communication is through language or symbols; the most obvious example is television. The nonverbal form of communication includes body movements and facial expression, voice tone and quality, allocation of personal space, touch, and personal expression such as style of dress.

Human communication is generally carried out for the following purposes: (1) to give information; (2) to obtain information; (3) to release tension; and; (4) to solve problems. Variables that affect success for the communicators include (a) their relationship; (b) their perceptions of the topic; and (c) their beliefs, values, and attitudes.

Advantages and Disadvantages

The communication model describes how messages are sent and received. It is easy to understand and use. This model's effectiveness can be readily assessed by evaluating whether the message was accurately received. A disadvantage is that not all communication models take into account the effect of the environment on message sending and receiving. For example, a simple message sent in the presence of distracting background can be received differently than

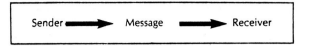

FIGURE 8-2

Linear model of communication.

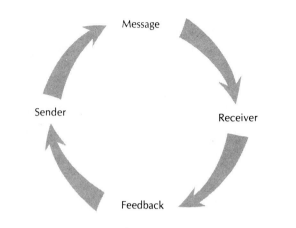

FIGURE 8-3

Circular model of communication.

the sender intended because the receiver may not realize he only heard part of the message.

Application to Community Health Nursing

The community health nurse is both the giver and receiver of information. When teaching, the nurse is the provider of information. When assessing individuals, families, groups or communities, the nurse is the receiver of information.

Some general guidelines or techniques for more effective communication are the following:
1. Attend and receive the message as an active listener.
2. Clarify the message by asking for an illustration.
3. Reflect and paraphrase to check the accuracy of the message received.
4. Validate and summarize at the close of the session.

Leadership

Leadership is the process of influencing people to accomplish goals. Leadership may be described by style or theory. Style refers to the way in which a person practices leadership. The three most recognized styles of leadership are autocratic, democratic, and laissez-faire. The purpose of a theory is to describe, explain, and predict. Thus theories on leadership attempt to describe the concepts in leadership and the relationships among them. They attempt to determine what elements constitute leadership or, in some cases, what elements constitute a leader.

Chief Characteristics

Style refers to the amount of control the leader exerts over subordinates. In the autocratic style, the leader uses maximum control, makes decisions, and tells subordinates what to do, and when and how to do it. The autocratic leader then indicates how well it was done either in the form of praise or criticism. The democratic leader invites input from the group in decision making and allows some flexibility in how and when to implement the decision. The group receives feedback from the leader in a factual way rather than in a judgmental way. The democratic group members also receives feedback from each other. The laissez-faire leader gives the group total freedom and is sometimes seen as a person who abdicates leadership responsibility. Stogdill (1974, pp. 365-370) reported that autocratic and democratic groups achieve about the same level of productivity. The democratic group showed more group cohesiveness, and the autocratic group demanded more attention from the leader. The laissez-faire group showed less productivity, less satisfaction, and less cohesiveness.

Earlier theories of leadership described a single factor as the key to effective leadership. The first of these was the "great man" theory, which postulated that some people are "born leaders." This was consistent with the practice of passing the leadership role from the king to his son. A second descriptive theory of leadership was trait theory. This theory combined all the traits that make a good leader. These traits included physical stature, intelligence, education, personality, charisma, and socioeconomic status. A third theory of leadership, called situation theory, used the idea of the right person being in the right place at the right time. For example, did Napoleon make history or did history make Napoleon? According to situation theory, history made Napoleon. A fourth theory was called interaction theory, which postulated that it was neither the person's personality nor the situation alone, but a combination of the two. Thus anyone could become a leader in the right situation.

Since the early 1960s, theories of leadership have evolved that emphasize consideration of multiple factors in determining effective leadership. These reflect influence from motivation theories, but they also consider the styles of leadership, the nature of the followers, and the situation. Studies at the University of Michigan identified two important aspects of leadership, which they called employee orientation and production orientation. Leadership studies at Ohio State University identified the two dimensions of leadership as initiation of structure and consideration. Structure was concerned with task behavior, and consideration was concerned with relationship behavior. The outcome of these and other studies led Hersey and Blanchard (1977, p. 100) to conclude that it was unrealistic to think of a single ideal type of leadership behavior. The effectiveness of leadership behavior demands that the leader use the appropriate style of leadership for the situation, meaning that a leader's style must vary from one situation to another. This has led to the general acceptance that effectiveness of leadership depends on the leader's ability to behave according to the situation and the followers.

Advantages and Disadvantages

People can learn leadership skills through study or by observing role models. Some people, by virtue of their personality and interests, are more likely to become leaders. Every nurse is a leader in some arena and will be a more effective leader if she can take into consideration all the variables that influence leadership effectiveness.

Application to Community Health Nursing

A large number of health professionals are involved in the delivery of health care, and the nurse is often expected to offer the needed leadership. The leader must consider the task or goal to be accomplished, group needs, including their relationship needs, and the situation. The nurse brings to the situation knowledge about change theory, motivation theory, group process skills, and interactional skills. All of these are needed for effective leadership.

CLINICAL APPLICATION OF THE NEUMAN SYSTEMS MODEL

The Neuman Systems Model is frequently used in community health nursing in the United States and Canada because its breadth and open structure make it applicable to individuals, families, groups, and communities. The model is supported by many theories and is a useful tool in community health nursing for organizing data and guiding practice.

Community health care emphasizes health promotion and maintenance of large groups of associated individuals (aggregates), rather than solely focusing on the health of individuals (Beddome, 1989). Frequently the community-as-client must be assessed for program planning, taking into account community resources and resource utilization patterns (Beddome. 1989).

The Neuman Systems Model, based on systems theory, enables community health nurses to describe the paradigm of nursing in terms appropriate to the community; that is, the person, family, group, or community can be the target of service. Environment is defined as all internal and external factors or influences that affect the community. Factors may be positive or negative. Negative factors are usually referred to as stressors. Emphasis is placed on the dynamic interaction between community and environment, as in Gestalt theory (Neuman, 1989). Health for the community is an optimal wellness or stable state. When a community system generates more energy than is being used, the wellness state moves toward negentropy (ideal wellness). When more energy is used than produced, the community moves toward entropy or death (Neuman, 1989, p. 33).

Community health nurses create linkages between the community, or aggregates within it, and health practices and ideals to assist the community in creating and shaping reality. This is accomplished through three levels of prevention: primary, secondary, and tertiary (Neuman, 1989). The function of primary prevention is to identify community risk factors and assist the community in health promotion and health education activities. Secondary prevention interventions are initiated when the community's normal defenses have been invaded and health related problems have developed. At this point, the community health nurse would initiate early case finding and treatment to strengthen lines of resistance, thus assisting the community to attain wellness. The focus of tertiary prevention is to maintain wellness after some system stability has returned, following stressor

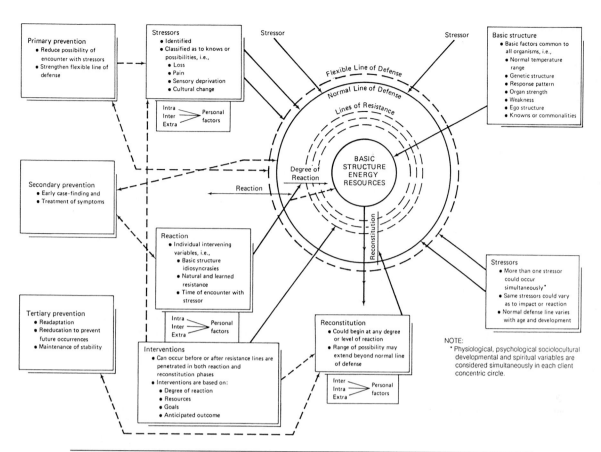

FIGURE 8-4 The Neuman Systems Model. From Neuman, B.: The Neuman systems model, ed 2, Norwalk, Conn, 1989, Appleton-Lange.

invasion. The nurse helps with readaptation and reeducation to prevent further occurrences (Neuman, 1989, p. 35).

The Neuman Systems Model graphically depicts the person (defined as community) as an open system with a central core of energy resources and survival factors surrounded by three layers of concentric circles (Fig. 8-4). When applied to community-as-client, the core represents the energy resources and survival factors within the intrastructure of the community. These can be classified according to the physiological, psychological, sociocultural, developmental and spiritual variables described by Neuman. The five variables are interdependent within the community, as they are within a person. Thus a change in one influences change in another, and items identified within one variable may fit into other variable categories as well. Categorizing data by variables is reductionistic, in contrast to a holistic, gestalt approach. However, using the Neuman model provides a means by which nurses can organize data in a comprehensive way, thus eliminating the possibility of overlooking any area. Following the assessment, the nurse must interpret the meaning of the parts to the community as a whole. Table 8-2 describes definitions and examples of community data within the five variables.

Surrounding the infrastructure (core) of the community, the Neuman Systems Model depicts three layers of defense against stressors; that is, lines of resistance, a normal line of defense, and a flexible line of defense. Although the

ultimate goal of all three defense lines is protection against stressors that can break down the community, when and how each line of defense is activated differs. For example, police and fire protection, health and illness services, and the penal system are lines of resistance established to protect, stabilize, and maintain the normal state of the community. The normal line of defense represents the usual range of responses of the community which have developed over time and mark the uniqueness of the community. Examples of the lines of defense could be the government and political structure, ways of doing business, and communications within the community among groups and organizations. In other words, the normal line of defense is the way the community copes with life's stressors to maintain balance. The number and intensity of stressors fluctuate on a daily basis. Thus the flexible line of defense acts as a buffer zone that contracts and expands to maintain the normal state of wellness for the community. Examples of expansion could be increases in services for citizens, opportunities for industrial or economic growth, or the proliferation of recreational parks within the community. Contraction of the flexible line of defense could occur in a minor state of emergency, such as a power failure or fire, or in the case of a major disaster, such as a flood, tornado, or an epidemic. In any case, lines of resistance would need to be mobilized and augmented to protect the infrastructure of the community.

TABLE 8-2
Definitions and examples of community variables

Variable	Definition	Examples
Physiological	Structures and functions of community	Urban, rural, suburban Geographical boundaries/location Water, sewage systems Safety systems (police, fire) Government Transportation system
Psychological	Cognitive, affective, and communication characteristics	Happy/depressed town Intelligence level Communication patterns Liberal vs. conservative Isolation vs. sensory overload
Sociocultural	Pattern of social, economic, demographic, political, recreational, and health characteristics	Poor/middle class/affluent Race, ethnicity Type of industry Day care for elderly/children Ambulance service Clinics/hospitals
Spiritual	Moral, religious, and value systems of community	Churches Health beliefs Burial practices X-rated book stores
Developmental	History, stage, and evolution of subsystems and aggregates in community	National registry of homes Aging and/or adolescent population Deteriorating city

TABLE 8-3
Stressors affecting community-as-client variables

Physical	Psychological	Social/cultural	Developmental	Spiritual
Intra-Community				
Increased infant mortality Hazardous waste dump Water supply contaminated Hospital old and obsolete	Insufficient health education about AIDS Increased divorce rate Potential for decreased emotional health in public housing areas	Homes crowded in downtown Park land bought by developer Decreased family income	High teen pregnancy rate Potential need for more child care centers Deteriorating inner city community	Many sect churches Health beliefs influenced by folk wisdom
Inter-Community				
Poor roads connecting town or regional medical center Distribution of physicians uneven	Anger between political parties Potential for isolation of elderly rural Inadequate communication system between rural and urban areas	Racial tension between migrants and townspeople Bussing students grades 4-6	Historical significance of town Age of community	Diverse value system between rural and urban sectors
Extra-Community				
Interstate highway system planned through town Nuclear power plant site outside town Flu epidemic Decreased state funding for services	Belief system of national political party in opposition to community's beliefs Fear of environmental contamination	Potential for unemployment related to industrial plant closing Influx of ethnic groups	New industry encroaching on farm land Potential for increase in young families to support new industry Potential growth in schools	New morality in opposition to community values Community selected as headquarters site for national denomination

TABLE 8-4

Nursing interventions using the Neuman system model

Prevention mode	Primary	Secondary	Tertiary
Prevention level	Before a stressor occurs	Following stressor invasion	After treatment/readaptation
Stressor nature	Mainly covert	Mainly overt or known	Mainly overt or residual
Degree of reaction	Hypothetical	Identified by symptomatology or known factors	Hypothetical or known—residual symptoms or factors
Aim of intervention	• Prevent stressor invasion • Reduce possibility of stressor encounter • Retain client stability	• Protect basic structure • Attain client stability	• Attain/maintain maximum level of wellness and stability
Nursing actions	• Educate/re-educate • Provide information to maintain or build on client strengths. • Motivate toward wellness. • Desensitize existing or potential noxious stressors; e.g., immunize, modify environment. • Support positive coping abilities. • Use stress as a positive intervention strategy; e.g., anticipatory counseling such as premarital or pre-retirement. • Advise regarding avoidance of hazards.	• Screening/early case finding • Mobilize and maximize internal/external resources toward stability and energy conservation; e.g., sleep/rest patterns, nutrition, pacing of activities. • Facilitate purposeful manipulations of stressors and reaction to stressors; e.g., counselling about high risk behaviors and avoidance of same, use of medications. • Motivate and educate client and significant others. • Facilitate appropriate treatment interventions; e.g., referral to diagnostic and treatment services. • Support positive factors toward wellness. • Advocacy	• Educate/reeducate and/or reorient as needed to prevent future occurrences or further deterioration. • Support client/client system in achieving goals. • Coordinate and integrate health resources; e.g., refer to self-help groups or to therapeutic counselling and rehabilitation services, assist in obtaining financial assistance. • Use of treatment modalities, such as behavior modification, reality orientation. • Client advocacy.

From: Neuman B: *The Neuman Systems Model*, ed 2, Norwalk, Conn., 1989, Appleton-Lange.

Table 8-3 provides examples of stressors that can affect the variables of Community-as-Client. Intracommunity stressors are those which are present within the community and may represent aggregates or the entire geopolitical community. For example, a community with a developmental variable of an aging population will have different needs than a community of young, upwardly mobile families. The intracommunity stressors interact with both the intercommunity (communication lines among groups and adjacent geopolitical areas) and the extracommunity stressors (factors imposed from without the community). Within the five variables, subsystems can be identified for assessment, such as education, politics, health, safety, and recreation. In this way comprehensive knowledge of the community can be obtained.

Actual examples of application of the Neuman Systems Model in a public health department, an aggregate population, and an individual community health nurse practice follow. The Kent-Chatham Health Unit in Ontario, Canada

has developed a record system for the nursing department based on the model and in accordance with the Standards of Practice set forth by the College of Nurses of Ontario (Allison, 1989). The records provide written evidence of the use of the nursing process and a nursing model. Prior to use, nurses are introduced to the model and are provided with guidelines on how to complete the forms. Appendix O provides an example of the Family Assessment Record in current use. Table 8-4 illustrates nursing interventions using the Neuman model (Allison, 1989).

An aggregate population of diabetics provides the second example. Veterans Administration Medical District 27 is the population from which the diabetic subjects were identified. A needs assessment of retrospective chart review provided data concerning educational needs of diabetic clients in this district. The Neuman Systems Model was used to categorize the stressors identified by the assessment (Table 8-5) and to design nursing interventions to reduce the number of com-

Text continued on p. 148.

TABLE 8-5

Stressors affecting VA diabetic population

	Sources of stressors		
	Intracommunity	**Intercommunity**	**Extracommunity**
Physiological	Age Diabetes Other illness	Staffing	
Psychological	Compliance Divorced/widowed	Stress	
Sociocultural	Distance from care Divorced/widowed Age Sex	Distance from care Funding Referrals Policy	Funding cuts Federal mandates
Developmental	Aging process Diabetes knowledge	Funding Program cutbacks	Low priority
Spiritual	Desire for health care	VA philosophy	Health care attitudes

From Nelson, PR: Needs assessment of diabetic education in veterans administration medical district 27, University of Portland, Portland, Ore, unpublished manuscript.

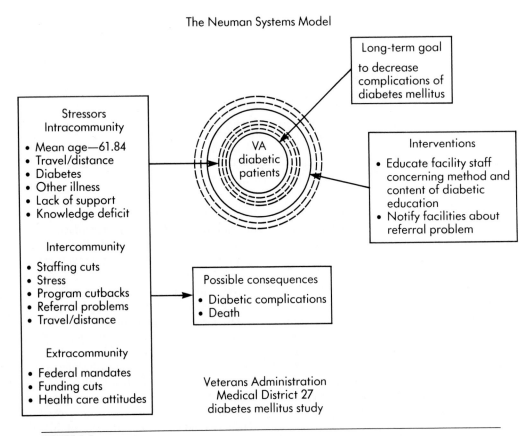

FIGURE 8-5

The Neuman Systems Model is applied to an aggregate population of diabetics. From Nelson, P.R. (1989) Needs assessment of diabetic education, Veterans Administration Medical District 27, University of Portland, Portland, Ore.

Hewitt Assessment Tool

Stressor List

Client's Perception of Stressor(s)	Actual	Potential	Stressor(s) as Perceived by Pract.	Actual	Potential

Stressors, Collaborative	Eniv. Factors	Nursing Diagnoses
	Intra, Inter, Extra	
	Intra, Inter, Extra	
	Intra, Inter, Extra	
	Intra, Inter, Extra	
	Intra, Inter, Extra	
	Intra, Inter, Extra	

FIGURE 8-6

The Hewitt assessment tool. **A,** Stressor List. From Hewitt, N.S. (1989): Assessment Tool/NSM. Unpublished manuscript, University of Portland, Portland, Ore.

plications experienced by diabetic clients (Nelson, 1989). Figure 8-5 shows the model that guided the study.

Many individual community health nurses have adapted the Neuman Systems Models Assessment Tool (Neuman, 1989, p. 61-63). One adaptation is illustrated in Figure 8-6. This is excerpted from a tool developed and tested in a precepted health clinic. The tool is multidimensional and provides a rich source of information from both the client's perspective (subjective) and the practitioner's perspective (objective). Stressors are identified by both the patient and the nurse in terms of actual and potential stressors. Collaborative stressors are also taken into account, as are the environmental factors. (Hewitt, 1989, p. 2). Nursing diagnoses, goals, interventions, and outcomes flow from the

Prevention as intervention

Primary	Secondary	Tertiary
Nursing Diagnosis: ___ Priority ___ Date	Nursing Diagnosis: ___ Priority ___ Date	Nursing Diagnosis: ___ Priority ___ Date
Goals:	Goals:	Goals:
Intervention:	Intervention:	Intervention:
Outcome:	Outcome:	Outcome:

FIGURE 8-6 cont'd

B, Prevention as intervention.

assessment and are recorded on a form as shown in Figure 8-6, *B*. A major disadvantage of using a comprehensive assessment tool is the time factor. When time is limited, the presenting stressor(s) can be identified, mutually agreed upon, and recorded on a form like Figure 8-6, *A*. Prevention as intervention can then be initiated. Further data can be elicited on future visits (Hewitt, 1989).

SUMMARY

This chapter has described the use of conceptual models in community health nursing. The chapter emphasized the importance to nursing of model development and scientific inquiry. The ANA and APHA conceptual models specific to community health nursing, as well as interdisciplinary and psychological models, were included.

Finally, the Neuman Systems Model was explicated from the perspective of Community-as-Client, since this nursing model is the one most widely used by community health nurses. Three actual examples of the use of the Neuman Model was provided.

KEY CONCEPTS

Community health nursing has historically reflected the qualities of both art and science; however, for nursing to advance it must develop as a theory-based profession.

Many conceptual models in nursing are mistakenly referred to as theories.

A conceptual model is a "set of concepts and those assumptions that integrate them into a meaningful configuration."

Conceptual models of nursing specify varying relationships and interactions among four essential components: person, environment, health, and nursing.

Conceptual models having the greatest application to community health nursing view people as being in continuous interaction with their environment.

In nursing practice, education, and research, conceptual models give direction and simplify and help organize information.

Both the ANA and APHA definitions of community health nursing emphasize the blending of nursing and public health knowledge as a foundation for determining the scope of practice. Both models acknowledge that community health nursing efforts are directed toward all people, emphasize a multidisciplinary role for nurses, and focus on the increasing priority of health promotion.

Interdisciplinary conceptual models with applications to community health nursing are systems theory, developmental theory, and interaction models.

Conceptual models specific to nursing have been developed by Roy, Rogers, Johnson, Orem, and King.

Among the psychosocial theories applicable to nursing, the writings of Maslow have been most widely used. Maslow's theory states that the basic motivations of individuals arise from a hierarchy of needs.

Change is an important concept in community health nursing. According to Lewin's application of field theory to the change process, change occurs in three steps: unfreezing, moving, and refreezing.

Along with change, communication and leadership are important psychosocial concepts with applications to community health nursing.

The Neuman systems model has many useful applications to community health nursing.

LEARNING ACTIVITIES

1. Write down what you consider to be the major themes in nursing. Compare them with the general themes cited in this chapter. How are they alike? How do they differ?

2. Select one of the conceptual models used in nursing and evaluate its potential usefulness to community health practice.

3. Identify several concepts in nursing that you think are related

and that guide actions. Using the concepts, try to construct a conceptual framework for your practice.

4. Debate one of these issues: (1) conceptual models should/ should not guide nursing practice, or (2) conceptual models help/hinder community health nursing practice.

5. Take one CHN experience and analyze it using the Neuman systems model.

BIBLIOGRAPHY

Allison EM: Family assessment recording, Kent-Chatham Health Unit, 1989, Chatham, Ontario Canada.

American Nurses' Association: A conceptual model of community health nursing practice, Kansas City, Mo, 1980, The Association.

American Public Health Association: The definition and role of public health nursing in the delivery of health care, Washington, DC, 1981, The Association.

Beddome G: Application of the Newman Systems Model to the assessment of community-as-client. In Neuman, B, editor: The Neuman systems model, ed 2, Norwalk, Conn, 1989, Appleton-Lange.

Bennis WG et al, editors: The planning of change, New York, 1976, Holt, Rinehart and Winston.

Bernhard LA and Walsh M: Leadership—the key to the professionalization of nursing, New York, 1990, Mosby-Year Book, Inc.

Bertalanffy LV: Problems of life: An evaluation of modern biological and scientific thought, New York, 1952, Harper Brothers.

Broncatello KF: Augur in action: application of the model, Advances in Nursing Science, 22, 13-23, 1980.

Burr WR et al, editors: Contemporary theories about the family, New York, 1979, Free Press.

Chance KS: Nursing models: A requisite for professional accountability. Advances in Nursing Science, 4, 2, 57-65, 1982.

Chinn PL and Jacobs MK: Theory and nursing (3rd ed). St. Louis, 1991, Mosby-Year Book, Inc.

Chinn R: The utility of system models and developmental models for practitioners. In Riehl JP and Roy SC, editors: Conceptual models for nursing practice, ed 2, New York, 1980, Appleton-Century-Crofts.

Chin R and Benne KD: General strategies for effecting changes in human systems. In Bennis WB et al, editors: The planning of change, New York, 1976, Holt, Rinehart and Winston.

Cooley CH: Social organization, New York, 1909, Scribner's.

Duvall EM: Marriage and family development, ed 5, Philadelphia, 1977, JB Lippincott.

Falco SM and Lobo MLL In George, J: Nursing theories: the base for professional nursing practice, Englewood Cliffs, NJ, 1980, Prentice-Hall, Inc.

Fawcett J: Analysis and evaluation of conceptual models of nursing, ed 2, Philadelphia, 1989, F.A. Davis.

Fawcett J and Downs FS: The relationship of theory and research, Norwalk, Conn, 1986, Appleton-Lange.

Heidt P: Effect of therapeutic touch on anxiety level of hospitalized patients, Nurs Res 30(1):32, 1981.

Hewett NS: Assessment tool using the Neuman systems model. Unpublished manuscript. University of Portland, 1989, Portland, Ore.

Hersey P and Blanchard KH: Management of organizational behavior, utilizing human resources, ed 3, Englewood Cliffs, NJ, 1977, Prentice-Hall, Inc.

Herzberg F: The managerial choice: to be efficient and to be human, Homewood, Ill, 1976, Dow Jones-Irwin, 1976.

Johnson DE: The behavioral system model for nursing. In Riehl JP and Roy SC: Conceptual models for nursing practice, ed 2, New York, 1980, Appleton-Century-Crofts.

Kerlinger FN: Foundations of behavioral research, ed 2, New York, 1973, Holt, Rinehart & Winston.

King I: A conceptual frame of reference for nursing, Nurs Res 17(1):27, 1968.

King I: A theory for nursing: systems, concepts, process, New York, 1981, John Wiley & Sons.

King, I: The "why" of theory development. In National League for Nursing: theory development, what, why, how? New York, 1978, National League for Nursing.

Krieger D: Foundations for holistic health nursing practices: the renaissance nurse, Philadelphia, 1981, JB Lippincott.

Lancaster J and Lancaster W, editors: Concepts for advanced nursing practice: the nurse as change agent, St. Louis, 1982, The CV Mosby Co.

Lewin K: Field theory in social science, New York, 1951, Harper.

Lewis M: Clinical aspects of child development, ed 2, Philadelphia, 1982, Lea & Febiger.

Maslow AH: Motivation and personality, ed 2, New York, 1970, Harper & Row.

McGregor D: The human side of enterprise, New York, 1960, McGraw-Hill Book Co.

Mead GH: Mind, self, and society, Chicago, 1934, University of Chicago Press.

Nelson MJ: Utilizing nursing models in nursing service. In J Reihl-Sisca, editor, Conceptual models for nursing practice, 1989, Norwalk, Conn, Appleton-Lange.

Nelson PR: Needs assessment of diabetic education in Veteran's Administration Medical District 27, 1989, University of Portland, Portland, Ore. Unpublished manuscript.

Neuman B: Family intervention using the Betty Neuman Health care. In Clements IW and Roberts FB: Family health: a theoretical approach to nursing care, New York, 1983, John Wiley & Sons.

Neuman B and Young RJ: A model for teaching total person approach to patient problems, Nurs Res 21:264, 1972.

Neuman B: The Betty Neuman health care systems model: a total person approach to patient problems. In Riehl JP and Roy SC, editors: Conceptual models for nursing practice, ed 2, New York, 1980, Appleton-Century-Crofts.

Neuman B: The Neuman systems model: application to nursing education and practice, ed 2, Norwalk, Conn, 1989, Appleton & Lange.

Nursing Development Conference Group: Concept formulation in nursing: process and product, Boston, 1973, Little, Brown & Co.

Orem D: Guides for developing curriculum for the education of practicing nurses, Washington, DC, 1959, US Government Printing Office.

Orem D: Nursing: Concepts of practice, New York, 1971, McGraw-Hill Book Co.

Orem D: Nursing: Concepts of practice, ed 3, New York, 1985, McGraw-Hill Book Co.

Riehl JP and Roy C: Conceptual models for nursing practice, ed 2, New York, 1980, Appleton-Century-Crofts.

Rogers ME: An introduction to the theoretical basis of nursing, Philadelphia, 1970, FA Davis.

Rogers ME: Nursing: a science of unitary man. In Riehl JP and Roy CS, editors: Conceptual models for nursing practice, New York, 1980, Appleton-Century-Crofts.

Rose A, editor: Human behavior and social processes an intractionist approach, Boston, 1962, Houghton Mifflin.

Roy C: Introduction to nursing: an adaptation model, Englewood Cliffs, NJ, 1976, Prentice-Hall, Inc.

Roy C: Introduction to nursing: an adaptation model, ed 2, Englewood Cliffs, NJ, 1984, Prentice-Hall, Inc.

Roy SC and Roberts SL: Theory construction in nursing: an adaptation model. Englewood Cliffs, NJ, 1981, Prentice-Hall, Inc.

Stogdill RN: Handbook of leadership: a survey of theory and research, New York, 1974, Free Press.

Walker LO and Avant KC: Strategies for theory construction in nursing, ed 2, Norwalk, Conn, 1989, Appleton & Lange.

Whall AL: Family therapy theory for nursing: Four approaches, Norwalk, CT, 1986, Appleton-Century-Crofts.

Whelton BJ: An operationalization of Martha Rogers' theory throughout the nursing process, Int J Nurs Stud 16:7-20, 1979.

9

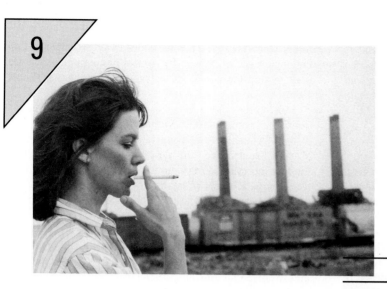

The Epidemiological Model Applied in Community Health Nursing

Linda Shortridge

Barbara Valanis

OBJECTIVES

After reading this chapter, the student should be able to:

Describe the history and components of the science of epidemiology.

Illustrate the use of a model of the natural history of a disease as the basis for community intervention.

Describe the common epidemiological methods.

Illustrate the general uses of epidemiology.

Describe the steps of an epidemiological investigation.

Interpret the relevance of epidemiological research findings to community health nursing practice.

KEY TERMS

advanced disease	immunity	prepathogenesis
agent	incidence	prevalence
attack rates	incubation period	rate
causality	inherent resistance	relational studies
confounding variable	levels of prevention	risk
ecological fallacy	morbidity	specific protection
ecological studies	mortality	surveillance
endemic	natural history	susceptibility
environment	pandemic	transmission cycle
epidemic	pathogenesis	web of causation
epidemiology	person-year	

E pidemiology is a community health science and is essential to nursing practice. Whereas a physician uses the basic medical science of physiology in diagnosing and treating an individual patient, the community health practitioner uses epidemiology in diagnosing and treating a community.

DEFINITION AND HISTORY

The term *epidemiology* is derived from three Greek words: (1) *epi,* upon; (2) *demas,* the people; and (3) *logos,* science. Thus it is the science of events that occur in a community of people. The following definition reflects the major components of the modern discipline: "Epidemiology is the study of the distribution of states of health and of the determinants of deviations from health in populations." The purpose of epidemiology is twofold: first, to identify the etiology of deviations from health and, second, to provide the data necessary to prevent and control disease through community health intervention.

Epidemiologists study a variety of factors related to the environment and the people in that environment in an attempt to identify the causes of observed patterns of health. They function as detectives concerned with the entire spectrum of health status from health to serious illness. They seek to identify the who, what, where, when, and how of disease causation. By comparing the characteristics of persons, places, and times associated with a particular illness against these same characteristics for persons who do not have the illness, they are able to narrow down the suspected causal agents of that illness. Once the agent and the susceptible population have been identified, epidemiologists attempt to determine how the agent is transmitted. This information provides a basis for intervention. Community health officials can act to prevent or control occurrence of the disease by removing the agent, by reducing the susceptibility of the population, or by preventing transmission of the agent to the population.

Epidemiology is an ancient and, for the most part, observational science. People have been trying for thousands of years to determine what causes disease. Supernatural events were one of the first factors used to explain the occurrence of illness. As long ago as 460-377 B.C., Hippocrates (considered by some to be the first epidemiologist) tried to explain disease occurrence on a rational rather than a supernatural basis. He pointed out that environment and life-style are related to the occurrence of disease.

During Biblical times, public health measures were based on observations about occurrence of disease, even when the actual disease agent was unknown. For example, the ancient practice of isolating lepers arose from the observation that the disease often developed in persons who came in close physical contact with a leper.

In the 1850s the investigative observations of John Snow in England resulted in the initiation of measures to prevent the use of certain water supplies. His work led him to suspect contaminated water as the source of cholera outbreaks. By measuring the frequency of cholera deaths in people living in a geographical area, he determined that rates of cholera mortality were much higher in certain parts of the city with a common water supply than in other sections with a different water supply. Thus measures could be taken to limit the occurrence of cholera by control of contaminated water even though the actual agent was as yet unknown (Snow, 1936).

Most early epidemiological observations and investigations were related to descriptions of outbreaks of infectious disease but lacked the rates to measure the frequency of disease occurrence. The development of rates, such as Snow's mortality observations, provided a scientific basis for systematic study of health and illness distributions. As data on infectious diseases accumulated and led to public health intervention, infectious diseases were largely controlled. After that, diseases of a chronic nature with noninfectious origins became more common, taking over as major causes of morbidity and mortality, particularly in industrialized nations (Figure 9-1). In 1900, infectious diseases accounted for over 40% of all deaths whereas heart disease, cancer, and stroke accounted for less than half of deaths from noninfectious diseases. By 1987, death from infectious disease was uncommon but heart disease, cancer, and stroke respectively accounted for 36%, 23%, and 7% of all deaths, a total of 66% (NCHS, 1989). However, infectious diseases are again becoming a focus of attention. Acquired immune deficiency syndrome (AIDS) has been a major focus of epidemiology in the last decade. In 1987, it moved up to the 15th most common cause of death, replacing congenital anomalies. By 1990, it was the fifth leading cause of death. The natural history of AIDS has now been established. Modes of transmission, susceptible population groups, and prevention strategies have been investigated, and information has been disseminated to the population at large.

The advent of procedures such as organ transplants, requiring concurrent use of immunosuppressive drugs, and the widespread use of chemotherapy for cancer have resulted in immune-suppressed or immune-impaired patients, who are highly susceptible to infection. For these patients common organisms in the hospital environment, including staphylococci, gram-negative bacteria, and fungal organisms, can be lethal. Elderly persons and others whose resistance is lowered by their disease process are also at risk. As a result infection control has become a major program in most hospitals. Similarly, infectious disease has emerged as a community problem. For example, gonorrhea incidence has risen dramatically. Genital herpes is on the rise. Other infectious diseases in the news during the past 15 years include Legionnaire's disease, toxic shock syndrome, tuberculosis, and measles.

Epidemiological investigations today focus on infectious diseases; chronic conditions such as heart disease, cancer, and stroke; acute events such as spontaneous abortion or accidents; and a wide spectrum of emotional and mental health conditions such as depression or alcoholism. In addition, epidemiology is no longer limited to the study of diseases or patterns of ill health. It also focuses on descriptions of the normal characteristics of populations, such as studies of body weight in relation to height and of blood group subtypes in different population segments. By extending its scope to include mental and social conditions in addition to disease, epidemiology has helped behavioral sci-

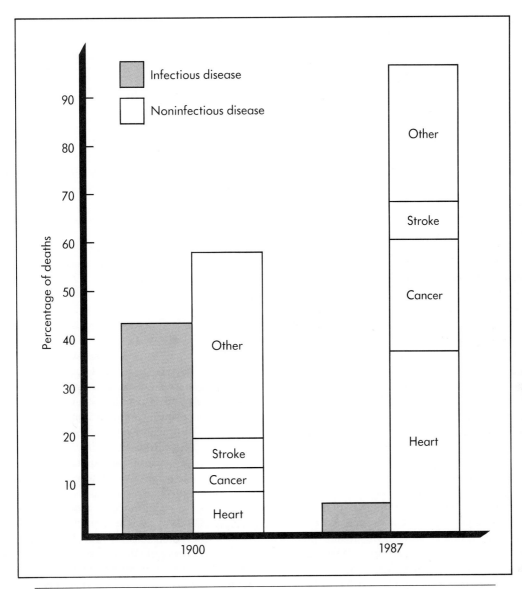

FIGURE 9-1

Proportional distribution of deaths from infectious and major noninfectious diseases, United States, 1900 and 1987.

entists, social workers, community health planners, and all those concerned with the health and well-being of human populations. It is truly multidisciplinary, both providing information to the medical, social, and behavioral sciences and drawing on these sciences in its research.

COMPONENTS OF EPIDEMIOLOGY

The term *epidemiology* refers both to the particular methods employed to study the causes of disease and to the body of knowledge that results from such investigations. The methods utilized by epidemiologists to study disease include observations and recordings of the existing patterns of a disease occurrence and examination of the probabilities and averages of demographic and physiological characteristics that are most common in the diseased population. Hence statistics are a crucial tool for the epidemiologist. Epidemiology also includes the body of knowledge on known epidemio-

logical characteristics of a particular disease or illness resulting from epidemiological studies. The epidemiological characteristics of a disease include its natural history, patterns of occurrence, and factors associated with high risk for developing the disease (risk factors).

A disease can be characterized in two ways—the clinical or physiological description and the epidemiological description (see Table 9-1). The clinical description relates to the onset and progression of symptoms in individuals. The epidemiological description relates to characteristics of the occurrence of disease in populations.

An episode of food poisoning illustrates the distinction between a clinical and an epidemiological approach to illness.

Clinicians (nurses, physicians) record the signs and symptoms such as elevated temperature, nausea and vomiting, or diarrhea that the patient experiences. They take a

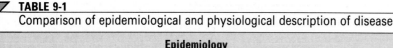

TABLE 9-1

Comparison of epidemiological and physiological description of disease

	Epidemiology	Physiology
Tools	Epidemiological methodology	Physiological methodology
Knowledge	Trends in disease occurrence	Physiology of human body
Outcome	Distribution of populations at high risk of disease	
	Social, economic, biological and genetic determinants of disease	
	Natural history of disease	
Purpose	Diagnosis and treatment in community health practice	Diagnosis and treatment decisions in medical practice
Focus	Group	Individual

careful history and perform a thorough physical examination, supplemented if necessary by laboratory tests. They then consider the differential diagnoses and come to the conclusion that the most likely diagnosis is gastroenteritis attributable to food poisoning. Then they institute treatment and record the patient's progress in terms of when the symptoms are relieved.

Epidemiologists describe this event in terms of how it affects the group. They note the time and place of onset of symptoms in all the sick individuals who can be identified, preferably including those with symptoms too mild to require medical treatment. They also assemble data on the circumstances related to the illness for all individuals to determine if they share a common circumstance. This may lead to a suspected common source of infection, such as food at a church supper. To identify the likely food item responsible for the poisoning, precise information is gathered on all the various foods eaten by those present. A comparison is made of illness rates among all those present at the supper who ate each food and those who did not. Once the contaminated food is identified, attempts are made to determine the source of the contamination. Often the source is someone involved in the food preparation. Once the source is identified, community health measures such as treatment of the person carrying the disease organism and instruction in hygienic food practices must be instituted to assure that the event does not recur.

BASIC EPIDEMIOLOGICAL CONCEPTS

Underlying the science of epidemiology are basic concepts and principles used to organize and analyze patterns of disease occurrence. The disease process involves the interaction of three kinds of factors: the causative agent(s), the susceptible host (man), and the environment. Any change in one of these three factors has the potential of affecting the balance of health. The natural history of a disease describes the interaction of a susceptible host, an agent, and an environment that may or may not enhance the development of disease. By understanding the natural history of disease, preventive measures can be initiated that will prohibit or prevent the development of the disease process. A major goal of epidemiology is to assist in the prevention and control of disease and the promotion of health by discovering the causes of disease and the ways in which these

causes can be modified. The concept of causality is basic to the study of epidemiology.

The Agent

An agent is a factor whose presence or absence causes a disease. For example, the presence of gonococcus causes gonorrhea; insufficient intake of vitamin C may lead to scurvy. Categories of causative agents include physical, chemical, nutrient, biological, genetic, and psychological agents. *Physical* agents include various mechanical forces or frictions that may produce injury as well as atmospheric abnormalities such as extremes of temperature or excessive radiation. *Chemical* agents include substances such as dusts, gases, vapors, fumes, and liquids. *Nutrient* agents are the specific basic dietary components that we need to survive. All living organisms, including insects, worms, protozoa, fungi, bacteria, rickettsia, and viruses, are *biological* agents. This class is infectious. *Genetic* agents are transmitted from parent to child through the genes. *Psychological* agents are stressful circumstances in the environment.

Certain characteristics of agents affect their ability to produce disease in the host. For infectious agents these characteristics are infectivity, pathogenicity, and virulence. Measures of these characteristics (i.e., the infection rate, pathogenicity rate, and case fatality) allow public health officials to assess the nature of the problem they are dealing with in order to plan for intervention. These characteristics are discussed further in Chapter 19. Important characteristics of the noninfectious agents include toxicity (for chemical agents), size and shape (for physical agents), chronicity or suddenness (for psychological agents), and homozygosity or heterozygosity (for genetic material).

The Environment

Environment is all external conditions and influences affecting the life of living things. Physical, socioeconomic, and biological environments provide reservoirs and modes of transmission for agents.

The physical environment includes the geological structure of an area and the availability of resources such as water and plants. Weather, climate, and season are important influences on these factors.

The socioeconomic environment contributes to the types of infectious agents in a location. Social and economic conditions include environmental sanitation, pasteurization of milk, disposal of garbage and excreta, and the availability of medical facilities for immunization and medical care. The socioeconomic environment may also influence non-infectious agents. For example, more psychological stressors may be found in low-income neighborhoods than in higher-income neighborhoods. Low-income neighborhoods are more likely to be near industrial plants, which may produce noninfectious agents such as dangerous chemicals, asbestos, or coal tar.

The biological environment includes other living plants and animals that may serve as either the reservoir or the vector for transmission of an infectious agent. Because these agents are living organisms, they require a place to live and multiply. The habitats of these agents are called reservoirs and may be any human, animal, insect, plant, soil, or in-animate matter that provides an environment for survival or reproduction. The reservoir is thus intimately related to the *transmission cycle* of the agent in nature. The trans-mission cycle, or life cycle, refers to where the agent resides and how it is transported to a susceptible host.

The Host

Disease can occur only in a susceptible human host. The concept of immunity is important to the understanding of resistance to disease caused by infectious agents. *Immunity* refers to the increased resistance on the part of a host to a specific infectious agent. Immunity can be humoral (anti-bodies in the blood) or cellular (specific to each type of cell). The role of each of these types of immunity varies with the infectious agent and with the immune response of the host. Immunity can also be passive or active. Passive immunity is attained either naturally (maternal transfer of antibodies to the fetus) or artificially (inoculation of specific protective antibodies). Passive immunity is temporary. In neonates it usually lasts 6 months, during which time the infant is protected only against infection experienced by the mother and for which she has made antibodies. By contrast, active immunity is long lasting and may protect an individual for life. Active immunity is attained naturally by infection or artificially by the inoculation of vaccine. This vaccine is obtained from fractions or products of the infectious agent or of the agent itself in killed, modified, or variant form. Major vaccination programs such as those for diphtheria and polio are based on the principle of active immunity. This principle was also the basis for the successful program to eradicate smallpox through an international vaccination and surveillance program.

In contrast to immunity, *inherent resistance* is the ability to resist disease independently of antibodies or of specifi-cally developed tissue responses. Anatomical or physiolog-ical characteristics usually provide resistance. Inherent re-sistance may be genetic or acquired, permanent or tempo-rary. The concept of inherent resistance is useful in understanding host resistance to both infectious agents and other types of agents. For example, factors such as general health status or nutrition may affect resistance to disease. Someone in good health who maintains good nutrition and a regular schedule of rest and exercise may be exposed to the tubercle bacillus and resist infection even though he is not immune to the organism. Similarly, this individual, if exposed to psychological stress, may resist ulcers better than someone in poorer general health.

Natural History of Disease

Table 9-2 gives the stages of the *natural history* of any disease and lists interventions specific for each stage. Ba-sically, there are two stages in the natural history (Leavell and Clark, 1968).

The first of these is the stage of *prepathogenesis, or susceptibility.* In this stage disease has not developed, but factors that favor its occurrence are present. For example, the poor eating habits and fatigue typical of college students during exam week represent risk factors that favor the oc-currence of the common cold.

The second stage in the natural history is *pathogenesis.* Within this stage there are three substages. In the first sub-stage, *presymptomatic disease* (sometimes called *early pathogenesis)*, the individual has no symptoms indicating the presence of illness. However, pathogenic changes have begun. In the second substage, *discernible early lesions,* changes may be detectable through sophisticated laboratory tests. During this period the early signs and symptoms of disease are developing. For example, premalignant changes in the cervix may be detected by a Pap smear long before the woman experiences symptoms and before signs become visible on visual examination. In the third substage of the natural history *advanced disease* occurs. By this stage suf-ficient anatomical or functional changes have produced rec-ognizable signs and symptoms. This stage includes disease so advanced that death is inevitable. The possible outcomes are complete recovery, a residual defect that produces some degree of disability, or death.

Exposure of the host to an agent occurs during the first stage, the stage of prepathogenesis. In the case of infectious agents exposure is followed by an *incubation period,* a time when the organisms multiplies to produce a host reaction and clinical symptoms. This period is relatively brief, usu-ally hours to months. For diseases caused by noninfectious agents the time from exposure to onset of symptoms is called the *induction* or *latency period.* This may last for years or decades. Accidents resulting from a severe psychological stressor may occur shortly after initial exposure to the stressor, by contrast, ulcers as a consequence of psycho-logical stress may require years to develop.

One of the shorter known latency periods for cancer is the 5-year latency period of leukemia in children resulting from radiation exposure. On the other hand, lung cancer resulting from asbestos exposure may have a latency period of 40 years. Exceptions to the general rules governing la-tency periods do occur—for example, some chemical agents cause almost instantaneous acute episodes of poi-soning.

Most diseases caused by infectious agents are of rela-tively short duration. The patient is usually ill for a few days to several months and generally recovers without any residual disability. If the illness has been severe the patient may die. The patient who has recovered rarely requires long-term follow-up, although there are exceptions. Tuberculosis and rheumatic heart diseases are examples of diseases caused by infectious agents that are chronic in nature.

In contrast to diseases caused by infectious agents, diseases caused by noninfectious agents or by unidentified agents are more likely to be of a chronic nature. With chronic diseases there is often residual disability requiring ongoing medical treatment and rehabilitation programs. For example, patients with cardiovascular disease are likely to require supervision of prescribed medications, control of diets, and modification of life-style.

Levels of Prevention

The natural history of a disease provides the basis for community health intervention. A disease evolves over time, and pathological change becomes less reversible as the disease process continues. The ultimate aim of intervention programs is to halt or reverse the process of pathological change as early as possible, thereby preventing further damage. A three-level model for intervention, based on the stages of disease natural history, has been developed (see Table 9-2). The goal of intervention at each of the three levels is to prevent the pathogenic process from evolving further. The three levels of prevention are called primary, secondary, and tertiary prevention.

Primary Prevention

Primary prevention is aimed at intervention before pathological changes have begun during the stage of susceptibility. Primary preventive efforts include both general health promotion and specific protection.

General health promotion includes all activities that improve the environment and favor healthy living. Thus efforts to improve the physical environment, whether that of the outdoors, home, school, or work, would be included. Health education aimed at educating the population about good nutrition, the need for rest and recreation, the preparation for retirement, hygiene, or the harmful effects of smoking or drug use is another form of general health promotion.

Efforts aimed at primary prevention of chronic noninfectious diseases (e.g., heart disease) must focus on such things as maternal diet during pregnancy, the diet of the child during early life, regular exercise, and education programs regarding the hazards of smoking. Although success cannot be guaranteed, the chances of achieving it are greatest if intervention occurs early in life, before physiological risk factors like obesity and elevated cholesterol levels develop. These physiological states involve cellular changes that are steps in the development of disease. Therefore the reduction of risk factors is actually secondary prevention.

TABLE 9-2
Natural history of disease and application of preventive measures

Stage	Events	Level of application of preventive measures	Specific interventions
I Prepathogenesis or susceptibility	1. Interrelations of various host, agent, and environmental factors bring host and agent(s) together 2. Disease-provoking stimulus is produced in the known host	Primary prevention	Health promotion (health education, nutrition counseling, adequate housing, personal hygiene, etc.) Specific protection (immunizations, sanitation, removing occupational and environmental hazards, use of specific nutrients, etc.)
II Pathogenesis Early pathogenesis	1. Interaction of host and stimulus 2. Stimulus or agent becomes established (if infectious agent, increases by multiplication) 3. Beginning tissue and physiological changes	Secondary prevention	Early diagnosis and prompt treatment (screening, case-finding, selective examination)
Discernible early lesions	1. Clinical recognition of disease is possible through laboratory or other tests that detect early physiological changes 2. Patient develops early symptoms	Tertiary prevention	Disability limitation (treatment to arrest disease process)
Advanced disease	1. Disability 2. Defect 3. Chronic state 4. Death		Rehabilitation (retraining for maximum use of remaining capacities, facilitating reentry to the family unit and to the workplace)

Adapted from Leavell HR, Clark EG: Preventive medicine for the doctor in his community, New York, 1965, McGraw-Hill Book Co.

Specific protection refers to measures aimed at protecting individuals against specific agents. Examples of these measures include immunization against polio or attempts to remove agents from the environment, such as sewage treatment, pasteurization of milk, or chlorination of water. Infectious diseases can be prevented by destroying the agent or removing it from the environment or by protecting the host through vaccination programs. For chronic conditions caused by noninfectious agents there is no single necessary agent. For example, chronic obstructive pulmonary disease may result from smoking, from asbestos exposure, from air pollution, or from a variety of other agents. Each potential agent must therefore be eliminated to assure control of disease. Specific protection measures, such as removal of hazardous substances from the workplace, will reduce occurrence of the disease but will not eliminate it.

Effects of primary prevention since 1900 can be seen in the dramatic reduction of mortality from infectious disease resulting largely from environmental manipulation and immunization programs (Figure 9-1). This reduction in infectious disease mortality, particularly among infants, young children, young women, and the elderly, has led to an increase in the total population. It has also resulted in the advent of chronic disease as a major community health concern. Because fewer people die of infectious disease, more live to an older age, when chronic diseases are common. Also, industrialization and changes in life-style have increased exposure to potential causal agents for noninfectious disease.

Secondary Prevention

Secondary prevention efforts seek to detect disease early and treat it promptly. The goal is to cure disease at its earliest stage or, when cure is impossible, to slow its progression as well as prevent complications and limit disability. Thus secondary prevention is focused primarily on presymptomatic disease or very early clinical disease. Screening is the most common form of secondary prevention. Many screening tests can detect early physiological indicators of disease before the person experiences any symptoms. Examples include cervical cancer tests, hearing tests, the tuberculin test for tuberculosis, and the phenylalanine test for PKU in infants. Such screening programs have become popular in recent years with the development of numerous test procedures.

Detection and early treatment of conditions provide a wide range of benefits. Mental retardation can be prevented in children with PKU by use of a special diet maintained until adulthood. The life of a cancer patient whose disease is detected while in the early stage may be saved. In the case of communicable disease, not only do early detection and treatment (secondary prevention) benefit those who are affected but the screening program provides primary prevention for those who might have been exposed to the infectious agent. For example, the VDRL as a screen for sexually transmitted diseases identifies clients who are then referred for diagnostic follow-up and treatment. Once treated, they cannot transmit the disease to others.

A word of caution: screening tests are given to individuals who think of themselves as being well. Because the tests are not diagnostic, they merely separate persons who are more likely to have the disease from persons who probably do not. Individuals screened as positive require a diagnostic follow-up to determine if they actually have the disease. For example, in a routine physical examination a complete blood count may be performed to screen for potential health problems such as infection or anemia. This is called casefinding. A low hemoglobin count may require further diagnostic follow-up to ascertain the cause of anemia. A high white blood count may require further diagnostic follow-up to determine the location of the infection. Thus from an ethical point of view, certain criteria should be met before a screening test is indiscriminately administered:

1. An effective treatment that will change the course of the disease must be available.
2. There must be evidence that the test does, in fact, detect the disease at an earlier stage in the natural history than when symptoms are present.
3. The test must have the ability to screen as positive individuals with the disease *(sensitivity)* and the ability to screen as negative individuals without the disease *(specificity)*.
4. Follow-up services must be available, and persons who are screened as positive must be notified and referred to such services.

These criteria are necessary because the sensitivity of screening tests is always less than 100%. In other words, a certain proportion of people tested who actually have the disease will not have a positive result on a screening test and, conversely, a certain proportion without the disease will not necessarily be screened as negative (because the specificity of a screening test is never 100%). It is therefore useful to teach clients about early symptoms as a part of the screening program so they will be alerted to the significance of symptoms that might appear later.

Tertiary Prevention

Tertiary prevention includes limitation of disability for persons in the earlier stages of illness and rehabilitation for those persons who have already experienced residual damage. Tertiary prevention activities focus on the middle to later phases of the stage of clinical disease, when irreversible pathological damage produces disability. For a client recovering from a stroke, exercise therapy to preserve muscle tone, restore motion, and prevent contractures is a form of tertiary prevention. It both limits disability and begins the process of rehabilitation. Psychosocial and vocational services are also usually part of a rehabilitation program. Appendix J contains a description of the natural history of pregnancy-induced hypertension (PIH), a major prenatal disease contributing to maternal and neonatal morbidity and mortality. The natural history of the disease is traced and preventive measures applicable to each stage of the disease are addressed. Although interventions for all stages are presented, the community health nurse focuses primarily on primary and secondary prevention. Some tertiary interventions will be appropriate for clients with residual organ damage or poor fetal outcome.

TABLE 9-3

Distribution of blood pressure and weight as independent and nonindependent factors

Adult Weight	Independent factors			Nonindependent (associated) factors		
	High blood pressure (%)	Low blood pressure (%)	Total (%)	High blood pressure (%)	Low blood pressure (%)	Total (%)
Overweight	2	18	20	7	13	20
Not overweight	8	72	80	3	77	80
TOTAL	10	90	100	10	90	100

Causality

The term *cause* generally means a stimulus that produces an effect or outcome. In epidemiology, cause also deals with a factor that produces an effect or outcome. However, the epidemiologist studies causal relationships with statistical measures of association. By using statistical methods, epidemiologists are able to judge the strength of a causal relationship between a stimulus and an outcome. They must first determine whether a stimulus and a response are associated or independent.

Principles of Association

In statistical terms, two events are said to be independent if the probability that they occur together is equal to the probability that one occurs multiplied by the probability that the other occurs. For example, in Table 9-3 under *Independent factors,* the proportion of adults in a community who are both overweight and have high blood pressure is exactly 2%. Since 20% of all of the adults are overweight and 10% of all the adults have high blood pressure and 20% multiplied by 10% also equals 2% (.20 × .10 = .02), the events are considered statistically independent of each other. By contrast, in Table 9-3 under *Nonindependent Factors,*although the percent who are overweight remains at 20% and the percent who have high blood pressure remains at 10% of the population, the proportion of individuals who are overweight and also have blood pressure is 7%. This is more than three times the 2% that would be expected by chance alone. In this case the two factors are not independent; they are associated. A variety of statistical tests for independence of factors is used to analyze epidemiological data. The type of test depends on the structure of the data. Thus in statistical terms, before a relationship between two factors is considered for further investigation of *causality,* the distribution of the two factors must be such that they cannot be accounted for by chance alone. They must have a statistically significant association.

It is important to stress that statistical associations are determined for *categories or groups* and not for individuals. In the example given in Table 9-3, under Independent Factors, it is not possible to say that high blood pressure and being overweight caused any individual to have heart disease. However, the information under Nonindependent Factors may suggest the possibility of causal association in a particular instance. This is especially true if the association between two categories of events is strong.

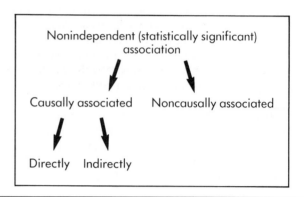

FIGURE 9-2

Types of statistical associations.

Causal Relationships

Once it has been determined that two factors are not independent but have a significant association, the next step is to determine whether the relationship is causal. As illustrated in Figure 9-2, nonindependent associations may be causally or noncausally related. *Direct causal associations* are those in which a factor causes a disease with no other variables intervening.

$$A \longrightarrow B$$

Apparent directness depends on the limitations of current knowledge. What is considered a direct association may become indirect if further studies of causal mechanisms reveal a new more direct cause for the association. For example, the early studies of toxic shock syndrome indicated tampons as the probable cause. Later research showed that the presence of staphylococcal organisms in the vagina was the actual direct cause. The tampons were a contributing cause in that they created an ideal environment for proliferation of the organism (Centers for Disease Control, 1980).

With *indirect causal associations* one or more variables, called *intervening variables,* occupy an intermediate stage between the cause and effect.

$$A \longrightarrow B \longrightarrow C \longrightarrow D$$

For example, breathing air polluted by cigarette or other smoke *(A)* causes damage to the respiratory epithelium (intervening variable *B*); this damage increases the susceptibility of the epithelium to infection (intervening variable

C), which results in chronic bronchitis (D).

Finally, as illustrated in Figure 9-2, although an association may be nonindependent, it may also be *noncausally associated*. In this case there is an illusion of an association between two variables when in fact no such association exists. The illusion is caused by a third variable (a confounder) that is correlated with the causal variable. The effect of the confounder cannot be distinguished from the effects of the hypothetical causal variable under study. An example of a confounding variable can be seen in studies of the effects of exposure to chemicals on menstrual function. An analysis looking at the duration of exposure to a chemical might show an increased occurrence of irregular menstrual cycles according to the duration of the exposure. However, menstrual cycle irregularity also increases with age and a close association between age and the duration of the exposure exists. One would expect the duration of exposure to the chemical to increase with age. Since age and duration of exposure increase together, the epidemiologist must use statistical methods to separate the effects of these two variables (age and duration of exposure). Age, if uncontrolled, is a confounding variable for the association between duration of exposure to a toxic chemical and its associated effect on menstrual function.

When there is sufficient evidence that a specific factor is causally related to an outcome effect, the experimental phase of epidemiology begins. In this phase, called a *randomized controlled trial*, the investigator determines who is exposed or not exposed to a causal factor.

Thus a factor is considered causal if reducing the amount or frequency of its occurrence reduces the frequency of the effect. For example, if treating hypertensive individuals to reduce their blood pressure reduces the frequency of stroke compared to the frequency of stroke in an equivalent untreated group of hypertensive individuals, hypertension would be considered a cause of stroke.

There are instances when an epidemiological experiment is not feasible or desirable. Then the investigator does not control exposure to a causal factor but makes a judgment as to causality based on events where the individual determines exposure. Because it would be unethical to expose human subjects to an agent thought to be harmful, such as tobacco smoke, studies are conducted comparing groups of individuals who normally smoke to groups that do not.

Criteria for Causality

The five criteria generally used for assessing causality in observational epidemiological studies are drawn from the 1964 Surgeon General's report. These criteria were used in that report to assess the causal relationship between smoking and a variety of health outcomes. The criteria were (1) evidence that exposure to the causal factor occurred before the disease process began, (2) the strength of the association, (3) the specificity of the association, (4) the consistency of the association among various epidemiological studies, and (5) the existence of a biological mechanism to explain how an agent could produce the disease. A cause can be any of a large number of characteristics relating to time, place, person, or events. Modern epidemiology has moved ahead from the "single-cause idea" and recognized

the presence of multiple causes in any biological phenomenon. However, the single-cause model of the past has its usefulness, particularly in the control of infectious diseases. Identification of the source of infection leads the way to isolation of the causal organism. This provides a means for eliminating or controlling the frequency of disease occurrence by restricting exposure of noninfected susceptible individuals to the pathogen. The tubercle bacillus, for instance, was identified as *the* cause of tuberculosis because it had to be present for tuberculosis to occur.

In the case of noninfectious disease agents the single-cause model is of limited usefulness, since no single factor or agent must be present to cause the disease. For example, even though smoking is recognized as a major cause of lung cancer, nonsmokers and individuals who have never been exposed to the cigarette smoke of others do get lung cancer. Clearly, there must be other substances that cause the disease. Nonsmokers exposed to asbestos may contract lung cancer. Also smokers who are exposed to other substances, such as asbestos, are much more likely to contract lung cancer than are smokers not exposed to these substances. Exposure to more than one causal factor may have an additional or multiplicative effect.

In a different example, home accidents may result from numerous factors such as clutter in the environment, loose throw rugs, curled edges of linoleum, electrical wires running across the room, wet floors, or poor lighting. Physical impairments such as problems with balance, musculoskeletal function, or eyesight may also cause a home accident. All of these factors can be addressed through public education, better engineering design and/or maintenance, or devices like corrective lenses or a walker. The presence of several factors increases the probability that an accident will occur. Such interrelationships between a multitude of factors constitute the *web of causation*. It is, fortunately, not necessary to understand completely the intricacy of relationships between factors to institute adequate preventive measures.

Numerous factors such as smoking, obesity, high blood cholesterol level, and stress are causes of heart attack. The more factors present in an individual, the greater will be the risk of an attack. Since the presence of these factors increases the risk for contracting a disease, they are called *risk factors*. Nurses can intervene and reduce the risk of heart attack by persuading individuals to give up smoking, lose weight, or change their diet to lower blood cholesterol. Planning of such interventions is based on understanding the natural history of disease.

The combined effects of two or more agents (synergism) are frequently seen in instances of causation by noninfectious agents. One of the classic examples of synergism was a study of the relationship between asbestos exposure and lung cancer. Nonsmoking workers exposed to asbestos do not have a statistically significant increase in the risk of dying from lung cancer when compared to nonsmoking nonexposed individuals. However, workers who smoke *and* are exposed to asbestos are estimated to have 92 times the risk of the nonsmoking nonexposed individuals (Kleinfeld et al. 1967). This is of concern because control efforts often must settle for minimizing rather than eliminating workplace exposures. The synergistic effect of other exposures could mean that substantial risk remains even with low-level exposures.

EPIDEMIOLOGICAL METHODS

Measuring the occurrence or frequency of disease is the basis of epidemiology. It is dependent on a source of data to provide the numbers of cases of disease or health outcomes and to furnish accurate information on the number of individuals at risk for a disease or health outcome. With accurate data sources, rates can be compiled with which comparisons between populations can be made.

Sources of Data

Epidemiological investigations use data from a variety of existing sources, such as census or hospital records. In other instances the data may be generated for a specific study through surveys that include interviews and physical examination. Four types of data commonly used by epidemiologists are (1) population statistics, (2) frequency of health events (morbidity and mortality data), (3) lists of causal factors or exposures to risk factors for disease, and (4) linkages that permit researchers to track subjects over time.

A population census, carried out every 10 years in many countries, is the main source of population statistics. Census data include information about the geographical and economic characteristics of the population and the personal and demographic characteristics of individuals and households. Certain of these data provide the denominator for routine health statistics.

Mortality statistics are generally based on the numbers and causes of death listed on death certificates. Since registration of deaths is required by law in most countries, this provides a fairly complete record of the number of deaths. Accuracy of the reported cause of death varies from place to place, but the reported data are probably adequate indicators of the mortality count for major causes of death. As a rule, morbidity statistics are not routinely recorded and therefore are less readily available and less accurate than mortality statistics. The two major sources of morbidity data are hospital records and notification systems like the nosology of some 37 infectious diseases decreed as reportable in the United States and the disease registries for cancer and birth defects.

The U.S. Centers for Disease Control systematically collects data on abortions, congenital anomalies, nosocomial infections, and other health conditions. Surveys are often conducted when data are not otherwise available. Summary statistics for a community can frequently be obtained from organizations that routinely use them for health planning purposes. These organizations include the community health department, regional planning agencies, hospitals, and a variety of government offices.

Data on causal or exposure factors are sometimes available from existing sources such as hospital records. Information on patients' smoking history, reproductive history, use of drugs, and occupation can sometimes be gained from them. Unfortunately, however, completeness and accuracy vary widely. Employer records are often used to gain information on exposures to toxic substances in the workplace.

The National Health Survey, established by Congress in 1956 and conducted by the National Center for Health Statistics (NCHS), provides a continual source of information on the health status of the United States.

Linkage data are often needed by epidemiologists to follow subjects over a particular length of time. They are frequently used in studies in which exposure to a specific factor is determined and researchers follow subjects over many years to measure the frequency of development of disease. Sources of data such as Social Security records, state motor vehicle records, postal records, and town registries can be used to locate subjects.

Rates in Epidemiology

In epidemiology a count or frequency of events is of limited interest by itself. However, when frequency is used as the numerator of a fraction that expresses a proportion and specifies time, it is of great value and is called a rate. Rates are expressed by a *numerator,* a *denominator,* and a specification of *place* and *time*. Both the numerator and the denominator have to be similarly restricted by population characteristics (age, sex, and race) and by time.

When the denominator refers to a population that includes the numerator, the relative frequency is expressed as a *rate*:

$$\frac{\text{No. of new cases of cervical cancer in Cincinnati in 1990}}{\text{No. of women in Cincinnati in 1990}} \times 100,000$$

Because cervical cancer can occur only among women, only women are included in the denominator. The women in both the numerator and the denominator are those living in Cincinnati in 1990. The resulting rate is generally multiplied by some constant value, usually 100,000 so that rates for different-sized populations can be compared.

By contrast, if the numerator is not included in the denominator, a *ratio* is obtained. The annual fetal death rate is the number of fetal deaths in a year related to the total number of annual births plus fetal deaths. The annual fetal death *ratio* is the number of fetal deaths in relation to the total population of live births. Here the denominator does not include the population of both affected and unaffected persons (live births and fetal deaths) but only of unaffected persons.

The numerator and denominator of rates may be *general* or *specific*. General rates include the total population whereas specific rates apply only to the population subgroup specified (e.g., women, children under 17 years of age, or black males). The rates most commonly used as indexes of community health are listed in Table 9-4.

Rates summarize large amounts of information in a way that allows comparisons to be made between populations in different places and at various points in time. This facilitates the assessment of trends, the identification of excesses of disease occurrence, and the evaluation of progress in control efforts. For example, public health officials have observed that the rates of lung cancer deaths among females have been increasing rapidly since 1965 (Figure 9-3). It has been estimated that if these rates continue to rise at the present rate lung cancer will overtake breast cancer as the leading cause of cancer mortality in women. In an attempt to reduce these preventable deaths, public health officials have instituted antismoking campaigns aimed heavily at young women.

The increase in female lung cancer mortality represents an epidemic. *Epidemics* are defined as rates of disease significantly higher than the usual frequency. The usual frequency represents the *endemic* level. A third term, *pandemic,* is used to describe epidemics that include large areas of the world—a worldwide epidemic. Figure 9-4 illustrates the endemic fluctuation of rates. The peak, in 1976, represents an epidemic since it is clearly in excess of normal rates, which in this example are between 10 to 20 cases per 100,000 population.

Death Rates (Mortality)

General mortality rates are called *crude rates*. The numerator of the crude rate includes all relevant deaths in the entire population of the geographic area of interest. The denominator is the number of persons in the population. When the numerator includes only deaths from a particular cause, for example coronary heart disease (CHD), the rates are called disease-specific or cause-specific. Cause-specific rates are expressed as the number of deaths from a cause in a year, divided by the average (midyear) population. Such rates provide only an average rate (maybe for the entire population, including men, women, whites and nonwhites, young and old). Thus there may be a problem in interpreting comparisons of such rates. The resulting rate is dependent on the distribution of population subgroups. For example, if young persons have low rates of mortality and elderly persons have high rates, then the crude rate for a population consisting mostly of older persons will be high whereas that for a population of mostly young persons will be low. This would be true even if the rates for each age group were identical in the two populations. We might observe such a situation when comparing crude rates for a state with a young population, such as Alaska, against those for a state with a substantial elderly population, such as Florida.

When comparing only two or three locations, it may be feasible to look at *specific rates* for subgroups, for example,

TABLE 9-4
Rates most frequently used as indexes of community health

Type of rate		Usual population factor
GENERAL MORTALITY		
Crude rate =	$\dfrac{\text{No. deaths during a yr}}{\text{Average (midyear) population}}$	Per 100,000 population
Cause-specific rate =	$\dfrac{\text{No. deaths from a stated cause in a yr}}{\text{Average (midyear) population}}$	Per 100,000 population
Age-specific rate =	$\dfrac{\text{No. deaths among persons in given age group in a yr}}{\text{Average (midyear) population in same age group}}$	Per 100,000 population
Proportional rate =	$\dfrac{\text{No. deaths from a specific cause in given time period}}{\text{Total deaths in same time period}}$	Per 100 population
MORBIDITY		
Incidence =	$\dfrac{\text{No. new cases disease in a place from time}_1 \text{ to time}_2}{\text{No. persons in a place at midpoint of time period}}$	Per 100,000 population
Prevalence =	$\dfrac{\text{No. existing cases in a place at given time}}{\text{No. persons in a place at same time}}$	Per 100,000 population
MATERNAL AND INFANT MORTALITY		
Maternal (puerperal) rate =	$\dfrac{\text{No. deaths from puerperal causes in a yr}}{\text{No. live births in same yr}}$	Per 100,000 live births
Infant rate =	$\dfrac{\text{No. deaths of children less than 1 yr of age during a yr}}{\text{No. live births in same yr}}$	Per 1000 live births
Neonatal rate =	$\dfrac{\text{No. deaths of infants less than 28 days of age in a yr}}{\text{No. live births in same yr}}$	Per 1000 live births
Fetal rate =	$\dfrac{\text{No. fetal deaths during yr}}{\text{No. live births and fetal deaths in same yr}}$	Per 1000 live births and fetal deaths
Perinatal rate =	$\dfrac{\text{No. fetal deaths at 28 wk or more and infant deaths under 7 days of age during a yr}}{\text{No. live births and fetal deaths at 28 wk or more in same yr}}$	Per 1000 live births and fetal deaths
FERTILITY		
General fertility rate =	$\dfrac{\text{No. live births during a yr}}{\text{No. females aged 15-44 at midyear}}$	Per 1000 population

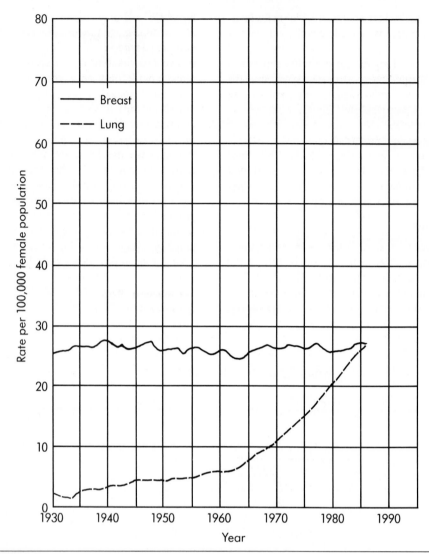

FIGURE 9-3

Age-adjusted death rates for women with breast cancer in the United States from 1930 to 1986. American Cancer Society (1990). Cancer statistics 1990. *Ca-A Cancer Journal for Clinicians*, 40, 1, 16.

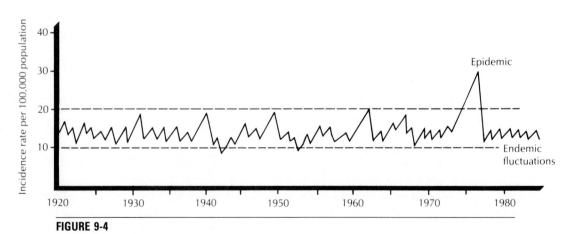

FIGURE 9-4

Schematic representation of endemic and epidemic rates.

sex-specific mortality for men and women or age-specific mortality for various age subgroups. These rates contain the number of deaths from a particular cause among the subgroup (e.g., number of CHD deaths among males) in the numerator and the number of persons comprising the subgroup (men) in the denominator. However, if we want to compare mortality for a large number of geographical locations or a large number of time periods, the use of specific rates becomes confusing because so many rates are involved. Imagine that you wanted to compare CHD rates for all 50 of the United States. Even if you compared only four age groups, you would be dealing with 200 different rates. Using a standardized or adjusted rate for each population being compared reduces the number to 50.

Adjusted rates have statistically accounted for the differences in distribution of age, sex, race, or other pertinent factors in the populations being studied. For example, most diseases show a strong relationship with age. Therefore any comparison of populations is considerably strengthened by correcting for the differences in age distribution. Use of age-adjusted rates allows you to answer the question "If these populations had the same age distribution how would their overall experience with this disease compare?" As in the example of comparing CHD rates in all 50 United States, comparison of the 50 age-adjusted rates would allow you to determine which states had excessively high or excessively low rates of mortality relative to the others.

In some cases the age-specific rates for a study population are unknown, or the population may be too small to determine reliable age-specific rates. The more stable rates of a larger population can be applied to the smaller study group. Comparison of the number of expected deaths in the smaller study population with the number actually observed will yield the standardized mortality ratio, or SMR:

$$\frac{\text{Observed deaths}}{\text{Expected deaths}}$$

An SMR of 1.0 indicates that the actual number of observed deaths in the study population is the same as the expected number based on standard population rates.

Another kind of mortality rate often used is the *proportional mortality rate* (PMR):

$$\frac{\text{Number of deaths from a specific cause}}{\text{Total number of deaths}}$$

This rate reflects the relative contribution of different causes of death to total mortality. Figure 9-1, showing the proportional distribution of death from various causes, is based on proportional mortality rates. The rates in the figures are general—and include the total population—but they may also be specific to subgroups such as men or women. The PMR requires no knowledge of the population at risk, only mortality data. The strength of the PMR is that it can be applied in situations in which only minimal data are available. Its weakness is that when it is high, due to a specific disease, it may reflect more deaths from the disease of interest but may also reflect fewer deaths from other causes.

Morbidity Rates

The two most commonly used morbidity rates are incidence and prevalence.

Incidence is a measure of all new cases arising during a defined period, usually 1 year, in a population at risk. Since it covers a specific length of time, the number of persons at risk is likely to change during that period. The simplest method to handle this potential change in the denominator is to let the population at the midpoint of the time period represent the average population at risk. Incidence is calculated as follows:

$$\frac{\text{No. of new cases of disease in a place from time to time}}{\text{No. of persons in a place at midpoint of time period}}$$

Incidence represents the risk of being afflicted with a particular disease. Thus these rates are useful in studies of disease etiology in which the incidence for groups exposed to a certain agent is compared with the incidence for groups not exposed. This measure of the risks for two groups is the *relative risk ratio*.

$$\text{Relative Risk Ratio} = \frac{\text{Incidence in exposed group}}{\text{Incidence in unexposed group}}$$

A relative risk ratio of 1.0 (1:1) means that the risk is the same for both groups. A ratio greater than 1.0 indicates an increased risk for the exposed group. Statistical tests are used to determine whether any increase in risk is greater than would be expected by chance alone.

Incidence is useful for monitoring the occurrence of a disease in defined populations over time. It is preferable to mortality for this purpose, since it reflects only diagnosed occurrences of the disease. Unlike mortality, however, incidence does not reflect additional factors such as improvements in treatment leading to improved survival. Such monitoring of disease can alert community health personnel to the presence of new hazards in the environment. For example, a sudden increase in a particular congenital malformation could indicate a recently introduced environmental hazard.

Special rates expressing incidence, called *attack rates*, are frequently used in surveillance and control of infectious disease. Attack rates are calculated when a clearly defined population has been exposed to an infectious agent. The rate represents the incidence of illness among that exposed population. An example is the incidence of hepatitis B among a class of children who were exposed to a contagious classmate. Changes in attack rates may indicate a change in the immune status of a population or may be an indication of a more virile strain of organism. These rates are discussed further in Chapter 19.

Prevalence is a measure of the existing number of cases present in a population at a give time:

$$\frac{\text{No. of existing cases in a place at given time}}{\text{No. of persons in a place at given time}}$$

This ratio is a function of the incidence and duration of a disease. The number of cases of chronic disease with low mortality tend to accumulate and will result in an increasing prevalence. Death and recovery are the two most common factors that reduce the number of cases. A less common factor is the relocation of affected individuals.

A major difference between incidence and prevalence is that knowledge of the time of onset of the disease is not required to determine prevalence. Prevalence rates are particularly useful when planning the provision of services, because they reflect both the incidence of new cases and the proportion of the population currently living with the disease. To evaluate the adequacy of existing services and to plan for future needs, public health officials require a measure of the case load requiring care. Prevalence is the measure generally used. In addition, future prevalence can be projected by using incidence, recovery, and mortality to estimate changes in prevalence over time.

THE SEQUENCE OF EPIDEMIOLOGICAL INVESTIGATION

Epidemiological investigations generally begin with descriptive epidemiology, move to analytical epidemiology, and conclude with experimental epidemiology.

Descriptive Epidemiology

This first step of investigation begins with observing and recording the existing patterns of occurrence for the condition under study. These observations are recorded in terms of person, place, and time, and they lead to a description of which specific characteristics are associated with a high versus those associated with a low frequency of disease occurrence. This phase of investigation suggests several hypotheses concerning etiology.

Consider the approach of investigators trying to learn what causes breast cancer. The first step is to obtain the rates of breast cancer for groups of people with different characteristics, rates in different geographical locations, and rates at various points in time. Epidemiologists would prefer to have the rates of newly occurring cases, *incidence*. However, since these are not generally available without a special survey or a disease registry, the rates of death from the disease *(mortality)* are used in early stages of the investigation.

When examining these rates, investigators note the following patterns about breast cancer:

◊ Rare among men compared to women
◊ More frequent among whites than nonwhites
◊ More frequent among single women versus married women
◊ More frequent among higher versus lower socioeconomic groups
◊ More frequent in successively older age groups
◊ Less frequent as the number of liveborn children increases
◊ Less frequent as age at the first full-term pregnancy decreases
◊ More frequent in developed Western countries than in less developed countries
◊ Less frequent in Asian countries such as Japan.

Analytical Epidemiology

Hypotheses suggested by the descriptive epidemiology of a condition are tested in the second investigative phase, called analytical epidemiology. The observed patterns regarding breast cancer have suggested hypotheses to epidemiologists, for example, that hormonal factors may be operating as a causal mechanism. Recently an association between the use of exogenous hormones and the occurrence of breast cancers has been proposed and tested by several investigators, with conflicting results (Trichopoulos et al., 1989; Olsson et al., 1989; Dupont et al., 1989). Differences in cell type have been explored in relation to the observed differences in breast cancer rates among whites and blacks. The role of diet has also been investigated as a possible causal factor. The results of these investigations have not been conclusive, and additional analytical work is needed.

Such analytical studies may be done on either an ecological or a relational level.

Ecological studies compare a large aggregate of people, usually in some defined geographical area, to another similarly large population. For example, cancer rates for the populations of towns with polluted drinking water may be compared to those for towns with pure drinking water to assess whether water pollution is associated with the elevated rates; or per capita data on fat consumption may be compared for countries with high and low rates of colon cancer to investigate the hypothesis that fat consumption influences the development of colon cancer. Such studies, while a useful first step in the analytical phase of investigation, are subject to the *ecological fallacy*. There is a fallacy in assuming that relationships observed among groups will be the same as among individuals. Although there may be a striking relationship between high cancer rates and polluted water in the populations studied, the same relationship will not necessarily be observed on individual levels. Imagine, for example, that the majority of residents in whom cancer developed in a town with polluted water were men who worked in other towns where they were exposed to carcinogens in the workplace. They likely drank less of the polluted water in their home town than did the other individuals in that town.

Relational studies, on the other hand, do relate exposure and disease in the same people. The presence or absence of exposure and disease is determined for each individual. Then the frequency of the presence of disease and exposure is assessed.

Four basic types of studies are commonly used in analytical epidemiology: (1) cross-sectional studies, (2) case-control studies, (3) cohort studies, and (4) historical cohort studies. Other names used synonymously with these terms are listed in Table 9-5, along with the design of each when used in either an ecological or a relational investigation.

Cross-sectional and case-control studies are generally used as a first step in the analytical phase of investigation because they can be done quickly, require small samples, and are relatively inexpensive. These studies provide preliminary evidence of an association between a hypothesized causal variable and a particular health outcome. Cohort and historical cohort studies generally require large samples, take longer to complete, and are expensive. They are not a practical design for investigating rare diseases because of the size of the population that must be followed to generate incidence cases. On the other hand, they do yield measures of incidence or risk. No incidence can be derived from cross-sectional or case-control studies, and any risk measures must be obtained by indirect means.

Because these analytical efforts are based on observa-

TABLE 9-5
A comparison of ecological and relational studies

Level of studies	Types of studies	Other common terms for study design	Basic design
Ecological	Cross-sectional	Correlational Ecological correlational	Rates of disease frequency are correlated with the frequency of a factor at various points in time
	Case-control	Retrospective	Places with high rates of a disease are compared to places with low rates for levels of factors thought to be related to causing that disease
	Cohort	Prospective Longitudinal	Rates of disease occurrence are compared into the future for places with current environmental exposure and places known not to have such exposure
	Historical cohort	Retrospective-prospective Nonconcurrent cohort	Rates of disease occurrence are compared for places with known past environmental exposure and places known not to have such exposure; tracking of rates begins at the time of exposure in the past and continues to the present
Relational	Cross-sectional	Correlational	Current rates of exposure among individuals are correlated with current rates of disease frequency among these same individuals
	Case-control	Retrospective Case comparison	Individuals with the study disease are compared to individuals without the disease, who are similar in regard to other characteristics, for frequency of prior exposure to the study factor
	Cohort	Prospective Longitudinal Prospective population	A group of individuals known to be exposed to a factor and a group of similar individuals not exposed are followed into the future for occurrence of the disease and comparison of its incidence
	Historical cohort	Retrospective-prospective Nonconcurrent cohort Retrospective cohort Retrospective mortality Retrospective incidence	A group of individuals known to be exposed to a factor at a time in the past is compared to a group of individuals not exposed and their disease incidence or mortality is compared from the time of exposure to the present

tional data, the possibility exists that the observed association of a suspected causal factor with the occurrence of a particular disease may be caused by other factors that interact in some unknown way with the factor under study. An example would be genetic self-selection of individuals for use of harmful substances. *Genetic self-selection* refers to a hereditary chemical "imbalance" that is thought to predispose a person to craving substances like alcohol and cigarettes. Confounding variables such as this may be identified at a later stage of investigation. Suppose that a researcher notes that rates of spontaneous abortion increase with the number of pregnancies. The number of pregnancies might not be a causative factor, but rather might be related to the age of the mother. If physiological aging decreases a woman's capacity for carrying a pregnancy to term, then age will confound the original association between parity and spontaneous abortion rates.

Experimental Epidemiology

When sufficient evidence from analytical studies supports the causal relationship of a specific factor to the occurrence of a particular disease, the experimental phase of epidemiological investigation is begun. This is the third phase of the investigation, which uses an experimental design to con-

firm the causal nature of relationships identified through observational studies.

Because it would be unethical to expose humans to an agent thought to be harmful, in most epidemiological experiments the study sample is chosen from individuals already exposed to the causal agent under study. The suspected causal factor is then removed from one study group. Their disease experience is compared to that of the group that continues to be exposed to the suspected factor. For example, if a high-lipid diet is thought to be a causal agent for stroke, patients may be randomly assigned to a treatment group that is given a special diet to reduce the intake of lipids while the remaining subjects continue with their usual dietary intake. The two groups are then compared for the incidence of stroke.

In the experimental phase of epidemiological study the investigator has control over who is or is not exposed as well as what the experimental conditions will be. Therefore the problems of the analytical studies are not generally present. As a result, data from experimental studies are typically used to prove causal relationships.

Ideally, experimental data demonstrating cause would be available before a decision was made on whether to set up programs to reduce or eliminate a particular exposure or to answer clients' questions about a particular risk. Often this is not possible.

Epidemiological research is proliferating. Results of studies are discussed in the lay press, sometimes before the relevant issue of a journal has arrived in the library. Health professionals are often besieged by clients who want interpretation and guidance about what to do. Should they ask their doctor to take them off oral contraceptives in view of a report showing an association of oral contraceptive use with breast cancer? What about all the advertisements the client has been seeing for mammography? Is it important to have mammograms? How often? Should all women have them regularly or only women in specific age and risk groups? What about school nurses teaching breast self-examination to high school girls? Is this a good idea? Why? Why not? Epidemiological research provides data for answering these questions, but results must be studied carefully. The quality of study designs varies, and results may be conflicting or attributable to biases in the study design. Thus to reach appropriate conclusions to guide practice, nurses should have sufficient understanding of epidemiological methods to allow them to read the literature critically.

The following discussion of a published study that generated national attention illustrates the type of critical analysis required when reading the literature. The case control study by MacMahon et al. (1983) involves biases inherent in research design that may affect the validity of results. These researchers reported a finding that coffee drinking was associated with the occurrence of pancreatic cancer. Cases were pathologically documented incidences of pancreatic cancer treated at the study hospital during a defined period. Control subjects were other patients with gastrointestinal disease treated by the same physicians at the same hospital during the same time. Use of coffee was assessed for the period immediately before diagnosis. This, together with the use of gastrointestinal disease patients as controls, may have introduced a bias that led to the findings reported. Because of the slow onset of many gastrointestinal diseases, the control patients may have experienced mild gastrointestinal discomfort for an extended period before being diagnosed. Because coffee drinking tends to produce gastrointestinal discomfort for many people, it is quite likely that these control subjects had considerably decreased or even eliminated their use of coffee before diagnosis. If so, the finding that pancreatic cancer patients drank more coffee than control subjects is not surprising.

USES OF EPIDEMIOLOGY

Epidemiological methods and the body of knowledge generated from epidemiological studies are basic to the practice of community health nursing. It is essential to have community health officials who are capable of both conducting epidemiological investigations or studies and also integrating the findings into the practice of community health.

Investigation of the Natural History of Disease

The purpose of epidemiological investigation is to determine the cause of disease, thus providing the data needed for control or eradication. Etiological studies represent a major use of epidemiological methods. For effective disease prevention, the cause(s) of disease must be identified and the means by which causal agents are transmitted to the human host understood. Epidemiological studies emphasize the prepathogenic or early pathogenic state. By contrast, clinical researchers are largely concerned with patient responses to treatment (physiological and psychological) during the later stages of a disease since the patients studied usually have sought treatment for the symptoms of illness.

Although there are numerous epidemiological studies based solely on hospitalized causes, it is essential to look at studies that are concerned with all cases of a disease in a population, regardless of their location. Without this spectrum of disease severity, it is impossible to understand the natural history. Thus epidemiological research often produces a different picture of the disease from that derived only by hospital data.

As an example, the study of acquired immunodeficiency syndrome (AIDS) or human immunodeficiency virus (HIV) has been a major focus of epidemiology in the last decade. Initially the majority of what was known about AIDS and HIV stemmed from the care of patients with advanced stages of the disease (e.g., Kaposi's sarcoma) or with an opportunistic infection (*Pneumocystis carinii* pneumonia). The severity of these symptoms and the vast amount of uncertainty regarding the transmission of AIDS led to a high degree of public hysteria. Only by studying populations at risk for the disease and patients in the early stages have we been able to increase our knowledge level to the point that public hysteria is reduced and the true impact of the disease being assessed. By studying persons in the early pathogenic stages researchers now know that AIDS is a syndrome ranging from early and silent infections to mild illnesses manifested by swollen lymph glands and weight loss to rare but lethal infections and cancer.

Identification of Risks

Risk refers to the probability of an unfavorable event. In epidemiology it generally means that there is a high likelihood that people who do not have a disease will acquire it if they come in contact with certain factors thought to increase its risk. Generally the risk to an individual of contracting a particular disease can be estimated only on the basis of the experience of a whole population. Once this experience is known, the relevant risks can be calculated for persons who are similar to those in that population. Further, population data on disease occurrence can provide information for estimating the effect on disease rates of a community intervention. Epidemiological methods are used to collect the appropriate data and to estimate these risks.

An individual's risk of contracting a disease caused by a particular exposure is determined by comparing the occurrence of the disease in a population exposed to the causal agent with the occurrence in a nonexposed population. The *relative risk ratio* estimates how much the risk of acquiring a disease increases with exposure to a particular causal agent or known risk factor. Thus a relative risk ratio of 5:1 implies that the risk of acquiring the disease is five times greater for someone exposed to an etiological agent than for someone not exposed.

Relative risk ratios are useful for identifying factors that represent increased risk of contracting a disease. Diabetes, obesity, hypertension, and smoking are considered risk factors for cardiovascular disease because populations with these characteristics show a rate of that disease several times greater than the rate in populations without these conditions or behaviors. Once the risk factors are identified, community health programs can be instituted to change high-risk behaviors and identify high-risk individuals through comprehensive screening programs. Such programs ensure medical treatment to reduce the risk. In addition, nurses and other clinicians can counsel individuals regarding methods to reduce their risk by adopting healthier life-styles.

The effect of community intervention to eliminate exposure to a causal agent on disease occurrence is estimated by a measure called *attributable risk*. This measure subtracts the rate of disease occurrence (incidence) in the nonexposed population from the rate of disease occurrence (incidence) in the exposed population. If cardiovascular disease develops in a nonsmoking population at a rate of 350 cases per 100,000 population and in a smoking population at a rate of 685 cases per 100,000 then 335 cases per 100,000 may be attributable to cigarette smoking and should be preventable if cigarettes are banned.

Identification of Syndromes and Classification of Disease

Identifying syndromes and classifying diseases relate directly to clinical medicine. Broad descriptive clinical and pathological categories often include widely varying elements. Their differing statistical distributions and the different ways in which the disease progresses or behaves in a population may make it possible to distinguish one element from another and thus identify characteristic syndromes. For example, all vascular diseases were once classified together; but as epidemiological data accumulated, it became clear that cerebrovascular disease and cardiovascular disease were distinct conditions, though both shared the characteristic narrowing or occlusion of a blood vessel as a preceding mechanism. However, populations with high rates of cerebrovascular disease, such as the Japanese, have low rates of cardiovascular disease, and the converse is true (Morris, 1975). Another example, the rubella syndrome was identified as a collection of malformations and functional problems common to offspring of mothers infected with German measles during pregnancy, particularly during the first trimester (Gregg, 1941). More recent examples include the identification of toxic shock syndrome as a definable group of symptoms and the identification of AIDS among homosexual men and other high-risk groups (MMWR, 1981).

Differential Diagnosis and Treatment

Descriptive data on, for example, the age and sex incidence of a disease aid clinicians in understanding the condition and in sorting through multiple possible diagnoses with the same or similar symptoms. Recognizing the association of age with prognosis for long-term survival in breast cancer will probably influence treatment and may influence control programs. Breast cancer diagnosed premenopausally tends to be more lethal than postmenopausal breast cancer, requiring more aggressive treatment and closer follow-up. Mumps may be a mild self-limiting disease in childhood,

but in adult men it can lead to infertility. Thus community health intervention to reduce susceptibility or prevent exposure of adult males who did not acquire infection during childhood is important.

Surveillance of the Health Status of Populations

Surveillance means keeping watch over. Epidemiological descriptions of diseases provide data about who is at risk of contracting a disease, where geographically the disease is more likely to occur, and when it is most often observed. This information alerts health workers to situations that should be monitored for early indication of a disease outbreak. Early detection programs can be set up and intervention promptly instituted.

For example, influenza rates tend to increase during late fall and early winter. Specific types of influenza are likely to recur in 2-to-3-year or 4-to-6-year cycles (Benenson, 1985). Groups at high risk of becoming seriously ill and dying of influenza are infants, young children, and elderly persons. Public health officials can monitor the population for early indications of an outbreak through reports of deaths from influenza, of increases in cases seen at emergency rooms, or of increased rates of absence from school or work because of respiratory illness. They can identify the signs of an influenza outbreak early and can take steps to immunize susceptible high-risk populations to prevent occurrence of the illness.

In another example, the epidemiology of measles indicates that it occurs most frequently among school-age children, that its rates vary by season (being highest in the fall), and that there are long-term cycles with increased outbreak every other year in large communities (and at less frequent intervals in smaller communities). Measles is transmitted from person to person by close contact; it therefore tends to occur in locations where children congregate (Benenson, 1985). Armed with this information, the school nurse can be alert to signs and symptoms of measles during the fall and can follow up on absences to determine if they were due to measles. Numerous such absences may indicate a need to review the immunization status of the school population. Although most schools require up-to-date immunizatons for a child to enter, all too often monitoring does not occur and follow-up programs must be instituted to ensure immunizations for the susceptible children.

Diagnosis, Planning, and Evaluation of Community Health Services

Epidemiology provides facts about community health. It describes the nature and relative size of the health problems to be dealt with, as well as how they are distributed in terms of geographical location, age group, socioeconomic group, and so on. This kind of information forms the basis for planning the number and types of services required to meet the needs of a particular community. A neighborhood with a high proportion of elderly individuals is likely to have high rates of cardiovascular disease, cancer, and other chronic debilitating diseases. If it is a low-income neighborhood, elderly residents may lack the financial resources to travel to a distant location for medical care. Thus health planners need to consider setting up a satellite clinic in the neighborhood or providing transportation or home services. Maternity and child health services can be planned to meet the needs of a community with a young population and high birthrate. Family planning facilities, well-child centers that include immunization services, and health education programs aimed at preventing disease through promotion of good health habits may be appropriate.

Evaluation of Health Services

Since many health services are initiated as an effort to treat a community problem identified by epidemiological data, these same data can be used as a monitoring device to evaluate the services. For example, one means of evaluating the effectiveness of a maternity and child health center established to reduce morbidity and mortality rates among mothers and children is to observe whether these rates drop and remain low after the health center is in operation.

APPLICATIONS OF EPIDEMIOLOGY IN COMMUNITY HEALTH NURSING

Most community health nurses are employed by agencies that interact directly with individual clients and families. These agencies include visiting nurse associations, community-based maternity and child health or mental health centers, alcohol and drug intervention programs, health maintenance organizations, and nursing centers. Nursing in occupational health settings, though usually limited to contact with the individual client, requires a consideration of the family's resources and needs in planning care. Some nurses will be employed as health planners or administrators. For example, the director of a visiting nurse association may be involved in planning and evaluating services of the agency, nursing administrators in a health department, by contrast, may be involved both in planning services of that agency and in coordinating the services of a variety of community agencies, similarly, nurses serving on community boards will need to be concerned with coordination of existing services and planning to meet currently unmet needs. Regardless of the agency or the nurses' position, they will be involved in some phase with the epidemiological process.

Care of patients and families is based on the following steps of the nursing process: (1) assessment, (2) planning, (3) implementation, and (4) evaluation. The same process is used in providing care for communities. In both instances, epidemiology furnishes the baseline information for assessing needs, identifying problems, setting priorities in development of a plan of care, and evaluating the effectiveness of care.

Agencies that provide care to communities interface through referrals, required reporting, and feedback mechanisms with agencies whose primary purpose is the provision of direct services to clients. Observations of need based on a common baseline of information are necessary if nurses at various levels and in various settings are to provide appropriate care. If such a baseline of information is not shared, each nurse will collect only the data he or she considers important and interpretations of the data will vary from nurse to nurse. Epidemiological concepts, such as the natural history of disease and primary, secondary, and ter-

tiary prevention, provide a unifying approach for defining which data should be collected and how they should be interpreted.

If such information is available at all levels and common interpretation is likely, then the referral and reporting system within a community will be facilitated and the system should respond effectively to a need. To assess needs, the nurse providing direct care requires data on the presence or absence of risk characteristics, including family composition and relationships, socioeconomic and cultural factors, environmental factors, and medical and health history (incidence, prevalence, and mortality, both current and over time). The nurse involved in planning services for the community requires parallel data—including the presence and distribution of risk characteristics, population composition by age, race, and socioeconomic and cultural factors, environmental factors, and medical and health histories.

CLINICAL APPLICATION

The following situation illustrates the use of epidemiological data by nurses providing direct services and involved in planning at the community level:

A nurse in the Visiting Nurse Service receives a referral for a home visit to a 15-year-old mother whose premature infant has just been discharged from the hospital. The mother of the infant lives with her 40-year-old mother and her 45-year-old father. On her way from the bus stop to the house, the nurse passes overturned trash cans with garbage strewn in the street and numerous teenagers lounging on the doorstep of a neighboring house. When she arrives, she notes that the apartment is hazy with cigarette smoke but appears clean and tidy. Upon assessing the infant, she finds that the baby has a temperature of 39° C and diarrhea but no signs of upper respiratory infection. The grandmother reports that the temperature was normal late yesterday when the infant was discharged from the hospital. The baby's mother has returned to school and the grandmother is caring for the baby. She states that she quit a part-time job so she could do this and that they can just scrape by on her husband's salary of $16,000 a year. The baby's mother is doing poorly in school and the family agrees that when she turns 16 it would be wise for her to quit school and obtain a part time job to help with family expenses and caring for the baby. The nurse learns that the baby's mother is continuing to see the baby's father and that she is irritable and impatient when the baby cries.

The nurse relies on epidemiological facts to interpret the assessment and plan appropriate nursing care. For example, the baby has an elevated temperature accompanied by diarrhea. He was fed once during the night and once in the morning with bottles of milk sent home from the hospital. Only the afternoon feeding was from formula mixed in the home. The nurse's knowledge of the natural history of infectious diseases reveals these important facts: (1) an elevated temperature and diarrhea in the absence of respiratory symptoms suggest a milk-borne infection and some other infection transmitted or oral-entry. Since the temperature is elevated, the symptoms are probably caused by an infection rather than a toxin. (2) Most gastrointestinal infections have an incubation period longer than 24 hours and most feedings were from hospital-supplied formula. The nurse concludes that the infection may have originated in the hospital and initiates a referral of the baby to a pediatrician for culture and treatment. Because of the nature of community health nursing, the care by this nurse does not stop at this individual level but continues with a report to health department nurses of a possible hospital-related infection in the premature nursery. These personnel will need to follow up on other recent discharges and to work with hospital epidemiologists to identify the source of infection.

The nurse also applies principles of epidemiology in the assessment of other high-risk factors present in this family. Teenage pregnancies are at increased risk for low birth weight and perinatal and infant mortality. Close spacing of pregnancies increases the risks to physical health of both the mother and the fetus. This teenage mother appears likely to become pregnant again. Such a pregnancy would probably be attended with complications. Additional infants in this family would increase pressures on the mother and her parents and disrupt family interactions, creating an environment conducive to child abuse. Nursing interventions include counseling the mother regarding birth control options and referral to a family-planning center. Plans should encompass teaching the mother about normal behaviors and growth and development of the infant.

In a broader sense, the nurse is also concerned for the need for assessible community services to support this family and others with similar needs. For example, the referral for family-planning services should be made to a facility that is accessible, affordable, and sensitive to the special needs of adolescents. If these types of facilities are not available for referral, the community health nurse acts as an advocate for the teenage population by participating in health boards responsible for the planning of community health services.

The mother's plan to terminate her education is another indication of a high-risk situation. Epidemiological data provide evidence of the long-term impact of educational level on the health of the teenage mother and infant. The teenager experiences a developmental crisis when the tasks of parenthood are superimposed on the normal development tasks of the adolescent. The nurse counsels the mother regarding the need to continue her education, continues to act as an advocate for the client by contacting the school nurse for counseling with the mother, and refers the mother to a community teen mothers' group for support. If programs are not available in the schools or community to support teenage mothers, then many clients will be faced with the same dilemma occurring in this family. The nurse assesses the need for such services and plans appropriate community-based interventions to provide them to the teenage population.

In this clinical situation the nurse is providing individual care to the teenage mother and family. These interventions will bring the mother into contact with nurses in other community agencies—the health department nurse, the family-planning clinic nurses, and the school nurse. If appropriate services are not available to meet the needs of the client, the nurse plans interventions directed to all similar clients with similar needs. Facilities such as family-planning centers and adolescent mothers' groups are available for refer-

rals because nurses and other professionals engage in health planning. This process includes monitoring births in the community. If the rate of illegitimate births is increasing, particularly among adolescents, family-planning centers in high-risk neighborhoods may be established. The health planning process also includes monitoring rates of school dropout, including high-risk groups such as teenage mothers. In high-risk communities, school-based services may be indicated that can provide educational counseling, information on growth and development, and in some cases assistance with child care. When nurses monitor appropriate epidemiological indicators and participate in the health planning process, the services needed for appropriate intervention with young clients will be available and the nurse providing direct services can make appropriate referrals. Ongoing monitoring of these indicators provides feedback as to the effectiveness of the services.

SUMMARY

Epidemiology, the study of the distribution of states of health and of the determinants of deviations from health in populations, is a community health science essential to nursing practice. It refers to both the methods used in the study of disease causation and the body of knowledge that arises from such investigations. Knowledge of the methods of epidemiology is useful to the community health nurse, both as a tool in conducting the investigation to evaluate and explain phenomena observed in the course of work and as a basis for interpreting and evaluating the epidemiological research literature. Epidemiological methods, such as measures of health, serve as tools for assessing community needs, monitoring changes in health status of the community, and evaluating the impact of community programs of disease prevention and health promotion.

The body of knowledge dervied from epidemiological studies, including the natural history of diseases, patterns of disease occurrence, and factors associated with high risk for developing disease, serves as an information base for community health nursing practice. This knowledge provides a framework for planning and evaluating community intervention programs aimed at primary, secondary, and tertiary prevention (i.e., prevention of illness, early detection and treatment of disease, and minimization of disability). Programs of *primary* prevention focus on distancing disease agents from susceptible hosts, decreasing agent viability, increasing host resistance, and altering the established host-agent-environment relationships. Screening and risk factor reduction programs are examples of *secondary* prevention. Vocational retraining and rehabilitative exercises for the disabled are *tertiary* prevention strategies. For the individual nurse the body of knowledge derived from epidemiological research serves as a basis for assessing individual and family health needs and for planning nursing interventions. It also provides tools for evaluating the success of the interventions.

KEY CONCEPTS

Epidemiology is the study of the distribution of health and illness in populations.

In the epidemiological approach to illness, the event is described in terms of how it affects the group.

Epidemiologists investigate causality based on relationships between a stimulus and an outcome by using statistical measures of association.

Concepts important to epidemiology are causality, natural history, agent, environment, host, disease process, and levels of prevention.

Natural history is the process by which a disease occurs and progresses in humans. The natural history of a disease involves three factors: a causative agent, a susceptible host, and the environment.

There are three stages to the natural history of a disease: prepathogenesis, or susceptibility; pathogenesis; and advanced disease.

Three levels of prevention are primary, secondary, and tertiary. Primary prevention involves prevention of illness; secondary prevention involves early detection

and treatment of disease, and tertiary prevention involves minimization of disability.

Epidemiological methods involve use of data from existing sources, such as census data, and data generated for specific studies. The three types of data required are population statistics, mortality data, and morbidity data.

Rates used in epidemiology include attack rates, incidence, and prevalence. Incidence is a measure of all new cases of illness arising during a given period in a population at risk; prevalence is a measure of the number of existing cases of illness in a population at a given time; and attack rates represent the incidence of illness among an exposed population.

Two kinds of causal associations are direct causal associations and indirect causal associations.

The knowledge derived from epidemiological studies provide a framework for planning and evaluating community health intervention programs.

LEARNING ACTIVITIES

1. Choose one of the major causes of morbidity and mortality, such as cardiovascular disease.
   a. On the basis of current epidemiological research evidence, outline the natural history, including known risk factors.
   b. Based on the natural history specify interventions for primary, secondary, and tertiary prevention of this disease.

2. Choose one of the interventions identified in activity B of number 1.

   a. Define the parameters of a community population in which such an intervention would be useful.
   b. Decide which measurements of disease would reflect the impact of your intervention on this population, e.g., incidence, prevalence, mortality, survival, complication rates.

3. Decide how the natural history of this disease will affect your own nursing care of patients or families.

BIBLIOGRAPHY

Benenson, A, editor: Control of communicable diseases in man, 1985, Washington DC, American Public Health Association.

Centers for Disease Control: Follow-up on toxic shock syndrome, MMWR 29:441-444, 1980.

Dupont WD, et al: Influence of exogenous estrogens, proliferative breast disease, and other variables on breast cancer risk, Cancer 63(5):948-57, 1989.

Gregg NM: Congenital cataract following German measles in the mother, Trans Ophthalmol Soc Australia 3:35-46, 1941.

Kleinfeld, M, Messire, J, and Kooyman, O: Mortality experience in a group of asbestos workers, Arch Environ Health 15:177-180, 1967.

Leavell, HR, and Clark, EG: Preventive medicine for the doctor in his community, New York, 1968, McGraw-Hill Book Co.

MacMahon, B, Yen, S, Tuchopoulos, D, Warren K, and Nardis, G: Coffee and cancer of the pancreas, N Engl J Med 304:630-633, 1981.

Morbidity and Mortality Weekly Reports (MMWR), Centers for Disease Control, 30:305-307, 1981.

Morris, JN: Uses of epidemiology, ed 3, London, 1975, E & S Livingstone, Ltd.

National Center for Health Statistics (NCHS), Advanced Report on Final Mortality Statistics, 38(suppl) Sept. 26, 1989.

Olsson, H, et al (1989). Early oral contraceptive use and breast cancer among premenopausal

women: Final report from a study in southern Sweden. J Natl Cancer Inst, 81(13), 1000-4.

Smoking and Health: Report of the advisory committee to the Surgeon General of the public health service, USDHEW, Pub. No. (PHS) 1103, Washington, D.C., 1964, U.S. Government Printing Office.

Snow, J: On the mode of communication of cholera, New York, 1936, The Commonwealth Fund, pp. 1-175.

Valanis, B: Epidemiology in nursing and health care, East Norwalk, Conn., 1986, Appleton-Century-Crofts.

Trichopoulos, D, et al (1989). Oral contraceptives, tobacco smoking, and breast cancer risk. Lancet, 2(8655), 158.

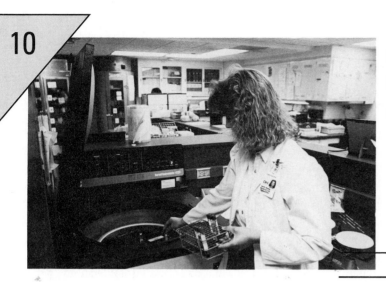

10

Research as a Guide to Community Health Nursing Practice

Beverly C. Flynn

OBJECTIVES

After reading this chapter, the student should be able to:

Discuss priority areas for research in community health nursing with considerations of the WHO and UNICEF (1978) definition of primary health care.

Describe the stages of the research process.

Describe roles and issues in research.

Cite several community health nursing research studies.

Identify ways the practicing community health care nurse can participate in research.

KEY TERMS

accessible health care	data gathering	inductive approach
action	deliberate sampling	multisectoral approach
appropriate technology	disease prevention	planning
assessment	evaluation	primary health care
communication	health promotion	random sampling
community involvement	implementation	

R| esearch for community health nursing practice has developed over the years and must continue to expand. Although increasing efforts are devoted to nursing research, community health nurses need to increase their scientific knowledge of what has worked and what has not worked in practice. Community health nurses are committed to improving the health of the community and are challenged to search for creative yet scientifically oriented solutions to today's health problems. Through research, community health nurses are developing the knowledge needed to meet this challenge.

This chapter focuses on the development of practice-based research in community health nursing. Primary health care as defined by the World Health Organization (WHO and UNICEF, 1978) is proposed as an appropriate approach to guide research and to develop concepts in community health nursing. An overview of the research process is presented. Questions for research that are generated from practice are linked with the key concepts of primary health care. Selected research issues and the roles and functions of the researcher and collaborators are discussed. Examples from community health nursing practice are provided throughout the chapter.

RELATIONSHIP OF COMMUNITY HEALTH NURSING TO PRIMARY HEALTH CARE

Primary health care was endorsed by all countries attending a World Conference in Alma Ata, Russia as the approach to reach the goal of "health for all by the year 2000" (WHO and UNICEF, 1978). "Primary health care is essential health care based on practical, scientifically sound and socially acceptable methods and technology made universally accessible to individuals and families in the community through their full participation and at a cost that the community and country can afford to maintain at every stage of their development in the spirit of self-reliance and self determination" (WHO and UNICEF, 1978, p. 16).

The contribution of nursing to primary health care has been considered by these countries. The International Council of Nurses (ICN) and WHO have provided leadership in supporting national nursing associations in their exploration of the contributions nurses make in primary health care.*

There is a link between community health nursing and primary health care. Both incorporate community-based practice, involvement of the community in health care decisions, a focus on disease prevention and health promotion, and use of an interdisciplinary approach in planning and implementing appropriate solutions to health problems. Thus community health nursing and primary health care are complementary. Consequently, research conducted by community health nurses can make a significant contribution to primary health care practice.

THE RESEARCH PROCESS

The research process is a problem-solving process involving assessment, planning, implementation, evaluation, and action. The action leads to reassessment, more planning and implementation, and so on.

The stages of the research process are summarized in the box below. Although the listing is sequential, the researcher actually works back and forth among the various stages of the research process. Decisions made in any one stage must be consistent with decisions made in other stages. All stages are viewed as part of the total study and are arrived at logically and systematically. To clarify each stage of the research process, common examples from nursing practice are presented.

Assessment

Assessment involves translating a hunch or a curiosity about a clinical problem into a question that can be researched. For example, a community health nurse may be curious about why some elderly in the community are able to live independently while others are institutionalized. The nurse reviews the research and related literature to gain an overview of the situation and its current stage of research. The initial literature review helps the nurse decide on the purpose

---

STAGES OF THE RESEARCH PROCESS

ASSESSMENT PHASE

Initiating the idea
Initial review of literature
Identifying the purpose of the research
Delineating the population

PLANNING PHASE

Sorting specific research problem
Key terms defined
Extensive review of literature
Delineating the conceptual framework
Delineating research questions and hypotheses
Selecting research approach and research design
Selecting data-gathering method
Developing data analysis plan (including use of computer software)
Selecting sample
Pilot studies to test instruments and apply data analysis
Human subjects approval process
Identifying limitations of research

IMPLEMENTATION PHASE

Inviting sample to participate in research
Implementing data gathering plan
Implementing data analysis plan

EVALUATION PHASE

Analyzing findings
Drawing conclusions
Preparing research reports
Presenting research

ACTION PHASE

Applying results
Taking action for social change

Selected stages of the research process are modified from Fox (1982), pp. 26-27.

---

*ICN and WHO, 1979; PAHO, 1977; WHO, 1982; WHO, 1984; WHO, 1985.

and population for the study. In the example of the elderly, the community health nurse decides that the purpose of the study is to determine whether or not community health nursing services are assisting them to live in the community. The group to be studied must be clearly defined by selecting a specific age minimum.

Planning

In *planning,* the specific research problem is stated. In the example above, the community health nurse decides that the problem to be investigated is a lack of information about the relationship between community health nursing services and the ability of the elderly to live independently in the community.

Next, key terms in the problem are defined. For example, in the study the elderly will be defined as persons 75 years or older. Information obtained from reviews of the literature can be used to define terms and assist in further developing a scientific body of knowledge for nursing practice.

Through an extensive literature review the nurse identifies conceptual frameworks and how research and data analyses were done and examines the results of previous research. Of particular concern at this point is what has and has not worked in previous studies.

The nurse also must select a conceptual framework that is appropriate for the problem to be investigated. In the example, the nurse selects a conceptual framework that can be adapted from the health services research field, incorporating environmental services, health services, and client characteristics (Aday and Anderson, 1974).

Next, the nurse delineates specific research questions or hypotheses or both for the research. These statements include the key variables of the study. In the example, the nurse questions if the range of community health nursing services for the elderly is appropriate for this population. It is hypothesized that the greater the range of community health nursing services the more the elderly are able to live independently in the community. The key variables are the range of community health nursing services and the ability to live independently in the community.

The nurse next selects a research approach; it may be historical, survey, or experimental. Each approach creates different requirements for a research design. Considerations include whether the data will be collected at one point in time or longitudinally, (meaning at various time points), and whether the data will be collected cross-sectionally or across various groups in the population. In the example, the nurse decides that a historical approach, or a review of past information, will not adequately address the problem. Nor is an experimental approach feasible because the study cannot be conducted under controlled conditions. Instead, the nurse decides that a survey is the most appropriate approach for comparing the elderly with different living arrangements. This approach permits a research design for collecting data at one time period.

The next stage involves selecting a *data gathering* method, such as observing, measuring, or questioning. Specific techniques and instruments are identified. For example, within the questioning method the interview or questionnaire technique might be considered and a specific instrument could be selected for the technique. Decisions need to be made about a data-gathering method, technique, and instrument for each of the major variables in the research questions or hypotheses. In the example the nurse decides to use the observing and questioning methods. She plans to observe community health nurses providing services to the elderly to delineate the range of services provided. To avoid a situation in which the nurses and the elderly feel uncomfortable about being observed, the nurse researcher plans to be a participant observer and work with the community health nurses. This allows the nurse researcher to participate in a natural situation for data collection. In addition to observation, the nurse researcher will use the questioning method and select an interview questionnaire that determines the level of physical functioning of the elderly. This interview may be completed with the elderly person or the elderly person's care giver.

The plan for data analysis is guided by the research questions or hypotheses. It is useful to identify the statistics to be used, computer software available to assist with data analysis, and also to design sample tables that will contain the data once they are collected. This will help ensure that all the data necessary to answer the research questions and to test the hypotheses are being collected. In the example it is decided to use descriptive statistics, for example, means, ranges, percents, and chi square. Figure 10-1 shows a sample table that can be used after data are collected in the research example.

The research questions and plan for data analysis guide sample selection. The statistics to be used direct the sample

Ability to live independently	Range of community health nursing services	
	High	Low
High		
Low		

FIGURE 10-1

Sample Table.

size. There are many methods of sample selection, but two will be considered here—random and deliberate sampling. *Random sampling* means that every case or subject has an equal opportunity of being included in the study. The second method is *deliberative* selection, in which specific cases or subjects are invited to participate in the study.

In the example, the nurse decides to study elderly persons in the county in which she works. She consults a statistician and together they decide that the sample should consist of 100 elderly persons over 75 years living in the community. This figure is based on an estimated sample size required for the statistics selected. It is impossible to know the exact number living in the community. The nurse therefore estimates the total elderly population based on census data. A deliberate sample of persons 75 years and older is selected until 100 are included in the sample.

Important in the planning phase is approval of the research by the institutional human subject review committee. These are groups of representatives of various disciplines or departments brought together for the purpose of reviewing research proposals. Their major concerns are protecting human participants in research from physical or mental harm as well as the researcher from undue complaints.

In the example, the local health department has a committee that covers research on health department services. The nurse researcher obtains approval from the committee. Usually an application is submitted to the committee to ensure the study subjects will not be physically or mentally harmed by the research. This process also protects the researcher from undue complaints, providing the subject's informed consent is obtained prior to the study.

The role of the researcher here is to communicate clearly in writing to the review committee what is planned, how subjects will be used in the research, and whether or not they are at risk to injury as a result of participating in the research. The researcher is ethically responsible for carrying out these plans as directed or approved by the committee. Changes that occur in the plans need to be reported to the committee for further sanctioning.

Pilot studies can be used to test data-gathering methods and to apply the data-analysis plan. A pilot study is especially important when the data-gathering technique is unfamiliar to the researcher, for example, if the instrument is new, if the instrument has not been used with the population under study, and if the study is conducted in an unfamiliar environment. The nurse researcher decides to pilot test her study with five elderly clients from a neighboring county. She obtains permission from both the nurse and the clients.

The assumptions and limitations of the research need to be identified. Assumptions are characteristics of the research situation that are not explored, usually because they have been well demonstrated in previous research. An assumption of the study is that some community services help the elderly to live in the community. The limitations are uncontrollable elements of the research, which limit the certainty of the findings or the applicability of the findings to the population in general. In the study a limitation is that deliberate sampling does not ensure that all the elderly are equally represented. As a result the study findings are not generalized beyond the study sample.

Implementation

Implementation of the research plan refers to carrying out the research procedures. This includes inviting the sample group to participate, obtaining their informed consent, collecting and verifying the data, entering the data for computer analyses, and analyzing the data. Prior to meeting the elderly, the nurse researcher sends a letter inviting them to participate in the study. She follows-up with phone calls and arranges appointments with the clients and community health nurse. After meeting the clients, the clients and/or caregivers are asked to give their signed consent to participate in the study. The nurse researcher collects the data through observation and interview with the clients and/or caregivers. She validates any conflicting information and reaches consensus with the clients and/or caregivers. After the data collection is complete, the researcher enters the data for computer analyses. The data are then analyzed.

Evaluation

Evaluation includes analyzing the findings and comparing them with previous research results. The conclusions are then drawn, building on a body of previous knowledge. Research reports should provide a clear documentation of what was done and when. The results of the research are presented for the specific problem, research questions, or hypotheses under study. What was found and what was not found in the study need to be reported. Recommendations for future research should be clear and consistent with the study results. The need for replication studies should be specified. Replication studies validate findings, especially in other samples or populations, because recommendations for practice must be based on more than one set of study results. The research should be presented to professional colleagues, to persons in decision-making positions, such as administrators, policymakers, and legislators, and to the general public, who might be affected by any decisions made. The worth of the research is judged by persons in these groups.

In the research example, the study findings indicated that the greater the range of community health nursing services the greater was the ability of the elderly to live independently. It was recommended that future research should include the elderly's problem severity. This was not part of the study but was found to affect the services delivered by the community health nurses. The nurse researcher presented her findings to the administrators and staff at the local health department, to the county-wide senior citizen organization, and to professional colleagues at their annual meeting. She also was interviewed by a reporter for an article in a local paper.

Action

The results of nursing research should be used in practice. Nurses must make specific recommendations of reliable or valid research findings from nursing practice to improve the health of the community. By applying research results in practice, nurses can take action for social change. This demonstrates to policymakers, other professionals, and the community that the research findings are relevant and applicable to practice.

In the example, the nurse may learn that a significant finding was the presence of a support person. The research may indicate that clients who are regularly visited by a community health nurse may be able to maintain independent living rather than being institutionalized.

The results of such a study could support the expansion of community health nursing services. The economic difference between maintaining an elderly client or married couple in the home versus placing one or both in an institution could be a compelling argument in support of home health care. Research documenting the effectiveness of nursing care is vitally needed. Effectiveness is measured in many ways, including cost, quality, and client satisfaction.

In addition to the obvious benefits to nursing practice, relevant research findings must be reported to community groups. This information can become part of the community's educational experience and help the community to make appropriate decisions based on local needs.

PRACTICE QUESTIONS FOR RESEARCH

Significant questions for research can be generated from community health nursing practice. Beginning community health nurses often have difficulty identifying potential questions for research arising from their practice. The following discussion focuses on examples of questions for research that are generated in practice. These questions are grouped by the concepts of primary health care: accessibility, community involvement, disease prevention and health promotion, appropriate technology, and multisectoral approach.

Accessible Health Care

Accessibility of health services is an issue concerning the extent to which community health nursing services reach people who need them the most or how equitably these services are distributed throughout the population.

A question for research related to this concept is whether the community health nursing services are accessible to those in greatest need. For example, are these services available in both urban and rural areas? Are the services available to groups of people most in need of them, in terms of time, location, and personnel? Other questions related to the use of services include the following: Who uses and who does not use the community health nursing services? What are their characteristics? What are the health care needs of the people who use the service compared with those who do not? What are barriers to the use of services? Are the costs too high? Are the services irrelevant to consumers' perceived needs? Are community health nurses sensitive to the concerns of consumers? Do consumers have transportation to reach the services?

Community Involvement

Community involvement is concerned with the level of community resident participation in health decision making. To promote the development of the community and the community's self-reliance, residents themselves need to participate in decisions about the health of the community. Residents and health providers need to work together in partnership to seek solutions to the complex problems facing communities today.

Questions for research generated from practice relate to the level and mechanism of community involvement in health decision making. For example, to what extent is the community involved in the various stages of assessing health care needs, planning, management, and monitoring community health nursing services? What mechanisms and processes exist to enable people to be actively involved and to take joint responsibility, along with community health nurses, for decisions? In particular, what decisions involving the community have been implemented? Are the community health nursing services better used as a result?

Disease Prevention and Health Promotion

Emphasis in community health care is directed toward health promotion and prevention of disease rather than being focused on curative services. Examples are activities that include physical exercise, seat belt use, smoking cessation, and other healthful life-style changes.

Priority questions for research include the following? What are the major preventable health problems in the community? Are there high rates of automobile accidents or high rates of heart disease? Are problems being addressed by preventive and health-promoting measures? What measures are being taken to reduce or control these problems? Do the community health nursing services include recommendations for infant car seat use, programs to reduce alcohol intake among drivers, smoking cessation programs, and programs that promote health in schools?

Appropriate Technology

Appropriate technology refers to health care that is relevant to people's health needs and concerns, as well as being acceptable to them. It includes issues of costs and affordability of services within the context of existing resources, such as the number and type of health professionals and other workers, equipment, and supplies and their pattern of distribution throughout the community. The National Science Foundation's definition (1979, p. 1) of appropriate technology summarizes these considerations: "Appropriate technologies are defined as those which are decentralized, require low capital investment, conserve natural resources, are managed by their users, and are in harmony with the environment."

The overriding questions to be answered by research are: Do the services use the simplest and least costly technology available? Are the services acceptable to the community? Are they affordable? What is the cost effectiveness of alternative approaches or strategies for community health nursing services? Are family home visits as effective as working with families in groups? Are nonprofessionals, such as home health aides, effective in providing some aspects of community health nursing services? What are the most effective management and supervisory techniques for nonprofessionals and professionals within a community health nursing agency?

Multisectoral Approach

It is recognized that the health of a community cannot be improved by intervention within just the health sector; other sectors are equally important in promoting the community's health and self-reliance. For example, education, environment, industry, housing, and nutrition are interrelated with health. Therefore these sectors need to work together in a *multisectoral approach* to coordinate their goals, plans, and activities to ensure that they contribute to the health of the community and to avoid conflicting or duplicating efforts.

Relevant questions for research include the following: What mechanisms exist that promote or hinder multisectoral collaboration? Do the committees or task forces that address community-wide concerns represent various fields, such as education, industry, housing, transportation, and health? What are examples of multisectoral efforts in seeking solutions to community problems? How were successful solutions derived? How are conflicting activities across the various sectors resolved? What are the gaps in efforts across the various sectors in solving community health problems?

ROLES AND ISSUES IN RESEARCH

Although some of the roles of the community health nurse researcher and issues related to research are implied in other sections of this chapter, additional aspects are worthy of consideration.

Relationships

The practicing community health nurse may conduct research or work with a researcher within an organization in carrying out a study. The practicing nurse, the administrator of nursing services, and the researcher are partners in a joint endeavor. Partners each have their own areas of expertise, yet benefit from the expertise of the others. The community health nurse, as an expert in practice, can identify problems needing to be researched and the feasibility of various research designs. The administrator can help identify policy issues related to the research and can provide organizational support. The researcher can help develop practice problems into researchable questions, suggest appropriate research methods, and design data analyses.

In conducting practice-based community research, the nurse may also work with the community group concerned with the research problem. Citizens, professionals, and other persons interested in the health of the community may identify a priority problem needing research. In this case, persons in the group have expertise about the community, and the researcher and the community health nurse work as resources to the group in conducting the research.

Involving others in the research process is not without problems. Perhaps the most difficult for researchers is the sharing of activities usually under their domain. An example is involving others in identifying the important questions to be researched. Because community health nursing research often takes place in a dynamic setting in which the chief responsibility is health care (e.g., a neighborhood clinic), priority may be given to clinical commitments rather than to research. For example, access to records and files may be controlled by others, and client information may be withheld by the agency. As a result, the research itself may become part of the politics of the situation. Researchers will need to be aware of these dynamics and use their expertise to ensure that the research is conducted with proper attention to sound principles of research.

Communication

Communication is important throughout the research process. This involves communicating with subjects, co-researchers, community health nursing practitioners, administrators, community residents, and policy makers. Communication can take many forms. The researcher needs to consider the appropriateness of verbal, written, and visual aids in clarifying information being presented. Often the researcher has an academic background and appointment and has been educated differently from practitioners and community citizens. The fact that researchers in nursing are often practitioners first may help close this gap. Even so, the researcher must carefully consider how the information is presented, including the level of understanding of the reader or listener, and be attentive to issues of concern to the audience being addressed. The format of presentation will vary depending on whether the audience is a group of academic researchers, practicing community health nurses, policymakers, or community citizens. However, some of the same material is applicable to all groups.

Information needs to be disseminated about the research early in the study and throughout the project. Negative findings must be presented along with positive results. A focus on concepts rather than on the specific program being studied may facilitate the acceptance of negative findings.

Ethics and the Researcher Role

Ethical issues need careful attention when research of any type is conducted. Ethical issues arise out of conflicting social pressures between the profession and the larger society. For example, there is the dilemma of whether or not to publish the results of research when the findings reflect negatively on a particular group. For example, the concern may arise that this information will be taken out of context and used to limit government funding of services to that population.

Ethical issues also need to be considered in designing a study. For example, community health nurses may wish to evaluate the effectiveness of the home health agency's policies for the care of AIDS patients. It would be unethical to assign a group of patients having AIDS as a control group if that meant withholding information about the diagnosis from the community health nurses providing nursing services to these patients.

Dilemmas may arise over ensuring the confidentiality of responses, disclosing the actual purpose of the research to the respondents, or even over disseminating results of the research to the respondents. As noted earlier, research plans are under close scrutiny by human subject review committees in most institutions today. The researcher is ethically responsible for carrying out these plans as directed or approved by the committee. Changes that occur in the plans need to be reported to the committee for further sanctioning.

There are also ethical considerations in data reporting. Fraudulent research data and results of health-related research have been published. This issue is important in nursing research because few replication studies exist. The effects of publishing false findings can be widespread, affecting not only the profession but also, perhaps more importantly, persons in the community.

Position of Researcher in Employment Setting

The issue of who employs the researcher and potential uncertainties about the authority structure are often major sources of concern for the nurse researcher. In an academic setting the researcher may be a faculty member who also has responsibilities for classroom teaching, clinical supervision of students, academic advising, and committee work. To be involved in a major research effort, the faculty member typically will need to be relieved of some of these responsibilities. Consideration can be given to a semester of full-time research, a reduction in teaching responsibilities and committee work, or some combination of these for the duration of the project.

It may be possible to establish more innovative employment opportunities in research. These could include status as visiting scholar or visiting researcher within a community organization or university, shared positions between universities and other organizations, or the promotion of sabbatical leave opportunities between service and university institutions. When researchers are hired by community organizations they should clarify their functioning in research. Questions should include the following: What are the other expectations for this position, for example, service, administration, or other research? How will the results be disseminated if they reflect negative features of a service program or a professional group? If the organization chooses not to disseminate a research report, what happens to the researcher's work? Does the researcher have continued access to the data? Can the researcher prepare papers for presentation at professional meetings and in the professional literature? Researchers need a clear understanding with their employers and administrators about the organization and expectations for their work, as well as the organization's authority in relation to publication and the investigator's access to data for professional purposes.

Another aspect that needs to be reemphasized relates to the action phase of the research process. If, after completing an investigation, it is concluded that the results are significant for community health nursing practice, the investigator needs not only to use the results in practice but also to see that the findings are clearly understood by relevant others, whether they be administrators, community health nurses, legislators, or citizens in the community. The community health nurse researcher may need to lobby for his or her research conclusions so that appropriate policies or legislation are enacted. At this point the link between research and practice can best become reality.

Funding of Research

A final issue is related to obtaining funds for research. Federal money for research is competitive in the 1990s. Researchers and others need to explore alternative funding sources and to use creative financing options. For example, employers could grant release time from work so that educators, administrators, consultants, and practitioners could conduct research. Joint financing could be arranged between the community group, the service agency, and university for the research. The pursuit of funding from voluntary foundations and organizations should not be overlooked. Likewise, state and local funding should be considered.

In addition to funding for specific research projects, mechanisms for collaborative research need to be established and similarly funded. Research institutes and centers with joint connections between community groups, health care organizations, industries, and universities can facilitate research in community health nursing. Such institutes can promote interdisciplinary collaboration to study community health problems and practice issues. The institutes also provide a unique environment for the delineation and articulation of the various roles in research and afford collaborative opportunities for community residents, students, educators, and service personnel in seeking solutions to community health problems.

SUGGESTIONS FOR PARTICIPATION IN RESEARCH

Practicing nurses can participate in each stage of the research process. They are in a key position to identify clinical problems that need research. Nurses can take anecdotal notes about clinical situations that will help in identifying not only key variables for study but also factors that might be controlled. They also can read research on the topic of concern and discuss observations with other nursing colleagues, including researchers. Frequently, nurse researchers work in universities and are more than willing to collaborate in joint research efforts. Practicing community health nurses have access to populations for study and can assist researchers in securing institutional approval to collect data. They also may be involved in data collection, whether it be for pilot studies, replication studies, or original research. The nurse may be a subject in research, through answering questionnaires and interview questions or being observed in practice.

Community health nurses can provide valuable insights into study findings, often explaining relationships, or lack thereof, to researchers. They can use relevant study findings in practice. They can also explain or report on findings of research to community people, administrators, policymakers, and others, thus taking action for social change.

Community health nurses work with community members in improving their health. They can help seek and identify scientifically oriented solutions to health and nursing problems; thus they are in a key position for the development of knowledge for practice.

CLINICAL APPLICATIONS

Selected examples of research studies are presented here because they are generated by community health nursing practice, involve a community health nurse as an investigator, or have implications for the use of research findings in community health nursing practice.

Although the first study is relatively old, it is a useful example of research relevant to questions of accessibility of health care services and appropriate technology. The nursing division of the DuPage County Health Department in Illinois undertook a survey of noninstitutionalized older adults to determine their needs for services (Managen et al., 1974). The study described the elderly in terms of their health condition, physical functioning, access to medical care, social isolation, and service needs. The major problems found were functional impairment, lack of a family physician, and social isolation. The results indicated that a 10.8% increase in services was needed by the elderly population. The services needed were intensive case finding, well-adult conference, and programs providing friendly visitors. The findings also were beneficial because they provided baseline information for evaluation of future services.

A second example deals with home care. In home care the amount and type of nursing care patients required are difficult to predict, yet are key issues in determining the accessibility of community health nursing service. Reliable and valid patient classification systems are needed to help determine nursing care requirements. Staff nurses in the Visiting Nurse Association of Los Angeles, Inc. were involved in testing a home health patient classification system (Churness, V.H. et al, 1988). They completed patient classification forms for 408 home visits. Seventy-five of these were scored by another nurse using the patients' medical records. Interrater reliability (where two raters' observations were compared) ranged from 33% to 100% for specific ratings. The predicted length of visits determined by the patient classification system were compared with the actual length of visits. It was found that actual visits were correctly predicted 69 percent of the time. The findings verified the complexity of measuring service requirements and were useful in revising the instrument which was tested further in the agency.

The effectiveness of self-care education for persons with arthritis was studied by Goeppinger and Others (1989) and addressed both the concepts of prevention and appropriate technology. This study examined the effectiveness of two intervention models, the home study and small group education, that covered the same content. The home study model was a correspondence course and included an audiotape. The small group model included an informal class led by trained persons and were held in community sites. A pretest-posttest control group design was used in the initial study and comparison group designs were used in the twelve months of follow-up studies. In their analysis of 374 patients that were randomly assigned to three groups, it was found that both intervention models significantly affected arthritis knowledge, self-care behavior, perceived helplessness, and pain. The home study model was more effective in maintaining improvements in perceived helplessness and the small group model was more effective in bringing about initial improvements in pain and depression. This study provides evidence that arthritis self-care education has positive clinical applications.

A review of research on the effectiveness of community health nursing home visits is related to the concept of appropriate technology (Combes-Orme et al, 1985). Eight studies concerned with maternal and child health were compared and it was concluded that within the studies' methodological limitations there was supporting evidence of the effectiveness of home visits to the maternal child population. Evidence of effectiveness was based on an increase in health knowledge in high-risk mothers and positive changes in maternal attitudes and parenting practices. These outcomes also were found to be associated with positive changes in infant health and development.

SUMMARY

It is suggested that the major concepts of primary health care can guide the research conducted by community health nurses and make a significant contribution to the development of a scientific knowledge base for practice. An overview of the research process is presented, applying an example from community health nursing research. Selected roles and issues in research are discussed followed by examples of community health nursing research studies. Finally, several suggestions are made as to how community health nurses may become involved in the research process.

KEY CONCEPTS

Research for community health nursing practice has developed over the years. Although increasing efforts are devoted to nursing research, community health nurses need to increase their scientific knowledge base for practice.

Community health nursing and primary health care are complementary; research conducted by community health nurses can make a significant contribution to nursing practice and also to primary health care practice.

The research process is a problem-solving process. It involves assessment, planning, implementation, evaluation, and action.

Significant questions for research can be generated from community health nursing practice and linked with the key concepts of primary health care.

Community involvement is a key concept of primary health care. It is concerned with the level of citizen or community resident participation in health decision making.

The overriding questions to be answered by research are: Do the services use the simplest and least costly technology available? Are the services acceptable to the community? Are they affordable? What is the cost effectiveness of alternative approaches or strategies for community health nursing services? Are family home visits as effective as working with families in groups? Are nonprofessionals, such as home health aides, effective in providing some aspects of community health nursing services? What is the most effective management and supervision for nonprofessionals and professionals within a community health nursing agency?

The issue of who employs the researcher and potential uncertainties about the authority structure are often major sources of concern for the nurse researcher.

Federal money for research is competitive in the 1990s. Researchers and others need to explore alternative funding sources and to use creative financing options.

LEARNING ACTIVITIES

1. Read the newspaper and identify one priority problem that could be researched in the community and has relevance to community health nursing practice.

2. From your community health nursing experiences specify a research question in which you could relate to one of the concepts of primary health care.

3. Identify a research study relevant to community health nursing in the literature and identify the strengths and limitations of the research.

4. Talk with a community member, a community health nurse, a researcher, and an administrator who have been involved in research and ask them about their roles and functions in research. What were the sources of role strain?

5. Identify from the literature three funding sources for research in community health nursing.

6. From the literature find one research study in which the findings can be used in community health nursing practice.

BIBLIOGRAPHY

Aday LA and Anderson R: A framework for the study of access to medical care, Health Services Research 9(13):208-220, 1974.

Churness VH, Kleffel D, Onodera ML, and Jacobson J: Reliability and validity testing of a home health patient classification system, Public Health Nursing 5(3):135-139, 1988.

Combes-Orme T, Reis J, and Dantes L: Effectiveness of home visits by public health nurses in maternal and child health: an empirical review, Public Health Rep 100(5):490, 1985.

Fox DJ: Fundamentals of research in nursing, ed 4, Norwalk, Conn, 1982, Appleton-Century-Crofts.

Goeppinger J, Arthur MW, Baglioni AJ, Brunk SE, and Brunner CM: A reexamination of the effectiveness of self-care education for persons with arthritis, Arthritis and Rheumatism 32(6):706-716, 1989.

ICN WHO: Report of the workshop on the role of nursing in primary health care, Geneva, 1979, World Health Organization.

Managan D, et al: Older adult: a community survey of health needs, Nurs Res 23(5):426, 1974.

National Science Foundation: NSF announcements for December, NSF bulletin, Washington, DC, 1979, The Foundation.

Pan American Health Organization: The role of the nurse in primary health care, Washington, DC, 1977, World Health Organization.

WHO and UNICEF: Primary health care: a joint report, Geneva, 1978, World Health Organization.

World Health Organization: Nursing in support of the goal health for all by the year 2000, Geneva, 1982, Division of Manpower Development, World Health Organization.

World Health Organization: Education and training of nurse teachers and managers with special regard to primary health care, Technical Report Series, 708, Geneva, 1984, World Health Organization.

World Health Organization: A guide to curriculum review for basic nursing education. Orientation to primary health care and community health, Geneva, 1985, World Health Organization.

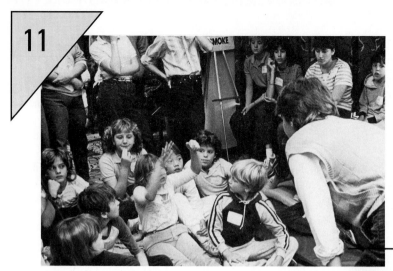

11

Education Models and Principles Applied to Community Health Nursing

Jeanette Lancaster

OBJECTIVES

After reading this chapter, the student should be able to:

Discuss the importance of health education in community health nursing.

Describe the theories of learning that are most influential in community health nursing.

Describe each of the three domains of learning.

Discuss three characteristics of adult learning that influence the development of community health programs.

Identify at least 10 factors that facilitate effective teaching.

Describe three models for effective health education: PRECEDE, Health Belief, and Health Promotion Models.

Describe three factors to consider when organizing effective learning experiences in the community.

Discuss criteria for selecting appropriate audiovisual and teaching-learning formats for community health programs.

KEY TERMS

affective domain	Gestalt theory	operant conditioning
andragogy	health education	perception
client-centered learning	health belief model	PRECEDE model
cognitive domain	health promotion model	psychomotor domain
conditioning		reinforcement
culture	humanistic theory	self-concept
evaluation	learning	stimulus-response theory
	motivation	

H ealth education is a vital part of community health nursing because the promotion, maintenance, and restoration of health require that clients understand health care requirements. Early nursing leaders like Florence Nightingale and Lillian Wald demonstrated creativity, initiative, and an understanding of the educational needs of their clients. Health education is equally vital today and community health nurses are in key positions to provide education because they see clients with varying needs and abilities in many settings.

Health education is an approach for teaching patients and their families to deal with past, present, and future health problems. This knowledge enables them to make informed decisions, to cope more effectively with temporary or long-term alterations in their health and lifestyle, and to assume greater personal responsibility for health (Speers, 1989). In an era of growing health costs and consumer demands for better health care, patients are increasingly expected to share responsibility for their own health maintenance (Higgins, 1988).

As people live longer, they are likely to experience chronic illnesses requiring complex changes in diet, exercise, and treatment. With a predominance of two-career families, there are often fewer family supports than in previous generations. Health education becomes more important in light of these social changes. This chapter focuses on the nursing role in client education and is primarily directed toward adult learners. However, many of the theories and principles presented also apply to students and children.

THEORIES OF LEARNING

The study of learning is important for community health nurses. To promote the health of individuals, families, and communities it is necessary to teach self-care and health promotion skills. Learning is defined in a variety of ways. Most definitions include a change in behavior that persists over time, is practiced, and is repeatedly reinforced. Although many theories of learning are potentially applicable to community health nursing, only a sample of the most prominent ones is included. The selected theories are grouped into three major schools of thought: conditioning, cognitive, and humanistic theories.

Conditioning Theories

Behavioral theorists approach the study of learning by concentrating on behaviors that can be observed and measured. Conditioning seeks to change behavior. Famous behaviorists who used conditioning are Ivan Pavlov, Edward Thorndike, and B.F. Skinner.

Pavlov was best known for his work on the digestion of dogs that showed how a neutral stimulus (one that produced no particular response from the dog) could become a conditioned stimulus that made the dogs salivate if the stimulus always preceded food. For example, if a bell was rung right before the dogs were fed, then they salivated at the sound of the bell. They might also salivate at the sound of the feeder's footsteps if the footsteps always preceded food. The bell or footsteps became a conditioned stimulus that produced a specific conditioned response (Good and Brophy, 1990).

Thorndike viewed learning as a series of stimulus-response connections. His theory of learning dealt with ways to strengthen or weaken these connections. He described theory as a trial-and-error set of events. Thorndike defined three major laws of learning:

1. law of readiness—people learn when they are in a state of readiness to connect with new information.
2. law of exercise—the more any stimulus-response connection is used, the stronger it will become; conversely, the less a connection is used, the weaker it will become.
3. law of effect—when a connection is followed by a reward, it is strengthened. A connection followed by a punishment is weakened (Sprinthall and Sprinthall, 1990).

Reinforcement, a concept important in health education, has its roots in the law of effect. Responses that are reinforced are most likely to be repeated. A reinforcer is "anything that strengthens behavior and increases the probability of its recurrence" (de Tornyay and Thompson, 1987, p. 3). In the teaching-learning process both positive and negative reinforcers are incentives for clients. Examples of positive reinforcers include recognition (praise, certificate of accomplishment, publicity, private and public acknowledgement), tangible rewards (gift, prize), additional responsibilities (opportunity for more self-management) and status indicators (being made a peer-group leader). Essentially, negative reinforcement is punishment or the removal of a positive reinforcer and the addition or substitution of an unpleasant stimulus. Negative reinforcement is not often used deliberately in patient education.

Skinner, like Thorndike, believed that rewards encourage a response to recur, and punishment tends to extinguish the response. Skinner described respondents as those responses that were triggered automatically such as jerking a hand when stuck with a pin, raising the knee when a nerve is tapped, and constricting an eye in bright light. Operants are responses that occur spontaneously without being triggered by an unconditioned stimulus. For example, stretching your legs, raising your hand, or shifting in your seat can occur without a known stimulus.

Skinner thought that reinforcement was the key to controlling behavior. To test this view, Skinner developed what is known as the Skinner box and worked with rats and pigeons to demonstrate that actions followed by a reward are likely to be repeated, whereas those that went unrewarded were not likely to recur. From his experiments Skinner coined the term *operant conditioning* to describe the way the animals operated on the environment after certain behaviors were rewarded.

Based on his success in controlling the behavior of animals, Skinner concluded that his techniques would also work on people. He believed that it is the environment that changes behavior. All that a person does is a function of his history of reinforcements and punishments (Sprinthall and Sprinthall, 1990). From his observations of children in schools, he concluded that children turned in homework and studied to avoid negative reinforcements such as embarrassment, poor grades, or punishment. However, considerable time passes between the time the child turns in the homework and the return of the graded work to the child. Skinner subsequently developed programmed instruction in which learners received instant grading of their work. Essentially, programmed learning is a type of instruction in which material is organized into a series of small steps (frames) and feedback is given after the response to each frame.

Cognitive View of Learning

The cognitive view of learning describes the way learning occurs in concert with developmental stages. A leader in cognitive theory, Jean Piaget thought that intellectual development, although continuous throughout life, progressed from birth to 14 years through four definitive stages (Biehler, 1986).

According to Piaget, cognition or thinking is an active and interactive process. The mind is not a blank sheet of paper upon which the environment writes its message nor does the mind exist in isolation. Rather, cognition is the constant process of going back and forth between the person and environment (Sprinthall and Sprinthall, 1990). Piaget described four stages of cognitive growth:

Age birth to 2 years:	Sensorimotor stage
Age 2 to 7 years:	Intuitive or preoperational stage
Age 7 to 11 years:	Concrete operations stage
Age 11 to 16 years:	Formal operations stage

Each stage is a major transformation from the previous one, and children must move through these stages in sequential order. In the sensorimotor stage the child responds primarily to the environment through the senses. Responses are largely determined by the situation, e.g., crying due to hunger. In the intuitive or preoperational stage children are able to store images and to use language; their predominant mode of thinking is intuitive and highly imaginative. They say what they think, hence the term "from the mouths of babes" (Sprinthall and Sprinthall, 1990, p. 108). During the stage of concrete operations children learn to test things for themselves and become almost too literal in their thinking. Skills such as counting, sorting, building, and manipulating fit this level of thinking. In formal operations children learn to test hypotheses, to use self-reflection, and to include the perspective of others. Piaget described the developmental stages in which learning occurred and discussed readiness to learn.

A group of Gestalt psychologists described a cognitive structural approach to learning. This approach holds that meaningful learning involves not only understanding facts but also the relationships between them. *Gestalt* is the German word for configuration or organization. Gestaltists believe that people experience the world in meaningful wholes; they do not see isolated stimuli but rather stimuli gathered into meaningful groupings. They see people, animals, and furniture rather than lines and patches of color. The key principles of Gestalt theory are "the whole is more than the sum of the parts" and "to dissect is to distort" (Biehler, 1982).

Gestalt theorists are interested in the way in which people interpret what they sense and observe. When individuals are asked to look at illusions of various kinds, they interpret what they see in terms of the arrangement of stimuli. Gestaltists also decided that perceptions are influenced by both past experiences and current interests. For example, people may interpret the word *joint* differently, depending on their background and experiences. For some the word means a place, for others it means a body part, and still others think of it as something to smoke.

Gestalt theorists approach instruction by developing ways to teach or guide learners to discover key ideas that can be used to organize bodies of information. They believe that learning facts or memorizing lists of information is of little value.

Humanistic View of Learning

More diversity exists within the humanistic view of learning than in either the conditioning or cognitive theories of learning. Humanistic theorists come from varying backgrounds, and their concepts are based on observations, impressions, and speculations rather than on experimental data. Humanists agree with cognitive theorists that observing behavior is not sufficient to explain and predict responses; however, they place greater emphasis on the importance of feelings, emotions, and personal relationships in determining behavior.

Humanistic thinkers contend that it is a mistake to separate actual classroom behavior into categories such as cognitive (thinking), psychomotor (motor or movement), and affective (feeling). They agree that such categorizations are useful when discussing complex topics but should be avoided when dealing with actual behavior. They also believe that learners should be encouraged to explore their feelings and engage in varying forms of self-expression. Additionally, humanists support the belief that people need to be aware of and able to clarify their values. Notable humanistic theorists who have influenced education are Abraham Maslow and Carl Rogers.

Maslow devised what is known as *third force psychology,* which states that if people are given free choice, they will do what is best for themselves. Thus, educators are urged not to be overly controlling and restrictive with learners but rather to help them grow and develop according to their natural inclinations.

Maslow (1968) described a hierarchy of human needs arranged in the following order of priority:
1. Physiological needs (sleep, thirst)
2. Safety needs (freedom from danger, anxiety, or threat)
3. Love needs (acceptance from others)
4. Esteem needs (confidence in one's ability, ability to master tasks)
5. Needs for self-actualization (creative self-expression, attempt to satisfy one's curiosity)

According to Maslow, unless lower-order needs are met, higher needs may not even be appreciated, let alone motivate behavior (Good and Brophy, 1990). The well-rested, psychologically secure learner may seek new information while the exhausted or frightened learner will not. Anxious clients who are in pain or who are hungry are not good candidates for teaching. Community health nurses must constantly assess clients' readiness to learn in terms of their cognitive ability and their level of need fulfillment.

Carl Rogers developed client-centered therapy that focused entirely on the client. In client-centered therapy, the therapist is nondirective, warm, positive, accepting, and able to empathize with the client's feelings and thoughts. He believed that when clients are treated with warmth and sensitivity, they become more accepting of themselves. Rogers (1969) applied his beliefs about therapy to the learning situation and proposed that learning should be learner-centered. The outcome of learner-centered education is that students become more self-directed and capable of guiding their own education. Similarly, when community health nurses treat clients in this way, the clients are often better able to accept themselves and feel more positive about their accomplishments and abilities.

NATURE OF LEARNING

The goal of all teaching is learning. It is discouraging to prepare and implement a teaching plan that is followed by the question "I'm sorry, but I did not understand what you said; could you start over?" Giving information does not guarantee that learning takes place. One way of understanding the nature of learning is to examine the three domains of learning: cognitive, affective, and psychomotor (Bloom, 1969). Each domain has specific behavior components arranged in hierarchical levels with each level building on the one before.

Cognitive Domain

The *cognitive domain* deals with the "recall or recognition of knowledge and the development of intellectual abilities and skills" (Bloom, 1969, p. 7). It is divided into a hierarchical classification of behaviors that Bloom refers to as a *taxonomy*. Learners master each behavior in the following order of difficulty: knowledge, comprehension, application, analysis, synthesis, and evaluation. Table 11-1 describes the levels in the cognitive domain.

For health education to be effective, it is important to assess the cognitive abilities of the learner so that the nurse's expectations and plans are directed toward the correct level. Teaching above or below the client's level of understanding may lead to frustration and discouragement.

Affective Domain

The *affective domain* describes changes in attitudes, values, and appreciations. In affective learning nurses influence what clients, families, and students think, value, and feel. Because the values and attitudes of nurses may differ from those of clients, it is important to listen carefully to detect clues to feelings that would influence learning. For example, people from different cultures value foods in unique ways. Some cultural groups eat no meats, others eat no pork or beef. It is important to know how people think and feel about health-related topics before teaching begins.

As in cognitive learning, a series of steps comprises affective learning. Table 11-2 shows the steps of learning in the affective domain and correlates them with those in the cognitive domain.

It is difficult to change deep-seated values, attitudes, beliefs, and interests. To make such changes, people need support and encouragement from those around them. Praise is helpful. Group support also reinforces learning new behaviors.

Psychomotor Domain

The *psychomotor domain* includes the performance of skills that require neuromuscular coordination. Community health clients are taught a variety of psychomotor skills such as giving injections, taking blood pressure, measuring blood sugar, bathing infants, changing dressings, and walking on crutches.

Three conditions must be met before psychomotor learning occurs: (1) the learner must have the necessary ability;

TABLE 11-1
Cognitive domain: levels of mastery

Level	Description	Clinical example
Knowledge	Recalling facts, methods, procedures	Diabetic client is able to list symptoms of hypoglycemia
Comprehension	Combining recall and understanding; to grasp the meaning of the information	Client describes relationship among hypoglycemia, diet, and insulin
Application	Using information in new, specific, and concrete situation	Client describes 1200-calorie diabetic diet and specifies foods to use based on personal preference
Analysis	Distinguishing between parts of information and understanding relationship among them	Client is able to determine factors causing hypoglycemic reaction
Synthesis	Putting the parts of information together in a unified whole	On experiencing hypoglycemic reaction, client can describe precipitating factors and design a new way to handle such a situation
Evaluation	Judging the value of ideas, procedures, and methods by using appropriate criteria	Diabetic client would judge how effectively and quickly 4 oz. of orange juice relieves symptoms of hypoglycemia

TABLE 11-2
Steps in the affective domain compared to cognitive domain

Affective domain	Cognitive domain
1. Learner receives the information	Knowledge
2. Learner responds	Comprehension
3. Learner values information	Application
4. Learner makes sense of the information	Analysis
5. Learner organizes information by adopting behavior consistent with new value system	Evaluation

(2) he or she must have a sensory image of how to carry out the skill; and (3) he or she must have opportunities to practice the learning. To facilitate learning, demonstrate the skill either in person, or with a video or pictures; allow the learner to practice and correct immediately any errors in performing the task.

In assessing a client's ability to learn a skill, evaluate his or her physical, intellectual, and emotional ability. A tremulous person with poor eyesight may be incapable of learning insulin self-injection. Similarly, some clients do not have the intellectual ability to learn the steps of a complex procedure. Teach at the level of the person's ability, neither above nor below the person's level of comprehension.

Each of the three learning domains must be taken into account for effective health education. Teaching strategies must be based on an assessment of learner needs, abilities, beliefs, values, and readiness to learn.

PRINCIPLES OF TEACHING AND LEARNING

Community health clients vary in age, background, learning needs, and the ability to learn. Nurses must be knowledgeable about the varying needs, goals, and abilities of learners in order to select appropriate instructional content and teaching strategies. Because a considerable amount of the teaching done by community health nurses is directed toward adult learners, emphasis is placed on the unique needs of this group.

Knowles, an authority in adult education, emphasizes participation in learning. He proposes a concept called *andragogy* or the art and science of helping adults learn (Knowles, 1980). According to Knowles, andragogy is based on four assumptions that differentiate it from techniques directed specifically toward children (*pedagogy*). These assumptions are: (1) as people grow older their concept of self shifts from one of dependency to one of self-direction; (2) they accumulate a growing supply of experiences that serve as resources for their own learning; (3) their readiness to learn is consistent with their developmental level; and (4) their orientation to learning shifts from future to present and from subject to problem. Adult learners tend to have a greater investment and interest in what they are learning; they see immediate relevance in the information.

Self-Concept

As people grow and mature, their self-concept or the personal view they hold of themselves moves from that of total dependency to one of increasing self-direction (Gleit, 1986). In contrast to children, adults view themselves as doers rather than passive receivers of information. The adult role is one of productivity, self-sufficiency, and independent decision making. The adult self-concept is enriched when the person is treated with respect, allowed to make his own decisions, and treated as a unique person. Adults tend to resist situations in which they perceive that they are being treated like children and are being told what to do. They want to be active participants in determining the type of health education that they need.

Experience

One's past experiences affect one's learning (Gessner, 1989). Previous education, interaction with the health care system, and knowledge of people with a similar condition influence learning. In completing an assessment, it is important to ascertain the patient's feelings, knowledge, and experiences that relate to the current health problem.

To enhance adult learning, greater emphasis can be placed on approaches that draw on their unique experiences, such as group discussions, case presentations, projects, and seminars. The nurse encourages adult learners to participate in establishing their own learning objectives and specific activities for fulfilling them. Adults can be assisted in identifying people who have met similar goals and in using these people as role models. Nurses should provide educational settings that are flexible and encourage the use of a variety of educational goals and objectives. The experiences of adults may also require the use of "unfreezing" techniques that help people break away from old ways of thinking and acting. Activities are directed toward helping adults look at themselves more objectively and correcting misconceptions that are based on previous experiences. Adults come to new learning situations with many experiences that influence their motivation to seek additional learning. If past experiences were rewarding and if the learning event made them feel better about themselves, they will bring a far more positive attitude than if they were previously bored, angered, or embarrassed. For example, if a young woman previously attended a preparation for childbirth class in which she thought the leader perceived her to be dumb and clumsy, she is not likely to be highly motivated to attend parenting classes conducted by the same agency.

What can be done if it is perceived that some of the learners have had poor experiences in the past? Initially, an attitude of warmth and acceptance helps learners feel that their presence is valued and their needs are important to the leader. Also, begin the first session by asking participants what they hope to obtain from the class(es), what format they prefer (if the leader is willing and able to be flexible), and what kind of educational programs they have participated in previously. An attitude of acceptance and interest in meeting learner needs can be built by responding honestly to questions even when the answer is "I don't know".

Readiness to Learn

Narrow (1979) describes readiness to learn as the state or condition of being both able and willing to make use of instruction. Motivation is a prerequisite to learning. Often, people are willing to learn about health-related topics because they see a benefit for themselves. Major life events stimulate adult learning. An illness brings about change and motivates many to learn especially when the illness is not severe. Many factors affect readiness to learn such as the timing of the instruction (in relation to need and desire to know and in relation to what other things are happening), awareness of diagnosis and scope of illness, previous experience, knowledge, self-concept, fear and anxiety, beliefs about health and illness, values, and available energy.

Time Orientation

Adults have a different time perspective for learning than children. Children usually do not perceive any immediate value for what they learn whereas adults generally recognize an immediate application. Although children learn with a subject-centered orientation, adults tend to be problem centered. Adults engage in learning largely in response to stimuli or pressures. Because of their problem-centered orientation, adults are motivated by immediate application of learning that provides direct feedback and further reinforces learning.

Individual Differences

People vary not only in experience and motivation but also in perception, culture, and language, all of which influence learning. The *perceptions* people have of their opportunities affects their learning. Often, potential learners simply are unaware of needs or refuse to learn information or skills that would assist them in promoting or at least maintaining health. Diabetics may refuse to learn to self-inject insulin. It is as if they were saying, "If I don't take insulin, I must not have diabetes." Denial often interferes with accurate perception.

Many other factors affect perception including values, culture, age, past experiences, education, emotional status, religion, and socioeconomic status. Rarely do two people perceive a situation in the same way. The characteristics of the neighborhood in which an adult was raised would influence his or her reactions to a house that had no running water or heat and was roach infested. Similarly, the way in which nurses and clients view illness and the forms of assistance available to alter the course of the illness often is dramatically different. For example, the nurse who is teaching a person with chronic obstructive pulmonary disease about how to use oxygen at home may see the potential benefits of the oxygen very differently than the patient. The client sees the oxygen as a symbol of the losses that he has experienced from his chronic illness. He hates being dependent on a machine for life-sustaining oxygen. The oxygen represents dependency, restriction, and a lasting change in his life; for him, the machine is not something that keeps him alive but rather it is something to be hated.

Culture also affects learning. Each cultural group has unique values, beliefs, and perceptions that must be considered when planning health education. In particular, diets and health attitudes vary considerably. The specific foods recommended on a 1200-calorie diet would be different for middle-aged women who were black, Hispanic, native American, or Italian. Their food preferences would differ as would their styles of cooking.

Similarly, cultural groups have specific views about health practices, including the role of health care providers. In many cultures medicine men or other traditional healers still provide health care. The potential contribution of these healers should not be ignored. Nurses should collaborate and consult with them to ensure that consistent and acceptable health advice and care is provided.

Barriers to Teaching and Learning

Barriers to learning can be due to the skills of the teacher, the ability of the learner, or the environment in which learning occurs. Many of these barriers can be overcome and a positive environment for learning maintained. For example, *teacher barriers* include failure to identify the learning need, lack of teaching ability, lack of confidence in teaching ability, poor communication skills, impatience with learners who progress at different rates, or preoccupation with personal concerns that interfere with paying adequate attention to the learner. Some teachers fail to match their teaching style to the needs of the learner. For example, many people are better able to learn when they see information rather than when they hear it. Giving such people written instructions, showing them pictures, or drawing diagrams is more effective than telling them the information. Teachers may also talk too fast, use language that is unfamiliar to the learners, speak too softly to be heard, or speak with an accent that is foreign to the learner.

Learner barriers include lack of motivation to learn, fear of what might be learned and the implications of the new information, or readiness to learn at that time. People do not learn effectively when they are in pain or are anxious, afraid, depressed, or angry. Learning is impaired when the person being taught cannot read or cannot understand what the teacher is saying and hesitates to acknowledge this lack of ability. As society becomes more culturally diverse, nurses do not always speak the same language as the client. Be sure the patient understands English or have someone translate your message into a language the patient can understand.

Environmental barriers include noise, excessive heat or cold in the room, lack or privacy when sensitive information is being presented, and interruptions from family members, health care providers, or other clients. Time constraints pose another barrier. For example, when the client is to be picked up by someone and is feeling rushed, little, if any, learning can occur.

Keen observational skills help to detect if learning barriers are present. Watch for facial expressions such as a frown or a sign of confusion to determine if the message being sent by the teacher is being received by the learner. If clients talk to one another during the teaching session, it may mean that they do not understand and are relying on one another for a clear explanation. Make sure that clients have understood the information, such as by asking them how they can apply the information at home. For example, if the discussion is on exercise and six different types have been described, ask the clients to talk about which type might work best for them considering where they live, the time they have available, their skill level, and their family obligations, all of which would affect their being able to exercise. You can also ask learners to make a list of ways they can incorporate what has been taught into their lives and to turn the list in at the end of the session. This is a more private way to get feedback on the learning than a group discussion would be.

Occasionally, teachers also need to get peer feedback on their skills. For example, most people who talk fast are unaware of it. Videotaping is an effective way to clearly see oneself as others do. Asking another nurse to sit in on the class and tell exactly how clearly the message was communicated is also helpful. Both these techniques can provide information about whether the teacher talked too fast, had a pronounced accent, used jargon or technical language, or responded to questions impatiently and discouraged the learners from active participation.

LEARNER NEEDS

The first and often overlooked step in health education program planning is determining learner needs. Often, health educators enthusiastically think of and develop an exciting program only to have it poorly received by potential learners. This may result from many factors but often occurs when the needs-assessment step is overlooked. Frequently, educators fall into the trap of teaching what they think the learners ought to know rather than what the learners want to know or are willing to learn at that time.

Nature of Needs

In general, adult learners have two types of needs: (1) basic needs, and (2) educational needs. Although different theorists define basic needs in various ways, the common themes include physical safety, security, love and affection, self-esteem, and recognition. This was discussed previously in the section on the humanistic view of learning.

In contrast, an educational need is ''something a person ought to learn for his own good, for the good of the organization, or for the good of society'' (Knowles, 1980, p. 88). An educational need represents a gap between what a person knows and the knowledge that is needed to effectively meet personal, organizational, or societal expectations. The goal of health educators is to help people assess their educational needs and determine ways to fulfill them.

Nature of Interests

Interests are related to needs in that they reflect personal preferences for learning. People may have multiple educational needs, yet only be interested in one or two of them. For example, a patient may be diabetic and need to learn how to prepare foods according to a prescribed diet, how to self-inject insulin, and how to give foot care. The person may be interested only in foot care, which is seen as the least intrusive new behavior.

Interests are highly personal and vary considerably from one person to another and within a person from time to time.

Interests, like needs, change as people move through the life stages. Eighteen year olds generally are not interested in the same topics as 50-year-olds. When teaching a 16-year-old and a 50-year-old person with diabetes, the nurse must be aware of the developmental needs of each and tailor the teaching according. The 16-year-old will be more interested in learning how to fit the diabetes into his lifestyle so that he will not be different from his peers while the 50-year-old is more likely to be interested in learning about the complications of the disease.

Also, what is happening at a given time influences interests. If a person is in pain, he is not likely to be interested in anything until the pain is relieved. Similarly, a new mother may need to learn how to bathe and nurse the baby and take care of her own needs. Since the baby's grandmother plans to assist during the first week home from the hospital, the new mother initially is more interested in the needs of the baby rather than her own. She listens intently to the information that the nurse provides about breastfeeding, all other teaching seems less important because she perceives that she can learn it later.

Assessing Needs and Interests

Three sources of needs and interests should be considered when planning adult education programs: those of the people being served, those of the sponsoring agency, and those of the community or society (Knowles, 1980). Since community and agency assessment is covered in Chapter 16, this discussion is limited to individual needs assessment.

According to Roberts (1981), assessment of needs can be done through a conscious evaluation process, either intuitively or systematically, or a combination of the two. The first question to be asked is "What should be taught?" There are many answers to this question, including surveys, verbal or written questionnaires, interviews, task forces, reading the professional literature, or watching, reading, or listening to the media.

Needs assessment also includes learning about the participant's backgrounds including his or her ability, skill, and experience. Nothing is worse than developing a program that is too complex for the learners. Likewise, if a program is too simple, learners may become restless and bored or feel insulted. Principles of needs assessment apply to developing teaching programs both for individuals and groups. Objectives for educational programs are discussed in the following section.

Developing Objectives for Educational Programs

Once the needs of the learners are determined, the nurse identifies the objectives that will guide the teaching. The identification of objectives can be done by the teacher alone or the teacher can be assisted by an advisory group of professionals and community members, by an entirely professional group, or by a task force established for putting together a specific program. Once the overall goals and objectives of the program are established, the specific learning objectives for the program should be developed. These objectives must be stated clearly and the expected outcomes must be defined in measurable terms. Objectives are written statements of the intended outcome or expected change in behavior. The four parts of an objective are addressed in these questions:

1. Who (person, group) is to exhibit the behavior?
2. What behavior is expected? Who is expected to do what?
3. What are the conditions? What experience, skill, etc, will the person bring to the learning situation?
4. What are minimally accepted performance standards? Is there a time limit? Does the performance have to be entirely accurate?

MODELS FOR HEALTH EDUCATION

Conceptual models are used to organize global ideas about individuals, groups, and situations in a meaningful way to guide the thinking, observations, and interpretations of people. Chapter 8 discusses the key terms used in understanding models and also describes several nursing and psychosocial models that are often used in community health nursing. Three models are described here: the PRECEDE Model, the Health Belief Model, and the Health Promotion Model. These three models are especially applicable to the educator role in community health nursing.

PRECEDE Model

Green et al (1980, p. 7) describe health education as any combination of learning experiences designed to encourage people to adapt their behavior so that they practice healthy habits. They have devised a model called PRECEDE, which is an acronym for "predisposing, reinforcing, and enabling causes in educational diagnosis and evaluation" (p. 11). Two basic propositions underscore the outcome-oriented PRECEDE model: (1) health and health behaviors are caused by multiple factors, and (2) health education designed to influence behavior must be multidimensional. The seven phases of the model are shown in the box at right.

The advantages of the PRECEDE model are that it uses a problem-solving approach and focuses on helping groups change behaviors. It begins by evaluating the environment in which the group lives and considers the social factors that influence health behaviors. The model then goes on to look at the factors within the group and its environment that predispose people to certain behaviors or health problems, followed by an examination of the factors that will be of assistance in adopting healthy actions. Priorities are set, the program is developed, implemented, and finally evaluated. This model is easy to use; its steps serve as a checklist to make sure that all stages of the problem-solving process are followed.

Health Belief Model

The Health Belief Model (HBM) was developed to provide a framework to explain why some people take specific actions to avoid illness while others fail to protect themselves (Hochbaum, 1958; Kegeles 1965; Rosenstock, 1974). When the model was developed there was concern in both the public and private health sectors that people were reluctant to be screened for tuberculosis, to have Pap smears to detect cervical cancer, to be immunized, or to take other preventive measures that were either available free or for a nominal cost (Pender, 1987) The model was designed to predict

---

PHASES OF THE PRECEDE MODEL

Phase 1: Consideration of quality of life. What are the major social problems of concern?

Phase 2: Identify specific health problems contributing to the social problem identified in phase 1.

Phase 3: Identify the specific health-related behaviors that seem linked to the selected health problem.

Phase 4: Sort and categorize into: predisposing factors (attitudes, beliefs, values, perceptions); enabling factors (barriers such as limited facilities, inadequate personnel or community resources, lack of income or insurance or restrictive laws and reinforcing factors (related to the feedback the learner receives from others which may encourage or discourage behavioral change).

Phase 5: Decide which factors make up the three classes on which the intervention will focus.

Phase 6: Develop and implement the program.

Phase 7: Evaluate the program.

Modified from Green L et al: Health education planning: a diagnostic approach; Palo Alto, Calif, 1980, Mayfield Publishing Co.

---

which prople would and which would not use preventive measures and to suggest interventions that might reduce their reluctance.

The model is divided into three major components: individual perceptions, modifying factors, and variables affecting the likelihood of initiating actions (Figure 11-1). A person's perceptions or view of susceptibility to disease and the seriousness of the disease combine to form his or her perceived threat of an illness. Contributory factors include such demographic variables as age, sex, race, and ethnicity, as well as personality, social class, and pressure from a reference group. Other factors include knowledge about the disease and prior contact with the disease. The likelihood that the person will take any action is influenced by the perceived benefits of the action weighed against the barriers to acting. Examples of barriers are costs, inconvenience, unpleasantness, or how much change it requires.

The model is useful in looking at health-protecting or disease-preventive behavior. It is useful in organizing information about clients' view of their state of health and what factors would influence them to change their behavior. Health education can be developed based on the data gathered from the use of the Health Belief Model as an organizing framework for looking at client status. For example, if an entire ethnic group in a neighborhood refuses to have their children immunized against measles, the Health Belief Model could be used to determine their perceptions of risk of the disease, their knowledge of the disease, and their views of what might be the advantages and disadvantages of being immunized. Group or individual instruction could be instituted that would clarify any misperceptions, reduce any inconveniences, and provide essential health information that is found to be lacking in the assessment of perceptions and benefits of actions.

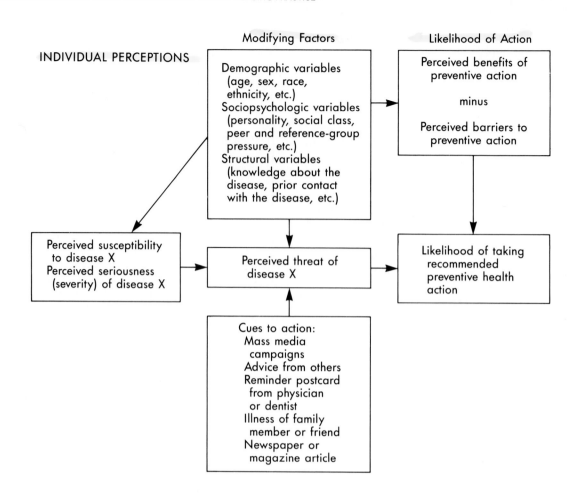

FIGURE 11-1

Rosenstock's Health Belief Model. *(From Becker MD et al: Selected psychosocial models and correlates of individual health-related behaviors, Med Care 15(5):24, 1977. Reprinted with permission.)*

Health Promotion Model

Pender (1987) developed a health promotion model to be used as a complement to health-protecting models like the HBM. Health promotion is "directed toward increasing the level of well-being and self-actualization in a given individual or group" (Pender, 1987, p. 57). This model is organized much like the HBM. Determinants of health-promoting behavior are organized into cognitive-perceptual factors, modifying factors, and variables affecting the likelihood of action (Figure 11-2). The *cognitive-perceptual factors* include: the importance of health, perceived control of health, perceived self-efficacy, definition of health, perceived health status, and perceived benefits of and barriers to health-promoting behavior.

The *modifying factors* include: demographic factors such as age, sex, race, ethnicity, education and income; biological characteristics such as body weight; interpersonal influences, including the expectations of significant others, family patterns of health care, and interactions with health professionals; situational factors or those present in the environment; and behavioral factors such as cognitive and psychomotor skills necessary to carry out healthy behaviors (Pender, 1987).

Variables affecting the likelihood of action depend on internal and external cues such as "wanting to feel good", mass media health messages, e.g., that regular exercise helps to prevent heart disease, or conversations with others. This model and the HBM are useful in community health nursing because they serve as frameworks for client assessment.

STRATEGIES FOR EFFECTIVE TEACHING

To facilitate the teaching-learning process the nurse should be aware of applicable models and strategies. Models as conceptualizations of reality provide a framework to guide the selection of appropriate interventions. Chapter 8 provides a detailed description of many conceptual models and theories that are currently used in community health. Also, knowledge of strategies that are important in promotion of learning will increase the nurse's ability to provide useful client-centered teaching. Various strategies can be employed to enhance the effectiveness of teaching efforts. These strategies include group education, communicating clearly, and selecting an appropriate learning format and climate. Also, the learning environment must be properly organized and the learners must be encouraged to participate. Creativity

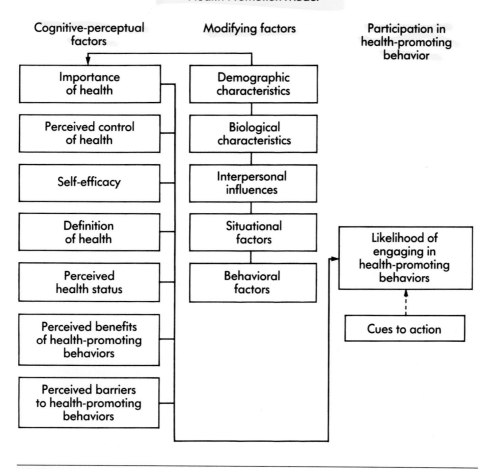

FIGURE 11-2

Pender's Health Promotion Model. *(From Pender NJ:* Health promotion in nursing practice, *Norwalk, Conn, 1987, Appleton & Lange. Reprinted with permission.)*

also enhances teaching effectiveness. Creativity consists of to providing information in ways that increase the learner's curiosity. The creative educator is open to new ideas, encourages learner input regarding teaching strategies, and is willing to try new ways of doing things.

The key to effective teaching lies in adopting a situation-specific approach. Although no hard and fast rules exist for effective teaching, the suggestions in the box on p. 190 are guidelines for implementing the educational role in community health nursing.

If the nurse suspects that a patient does not understand the information being taught because of a poor grasp of the language, the following steps may be helpful:

1. Speak slowly
2. Use simple sentences
3. Avoid technical terms
4. Give instruction in the same sequence in which he or she will carry it out
5. Do not assume the learner has understood (Tripp-Reimer and Afifi, 1989).

Explaining is an essential part of teaching. One of the most common ways to explain is to use examples. Examples

are helpful in clarifying material that is difficult to understand; de Tornyay and Thompson (1987) offer the following suggestions for using examples:

1. Begin with simple examples and progress to more complex ones
2. Select examples that are relevant to the patient's experiences
3. Relate examples to the ideas to be taught
4. Make sure the listener understands the example.

Group Education

Although the first portion of this chapter focuses on principles of teaching and learning that can be applied to both individuals and groups, it should be noted that groups do have unique characteristics that must be considered when educational activities are being planned. Information on working with groups in the community is given in Chapter 17.

Planning educational activities for groups of learners offers several advantages to the nurse. First, it may be an economical way to present the same material to more than one individual. By using the same teaching plan for more

TEACHING TIPS

1. Be consistent and trustworthy.
2. Be enthusiastic and let the learner know there is something of value being offered.
3. Be careful not to discuss your personal life with the learner.
4. Pay attention to the image you present and the messages given by your posture, clothes, gestures, hair, and tone of voice.
5. Be organized; it helps to convey a sense of competence to the learner.
6. Evaluate the effectiveness of teaching methods routinely.
7. Vary teaching strategies and resources as appropriate.
8. Record teaching experiences, successes, and failures because this information may be helpful to others in similar situations.
9. Expect good and bad days in teaching and learning.
10. Remember that the learner is an individual worthy of respect and not a disease process or procedure.
11. Give reasons when you ask the learner to do something.
12. Never equate intelligence with educational level. Cultural, religious, and ethnic variables, as well as lack of intelligence, may contribute to misunderstandings.
13. Attempt to motivate learners through recognition of need, not outward pressure.
14. Sense the appropriate moment for learning and act on it.
15. Write instructions legibly.
16. Allow time for interruptions.
17. Be careful not to overwhelm the learner with technical terms.
18. Provide feedback about learner progress.
19. Correct errors with information, not judgments.
20. Be careful not to allow racial bias to interfere with the learning process.
21. Focus on constructive thoughts.

From Murray R and Zentner J: Nursing concepts for health promotion, ed 3, Englewood Cliffs, NJ, 1985, Prentice Hall Press.

DO'S AND DON'TS FOR EFFECTIVE COMMUNICATION IN TEACHING

DO

- Watch for learner clues indicating the message is unclear.
- Rephrase the message, repeat the content, and ask for feedback until you are certain the learner has received the intended message.
- Be familiar and comfortable with the content before attempting to teach it.
- Speak the learner's language.
- Be specific when giving information.
- Stick to the point and be brief.
- Discuss key points first.
- Be careful about teasing and joking with clients.

DON'T

- Be afraid to ask clients to teach you the terms with which they are comfortable.
- Be condescending. Clients quickly pick up such an attitude and resent it.
- Allow language to alienate you from the learner.

Modified from Archer S and Fleshman R: Community health nursing: patterns and practice, ed 2, North Scituate, Mass, 1979, Duxbury Press; Narrow BW: Patient teaching in nursing practice, New York, 1979, John Wiley & Sons, Inc; and Miller A: When is the time ripe for teaching? Am J Nurs 85(7):801, 1985.

than one client, resources in terms of time and money are preserved. In addition, by reducing the number of identical individual teaching plans produced, the nurse can greatly increase efficiency in client teaching. No longer must the nurse "reinvent the wheel" each time client teaching is attempted; several learners can be reached with one teaching plan.

Next, group teaching provides the nurse with a mechanism for ensuring that education is implemented through the nursing care plan. Group activities offer the nurse and client a structured time for the teaching aspect of the care plan (Evans, 1980).

Group teaching can increase the relevance of educational programs. Because group instruction often allows the nurse to plan the content well in advance, programs are frequently based on identified rather than presumed learning needs. The leader can assess through interviews, surveys, or other means the learning needs that the participants think are

important. Programs can then be planned to meet those identified needs.

Another advantage of group teaching is that people do not feel alone or different. The group setting allows each client an opportunity to talk with others who have similar problems and needs. In groups clients can assume an active role in helping one another and serve as role models for changed behaviors (Lorig, 1985).

Clear Communication

Often the messages that nurses hope to deliver to clients never reach them. Before presenting educational programs, the nurse should assess learner readiness and be aware of possible barriers to effective communication. Emotional stress and physical illness are only two of the many factors that may limit the amount of information a learner is able to absorb. The nurse must be aware of limitations affecting the learner and plan educational activities accordingly.

The community health nurse must assume the responsibility for offering information that is understandable. Medical jargon and technical terms may interfere with the clarity of the intended message. For example, in helping clients understand the need for diet control in hypertension, the nurse might use the term *high blood pressure* rather than *hypertension* to make certain that the learner understands. Thus, skill must be developed in fitting the message to the learner. The box offers do's and don'ts that may be helpful to the nurse in developing communication skills (Archer and Fleshman, 1979; Narrow, 1979; Miller, 1985).

Selecting the Learning Format

Simply stated, the learning format describes the way participants are organized for an educational activity. A wide variety of formats (or methods) is available and selection of the most effective method can be difficult. To choose the best format, the objectives of the teaching program should be kept firmly in mind and the advantages and limitations of each method must be weighed carefully. Selection of an optimal learning format can help meet program objectives, heighten learner interest, and encourage active participation.

Although formats or methods of learning can be designed for both individuals and groups, the nurse practicing in the community most often works with groups. Table 11-3 describes the most commonly used group formats and lists the potential advantages and disadvantages of each.

Learning Climate

Carefully planned programs quickly lose their effectiveness if the environment is not conducive to learning. The nurse can take simple measures to manipulate the learning climate of the program.

The nurse can first start to set the learning climate for an educational endeavor when the program is announced. The tone and appearance of the letters, fliers, and media messages that announce the program give participants a mental picture of what the activity will be like. By carefully considering the program objectives and information gained in the assessment phase about the culture, beliefs, and educational level of the learners, the nurse can develop preparatory materials that are appealing to the target population.

Creativity can improve the physical setting, e.g., chairs can be moved from traditional rows into circles or semicircles to facilitate interaction. They may be discarded completely and pillows, mattresses, or sofas used as substitutes. The nurse should arrive early enough to arrange the seating, adjust the temperature and lighting, and organize audiovisual materials. A coffee pot and soft music often convey to learners that their comfort is important (Knowles, 1980).

The opening session of any educational activity affects the learning climate. Each participant should be greeted cordially and oriented to the objectives. Attention should be paid to unique learner characteristics. The degree of formality and privacy created in the learning environment should reflect the information gathered in the needs assessment.

Organizing Learning Experiences

Planning a teaching program requires that the nurse make decisions about the sequence of the learning activities. The nurse must consider the traits of the learner rather than have a preconceived notion of how to organize and present the material. The principles of continuity, sequence, and integration aid nurses in organizing educational programs.

The concept of continuity involves placing repeated emphasis on particular components of the educational experience. For example, a community health nurse working with a group of obese people may wish to emphasize the concept of individual responsibility in weight control. Learning activities would then be planned to ensure that the concept was repeated or reinforced as the group progressed.

Sequence means that each learning experience builds on the previous one and requires a higher level of functioning. This principle is consistent with Bloom's taxonomy of learning domains. For example, when teaching exercises to a weight-control group, the nurse should sequence the learning activities so that participants start with simple exercises and progress to the more complex exercises that require greater skill or coordination.

Finally, the concept of integration is helpful in organizing learning experiences. Integration of the various components of the teaching plan demonstrates how each aspect fits into the big picture. Participants in a weight-control class may find it helpful to understand how proper diet and exercise are related in controlling weight. Thus, basic principles of organization allow individualization of the plan so that the objectives of the program match the learning situation (Knowles, 1980).

Participative Learning

Learning in either the psychomotor domain or at the application level demands that the instructor use action or participative learning as a teaching strategy. In participative learning, learners are responsible for acquiring and implementing affective, cognitive, and behavioral changes. The instructor provides the means for this process to take place (Tarnow, 1979). It is the leader's responsibility to structure the learning activities and teaching strategies to involve the learner actively. For example, learning the proper technique for injecting insulin requires that the learner observe the demonstration (cognitive domain), practice the skill (psychomotor domain), and repeat the demonstration (psychomotor domain).

The nurse, on the other hand, is responsible for ensuring that proper teaching materials are available and that the learner is provided with adequate information in the demonstration to repeat the procedure. By structuring the learning environment, the nurse is able to allow learner participation which makes the learning more effective than lectures, films, or reading materials (Tarnow, 1979).

Audiovisual Materials

Audiovisual materials are teaching aids such as printed materials, films, videotapes, television, radio, records, and audiotapes. When used properly, audiovisual materials can facilitate learning by creating interest and motivating and stimulating learning. They can also make use of otherwise nonproductive time, such as time spent in the waiting area of an outpatient clinic. Used inappropriately, however, audiovisual materials may inhibit or interfere with learning by overloading the learner with stimuli. Proper selection of audiovisual materials requires consideration of the characteristics of the audiovisual materials.

Characteristics of the Learner

The audience must be considered when selecting audiovisual materials. Possible physical handicaps, age, educational level, knowledge of the subject, and size of the group must be taken into account. Any sensory deficit must be carefully considered when selecting educational media. For example, learners with poor vision require different audio-

TABLE 11-3
Common formats used with groups

Format	Brief description	Advantages	Limitations
Open forum	Public meeting in which participants are provided with opportunity to air their views	1. Allows audience participation 2. Stimulates thought 3. Raises questions 4. Identifies concerns	1. May delay reaching consensus by group 2. Success often rests on ability of moderator
Role playing	Acting out situations; usually done in front of group with time allotted at conclusion for discussion	1. Provides concreteness to learning situation 2. Encourages use of problem-solving skills 3. Requires learner participation	1. Group members may be too shy to participate 2. Intended content (or points) may or may not surface
Skits	Brief, rehearsed, dramatic presentation	1. May evoke emotional involvement 2. Stimulates discussion	1. May distract from intended message 2. Requires rehearsal time
Field trip or tour	Visit by group to object or place for first-hand observation and study	1. Entertains learner 2. Enables learner to view object or place in context of larger community 3. May motivate learners to seek additional learning experiences 4. Sharpens observational skills 5. Traveling time facilitates participant interaction	1. Time is required to make advance arrangements 2. Cost may be prohibitive 3. Time required may not be available 4. Finding appropriate site may be difficult 5. Schedules are difficult to maintain
Interview	Presentation in which one or more individuals answer questions posed by one or more interviewers	1. Provides common learning experience for all participants 2. Allows audience to hear differing points of view 3. May be used in eliciting audience involvement 4. Requires less preparation time than formal presentation	1. Requires skill on part of interviewer 2. Interviewer must possess knowledge of subject at hand
Lecture	Formal, oral presentation of subject	1. May be organized easily 2. May be used with groups of any size 3. Can convey enthusiasm	1. Requires speaking ability and expertise 2. Audience is passive 3. Feedback is limited
Committee or task force	Small group organized to achieve goal that cannot be efficiently reached by larger group or individual	1. Relieves members of larger group of tasks at hand 2. Permits variety of interests to be represented 3. Facilitates communication and decision making 4. Provides leadership opportunity for group members	1. Members of committee may be unable to work together effectively 2. Committee members may not have necessary time 3. Larger group may not support actions of committee
Discussion group	Group that meets to discuss predetermined topic	1. Permits participation of all members 2. Pools abilities and expertise toward reaching common goal	1. Time consuming 2. One member may dominate group 3. Extraneous discussions may divert group's efforts

TABLE 11-3
Common formats used with groups—cont'd

Format	Brief description	Advantages	Limitations
Demon-stration	Presentation that shows in detail how to perform certain act or procedure	1. Learners may be more likely to retain and understand what they see as opposed to what is read or heard 2. Pace is flexible and permits instructor to repeat if necessary	1. Materials needed for demonstration may be expensive, limited, or difficult to transport 2. Number of participants is limited by space and materials available
Brain-storm-ing	Participants "throw out" as many ideas as possible on given subject; ideas are recorded as they are given and are discussed later	1. Allows participation by all members 2. Allows freedom of expression 3. Encourages creativity 4. May present solutions to previously unsolved problems	1. Suggested ideas may be impractical for implementation 2. Ideas may be criticized during following discussion period 3. Participants may be unable to develop novel approaches to identified problem
Buzz ses-sions	Large group is divided into several small groups to simultaneously meet and discuss assigned topic; may report back to large group at end of session	1. Allows participation of each member 2. Encourages thought about assigned topic 3. Provides mechanism for generation of "fresh ideas"	1. Reports of small groups may be tedious or contradictory 2. Time may limit contributions each individual may make 3. May be time-consuming to organize small groups 4. Small groups may not discuss assigned topic
Case study	Detailed account of one or more events that is presented to group of learners; discussion or written activity usually follows	1. Assists in developing problem-solving skills 2. Enables learner to consider alternative solutions 3. Presents many concepts on several levels in interesting fashion	1. Learner may not find case study relevant 2. Requires considerable time to prepare 3. Does not require all learners to participate in discussion 4. Requires skill in preparation
Mass media	Messages conveyed through television, radio, films, slides, videotapes or audiotapes, as well as charts, books, posters, teaching manuals	1. Reaches large audience 2. Efficient 3. Low cost per volume	1. Message is not individualized 2. Can be expensive for initial outlay

visual aids than those with hearing deficits. In teaching people with auditory deficits, visual and tactile aids such as films, printed materials, and live or video demonstrations are helpful. For people with visual deficits, auditory and tactile aids such as audiotapes, demonstrations that rely on verbal explanations, and large-print materials with bold lettering and generous spacing should be used instead.

Many clients cannot read at the level at which educational materials are printed. A person's level of education may not be an accurate indicator of reading level. In misjudging the reading ability of the learner, the nurse risks not only embarrassing the client but also closing the door to any future teaching. Thus, the community health nurse must be con-

stantly alert for any client feedback indicating an inability to comprehend the material presented.

When selecting visual aids requiring reading for a group, the task becomes more complex. The educational level and the occupations of group members as well as the reading level of the local newspaper enables educators to determine with some degree of accuracy the level at which the program should proceed.

The readability of educational materials can be affected by the legibility of the printed words, as well as by illustrations. The size of the type used, the shape of the letters, the amount of space between letters, and supplemental illustrations can enhance the readability of printed materials.

Objectives of the Program

The materials selected will depend upon the objectives of the program. Well-written objectives are invaluable to the nurse when selecting audiovisual materials. Because behavioral objectives specify the learning domain and the relative complexity of behavior, they are therefore an effective tool in selecting educational media. For example, if the objective is for the client to demonstrate a dressing change, the audiovisual aid would include a live or video demonstration followed by a repeat performance by the learner.

Characteristics of the Materials

Audiovisual materials are often selected on the basis of what the instructor is comfortable using or what is currently available rather than by considering the specific advantages and disadvantages of each material. Table 11-4 outlines the various audiovisual materials available and compares the advantages and disadvantages of each type. No presentation should begin until the material has been previewed, the equipment checked, and the nurse is familiar and comfortable with using it.

In selecting audiovisual aids for a specific presentation, the following questions should be asked:

1. Is the audio and/or visual aid necessary? if so, why?
2. Is color or motion necessary? How will it help the presentation?

Because of the cost and time involved, audiovisual materials should be used only when they are essential for conveying a message.

Mass media (radio, television, and newspapers) are especially effective in community health. The same process is used in preparing information for dissemination through the mass media as for selecting media for individual presentations. Characteristics of the intended audience must be assessed, objectives written, and a vehicle for the message selected. The nurse must recognize that the use of media in community settings is not the answer to every teaching need. It can be effective in delivering new information, setting agendas, and producing simple behavior changes. Improper use of mass media, as of any audiovisual aid, may not only fail to communicate the intended message to the target audience, but may also deter any future participation in desired health-related activities.

RESOURCES FOR COMMUNITY HEALTH NURSING

Resources for planning and implementing education programs include libraries, health departments, and chapters of national organizations (e.g., the American Cancer Society and the American Heart Association). Such agencies offer books and printed materials as well as films, videotapes, and slide presentations that can be borrowed. It is essential that the community health nurse keep abreast of the audiovisual materials available for use and the means for obtaining them.

Some communities publish a community resource directory that provides information about the purpose of an agency, the services offered, eligibility requirements, and referral procedures.

BARRIERS TO COMMUNITY HEALTH EDUCATION

Successful implementation of the educational aspect of community health nursing requires that the nurse be aware of and plan for potential barriers. Such barriers include lack of time, money, space, energy, confidence, organizational support, and equipment.

In planning a teaching program the nurse must establish a schedule that allows flexibility yet ensures that deadlines are met. A good rule is to allow an extra 2 weeks in any schedule to accommodate unforeseen delays. Time management is essential to successful program planning.

Lack of money to implement a desired program is a common obstacle. Organizations, businesses, and industries in the community may grant funds for educational projects if benefits to them in terms of employee health can be demonstrated. The assessment phase of the educational process provides nurses with valuable information regarding individual learners' willingness and ability to pay for educational activities.

The amount and type of space available for teaching are another barrier to the nurse. Problems of space limitations can be resolved in several ways. Small rooms may require that programs be repeated so all interested learners can attend. Nurses must become increasingly assertive in negotiating for space. The educational aspect of nursing is too important; it must not be sacrificed because of space limitations. Finally, nurses must be involved in planning new facilities to meet the educational needs of the community.

Most programs require considerable energy and the nurse must have sufficient energy to devote to the task without feeling overwhelmed by the magnitude of the program. Often, the teaching can be divided among team members to conserve the energy of all involved. Self-confidence is also required.

Self-confidence can best be acquired by performing the role of teacher. In order to overcome initial discomfort, however, the nurse can role-play with a colleague. It is important to select a person who will provide honest and helpful feedback. Videotaping and self-critiquing one's performance in a lecture format may be another useful tool for increasing confidence in one's ability as a teacher. Possibly the biggest boost to the nurse's self-confidence, however, is seeing the successful outcome of teaching in the positive effects it has on a client's life.

With the current emphasis on cost effectiveness, the nurse may encounter a lack of organizational support in implementing teaching projects. Many agencies encourage their staff to see as many clients as possible within a given period of time. The educational component of care is often seen as a nice extra that is to be included only if time permits. The nurse must devote careful attention in the assessment phase to demonstrating the need for educational endeavors. For example, if an industry is reluctant to grant employees time off from work to participate in preventive or health-promotion activities, the nurse can gather information to demonstrate that such activities are cost effective in terms of fewer days lost as a result of illness. The nurse can involve key people from each agency in the planning process. Such participation often promotes support of educational endeavors.

TABLE 11-4

Advantages and limitations of selected audiovisual materials

Audiovisual material	Advantages	Limitations
Books and other printed material	1. May be used for individual instruction 2. Allow learner to proceed at individual pace 3. Require no special equipment or setting for use 4. May be used to supplement other media	1. Useful only with literate learners 2. Reading level of printed material must match that of learner 3. Not suitable for use with groups 4. Useful only when in language of learner
Chalkboard	1. May be used for large audiences 2. Requires no advance preparation 3. Enhances verbal communication 4. Is inexpensive 5. Is reusable	1. Learner cannot control pace of presentation 2. No way of preserving images
Photographic print series	1. Is inexpensive 2. Is widely available 3. Is easily manipulated 4. Permits close-up study 5. Allows learner to progress at individual pace 6. Requires no equipment for use 7. May be used for self-study	1. Black and white pictures may limit proper interpretation 2. Sizes and distances may be distorted 3. Difficult to use with large groups 4. Photographic skill and equipment required for preparation
Slide series	1. Sequence can be altered to meet specific needs 2. Can be easily revised 3. Is convenient to handle, store, and use 4. Is appropriate for individual or group instruction 5. Is easily prepared with 35 mm camera 6. Presentation can be upgraded over period of time by gradually replacing single slides 7. Provides sharp image to learner	1. Special equipment is required for preparation and projection 2. Slides may get out of sequence and be inappropriately projected
Filmstrips	1. Are in same sequence 2. Can be held on screen as long as desired 3. Handle easily; compact 4. May be used for individual or group instruction 5. Projected with simple equipment 6. Learner controls projection rate	1. Fixed sequence limits revision 2. Difficult to produce
Audiotapes	1. Can be used in individual or group instruction 2. Prepared and played back easily with simple inexpensive equipment 3. Economical to duplicate 4. Can be used alone or in conjunction with video materials 5. Stored easily 6. Selected easily (reel-to-reel tapes)	1. Fixed rate for information giving 2. Possible to erase recording if tape is mishandled 3. May be difficult to locate specific portions of tape for playback purposes
Overhead transparencies	1. May be used in front of room, thus permitting eye contact between instructor and learner 2. Prepared easily and inexpensive 3. Operated and maintained easily 4. Are especially effective with large groups 5. Require limited planning; can be written on during presentation 6. May highlight, reinforce, or supplement verbal presentation 7. May be used in lighted or semidarkened room 8. Can be produced for minimal cost 9. Can be used repeatedly 10. Instructor can control speed of presentation 11. May be easily filed for future reference	1. Storage of equipment may be problematic 2. Equipment may block learner's view 3. Ordinary typewriters may produce images too small to be seen 4. Many people put too much detail in transparency

Continued.

◣ **TABLE 11-4**
Advantages and limitations of selected audiovisual materials—cont'd

Audiovisual material	Advantages	Limitations
Films or video-tapes	1. May be used with individual or groups 2. May be used in demonstrating motion or relationships 3. Ensure consistency of presentation 4. Enable learner to transcend limitations of time, space, and human body 5. Provide realism in terms of shapes and structures	1. Expensive to prepare, maintain, and purchase 2. Difficult to revise 3. Expense may limit accessibility and cause material to become dated 4. Subject to damage with each use 5. Projection equipment may be cumbersome or difficult to operate 6. Different sizes of reels require special projectors (i.e., 8 mm, 16 mm) 7. Difficult to keep updated

A final barrier nurses frequently encounter is the lack of necessary equipment for implementing programs. The nurse should be aware of organizations in the community that are willing to loan or donate the needed equipment. Grants are often available for the purchase or development of audiovisual materials, and the nurse should be familiar with application procedures. In any event, the planning phase of the teaching project must include taking into account the equipment available and developing teaching strategies accordingly.

EVALUATION OF EFFECTIVENESS

Never take for granted that because an individual has attended an educational program, learning has taken place! All too often nurses and other health professionals assume that because the information has been transmitted to the learner, all program objectives have been met. Evaluation is necessary throughout the teaching-learning process to ensure that program objectives are met.

Evaluation is as important in teaching as it is in the nursing process. Evaluation can range from simple to sophisticated—its type and complexity should be based on what is being evaluated. For example, when considering a client's ability to perform a psychomotor skill, viewing the actual performance of the skill is the most appropriate means of assessment. In evaluating a teaching program, a more complex procedure that includes many people and a variety of data collection methods will be necessary. Without a process of evaluation, systematic decisions regarding improvement of client teaching or program quality are impossible.

Evaluation of Teacher Effectiveness

Ongoing feedback and evaluation are valuable to the learner and teacher alike. For the learner, feedback reinforces desired behaviors and allows for the correction of misinformation. Feedback to the instructor allows for modifications in the teaching process to better meet the learner's needs. Because feedback is most effective when it is immediate, it is a learning tool for both the instructor and the learner (Tarnow, 1979).

Evaluation of the teaching process occurs continuously. The instructor may receive feedback from the learner in written form, such as a test or evaluation sheet; verbally in the form of questions asked or responded to; or nonverbally as in return demonstrations and facial expressions. If evaluation is done as teaching is in progress, the nurse will be able to predict with a large degree of accuracy the extent to which the program objectives will be met and the time required for their attainment. Ongoing evaluation also allows the teacher to correct misinformation or confusion.

Redman (1984) suggests that it is unwise to teach for a long period of time without requiring learners to respond. If evaluation reveals that the learning objectives have not been met, the nurse must determine why the teaching was not effective. Was the instructor familiar and comfortable with the subject matter? The learner may perceive that the instructor does not understand the subject. Clients may think that if the nurse could not understand the subject matter, how could they?

The frequency of evaluation depends on the subject matter, the amount of time available, the amount of material to be presented, and the nature of the learners. For example, a nurse wishing to assess the effectiveness of teaching insulin injection skills may include different evaluative "check points" in the teaching plan than would a nurse attempting to teach the physiology of human reproduction. Whatever form of evaluation is used, the nurse is responsible for communicating to the learner in advance how and when evaluation is to take place (Narrow, 1979). Often, the nurse chooses not to use the word "evaluation" when talking to clients but instead may say something like, "I'll demonstrate a breathing exercise, and then you can show me how to do it."

Factors that influence learner readiness and motivation have already been discussed in this chapter and must be reassessed if teaching seems to be ineffective. Finally, the nurse must ask if the desired behavior change is really necessary. Such a question inevitably leads back to the original learning objectives and encourages the nurse to rethink the practicality and merit of each of the unattained objectives (Redman, 1984).

TABLE 11-5
Advantages and disadvantages of common data collection methods

Method	Advantages	Disadvantages
Direct observation of behavior	1. Product and process of learned behavior can be observed	1. Time consuming 2. Does not evaluate cognitive skills underlying psychomotor acts
Interview	1. May be formal or informal, structured or unstructured 2. Data obtained from structured interview may be uniform and easy to analyze 3. Allows for full range of views	1. Time consuming 2. Unstructured interview may be difficult to analyze 3. Interviewer bias may affect results
Questionnaires	1. Obtain reliable information from specific questions 2. Avoid interviewer bias	1. May be misinterpreted by respondent 2. May interfere with activity 3. Time consuming 4. Answers may be misinterpreted by evaluator
Standardized tests	1. Provide an opportunity to compare data from one group with national norms	1. May remind adult learner of childhood schooling 2. Group may not be representative of national norm
Tailor-made tests	1. Produce data about changes for which tests were designed 2. May demonstrate student progress	1. May lack validity and reliability

Evaluation of Program Effectiveness

It is helpful for the nurse to become familiar with the purpose of program evaluation before attempting to judge the effectiveness of a teaching endeavor. Knowles (1980) identifies two main purposes of program evaluation: (1) to improve the organization of the operation, including the physical facility, personnel, planning process, and decision-making process, and (2) to improve the actual program, which involves the objectives, teaching strategies, and materials. Both purposes serve to stimulate the learner and promote growth and improvement.

Once the purpose and focus of the program evaluation are determined, the evaluation process follows in a series of several simple steps. First, the questions to be answered must be developed and if possible, pretested. These questions are identified during the program planning stage and relate to the desired outcomes.

Rankin and Duffy (1983, p. 62) list seven outcomes of patient education programs. These are:

1. Patient compliance with treatment plan
2. Cessation of certain behaviors (e.g., smoking)
3. Knowledge acquisition
4. Patient satisfaction with health care and/or health care provider
5. Reduction in certain emotions such as patient anxiety, fear, or feelings of helplessness
6. Increased confidence levels (e.g., of ability to self-administer insulin)
7. Ability to present self at most propitious time for early diagnosis and treatment

Next, data must be collected to answer the questions that are identified.

A variety of data collection methods is available to the nurse, and the specific method used is determined by the objectives of the program being evaluated, the variables to be measured, and the time and cost involved. The most common methods of data collection have been summarized in Table 11-5 along with some of the advantages and disadvantages of each. Because each method is subject to error and bias, an ongoing evaluation program requires a combination of methods.

Whichever method of evaluation the nurse chooses to use to determine teaching and program effectiveness, it is helpful to keep in mind the curve of normal distribution. In any group of learners, about 2% will be extremely negative and 2% will be extremely positive in their evaluation of the program. Another 14% will be fairly negative with 14% quite enthusiastic. The majority of participants (68%) will be somewhat neutral in their responses (Knowles, 1980). Therefore, even though the nurse should consider the extremely negative responses, he or she should not become alarmed or discouraged unless the proportion of extremely negative criticism goes above 16%.

Now the data can be analyzed by all who participated. The learners and instructors, the program director and management personnel, outside experts, and community representatives provide unique observations, perceptions, and suggestions about the program. The nurse seeking to determine the adequacy of a program for a given community would do well to collect data from as many sources as possible and to include the evaluators in the process of analyzing the data and modifying the program accordingly.

CLINICAL APPLICATION

A community health nursing goal is to promote the health of client groups. Often the aim of health promotion is to reduce the risk of a health-disrupting incident. One target group for health education would be clients attending a cardiac rehabilitation clinic. Essentially, the nursing process is used to assess learning needs, plan and implement a group-specific teaching program, and continuously evaluate program effectiveness.

For example, 10 post-cardiac surgery patients between the ages of 39 and 64 years are enrolled in a health education class at an HMO. All the patients are white males who were previously employed full-time before their surgery. Each one wants to return to work as soon as possible. Each has a good chance for recovery if he pays close attention to diet, exercise, stress management, physical activity, and medication.

The most appropriate format for teaching these patients about their diet, kinds and amount of exercise, ways to manage stress, and how to take their medications is through small group lectures and discussions. The group approach is convenient and economical. All 10 patients need to receive the same core information about rehabilitation. Because the group is small, there will be time for individual questions and small group discussions. Group members can also learn from one another about ways to cope with any restrictions on their previous level of activity, any new dietary priorities, and so on. The group format also allows members to recognize that others have similar health needs and requirements for activity changes.

The advantages of group discussion for these 10 patients outweighs the disadvantages. It is not always possible to personalize small group instruction as much as individual teaching. If the nurse is attentive to nonverbal behavior and recognizes when participants have questions or concerns, she can offset the potential disadvantage of group instruction that arises when not everyone is allowed to receive one-on-one teaching.

In planning a teaching program for these clients, several factors must be kept in mind including attitudes, beliefs, values, knowledge, motivation, family support, aspirations, readiness to learn, and type of job previously held. Before beginning a teaching program, find out what past experiences the individuals have had with heart disease. For example, if one person in the group knew someone who had heart disease and died, this person would have a different attitude toward health education than another group member whose contacts with cardiac patients have all been positive. One method for gathering this type of background information is to use the initial one or two group meetings to set goals. For example, members might be asked to develop a list of eight concerns they wish to discuss. The group then can set priorities within the list. If the group-generated essential information is left off the list, the nurse can suggest its addition.

Once a comprehensive list is generated, plan the format and style for offering the classes. The way in which the course is conducted will depend upon the characteristics of the group. Some groups will respond to lecture, others to lecture and discussion, and still others can benefit from a question-and-answer format. Regardless of the format chosen, the leader should make certain that all members understand the material being taught. The nurse will also want to use all available community resources, especially materials from the American Heart Association. Evaluation occurs throughout the program and may include a participant survey in the last session. This could be a questionnaire mailed to participants at a later date or a telephone survey about how effective the classes were.

SUMMARY

This chapter has described several components of the educational aspects of the role of community health nursing. Educational strategies are important for health promotion and disease prevention. To provide effective education to students, clients, and colleagues, community health nurses must understand the nature of learning. Not all learning experiences require participants to synthesize the information provided. In a number of instances it is appropriate for learners to comprehend or apply information without being accountable for higher levels of cognition. Learning also has cognitive, affective, and psychomotor components. It is insufficient simply to give clinic clients a sheet of diet instructions without paying some attention to their cognitive ability to understand the material and accept the implications of the instructions.

Planning effective health education programs necessitates drawing on theories of learning. People learn in different ways, and beliefs vary about how learning occurs. In some situations the most effective mode for health education follows SR tenets. Other learners and educators are more comfortable with cognitive-discovery, Gestalt, or humanistic views of learning, or some combination thereof.

Effective health education programming takes into account a variety of principles of teaching and learning. The majority of clients seen by community health nurses are adults; hence, special characteristics of adult learners have been noted as have other learner qualities such as self-concept, experience, readiness to learn, assumptions about learning and teaching, motivation, and individual differences.

Assessment of learner needs and interests follows the section of principles of teaching and learning. Without a careful assessment, how can educators plan? Occasionally, educators develop splendid programs that are of no interest to learners. Whose time is wasted? To develop educational programs suited to learner needs and wants, a thorough assessment is required. What do learners want or need? How can these needs and desires be met cost-efficiently and effectively? When, where and how can an effective program be developed and by whom? These questions are answered through careful assessment, planning (including development of purposes and objectives), implementation, and evaluation.

KEY CONCEPTS

Health education is a vital component of community health nursing because the promotion, maintenance, and restoration of health rely on client understanding of health care requirements.

One person cannot promote the health of another. People are responsible for working toward higher levels of health through their behavior both as individuals and in groups.

Three prominent theories of learning applicable to community health nursing are stimulus-response, cognitive, and humanistic theories.

Stimulus-response theorists believe that students should learn in a structured, systematic manner with stimulus situations planned to arouse specific types of responses.

The most effective technique for teaching adults is andragogy, which means helping people to learn. In this technique, education helps the learner discover what is not known.

The key to effective teaching is planning the appropriate approach for the specific situation. Effective planning necessitates drawing on theories of learning.

Adults learn differently from children; such factors as self-concept, readiness to learn, motivation, and individual differences should be taken into account when planning health programs for adults.

Learners have different needs and their needs should be carefully assessed before program planning begins.

Three current and useful models for organizing health education are: the PRECEDE Model, the Health Belief Model, and the Health Promotion Model.

Evaluation is a vital part of the learning process. It helps to determine effectiveness of the teaching and the extent to which program objectives have been met.

LEARNING ACTIVITIES

1. Review the theories of learning summarized in the chapter and decide which one would most effectively fit the learning needs of your class.

2. Imagine that you are going to plan a class on weight reduction for your classmates. Develop a plan that incorporates one theory of learning, the learning domain most important to your strategy, and that takes into account the needs of adult learners and the specific characteristics you have observed in the class.

3. Recall a conversation with a client that did not seem to go well. Identify what might have been the problem. Was the com-

munication too advanced, too elementary, or poorly timed?

4. In order to start an exercise class for 10 of your classmates, which model for health education would be most useful? Outline the proposed program using that model.

5. Recall a learning experience in which the content, style, timing, or understanding of learner needs was not effective. Once you determine what was wrong, develop a plan for overcoming the problem and turning a negative or neutral learning situation into a positive one.

BIBLIOGRAPHY

Archer S and Fleshman R: Community health nursing: patterns and practice, ed 2, North Scituate, Mass, 1979, Duxbury Press.

Biehler RF: Psychology applied to teaching, ed 5, Boston, 1986, Houghton Mifflin Co.

Biehler RF: Psychology applied to teaching, ed 4, Boston, 1982, Houghton Mifflin Co.

Bloom B: Taxonomy of educational objective, handbook 1: cognition domain, New York, 1969, David McKay Co Inc.

de Tornyay R and Thompson MA: Strategies for teaching nursing. New York, 1987, John Wiley & Sons.

Evans LK: Health education from a group perspective, Top Clin Nurs 2(2):45, 1980.

Gessner BA: Adult education: the cornerstone of patient teaching, Nurs Clin North Am 24(3):589, 1989.

Gleit C: Theories of learning. In Whitman NI, et al: Teaching in nursing practice, Norwalk, Conn, 1986, Appleton-Century-Crofts.

Good RL and Brophy JE: Educational psychology: a realistic approach, ed 4, New York, 1990, Longman, Inc.

Green L et al: Health education planning: a di-

agnostic approach, Palo Alto, Calif, 1980, Mayfield Publishing Co.

Higgins MG: Learning style assessment: a new patient teaching tool? J Nurs Staff Development, 4:14, 1988.

Hochbaum GM: Public participation in medical screening programs: a sociological study, US Public Health Service Pub No 572, Washington, DC, 1958, US Government Printing Office.

Kegeles SS et al: Survey of beliefs about cancer detection and taking Papanicolaou tests, Public Health Reports, 80(9): 815, 1965.

Knowles MS: The modern practice of adult education: andragogy versus pedagogy, ed 2, Chicago, 1980, Follett Publishing Co.

Lorig K: Health education: beyond health teaching. In Archer SE and Fleshman RP, editors: Community health nursing, ed 3, Monterey, Calif, 1985, Wadsworth Inc.

Maslow A: Toward a psychology of being, ed 2, New York, 1968, Van Nostrand Reinhold Co Inc.

Miller A: When is the time ripe for teaching? Am J Nurs 85(7):801, 1985.

Narrow BW: Patient teaching in nursing practice, New York, 1979, John Wiley & Sons, Inc.

Pender N: Health promotion in nursing practice, ed 2, Norwalk, Conn, 1987, Appleton & Lange.

Rankin SH and Duffy KL: Patient education: issues, principles, and guidelines, Philadelphia, 1983, JB Lippincott Co.

Redman BK: The process of patient teaching in nursing, ed 5, St Louis, 1984, The CV Mosby Co.

Roberts FB: A model for parent education, Image 13:86, 1981.

Rogers C: Freedom to learn, Columbus, Ohio, 1969, Merrill Publishing Co.

Rosenstock IM: Historical origins of the health belief model. In Becker MH, editor: The health belief model and personal health behavior, Thorofare, NJ, 1974, Slack Inc.

Speers AT: Patient education: theory and practice, J Nurs Staff Development, 3:121, 1989.

Sprinthall NA and Sprinthall RC: Educational psychology: a developmental approach, ed 5, New York, 1990, McGraw Hill Inc.

Tarnow KG: Working with adult learners, Nurs Ed 4(5):34, 1979.

Tripp-Reimer T and Afifi LA: Cross-cultural perspectives on patient teaching, Nurs Clin North Am 24(3):613, 1989.

Program Management

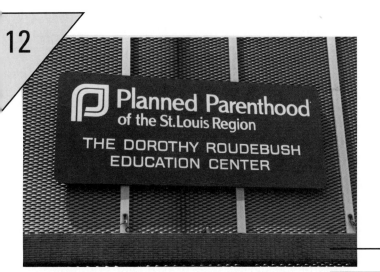

Marcia Stanhope

Gwendolen Lee

OBJECTIVES

After reading this chapter, the student should be able to:

Compare the program management process to the nursing process.

Analyze the program planning process and its application to community health nursing.

Compare and contrast a program planning method to use in community health nursing practice.

Identify the benefits of program planning.

Analyze the components of program evaluation and application to community health nursing.

Identify evaluation methods and techniques.

Name program evaluation sources.

Describe types of program evaluation measures.

Describe types of cost studies applied to program management.

KEY TERMS

assessment of need	evaluation	process
case register	evaluation of program effectiveness	program
case studies		program evaluation
census data	evaluative research	statistical indicators
community forum	formative evaluation	strategic planning
community resident survey	health index	structure
	health planning	summative evaluation
cost accounting	health systems agency	systems model of evaluation
cost effectiveness	key informants	
cost benefit	outcome	tracer method
estimation of risk	planning	

P rogram management consists of assessing, planning, implementing, and evaluating the processes involved in the life of a program. The program management process parallels the nursing process. One is applied to a program whereas the other is applied to clients. This chapter will focus primarily on planning and evaluation. Although presented in separate discussions, these factors are interrelated, dependent processes that work together to bring about a successful program (USDHHS, 1989). This chapter will not deal with implementation because most chapters in the text focus on implementation.

The process of program management, like the nursing process, consists of a rational decision-making system designed to help nurses know when to make a decision to develop a program (problem identification), to know where they want to be at the end of the program (assessment), how to decide what to do to have a successful program (planning), how to develop a plan to go from where they are to where they want to be (implementation), how to know they are getting there (formative evaluation), and what to measure in order to know that what they are doing is appropriate (summative evaluation) (USDHHS, 1989).

With more emphasis on accountability for nursing actions toward clients and the introduction of prospective payment systems, the focus of nursing is changing. Planning for nursing services is essential today if the nursing discipline is to survive in the field of health care delivery.

This chapter examines how nurses can act instead of react by planning programs that can be evaluated for their effectiveness in meeting their social purpose. This discussion focuses on the historical development of health planning and evaluation, a generic program planning and evaluation method, the benefits of planning and evaluation, the elements of planning and evaluation, and cost studies applied to program evaluation. Appendix L provides an overview of specific program management models that are applied in community health nursing practice.

DEFINITIONS AND GOALS

A *program* is an organized response designed to meet the assessed needs of individuals, families, groups, or communities by reducing or eliminating one or more health problems. Examples of specific programs in community health nursing are home health programs, immunization programs, health-risk screening programs for industrial workers, and family planning clinic programs. These specific programs are usually conducted under the direction of a total program plan of the local health department. More broadly based group and community programs are the community school health program, the occupational health and safety program, the environmental health program, and community programs directed at specific illnesses through special-interest groups (e.g., American Heart Association, the American Cancer Society, and the March of Dimes).

Planning is defined as the selecting and carrying out of a series of actions designed to achieve stated goals (Kropf, 1990). The *goal* of planning is to ensure the acceptability, equality, efficiency, and effectiveness of services. *Evaluation* is defined as the methods used to determine whether a service is needed and likely to be used, whether it is

conducted as planned, and whether the service actually helps people in need (Posavac and Carey, 1980, p. 6). Evaluation for the purpose of assessing whether objectives are met or planned activities are completed is referred to as *formative evaluation*. This type of evaluation begins with an assessment of the need for the program. At this stage an evaluation of need has occurred. Evaluation to assess program outcomes or as a follow-up of the results of the program activities is called *summative evaluation*.

Program evaluation is an ongoing process from the initial planning phase until the program is terminated. The major goals of program evaluation are to determine the relevance, progress, efficiency, effectiveness, and impact of program activities to the clients served (Veney and Kaluzny, 1984).

HISTORICAL OVERVIEW OF HEALTH CARE PLANNING AND EVALUATION

As the health care delivery system has grown in the past 60 years, emphasis in health planning and evaluation has increased. Factors that have fostered increased interest in planning and evaluation are advances in health care technology and consumer education, increased health care expectations, third-party payers, budget pressures, increased professional conflicts, focus on preventive care, new focus on health care as a business, unionization of health care workers, urbanization, increased health risks, personnel shortages, and increased health care costs.

In the 1920s the American Public Health Association's Committees on Administrative Practice and Evaluation emphasized the need for public health officers to engage in better program planning to change the haphazard method by which public health programs were begun (Pickett and Hanlon, 1990). During this period, the Committee on Costs of Medical Care studied the economic and social aspects of health services. The committee recognized the need for comprehensive health care planning, citing the rising costs and the unequal distribution of health services across the nation (Anderson, 1966; Committee on the Costs of Medical Care, 1970). As a result of the committee report, a few states began to coordinate medical services for their residents. However, regionalized planning for health services nationwide was not attempted until the American Hospital Association established its Committee on Postwar Planning in 1944.

The post–World War II era also brought an interest in evaluating program effectiveness. As government and third-party payers began to finance health care services and money became more plentiful, public demand for health services grew. As a result, numbers and kinds of health care agencies increased; laws were passed to increase the scope of and control over health care, and the health care delivery system was beginning to be held accountable for its actions (Pickett and Hanlon, 1990). The federal government's first attempt to legislate health planning was the passage of the Hospital Survey and Construction Act in 1946 (also called the Hill-Burton Act).

The 1960s were marked by the Great Society programs of President Johnson. The social, economic, and health programs that grew out of the Great Society concept were designed primarily to meet peoples' needs and to show that the federal government could deliver services to the public efficiently. For example, the *Community Mental Health Centers Act* of 1963 (P.L. 88-464) gave state governments the authority to plan mental health programs to meet population needs. This legislation clearly defined the roles of consumers and professionals as advisors in the planning process for all future health planning legislation. In 1965 the Regional Medical Program legislation (P.L. 89-239) was passed to upgrade the quality of tertiary health care services to consumers. This legislation required health providers and consumers to work together in planning groups to address a number of issues in health care, such as heart disease, cancer, kidney disease, and cerebrovascular accidents. Thus, the phrase "partnership for health" was coined.

During this time the Office of Health Planning was established in the Department of Health, Education, and Welfare (now the Department of Health and Human Services, or DHHS). Because the scope and functioning of the Office of Health Planning was limited and had no direct authority for national health planning, the Eighty-Ninth Congress passed the Comprehensive Health Planning (CHP) and Public Health Services amendments in 1966, P.L. 89-749 (McCarthy and Jonas, 1986) in an attempt to develop a national health planning system. This was the law and provided grants for planning, development, and implementation of a variety of public health services.

The CHP amendments also provided a format for the development of later planning legislation. From the CHP experience, the states and federal government developed a method for organizing planning within states. Data on existing needs and resources were collected, procedures for reviewing facilities and program changes were established, and methods for cooperation between governmental and health care agencies were developed.

Although the CHP legislation proved inadequate for comprehensive health planning, the strengths of the planning legislation led Congress to pass the National Health Planning and Resources Development Act (P.L. 93-641) in 1974. This act was a landmark in health care legislation because of its specific directions regarding the structure, process, and functions of a national health planning system.

Although P.L. 93-641 provided a more comprehensive structure and more power over federal program funds than the CHP amendments of 1966, there still existed limited authority to carry out some of the more critical tasks of improving the health of residents, increasing accessibility and quality of services, restraining costs, and preventing unnecessary duplication of services. Power over the private health care sector continued to be essentially nonexistent.

As "new federalism" became the catch phrase of the 1980s and emphasis was placed on cost shifting, cost reduction, and more competition within the health care system, President Ronald Reagan proposed doing away with the federal government's role in health planning. In 1981, with cutbacks in federal spending, states began the takeover or dismantling of their own health planning systems as established under P.L. 93-641 (Institute for Health Planning, 1981). Today the national health planning system has come to a halt. The macrolevel federal, state, and consumer partnership for health is nonexistent.

The process of health planning today is in the control of hospitals, physicians, HMOs, pharmaceutical companies, equipment companies, and insurance companies (Kropf, 1990; Sofaer, 1988). The outcome of the national health planning effort is often influenced by the political party in power. The community health nurse must be involved in aspects of health planning for the community in which he or she lives.

In addition, internal health care agency planning is necessary to meet the goals and objectives of providing efficient, effective health care services to the consumer at reasonable cost. Pickett and Hanlon (1990) emphasized the responsibility of community health personnel to participate in internal planning and evaluation to solve the problems of a client population. Internal health care agency planning is often affected by the health care planning within the community as well as national health care planning.

BENEFITS OF PROGRAM PLANNING

Systematic planning for meeting client needs benefits clients, nurses, and the employing agencies. Planning focuses attention on what the organization and health provider are attempting to do for clients. Planning assists in identifying the resources and activities that are essential in meeting the objectives of client services. Planning reduces role ambiguity by assigning responsibility to specific providers to meet program objectives.

Planning also reduces uncertainty within the program environment and enhances the abilities of the provider and the agency to cope with the external environment. Everyone involved with the program can anticipate what will be needed to implement the program, what will occur during implementation, and what the program outcomes will be. Planning assists the provider and the agency to anticipate events. Finally, planning allows for quality decision making and better control over the actual program results. Today this type of planning is referred to as *strategic planning* and involves the successful matching of client needs with specific provider strengths and competencies and agency resources.

Planning usually reflects the planner's desire to reduce the gap between the program goals and the realities of program implementation and to minimize unanticipated occurrences during program implementation. Inherent in the planning process is the desire to implement a reality-based program that can be readily evaluated.

THE PLANNING PROCESS

Health program planning is affected by governmental control over licensure and funding, by the social structure, and by the cultural and belief system in which the program must function. Program planning is essential to meet federal, state, and local government mandates for funding, philanthropic organization funding guidelines, and internal organizational planning requirements.

Nutt (1984) describes a basic planning process that is reflected in the steps of most planning methods. The process includes five planning stages for program development: formulation, conceptualization, detailing, evaluation, and implementation (Table 12-1).

TABLE 12-1
Basic planning process

Basic planning	Elements
1. Formulation	Client identifies problems
2. Conceptualization	Provider group identifies possible solutions
3. Detailing	Client, provider analyze available solutions
4. Evaluation	Clients, providers, administrators select best plan
5. Implementation	Best plan presented to administrators for funding

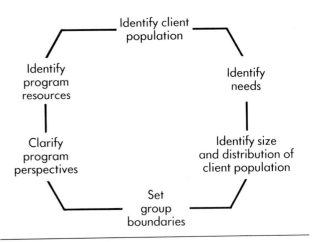

FIGURE 12-1

Steps in needs assessment process.

Formulation

The initial and most critical step in planning for a health program is defining the problem and assessing client need. This stage in the planning process can be *preactive*, projecting a future need; *reactive*, defining the problem based on past needs identified by the consumer or the sponsoring agency; *inactive*, defining the problem based on the existing health state of the population to be served; or *interactive*, describing the problem using past and present data to project future population needs (Achoff, 1982).

Program planners must verify the existence of a current health problem that is being ignored or being unsuccessfully treated in a client group. These data will provide the rationale to establish a new program or revise existing programs to meet the needs of the client group. The *assessment of need* is defined as a systematic appraisal of type, depth, and scope of problems as perceived by clients, health providers, or both.

The needs assessment process includes six steps (Figure 12-1): (1) identify the client population, (2) identify the needs to be met, (3) specify the size and distribution of the client population, (4) set boundaries for the client group, (5) clarify the perspectives on the program target, and (6) identify the program resources (Posavac and Carey, 1980; Rossi and Freeman, 1985).

The *client population* may be identified as a community or group, as families or individuals. The client population should be defined specifically by its biological and psychosocial characteristics, by geographical location, and by the problems to be addressed. For example, in a community with a large number of preschool children who require immunizations to enter school, the client population may be described as all children between the ages of 4 and 6 years residing in Central County who have not had up-to-date immunizations.

The *needs to be met* for the client population must be identified by both the client and by the health provider. *If the client population does not recognize the need, the program will usually fail.* A health education program may be necessary to alert the population to the existing need. In the example of the need for immunization of preschool children, public service announcements on television and radio and in newspapers may be used to alert parents to laws requiring immunizations, to the continued existence of communicable diseases, and to communicable diseases, such as smallpox,

that have been successfully eradicated by immunization programs. A good example of this is the 1990 outbreak of rubella in Los Angeles. Local and national television was used to bring attention to the problem, to encourage parents to have children immunized, and to encourage other communities to launch campaigns to prevent other outbreaks.

Specifying the size and distribution of a client population for a program involves more than counting the number of persons in the community who may be eligible for the program. The number of persons with the problem who are unserved by existing programs and the number of eligible persons who have and have not taken advantage of existing services must also be determined. In planning the preschool immunization program, the estimates of numbers of preschool children in the county may be obtained from census data or birth certificates. One then must determine the number of children unserved and the number of children who have not used services for which they are eligible.

Boundaries for the client population are primarily established by defining the size and distribution of the client population. The boundaries will stipulate who is included and who is excluded in the health program. If the immunization program was designed to serve only preschool children of low-income families, all other preschool children would be excluded.

Perspectives on the program might differ among health providers, agency administrators, policymakers, and potential clients. Collecting data on the opinions and attitudes of all persons directly or indirectly involved with the program's success is essential to determining the program's feasibility, the need to redefine the problems, or the decision to abandon a new program or expand an existing program. For example, policymakers in the 1970s determined that neighborhood health clinics were the answer to providing service for low-income residents. They discovered that their perspectives were not the same as most health providers or clients. The neighborhood health clinic concept failed. If the policy makers had explored the perspectives of the clients when planning the program, they might have chosen another option.

TABLE 12-2
Summary of needs assessment tools

Name	Definition	Advantages	Disadvantages
Community forum	Community, group, organization, open meeting	Low cost Learn perspectives of large number of persons	Limited data Limited expression of views Discourages less powerful Becomes arena to discuss political issues
Key informant	Identify, select, and question knowledgeable leaders	Provides picture of services needed	Bias of leaders Community characteristics may be incorrectly perceived by informants
Indicators approach	Existing data used to determine problem	Excellent data on problems and location of client groups Observations made at regular intervals show trends New problems can be identified	Data may be obsolete Growth and change in population may make data outdated
Survey of existing agencies	Estimates of client population via services used by similar community	Easy method to estimate size of client group Know extent of services offered in existing programs	Records and data may be unreliable All cases of need may not be reported Exaggeration of services may occur
Surveys/census	Measurement of total or sample client population by interview or questionnaire	Direct and accurate data on client population and their problems	Expensive Technically demanding Need large number of interviews or observations

Before implementing a health program, one must also *assess available resources*. Program resources include personnel, facilities, equipment, and financing. The numbers and kinds of personnel available to implement a program must be determined. The availability of supplies and up-to-date equipment is as essential a resource for implementing a program as are the source and amount of funds. If any one of the essential resources is unavailable, the program is likely to be inadequate to meet the needs of the client population.

Needs Assessment Tools

A number of tools exist to assist the program planner in the needs assessment process (see Chapter 16). The major tools, summarized in Table 12-2, used for needs assessment, are census data, key informants, community forums, surveys of existing community agencies with similar programs, surveys of residents of the community to be served (client population), and statistical indicators (Jury, 1984; Rossi and Freeman, 1985).

Conceptualization

The need and demand for a program are determined through the formulation process. This stage of planning creates options for solving the problem and considers several solutions. Each option for program solution is examined for its uncertainties and consequences leading to a set of outcomes.

When considering alternative solutions to the problem, some will have more risk or uncertainties than others. One must decide between the solution that involves more risk and the solution that is free of risk. A "do nothing" decision is always the decision with the least risk to the provider. When choosing a solution one looks at the probability of achieving the desired outcome. After careful thought about each possible solution to the problem, one should rethink the solutions (Behn and Vaupel, 1982). The information collected from census data, key informants, community forums, surveys of existing community agencies, and statistical indicators should be used to develop these alternative solutions.

Decision trees are useful graphical aids that will give a picture of the solutions and the consequences and risks of each. Such a pictorial graph of the process of identifying a solution helps clients and administrators to understand why one solution may be chosen over another. Figure 12-2 shows the process of conceptualization using a decision tree.

Although in this example the best consequence would be for families to provide for immunizations, one must consider the value of this action to the parents, the odds that immunizations will occur if a formal clinic is not established, the cost to the parents vs. the taxpayer, and the cost to the community. Costs to the community include the possibility of increased incidence of communicable disease or mortality, and increased need for more expensive services to treat

Solution	Alternatives	Uncertain risks	Consequences

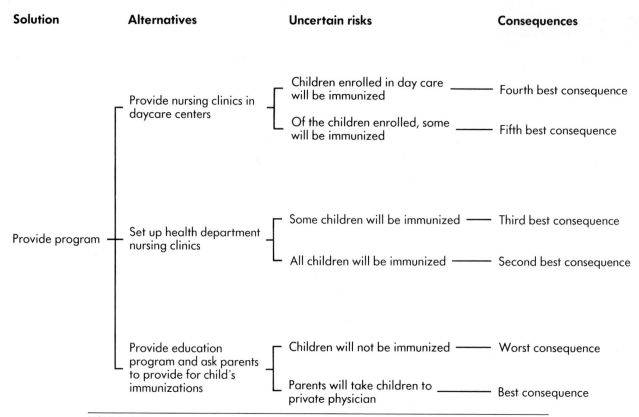

FIGURE 12-2

Ranking of solutions to problem: providing preschool immunization program to low-income children, using a decision tree.

the diseases if children are not immunized. If the parents provide the immunizations, costs to the taxpayer and to the community are low.

Detailing

In this phase the provider, with client input, determines the possibilities of solving a problem using one of the solutions identified. The provider details the costs, resources, and program activities needed to choose one of the solutions from the conceptualization phase. For each of the solutions the program planner must list activities that will need to be implemented to use one of the solutions. Examples of activities include developing a script for a health education program, implementing a TV program, offering a clinic 8 hours per day, and providing a mobile clinic to each day care center for 4 hours each day in order to provide the immunizations.

For each of the alternatives, the program planner lists the resources needed to implement each activity. The resources to be considered include all costs of personnel, supplies, equipment, facilities, and acceptability to the clients and the administrators of the program. Personnel could include nurses, volunteers, and clerks; supplies might include handouts, bandaids, medications, records, and consent forms; equipment might include syringes, needles, stethoscopes, and blood pressure cuffs; facilities might include a TV studio

for a media blitz on the education program, examination tables, chairs, and emergency carts. Finally, the costs of each solution must be considered by determining the costs of personnel, supplies, equipment, and facilities for each solution. As indicated, clients should review each solution for acceptability to them.

Evaluation

In the evaluative phase each alternative would be weighed to judge the costs, benefits, and acceptability to the client, community, and provider. The information outlined in the detailing phase would be used to rank the solutions for choice by client and provider based on cost, benefit, and acceptance. Consideration must be given to the solution that will provide the desired outcomes. Looking at available information might suggest whether each of the options had been tried before in another place or by someone else. The results from other sources would be helpful in deciding whether a chosen solution would be useful.

Implementation

In the implementation phase the clients, providers, and administrators select the best plan to solve the original problem. In this phase change theory is useful to help to create an environment in which the best solution may be supported by funding. Providing reasons why a particular solution was

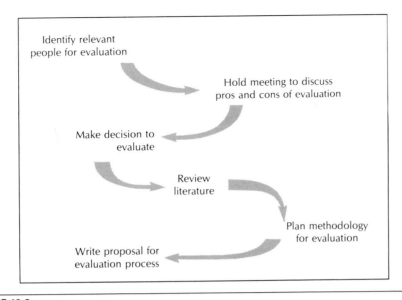

FIGURE 12-3

Six steps in planning for program evaluation.

chosen will help the provider to get the approval of the administration for the plan. Involving clients and administrators throughout the planning process will help to promote acceptance of the plan.

PROGRAM EVALUATION
Benefits of Program Evaluation

The major benefit of *program evaluation* is that it determines and demonstrates whether the program is fulfilling its purpose. It should answer the questions: Are the needs for which the program was designed being met? Are the problems it was designed to solve being solved? This is critical information for funding agencies, top-level decision makers, accreditation reviews, and the community-at-large. Evaluation data may be used to justify expanding the program, reducing the program, or even closing it.

Planning for the Evaluative Process

Planning for the evaluative process is an integral part of program planning. Program evaluation begins with the initial program planning phase, as formative evaluation is the assessment of need. The basic questions to be answered, after careful consideration of the data collected from census, key informants, community forums, surveys, or health statistics indicators are: Will the objectives and resources of this program meet the identified needs of the client population? Is the program relevant? Once need has been established and the planning process for designing the program has been instituted, the community health nurse must plan for program evaluation. As a part of the planning process, Posavac and Carey (1980) describe six steps to use for program evaluation (Figure 12-3).

The *first step* is to identify the relevant people for evaluation. Program personnel, program sponsors, and the clients of the program should be included in planning for evaluation.

The *second step* is to arrange preliminary meetings to discuss the questions of whether the group wants an evaluation, and if so, why, what kind, and when. If the program planners and others agree on an evaluation, the resources for conducting the program evaluation must be identified. It should be noted that evaluation is necessary even though some may not be interested in it. Community health nurses can be instrumental in helping others to see that without evaluation money to support programs will not be available or need for a new nurse to help with the work cannot be justified.

The *third step* comes after the relevant people have met and considered the questions in the previous steps. They are ready to decide whether the evaluation should be carried out. Even though evaluation may be desired, the decision to conduct the evaluation may be an administrative one, based on availability of resources, or determined by the existing circumstances. For example, if a program evaluation were attempted in a situation where program personnel wanted it and clients chose to be uncooperative, evaluation efforts would fail.

The *fourth step* is to examine the literature for suggestions about the appropriate methods and techniques and their usefulness in program evaluation. This step is particularly helpful if the organization has chosen an evaluator who is external to the program. If the evaluation is internal, the evaluators may be familiar with the literature.

The external evaluator may make suggestions regarding the questions to be answered in the evaluation process. If the literature has been reviewed by the community health nurse and others affected by the evaluation, they can determine whether the evaluation suggestions are appropriate for their situation.

The *fifth step* is to plan the methodology, including decisions about what items will be measured, how they will be measured, and on what population.

The *sixth* and final step is to write a proposal that outlines the purpose and goals of the overall program, the type of evaluation to be done, the operational measure to be used to evaluate the program goals, the choice of internal or external evaluators, the available resources for conducting the evaluation, and the readiness of the organization, personnel, and clients for program evaluation.

Types of Evaluation

The types of program evaluation include the following: (1) evaluation of *relevance,* the need for the program; (2) *progress,* the tracking of program activities to meet program objectives; (3) *efficiency,* the relationship between program outcomes and the resources expended; (4) *effectiveness,* the ability to meet program objectives and the results of program efforts; and (5) *impact,* the long-term changes in the client population (Kaluzny and Veney, 1984).

Relevance. Evaluation of relevance is an important component of the initial planning phase. As money, providers, facilities, and supplies for delivering health care services are more closely monitored, the automatic assumption that all health care delivery programs are needed is an error. The needs assessment done by the community health nurse will determine whether the program is needed.

Progress. The monitoring of program activities, such as hours of services, numbers of providers used, numbers of referrals made, and amount of money spent to meet program objectives, provides an *evaluation of the progress* of the program. This type of evaluation is an example of *formative evaluation* and occurs on an ongoing basis while the program is in existence. This provides an opportunity to make effective day-to-day management decisions about the operations of the program. Progress evaluation occurs primarily during implementation. The community health nurse who completes a daily or weekly log of clinical activities (i.e., number of clients seen in clinic or visited at home, number of phone contacts, number of referrals made) is contributing to progress evaluation of the nursing service.

Efficiency. If the reason for evaluation is to examine the *efficiency* of a program, it may occur on an ongoing basis as *formative evaluation* or at the completion of the program as a *summative evaluation.* The evaluator may be able to determine whether the program provides better benefits at a lower cost than a similar program or whether the benefits to the clients or numbers of clients served justify the cost of the program.

Effectiveness and Impact. An *evaluation of effectiveness* may help the community health nurse evaluator determine both client and provider satisfaction with the program activities, as well as whether the program met its stated objectives. However, if *evaluation of impact* is the goal, then long-term effects, such as changes in morbidity and mortality, must be investigated. Both effectiveness and impact evaluations are usually *summative evaluation* functions primarily performed as end-of-program activities.

The Evaluative Process

The evaluative process described by Suchman (1967) is modified and explained here. It is very similar to steps in the planning process. The first step in the evaluative process is *goal setting.* The value and beliefs of the agency, the

providers, and the clients provide the basis for goal setting and should be considered at every step of the evaluation process. The fact that children should not be exposed to early childhood diseases would lead to a program goal to decrease the incidence of early childhood diseases in the county where the program is planned.

The second step is *determining goal measurement.* In the case of the previous goal, disease incidence would be an appropriate goal measurement. The third step is *identifying goal-attaining activities.* This would include such activities as media presentations urging parents to have their children immunized. The fourth step is *making the activities operational,* i.e., actually administering the immunizations. The fifth step is *measuring the goal effect,* which consists of reviewing the records and summarizing the incidence of early childhood disease before and after the program. The final step is *evaluation of the program,* determining whether the program goal was achieved. Keep in mind that only one program goal is used in this example. Most programs have multiple goals (Figure 12-4).

Formulation of Objectives

The most important step in the evaluative process is the formulation of program objectives. The objectives set the stage for conducting the program and provide the mechanism for evaluating the activities and the total program. The following discussion will help in the development of clear, concise objectives. Development of program objectives coincides with the initial phases of program planning.

Specification of Objectives (Goals). If the objectives are too general, program evaluation becomes impossible. The objectives must be specific and stated so that anyone reading them could conduct the program without further instruction. To be truly effective, objectives must be very specific and should begin with a general program goal and move on to specific objectives that will help meet the program goal.

Shortell (1978) indicates that useful program objectives include a statement of the specific behaviors, accomplishments, and success criteria for the program. Each program objective requires a strong, action-oriented verb to specify the behavior, a statement of a single purpose, a statement of a single result, and a time frame for achieving the expected result. For example, a program objective that meets these criteria may be to decrease (action verb) the incidence of early childhood disease in Center County (result) by providing immunization clinics in all schools (purpose) between August and December of 1994 (time frame).

As objectives are developed, an operational indicator for each objective should be considered so the evaluator knows when and if the objective has been met. For instance, an operational indicator for the above objective would be: a 10% to 25% decrease in the incidence rates of the most commonly occurring childhood vaccine-preventable illnesses in Center County. Such indicators provide a target for persons involved with program implementation.

Levels of Program Objectives. It is customary for objectives to be stated in levels from general to specific. The first level consists of general and broad objectives that are sometimes called goals. Their purpose is to focus on the major reason for the program.

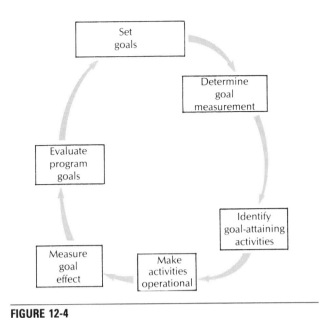

FIGURE 12-4

The evaluative process.

A *general program objective (goal)* may be to reduce the incidence of low-birth-weight babies in Center County in 1995 by improving access to prenatal care. The specific objectives, or subgoals, describe a measurable behavior, the circumstances under which the behavior is observed, and the minimal acceptable standard for the performance of the behavior. A specific objective for this program may be to open a prenatal clinic in each health department within the county by January 1992 to serve the population within each census tract of the county.

Specific program activities are then planned to meet each specific objective; resources, like number of nurses, equipment, supplies, and location, are planned for each of the objectives. It is assumed that as each specific objective is met, the general program objective will also be achieved. Remember that several specific objectives are required to meet a general program objective or goal.

Sources of Program Evaluation

Major sources of information for program evaluation are program participants, program records, and community indexes. The program participants, or consumers of the service, have a unique and valuable role in program evaluation. Whether the clients, for whom the program was designed, accept the services will determine to a large extent whether the program achieves its purpose. Thus, their reactions, feelings, and judgements about the program are very important to the evaluation.

To assess the response of participants in a program, the evaluator may use a written survey in the form of a questionnaire or an attitude scale. Interviews and observations are other ways of obtaining feedback about a program. Attitude scales are probably used most often, and they are usually phrased in terms of whether the program met its objectives. The client satisfaction survey is an example of an attitude scale often used in the health care delivery system

to evaluate the attainment of program objectives (see Appendix A1).

The second major source of information for program evaluation is program records, especially clinical records. Clinical records provide the evaluator with information about the care given to the client and the results of that care. To determine whether a program goal has been met one might summarize the data from a group of records. For example, if one overall goal is to reduce the incidence of low-birth-weight babies through prenatal care, records would be reviewed to obtain the number of mothers who received prenatal care and the number of low-birth-weight babies born to them.

A third major source of evaluation is community indexes. Doster (1979, p. 79) defines a *health index* as a "summary of the health features of a community that enable us to determine health care delivery needs." Doster further divides the health index into six categories: definition of community, people, environment, communication, health and illness indicators, and health provider resources and services. However, the evaluator must examine the community indexes in light of other variables or events in the community that may also affect the achievement of the program's purpose.

Health and illness indicators, such as mortality and morbidity data, are probably cited more frequently than any other single index for program evaluation. Health and illness indicators are useful in evaluating the impact of health care programs. Incidence and prevalance are also valuable indexes used to measure program effectiveness and impact (see Chapter 9 for further discussion of rates and ratios).

COST STUDIES APPLIED TO PROGRAM MANAGEMENT

Although cost must be considered in planning and evaluating, it is particularly significant in programs involving nursing services. The major types of cost studies primarily applied in the health care industry are cost accounting, cost benefit, cost efficiency, and cost effectiveness studies. A discussion of types of cost studies is presented to give the reader an idea of the kinds of questions that can be answered with such studies. Nurses must be willing to answer these questions to help show the actual costs of nursing programs and the relevance of the program to the clients it served.

Cost Accounting

Cost accounting studies are performed to find the actual cost of a program. A question answered by this method could be, "What is the cost of providing a family planning program in Anytown, USA?" To answer the question, the total costs of equipment, facilities (rental), personnel (salaries and benefits), and supplies used over a period of time are calculated. The total program costs are divided by the number of clients participating in the program during that time. The total program cost per client is the end product. Thus, a cost accounting study can provide data about total program costs and about total cost per client, which makes program management easier. A simple example of cost accounting is what one does each month when balancing a checkbook. One looks at the costs of providing food, shelter, and clothing for a family vs. the family income.

Cost Benefit

Cost benefit studies are a way of assessing the desirability of a program by placing a specific dollar amount on all costs and benefits. If benefits outweigh the costs, then the program is said to have a *net positive impact*. The major problem with cost benefit analysis is placing a quantifiable value on all benefits of the program. The question is, can a dollar value be placed on human life, on safety, on the relief of pain and suffering, or on prevention of illness? These are all program benefits. If an attempt is made to perform cost benefit analysis of a hospice program, can a dollar amount be placed on the family and client support and comfort provided or on the relief of pain of the terminally ill? Can such benefits be weighed against costs to justify continuing the program? Or should the program be continued in spite of costs?

It is recognized that public health programs have net positive impacts because preventing morbidity with illness-prevention programs such as hypertension screenings averts or reduces the future cost of chronic long-term illnesses like stroke or cardiovascular disease. To initiate a cost benefit study for a program, it must be decided which costs and which benefits are to be included, how the costs and benefits are to be valued, and what constraints are to be considered — legal, ethical, social, and economic. For example, in a home health care program funded by the state health department to offer care to AIDS clients, the mortality rate would continue to be high because a cure is not available. Would the program be considered to have a low cost benefit ratio (negative impact) because clients cannot be cured? The program would be considered to have a high cost benefit ratio (positive net impact) if the cost of home health care services was less expensive than providing similar care in the hospital. The benefits of the program would include the reduction in costs to the client and reduction in need for hospital services (Rossi and Freeman, 1985).

Cost Effectiveness

Cost effectiveness analysis, a measure of the quality of a program as it relates to cost, is the most frequently used analysis in nursing. Cost effectiveness is a subset of cost benefit analysis and is designed to provide an estimate of costs incurred in achieving a given outcome. A cost effectiveness study can answer several questions: did the program meet its objectives? were the clients and nurses satisfied with the effects of the interventions? Are things better as a result of the interventions? (Kaluzny and Veney, 1984). In cost benefit analysis both costs and outcomes are quantitative, whereas in cost effectiveness analysis the outcomes are qualitative. Outcome measures addressed by cost effectiveness might be increased client knowledge after health teaching, changes in client's condition after treatment, differences in graduates of two nursing programs with similar goals, and the ability of two hearing screening programs to detect hearing loss.

A cost effectiveness study requires collection of baseline data on clients before the program is implemented and evaluation after the program is completed. The boxed material below shows the procedure for completing a cost effectiveness study.

STEPS IN COST EFFECTIVENESS ANALYSIS

Step I	Identify the program goals or client outcome to be achieved.
Step II	Identify at least two alternative means of achieving the desired outcomes.
Step III	Collect baseline data on clients.
Step IV	Determine the costs associated with each program activity.
Step V	Determine the activities each group of clients will receive.
Step VI	Determine the client changes after the activities are completed.
Step VII	Combine the costs (Step IV), amount of activity (Step V), and outcome information (Step VI) to express costs relative to outcomes of program goals.
Step VIII	Compare cost outcome information for each goal to present cost effectiveness analysis.

There are several potential outcomes of a cost effectiveness study. For example, a community health nurse is interested in comparing two methods for implementing a program to teach diabetic clients self-care techniques. The nurse chooses self-teaching modules and a group formal instruction program for comparison. There are several potential outcomes of comparing the two teaching methods. Of the potential outcomes in a cost effectiveness study, the program of choice would be the most effective teaching method for the least cost. However, if the most costly program demonstrates superior effectiveness it may be chosen. If the least costly program is of poor quality, a more costly program would be appropriate.

Cost Efficiency

Cost efficiency analysis is the actual cost of performing a number of program services. To determine cost efficiency of a program, its productivity must be analyzed. Productivity is the relationship between what the nurse does and how much it costs for him or her to do it.

To determine the nurse's activities with a group of clients, one is primarily concerned with a nurse's workload, including direct client care and indirect care activities such as charting, phone calls, client care conferences, and travel. The functions are then related to the client load, client need, and the number of nurses available to meet the needs of all clients served by a program.

Figure 12-5 shows an example of the cost efficiency of a home health agency. The graph indicates that as the number of client visits per year increases, the cost per client visit decreases. The graph assumes that the number of nurses from the beginning to the end of the time period is the same, that the nurses' workloads were essential to provide home health services, that caseloads were assigned based on staff mix and client need, and that organizational structure was conducive to nurses being highly productive.

All cost studies have three major tasks: financial, research, and statistical. The financial tasks involve identi-

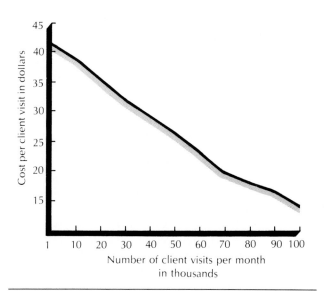

FIGURE 12-5

Cost per client visit at home health agency.

fying total program costs and breaking them down into smaller parts. To identify the costs of a nurse's participation in a teaching program, the costs for facilities, equipment, supplies, and salaries would have to be examined. All costs associated with the program, such as the nurse's time and use of facilities, equipment, and supplies, should be compared to the total program costs. The statistical tasks involve the identification of appropriate quantifiable measures for analyzing data, and the research tasks involve setting up an appropriate study design to answer the questions of benefit, efficiency, or effectiveness.

Nurses with varying educational backgrounds may be involved in cost studies with the assistance of people knowledgeable in research statistics and accounting techniques. Nurses with undergraduate degrees may be involved in the actual implementation of a cost study, whereas nurses with graduate degrees may be involved in planning, designing, implementing, analyzing, and evaluating study results related to program management.

Cost studies are essential to show the worth of nursing in the marketplace of the future and nurses should be familiar with the results of cost studies so that sound decisions may be made about future program management. Nurses must be ready to identify appropriate program outcomes, client outcomes, total dimensions of roles of graduates, and total dimensions of nursing procedures so that appropriate decisions about program management will be made based on adequate information.

CLINICAL APPLICATION

The following is a real-life example of the application of the program management process by an undergraduate community health nursing student. This activity resulted in the development and implementation of a nurse-managed clinic for the homeless. This example shows how students as well as providers can make a difference in health care delivery. It also shows that there is no mystique in the program management process.

Eva was listening to the radio one Sunday afternoon, only to hear an announcement about the opening of a soup kitchen within the community for the growing homeless population. She was beginning her community health nursing course and wanted to find a creative clinical experience that would benefit herself as well as others.

The announcement gave her an idea. Although it mentioned food, clothing, shelter, and social services, nothing was said about health care. She contacted the pastor of the church who was planning to open the soup kitchen to discuss the issue *(formulation and assessment)*. She found him most receptive to the idea of developing a solution to the health care needs of the homeless. In her assessment, Eva found that no other health services were available to the homeless in the community. She looked at national data to estimate needs and size of the population. She talked with the community health nursing faculty to discuss potential solutions to the problem. She talked to members of the homeless population to get their perceptions of their needs.

Upon completing her assessment she *conceptualized* the solutions. Several solutions were possible: work with the health department, attempt to provide better care through the local medical center, or open a clinic on site at the soup kitchen where most of the people gathered, so that transportation would not be a problem.

After considering the solutions she *detailed* the plan looking at the resources needed for opening a clinic at the soup kitchen. She considered supplies, equipment, facilities, and acceptability to the clients. She also considered the time involved, the activities required to implement a program, and funding sources.

In *evaluating* the possibilities she considered the cost, the client and community benefits, and acceptability to clients, self, faculty, and the church. Although it would have been easier for her to choose to work with the health department or the medical center, she knew that the solution most acceptable to the clients would be to have a clinic located at the soup kitchen. The clinic would be more accessible, transportation would not be needed, and health services through the clinic could possibly prevent more costly hospital and emergency care (value).

Eva presented her plan to the faculty and the church. She convinced them that it would not be a costly endeavor. She had nurses in the community who volunteered to help, she had a carpenter who would donate his time to build an examining room in the back of the soup kitchen, and she had equipment promised to her by community physicians. The client assessment indicated that a first-aid and health assessment clinic was what was needed most. With approval from all, *(implementation)* Eva began the clinic in 1981 seeing 25 to 35 clients a week, 1 hour per day for 5 days per week.

Eva evaluated the *relevance* of the program via the needs assessment process. She tracked the *progress* of the program by keeping records of her activities. She kept track of the resources in relation to the number of persons served *(efficiency)* and used this data to convince the church and the College of Nursing to fund the ongoing clinic operation after she graduated. A *summative evaluation* of the clinic was completed by the faculty at the end of 4 years. The program's *impact* was outstanding. The clinic had grown. The client demand was high, most of the health problems could be handled at the clinic, which eliminated the cost burden to the community for more expensive health care, and it was highly acceptable to the clients *(effectiveness)*. This clinic began as a service to 25 people for 1 hour per day. Today this clinic is open all day, 5 days per week, has over 900 clients per year, and provides for over 5000 client visits per year. The success of this clinic shows the effect one community health nursing student can have on a community.

SUMMARY

Planning programs and planning for the evaluation of programs are two of the most important activities for community health nurses to ensure successful program implementation. Whether the program being planned is a national health insurance program like Medicare, a state health care program like early childhood developmental screening programs, or a local program like vision screening for elementary school children, the essential elements of planning are applicable.

Needs assessment is a key ingredient in the planning process. The target population for any program must be identified and involved in program development. If the client population does not recognize the need for a health services program, that program is destined to fail regardless of the commitment of health providers and the program's resources.

A number of tools are available for assisting planners in needs assessment. Some of the major tools used for needs assessment are census data, key informants, community forums, surveys of existing community agencies, surveys of community residents, and statistical indicators.

Several procedural methods can be applied to plan program offerings. A few of these methods are the Planning, Programming, and Budgeting System; Program Evaluation Review Technique; the Critical Path Method; the Multi-Attribute Utility Method; and the Program Planning Method (see Appendix L).

The application of the planning process to program development is an indication that the planners wish to reduce the gap between program goals and the realities of program implementation and the likelihood of unanticipated occurrences during program implementation.

When plans for program implementation are being developed, the plan for program evaluation should also be developed. All persons involved in program implementation should be a part of the plan for program evaluation. The major benefit of program evaluation is to determine whether the program is fulfilling its stated goals. Quality assurance programs are prime examples of program evaluation in health care delivery. Evaluation data are used to justify the continued existence of programs in community health.

Program evaluation focuses on goal attainment and the efficiency and effectiveness of program activities. Many methods of program evaluation are described in the literature. The primary method of evaluation used in health care today is Donabedian's Evaluative Framework. The systems model, tracer method, and case register are other methods applied to program evaluation (see Appendix L).

Program records and community indexes serve as the major source of information for program evaluation. Surveys, interviews, observations, and tests are ways to assess consumer and participant response to health programs. Cost studies help identify program benefits and effectiveness.

Planning for the evaluative process is an integral part of program planning and should not be initiated after the program has been in operation for several months. As economic resources become scarce, nursing and the health care system must be able to justify their existence, prove that their services are responsive to consumer needs, and show their professional concern for accountability. Planning and evaluation will assist in meeting these objectives.

KEY CONCEPTS

Planning and evaluation are essential elements of program management and vital to the survival of the nursing discipline in health care delivery.

A program is an organized response designed to meet the assessed needs of individuals, families, groups, or communities by reducing or eliminating one or more health problems.

Planning is defined as selecting and carrying out a series of actions designed to achieve a stated goal.

Evaluation is defined as the methods used to determine if a service is needed and will be used, whether a program to meet that need is carried out as planned, and whether the service actually helps the people it intended to help.

To develop quality programs, planning should include four essential elements: problem diagnosis and assessment of need, identification of problem solutions, analysis and comparison of alternative methods, and selection of the best plan and planning methods.

The initial and most critical step in planning a health program is assessment of need.

Some of the major tools used in needs assessment are census data, community forums, surveys of existing community agencies, surveys of community residents, and statistical indicators.

The major benefit of program evaluation is to determine whether a program is fulfilling its stated goals. Quality assurance programs are prime examples of program evaluation.

Plans for program implementation and program evaluation should be developed at the same time.

Program records and community indexes serve as major sources of information for program evaluation.

Planning programs and planning for their evaluation are two of the most important ways in which community health nurses can ensure successful program implementation.

Cost studies help identify program management benefits, effectiveness, and efficiency.

LEARNING ACTIVITIES

1. Choose the definitions that best describe your concept of programs, planning, and evaluation.

2. Apply the program planning process to an identified clinical problem for a client group with whom you are working in the community.
   a. Assess the client need.
   b. Choose tools appropriate to the assessment of needs.
   c. Analyze the overall planning process of arriving at decisions about program implementation.
   d. Summarize the benefits for program planning that are applicable to your situation.

3. Given the situation just described, choose three or four of your classmates to work with on the following projects.
   a. Plan for evaluation of the above program.
   b. Apply the evaluative process to the situation.
   c. Name the measures you will use to gather data for evaluating your program.
   d. Name the sources you will tap to gain information for program evaluation.
   e. Analyze the benefits of program evaluation that are applicable to your situation.

4. Talk with a community health nurse or administrator about the application of program planning and evaluation processes at the local agency. Compare their answers to your readings.

BIBLIOGRAPHY

Achoff R: Our changing concept of planning, J Nurs Adm 35:40, 1982.

Anderson O: Influence of social and economic research on public policy in the health field: a review, Milbank Mem Fund Q 44:11, 1966.

Barentson P: Critical path planning: present and future technique, Princeton, NJ, 1970, Brendon Systems Press.

Begley C et al: Evaluation of a primary health care program for the poor, Community Health 14(2):107, 1989.

Behin R and Vapel J: Quick analysis for busy decision makers, New York, 1982, Basic Books.

Blaney D and Hobson C: Cost-effective nursing practice: guidelines for nurse managers, Philadelphia, 1988, JB Lippincott Co.

Bloch D: Interrelated issues in evaluation and evaluation research, Nurs Res 29(69):69-73, 1980.

Budgen C: Modeling a method for program development, J Nurs Adm 17(12):19, Dec 1987.

Clemmesen J: Registration in the study of human cancer. In Holland WW and Karhausen L, editors: Health care and epidemiology, Boston, 1979, GK Hall & Co.

Commission on Hospital Care: Hospital care in the United States, New York, 1947, The Commonwealth Fund.

Committee on the Costs of Medical Care: Medical care for the American people, Chicago, 1932, University of Chicago Press. Reprinted, Washington, DC, 1970, Department of Health, Education, and Welfare.

Dean D et al: A report of a collaborative process between a university and a church, Family and Community Health 10(4):13, 1988.

Delbecq A and Van de Ven A: A group process model for problem identification and program planning, J Appl Behav Sci 7(4):466-492, 1971.

Donabedian A: Explorations in quality assessment and monitoring, vol 2, Ann Arbor, Mich, 1982, Health Administration Press.

Doster C: Health index of a community. In Community health today and tomorrow, NLN Pub No 52-1768, New York, 1979, National League for Nursing.

Downey A et al: Health promotion model for 'heart smart': the medical school, university, and community, Health Values 13(6):31, 1989.

Edwards W, Guttentag M, and Snapper K: A decision-theoretic approach to evaluation research. In Struening E and Guttentag M, editors: Handbook of evaluative research, Beverly Hills, Calif, 1975, Sage Publications Inc.

Fagin C: Strategic planning—outline of plan, J Prof Nurs 3(2):79, 1987.

Fralic M: Using a PERT planning network to manage a nursing service computer system installation, J Nurs Adm 29-31, 1984.

Friedman L et al: Cost-effectiveness of a self-care program, Nurs Econ 6(4):173, 1988.

Hargreaves M et al: Changing community health behaviors: a model for program development and management, Health Values 10(6):34, 1986.

Hegyvary ST: An evaluator's perspective, Nurs Res 29:91, 1980.

Helbig D, O'Hare D, and Smith N: The care component core—a new system for evaluating quality of inpatient care, Am J Pub Health 62:540-546, 1972.

Horwitz O: Epidemiological parameters for public health evaluation of a chronic disease. In Holland WW and Karhausen L, editors: Health care and epidemiology, Boston, 1979, GK Hall & Co.

Johnson J et al: Writing a winning business plan, J Nurs Adm 18(10):15, 1988.

Jones K: Feasibility analysis of preferred provider organizations, J Nurs Adm 20(1):28, 1990.

Jury J: Practical tips for establishing a coordinated community wellness program, Health Values 8(5):3-5, 1984.

Kaluzny A and Veney J: Evaluating health care programs and services. In Williams S and Torrens P, editors: Introduction to health services, New York, 1984, John Wiley & Sons Inc.

Keil U: Community registers of myocardial infarction as an example of epidemiological register studies. In Holland WW and Karhausen L, editors: Health care and epidemiology, Boston, 1979, GK Hall & Co.

Kessner DM and Kalk CE: Contrasts in health status: a strategy for evaluating health services, vol 2, Washington, DC, 1973, Institute of Medicine, National Academy of Sciences.

Kropf R: Planning for health services. In Kovner A, editor: Health care delivery in the United States, New York, 1990, Springer Publishing Co Inc.

Krueger JC: Establishing priorities for evaluation and evaluation research, Nurs Res 29:115, 1980.

Litwack L, Linc L, and Bower D: Evaluation in nursing: principles and practice, New York, 1985, National League for Nursing.

Lowe J et al: Quality assurance methods for managing employee health-promotion programs: a case study in smoking cessation, Health Values 13(2):1, 1989.

Lukas J: Strategic planning in hospital: applications for nurse executives, J Nurs Adm 11-17, 1984.

Martin J: The array of community services for people with AIDS, Caring 8(11):18, 1989.

McAlvanah M: Long range planning—who has the time? Pediatr Nursing 14(3):247, 1988.

McCarthy C and Jonas S: Planning for health services. In Jonas S, editor: Health care delivery in the United States, ed 2, New York, 1981, Springer Publishing Co Inc.

Morris F: A comparison of three allied health manpower projection methodologies, J Allied Health 16(1):59, February 1987.

Nash M: Strategic planning: the practical vision, J Nurs Adm 18(4):12, 1988.

Nutt P: Planning methods for health and related organizations, New York, 1984, John Wiley & Sons Inc.

Pentz M: Community organizations and school liaisons: how to get programs started, J Sch Health 56(9):382, 1986.

Phaneuf MC: Future direction for evaluation and evaluation research in health care, Nurs Res 29:123, 1980.

Posavac EJ and Carey RG: Program evaluation: methods and case studies, Englewood Cliffs, NJ, 1980, Prentice Hall Press.

Public Law 89-749: Comprehensive health planning and public services amendments of 1966, Nov 3, 1966.

Public Law 79-725: Hospital survey and construction act, Aug 13, 1946.

Public Law 93-641: National health planning and resources development act, Jan 4, 1975.

Roman D: The PERT system: an appraisal of program evaluation review technique. In Schulberg H, Sheldon A, and Baker F, editors: Program evaluation in the health fields, New York, 1969, Behavioral Publications Inc.

Rossi P and Freeman H: Evaluation: a systematic approach, Beverly Hills, Calif, 1985, Sage Publications Inc.

Schultz P and Magilvy J: Assessing community health needs of elderly populations: comparison on three strategies, J Adv Nurs 13(2):193, March 1988.

Shortell S and Richardson W: Health program evaluation, St Louis, 1978, The CV Mosby Co.

Smith J and Sorrell V: Developing wellness programs: a nurse-managed stay well center for senior citizens, Clin Nurse Specialist 3(4):198, 1989.

Sofaer S: Community health planning in the US: a post mortem, Family and Community Health 10(4):1, 1988.

Suchman EA: Evaluative research, New York, 1967, Russell Sage Foundation.

US Division of Health and Human Services: Program management: a guide for improving program decisions, Atlanta, 1989, Centers for Disease Control.

Valdiserri R: Applying the criteria for the development of health promotion and education programs to AIDS risk reduction programs for gay men, J Community Health 12(4):199, Winter 1987.

Veney J and Kaluzny A: Evaluation and decision making for health service programs, Englewood Cliffs, NJ, 1984, Prentice Hall Press.

Warner K and Luce B: Cost-benefit and cost-effectiveness analysis in health care, Ann Arbor, Mich, 1982, Health Administration Press.

Wiest J and Levy F: A management guide to PERT.CPM, Englewood Cliffs, NJ, 1969, Prentice Hall Press.

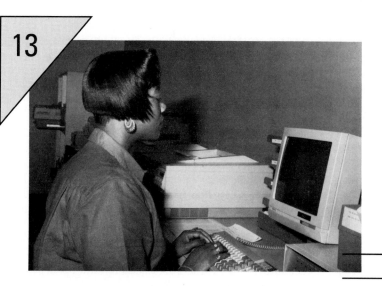

13

Promoting Quality in Community Health Nursing

Marcia Stanhope

OBJECTIVES

After reading this chapter, the student should be able to:

Define quality assurance.
State the goals of quality assurance and record keeping.
Discuss the historical development of quality assurance in nursing.
Evaluate approaches and techniques for implementing a quality assurance program.
Describe a model quality assurance program.
Identify the purposes for the types of records kept in community health agencies.
Explain a method for documentation of client care in community health nursing.

KEY TERMS

accountability	institutional licensure	provider service records
accreditation	licensure	
audit process	malpractice litigation	quality assurance
certification	mandatory nurse licensure	quasi-voluntary
competitive medical plans	permissive licensure	reciprocity
concurrent audit	Phaneuf Nursing Audit	retrospective audit
evaluative studies	Professional Review Organizations (PROs)	staff review committees
health maintenance organizations	Professional Standards Review Organization (PSRO)	utilization review
		voluntary credentialing

*Contents in this chapter may reflect contributions by Kathleen Blomquist from edition 2 of this text.

T oday's society demands greater accountability and increased efficiency and effectiveness from the health care system. Quality assurance, or quality control, is the tool used to assure the public that it is getting top value for money spent.

Both consumers and providers have a vested interest in the quality of the system. According to Jonas (1986), the health care provider has three basic reasons to be concerned about health care quality:

1. The principle of nonmaleficence—above all, do no harm—has been a basic principle of the health care system since the writing of the Hippocratic Oath.
2. The principle of beneficence—do good work—is a basic principle of professionalism.
3. The strong social work ethic in our culture, which places a high value on "doing a good job in and of itself."

Jonas says that in health care there is a direct link between doing a good job and individual and professional survival.

Objective and systematic evaluation of nursing care has become a priority within the nursing profession because of prospective payment mechanisms and consumer demands for quality nursing. Nursing's commitment to direct accountability, its evolution as a scientific discipline, and concerns about how costs of health services limit access, demand quality assurance (Lang and Clinton, 1984; Maciorowski, Larson, and Keane, 1985).

Records are maintained on all clients of the health care system to provide complete information about the client and to show the quality of care being given to the client within the system. Records are a necessary part of a quality assurance program, as are the tools and methods for evaluating quality.

DEFINITIONS AND GOALS

Quality assurance is the promise or guarantee that certain standards of excellence are being met in care delivered (Lalonde, 1988). The quality assurance or quality control process (1) sets standards for care, (2) evaluates care provided, based on the standards, and (3) takes action to bring about change when care does not meet standards (Bull, 1985; Maibusch, 1984). Quality assurance is concerned with the accountability of the provider. *Accountability* means being responsible for care and answerable to the client (Meisenheimer, 1989).

The goals of quality assurance are (1) to ensure the delivery of quality client care and (2) to demonstrate the efforts of the health provider to provide the best possible results (Jonas, 1986). The process of health care includes two major components: technical interventions and interpersonal relationships between practitioner and client. Both are important in providing quality care, and both can be evaluated (Donabedian, 1985). A variety of approaches and techniques are used in quality assurance programs. Approaches are methods used to ensure quality, and techniques are tools for measuring quality (Weitzman, 1990).

Although the term *quality assurance* has traditionally been used, it has recently been called into question, as one cannot actually assure or guarantee quality. Newer terminology designed to more accurately reflect the nature of such activities includes *quality management* or *quality improvement*. However, because these terms are not yet in widespread use, this chapter will continue to use the traditional terminology.

HISTORICAL DEVELOPMENT OF QUALITY ASSURANCE IN NURSING AND HEALTH CARE

Quality assurance approaches have been evident in nursing since the days of Florence Nightingale. In 1860 Nightingale called for the development of a uniform method to collect and present hospital statistics to improve hospital treatment. Nightingale was a pioneer in setting standards for nursing care. The impetus for establishing nursing schools in the United States came in the late 1800s from a desire to set standards that would upgrade nursing care. In the early 1900s efforts were begun to set similar standards for all nursing schools. From 1912 to 1939 the interest in quality nursing education led to the development of nursing organizations involved in accrediting nursing programs. Licensure has been a major issue in nursing since 1892. By 1923 all states had permissive or mandatory laws directing nursing practice.

After World War II the attention of the emerging nursing profession focused on establishing a scientific method of practice. The nursing process was the chosen method and included evaluation of how the activities of nurses helped clients (Maibusch, 1984). Quality assurance involves the evaluative step in the nursing process.

The 1950s brought the development of tools to measure quality assurance. One of the first tools created was the *Phaneuf Nursing Audit* (1952, 1965), which has been used extensively in community health nursing practice.

In 1966 the American Nurses Association (ANA) created the Divisions on Practice in its bylaws. As a result of this, in 1972 the Congress for Nursing Practice was charged with developing standards to be used to institute quality assurance programs. The Standards for Community Health Nursing Practice were distributed to ANA Community Health Nursing Division members in 1973. In 1986 the standards were revised; these revised standards can be found in Appendix F1.

In 1972 the Joint Commission on Accreditation of Hospitals (JCAH) clearly stated the responsibilities of nursing in its description of standards for nursing services. The JCAH called on the nursing industry to clearly plan, document, and evaluate nursing care provided. In the mid 1980s JCAH became the Joint Commission on Accreditation of Health Care Organizations (JCAHCO) and began developing quality control standards for home health nursing and for hospital nursing.

Also in 1972, the Social Security Act (Public Law 92-603) was amended to establish the *Professional Standards Review Organization (PSRO)* and to mandate the review of the delivery of health care to clients of Medicare, Medicaid, and maternal and child health programs. The PSRO program was modified to become the *Professional Review Organizations (PROs)* by 1983 Social Security Amendments. The purpose of the PROs is to monitor implementation of the prospective reimbursement system for Medicare clients (see Chapter 4). PSRO and PROs have made quality assurance a primary issue for all health care professionals.

Efforts to ensure quality nursing care continue. Past efforts include the quality assurance model developed by the

ANA (1977), the study by Jacobs et al. (1978) to define critical requirements of safe practice, the ANA study of nurse credentials (1979), and the National League for Nursing (NLN) study of accreditation (1979).

Efforts specifically directed toward strengthening community health nursing practice have been the development of frameworks for community health nursing practice by both the ANA (1982) and the American Public Health Association (1980). A discussion of these two models and of the Consensus Conference on the Essentials of Public Health Nursing Practice and Education, 1984 can be found in Chapter 8. The quality of community health nursing education is of major concern to the Association of Community Health Nursing Educators, which was established in 1978. In 1991 two reports were published by this organization that identified the curriculum content required to prepare community health nursing students for practice (ACHNE, 1991).

APPROACHES FOR A QUALITY ASSURANCE PROGRAM

Two major categories of approaches exist in quality assurance today: general and specific. The general approach examines the ability of the person or agency to meet criteria or standards. Specific approaches to quality assurance are methods used to evaluate provider and client interaction.

General Approaches

Credentialing mechanisms are general quality assurance approaches often used in the health care system. Credentialing generally is defined as the formal recognition of a person as a professional with technical competence (Cary, 1989) or of an agency that has met minimum standards of performance. These mechanisms are used to evaluate the agency structure through which care is provided and the outcomes of care given by the provider.

According to Hinsvark (1985), the credentialing process has four goals: (1) to produce a quality product; (2) to confer a unique identity, for example, registered nurse; (3) to protect the provider and the public; and (4) to control the profession. Credentialing can be mandatory or voluntary. *Mandatory credentialing* requires statutory law. State nurse practice acts are examples of mandatory credentialing. *Voluntary credentialing* is performed by an agency or institution. Certification examinations offered to nurses by the ANA are examples of voluntary credentialing. *Licensing, certification,* and *accreditation* are all examples of credentialing.

Licensure

Licensure is one of the oldest general quality assurance approaches in the United States and Canada. Individual licensure is a contract between the profession and the state in which the profession is granted control over entry into and exit from the profession and over quality of professional practice.

The licensing process requires that regulations be written to define the scope and limits of the professional's practice. Job descriptions based on these regulations set minimum and maximum limits on the functions and responsibilities of the practitioner.

Licensure of nurses has been mandated by law since 1903, when North Carolina, New York, New Jersey, and Virginia enacted laws regarding nurse registration. Today all 50 states have mandatory nurse licensure. *Mandatory nurse licensure* requires all who practice nursing for compensation to be licensed.

Accreditation

Accreditation, a voluntary approach to quality control, is used for institutions. Since 1954 the National League for Nursing (NLN), a voluntary organization, has established standards for inspecting nursing education programs. In 1966 community health home-health program standards were established by the NLN for the purpose of accrediting these programs. In addition state boards of nursing accredit basic nursing programs so that their graduates are eligible for the licensing examination.

The accreditation function may be classified as *quasi-voluntary.* Although appearing to be a voluntary participatory program, accreditation often is linked to governmental regulation that encourages programs to participate in the accrediting process. Examples include the federal Medicare regulations restricting payments to accredited public health and home health care agencies.

Accreditation provides a means for effective peer review and an opportunity for an in-depth review of program strengths and limitations (Cary, 1989). In the past the accreditation process primarily evaluated an agency's physical structure, organizational structure, and personnel qualifications. However, beginning in 1990 more emphasis was placed on evaluation of the outcomes of care and on the educational qualifications of the person providing the care.

Certification

Certification, another general approach to quality, combines features of licensure and accreditation. Certification usually is a voluntary process within professions. Educational achievements, experience, and performance on an examination determine a person's qualifications for functioning in an identified specialty area such as community health nursing.

In 1958 the ANA began to study reasons for establishing a certification program in nursing. The ANA determined that such a program was needed to provide peer recognition to nurses involved in direct client care and to provide the health care consumer with further evidence of nursing's ability and willingness to accept increasing responsibilities in health care delivery. In 1966 five clinical units were established within the ANA to determine standards of nursing excellence: medical-surgical, geriatric, community health, psychiatric and mental health, and maternal-child health. These units functioned to develop certification criteria, applicant eligibilty, and certification mechanisms. In 1990, 21 certification areas existed, and 2761 community health nurses had been certified by ANA since the program's inception (ANA, 1990). To become a certified community health nurse, one must have a baccalaureate degree in nursing and 2 years of practice as a community health nurse immediately before application.

Although usually a voluntary process, certification can be a quasi-voluntary process. For example, to function as a nurse practitioner in some states, one must show proof of educational credentials and take an examination to be "certified" to practice within the boundaries of the state.

There are major concerns about certification as a quality assurance mechanism. Data are lacking about the clinical competence of the practitioner at the time of certification because clinical competency usually is measured by written test. There also is insufficient data about the quality of the practitioner's work following the certification process. Except for occupational health nurses and nurse anesthetists, certification has not been recognized by employers as an achievement beyond basic preparation, so financial rewards are few. Although the nursing profession has accepted the certification process as a mechanism for recognizing competence and excellence, certifiers must help nurses communicate to the public the significance of certified nurses in health care delivery.

Charter, Recognition, and Academic Degrees

Other general approaches to quality assurance involve charter, recognition, and education degrees. **Charter** is the mechanism by which a state governmental agency, under state laws, grants corporate status to institutions with or without rights to award degrees, for example, university-based nursing programs. **Recognition** is defined as a process whereby one agency accepts the credentialing status of and the credentials conferred by another, for example, when state boards of nursing accept nurse practitioner credentials that are awarded by the ANA or by one of the specialty credentialing agencies. **Academic degrees** are titles awarded to individuals recognized by degree-granting institutions as having completed a predetermined plan in a branch of learning. There are four academic degrees awarded in nursing, with some variations at each degree level: Associate of Arts/Science; Bachelor of Science in Nursing; the master's degrees—Master of Science in Nursing and Master of Nursing; and the doctoral degrees—Doctor of Philosophy, Doctorate of Nursing Science, Doctorate of Science in Nursing, and Doctorate of Nursing.

Specific Approaches

The overall goal of specific quality assurance approaches is to monitor the process and outcomes of client care. The goals are (1) to identify problems between provider and client, (2) to intervene in problem cases, (3) to provide feedback regarding interaction between client and provider, and (4) to provide documentation of interactions between provider and client.

The specific approaches often are implemented voluntarily by agencies and provider groups interested in the quality of interactions in their setting. However, the state and federal governments require mandatory programs within public health agencies. For instance, regulations require periodic utilization review, peer reviews (audits), and other quality control measures within public health agencies that receive funds from state taxes, Medicaid, Medicare, and other public funding sources. Examples of specific approaches to quality control are agency staff review committees (peer review), utilization review committees, research studies, PRO monitoring, client satisfaction surveys, risk management, and malpractice litigation.

Staff review committee

Staff review committees are the most common specific

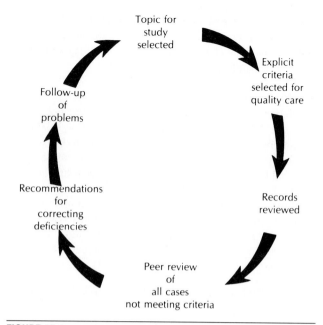

FIGURE 13-1

The audit process.

approach to quality assurance in the United States. Staff, or peer review, committees are designed to monitor client-specific aspects of certain levels of care. The audit is the major tool used to ascertain quality of care.

The ***audit process*** (Figure 13-1) consists of six steps: (1) selection of a topic for study; (2) selection of explicit criteria for quality care; (3) review of records to determine whether criteria are met; (4) peer review of all cases that do not meet criteria; (5) specific recommendations to correct problems; and (6) follow-up to determine whether problems have been eliminated (LoGerfo and Brook, 1984).

Two types of audits are used in nursing peer review: concurrent and retrospective. The ***concurrent audit*** is a method for evaluating quality of ongoing care through appraisal of the nursing process. Concurrent audit currently is used by Medicare and Medicaid to evaluate care being received by public health/home health clients. The advantages of this method are (1) identification of problems at the time care is given, (2) provision of a mechanism for identifying and meeting client needs during care, (3) implementation of measures to fulfill professional responsibilities, and (4) provision of a mechanism for communicating on behalf of the client. The disadvantages of the concurrent audit are that (1) it is time consuming; (2) it is more costly to implement than the retrospective audit; and (3) because care is ongoing, it does not present the total picture of care that the client ultimately will receive.

The ***retrospective audit*** evaluates quality of care through appraisal of the nursing process after the client's discharge from the health care system. The advantages of the retrospective audit are that it provides (1) comparison of actual practice to standards of care, (2) analysis of actual practice findings, (3) a total picture of care given, and (4) more accurate data for planning corrective action. Disadvantages of the retrospective audit method are (1) the focus of evaluation is directed away from ongoing care and (2) client problems are identified after discharge, so corrective action can only be used to improve the care of future clients.

Utilization Review

The purpose of *utilization review* is to assure that care actually is needed and that the cost is appropriate. LoGerfo and Brook (1984) described three types of utilization review: (1) prospective—an assessment of the necessity of care before giving service (2) concurrent—a review of the necessity of services while care is being given and (3) retrospective—an analysis of the necessity of the services received by the client after the care has been given. Each of these reviews provides an assessment of the appropriateness of the cost of care. Prospectively, care can be denied and money saved. Concurrently, services can be cut if they are not deemed essential. Retrospectively, payment can be denied to the provider if the care was not necessary.

Utilization review grew in the mid-twentieth century out of concern for increasing health care costs. The first committees were developed by insurance companies and professional groups. Utilization review committees became mandatory under the 1965 Medicare Law as a control measure for hospital costs (LoGerfo and Brook, 1984).

The utilization review process includes the development of explicit criteria regarding the need for services and the length of service. Utilization review has been used primarily in hospitals to establish the need for client admission and to determine the length of hospital stay. In community health, especially home health care, utilization review establishes criteria for admission to agency service, the number of visits a client may receive, the eligibility for client services such as a nursing aide or physical therapist, and discharge.

Utilization review has several advantages: (1) it assists clients to avoid unnecessary care, (2) it may encourage the consideration of alternative care options such as home health care rather than hospitalization, (3) it can provide guidelines for staff and program development, and (4) it provides for agency accountability to the consumer. The major disadvantage of utilization review is that not all clients fit the classic picture presented by the "explicit criteria" used to determine approval or denial of care. For example, an elderly female client was admitted to a home health care agency for management after hospital discharge. The client was paraplegic as a result of a cerebrovascular accident. After several weeks of physical and speech therapy, the client showed little sign of progress. The utilization review committee considered the client's condition to be stable and did not recognize the continued need for management to prevent future complications; therefore, Medicare payment was denied.

Appeal mechanisms have been built into the utilization review process used by Medicare and Medicaid. The appeal allows providers and clients to present additional data that may help to reverse the original decision to deny payment.

Risk Management

Risk management committees often are a part of the quality assurance program of a community agency. The goal of risk management is to reduce the liability on the part of the agency and the number of grievances brought against the agency. The risk management committee reviews all risks to which an agency is exposed. It reviews client and personnel safety policies and procedures and determines whether personnel are following the rules. Examples of problems reviewed by a risk managment committee would include administering incorrect medication dosage, intravenous infiltration, client injury caused by a malfunctioning machine, or injury to the nurse as a result of a needle puncture. Incident reports are reviewed by the risk management committee for appropriate, accurate, and thorough documentation of any problem that occurs relating to clients or personnel. In addition patterns are identified that may require changes in policy or staff development to correct the problem. As a part of risk management, grievance procedures are established for both clients and personnel.

Professional Review Organizations

The PSRO program was established in 1972 in an amendment to the Social Security Act (Public Law 92-603) as a publicly mandated utilization and peer review program. This law provided that medical, hospital, and nursing home care under Medicare, Medicaid, and Title V Maternal and Child Health Programs would be reviewed for appropriateness and necessity and such care would be reimbursed accordingly.

In 1984 Congress passed the Peer Review Improvement Act (PL 97-248), creating **PROs.** PROs replaced PSROs and are directed by the federal government to (1) reduce hospital admissions for procedures that can be performed safely and effectively in an ambulatory surgical setting on an outpatient basis, (2) reduce inappropriate or unnecessary admissions or invasive procedures by specific DRGs, and (3) reduce inappropriate or unnecessary admissions or invasive procedures by specific practitioners or hospitals. Quality measures include reduction of unnecessary admissions caused by previous substandard care, avoidable complications and deaths, and unnecessary surgery or invasive procedures (Gremaldi and Micheletti, 1985).

Institutions contract with PROs for quality reviews. PROs are local (usually state) organizations that establish criteria for care based on local patterns of practice. They can be for-profit or not-for-profit organizations. They have access to physicians or may include physicians in their membership. PROs must define their operational objectives and are required to consult with nurses and other nonphysician health care providers when reviewing the activities of those professionals. PROs monitor access to care and cost of care. Professionals working under the regulation of PROs should develop accurate and complete documentation procedures to ensure compliance with the criteria of the PRO.

The federally mandated quality review process has produced much debate regarding limitations and benefits. Limitations of the process include jeopardizing professional autonomy because decision making regarding care includes professionals, consumers, and government representatives. Another limitation of this process is the development of a costly control mechanism whereby client care activities may be determined by cost rather than by professional criteria. The PSRO/PRO system has challenged health care professionals to develop standards and to institute peer review mechanisms to increase accountability for care provided. This has been a benefit of the system (Bull, 1985; Gremaldi and Micheletti, 1985; Lieski, 1985).

In 1985 PRO authority was expanded to include review of services offered by health maintenance organizations and competitive medical plans. In addition the Medicare Quality Assurance Act was passed to strengthen quality assurance programs and to improve access to posthospital care. This act required hospitals receiving Medicare payments to provide discharge planning supervised by registered nurses and social workers to Medicare beneficiaries.

Evaluative Studies

Evaluative studies for quality health care have increased throughout the twentieth century. The purpose of such studies is to show the effect of nursing and health care interventions on client populations. Three major models have been used to evaluate quality: Donabedian's structure-process-outcome, the tracer, and the sentinel.

Donabedian's (1982) *model* introduced three major methods for evaluating quality care. The first method is structure, evaluating the setting and instruments used to provide care, for example, facilities, equipment, characteristics of the administrative organization, client mix, and the qualifications of health providers. The second is process, evaluating activities as they relate to standards and expectations of health providers in the management of client care. The third is outcome, the net change that occurs as a result of health care or the net result of health care. The three methods may be used separately to evaluate a part of care. However, to get an overall picture of quality of care they should be used together.

The *tracer method* described by Kessner and Kalk (1973) is a measure of both process and outcome of care. This method is more effective in evaluating health care of groups rather than of individual clients, and it is more effective in evaluating care delivered by an institution rather than by an individual provider.

Kessner and Kalk (1973) described the following essential characteristics for implementing the tracer method. A tracer, or a problem, should have a definite impact on the client's level of functioning; well-defined and easily diagnosed characteristics; population prevalence high enough to permit adequate data collection; a known variation resulting from use of effective health care; well-defined management techniques in either prevention, diagnosis, treatment, or rehabilitation; and understood (documented) effects of nonmedical factors on the tracer. Stevens (1985) provided a taxonomy for selecting client groups for tracer outcome studies in nursing: (1) a particular disease, (2) similar treatment, (3) similar needs, (4) similar community, (5) similar life-style, and (6) similar illness stage. The tracer method seemingly could provide nurses with data to show the differences in outcomes as a result of nursing care standards.

The *sentinel method* of quality evaluation is based on epidemiological methods (Rutstein et al., 1976). This method is an outcome measure for examining specific instances of client care. The characteristics of this method are as follows: (1) cases of unnecessary disease, disability, complications, and death are counted; (2) the circumstances surrounding the unnecessary event, or the sentinel, are examined in detail; (3) a review of morbidity and mortality is used as an index to determine a critical increase in the untimely event, which may reflect changes in quality of care; and (4) health status indicators such as changes in social, economic, political, and environmental factors which may have an effect on health outcomes, are reviewed. Changes in the sentinel indicate potential problems for others. For example, increases in encephalitis in certain communities may result from increases in mosquito populations.

Client Satisfaction

Client satisfaction is another approach to measuring quality of care. Client satisfaction can be assessed using in-person or telephone interviews and mailed questionnaires. In community health nursing satisfaction surveys are used to assess care received during a specific agency admission, to assess the client's personal nursing care, or to assess the total care that the client received from all services.

Satisfaction surveys may measure the interventions of client care, attitudes about the care received and the providers of care, and perceptions of the situation (environment) in which the care was received. Clients often are more critical of interpersonal and situational components of care than of the interventions of care.

Satisfaction surveys are an essential aspect of quality assessment. The survey data provide clues to reasons for client compliance or noncompliance with plans of care. The surveys also provide data about health-seeking behaviors, the probability of malpractice litigation, and the likelihood of continuing client-provider-agency relationships. The NLN (CHHA/CHS, 1985) provides an example of a client satisfaction survey (Discharged Patient Questionnaire) that can be used in a community health agency (Appendix A1).

Malpractice Litigation

Malpractice litigation is a specific approach to quality assurance imposed on the health care delivery system by the legal system. Malpractice litigation typically results from client dissatisfaction with the provider and with the content of the care received. Nursing is not immune from malpractice litigation. A discussion of legal issues affecting community health nurses can be found in Chapter 7. If community health nursing continues to have a sound quality assurance program, thereby policing its own client-care quality, the risk of quality control measures being imposed by an external source such as the legal system will continue to be reduced.

MODEL QUALITY ASSURANCE PROGRAM

The primary purpose of a quality assurance program is to ensure that the results of an organized activity are consistent with the expectations. All personnel affected by a quality assurance program should be involved in its development and implementation. Although administration and management are responsible for the quality of services, the key to that quality is the knowledge, skills, and attitudes of the personnel who deliver the service (Porter, 1988).

In 1977 the ANA introduced a model for a quality as-

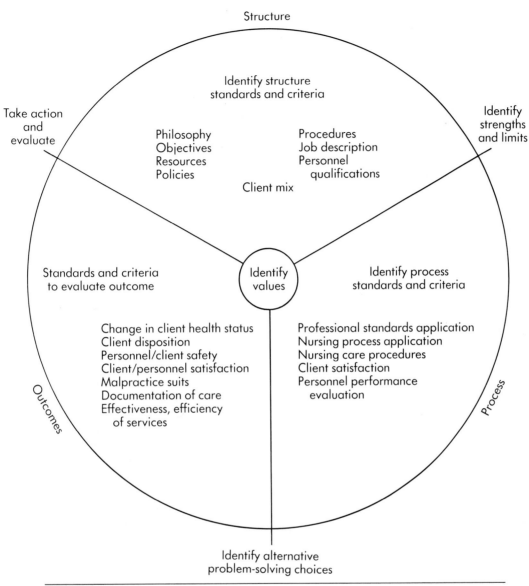

FIGURE 13-2

Model quality assurance program.

surance program. Figure 13-2 depicts the model, which identifies seven basic components of a quality assurance program. A quality assurance program answers the following questions about health care services and nursing care: (1) What is being done now? (2) Why is it being done? (3) Is it being done well? (4) Can it be done better? (5) Should it be done at all? (6) Are there improved ways to deliver the service? (7) How much is it costing? (8) Should certain activities be abandoned and/or replaced? (Gottlieb, 1988).

The ANA model and Donabedian's framework for evaluating health care programs using the components of structure, process, and outcome can be used actively in developing a quality assurance program. Today outcome is the most important ingredient of a program. Outcome now is the key to evaluation of providers and agencies by accrediting bodies, by insurance companies, and by Medicare and Medicaid through PROs and other accrediting agencies.

Structure

Values identification, the first step in a quality assurance program, serves to define the beliefs of the agency about humanity, nursing, the community, and health. The beliefs of the community, the population to be served, and the providers of care are equally important to the agency beliefs, and all need to be considered to provide quality service.

Identification of standards and criteria for quality assurance begins with the writing of the philosophy and objectives of the organization. These program objectives are being written in the 1990s to define the intended results of nursing care, descriptions of client behaviors, and/or change in health status to be demonstrated on discharge (Rinke and Wilson, 1988).

Once objectives are formulated, the required resources are identified to accomplish the objectives. Need for the resources of personnel, supplies and equipment, facilities, and finances are described. Once resources are determined, policies, procedures, and job descriptions are formulated to serve as behavioral guides to the employees of the agency. These documents should reflect the essential nursing and other health provider qualifications needed to implement the services of the agency.

The philosophy and objectives of an agency serve to define the structural standards of the agency. Evaluation of structure is a specific approach to quality appraisal. In evaluating the structure of an organization, the evaluator determines whether the agency is adhering to the stated philosophy and objectives. Is the agency providing services to populations across the life span? Are primary, secondary, and/or tertiary preventive services offered? Standards of structure are defined by the licensing or accreditating agency, for example, the NLN standards for accrediting home health agencies (CHHA/CHS, 1986).

Standards of structure are evaluated internally by a committee composed of administrative, management, and staff members for the purpose of doing a self-study. Standards of structure also are evaluated by a utilization review committee often composed of an external advisory group with community representatives for all services offered through an agency, such as a nurse, a physical therapist, a speech pathologist, a physician, a board member, and an administrator from a sister agency. The data from these committees identify the strengths and weaknesses of the agency structure.

Process

The evaluation of process standards is a specific appraisal of the quality of care being given by agency providers such as nurses. Agencies use a variety of methods to determine criteria for evaluating provider activities: conceptual models such as a developmental model or Neuman's Systems Model, the standards of care of the provider's professional organization such as the ANA community health nursing standards, or the nursing process. The activities of the nurse are evaluated to see whether they correspond with nursing care procedures defined by the agency.

The primary approaches used for process evaluation include the peer review committee and the client satisfaction survey. The techniques used for process evaluation are direct observation, questionnaire, interview, written audit, and videotape of client and provider encounters.

Although many audit instruments have been developed, Schmele recently has developed and tested an instrument based on the nursing process and applied in the community setting: The Schmele Instrument to Measure the Process of Nursing Practice in Community Nursing Service. This is a three-part instrument that includes data from direct observation, from the record audit, and from the client by means of survey questionnaire. Each technique involves evaluation of the four steps of the nursing process (Schmele, 1985; Meisenheimer, 1989). A copy of a second instrument developed by Schmele to measure the process of nursing practice in Home Health (SIMP-H) appears in Appendix E2.

Once data are collected to evaluate nursing process standards, the peer review committee reviews the data to identify strengths and weaknesses in the quality of care delivered. The peer review committee usually is an internal committee composed of representatives of the nursing staff who are trained to administer audit instruments and conduct client interviews.

Outcome

The evaluation of outcome standards, or the end result of nursing care, is one of the more difficult tasks facing nursing today. To be able to identify changes in the client's health status as a result of nursing care will give nursing data that show the contribution of nursing to the health care delivery system. Research studies using the tracer method or the sentinel method to identify client outcomes and client satisfaction surveys are approaches that may be used to measure outcome standards. Techniques that can be used to measure outcome standards are client admission data on the level of dependence, the acuity of problems, and discharge data that may show changes in levels of dependence and activity.

From these data strengths and weaknesses in nursing care delivery can be determined. The most common measurement methods used are direct physical observations and interviews. Rissner (1975) developed a client satisfaction survey to evaluate client attitudes and the content of nursing care in a primary setting. The survey has been adapted for use in home health by Reeder (Meisenheimer, 1989).

Instruments also have been developed to measure general health status indicators in home health (Choi et al., 1987; Gould, 1985; Padilla and Grant, 1987). The Omaha Visiting Nurses Association Problem Classification System includes nursing diagnosis, protocols of care, and a problem rating scale to measure nursing care outcomes. Community health nursing has been involved primarily in evaluating program outcomes to justify program expenditures rather than in evaluating client outcomes.

Outcome evaluation assumes that health care has a positive effect on client status. The major problem with outcome evaluation is determining which nursing care activities are primarily responsible for causing changes in client status. In community health nursing there are multiple uncontrolled factors in the field, such as environment and family relationships, that have an effect on client status, and often it is difficult to determine whether these factors are the cause of changes in client status or whether nursing interventions have the most effect. NLN recently has published useful guides for developing outcome criteria (Rinke, 1987).

Types of problems studied in a quality assurance program include: reasons for client death, client injury, personnel and client safety and agency liability, causes of increased costs, denied reimbursement by third-party payers, client complaints, inefficient service, staff noncompliance with standards of structure, lack of resources, unnecessary staff work and overtime, documentation of care, and client health status. The box on p. 223 summarizes quality assurance measures.

Evaluation, Interpretation, and Action

Interpreting the findings of a quality care evaluation is an essential component of the process. It allows for the identification of discrepancies between the quality care standards of the agency and the actual practice of the nurse or other health providers. These patterns reflect the total agency's functioning over time and generate information for decisions

QUALITY ASSURANCE MEASURES		
STRUCTURE Internal agency committees	**PROCESS** Peer review committees	**OUTCOME** Internal agency
Self-study Review agency documents	Prospective audit Concurrent audit Retrospective audit	Evaluative studies Survey health status change
External agency		Client
Regulatory audit Utilization review	Client Satisfaction survey	Satisfaction survey Malpractice suits

to be made about the strengths and limitations of the agency.

Regular intervals for evaluation should be established within the agency, and periodic reports should be written so that the combined results of structure, process, and outcome efforts can be analyzed and health care delivery patterns and problems can be identified. These reports should be used to establish an ongoing picture of changes that occur within an agency to justify community nursing services.

Identification and choices of possible courses of action to correct the weaknesses within the agency should involve both the administration and the staff. The courses of action chosen should be based on their significance, economic benefit, and timeliness. For example. if there is a nursing problem dealing with the recording of client health education, the agency administration and staff may analyze the problem to see why it is occurring. If the reasons given by the nurses include lack of time to do paperwork properly, case overloads that reduce the amount of time spent with clients, or lack of available resources for health education, it would not be appropriate to deal with the problem by providing a staff development program on the importance of doing and recording health education. It would be more important to assess how to provide the time and resources necessary for the nurses to offer health education to the clients. Economically it may be more beneficial to provide dictating equipment and clerical assistance so that nurses can dictate notes and other paperwork, thereby providing more client contact time, or it may be more beneficial economically to employ an additional nurse and reduce caseloads.

Taking action is the final step in the quality assurance model. Once the alternative courses of action are chosen to correct problems, actions must be implemented for change to occur in the overall operation of the agency. Follow-up and evaluation of actions taken must occur for improvement in quality of care to occur. Health care provider evaluation and documentation are essential to the evaluation of quality care in any organization. The following sections focus on the methods of provider evaluation and the kinds of documentation that normally occur in a community health agency.

HEALTH PROVIDER EVALUATION

Inherent in any quality assurance program should be the individual evaluation of health providers. Although the overall agency structure, the process of care delivered by health provider groups, and client outcome may be evaluated, it is also essential to determine the individual provider's contribution to the overall quality of the agency to protect the clients who are recipients of the provider's care.

The history of the evaluative process indicates that personnel evaluation often has been based on traditional trait ratings of personality and performance traits. Examples of trait rating measures are personal appearance, leadership, responsibility, accuracy, creativity, and ability to communicate.

The present trend in personnel evaluation is to use appraisals based on specific performance: single global ratings, behaviorally anchored ratings, and objectives-oriented ratings (Wiatrowski and Palkon, 1987).

The single global ratings scale includes a number of behaviors that are all-inclusive of the performance expected of a nurse in community health. Supervisors rate nurses on all the behaviors and assign a total score or single rating for overall job performance. This type of performance evaluation technique allows for comparison of a nurse with peers and offers a mechanism for effectively getting agreement among separate supervisor ratings.

Behaviorally anchored ratings are criterion-referenced evaluation tools that include direct observation of a list of behaviors that the nurse should perform in delivering quality care. Such a scale allows the supervisor to rate the nurse on a list of behaviors that can be generalized to all nurses based on specific criteria. This type of scale provides a better rating method than the single global ratings scale because certain individual nurse behaviors can be assessed. Development of better job descriptions can result from the assessment of nurse behaviors in a specific setting such as community health.

The objectives-oriented rating tools are developed jointly between the supervisor and the nurse. These tools reflect agreement on specific performance objectives to be met by the nurse as well as agreement on how these objectives are to be measured. This type of performance rating is said to be both more objective and more explicit to the nurse, and it allows the supervisor to pinpoint specific accomplishments of individuals and allows these persons to say how they have met their goals (self-evaluation).

Instances occur when different performance evaluation measures may be used more appropriately. The advantages and disadvantages of each method are outlined in Table 13-1 on p. 224.

Regardless of the evaluation method used, performance evaluation should be an ongoing process that includes: a

TABLE 13-1
Select advantages and disadvantages of health provider evaluation methods

Method	Advantages	Disadvantages
Trait ratings	Inexpensive Less time consuming	Permit subjective interpretation by evaluator Examine nonspecific behaviors
Single global ratings	Provide comparative measures for group Inexpensive Collect data from records Less time consuming	Unable to pinpoint behaviors specific to provider Nonmotivating Unable to pinpoint specific deficiencies Unable to use to develop job descriptions
Behaviorally anchored ratings	Collect data specific to group, such as nurses Give better overall performance rating Pinpoint deficiencies for staff development Provide comparative measures for groups Useful for evaluating merit	Expensive Require direct supervisor observation, therefore time consuming Ratings nonspecific to individual behavior
Objectives-oriented ratings	Pinpoint performance deficiencies Provide self-evaluation Collect data specific to evaluatee Motivate personnel	Expensive Time consuming Difficult to compare groups of providers Evaluation of merit difficult

staff development program to teach the nurse new interventions and types of care to be provided; the methods of evaluation to be used; a system of accountability based on job descriptions and standards of care; and a reward and sanction system.

RECORDS
Purposes of Records

Records are an integral part of the communication structure of the health care organization. Accurate and complete records are required by law and must be kept by all agencies, governmental and nongovernmental. In most states, the state departments of health stipulate the kind and content requirements of records for community health agencies.

Records provide complete information about the client, indicate the extent and quality of services being rendered, resolve legal issues in malpractice suits, and provide information for education and research.

Community Health Agency Records

Within the community health agency many types of records are kept and are used to predict population trends in a community, to identify health needs and problems, to prepare and justify budgets, and to make administrative decisions. The kinds of records kept by the community health agency may include reports of accidents, births, census, chronic disease, communicable disease, mortality, life expectancy, morbidity, child and spouse abuse, occupational illness and injury, and environmental health.

Other types of records kept within the agency are records used to maintain administrative contact and control of the organization. Three types of records make up this category: clinical, service, and financial. The clinical record is the client health record. The provider service records include information about the numbers of home visits made daily, transportation and mileage, the provider's time spent with the client, and the amount and kinds of supplies used. The service record is completed on a daily basis by each provider

and is summarized monthly and annually to indicate trends in health care activities and costs relative to personnel time, transportation, maintenance, and supplies. The provider service records are used to correlate with the agency's financial records of salaries, overhead, and transportation costs, and they serve as the basis for the cost accounting system (Pickett and Hanlon, 1990). These records are basic to peer review and audit.

Three additional kinds of service records seen in the community health agency are the central index system, the annual implementation plan, and the annual summary of agency activities. The central index system is a data filing system that indicates the services requested, services offered, active and inactive clients of the agency, and a profile of the agency's clients.

The annual implementation plan is developed at the beginning of each fiscal year to define the short-term and long-term goals of the agency. The annual implementation plan serves as the basis for the agency's annual summary. The annual summary reflects the success of the agency in meeting the annual objectives, changes in population trends and health status during the year, the actual versus the projected budget requirements, and the number of services offered, the number of clients served, and the plans and changes recommended for the future. This plan serves as the basis for the evaluation of agency structure.

As an outgrowth of quality assurance efforts in the health care system, comprehensive methods are being designed to document and measure client progress and client outcome from agency admission through discharge. An example of such a method is the client classification system developed at the Visiting Nurses' Association of Omaha, Nebraska (Martin, 1982). This comprehensive method for evaluating client care has several components: a classification system for assessing and categorizing client problems, a data base, a nursing problem list, and anticipated outcome criteria for the classified problems. Such schemes are viewed as having the potential to improve the delivery of nursing care, documentation, and the descriptions of client care. Briefly, implementation of comprehensive documentation methods will enhance nursing assessment, planning, implementation and evaluation of client care, and it will allow for the organization of pertinent client information for more effective and efficient nurse productivity and communication. (See Chapter 14.)

CLINICAL APPLICATION

Catherine, a community health nursing student, has been asked to be a member of the health care team designated to monitor the quality of service provided to the clients and community of the health care agency. As a member of this committee she is interested in identifying the current system used to monitor quality.

To prepare for her role in planning and implementing a quality assurance program she reads the federal and state regulations to identify those elements which, by law, must be included in the quality assurance program. She finds that Medicare now has specific tools to measure outcomes of client care. She learns that when the Medicare evaluator visits the agency, Catherine will be making home visits with the evaluator to observe directly the physical appearance of the client.

At the first meeting, the student is interested in the relationship between the philosophy and objectives of the agency. Does the philosophy reflect beliefs about the clients to be served by the agency, the type of nursing care and services to be delivered, the population or the community to be served and, finally, beliefs about health care versus illness care? Are the objectives of the agency reflective of the stated beliefs in the philosophy? For example, does the philosophy indicate beliefs about client education or research? If so, are there agency objectives that address providing health education or enhancing research related to better client care?

Once the committee establishes from the philosophy and objectives that the agency's goal is to deliver primary health care services to the total population of the community, Catherine is interested in the standards of care used to deliver quality health care. In nursing, are the ANA standards for community health nursing used to evaluate nursing care given? Are the nurses employed by the agency qualified to fulfill their job description through education, experience, or both?

Then the committee looks at the employment criteria of the agency. Do the criteria reflect the beliefs of the agency about nursing and the agency goals? Do the agency's policies and procedures assist the nurse in meeting the stated standards of care?

Given the structure of the agency, how is the process of care evaluated? Does the agency use prospective, concurrent, or retrospective audits to evaluate the process of care given? Are the audits designed to measure the standards of care used by the agency? How is the data used after it is collected? Is there any evidence that the evaluation makes a difference? Has the process of care changed as a result of the evaluation?

After the structure and process elements are identified, the committee members and the student are interested in outcome elements. How is health outcome defined by the agency: client satisfaction, change in health status, number of malpractice suits, or number of Medicare payments received? How is the data used to make a difference in future quality outcomes?

After answering these questions with the committee, Catherine decides she would like to perform a self-evaluation or, preferably, have a peer review by fellow students to determine the quality of care she has given through the semester. She uses the client satisfaction survey in Appendix A1 to determine how the clients feel about the services she has delivered. She applies the SIMP audit instrument (see Appendix E2) to review and evaluate several records of clients she has cared for. She interprets the data, makes adjustments in her care, and shares findings with her faculty advisor. Catherine feels good about the process and outcomes of her clients' care. She has functioned under the agency policies and knows that she has contributed to the overall quality of care as defined by the agency structure.

SUMMARY

Quality assurance programs in health care delivery maintain control over the system and demand accountability from the individual providers within the system. A quality assurance program consists of varying general and specific approaches and techniques used to evaluate the structure, process, and outcomes of client care. The ANA has put forth a model quality assurance program that reflects the components of the nursing process in the evaluation of client care activities.

Records kept by community health agencies are instrumental in identifying elements of health care delivery that establish a total picture of the contribution of the agency to the client community.

The beneficiaries of quality assurance programs are (1) the recipients of care, who receive safe, effective, satisfying service; (2) the providers of care, because evaluation offers opportunity to promote personal and professional growth; (3) the agencies, which obtain data for planning, cost containment, and legal protection; and (4) the profession, because quality assurance programs promote development of standards and protocols and the generation of new knowledge (Bergman, 1982).

KEY CONCEPTS

The health care delivery system is the largest employing industry in the United States; society is demanding increased efficiency and effectiveness from the system. Quality control is the tool used to ensure effectiveness and efficiency.

Objective and systematic evaluation of nursing care has become a priority within the profession for several reasons, including the effects of cost on health care accessibility, consumer demands for better quality care, and increasing involvement of nurses in public and health agency policy formulation.

Quality assurance is the monitoring of the activities of client care to determine the degree of excellence attained in implementation of the activities.

Quality assurance has been a concern of the profession since the 1860s, when Florence Nightingale called for a uniform format to gather and disseminate hospital statistics.

Licensure has been a major issue in nursing since 1892.

Two major categories of approaches exist in quality assurance today—general and specific approaches.

Accreditation is an approach to quality control used for institutions, whereas licensure is used primarily for individuals.

Certification combines features of both licensing and accreditation.

Three major models have been used to evaluate quality: Donabedian's structure-process-outcome model, the sentinel model, and the tracer model.

Seven basic components of a quality assurance program are (1) identifying values; (2) identifying structure, process, and outcome standards and criteria; (3) selecting measurement techniques; (4) interpreting the strengths and weaknesses of the care given; (5) identifying alternative courses of action; (6) choosing specific courses of action; and (7) taking action.

Records are an integral part of the communication structure of a health care organization. Accurate and complete records are by law required of all agencies, whether governmental or nongovernmental.

Quality assurance mechanisms in health care delivery are the mechanisms for controlling the system and requesting accountability from individual providers within the system. Records help establish a total picture of the contribution of the agency to the client community.

LEARNING ACTIVITIES

1. Write your own definition of quality assurance; compare your definition with the one given in the text. Are they the same or different? Give justification for your answer.

2. List the goals of quality assurance.

3. Interview a nurse who is a coordinator of (or is responsible for) quality assurance in a local health agency. Ask the following questions and add others you may wish to have answered:

   a. What is quality assurance?

   b. What are the goals the organization hopes to attain by having a quality assurance program?

   c. How are records used for quality assurance?

   d. Describe the components of the quality assurance program.

   e. Discuss the approaches and techniques that are used to implement the quality assurance program.

   f. How has the quality assurance program changed in the health agency over the past 20 years?

   g. What influence has the quality assurance program had on provider accountability?

4. List and describe the types of records usually kept in a community health agency. Explain the purpose of each type of record.

BIBLIOGRAPHY

Ager J: Testing the quality patient care scale. In Wandelt M and Ager JW, editors: Quality patient care scale, New York, 1974, Appleton-Century Crofts.

American Nurses' Association Committee for the Study of Credentialing in Nursing: The study of credentialing in nursing: a new approach, vols 1 and 2, Kansas City, Mo, 1979, The Association.

American Nurses' Association: Quality model: a plan for implementation of the standards of nursing practice, Kansas City, Mo, 1977, The Association.

American Nurses' Association: A conceptual model of community health nursing, Kansas City, Mo, 1982, The Association.

American Nurses' Association: The key to your professional future: professional certification, Kansas City, Mo, 1990, The Association.

American Nurses' Association Congress on Nursing Practice: Standards of nursing practice, Kansas City, Mo, 1973, The Association.

American Nurses' Association: The measure of distinction among professionals, Kansas City, Mo, 1985, The Association.

American Nurses' Association: Facts about nursing, Kansas City, Mo, 1985, The Association.

American Nurses' Association and Sutherland Learning Associates: Workbook for nursing quality assurance committee members: community health agencies, Kansas City, Mo, 1982, The Association.

American Public Health Association: The definition and role of public health nursing in the delivery of health care, Washington, DC, 1980, The Association.

Association of Community Health Nursing Educators: Essentials of baccalaureate education, Louisville, Ky, 1991, The Association.

Bergman R: Evaluation of nursing care—could it make a difference? Int J Nurs Stud 19(2):53, 1982.

Bernherdt I and Schuette L: P.E.T.: a method of evaluating professional nurse performance, J Nurs Adm 5:18, 1975.

Brent N: Quality assurance and the home health care nurse: taking an active role, Home Healthcare Nurse 6(4):6, 1988.

Brief A: Developing a usable performance appraisal system, J Nurs Adm 9(10):7, 1979.

Bull MJ: Quality assurance: its origins, transformations, and prospects. In Meisenheimer CG, editor: Quality assurance: a complete guide to effective programs, Rockville, Md, 1985, Aspen Publishers, Inc.

Carter J: Standards of nursing care, New York, 1976, Springer Publishing Co, Inc.

Cary A: Credentialing: opportunities and responsibilities in nursing. In Lambert C and Lambert V: Perspectives in nursing, Norwalk, Conn, 1989, Appleton & Lange.

Chernin S and Ayer T: The outcome audit: assuring quality care, Caring 9(2):8, 1990.

Choi T et al: Health specific family coping index for noninstitutional care. In Rinke L, editor: Outcome measures in home care, vol 1, New York, 1987, National League for Nursing.

Chu N and Schmele J: Using the ANA Standards as a basis for performance evaluation in the home health setting, Journal of Nursing Quality Assurance 4(3):25, 1990.

Council of Home Health Agencies and Community Health Services: Accreditation of home health agencies and community nursing services: criteria and guide for preparing reports, New York, 1986, National League for Nursing.

Council of Home Health Agencies and Community Health Services: Administrator's handbook for the structure, operation, and expansion of home health agencies, New York, 1985 and 1988, National League for Nursing.

Daubert E: A system to evaluate home health care services, Nurs Outlook 25(3):168, 1977.

Decker F et al: Using patient outcomes to evaluate community health nursing, Nurs Outlook 27(4):278, 1979.

Decker CM: Quality assurance: accent on monitoring, Nurs Manag 16:20, 1985.

Dolbie S and Creason N: Outcome criteria for the patient using intravenous antibiotic therapy at home, Home Healthcare Nurse 6(4):23, 1988.

Donabedian A: The criteria and standards of quality, vol 2, Explorations in quality assessment and monitoring, Ann Arbor, Mich, 1982, Health Administration Press.

Donabedian A: Explorations in quality assessment and monitoring, vol 3, Ann Arbor, Mich., 1985, Health Administration Press.

Driever M: Interpretation: a critical component of the quality assurance process, Journal of Nursing Quality Assurance 2(2):55, 1988.

Dunn M: Development of an instrument to measure nursing performance, Nurs Res 19:502, 1970.

Ehrat K: The cost-quality balance: an analysis of quality, effectiveness, efficiency, and cost, JONA 17(5):6, 1987.

Eriksen L: Patient satisfaction: an indicator of nursing care quality, Nursing Management 18(7):31, 1987.

Fosbinder D: Setting standards and evaluating nursing performance with a single tool, JONA 19(10):23, 1989.

Goodspeed R and Goldfield N: Quality assurance in a preferred provider organization, Journal of Ambulatory Care Management 10(2):8, 1987.

Gottlieb H: Quality assurance: a blueprint for improved patient care and service, Home Healthcare Nurse 6(3):11, 1988.

Gould J: Standardized home health nursing care plans: a quality assurance tool, QRB 11(11):334, 1985.

Gremaldi PL and Micheletti JA: PRO objectives and quality criteria, Hospitals 59:64, 1985.

Harris M: The value of the clinical record, Home Healthcare Nurse 6(4):8, 1988.

Hastings C: Measuring quality in ambulatory care nursing, JONA 17(4):12, 1987.

Haussmann RKD and Hegyvary ST: Monitoring quality of nursing care: part III, Hyattsville, MD, 1977, USDHEW, PHS, HRA, B of HM, Division of Nursing.

Haussmann RKD, Hegyvary ST, and Newman JF: Monitoring quality of nursing care: part II, Bethesda, MD, 1976, USDHEW, USPHS, HRA, B of HM, Division of Nursing.

Health Care Financing Administration: HCF research report: PSRO program evaluation, Washington, DC, 1979.

Heyrman H: Home care quality assurance: dollars and sense or dollars and cents, Home Healthcare Nurse 5(2):8, 1987.

Hexum J: Monitoring standards instead of problems, Journal of Nursing Quality Assurance 1(3):8, 1987.

Hinsvark I: Credentialing in nursing. In McCloskey J and Grace H, editors: Current issues in nursing, Oxford, England, 1985, Blackwell Scientific Publications, Inc.

Horn BJ and Swain MA: Development of criterion measures of nursing care, vols I and II, Final report to the National Center for Health Services Research for HS D1649, Springfield, Va., 1977, National Technical Information Service.

Hough B and Schmele J: The slater scale: a viable method for monitoring nursing care quality in home health, Journal of Nursing Quality Assurance 1(3):28, 1987.

Jacobs A, Fivars G, Edwards DS, et al: Critical requirements for safe/effective nursing practice, Kansas City, Mo., 1978, Pub. No. 651, ANA Council of State Boards of Nursing.

Jonas S: Measurement and control of the quality of health care. In Jonas S, editor: Health care delivery in the United States, New York, 1986, Springer Publishing Co., Inc.

Jones F: Certification for specialization. In McCloskey J and Grace H, editors: Current issues in nursing, Boston, 1985, Blackwell Scientific Publications, Inc.

Kessner DM and Kalk CE: Assessing health quality—the case for tracers, N Engl J Med 288:189, 1973.

Kraft M: Quality monitoring in long term care, Journal of Nursing Quality Assurance 2(1):39, 1987.

Kreidler M et al: Developing standards and criteria: family health nurse specialists in a nursing center, Journal of Nursing Quality Assistance 4(1):73, 1989.

Lalonde B: Assuring the quality home care via the assessment of client outcomes, Caring 7(1):20, 1988.

Lang NM and Clinton JF: Assessment of quality of nursing care, vol 2, Annual review of nursing research, New York, 1984, Springer-Verlag.

Larson J and Williams N: Quality assurance, HMOs and home care, Caring 6(7):13, 1987.

Lawler T: The objectives of performance appraisal—or where can we go from here? Nursing Management 19(3):82, 1988.

Lieski AM: Standards: the basis of a quality assurance program. In Meisenheimer CG, editor: A complete guide to effective programs, Rockville, Md., 1985, Aspen Publishers, Inc.

LoGerfo J and Brook R: Evaluation of health services and quality of care. In Williams S and Torrens P, editors: Introduction to health services, New York, 1984, John Wiley & Sons, Inc.

Lohr K and Harris-Wehling J: Medicare: a strategy for quality assurance, a recapitulation of the study and definition of quality of care, QRB 17(1):6, 1991.

Maciorowski LF, Larson E, and Keane A: Quality assurance: evaluate thyself, J Nurs Adm 15:38, 1985.

Maibusch RM: Evolution of quality assurance for nursing in hospitals. In Schrolder PS and Maibusch RM, editors: Nursing quality assurance, Rockville, Md., 1984, Aspen Publishers, Inc.

Martin K: A client classification system adaptable for computerization, Nurs Outlook 30:515, 1982.

Martin K and Scheet N: The Omaha system: providing a framework for assuring quality of home care, Home Healthcare Nurse 6(3):24, 1988.

McCann B and Enck R: National standards in hospice care, Caring 5(10):28, 1986.

McCann B and Rooney A: Striving for excellence in home care: a quality assurance approach, Caring 7(10):15, 1988.

McCloskey J: ANA's Nursing accreditation. To what end? In McCloskey J and Grace H, editors: Current issues in nursing, Oxford, England, 1985, Blackwell Scientific Publications, Inc.

McCloskey J: The state board test pool exam: entrance to professional nursing. In McCloskey J and Grace H, editors: Current issues in nursing, Boston, 1985, Blackwell Scientific Publications, Inc.

McNeese B: Patient satisfaction: how is it being addressed? Home Healthcare Nurse 6(3):13, May 1988.

Meisenheimer C: Quality assurance for home health care, Rockville, Md., 1989, Aspen Publishers, Inc.

Miller J: Evaluating structure, process and outcome indicators in ambulatory care: The AMBUQUAL approach, Journal of Nursing Quality Assurance 4(1):40, 1989.

Mowry M and Korpman R: Automated information systems in quality assurance, Nursing Economics 5(5):237, 1987.

National League for Nursing: Historical perspective of NLN's participation in the ANA credentialing study, NLN accreditation update, Report No. 1, New York, Oct. 1979, The League.

National League for Nursing Accreditation Division for Home Health Care and Community Health: Accreditation criteria, standards, and substantiating evidences, New York, 1987, The League.

Nauright L: Toward a comprehensive personnel system: performance appraisal, Part IV, Nursing Management 18(8):67, 1987.

O'Brien N et al: A managerial perspective on controlling the quality of patient care, Dimensions in Health Services 64(4):22, 1987.

Office of Professional Standards Review: PSRO Program Manual, Washington, DC, 1974, Department of Health, Education, and Welfare.

Openshaw S: Literature review: measurement of adequate care, Int J Nurs Stud 21:295, 1984.

Padilla GV and Grant MM: Quality assurance programme for nursing, J Adv Nurs 7:135, 1982.

Padilla G and Grant M: Quality of life as a cancer nursing outcome variable. In Rinke L, editor: Outcome measures in Home Care, vol 1:169, 1987.

Peters D and Poe S: Using monitoring in a home care quality assurance program, Journal of Nursing Quality Assurance 2(2):32, 1988.

Phaneuf M: A nursing audit method, Nurs Outlook 5:42-45, 1965.

Phaneuf M: The nursing audit: profile for excellence, New York, 1976, Appleton-Century-Crofts.

Phaneuf MC and Wandelt MA: Quality assurance in nursing, Nurs Forum 13(4):329, 1974.

Phaneuf M and Wandelt M: Three methods of process oriented nursing evaluation, QRB 7(8):20, 1981.

Pickett G and Hanlon J: Public health administration and practice, St. Louis, 1990, Mosby-Year Book, Inc.

Pinkerton S: Legislative issues in licensure of registered nurses. In McCloskey J and Grace H, editors: Current issues in nursing, Oxford, England, 1985, Blackwell Scientific Publications, Inc.

Porter A: Assuring quality through staff nurse performance, Nurs Clin North Am 23(3):649, 1988.

Porter-O'Grady T: Credentialing, privileging, and nursing bylaws: assuring accountability, J Nurs Adm 15(12):23, 1985.

Public Law 97-248, Tax Equity and Fiscal Responsibility Act of 1982.

Rinke L, editor: Outcome measures in home care, vol 1 and 2, New York, 1987, National League for Nursing.

Rinke L and Wilson A: Client oriented project objectives, Caring 7(1):25, 1988.

Rissner N: Development of an instrument to measure patient satisfaction with nurses and nursing care in primary care settings, Nurs Res 24(1):45, 1975.

Rosser R, Watts V, Berenburg W, et al: The measurement of hospital output, Int J Epidemiol 1:361-368, 1972.

Rutstein DD et al: Measuring the quality of medical care: a clinical method, N Engl J Med 294:528, 1976.

Schmele J: A method for evaluating nursing practice in a community setting, QRB 11(4):115, 1985.

Schmele J and Foss S: A process method for clinical practice evaluation in the home health setting, Journal of Nursing Quality Assurance 3(3):54, 1990.

Schmele J and Allen M: A comparison of four nursing process measures of quality in home health, Journal of Nursing Quality Assurance 4(4):26, 1990.

Smeltzer C, Hinshaw AS, and Feltman B: The benefits of staff nurse involvement in monitoring the quality of patient care, Journal of Nursing Quality Assurance 1(3):1, 1987.

Smith RL: Internal properties of the C.A.S.H. nursing care evaluation instrument, Health Serv Res 10(2):136, 1975.

Stanhope M: A concurrent and retrospective evaluation of the effects of intrinsic and extrinsic motivating factors on nurse performance in home health care setting, unpublished doctoral dissertation, Birmingham, Ala., 1981, University of Alabama.

Stanhope M and Murdock M: A psychometric measure of the Phaneuf Nursing Audit. Paper presented at the American Public Health Association Annual Meeting, Los Angeles, November 1981.

Sudela K and Landureth L: Criterion referenced performance appraisal system: a blueprint, Nursing Management 18(3):54, 1987.

Stevens B: The nurse as executive, 1985, Contemporary Publishing.

Ulrich B, Fredin N and Cavouras CA: Assuring quality through a professional practice approach, Nursing Economics 4(6):277, 1986.

USPHS: Essentials of public health nursing practice and education consensus conference, Washington, DC, 1984, US Government Printing Office.

Wagner D and Cosgrove D: Quality assurance: a professional responsibility, Caring 5(1):46, 1986.

Wagner D: Quality assurance: issues and process, Caring 5(9):62, 1987.

Wagner D: Who defines quality: consumers or professional? Caring 7(10):27, 1988.

Wandelt M and Ager J: Quality patient care scale, New York, 1975, Appleton-Century-Crofts.

Wandelt M and Stewart D: Slater nursing competencies rating scale, New York, 1975, Appleton-Century-Crofts.

Weid L: Medical records, medical education and patient care, Chicago, 1970, Year Book Medical Publishers, Inc.

Weidmann J and North H: Implementing the Omaha Classification system in a public health agency, Nurs Clin North Am 22(4):971, 1987.

Weiser M: Tracking quality assurance activities: development of an administrative model, Journal of Nursing Quality Assurance 1(3):14, 1987.

Weitzman B: The quality of care: assessment and assurance. In Kovner A: Health care delivery in the United States, New York, 1990, Springer Publishing Co.

Werner J: PSROs and hospital accreditation. In McCloskey J and Grace H, editors: Current issues in nursing, Oxford, England, 1984, Blackwell Scientific Publications, Inc.

Whittaker A and McCanless D: Nursing peer review: monitoring the appropriateness and outcome of nursing care, Journal of Nursing Quality Assurance 2(2):24, 1988.

Wiatrowski M and Palkon D: Performance appraisal systems in health care administration, Health Care Manage Rev 12(1):71, 1987.

Wright D: An introduction to the evaluation of nursing care: a review of the literature, J Adv Nurs 9:457, 1984.

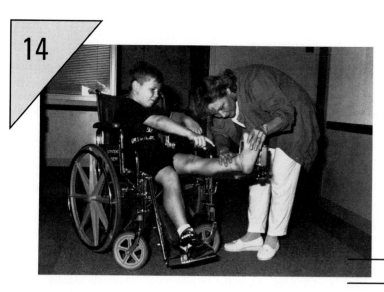

14

Nursing Diagnoses Applied to Community Health Nursing

Karen S. Martin

Nancy J. Scheet

OBJECTIVES

After reading this chapter, the student should be able to:

Define nursing diagnosis/client problem.

Describe the relationship between nursing diagnosis and nursing process, medical diagnosis, problem-solving process, and quality assurance.

Discuss the historical development of nursing diagnosis.

Compare and contrast current nursing diagnosis symptoms and frameworks.

Describe the organization and principles of the Omaha Problem Classification Scheme's nursing diagnoses.

Give examples of practice, documentation, and data management benefits derived from use of the Omaha Problem Classification Scheme by students and practitioners.

Summarize the process of applying the Omaha Problem Classification Scheme to client data.

KEY TERMS

accreditation	Functional Health Patterns	Omaha Problem Classification Scheme
Chronic Illness Diagnoses	inductive approach	Omaha System
client problem	modifier	Psychiatric-Mental Health Nursing Diagnoses
clinical judgement	North American Nursing Diagnosis Association (NANDA) diagnoses	Self-Care Diagnostic Approach
data management		signs/symptoms
documentation	nursing diagnosis	taxonomy
domain	nursing practice	third-party payors
	nursing process	trend

"E" ach year, innovators, gurus, and forecasters appear with new panaceas intended to solve people problems and meet organizational needs. Some of these innovations are simply old wine with new labels, some are passing fads, and others become trends that are adopted and implemented" (del Bueno, 1985). Into which category of innovation does the concept of nursing diagnosis fall? Is it a recycled version of previous concepts? Is it a fad that will vanish soon? Or is it a trend that will persist within nursing practice, education, and research?

Using del Bueno's humorous yet thoughtful method of analysis, nursing diagnosis can be designated as a trend. Nursing diagnosis is appropriate for the profession in general and for community health nursing in particular. A large number of nurses have enthusiastically integrated nursing diagnoses into their practice within a relatively short span of time. Nursing diagnoses are being implemented by virtually all specialty groups and in all practice settings.

Additional reasons why nursing diagnosis is a trend that will persist are described in this chapter. Nursing history is pertinent to nursing diagnosis and developments in community-based practice is also presented. This chapter also contains a review of current systems and frameworks of nursing diagnoses. Although all offer potential benefits to community health nurses, the Omaha Problem Classification Scheme is the only system developed *by* practicing community health nurses *for* practicing community health nurses. Narrative and tabular examples are included to illustrate the complex, extensive, and diverse information clients present to community health nurses. Nurses who practice in home health, public health, school health, ambulatory care, or emerging health-delivery settings need simple yet comprehensive tools to manage client data. The Omaha Problem Classification Scheme can assist in guiding practice decisions, sorting and documenting pertinent client data in a uniform manner, and providing a framework for a clinical data management information system.

DEFINITIONS

Although the terms *nursing diagnosis* and *client problem* have been defined in various ways, they will be used interchangeably and their similarities will be emphasized throughout this chapter. The nursing diagnosis definition was developed by members of the North American Nursing Diagnosis Association (NANDA) whereas the client problem definition was developed for the Omaha Problem Classification Scheme.

Nursing diagnosis is a clinical judgement about individual, family, or community responses to actual and potential health problems/life processes. It provides the basis for selection of nursing interventions to achieve outcomes for which the nurse is accountable (Carroll-Johnson, 1990). *Client problem* is a matter of difficulty or concern that historically, presently, or potentially adversely affects any aspect of the client's well-being; accurate problem identification enables the professional to focus interventions (Martin and Scheet, 1992a).

The evolution of nursing diagnosis and client problem share many similarities. Both terms can be adapted to apply to divergent situations and populations. Nursing diagnosis and client problem can be incorporated into community health programs as well as acute and long-term care programs. The concepts are applicable to the client as a single individual, family group, or community.

Nursing Diagnosis and Nursing Process

Nursing diagnosis is an essential, even pivotal component of the nursing process. Nursing diagnosis follows the data collection or assessment phase and precedes the planning, implementing, and evaluating phases. The identification of accurate nursing diagnoses or client problems is critical to the success of nursing care.

It is important for the community health nurse to recognize that the nursing process and its cornerstone, nursing diagnosis, exist within a larger perspective. In addition to

Problem-solving process	Medical diagnostic process	Nursing process
Information gathering	History and physical examination	Data collection
Problem	**Diagnosis**	**Nursing diagnosis**
Plan	Plan	Plan
Action	Treatment	Intervention
Evaluation	Evaluation	Evaluation

FIGURE 14-1

The relationship of the nursing process to the problem-solving and medical diagnostic processes.

nursing, other disciplines that require logical thinking and systematic nomenclature also employ a problem-solving approach. The problem-solving process includes generalized information gathering, problem identification, and analysis, as well as decision-making based on fact, intuition, and experiences. Physicians employ a medical diagnostic process that is similar to the nursing process and the problem-solving approach. Within the medical model, diagnosis is substituted for problem identification and nursing diagnosis. Figure 14-1 illustrates the relationship of nursing diagnosis to the broader concepts of nursing process, medical diagnosis, and the problem-solving process.

Nursing diagnosis and nursing process are related to the concepts of medical diagnosis and the problem-solving process. They also include quality assurance activities, which are referred to increasingly as *continuous quality improvement activities* (Deming, 1986; Walton, 1986). In addition to the obvious potential benefits of quality assurance activities to clients, the activities are important to community health nurses because they enable nurses to define and communicate the nurse's role and the contribution nurses make to clients. Such benefits are described in detail in Chapter 13.

Quality assurance programs must be based on two prerequisites regardless of the specific quality measurement tools involved. The first prerequisite is measurement. Nursing diagnosis provides a natural and appropriate point of reference for measuring client outcomes. Client status in relation to nursing diagnosis is a variable that can be examined over time. The second prerequisite is unity. A community health agency's quality assurance/improvement program should consist of multiple related yet diverse activities. These may include orientation, continuing education, staff-supervisory review sessions, record audit, peer review, utilization review, risk management, and shared staff-supervisory site visits. Incorporating nursing diagnoses throughout a quality assurance/improvement program provides an important link among the various activities.

HISTORICAL PERSPECTIVE OF NURSING DIAGNOSIS

Nursing diagnosis is not a recent innovation. Since the beginning of recorded history, many nurses, including community health nurses, have used systematic practice and problem-solving skills involving the diagnostic process. Only recently, however, has the term *nursing diagnosis* been applied. Milestones pertinent to the evolution of nursing diagnosis are described in this chapter and depicted in Table 14-1. (See Chapter 1 for a history of general community health nursing.)

Historians frequently credit Florence Nightingale with clearly demonstrating the benefits of the nurse's role in prevention and therapy, originating interest in the nursing process, and establishing the scientific basis of nursing. Almost 50 years lapsed before the scientific basis for community health nursing practice was established in the United States. At the beginning of the twentieth century, early community health nursing leaders such as Lillian Wald, Lavinia Dock, and Margaret Higgins Sanger made a commitment to provide preventive and therapeutic nursing services to the entire community. Their commitment resulted from humanitarian and democratic ideals and a pragmatic view of public health. As early leaders, they advocated autonomous practice and for nurses to increasingly apply the problem-solving approach and the concept of diagnosis related to the individual, family, and entire community.

Social changes and the advent of public health physicians served to hamper nursing autonomy in the decades that followed the turn of the century. Significant professional nursing advances occurred slowly until the 1950s. That decade was crucial to the concept of nursing diagnosis and advances in nursing research. Diagnosis was clearly identified in the literature as a function of nursing and a cornerstone of clinical research. Fry (1953) was one of the first to use the term nursing diagnosis. Other writers described the nurse's legal accountability for problem identification or diagnosis and delineated nursing as a process (Hornung, 1956; Lesnik and Anderson, 1955; McManus, 1951).

It was Abdellah's research study in 1957, however, that served as a turning point in the nursing profession's recognition of the value of diagnosis. In a study that included public health nurses and their clients, Abdellah defined nursing diagnosis as a "determination of the nature and extent of nursing problems by individual patients or families re-

<table>
<tr><td colspan="2">▷ TABLE 14-1
Milestones in the history of nursing diagnosis</td></tr>
<tr><td>19th century</td><td>Florence Nightingale applied the scientific method and originated interest in nursing process. She used and advanced theory, research, and the science of statistics.</td></tr>
<tr><td>Early 20th century</td><td>Lillian Wald, Lavinia Dock, and Margaret Higgins Sanger promoted the concept that serious health-related problems affected entire populations irrespective of socioeconomic, ethnic, cultural, or religious boundaries.</td></tr>
<tr><td>1953</td><td>Vera Fry was one of the first to use the term nursing diagnosis.</td></tr>
<tr><td>1957</td><td>Faye Abdellah conducted the first research study involving nursing diagnosis/client problems. She developed a list of 21 nursing problems addressing physical, emotional, and sociological client needs.</td></tr>
<tr><td>1960s</td><td>Nursing leaders introduced definitions and concepts pertinent to the diagnostic process and emphasized client focus. Community health leaders initiated projects that addressed evaluation.</td></tr>
<tr><td>1970s-1980s</td><td>Development of nursing diagnosis systems and frameworks including (a) Omaha Problem Classification Scheme, (b) North American Nursing Diagnosis Association Diagnoses, (c) Psychiatric-Mental Health Nursing Diagnoses, (d) Chronic Illness Diagnoses, (e) Self-Care Diagnostic Approach, and (f) Functional Health Patterns.</td></tr>
</table>

TABLE 14-2
Comparison of nursing diagnoses

Systems and frameworks	Taxonomic structure	Settings where especially applicable
Omaha PCS	Mutually exclusive domains (4), problems (40), modifiers (2 sets), and clusters of signs/symptoms	Community health that includes home/public health and schools, ambulatory care, and emerging community-based programs
NANDA diagnoses	Human response patterns (9), diagnostic categories (120) at three levels, and major/minor defining characteristics	Hospitals, ambulatory care, and nursing homes
Functional health patterns	Patterns (11) used to group/organize NANDA diagnoses	Hospitals, ambulatory care, and nursing homes
Psychiatric-mental health diagnoses	Human response patterns (8) and diagnostic categories (over 200) at two levels	Inpatient and outpatient psychiatric-mental health facilities
Chronic illness diagnoses	Client need categories (10) and diagnostic categories (51)	Nursing homes, ambulatory care, and home health
Self-care diagnostic approach	Self-care categories (7) and diagnostic categories (104) at three levels	Hospitals, anbulatory care, and nursing homes

ceiving nursing care" (Abdellah, 1957, p. 4). A nursing problem was defined as a "condition faced by the patient or family which the nurse can assist him or them to meet through the performance of her professional functions" (Abdellah, 1957, p. 4). Abdellah noted that "fundamental to the development of a nursing science is the nurse's ability to make a nursing diagnosis and prescribe actions or strategies that will result in specific responses in the patient" (Abdellah, 1969). Clinical judgement was finally identified as a basic responsibility of nurses.

Nursing leaders expanded the theoretical base of the profession and clarified the diagnostic responsibility of nurses early in the 1960s. Chambers' definition of nursing diagnosis was widely cited as a "careful investigation of the facts to determine the nature of a nursing problem. A nursing problem is a specific need of the patient that requires nursing action to meet the needs" (1962, p. 102). Chambers' efforts helped to differentiate nursing diagnosis from medical diagnosis. Komorita (1963) reviewed nursing diagnosis definitions and identified their benefits as the potential to increase nursing's body of knowledge and research and the quality of nursing care. Levine offered an alternative term, *trophicognosis,* for the diagnostic process (1966).

By the middle of the decade, nurses addressed nursing diagnosis beyond the definitional level and began to associate the term within a larger frame of reference appropriate for a practice-based discipline (Durand and Prince, 1966; Henderson, 1966). Henderson focused the diagnostic process on the client, not the nurse, when she identified 14 basic needs of clients. In their 1967 text, Yura and Walsh (1988) made the most comprehensive and earliest identification of the four phases of nursing process: assessing, planning, implementing, and evaluating.

Visionary community health leaders generated knowledge and advanced the science of nursing. By directing their efforts toward evaluation, they increased attention on the nursing process. Freeman (1961), Roberts and Hudson (1964), and Phaneuf (1964) were among the community

health leaders who conducted evaluation research designed to measure client change and the effectiveness of public/community health nursing. These efforts set the stage for other community health nurses such as those involved with the Omaha Problem Classification Scheme to develop the concept of nursing diagnoses from the client's perspective.

SYSTEMS AND FRAMEWORKS OF NURSING DIAGNOSES

During the 1970s, many nurses began to participate in efforts to standardize language and to develop diverse nursing diagnosis systems. These efforts were focused on nursing in general as well as on specific practice areas including community health. Hinshaw supported pluralism; her conclusion was that "diversity is the spice of nursing" (1989). Differences in the approaches included methods for developing nursing diagnoses, ways in which the diagnoses were organized, and specialties to which the diagnoses were applicable. Similarities in the nursing diagnosis approaches included time of initiation, nursing focus, compatibility with the nursing process, nomenclature, and potential as a mechanism for reimbursement.

When considered as a whole, the approaches to nursing diagnosis increased the credence of nursing as a profession. Thus, the concept of nursing diagnosis, considered radical in previous decades, gained acceptance as an integral part of the nursing profession. The publication of the American Nurses' Association *Social Policy Statement,* a significant milestone of the era, served to advance the nursing diagnosis movement. Nursing was defined as "the diagnosis and treatment of human responses to actual or potential problems" (ANA, 1980, p. 9).

Six systems and frameworks of nursing diagnoses have been selected for presentation in this chapter (see Table 14-2). Each has been disseminated through publications and presentations. Each can assist the nurse who applies nursing diagnoses. Each has been implemented in a variety of settings and is potentially applicable to community-based nursing practice. The Omaha Problem Classification Scheme, however, is uniquely the only system developed *by* practicing community health nurses *for* practicing community health nurses. It will be discussed in detail later in the chapter.

NANDA Diagnoses

The origins of the North American Nursing Diagnosis Association (NANDA) diagnoses lie in documentation, just like those of the Omaha Problem Classification Scheme. In the early 1970s, automated recordkeeping was introduced at the hospitals associated with St. Louis University School of Nursing. Nurses wanted to articulate why they were providing patient care and what services they were providing. Colleagues were demanding that nurses provide relevant language.

Based on the conclusion that nurses in other hospitals and health care centers were experiencing similar concerns, faculty nurses and those employed in the hospitals decided to host a national conference. Approximately 100 nurses attended the First National Conference on Classification of Nursing Diagnoses held in St. Louis in 1973 (Gebbie and Lavin, 1975). Participants worked in small groups to develop nursing diagnoses based on their knowledge and experience. Diagnoses were presented to all participants for discussion and voting. By the conclusion of the first conference, an alphabetized list of 30 major diagnoses was approved.

The publication and use of nursing diagnoses led to the establishment of bylaws and a change in the organization's name and structure in 1982. Taxonomy and diagnosis review committees were established to screen submitted diagnoses before they were released to the members. To increase validity, members were encouraged to conduct research for new nursing diagnoses and to refine existing diagnoses.

Taxonomy I Revised represents the diagnostic structure currently approved by NANDA; Taxonomy II is in progress. Rules have been established for adding to or revising diagnoses according to the NANDA bylaws. The first level of Taxonomy I is based on patterns of unitary person, a framework developed by a group of nurse theorists. The first level is comprised of nine human response patterns that include (1) choosing, (2) communicating, (3) exchanging, (4) feeling, (5) knowing, (6) moving, (7) perceiving, (8) relating, and (9) valuing. The second, third, and fourth levels include approximately 120 diagnostic categories. Areas are designated for adding diagnoses in all response patterns. Diagnoses are accompanied by lists of major and minor defining characteristics. In addition, related factors are suggested for each diagnosis.

Functional Health Patterns

Gordon (1991) has been pivotal in the nursing diagnosis and NANDA movements since the early 1970s. She has developed and espoused a typology of functional health patterns as the organizing principle for nursing diagnoses in contrast to the human response patterns.

The functional patterns are intended to offer a logical assessment framework for nurses as they provide care to clients. The patterns consist of: (1) health-perception-health-management, (2) nutritional-metabolic, (3) elimination, (4) activity-exercise, (5) cognitive-perceptual, (6) sleep-rest, (7) self-perception-self-concept, (8) role-relationship, (9) sexuality-reproductive, (10) coping-stress-tolerance, and (11) value-belief.

Psychiatric-Mental Health Nursing Diagnoses

The ANA *Social Policy Statement* of 1980, which incorporates diagnosis in the definition of nursing, provided the impetus for developing a classification system of nursing diagnoses for psychiatric-mental health nurses (O'Toole and Loomis, 1989). The ANA Division of Practice specific to that specialty initiated a task force to develop a system that had clinical utility.

Task force members identified two major political and conceptual issues pertinent to psychiatric-mental health nursing diagnoses (Loomis et al, 1987). The *Diagnostic and Statistical Manual of Mental Disorders* (DSM-III), published by the American Psychiatric Association, has historically provided standard terminology for physicians, nurses, and others in the specialty. Nurses, however, needed diagnoses that would emphasize their domain and practice, focus on their contributions, and guide their interventions. The nurses on the task force gathered terminology representing pertinent nursing diagnoses. They developed a plan to establish validity and reliability and to disseminate the classification system among their members.

The 1987 draft of the psychiatric-mental health nursing diagnoses is organized according to eight human response patterns and is similar conceptually and organizationally to NANDA diagnoses. The patterns relate to the following processes: (1) activity, (2) cognition, (3) ecological, (4) emotional, (5) interpersonal, (6) perception, (7) physiological, and (8) valuation. More than 200 diagnoses are categorized under the eight processes.

Chronic Illness Diagnoses

A scheme of nursing diagnoses pertinent to chronically ill clients was developed through a research process. The research study was initiated because limited diagnoses existed pertinent to this client population and those that existed had not been sufficiently validated (Hoskins et al, 1986). Human need and motivation theories were used as the framework to assess clients and formulate diagnoses.

At the conclusion of the research project, 51 diagnoses were identified. These diagnoses were organized according to the following 10 categories of client need (a) air, (b) nutrition, (c) elimination, (d) sleep and rest, (e) activity/mobility, (f) safety and security, (g) love and belonging, (h) sexual integrity, (i) self-esteem, and (j) self-actualization.

Self-Care Diagnostic Approach

Jenny (1987, 1989) and others have written about the importance of organizing nursing diagnoses in terms familiar and acceptable to practicing nurses. Self-care has been suggested as an appropriate organizing principle for classifying nursing diagnoses. The principle of self-care is congruent with current nursing practice models, including Orem's self-care requisites, Roy's adaptive modes, Neuman's personal stressors, and Maslow's human needs.

Diagnoses that follow the holistic self-care philosophy

THE DOMAINS AND PROBLEMS OF THE OMAHA PROBLEM CLASSIFICATION SCHEME

I. Environmental domain
01. Income
02. Sanitation
03. Residence
04. Neighborhood/workplace safety
05. Other

II. Psychosocial domain
06. Communication with community resources
07. Social contact
08. Role change
09. Interpersonal relationship
10. Spiritual distress
11. Grief
12. Emotional stability
13. Human sexuality
14. Caretaking/parenting
15. Neglected child/adult
16. Abused child/adult
17. Growth and development
18. Other

III. Physiological domain
19. Hearing
20. Vision
21. Speech and language
22. Dentition
23. Cognition
24. Pain
25. Consciousness
26. Integument
27. Neuromusculoskeletal function
28. Respiration
29. Circulation
30. Digestion-hydration
31. Bowel function
32. Genitourinary function
33. Antepartum/postpartum
34. Other

IV. Health related behaviors domain
35. Nutrition
36. Sleep and rest patterns
37. Physical activity
38. Personal hygiene
39. Substance use
40. Family planning
41. Health care supervision
42. Prescribed medication regimen
43. Technical procedures
44. Other

are associated with health tasks and activities. The assumption is made that self-care requires a diversity of functional abilities and personal resources. Jenny identified nursing diagnoses in the following seven categories: (1) physiological homeostasis, (2) bodily care, (3) ego integrity, (4) social interaction, (5) health protection, (6) health restoration, and (7) environmental management. Jenny reorganized, clarified, and deleted some NANDA diagnoses and placed over 100 diagnoses in a taxonomy that had three levels of abstraction.

THE OMAHA PROBLEM CLASSIFICATION SCHEME

Early in the 1970s, the Visiting Nurse Association (VNA) of Omaha, Nebraska staff, supervisors, and administrators began the process of converting a narrative method of documentation to a problem-oriented approach. No systematic nomenclature or classification of client problems existed, however, that could be used with a problem-oriented record system. This realization provided the impetus for the first VNA of Omaha research project. With the assistance of community health nursing educators, the project was conducted in 1975 and 1976 and was funded through a contract with the Division of Nursing, US Department of Health, Education, and Welfare. It was designed to produce a valid and reliable scheme of client problems or nursing diagnoses applicable in the community health setting. The VNA of Omaha staff conducted two more research projects, funded

by the Division of Nursing, between 1977 and 1980 and 1984 and 1986. The validity and reliability of the Problem Classification Scheme and the other two components of the Omaha System were established during these projects. The fourth research project, funded by a 3-year grant from the National Center for Nursing Research, National Institutes of Health, was initiated in 1989. It was designed to collect and analyze data about relationships within the Omaha Problem Classification Scheme; it was also designed to suggest revisions if needed, and to explore the potential for implementation in diverse settings (Martin and Scheet, 1992a, 1992b).

An inductive approach was used throughout the research projects. Empirical data generated by practicing community health nurses provided the basis for the development and refinement processes. Approximately 600 nurses who provided home health, public health, and clinic services and who were employed by eight geographically and organizationally diverse community health agencies were involved.

Organization

The Omaha Problem Classification Scheme is a client-focused taxonomy of nursing diagnoses in clear and concrete language. Concepts included in the nursing process and clinical judgement provide its theoretical framework.

The language of the Scheme is organized at four discrete

levels, a characteristic that increases the power of the Scheme. The vocabulary of each of the four levels of the Omaha Problem Classification Scheme is consistent and parallel. The levels of the Scheme are (1) Domains, (2) Problems, (3) Modifiers, and (4) Signs/Symptoms. The box illustrates the content and relationship of the domain and problem levels. The case example that appears later in the chapter, the box, and Table 14-3 further illustrate the organization of the Problem Classification Scheme.

The four domains, the first levels of the Problem Classification Scheme, define the scope of community-based practice. These domains are (1) Environmental, (2) Psychosocial, (3) Physiological, and (4) Health Related Behaviors. Understanding the meaning of and relationship among the domains is a prerequisite to accurately implementing the Scheme. The community health nurse does not, however, document the domains in the client record.

The 40 client problems are the second level of the Problem Classification Scheme. These client problems or nursing diagnoses are the most critical portion of the Scheme. Problems identified by the nurse are always documented in the client record.

Two sets of modifiers represent the third level of the Scheme and are used in conjunction with each client problem. Modifiers selected by the community health nurse are (1) Family or Individual, and (2) Actual, Potential, or Health Promotion. Using two modifiers with a problem enhances application across the health-illness continuum and adds an important degree of specificity and precision. Some nurses have expanded the Individual and Family modifiers to include groups and communities.

The fourth level of the Problem Classification Scheme involves a cluster of signs and symptoms specific to each problem. Clues and cues are produced as the home health or public health nurse gathers, sorts, and prioritizes data. These suggest signs and symptoms which, in turn, suggest the presence of actual client problems.

The Problem Classification Scheme is the first component of the Omaha System. The other two components are the Problem Rating Scale for Outcomes, and the Intervention Scheme. These components were developed and refined following the same research procedures as those used for the Problem Classification Scheme. When the three components of the Omaha System are applied to client data, they offer a method of addressing nursing diagnoses, nursing interventions, and client outcomes. As a unit, the Omaha System provides the community health nurse with a tool whereby important nursing concepts can be applied. Through this method, decisions can be made about what constitutes nursing practice as well as how to evaluate that practice and measure the impact of that practice. The entire Omaha System, its associated definitions, and examples of its application in diverse multidisciplinary home and public health programs, schools, ambulatory care, and emerging community-based programs appear in other publications (Martin and Scheet, 1992a, 1992b).

Benefits

Community health nursing activities range from illness care to health promotion services. Support for these activities,

especially the amount of federal reimbursement, varies markedly over time. Financial support for home health services escalated with the advent of Medicare. Recently, increased support for preventive and health promotion programs can be traced to the popularity of the wellness movement and the escalating incidence of HIV, low-birth-weight infants, and neglect/abuse (APHA, 1990).

Areas where community health nurses practice include the home, clinic, school, and other health-delivery settings. The community health nurse's client may be an individual, family, group, or entire community. Because of the diversity and complexity of the specialty, it is crucial that community health nurses focus on areas of concern, organize their practice efficiently and effectively, articulate their professional contributions, and relate their value to third-party payers and the general public.

How can the Omaha Problem Classification Scheme assist the community health nurse who is functioning in a staff, supervisory, or administrative capacity? The Scheme is useful with practice, documentation, and data management across the entire range of community health nursing practice and settings (Martin and Scheet, 1992a, 1992b). By blending the art and science of community health nursing, the Omaha Problem Classification Scheme provides a tool for (1) completing uniform assessments, (2) sorting complex client data, (3) describing client data from a nursing perspective, (4) quantifying client concerns, (5) enhancing communication, and (6) limiting recording time. Classifying client problems is important for the community health student nurse, the novice, the experienced practitioner, and the agency. Examples in the rest of this chapter demonstrate how the Omaha Problem Classification Scheme can be applied to clinical data.

Practice

The systematic and flexible yet simple organization of the Omaha Problem Classification Scheme helps introduce newcomers to the world of community health practice. Many acute-care practitioners and students follow a medical model and equate nursing with sickness care. To introduce a nursing perspective, the Problem Classification Scheme can be applied to the community health client with physiological problems. For example, a nurse can obtain data from the client and use the Scheme to identify the signs and symptoms of *edema* and *discoloration of skin/cyanosis* that suggest the problem *29. Circulation: impairment/individual*. A community health nurse who receives a referral on a new patient with insulin-dependent diabetes might collect subjective and objective data to identify several problems such as *35. Nutrition* and *43. Technical Procedures*. Although signs and symptoms may exist suggesting that these problems are actual, it is also possible that no signs and symptoms are present. In the absence of signs and symptoms, the nurse may select Potential or even Health Promotion as an appropriate problem modifier. Using the Problem Classification Scheme's Potential and Health promotion modifiers is frequently a new experience for the nurse who previously worked in acute-care setting.

The Omaha Problem Classification Scheme is uniquely beneficial in orienting the new staff or student nurse to a more holistic, preventive, and client-controlled perspective of health care. Both home health and public health nurses serve clients whose environmental and psychosocial concerns have a significant effect on their physical health status. As noted previously, those clients may be individuals, families, groups, or communities. It is, therefore, important that the community health nurse identify and address all pertinent Actual, Potential, or Health Promotion problems. In contrast to clients served in acute-care settings, community health clients are primarily responsible for their own health status. Consequently, the community health nurse must assess the client's health behavior, identify Actual, Potential, and Health Promotion problems, and intervene appropriately. Such a comprehensive approach is needed when the nurse initiates visits to an expectant mother who had been abusing drugs until 2 years ago. The expectant mother expresses an interest in eating a nutritious diet and producing a full-term, healthy infant. Data collected by the nurse suggest the following: *14. Caretaking/parenting: potential/individual, 17. Growth and development: potential/family, 35. Nutrition: health promotion/family,* and *39. Substance use: potential/family.*

The Problem Classification Scheme helps the experienced as well as the new nurse identify patterns as the client copes with environmental, psychosocial, physiological, and health-related behavior problems (Cell, Peters, and Gordon, 1984; Weidmann and North, 1987). It is difficult for any community health nurse, even an experienced practitioner, to collect, sort, and analyze client data accurately and efficiently. This difficulty increases in direct proportion to a number of factors. Those include (1) the size of the client unit, (2) the severity and number of problems, (3) the willingness and ability of the client to share information with the nurse, and (4) the skill of the nurse. Community health nurses use the Scheme as a system of cues and clues to identify and record risk factors, signs/symptoms, and problems pertinent to clients accurately and concisely. This approach produces evidence of patterns that exist within the client data. The ability to identify discrete client problems enables the community health nurse to plan and implement interventions efficiently and effectively.

Community health nurses who work with antepartum clients may apply the Omaha Problem Classification Scheme to an individual, family, group, or community. An example of group application is a nurse conducting a series of prenatal classes for adolescents. Class members are young women and men who all live in a neighborhood with a high prevalence of crime and substance abuse. Some live with one parent, some with other teens, and several stay in a shelter for the homeless. They are therefore at risk because of their age, low economic status, and living conditions. Early in the series of classes, the nurse defines the group as a client and uses conclusions from the Problem Classification Scheme to guide development of the class outline. Eleven problems and modifiers identified by the nurse include: *O1. Income: actual; 03. Residence: actual; 04. Neighborhood/workplace safety: actual; 08. Role change: actual; 14. Caretaking/parenting: potential; 15. Neglected child/adult: potential; 16. Abused child/adult: potential; 33. Antepartum/postpartum: potential; 35. Nutrition: actual; 40. Fam-*

ily planning: actual; and *41. Health care supervision: actual.*

The nursing staff of an agency may address the community as the client by conducting a neighborhood assessment that focuses on pregnancy. The project is designed to count the number of expectant mothers, differentiate between those at high and low risk, and identify services that would benefit all. Data may be generated from the home visit program, prenatal classes, and a neighborhood survey. Data analysis would suggest target subgroups and intervention strategies for short- and long-term implementation. See Part III for more information about the community as the client.

Documentation

The Omaha Problem Classification Scheme provides a framework for documentation. After using the language and structure of the Scheme as an assessment tool, nurses identify and record areas of client interest and concern. Because the language of the Scheme is consistent and clear, nurses can transform their clinical judgement decisions into written entries on the client record and communicate pertinent client data to others. By examining data obtained from multiple client records, community health professionals and record reviewers can observe caseload or agency-wide trends (Schmele, 1986).

The taxonomic principles incorporated in the Problem Classification Scheme can be readily applied to client records. Using vocabulary that is organized into discrete categories minimizes overlap and redundancy. All these characteristics assist the nurse to document home, public, and school health services with speed, accuracy, and precision.

Documentation has always been an essential responsibility of the health care professional, especially in the community health setting. It has, however, become increasingly important. Currently administrators and supervisors recognize that they and others make many significant program, management, financial, and legal decisions on the basis of the content and quality of the agency's client records. Record reviews are a critical component of agency evaluations conducted by state accreditors as well as by national representatives from the Community Health Accreditation Program of the National League for Nursing and the Joint Commission on Accreditation of Healthcare Organizations. The purpose of these record evaluations is to determine compliance with state and federal regulations and with quality standards. Other decisions are made by reviewers for third-party payers including Medicare, Medicaid, health maintenance organizations, and private insurance companies. These reviewers examine client records for proof that clients' health care needs justify nursing service. As all external representatives conduct their reviews, they prefer brief yet comprehensive documentation of essential data.

Data Management

Information obtained from individual client records can and must be compiled into group or aggregate data. These data become essential components of an agency's manual, semi-automated, or automated management information

ILLUSTRATIONS FROM THE PROBLEM CLASSIFICATION SCHEME

03. Residence
Health promotion
Potential deficit
Deficit
    01. Structurally unsound
    02. Inadequate heating/cooling
    03. Steep stairs
    04. Inadequate/obstructed exits/entries
    05. Cluttered living space
    06. Unsafe storage of dangerous objects/substances
    07. Unsafe mats/throw rugs
    08. Inadequate safety devices
    09. Presence of lead-based paint
    10. Unsafe gas/electrical appliances
    11. Inadequate/crowded living space
    12. Homeless
    13. Other

33. Antepartum/Postpartum
Health promotion
Potential impairment
Impairment
    01. Difficulty coping with pregnancy/body changes
    02. Inappropriate exercise/rest/diet/habits
    03. Discomforts
    04. Complications
    05. Fears delivery procedure
    06. Difficulty breast-feeding
    07. Other

14. Caretaking/Parenting
Health promotion
Potential impairment
Impairment
    01. Difficulty providing physical care/safety
    02. Difficulty providing emotional nurturance
    03. Difficulty providing cognitive learning experiences and activities
    04. Difficulty providing preventive and therapeutic health care
    05. Expectations incongruent with stage of growth and development
    06. Dissatisfaction/difficulty with responsibilities
    07. Neglectful
    08. Abusive
    09. Other

41. Health care supervision
Health promotion
Potential impairment
Impairment
    01. Fails to obtain routine medical/dental evaluation
    02. Fails to seek care for symptoms requiring medical/dental evaluation
    03. Fails to return as requested to physician/dentist
    04. Inability to coordinate multiple appointments/regimens
    05. Inconsistent source of medical/dental care
    06. Inadequate prescribed medical/dental regimen
    07. Other

system. The Omaha Problem Classification Scheme provides a coding structure for transforming client data into information that is computer compatible. Various nurses, programmers, and software vendors have incorporated the Problem Classification Scheme into software developed for diverse programs (Martin and Scheet, 1992a; Simmons and Hailey, 1988; Zielstorff, Jette, and Barnett, 1990).

Accurate and timely aggregate data can provide many benefits to agency personnel. The staff member who has access to caseload data can observe trends and patterns in the number, type, and location of clients served. When the Problem Classification Scheme is the framework for documentation and data management, information can be obtained about the problems, modifiers, and signs/symptoms in relation to a caseload. These data are important as agency staff hire personnel, develop orientation schedules, and plan staff development programs.

Caseload data generated by one staff member can be combined in multiple ways with information generated by other direct delivery personnel. Data may be specific to a subgroup of clients, one program, or a geographic area. It may also represent the entire agency. Supervisors and administrators can examine and use client data trends generated from the Problem Classification Scheme. This information is critical for program planning, quality assurance activities, and costing analyses that lead to the development of sound community health services that can be reimbursed.

CLINICAL APPLICATION

The following case example depicts the relationship of the diagnostic process and the Omaha Problem Classification Scheme. Data collection, data assessment, and problem identification are illustrated for a typical family visited by a community health nurse. The diagnostic process is also applicable to the group and community levels. Data can be obtained from individuals and families within the group or community by using the Problem Classification Scheme as a framework. These data can be sorted, collated, and analyzed. Aggregate data can provide meaningful information about the degree of health or illness within a specific population.

Dhun Ziong and her children were referred to the VNA by Sue Michaels, a maternity nurse. Dhun, age 19, was the mother of a preschool-aged daughter, Lor, and a newborn son, Bo. Dhun spoke Vietnamese but very little English. The English-speaking staff at the hospital where Dhun had just delivered had difficulty communicating with her and reported that she demonstrated little bonding with her newborn.

Sue Michaels reported that Dhun Ziong had been exposed to a confirmed case of hepatitis B just prior to delivery and that Dhun and Lor were given injections of gamma globulin in the clinic. Dhun had an appointment to return after 6 weeks for her postpartum exam. She was scheduled to begin the HBV vaccination series after she weaned the baby and

TABLE 14-3
Case Example

Domain	Client data	Problems and signs/symptoms
Environmental	Dhun exposed to a confirmed case of Hepatitis B.	02. Sanitation: potential/family

	Renting small, two-room basement apartment. Apartment crowded and cold. House needs repairs, especially furnace.	03. Residence: deficit/family
		   02. Inadequate heating/cooling
		   05. Cluttered living space

Psychosocial	Moved to United States 8 months ago without extended family. Has church sponsor. Fluent in Vietnamese; little English.	06. Communication with community resources: impairment/family
		   01. Unfamiliar with options/procedures for obtaining services
		   05. Language barrier

	Mother held newborn, Bo, for part of visit. Handled adequately. Did not speak to newborn or toddler, Lor. Described adequate food and feeding techniques for both children. Dhun stated that Lor had a severe respiratory infection for 3 days.	14. Caretaking/parenting: actual/Dhun
		   01. Difficulty providing physical care/safety
		   02. Difficulty providing emotional nurturance
		   04. Difficulty providing preventive and therapeutic health care

	Children dressed warmly. Newborn assessment within normal limits—appears healthy. Breast fed q 3-4 hr. Wt 5 lb 11 oz, Ht 19″, HC 13¼″. Examined Lor—diminished breath sounds; rales R lower lobe. No other findings.	17. Growth and development: potential/family
Physiological	8-point check completed on Dhun—within normal limits. Episiotomy intact. No s/s of infection. Fundus firm at umbilicus. T 98.6, B/P 118/78. Denies headaches, generalized muscle aches. Urine and stool normal color. No signs of jaundice. Appetite adequate—eats traditional Vietnamese foods.	33. Antepartum/postpartum: potential/Dhun
Health related behaviors	Dhun will take Lor to clinic MD today. Dhun has clinic appointment in 6 weeks for pp exam. Will receive HBV vaccine series after discontinuing breastfeeding. Sponsor will provide transportation.	41. Health care supervision: potential/family

to receive the other two doses 1 and 6 months later. Sue Michaels also said that Dhun had a positive TB skin test at the clinic. After investigation confirmed the lack of any abnormality, the skin test results were attributed to the routine tuberculosis inoculation she had received as a child in Vietnam.

The community health nurse, Jan Smith, contacted a Vietnamese interpreter to accompany her on the initial home visit. During that visit, Jan Smith collected objective and subjective data according to the Environmental, Psychosocial, Physiological, and Health Related Behaviors domains of the Problem Classification Scheme. The nurse was continuously sensitive to Dhun Ziong's cultural values and recognized that parenting and bonding are culturally-defined processes. Family data were examined to identify signs, symptoms, and problems (see box on p. 234 and Table 14-3).

During the admission visit, Jan Smith identified seven problems in the Ziong family. When she considered these problems in relation to the modifiers, she recorded that five problems were modified by Family and two by Individual. She then considered the problems in relation to the second set of modifiers. For the three actual problems, one or more signs and symptoms were identified. Supporting data indicated risk factors for the four potential problems. The

Ziong case example was not written to include any problems modified by Health Promotion, which is the third option available in the Omaha Problem Classification Scheme. An experienced community health nurse, Jan Smith, considered problems in addition to the seven that she had already identified. She recognized, however, that insufficient data existed to document further problems. During subsequent visits, she planned to collect more objective and subjective data that would lead to documenting or ruling out additional problems.

The case example and the tables were written to depict the initial data collection, data assessment, and problem identification process. Use of the Omaha Problem Classification Scheme increased the meaning of that process and the potential to communicate it accurately to others. In Table 14-3, pertinent subjective and objective data appear in the Client Data column. Less pertinent data obtained during the visit are not recorded. After sorting, data are collapsed to generate appropriate problems and signs/symptoms that are listed in the right column. The corresponding domains are noted in the left column. For example, the family's current health status, need for regular medical care, and reliance on their sponsor for transportation suggested the potential problem of *41. Health care supervision,* which is in the domain of *Health Related Behaviors.*

During the initial home visit, Jan Smith completed far more of the nursing process than application of the Problem Classification Scheme. As soon as individual and family problems were identified, she initiated two more important activities. First, she was concerned about outcomes and established a baseline of degree of severity for the family. This baseline would become a method of comparison for measuring the family's progress at a later date. Second, she planned and intervened as suggested by the referral information and the data collected during the visit. Tools available to the community health nurse that assist with these nursing activities are the Omaha System's Problem Rating Scale for Outcomes and the Intervention Scheme.

SUMMARY

Nursing diagnosis offers benefits to nurses involved in practice, education, and research. Not only is it compatible with fundamental concepts important to the profession, it is an essential, even pivotal component of the nursing process. Nursing diagnosis is also compatible with the diagnostic components of more generalized concepts such as medical diagnosis and problem solving. While nursing diagnosis originated over a century ago, general acceptance and application increased steadily over the last 40 years. At present, most nursing students are introduced to the concept and a large proportion of practitioners use the concept in some manner. Because of these reasons and changes that are occurring throughout the health care system, the use of nursing diagnosis is a trend that is expected to continue and thrive.

A variety of nursing diagnosis systems and frameworks have been developed. Although six have been described in this chapter, the Omaha Problem Classification Scheme has been emphasized. The research-based Omaha Scheme is a taxonomy of client-focused problems or nursing diagnoses developed for use by practicing community health nurses. It is comprehensive and flexible, and can be adapted to diverse public, home, and school health programs. Examples of use and resulting benefits are described in relation to practice, documentation, and data management.

KEY CONCEPTS

Florence Nightingale is credited with originating interest in the nursing process and demonstrating diagnostic skills. Nursing diagnosis did not gain wide acceptance, however, until recent years.

Nursing diagnosis is a trend that will continue to flourish within nursing practice, education, and research. It is an important tool for the community health nurse.

Client problem and nursing diagnosis are similar in definition, use, and benefits.

Nursing diagnosis is an essential, even pivotal, component of the nursing process and community health nursing practice. Nursing diagnosis follows the data collection or assessment phase of the nursing process and precedes the planning, implementing, and evaluating phases.

The relationship between nursing diagnosis and the nursing process is comparable to the relationships between problem identification and the problem-solving process and diagnosis and the medical diagnostic process.

Various systems and frameworks of nursing diagnosis have been developed that increase the credence of the nursing profession. Included are the Omaha Problem Classification Scheme, NANDA Diag-

noses, Psych-Mental Health Diagnoses, Chronic Illness Diagnoses, Self-Care Diagnostic Approach, and Functional Health Patterns.

The Problem Classification Scheme of the Omaha System is unique in that it is the only nursing diagnosis system developed inductively by practicing community health nurses for practicing community health nurses.

The Omaha Problem Classification Scheme was developed and refined through a process of research. Reliability and validity were established for the entire Scheme.

The Omaha Problem Classification Scheme was designed to follow taxonomic principles. The Scheme consists of client-focused domains, problems, modifiers, and signs/symptoms. The four domains are Environmental, Psychosocial, Physiological, and Health Related Behaviors.

The Omaha Problem Classification Scheme offers benefits in three principal areas: practice, documentation, and data management. These areas are of concern to community health educators and students as well as community health staff, supervisors, and administrators.

LEARNING ACTIVITIES

1. Develop your own nursing diagnosis definition. Compare and contrast that definition with the client problem and nursing diagnosis definitions in the text.

2. Review the six systems and frameworks of nursing diagnoses described in the text. Evaluate their applicability to community health nursing.

3. Interview a community health staff nurse, supervisor, and administrator. Ask their opinion about current issues and expected changes involving practice, documentation, and data management.

4. Accompany an experienced home health, public health, or school health nurse on a home, clinic, or school visit. Observe and discuss if that nurse uses a nursing diagnosis system or framework.

5. Work with a partner or in a small group. Select a community health client whom you have visited *or* think of a fictitious client. List typical referral and first visit data. Independently apply the Omaha Problem Classification Scheme to the client data. Compare your problem, modifier, and sign/symptom selections with your partner or group members. Discuss.

BIBLIOGRAPHY

Abdellah F: Methods of identifying covert aspects of nursing problems, Nurs Res 6:4-23, 1957.

Abdellah F: The nature of nursing science, Nurse Res 18:390-393, 1969.

American Nurses' Association: Social policy statement, Kansas City, Mo, 1980; The Association.

American Public Health Association (APHA): Summary of healthy people 2000, Washington, DC, 1990, US Government Printing Office.

Andersen E and McFarlane J: Community as client: application of the nursing process, Philadelphia, 1988, JB Lippincott Co.

Barkauskas V: Home health care: responding to need, growth, and cost containment. In 1990, Chaska N, editor: The nursing profession, St Louis, 1990, Mosby–Year Book, Inc.

Carpenito L: Nursing diagnosis: application to clinical practice, ed 3, Philadelphia, 1989, JB Lippincott Co.

Carroll-Johnson R: Reflections on the 9th biennial conference, Nurs Diag 1:49-50, 1990 (editorial).

Carroll-Johnson R, editor: Classification of nursing diagnosis: proceedings of ninth national conference, Philadelphia, 1991, JB Lippincott Co.

Cell P, Peters D, Peter G et al: Implementing a nursing diagnosis system through research: the New Jersey experience, Home Healthcare Nurse 2:26-32, 1984.

Chambers W: Nursing diagnosis, Am J Nurs 62:102-104, 1962.

del Bueno D: Bandwagons, parades, and panaceas, Nurs Outlook 33:136-138, 1985.

Deming WE: Out of crisis, Cambridge, Mass, 1986, Massachusetts Institute of Technology.

Donabedian A: Evaluating the quality of medical care, Milbank Q 44(2):166-206, 1966.

Donabedian A: The quality of care: how could it be assessed? JAMA 260(12):1743-1748, 1988.

Donahue MP: Nursing—the finest art: an illustrated history, St Louis, 1985, The CV Mosby Co.

Durand M and Prince R: Nursing diagnosis: process and decision, Nurs Forum 5:50-64, 1966.

Freeman R: Measuring the effectiveness of public health nursing service, Nurs Outlook 9:605-607, 1961.

Fry V: The creative approach to nursing, Am J Nurs 53:301-302, 1953.

Gebbie K, editor: Summary of the second national conference: classification of nursing diagnoses, St Louis, 1976, The Clearinghouse—National Group for Classification of Nursing Diagnoses.

Gebbie K and Lavin MA, editors: Classification of nursing diagnoses, St Louis, 1975, The CV Mosby Co.

Gordon M: Nursing diagnosis: process and application, ed 3, St Louis, Mosby–Year Book, Inc.

Grobe S: Nursing intervention lexicon and taxonomy study: language and classification methods, Adv Nurs Sci 13:22-33, 1990.

Hannah K et al, editors: Clinical judgement and decision making: the future with nursing diagnosis, New York, 1987, John Wiley & Sons Inc.

Henderson V: The nature of nursing, New York, 1966, Macmillan Publishing Co.

Henderson V: Nursing process—a critique, Holistic Nurs Pract 1:7-18, 1987.

Hinshaw AS: Nursing diagnosis: forging the link between theory and practice. In Carroll-Johnson RM, editor: Classification of nursing diagnoses: proceedings of eighth national conference, St Louis, 1989, The CV Mosby Co.

Hornung G: The nursing diagnosis—an exercise in judgement, Nurs Outlook 4:29-30, 1956.

Hoskins L et al: Nursing diagnosis in the chronically ill: methodology for clinical validation, Adv Nurs Sci 8:80-89, 1986.

Hurley M, editor: Classification of nursing diagnoses: proceedings of the sixth national conference, St Louis, 1986, The CV Mosby Co.

Jenny J: Knowledge deficit: not a nursing diagnosis. Image 19:184-185, 1987.

Jenny J: Classification of nursing diagnosis: a self-care approach. In Carroll-Johnson RM, editor: Classification of nursing diagnoses: proceedings of eighth national conference, St Louis, 1989, The CV Mosby Co.

Jorgensen C and Young B: The supervisory shared home visit tool, Home Healthcare Nurse 7:33-36, 1989.

Kim MJ, McFarland G, and McLane A, editors: Classification of nursing diagnoses: proceedings of the fifth national conference, St Louis, 1984, The CV Mosby Co.

Kim MJ and Moritz DA, editors: Classification of nursing diagnoses: proceedings of the third and fourth national conferences, New York, 1982, McGraw-Hill Inc.

Komorita N: Nursing diagnosis. Am J Nurs 63:83-86, 1963.

Leavell H and Clark EG: Preventive medicine for the doctor in his community, ed 3, New York, 1965, McGraw-Hill Inc.

Lederer J et al: Care planning pocket guide, ed 3, Redwood City, Calif. 1990, Addison-Wesley Publishing Co. Inc.

Lesnik M and Anderson B: Nursing practice and the law, ed 2, Philadelphia, 1955, JB Lippincott Co.

Levine M, editor: Exploring progress in medical-surgical nursing practice, New York, 1966, American Nurses' Association.

Loomis M et al: Development of a classification system for psychiatric/mental health nursing: individual class response, Arch Psych Nurs 1(1):16-24, 1987.

Martin K: Research in home care, Nurse Clin North Am 23:373-385, 1988.

Martin K and Scheet N: The Omaha system: providing a framework for assuring quality of home care, Home Healthcare Nurse 6:24-28, 1988.

Martin K and Scheet N: The Omaha system: applications for community health nursing, Philadelphia, WB Saunders Co, (1992a).

Martin K and Scheet N: The Omaha system: a pocket guide for community health nursing, Phil-adelphia, WB Saunders Co, (1992b)

McCloskey J: Implications of costing out nursing services for reimbursement, Nurs Management 20:44-49, 1989.

McCloskey J and Grace H, editors: Current issues in nursing, ed 3, St Louis, 1990, Mosby-Year Book, Inc.

McCormick K: A unified nursing language system. In Marion Ball M et al, editors: Nursing informatics, New York, 1988, Springer-Verlag New York Inc.

McLane A, editor: Classification of nursing diagnoses: proceedings of the seventh national conference, St Louis, 1987, The CV Mosby Co.

McManus R: Action research, Am J Nurs 51:739-740, 1951.

Neufeld A and Harrison M: The development of nursing diagnoses for aggregates and groups, Public Health Nurs 7:251-255, 1990.

Nightingale F: Notes on nursing: what it is and what it is not, London, 1859, Harrison House Publishers.

O'Toole A and Loomis M: Classifying human response in psychiatric-mental health nursing. In Classification systems for describing nursing practice, Kansas City, Miss, 1989, American Nurses' Association.

Phaneuf M: A nursing audit method, Nurs Outlook 12:42-45, 1964.

Porter E: Critical analysis of NANDA nursing diagnosis taxonomy I, Image 18:136-139, 1986.

Porter E: The nursing diagnosis of population groups. In McLane A, editor: Classification of nursing diagnoses: proceedings of the seventh conference, St Louis, 1987, The CV Mosby Co.

Roberts D and Hudson H: How to study patient progress, US Public Health Service Pub No 1169, Washington, DC, 1964, US Government Printing Office.

Schmele J: Teaching nurses how to improve their documentation, Home Healthcare Nurse 4:6-10, 1986.

Simmons D and Hailey R: Management information systems. In Benefield L, editor: Home health care management, Englewood Cliffs, NJ, 1988, Prentice Hall.

Stewart M, Innes J, Searl S, et al, editors: Community health nursing in Canada, Toronto, 1985, Gage Educational Publishing Co.

Walton M: The Deming management method, New York, 1986, The Putnam Publishing Group Inc.

Weed L: Medical records that guide and teach, New Engl J Med 278:593-600, 652-657, 1968.

Weidmann J and North H: Implementing the Omaha classification system in a public health agency, Nurs Clin North Am 22:971-979, 1987.

Wold S, editor: Community health nursing: issues and topics, Norwalk, Conn, 1990, Appleton & Lange.

Yura H and Walsh M: The nursing process: assessing, planning, implementing, evaluating, ed 5, Norwalk, Conn, 1988, Appleton & Lange.

Zielstorff R, Jette A, and Barnett GO: Issues in designing an automated record system for clinical care and research, Adv Nurs Sci 13:75-88, 1990.

PART THREE

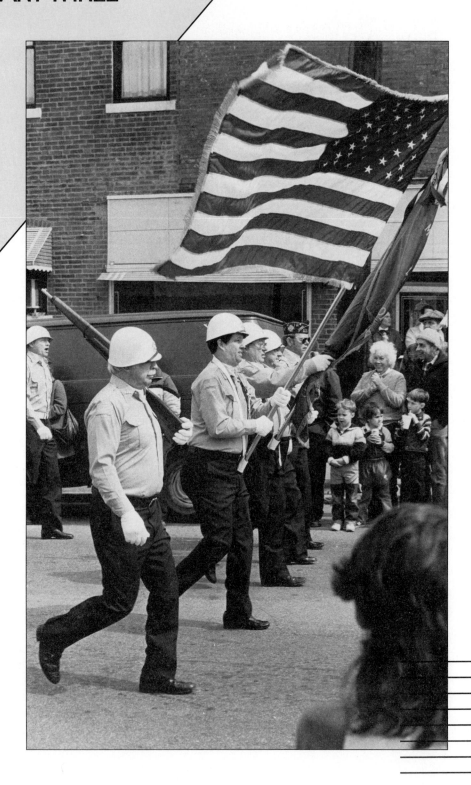

The Community as Client

T he primary orientation of health care delivery has been toward care and cure of the individual. There is increasing evidence that life-style and personal health habits influence the health of individuals, families, groups, and communities.

Although it is necessary to identify health-risk factors among individuals and groups in the community, it is of paramount importance that community health nurses learn to identify and work with health problems of the total community. Healthy communities provide greater resources for growth and nurturing of individuals and families than do their unhealthy counterparts.

Chapter 15 explains exactly what it is that makes community health nursing unique. Often people confuse community health nursing with community-based practice. There is a core of knowledge known as public health that forms the foundation for community health nursing. Working with people in the community may not be community health nursing if an individual or acute care focus is merely moved from the hospital to the community. Chapter 16 provides a framework for applying the nursing process to the community client.

Certainly, community health nurses using a public health approach work with individuals and families to promote health, intervene in disease onset or progression, and assist with rehabilitation. Likewise, nurses often find that strategies used to introduce health behaviors directed at illness prevention and lifestyle changes are applicable to groups in the community. Chapter 17 discusses group concepts that can be used to promote health behaviors of individuals through groups, to identify community groups and their contributions to community life, and to assist groups to work toward community health goals.

Concern currently exists about the environment's effects on health and social conditions causing an increase in the rate of infectious diseases. Community health nurses must be concerned with prevention, control, case-finding, reporting, and maintenance strategies as they relate to communicable and infectious disease processes and to environmentally related problems. Technological advances are increasingly influencing the environment and making the environment a potential threat to many aspects of health maintenance. As discussed in Chapter 18, nurses must help others recognize how their actions as individuals and in a composite group or community are destroying vital parts of the environment.

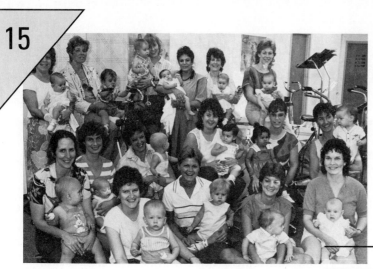

15

Community-Based Population-Focused Practice: The Foundation of Specialization in Public Health Nursing

Carolyn A. Williams

OBJECTIVES

After reading this chapter, the student should be able to:

Describe specialization in public health nursing and community health nursing and the practice goals of each.

Contrast clinical community health nursing practice with population-focused practice.

Describe what is meant by population-focused practice.

Name the barriers to acceptance of population-focused public health nursing.

KEY TERMS

body of knowledge	Consensus Conference of 1984	nursing roles
community-based population	epidemiology	population
public health nursing specialist	noninstitutional population	population-focused practice
community health nursing specialist	nursing process	public health nurse

Today more than at any time in our history, a community-based, population-focused approach to planning, delivering, and evaluating nursing care is important. This is a crucial period for public health nursing and community health nursing, a time of opportunity and challenge. Several trends and circumstances lead to this conclusion. The first is the emergence of modern-day epidemics and causes of mortality, many of which affect the young, infants, and teenagers, and many of which are preventable. The second is the concern of the public and of those in the corporate and business community about the continuously escalating cost of medical care. The third is the changing demography of the United States population, particularly the aging of the population and the resulting pressures on the resources available for health care. The fourth trend is the growing disenchantment of segments of the American public with the failure of the current health care system.

The main points made in this chapter are that: (1) in the decade of the 1990s and the beginning of the 21st century, strong public health-minded leadership will be needed to provide the direction for the development of a health care system in which prevention of dysfunction and disease are primary concerns, and (2) the specialties of public health nursing and community health nursing can and should have major roles in bringing about this new order. The argument to be presented is that although there are problems with the present status of the health care system and the roles that public health nursing and community health nursing currently play, there is great potential for a new flowering of the respective specializations. It is further suggested that whether or not this potential is realized depends on the extent to which the leadership in public health nursing is able to prepare and support nurses who have the knowledge and skills to design, manage, monitor, and evaluate systems of care (prevention included) that address the high importance and high-impact problems experienced by populations. To summarize, it is argued that nursing's future in community-based practice will be determined by the extent to which the profession takes seriously and moves forward with a population-focused approach to practice.

In this chapter the importance of population-focused practice will be discussed. It is based on the premise that the clear focus on free-living, community-based populations is what distinguishes public health nursing as an area of specialization from other areas of specialization in nursing. Although a more detailed discussion of population-focused practice will be presented later, it may be helpful at this point to define what is meant by the term "population" and to comment on what is meant by population-focused practice. A basic definition of a population is a collection of individuals who have in common one or more personal or environmental characteristics. Thus those who are members of a community defined either in terms of geography (e.g., county) or a special interest (e.g., children attending a particular school) can be seen as constituting a population. Frequently it is useful to identify subpopulations within the larger population. Examples include high-risk infants under 1 year of age, unmarried pregnant adolescents, or individuals exposed to a particular event such as a chemical spill. The basic notion in population-focused practice is that problems are defined (diagnoses) and solutions (interventions) are proposed for defined populations or subpopulations as opposed to diagnoses and intervention/treatment carried out at the patient or client level. The importance of this approach and how it relates to nurses working in community settings and to the specializations of public health nursing and community health nursing will be discussed later in the chapter.

THE RELATIONSHIP BETWEEN PUBLIC HEALTH NURSING AND COMMUNITY HEALTH NURSING

Is it important to distinguish between public health nursing and community health nursing? Diverse opinions abound as to what public health nursing and community health nursing are and how they relate to each other. Many individuals use the terms as though they were completely interchangeable. Some wish to miminize the differences because they feel that focusing on distinctions is trivial. However, some clarification is useful to grasp the importance of a population-focused approach, to understand its relationship to the success of nursing strategies directed toward community-based clients, and to be clear about the choices available in nursing roles.

The notion that the focus of community health nursing is ". . . the provision of health services among people of the community and the encouragement of health promoting behavior" described in a paper by de Tornyay (1980, p. 85) is held by many nurses. There de Tornyay emphasized that community health nursing places particular attention on the maintenance of health, the provision of services extending over time as opposed to episodic services, and the prevention of disease. She described the responsibilities of community health nurses in the area of long-term care, in primary care, in work with certain population groups, and in the provision of a range of services for people living in a specific area. In each of the descriptions the emphasis is on the direct care services provided by the nurse. Although population groups variously defined are mentioned, the basic message is that a community health nurse is primarily a direct care clinician, providing services to the members of various groups in the community. In de Tornyay's discussion only brief mention was made of the administrative and supervisory responsibilities of community health nurses.

Much of the material in current textbooks reflects a perspective similar to that of de Tornyay. The emphasis on providing clinical services in community settings is also the predominant focus of the American Nurses' Association's statement, A Conceptual Model of Community Health Nursing, which was developed by the Division of Community Health Nursing (1980).

Several distinctions relevant to this discussion are set forth in the ANA conceptual model. First, the statement identifies two categories of nurses in community health: generalists prepared at the baccalaureate level who practice in community health settings and specialists in community health nursing who have master's level preparation or beyond. The practice of the generalist is described as follows (ANA, 1980, p. 9):

> The nursing process is applied to the client, who may be an individual, family, group, or community. While working with individual clients, the nurse keeps the community perspective in mind.

In describing the scope of practice for community health nursing, the major objectives of the community health nurse are stated as "the preservation and improvement of the health of a community" (ANA, 1980, p. 11). One way to look at the relationship between public health nursing and community health nursing is to view public health nursing as a specialized field of practice with certain attributes within the broad arena of community health nursing. This view is consistent with recommendations developed at a Consensus Conference on the Essentials of Public Health Nursing Practice and Education, sponsored by the Division of Nursing and held in Washington, D.C., in September of 1984 (1985).

One of the most interesting outcomes of the conference was consensus on the use of the terms *community health nurse* and *public health nurse*. It was agreed that the term "community health nurse" could apply to all nurses who practice in the community, whether or not they have had preparation in public health nursing. Thus, nurses providing tertiary care in a home setting, school nurses, nurses in clinic settings, in fact, any nurse who does not practice in an institutional setting falls into the category of "community health nurse." Nurses with a master's degree or a doctorate degree who are practicing in community settings can be referred to as "community health nurse specialists" regardless of the area of nursing in which the degree was earned. According to the conference statement, "the degree may be in any area of nursing, such as maternal-child health, psychiatric-mental health, or medical-surgical nursing or some subspeciality of any clinical area" (p. 4).

In contrast to the focus on the setting as the key variable in defining the community health nurse, public health nurses were defined in terms of their educational preparation. The participants of the consensus conference agreed "that the term 'public health nurse' should be used to describe a person who has received specific educational preparation and supervised clinical practice in public health nursing" (p. 4). At the basic, or entry level, a public health nurse is one who "holds a baccalaureate degree in nursing that includes this educational preparation; this nurse may or may not practice in an official health agency but has the initial qualifications to do so" (p. 4). Specialists in public health nursing are defined as those who are prepared at the graduate level, either master's or doctoral, "with a focus in the public health sciences" (p. 4).

If one takes seriously the definitions of the community health nurse and the public health nurse agreed to in the 1984 consensus conference, it is clear that the setting in which one practices is viewed as the feature distinguishing community health nurses from other nurses. However, setting is not used to set apart public health nurses; here type of preparation is the distinguishing feature. However, using setting as a distinguishing feature for community health nursing is problematic for several reasons.

First, the way community is equated with "noninstitutionalization" leads to further confusion. According to the statement, an individual who has received preparation in any clinical or subclinical area and who practices in a noninstitutional setting can be seen as a community health nursing specialist. Such a broad view may indeed be consistent with the way things have been perceived, but it is not clear that the distinction of setting is very meaningful. For ex-

ample, two nurses could have completed a master's program in medical-surgical nursing with a subspecialization in nephrology. They both could be providing the same clinical services to similar populations, including home visits. But the nurse who is employed in a dialysis center would be viewed as a community health nursing specialist and the nurse working in the hospital-based dialysis center would not be seen as such a specialist.

Another problem with the use of setting as a distinguishing feature is that so much shifting and reorganization is occurring in the health care system that the institutional/noninstitutional distinction made in the consensus statement is outdated. Is a hospital-linked health maintenance organization an institutional setting? How does one define a hospital-based home care agency? Are not the more important distinctions the care needs of the populations or subpopulations being served and the types of decisions required by the professional nurses involved? For these reasons the use of setting to distinguish areas of specialization for nurses with graduate preparation has serious problems.

Public Health Nursing as a Field of Practice, an Area of Specialization

For the most part, the discussion to this point has focused on general definitions of the roles of community health nurses and public health nurses as opposed to the "field" of community health nursing and the "field" of public health nursing or the arenas encompassed by specialization in either "field." It is reasonable to ask, Is community health nursing really a speciality area? It was suggested by those participating in the consensus conference mentioned above that "the term 'community health nursing' came into broad use when the American Nurses' Association sought to create a unit within the organization to which nurses working in scattered community settings could belong. These settings included doctors' offices, work sites, schools, street clinics, and other similar community locations where nursing functions are carried out" (p. 3). The consensus conference report went on to elaborate that "the term 'community health nurse' is simply an umbrella term used for all nurses who work in the community, including those who have formal preparation in public health nursing. In essence, public health nursing requires specific educational preparation and community health nursing denotes a setting for the practice of nursing" (p. 4). If one accepts this view, it is difficult to see community health nursing as a discrete speciality. Thus, rather than calling graduate-prepared nurses who simply work in community settings community health nurse specialists, it might be more clear and more appropriate to refer to these nurses in a manner that is more in keeping with their area of practice specialization (e.g., ambulatory pediatrics, nurse midwifery, or school nursing). In contrast, a case can be made that public health nursing clearly is an area of specialization. What makes it so? Two characteristics are offered: the focus of practice, detailed below, and the specialized knowledge supporting the practice.

With regard to the nature of practice, four characteristics are particularly salient. Those are (1) the focus on populations that are free-living in the community as opposed to those that are institutionalized; (2) the predominant emphasis on strategies for health promotion, health maintenance, and disease prevention; (3) the concern for the connection between health status of the population and the living environment (physical, biological, sociocultural); and (4) the use of political processes to affect public policy as a major intervention strategy for achieving goals.

In 1981 the Public Health Nursing Section of the American Public Health Association put forth a statement on the Definition and Role of Public Health Nursing in the Delivery of Health Care, which clearly describes the field of specialization. Central elements of their definition were:

> Public health nursing synthesizes the body of knowledge from the public health sciences and professional nursing theories. The implicit over-riding goal is to improve the health of the community. . . . Public Health Nursing practice is a systematic process by which:

1. The health and health care needs of a population are assessed in collaboration with other disciplines in order to identify subpopulations (aggregates), families, and individuals at increased risk of illness, disability, or premature death;
2. A plan for intervention is developed to meet these needs, which includes resources available and those activities that contribute to health and its recovery, the prevention of illness, disability, and premature death;
3. A health care plan is implemented effectively, efficiently, and equitably; and
4. An evaluation is made to determine the extent to which these activities have an impact on the health status of the population (APHA, p. 3-4).

As far as preparation is concerned, as mentioned earlier, the specialist in public health nursing was defined by the 1984 consensus conference as one "prepared at the graduate level with a focus in the public health sciences; such a person holds a master's or doctoral degree, and may or may not practice in an official public health agency, but is qualified to do so" (p. 4). In the consensus statement it was specifically pointed out that the public health nursing specialist "should be able to work with population groups, and to assess and intervene successfully at the aggregate level" (p. 11). Areas deemed essential for the preparation of such specialists were "Epidemiology, Biostatistics, Nursing theory, Management theory, Change theory, Economics, Politics, Public health administration, Community assessment, Program planning and evaluation, Interventions at the aggregate level, Research, History of public health, and Issues in public health" (p. 11).

Population-Focused Practice Versus an Individual Focus

It is proposed that the fundamental factors that should distinguish public health nursing from other areas of specialization in nursing are practice which is community-based and population-focused. As described earlier, a population or aggregate is a collection of entities (usually individuals/persons) who share one or more personal or environmental characteristics. A population focus is historically consistent with public health philosophy and is reflected in the definition of public health nursing developed by the Public Health Nursing Section and officially adopted by the American Public Health Association (APHA, 1981). That state-

ment defines the goal of public health nursing as "improving the health of the entire community" (p. 4). Of particular significance is the APHA statement that: "Identifying subgroups (aggregates) within the population which are at high risk of illness, disability, or premature death and directing resources toward these groups is the most effective approach for accomplishing the goal of public health nursing" (p.4). Such practice is built on but is different from basic clinical nursing practice.

Basic professional education in nursing, medicine, and other clinical disciplines focuses primarily on developing competence in decision-making at the level of the individual client—assessing health status, making management decisions (ideally with the client), and evaluating the effects of care. This is at the level of the individual Xs, Os, and Ys in Figure 15-1. Little attention is given to defining problems and proposing solutions at the population or subpopulation level, the groups of Xs, Os, and Ys in Figure 15-1. Population-level decision-making is different from decision-making in clinical care and demands the specialized preparation described above. For example, in a clinical direct care situation the nurse may determine that a client is hypertensive and explore options for intervention. At the population level the questions would include the following:

◇ What is the prevalence of hypertension among various age, race, and sex groups?
◇ Which subpopulations have the highest rates of untreated hypertension?
◇ What programs could reduce the problem of untreated hypertension and thereby lower the risk of further cardiovascular morbidity and mortality?

Frequently, those who specialize in public health nursing are concerned with more than one subpopulation. Those concerned with the health of a given community must ul-

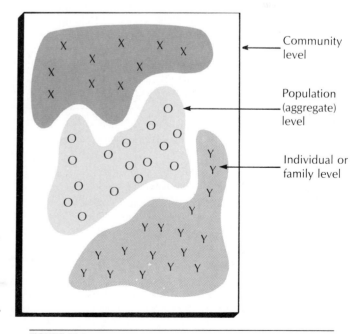

FIGURE 15-1

Levels of practice.

timately consider the health of multiple and sometimes over-lapping populations (e.g., adolescents at risk for unplanned pregnancy and all youth in a given school system). In addition a population focus requires consideration of those who may need particular services but have not entered the health care system (e.g., patients with untreated hypertension).

The Arenas for Specialization in Public Health Nursing and Community Health Nursing

A very broad understanding of public health should include some concern for all populations within the community, both free-living and institutionalized. Further, it would consider the match between the health needs of the population and the health care resources in the community, including those services offered in institutional settings. Although all direct care providers may contribute to the community's health in the broadest sense, not all are primarily concerned with the population focus, or the "big picture." Thus all nurses in a given community, including those working in hospitals, physicians' offices, and health clinics, theoretically would be contributing positively to the health of the community. However, the special contribution of public health specialists is to look at the community as a whole and raise questions about its overall health status and factors associated with that status.

The prevalent view of public health nursing historically and at present is to provide direct care services, including health education, to persons or family units outside of institutional settings. Such practice falls into the upper right quadrant (section B) in Figure 15-2. To accept the arguments made earlier for community-based, population-focused practice places specialization in public health nursing in the upper left quadrant of Figure 15-2 (section A). In addition to the population focus, there are three more reasons that the most important practice arena for public health nursing is represented in the upper left quadrant of Figure 15-2. First, preventive strategies can have the greatest impact on *noninstitutionalized populations*, which represent the majority of a community most of the time. Second, the major interface between health status and the environment (physical, biological, sociocultural) occurs in the noninstitutional population. Third, for philosophical, historical, and economic reasons population-focused practice is most likely to flourish in organizational structures that serve noninstitutionalized populations (health departments, health maintenance organizations, health centers, etc.).

What roles in the care system would public health nursing specialists have? Options include Director of Nursing for a health department, Director of the Health Department, State Commissioner for Health, or Director of Maternal and Child Health services for a state health department or a local health

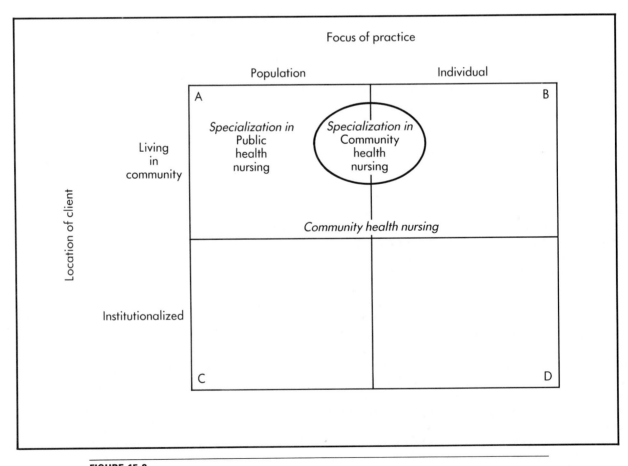

FIGURE 15-2

Arenas for practice.

department. Although nurses have in the past occupied and currently do occupy all of these roles, they are in the minority. Frequently, nurses who do occupy these roles are not seen as public health nursing specialists. Where does the staff public health nurse fit into the scheme? It is suggested that the staff public health nurse is not a public health nurse specialist. Although she or he works in the context of a public health program, the focus of the practice is in dealing with individual patients and individual families, thus the arena for practice is in section B of the diagram.

Figure 15-2 also shows that specialization in public health nursing as it has been defined in this chapter is a part of the broader field of community health nursing. In the middle of the diagram is a circle labeled specialization in community health nursing. It is partly in section A and partly in section B. It is suggested that there is a need and a place for specialization in community health nursing that is more focused than the definition put forth in the consensus conference discussed earlier in the chapter. Such specialization would include some responsibilities for providing direct care services and some responsibilities for dealing with subpopulations in the community. Preparation for such specialization would include master's preparation in a direct-care clinical area (e.g., family nurse practitioner) and some work in the public health sciences. Examples of roles such specialists might have include case manager, supervisor in a home health agency, school nurse, occupational health nurse, parish nurse, and a nurse practitioner who also manages a nursing clinic.

Sections C and D represent nurses who focus on institutionalized populations. Nurses who provide direct care in hospital settings fall into section D, and those who are responsible for the administration of nursing services in institutional settings fall into section C.

The Need to Think Broadly About Roles in Public Health Nursing

Within public health and community nursing circles there has been a tendency to talk about public health nursing and community health nursing from the point of view of a role, such as the public health nursing role or the community health nursing specialist. This is limiting. In discussing such roles there is an enormous preoccupation with a direct care provider orientation. Even in discussions about how a practice can become more population-focused, it is interesting that the focus frequently is on how an individual practitioner, such as a staff nurse in an agency, can adopt such a practice focus. Rarely is attention given to how nurse administrators in public health (one role for public health nursing specialists) might reorient their practice toward a population focus, which is more critical, useful, and possible for an administrator than for the staff nurse. This is because in many agencies nursing administrators, supervisors, or others (sometimes program directors who are not nurses) make the key decisions about how staff nurses will spend their time—what types of clients will be seen and under what circumstances. One can ask, to what extent are such decisions based on the types of data described earlier?

With regard to public health nursing administrators, those who are prepared to practice in a population-focused manner should be more effective than those who are not prepared to do so. On the other hand, staff public health nurses would benefit from having a clear understanding of population-focused practice for three reasons. First, it would give them professional satisfaction in being able to put their own clinical activities into perspective, to see how what they do clinically contributes at the population level. Second, it would help them understand and appreciate the practice of their associates who are population-focused specialists. Third, it would give them a firmer basis for providing clinical input to decision making at the program or agency level, a necessary contribution to effective and efficient population-focused practice. Clearly it is desirable that staff nurses have a population perspective, but the reality is that their ability to make decisions at that level is more limited than that of the nurse who has some administrative responsibility.

Another problem with thinking in terms of nursing roles is that present role conceptualizations are frequently too limited to allow for population-focused practice. Also, roles that might include the type of decision making being suggested may not be defined as nursing roles. Examples include directorships of health departments, state or regional programs, and units of health planning and evaluation. If population-focused public health nursing is to be taken seriously and strategies for its implementation (assessment, intervention, and evaluation) are to be applied at the population level, more consideration must be given to organized systems for assessing population needs and managing care. Such a view of public health nursing clearly places those who specialize in this area in the position of dealing with health care policy. In other words, public health nurse specialists must move into situations in which policy formation is a recognized component; however, to do this, some nurses may have to assume positions outside of what are usually considered nursing positions or nursing roles. This is true because, at present, much of the policy-making that directly affects whether nursing services are provided to certain populations and what services are rendered occurs outside the range of what are normally referred to as nursing roles.

Too much attention to defining nursing roles, particularly defining them in such a manner that they would fit into the present way of structuring nursing services, may have unfortunate limitations. For the immediate future it may be more useful to concentrate on identifying the skills and knowledge needed to make decisions in population-focused practice. The question can be raised of where in the broader community and health care system such decisions are made, and given the answers, the strategy should be to develop nurses with the substantive knowledge, skills, and political finesse necessary for success in such positions. Some of these positions are within nursing settings, particularly roles such as the administrator of the nursing service and top level staff nurse administrators, but as suggested earlier, other such positions may be outside of what are traditionally viewed as nursing roles.

CHALLENGES FOR THE FUTURE

There are several barriers to the full development of specialization in public health nursing, and our challenge is to address them. One of the most serious is the "mind-set" of many nurses that the only role for a nurse is at the bedside or at the client's side, the direct care role. Clearly, the heart of nursing is the direct care provided in personal contacts with clients. On the other hand, two things should be clear to the observant nurse. The first is that whether a nurse is able to provide direct care services to a given client is contingent on a number of decisions on the part of individuals within and without the care system. Second, nursing needs to be involved in those fundamental decisions. Perhaps the one-to-one focus of nursing and the cultural expectation of the "proper role" of women have influenced nurses to hesitate to view more positively indirect modes of contributing, such as administration, consultation, and research. Unfortunately, the mind-set of many nurses is reinforced and adopted by others who are not in nursing.

Another barrier to the type of practice implied in population-focused public health nursing is the structure within which nurses work and the process of role socialization that occurs within those structures. The fact that a particular role might not exist within the nursing unit may suggest that it is undesirable or impossible for nurses. For example, nurses interested in using political strategies to effect changes in health-related policy, an activity clearly within the practice domain of public health nursing, may run into a number of barriers if the goals disrupt the agenda of other groups within the health care arena. Such groups may use subtle but effective maneuvers to lead nurses to conclude that involvement takes them from the client and is not in their own or the client's best interests.

In response to the major changes in structuring the organizations through which care is given and how it is paid for, leaders in the medical community are saying some very interesting things. In one commentary it was suggested that physicians should consider taking the responsibility for health plans so that they could influence what happens. And, in the same commentary, it was pointed out that "assuming responsibility for a health plan means assuming financial, organizational, and clinical responsibility for the health of a population" (Kralewski et al., 1986, p. 342). In another commentary Hillman and his associates (1986) argued that physicians should become more involved in the design and management of care systems and that they should receive additional training for roles as physician-executives. The emergence of such interests in medicine presents a new challenge to nursing leadership and makes it urgent that we move forward in preparing nurses who can design nursing services that can effectively identify and respond to the needs of the many subpopulations in the community.

Another barrier is that relatively few nurses receive graduate level preparation in the concepts and strategies of disciplines basic to public health (e.g., epidemiology, biostatistics, community development, service administration, and policy formation). One of the problems mentioned earlier, which continues to be a problem in master's level preparation for public health nursing, is that in many programs the skills necessary for population assessment and management are not given the in-depth treatment accorded other components of the curriculum, particularly the direct care aspects. In short, with few exceptions, within the graduate programs in public health nursing and community health nursing, there is no aggressive effort to develop population-

focused skills that are commensurate with the need. The bias of many nurses seems to be that these skills are less important than clinical skills. However, these skills are as essential as direct care skills; they are just as difficult to develop and they should be given more attention in graduate programs that prepare nurses for specialization in public health nursing.

In view of the health and health care system problems facing this country; the need to move forward in meeting the year 2000 health objectives for the nation; the report from the Institute of Medicine on the Future of Public Health (1988), which argued that there is a compelling need for capacity building and for strong leadership in public health; and the prediction put forth in *Megatrends 2000* by Naisbitt and Aburdene (1990) that the decade of the 90s would be a decade of women in leadership, the time for new growth in public health nursing may be at hand. Nurses constitute the largest professional group in public health, but with few exceptions, they do not occupy major positions of leadership. However, there is a substantive match between (a) what has been put forth as the focus of specialization for public health nursing (dealing at the broad population level with policy and political issues and the development of strategies for health promotion, health protection, and disease prevention at the population level), and (b) what is called for by the Institute of Medicine's study as necessary to further the enterprise of public health.

The greatest need is for nurses to occupy top leadership roles, where the emphasis is on high-level management, making those decisions associated with top echelon leadership " . . . developing policy, setting priorities, allocating resources, and modifying and manipulating organizational structures" (Milbank, 1976, p. 39). Currently, the majority of the roles nurses occupy in organizations, whether in health departments, in other traditional public health structures, or in hospitals are at lower levels at which policy making is limited and the emphasis is on carrying out policy.

In addition to the need for attitudinal changes both within and without the field of nursing, changes need to occur in the educational process. There is a critical need to prepare nurses for leadership roles in policy making and in the design, development, management, monitoring, and evaluation of population-focused heath care systems. Masters and doctoral level preparation for such functions is necessary if public health nursing as defined by the American Public Health Association (1981) and described earlier in this chapter is to be practiced.

CLINICAL APPLICATION

The basic thesis of this chapter is that population-focused nursing practice is different from clinical nursing care delivered in the community. If one accepts the thesis of this chapter that specialization in public health nursing is population-focused and encompasses a unique body of knowledge, then it is useful to debate where and how public health nursing specialists practice and how their practice compares with what has been defined as specialization in community health nursing.

In your community health class, debate with classmates whether the following categories of nurses who typically function in the community are practicing population-focused nursing and classify them according to the definitions of specialization.

1. School nurses
2. Home health nurses
3. Discharge planners
4. Nurses in a health maintenance organization
5. Nurses in public health clinics
6. Nurses working in nursing homes

Which are (are not) public health or community health specialists? Why are they considered (not considered) specialists?

Interview three nurses working in one of the settings on the list. Determine what their scope of practice is. Are they carrying out population-focused practice? Could they? How?

SUMMARY

It has been suggested that preparation for practice in public health nursing should include graduate study in areas such as epidemiology, biostatistics, community development, policy formation, and administration. The relationship between the type of position held in an organizational structure and the potential to practice with a population focus has been discussed. A central point is that those in administrative roles in settings that provide community-based personal care services make decisions that affect populations; thus population-focused public health nursing is more directly relevant and applicable to their situation. Such administrators would profit from being prepared to practice in a population-focused manner and from having staff associates who are also prepared (e.g., specialists in planning, evaluation, and community development).

In view of the previous comments, the question of how baccalaureate level preparation fits in can be raised. There are various opinions on this topic. One is that at the baccalaureate level there should be two types of learning ob-

jectives. First, undergraduate students should be introduced to the earlier mentioned key concepts and strategies of the disciplines basic to public health. Second, baccalaureate students should be given opportunities to understand how (a) decision-making on the part of those responsible for population-level decisions differs from clinical decisions made by individual providers and that (b) such decision-making influences clinical decisions in a variety of ways (i.e., population-focused decisions determine what kinds of providers are hired (nurse practitioner or physician), what patients can be seen, what range of services are offered, and in what type of settings).

A key distinction between the focus of preparation at the baccalaureate level and at the master's and doctoral levels is that baccalaureate-level preparation should provide beginning insight into what population-focused practice is—both its benefits and some understanding of the knowledge and skills necessary for such practice. Preparing graduates to assume primary responsibilities as public health nursing specialists and community health nursing specialists should be left to graduate programs.

For several reasons it is important to emphasize that undergraduate programs introduce students to population-focused practice. First, as professionals, all baccalaureate graduates entering first-level staff positions should have an appreciation of the context of their practice—how what they do as clinicians relates to the populations served by the settings in which the nurses work. Second, such preparation should facilitate a better understanding of the reciprocal relationship that is desirable between direct care clinicians and population-focused specialists. Such reciprocity might lead to better collaboration and more effective and efficient nursing services. Finally, a good foundation in public health nursing at the undergraduate level can be extremely important in attracting students to this practice specialty.

KEY CONCEPTS

Setting is frequently viewed as the feature that distinguishes public health nursing from other nursing specialties. A more useful approach is to use characteristics such as the following: a focus on populations that are free living in the community; the emphasis on prevention; the concern for the interface between health status of the population and the living environment (physical, biological, sociocultural); and the use of political processes to affect public policy as a major intervention strategy for achieving goals.

According to the 1984 Concensus Conference sponsored by the Nursing Division for the Department of Health and Human Services, specialists in public health nursing are defined as those who are pre-

pared at the graduate level, either master's or doctoral, "with a focus in the public health sciences" (p. 4).

Specialization in public health nursing is seen as a subset of community health nursing.

Population-focused practice is the focus of specialization in public health nursing. This focus on community-based population is the fundamental factor that distinguishes public health nursing from other nursing specialties.

Population is defined as a collection of individuals who share one or more personal or environmental characteristics.

LEARNING ACTIVITIES

1. Define for your personal understanding (a) the specialist in public health nursing, and (b) the specialist in community health nursing.

2. State your opinion of the similarities and/or differences between the clinical role and the population-focused role of the public health nursing specialist.

3. Review the models of Community Health Nursing Practice of the ANA and APHA as described in this chapter.

4. With three or four of your classmates, debate the issue of a clinical nurse role versus population-focused practice.

BIBLIOGRAPHY

Acheson RM: Epidemiology: the training of community physicians in Great Britain. In White KT and Henderson MM, editors: Epidemiology as a fundamental science, New York, 1976, Oxford University Press, Inc.

American Nurses' Association, Division of Community Health Nursing: Conceptual model of community health nursing, Pub. No. CH-10, Kansas City, Mo., 1980, The Association.

American Public Health Association: The definition and role of public health nursing in the delivery of health care: a statement of the public health nursing section, Washington, D.C., 1981, The Association.

Consensus Conference on the Essentials of Public Health Nursing Practice and Education, Rockville, Md, 1985, U.S. Department of Health and Human Services, Bureau of Health Professions, Division of Nursing.

de Tornyay R: Public health nursing: the nurse's role in community-based practice, Ann Rev Public Health 1:83, 1980.

Flynn BC, et al: One master's curriculum in community health nursing, Nurs Outlook, 26:633, 1978.

Ginzberg E: The monetarization of medical care,

N Engl J Med, 310:1162, 1984.

Goeppinger J: Community health nursing: primary nursing care in society. In Flynn BC and Miller MH, editors: Current prospectives in nursing, II, St. Louis, 1979, The CV Mosby Co.

Highriter ME: A computerized nursing management information system for identification and community follow-up of high-risk infants. In Werley HH and Grier MR, editors: Nursing information systems, New York, 1981, Springer Publishing Co., Inc.

Hillman AL, et al: Managing the medical-industrial complex, N Engl J Med, 315:511, 1986.

Institute of Medicine: The future of public health, Washington, DC, 1988, National Academy Press.

Kralewski JE, et al: The physician rebellion, N Engl J Med, 316:339, 1986.

Milbank Memorial Fund: Commission on higher education for public health, (Cecil G. Sheps, Chairman), New York, 1976, Prodist.

Naisbitt J and Aburdene P: Megatrends 2000: ten new directions for the 1990's, New York, 1990, William Mouvoa and Company.

Skrovan C, Anderson ET, and Gottschalk J: Community nurse practitioner, an emerging role, Am J Public Health, 64:847, 1974.

Starr P: The social transformation of American medicine, New York, 1982, Basic Books, Inc., Publishers.

Williams CA: Nursing leadership in community health: a neglected issue. In McCloskey JC and Grace HK, editors: Current issues in nursing, Oxford, England, 1981, Blackwell Scientific Publications, Ltd.

Williams CA: Population-focused community health nursing and nursing administration: a new synthesis. In McCloskey JC and Grace HK, editors: Current issues in nursing, ed 2, Boston, 1985, Blackwell Scientific Publications, Ltd.

Williams CA and Highriter ME: Community health nursing: population focus and evaluation, Public Health Rep, 7:197-221, 1978.

Woods J and Ohlson V: Graduate preparation for community nursing practice. In Flynn BC and Miller MH, editors: Current perspectives in nursing: social issues and trends, St. Louis, 1977, The CV Mosby Co.

16

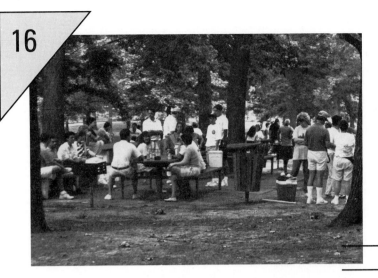

Community as Client: Using the Nursing Process to Promote Health

Jean Goeppinger

George F. Shuster III

OBJECTIVES

After reading this chapter, the student should be able to:

Decide whether nursing practice is community oriented.

Illustrate selected concepts basic to community-oriented nursing practice—community, community client, community health, and partnership for health.

Understand the relevance of the nursing process to community-oriented nursing practice.

Decide which methods of assessment, intervention, and evaluation are most appropriate in selected situations.

Develop a community-oriented nursing care plan.

KEY TERMS

aggregates
community
community health
community health
  problem
community health
  strength
community-oriented
  practice
confidentiality
data collection
data generation
early adopters
evaluation

goal
health policy
implementation
informant interviews
interacting group
intervention activities
lay advisors
mass media
mediating structures
objective
participant observation
partnership
practice setting
probability

problem analysis
problem prioritization
Program Planning
  Model
role negotiation
secondary analysis
survey
target of service
triangulation
typology
unit of service
value
windshield surveys

A lthough nurses have traditionally considered the community as a client (Anderson, 1983; Schultz, 1987; Williams, 1977), many community health nurses view the community as their most important client (USDHHS, 1985). This chapter provides both conceptual clarity and guidelines for nursing practice with the community as client, emphasizing the use of the nursing process to promote community health.

COMMUNITY DEFINED

The concept of community has a number of different meanings. Some authors define community very simply. Hanchett (1979, p. 7) defines it as "people in relationship with others." She views the community as a whole (1990). Others define it more elaborately. The Expert Committee Report on community health nursing of the World Health Organization (1974, p. 7) includes this definition: "A community is a social group determined by geographic boundaries and/or common values and interests. Its members know and interact with one another. It functions within a particular social structure and exhibits and creates norms, values and social institutions."

Still other theorists and writers present typologies rather than single definitions. One such typology of community was described by Blum in the 1974 edition of his classic text, *Planning for Health*. The categories or types of communities include communities defined by geopolitical, interactional, and problem-solving dimensions (see box).

Most definitions of community include three dimensions: people, place, and function. "People" are the community residents. "Place" refers to both spatial and time dimensions, and "function" refers to the aims and activities of the community. Community-oriented nurses need to examine regularly how the personal, spatial, and functional dimensions of the community shape their nursing practice. Using a conceptual definition of community and a set of indicators of the concept is helpful. In this chapter we use the following definition: community is a locality-based entity, composed of systems of formal organizations reflecting societal institutions, informal groups, and aggregates. These components are interdependent and function to meet a wide variety of collective needs (Goeppinger, Lassiter, and Wilcox, 1982). This definition includes personal, spatial, and functional dimensions and recognizes interdependence or interaction among the systems within a community. Indicators of the dimensions of this definition are listed in Table 16-1.

THE COMMUNITY AS CLIENT

The uniqueness of community health nursing has customarily been attributed to its practice setting. The idea of health-related care being provided within the community is not new. Indeed, at the turn of the century most persons stayed at home during illnesses. Consequently, the practice environment for community health nurses was the home rather than the hospital.

As the range of community nursing expanded, many different kinds of agencies were established, and their services often overlapped. For instance, both privately established voluntary agencies and official local health agencies worked to control tuberculosis. Nurses from both types of

agencies practiced in clients' homes and not in the hospital. Early community health nursing textbooks included lengthy descriptions of the home environment and tools for assessing the extent to which that environment promoted the health of family members. Health education about the domestic environment was frequently a major part of home nursing care.

By the 1950s, visiting nurse associations, health departments, schools, industries, and neighborhood health centers,

THE TYPES OF COMMUNITIES

Face to face community
Neighborhood
Community of identifiable need
Community of problem ecology
Community of concern
Community of special interest
Community of viability
Community of action capability
Community of political jurisdiction
Resource community
Community of solution

From Blum HL: Planning for health, New York, 1974, Human Sciences Press Inc.

TABLE 16-1
The concept of community specified

Dimensions	Indicators
Space and time	Geopolitical boundaries
	Local or folk name for area
	Size in square miles, acres, blocks, or census tracts
	Transportation avenues such as rivers, highways, railroads, and sidewalks
	History
	Physical environment such as land use patterns and condition of housing
People or person	Number and density of population
	Demographic structure of population such as age, sex, socioeconomic, and racial distributions; rural and urban character; and dependency ratio
	Informal groups such as block clubs, service clubs, and friendship networks
	Formal groups such as schools, churches, businesses, industries, governmental bodies, unions, and health and welfare agencies
	Linking structures
Function	Production, distribution, and consumption of goods and services
	Socialization of new members
	Maintenance of social control
	Adapting to ongoing and expected change
	Provision of mutual aid

and homes had all become areas of practice for community nurses. Many of the new community nurses did not consider the environments in which they practiced. Although their practices took place within the community, they focused on the individual patient or family seeking care. The care provided was not community oriented; rather, it was oriented towards the individual or family who lived—and was ill—in the community. Direct "hands on" clinical nursing care delivered to individuals or families in community settings was and is a more popular conception of community nursing practice than the idea of the whole community being the target of nursing practice. But when the location of the practice is in the community and the focus of the practice is the individual or family, the client is indeed the individual or family—not the whole community.

Therefore, the community is considered the client only when nursing practice is community oriented. Community-oriented practice seeks healthful change for the whole community's benefit. The focus is on the collective or common good instead of individual health. The units of service may be individuals, families or other interacting groups, aggregates, institutions, and communities. Change is intended to affect the whole community, including all units of service—not just the individual, family, or specific aggregate. For example, an occupational health nurse's target might be an entire work force. The nurse would not only help the disabled worker seeking service to achieve independence in activities of daily living, but also would become involved with promoting vocational rehabilitation and seeking reasonable employment policies for all disabled workers.

Community Client and Nursing Practice

The community client is relevant to nursing practice for several reasons. The concept of community client makes direct clinical care an aspect of community health practice. For instance, direct nursing care is provided to individuals and family members because their health needs represent common community-related problems rather than problems that are unique to their situations. Therefore changes in their health will affect the health of their communities. In such cases, decisions are made at the individual level because of their effect on community health. The improved health of the community is the overall goal of nursing intervention. Community health nursing intervention to stop abuse of the elderly and battering of women are two instances where nursing interventions would be undertaken primarily because of the social, not the individual, effects of abuse.

The concept of community client also highlights the complexity of the change process. Change for the benefit of the community often must occur at several levels, ranging from the individual to the societal. As Ryan (1976) points out, the victim cannot always be blamed and expected to correct the deficit without concurrent changes in the helping professions and public policy. For instance, lifestyle-induced health problems such as smoking, overeating, and speeding cannot be solved simply by asking individuals to choose health-promoting habits. Society must also provide healthful choices. Most individuals cannot change their habits alone; they require the support of family members, friends, com-

munity health care systems, and relevant social policies.

A commitment to the health of the community client requires a process of change at each of these levels. Specific nursing roles and collaborative practice models are required for each of the units of service (Pesznecker and McNeil, 1984). One nursing role emphasizes individual and direct personal care skills. Another nursing role focuses on the family and aggregate as the unit of service. A third nursing role focuses on the community as a unit of service, especially constituent community groups (Goeppinger, 1984; Chalmers and Kristajanson, 1989).

The definition of community client as the target of service includes two key concepts: community health and partnership for community health. Together these are the goal and means of community-oriented practice.

DEFINING GOALS AND MEANS OF COMMUNITY-ORIENTED PRACTICE

Community-oriented practice is targeted to the community. In this approach, the nurse and community seek healthful change together. The practice goal is community health, which is an ongoing series of health-promoting changes rather than a fixed state. The most effective method of achieving changes for health is partnership. Specific examples of partnership between the nurse and the community (Jefferson County) are provided throughout this chapter to illustrate community-oriented practice.

Community Health

Like the concept of community, community health has three common characteristics or dimensions. They are: status, structure, and process. These dimensions define community health as the goal of community-oriented practice in different ways.

Status

Community health as defined in terms of status or outcome is the most well-known and accepted approach. The physical component of community health is frequently measured by traditional morbidity and mortality rates, life expectancy indexes, and risk factor profiles. The emotional component can be measured by consumer satisfaction and mental health indexes. Crime rates and functional levels reflect the social component of community health. Other status measures such as worker absenteeism and infant mortality rates reflect the effects of all three components.

Structure

Community health as viewed from a structural perspective usually comprises community health services and resources as well as attributes of the community structure iself. Indicators used to measure community health services and resources include utilization patterns, treatment data from various health institutions, and provider-patient ratios. The problems with using these measures are serious. For instance, inequities in access to care and quality of care are well known. Less well known but equally problematic is the erroneous assumption that there is a direct causal relationship between the provision of service and improved health (Miller and Stokes, 1978; Mooney and Rives, 1978).

Such problems necessitate cautious use of health services and resources as measures of community health.

Attributes of the community structure are commonly identified as social indicators, or correlates, of health. Measures of community structure include demographic characteristics such as dependency ratios, socioeconomic and racial distributions, and educational levels. Their relationships to health status have been thoroughly documented. For instance, it has been found that health status is inversely related to age and directly related to socioeconomic level.

Process

The definition of community health as the process of effective community functioning or problem solving is well established. However, the definition is especially appropriate to community-oriented nursing because it directs the study of community health to the "promotion of effective community action or "wellness" (Wilson, 1976), which is an important aim of community-oriented nurses. Chalmers and Kristajanson (1990) have recently added a fourth model of community level practice to their typology; this model reflects the process dimension. They call it the "health promotion model" and describe it as "a mediating, enabling, and advocacy strategy that aims to develop community systems and make health a politically accountable issue."

The concept of community competence, defined originally by Cottrell (1976), provides a basic understanding of the process dimension of community health. Community competence is a process whereby the components of a community—organizations, groups, and aggregates—"are able to collaborate effectively in identifying the problems and needs of the community; can achieve a working consensus on goals and priorities; can agree on ways and means to implement the agreed-on goals; and can collaborate effectively in the required actions," (Cottrell, 1976, p. 197). Cottrell also proposed eight essential conditions of competence. These conditions are listed and defined in Table 16-2.

The term *community health* as used in this chapter is the meeting of collective needs through identifying problems and managing interactions within the community itself and between the community and the larger society. This definition emphasizes the process dimension but also includes the dimensions of status and structure. Indicators of all these dimensions are listed in Table 16-3.

Strategies to Improve Community Health

Strategies to improve community health depend, to some extent, on the dimension of community health that is emphasized. If the emphasis is on the status dimension, the most appropriate strategy is usually at the level of primary prevention. The objective is either to prevent a disease or treat it in its presymptomatic stages. Immunization programs are an example of a primary-level nursing intervention the effectiveness of which would be reflected in morbidity and mortality rates.

Nursing intervention strategies focused on the structural dimension would be directed to either health services or demographic characteristics. Intervention aimed at altering health services might include program planning. Intervention aimed at affecting demographic characteristics might

TABLE 16-2
The conditions of community competence

Condition	Definition
Commitment	The affective and cognitive attachment to a community "that is worthy of substantial effort to sustain and enhance" (Cottrell, 1976, p. 198).
Self-other awareness and clarity of situational definitions	The lucid and realistic perception of one's own and the other's community components, identities, and positions on issues.
Articulateness	The technical aspects of formulating and stating one's views in relation to the other's views.
Effective communication	The accurate transmission of information, based on the development of common meaning among the communicators.
Conflict containment and accommodation	The inventive and effective assimilation and management of true, or realistically, perceived differences.
Participation	Active, community-oriented involvement.
Management of relations with larger society	Adeptness at recognizing, obtaining, and using external resources and supports and, when necessary, stimulating the creation and use of alternative or supplementary resources.
Machinery for facilitating participant interaction and decision making	Flexible and responsible procedures, formal and informal, facilitating interaction and decision-making.

From Goeppinger J, Lassiter PG, and Wilcox B: Community health is community competence, Nurs Outlook 30(8):464-467, 1982.

include community development (Rothman and Tropman, 1987).

When the emphasis is on the process dimension, the most appropriate strategy is usually health promotion. For example, if family life education is lacking in a community because of ineffective communication among parents, children, school board members, religious leaders, and health professionals, then the most effective strategy may be to open discussion among these groups and assist community members to develop education programs.

Community partnership is crucial because community members and professionals who are active participants in a collaborative decision-making process have a vested interest in the success of efforts to improve the health of their community. Consequently, all strategies must include a community partnership as the basic means, or key, for improvement.

Partnership for Community Health

Most changes must aim at improving community health through partnerships between community residents and health workers from a variety of disciplines. Often, community residents are viewed as data sources and recipients

TABLE 16-3
The concept of community health specified

Dimensions	Indicators
Status	Vital statistics—live births, neonatal deaths, infant deaths, maternal deaths,
	Disease incidence and prevalence of leading causes of mortality and morbidity
	Health risk profiles of selected aggregates
	Functional ability levels
Structure	Health facilities such as hospitals, nursing homes, industrial and school health services, health departments, voluntary health associations, categorical grant programs, and prepaid health plans
	Health-related planning groups
	Health manpower such as physicians, dentists, nurses, environmental sanitarians, social workers, and others
	Health resource utilization patterns such as bed occupancy days and patient/provider visits
Process	Commitment
	Self-other awareness and clarity of situational definitions
	Articulateness
	Effective communication
	Conflict containment and accommodation
	Participation
	Management of relationships with the larger society
	Machinery for facilitating participant interaction and decision making

of intervention. This form of partnership is called *passive participation* (Feuerstein, 1980, p. 1). In contrast is the type of lay-professional partnership that emphasizes active participation in which power is shared among lay and professional persons throughout the assessment, planning, implementation, and evaluation process.

In the past, nurses have not been influential in initiating community changes. By the same token, however, nurses have generally been actively involved in the implementation phase. Intervention by the nurse, for the community's benefit, has been a common practice mode. This mode contrasts with a partnership approach, where all involved are assessing, planning, and implementing needed changes in the community.

Partnership is often equated with participation and involvement of the community or its representatives in healthful change. Partnership is defined here as the informed, flexible, and negotiated distribution (and redistribution) of power among all participants in the processes of change for improved community health. Its three main characteristics are that it is informed, flexible, and negotiated.

First, partnership is informed. Lay and professional partners must be aware of their own and the other's perceptions, rights, and responsibilities. Partnership is also flexible. Lay and professional partners must recognize the unique as well as similar contributions each can make to a given situation. Professionals often contribute substantive expertise that lay persons lack. On the other hand, a lay person's perceptions

of community health problems are often more accurate than those of a professional's. Because contributions vary and each situation is different, the distribution of power must be negotiated at every stage of the change process.

So defined, partnership is as essential a concept for community health nurses as are the concepts of community, community client, and community health. Partnership is important because health is not given, but rather is generated through new and increasingly effective forms of lay-professional collaboration. For example, maternal-child health in both developed and developing countries is affected more by wise grocery shopping and menu planning or improvements in home gardening than by the ingestion of vitamin and mineral supplements (Combs-Orme et al, 1985). Changes in grocery shopping and gardening practices require active participation of both lay and professional people. Partnership in identifying problems and setting goals is especially important because it elicits the commitment essential to successful change.

The significance and effectiveness of partnership in improving community health is supported by a growing body of literature. Classic studies document the utility of partnership models involving village health workers (Kingma, 1975), Latina opinion leaders (Lorig and Walters, 1980-1981), health facilitators (Salber, 1981), lay advisors (Salber, 1979; Salber, Beery, and Jackson, 1976), and health guides (Warnecke et al, 1976). The roles of these partners in health have included listening sympathetically, offering advice, making referrals, and instituting programs. More recently, the effectiveness of partnership models between nurses and communities has been demonstrated in situations involving arthritis self-care (Lorig, et al, 1989; Goeppinger et al, 1989), spouse abuse (Anderson, McFarlane, and Helton, 1986), migrant health (Smith and Gentry, 1987), child health (Armstrong-Esthen et al, 1987), Native Americans (Cleriver, Ratcliff, and Rogers, 1989), and care of the elderly (Jamieson, 1987 and 1990, Bremer, 1987). The latest work of Werner (1988) has demonstrated the continuing utility of partnership models to improved health in developing countries. In international health, partnership models are generally viewed as empowering people through their lay leaders to control their own health destinies and lives. In the United States partnership models have involved churches (Dean et al, 1988), as well as informal community leaders.

Despite supportive data, professional health workers have often challenged the notion of partnership. Unfortunately, passive compliance is more frequently sought than the true collaboration inherent in a partnership. Also, questions are frequently raised about the ability of health care consumers to determine health needs accurately and to evaluate professional practice.

The meaning of partnership, like the meanings of community, community client, and community health, is not fully understood, nor is any single meaning universally accepted. However, sufficient clarity and agreement do exist to consider these four concepts the basic elements of a conceptual framework for community-oriented nursing practice. In the following sections these concepts form the framework of the community-oriented nursing process.

Most nurses are familiar with the nursing process as it

applies to individually focused nursing care. Using the nursing process to promote community health means applying the nursing process to community-focused nursing care. The steps of the nursing process that directly involve the community client include assessment, planning, implementation, and evaluation. Figure 16-1 provides an overview of the nursing process as directed to the community client.

Application of the nursing process to the community client is illustrated in the following sections with case studies taken from the practices of two community health nurses. For clarity, infant malnutrition and the high prevalence of smoking are the only community health problems used to illustrate application of the nursing process. In reality, several community health problems were identified in each situation. Their relative importance was determined, and infant malnutrition and smoking behavior were designated the most important problems before continuing with intervention.

ASSESSING COMMUNITY HEALTH

Assessing community health requires gathering relevant existing data, generating missing data, and interpreting the data base. Gathering of the data and its initial interpretation are the first steps in the assessment phase of the nursing process.

Data Collection and Interpretation

The primary goal of data collection is to acquire usable information about the community and its health. The systematic collection of data about community health necessitates gathering or compiling existing data and generating missing data. These data are then interpreted, and community health problems and capabilities are identified.

Data gathering is the process of obtaining existing, readily available data. These data usually describe the demography of a community: age, sex, and socioeconomic and racial distributions; vital statistics, including selected mortality and morbidity data; community institutions, including health care organizations and the services they provide; and health manpower characteristics. Often these data have been collected by others via structured interviews and questionnaires and are available in published reports.

Other data, generally not statistical, are less easily available. Frequently they must be developed by the nurse/data collector through interaction with community members or groups. This process is termed *data generation*. Data that need to be generated include information about a community's knowledge and beliefs, values and sentiments, goals and perceived needs, norms, problem-solving processes, and power, leadership, and influence structures. These data are more apt to be collected via interviews and observation and to be qualitative.

A composite data base is created by combining the gathered and generated data. Data interpretation seeks to attribute meaning to the data. First, data are analyzed and synthesized and themes are noted. Community health problems, or needs for action, and community health strengths, or capabilities, are determined. Next, the resources available to meet the needs are identified. Problems are indicated by differences between the nurse's and community's concepts of community health and the available data. Strengths, on the other hand, are suggested by similarities between the nurse's and community's concepts of community health and available data. The nurse and community, working in a partnership, identify problems. Next, the resources available to meet the needs are identified. Active community participation is critical for the data interpretation process, particularly in identifying problems.

The Program Planning Model, initially proposed by Delbecq and Van de Ven (1971), is a widely accepted technique for encouraging lay participation in problem identification. The model illustrates active community participation in problem identification and program planning. It maximizes the contributions of various groups with diverse interests and expertise. This model depends heavily on nominal groups, "groups in which individuals work in the presence of one another but do not interact" (Delbecq and Van de Ven, 1971, p. 467), the separation of person from collective problems, and a round-robin procedure for listing problems without concurrently evaluating or elaborating on them.

The model, popularly known as the *nominal group process*, was compared in one early study with three other methods for identifying and prioritizing health needs (Scutchfield, 1975). The other methods were community diagnosis, random consumer survey, and comprehensive health planning ratings. The health care priorities of the consumer responding to the household survey were the cost of medical care, physician unavailability, and lack of specialty services. Health planning ratings emphasized service gaps and under-utilization. The community diagnosis method resulted in an emphasis on particular diseases. The nominal group process, which involved consumers as well as health professionals and health planners, resulted in a greater emphasis on lack of services and facilities and financing problems than did the community diagnosis method, which involved only health professionals. Flexner and Littlefield (1977, p. 246) note that the community diagnosis lacks the understanding that "what the consumer feels is important may in fact be important, even though this perspective may be alien to the objective information orientation" of the data gatherer. Conversely, the random consumer survey and comprehensive health planning ratings lack the provider's and planner's perspective. The nominal group process, involving health-care consumers as well as health-care providers and planners, offers the most balanced perspective.

Other consensus methods such as the Delphi technique are also used to define the extent of agreement among content experts, policymakers, and community members about the presence and importance of certain health problems. The recent literature suggests that consensus methods will produce useful and credible results if problems are carefully selected, participants in the process are deliberately selected and closely monitored, justifiable and reasonable levels of consensus are expected, and the findings are used as guides for decision making. (Fink et al 1984).

Data Collection Methods

A variety of methods should be used to collect data. Methods that encourage the nurse to consider the community's per-

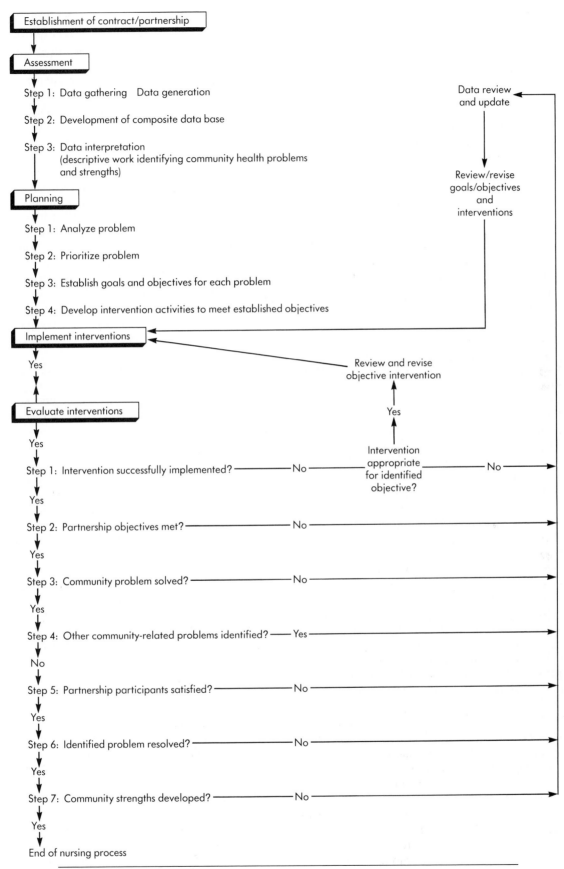

FIGURE 16-1

Flow chart illustrating the nursing process with the community client.

ception of its health problems and capabilities are as important as those methods structured to yield knowledge that the nurse considers essential.

Five methods of collecting data useful to the community health nurse are informant interviews, participant observation, secondary analysis of existing data, surveys, and windshield surveys. These methods can be clustered into two distinct but complementary categories: methods that rely on what is directly observed by the data collector and methods that rely on what is reported to the data collector.

Direct Data Collection

Informant interviews, participant observation, and windshield surveys are examples of direct data collection. Informant interviews, which consist of directed conversation with selected members of a community about community members or groups and events, are basic to effective data collection. Also basic is participant observation, the deliberate sharing, in so far as circumstances permit, in the life of a community. Informant interviews and participant observation are techniques particularly suitable for generating information about community beliefs, norms, values, power and influence structures, and problem-solving processes (Ruffing-Rahal, 1985). Such data can seldom be reported in numbers, so often they are not collected. Even worse, impressions—intuitive and unverified—are sometimes substituted for data.

In the example of the community with the infant malnutrition problem, informant interviewing with social workers and religious leaders provided data indicating a community with well-defined clusters of persons with low incomes, concerns about adolescent pregnancy, and worries about the health of its babies. The data reflecting concerns and worries would have been difficult to acquire without personal interviews.

Windshield surveys are the motorized equivalent of simple observation. The nurse, driving a car or riding public transportation, can observe many dimensions of a community's life and environment through the windshield. Common characteristics of street people, neighborhood gathering places, the rhythm of community life, quality of housing, and geographic boundaries can be readily observed. In the infant malnutrition example, the windshield survey suggested that the community had a significant number of unemployed persons because adults were observed "hanging out" at country crossroads in the daytime.

All three of these methods require sensitivity, openness, curiosity, and the ability to listen, taste, touch, smell, and see life as it lived in a community.

Collection of Reported Data

Two methods of collecting reported data are secondary analysis and surveys. In secondary analysis, the community health nurse uses previously gathered data, such as minutes from community meetings. This type of analysis is extremely valuable because it is efficient and economical. Many sources of data useful for secondary analysis — public documents, health surveys, minutes from meetings, statistical data, and health records — are readily available. In the Jefferson County infant malnutrition example, birth records noting low birth weights and health department clinic records of low-weight-for-height children provided information that reflected an infant malnutrition rate that was higher than average.

Surveys, which report data from a sample of persons, are equally useful but somewhat less efficient and economical than observational methods and secondary analyses because they require time-consuming and costly data collection. Thus the survey method is not often used by the community health nurse. However, surveys are necessary for identifying certain community problems. For example, a lack of accessible personal health services cannot be readily and reliably documented in any other fashion.

Because no data collection method is without bias, it is best to use several methods with different strengths and weaknesses. This is called *triangulation*. Using multiple complementary methods is essential to and consistent with community health nursing practices. Readers interested in further information about survey and secondary analysis methods should refer to *The Practice of Social Research* (Babbie, 1989). Readers interested in additional information about observational methods should refer to *Essentials of Nursing Research* (Polit and Hungler, 1989).

Nursing assessment of community health—data collection and interpretation—is focused. Focus, or perspective, can be provided by detailed assessment guides, which are built on a conceptual framework of definitions of community and community health.

Assessment Guides

Concepts stated in behavioral or observable terms can serve as assessment guides. The concepts of community and community health have already been defined in such terms. The concept of community has been specified (see Table 16-1). The original definition (see p. 254) includes three dimensions: place and time, people or person, and function. Each of these dimensions is specified by several indicators. For example, the spatial dimension is represented by indicators such as size and politcal boundaries.

The specifics of community health—its status, structure, and process dimensions—are presented in Table 16-3. In the infant malnutrition example, status dimension data were gathered from morbidity/mortality data. Structural dimension data were gathered from vital statistics and from informant interviews with social workers. Process dimension data were gathered from informant interviews with community religious leaders. In this way, the concepts of community and community health provide the framework for the Assessment Guide in Appendix E. Together, the concepts and Assessment Guide constitute the Community Health Assessment Model, which is the basis of the *Community-Oriented Health Record* (COHR; see Appendix E1). Data, problems, and capabilities are all organized by using the Community Health Assessment Model.

Assessment Issues

Gaining entry or acceptance into the community is perhaps the biggest challenge in assessment. The community health nurse is usually an outsider and often represents an established health care system that is neither known nor trusted by community members. They may therefore react with indifference or even active hostility. In addition, the community health nurse may feel insecure about his or her skills as a community worker, and the community may refuse to acknowledge its need for those skills. Because the nurse's success largely depends on the way he or she is viewed, entry into the community is critical. Often the nurse can gain entry by participating in community events, looking and listening attentively, visiting people in formal leadership positions, employing an assessment guide, and using a peer group for support.

Once the nurse gains entry at an initial level, role negotiation often becomes an issue. The concept of role involves the values, behaviors, or goals that govern an individual's interactions with others. The nurse must decide how long to separate the roles of data collector and intervenor. Effective implementation of the nursing process requires initial collection of an adequate data base. The danger of premature response to health needs and social injustice is great. Nurses can facilitate role negotiation by a thoughtful and consistent presentation of the reasons for their presence in the community and by sincere demonstrations of their commitment to the community. Keeping appointments, emphasizing the importance of clarifying community members' perceptions of health needs, and respecting persons' right to choose whether they will work with the nurse are often useful techniques.

Maintaining confidentiality is also important. Nurses must scrupulously protect the identity of community members who provide sensitive or controversial data. In some cases the nurse may consider withholding data; in other situations she may be legally required to disclose data.

Of a less personal nature is the issue of small-area analysis. This issue concerns the inappropriateness of reaching conclusions based on data gathered from small areas. For example, calculation of mortality rates in a rural county when the denominator is as small as 5000 may be skewed. This issue frequently compromises the validity of many identified health problems. It reinforces the usefulness of triangulation, because if similar health problems are identified using several assessment methods, the nurse can be more confident of their validity.

This section, *Assessing Community Health,* provided an overview of the data collection and interpretation required in the community assessment process. The Program Planning Model was described as a method for encouraging active community participation in this process. The result of this community assessment is the establishment of a composite data base. Five specific methods for collecting the data necessary for establishing a composite data base were presented along with a section on using assessment guides as a means for focusing this process. Finally, assessment issues encountered during data collection were discussed. Gathered data and generated data are combined to create a composite data base. This composite data base is used as a means of uncovering and identifying community health problems such as the infant malnutrition problem in Jefferson County. Remember, a community assessment will identify multiple community health problems. Each one of these must be analyzed and assigned a priority score to determine

which are the most serious problems. In the next sections, the infant malnutrition example is used to illustrate how an identified problem is analyzed and assigned a priority score.

PLANNING FOR COMMUNITY HEALTH

The planning phase includes analyzing the identified community health problems, establishing priorities among them, establishing goals and objectives, and identifying intervention activities that will accomplish the objectives.

Problem Analysis

Problem analysis seeks to clarify the nature of the problem. The nurse identifies the origins and impact of the problem, the points at which intervention might be undertaken, and the parties that have an interest in the problem and its solution. Analysis often requires the development of a problem matrix, in which the direct and indirect precursors and consequences are identified and interrelationships among the problems, precursors, and consequences are mapped. The matrix is important because the nurse can anticipate that several of the same precursors and consequences underlie many of the problems. The problem of highest priority may be among the common precursors and consequences.

Problem analysis should be undertaken for each identified problem. It often requires organizing a special group composed of the nurse, persons whose areas of expertise relate to the problem, persons whose organizations are capable of intervening, and representatives of the community experiencing the problem. Both content and process specialists must participate. Together they can identify the problem correlates and explain how they affect the problem.

This process is seen in the following example of Problem Analysis (Figure 16-2). Problem correlates (precursors and consequences) of infant malnutrition are listed in the first column. Correlates are from all facets of community life. Social or environmental correlates are as appropriate as those oriented to the individual. For example, teenage pregnancy is a social correlate of infant malnutrition, and high unemployment is an environmental correlate. In the second column the relationships between each correlate and the problem are noted. The third column contains data from the community and the literature that support the relationship, written in capsule fashion. The suspected infant malnutrition example and a few of its correlates are given. Infant malnutrition is thought to be correlated to inadequate diet, community norms, poverty, disturbed mother-child relationship, and teenage pregnancy.

Problem Prioritization

Infant malnutrition represents only one of several community health problems identified by the community assessment. In reality, several community-health problems besides infant malnutrition were identified. They included a mortality rate from cardiovascular disease that was higher than the national norm.

Each problem identified as part of the assessment process must be put through a ranking process to determine its relative importance. This ranking process, in which problems are evaluated and priorities established according to predetermined criteria, is termed *problem prioritization*. It

Problem analysis

Name of community: Jefferson County

Problem statement: Infant malnutrition in Jefferson County

Problem correlates	Relationship of correlates to problem	Data supportive to relationships (refer to appropriate sections of data base and relevant research findings in current literature)
1. Inadequate diet	Diets lacking in required nutrients contribute to malnutrition.	All county infants and their mothers seen by PHNs in 1990 referred to nutritionist because of poor diets.
2. Community norms	Bottle fed babies less apt to receive adequate amounts of safe milk containing necessary nutrients.	Area general practitioners and nurses agree that 90% of mothers in county bottle-feed.
3. Poverty	Infant formulas are expensive.	60% of new mothers in county are receiving welfare benefits.
4. Disturbed mother-child relationship	Poor mother-child relationship may result in infant's failure to thrive.	Data from nursing charts of 43 mothers with infants diagnosed as "failure to thrive."
5. Teen-age pregnancy	Teen-age mothers most apt to have inadequate diets prenatally, to bottle feed, to be poor, and to lack parenting skills.	90% of births in 1992 were to women 19 years of age or younger.
Column 1	Column 2	Column 3

FIGURE 16-2

Problem analysis: infant malnutrition.

involves the contributions of community members, substantive experts, administrators, and resource controllers.

Criteria that have been helpful in ranking problems include: (1) community awareness of the problem; (2) community motivation to resolve or better manage the problem; (3) nurse's ability to influence problem solution; (4) availability of expertise relevant to problem solution; (5) severity of consequences if the problem is unresolved; and (6) speed with which resolution can be achieved. These criteria are listed in the first column of Figure 16-3; once again the example of infant malnutrition is used.

Given an acceptable and comprehensive set of criteria and a list of community health problems, the process of assigning priorities is rather simple. Each problem is considered independently and a priority score is calculated. The criteria are weighted on a scale ranging from a low score of 1 to a high score of 10 (Column 2). These criteria are weighted jointly by the members of the partnership using the perceived importance of each criterion to the identified community health problem. For instance, when members of the partnership assigned a weight to the first criterion listed in Figure 16-3, they had to ask each other: "How important is community awareness of infant malnutrition in Jefferson County for problem resolution?" Each of the criteria is considered separately and independently, and then assigned a criterion weight.

Next, the importance of each criterion relative to the problem must be considered and rated relative to the partnership's ability to resolve it. In deciding the rating to be assigned, the members of the partnership answer questions related to their ability to influence and/or change the situation relative to the criterion. In the infant malnutrition example, they asked each other how widespread community awareness of the problem was. After questions about the criterion's significance have been discussed by the members of the partnership and there is agreement on its rating, the score is then recorded in column 4. In differentiating between the ideas of weight (Column 2) and rate (Column 4), it may be helpful to remember that a criterion could be extremely important in considering priorities, but rate low for a particular problem because the members of the community partnership feel it would be difficult to influence or change things relative to that particular criterion.

After this process has been repeated separately for each identified problem and a significance score has been determined, significance scores of all the problems are compared. Priorities are established. The most significant problems, those with the highest priority scores, are selected as the focus for intervention.

Establishing a priority score for each identified problem can appear complicated; however, it helps to recall that the criteria were established (Column 1) and weighted (Column

Problem prioritization

Criteria	Criteria weights (1-10)	Problem	Problem rating (1-10)	Rationale for rating	Problem significance (weight × rate)
1. Community awareness of the problem	5	Infant malnutrition in Jefferson County	10	Health service providers, teachers, and a variety of parents have mentioned problem.	50
2. Community motivation to resolve the problem	10		3	Most feel this problem is irresolvable because majority of those affected are indigent.	30
3. Nurse's ability to influence problem resolution	5		8	Nurse skilled at consciousness raising and mobilizing support.	40
4. Ready availability of expertise relevant to problem resolution	7		10	WIC program, nutritionist available. County extension agent interested.	70
5. Severity of consequences if problem is left unresolved	8		5	Effects on marginal malnutrition not too well documented.	40
6. Quickness with which problem resolution can be achieved	3		3	Extended time to mobilize rural community with no history of social action.	9
					Total: 239
Column 1	Column 2	Column 3	Column 4	Column 5	Column 6

FIGURE 16-3

Problem prioritization: infant malnutrition.

2) by participants in the community partnership before prioritization began. Also, problem rating (Column 4) and the rationale for rating (Column 5) are established via the participation of all members in the community partnership. Although the numerical scores are subjective, the active involvement of the nurse and representatives of different community interests, and the use of triangulation help ensure that the data used to establish the rationale are relevant as well as accurate. Community participation also helps ensure that the significance score established for each problem reflects its importance relative to other community health problems.

The process of establishing a total significance score for the problem of suspected infant malnutrition is called problem prioritization and is depicted in Figure 16-3. Community motivation to resolve the problem was the criterion weighted as most important to problem resolution. Yet most community residents believed the problem could not be solved because of the poverty of those affected. Therefore the relative significance of this criterion when applied to the problem of infant malnutrition was low.

A similar process with the remaining five criteria listed in Column 1 of Figure 16-3 yielded a total significance score of 239 for the suspected infant malnutrition problem. Assuming 239 is the highest significance score among the several identified community health problems, infant malnutrition is justified as the priority problem requiring intervention.

Establishing Goals and Objectives

Once high-priority problems are identified, relevant goals and objectives are developed. The goal is generally a broad statement of desired outcome. Objectives are the precise statements of the desired outcome.

An example of a goal and objectives relevant to the infant malnutrition problem is depicted in Figure 16-4. The goal presented is to reduce the incidence and prevalence of infant malnutrition. The objectives are more precise and are behaviorally stated, incremental, and measurable. They pertain to assessing infant developmental levels, determining eligibility for the Women, Infants and Children Program (WIC), implementing an outreach program, enrolling infants in the WIC program, and incorporating supplemental foods into existing diets.

As noted earlier, establishing these goals and objectives involves collaboration between the nurse and representatives of the community groups affected by both the problem and the proposed intervention. This often requires considerable negotiation among all participants in the planning process. One important advantage offered by the continuous active

Goals and Objectives

Name of community: *Jefferson County*

Problem/concern: *Infant malnutrition*

Goal statement: *To reduce the incidence and prevalence of infant malnutrition*

Present date	Objectives (number and statement)	Completion date
1-92	No. 1 *80% of infants seen by health department, neighborhood health center, and private physicians will have their developmental levels assessed.*	8-92
1-92	No. 2 *WIC program eligibility will be determined for 80% of infants seen by health department, neighborhood health center, and private physicians.*	5-92
1-92	No. 3 *An outreach program will be implemented to identify at-risk infants not now known to health care providers.*	8-92
1-92	No. 4 *WIC program eligibility will be determined for 25% of at-risk infants.*	1-93
1-92	No. 5 *75% of all infants eligible for WIC food supplements will be enrolled in the program.*	12-92
1-92	No. 6 *50% of the mothers of infants enrolled in WIC will demonstrate 3 ways of incorporating WIC supplements into their infants' diets.*	5-92

FIGURE 16-4

Goals and objectives: infant malnutrition.

involvement of people affected by the outcomes is that they have a vested interest in those outcomes and therefore are supportive and committed to the success of the intervention. Once goals and objectives are established, intervention activities to accomplish the objectives can be identified.

Identifying Intervention Activities

Intervention activities, the means by which objectives are met, are the strategies that achieve the objectives, the ways change will be affected, and the ways the problem cycle will be interrupted. Because alternative intervention activities do exist, they must be identified and evaluated. The process of sketching possible interventions and selecting the best set of activities to achieve the goal of documenting and reducing infant malnutrition are depicted in Figures 16-5 and 16-6.

To achieve the objective related to assessment of infant developmental levels (see Figure 16-4, Objective 1), five intervenor activities are listed in the second column of Figure 16-5. Each is relevant to the first objective: 80% of infants seen by the health department, neighborhood health center, and private physicians will have their developmental levels assessed. The first two activities involve WIC program personnel as the principal change agents. The last three involve the community nurse practitioner (CNP), WIC pro-

gram personnel, and the staff of the health department, neighborhood health center, and private physicians' offices as the change partners.

The probable effectiveness of each of the activities is considered in the third and fourth columns. The value,* or the likelihood that the activity will foster achievement of the objective and eventual resolution of the problem, is noted in Column 3. Clearly, it is more valuable in the long term to teach others to assess infant development (Activity 4) than to do it for them (Activity 1). It is also valuable to analyze the change process necessary to accomplish the objective (Activity 5). Consequently, Activities 4 and 5 have higher value scores than Activity 1.

On the other hand, the probability,* or the likelihood that the means can be implemented, is highest when only the CNP is involved, because the nurse has more control over her own behavior than over the behavior of others. Therefore Activities 1 and 3 have higher probabilities than Activities 2, 4, and 5. Probability is recorded in Column 4. Conditions explaining the numerical scores are noted

---

*The value and probability scores of intervenor activities may range from one (low) to ten (high). The range of one to ten was arbitrarily determined.

Plan: Assess Infants' Developmental Levels

Name of community: _Jefferson County_

Objective number 1. _80% of infants seen by health department, neighborhood health center, and private physicians will_

and statement: _have their development levels assessed._

Plan

Date	Intervenor activities/means	Value (1-10)	Probability (1-10)	Activity/means selected for implementation*
1-92	1. WIC program supplies personnel to assess infant developmental levels.	1	10 Total 10	Insufficient personnel and time. Existing community resources (potential) ignored.
1-92	2. WIC program provides in-service education to staff on assessment of infant development.	5	5 Total 25	Antipathy between WIC personnel and other health workers high. Need for education must be assessed first and enthusiasm for objectives created.
1-92	3. CNP provides in-service education to staff in assessment of infant development.	3	10 Total 30	CNP can't do it alone!
1-92	*4. CNP assists WIC personnel to identify in-service educational needs of area health care providers about assessment of infant development.	8	8 Total 64	Most likely to build on existing community strengths. CNP skilled in needs assessment and interpersonal techniques needed to decrease antipathy.
1-92	*5. CNP assists WIC personnel to identify driving and restraining forces relative to implementation of objective.	10	8 Total 80	Without this, change effort likely to fail.

FIGURE 16-5

Plan: assess infants' developmental levels.

briefly in the fifth column. The activities with the highest scores, computed by multiplying the value by the probability, are selected because it is important to be able to affect the objective (value) and carry out the means (probability). In this case, Activities 4 and 5, with total scores of 64 and 80 respectively, would be selected.

It is important to recognize that although the numbers assigned by the nurse to both Column 3 (value) and Column 4 (probability) are based on subjective judgement, the resulting totals are useful to establish a relative basis for judging which of the potential intervenor activities (Column 2) will be most effective in meeting the objectives. The activities with the highest scores, computed by multiplying the value by the probability, are selected because it is important to be able to both affect the objective (value) and carry out the means (probability).

A second example of plan development is also depicted (see Figure 16-6; Plan: Implement an Outreach Program). The activities relate to Objective 3 of the Goals and Objectives, (see Figure 16-4), implementation of an outreach program, and involve using lay advisors, hospital nurses, public health nurses, and WIC program personnel. Activities 1 and 2, with total scores of 48 and 40 respectively, were selected. Activity 1 builds on existing informal community leaders and Activity 2 addresses needed changes in the formal health care delivery system.

IMPLEMENTATION FOR COMMUNITY HEALTH

Implementation, the third phase of the nursing process, comprises the work/activities aimed at achieving the goals and objectives. Implementation efforts may be made by the person or group who established the goals and objectives, or they may be shared with or even delegated to others. The issue of centralizing implementation efforts is important, and the community health nurse's position on this issue can be influenced by a variety of factors.

Factors Influencing Implementation

Implementation is shaped by the nurse's chosen roles, the type of health problem selected as the focus for intervention, the community's readiness to participate in problem resolution, and characteristics of the social change process. The nurse participating in community-oriented intervention commands knowledge and skills not possessed by the other intervenors. The question is how the nurse uses the position, knowledge, and skills.

Nurse's Role

Nurses can act as content experts, helping communities to select and attain task-related goals. In the example of infant malnutrition, the nurse used epidemiological skills to determine the incidence and prevalence of malnutrition. The nurse also served as a process expert by increasing the

Plan: Implement an Outreach Program

Name of community: *Jefferson County*

Objective number 3. *An outreach program is implemented to identify at-risk infants*

and statement: *not now known to health care providers.*

Plan

Date	Intervenor activities/means	Value (1-10)	Probability (1-10)	Activity/means selected for implementation*
1-92	*1. CNP identifies and trains lay advisors in community as case finders.	8	6 Total 48	Lay leaders already known, proven to be effective change agents; can't however, be paid.
1-92	*2. Local hospital administrators alter job descriptions of nurses in maternity and pediatrics to include case finding and referral.	8	5 Total 40	All babies in Jefferson County born in hospital since 1978. Administrator interested in community. Administration powerful and can alter nurses' job descriptions.
1-92	3. CNP encourages public health nurses to do better job of case finding.	8	2 Total 16	Public health nurses have historic role in case finding. CNP not well known by PHNs. PHNs reported to be overworked.
1-92	4. WIC personnel devote 1 evening/week to case finding.	1	10 Total 110	One nurse (nonresident) eager to do this. Doesn't develop existing community resources.
Column 1	Column 2	Column 3	Column 4	Column 5

FIGURE 16-6

Plan: implement an outreach program.

community's own capabilities in documenting the problem rather than by contributing substantive expertise only.

Content-dominated roles are often considered *change agent roles,* while process roles are termed *change partner roles.* Change agent roles emphasize gathering and analyzing facts and implementing programs, while change partner roles include those of enabler-catalyst, teacher of problem-solving skills, and activist-advocate (Rothman, 1974, Bodenstein, 1974).

The Problem

The role the nurse chooses depends on the nature of the health problem and the community's decision-making ability, as well as on professional and personal preferences. Some health problems clearly necessitate certain intervention roles. If a community lacks democratic problem-solving abilities, the nurse may select teacher, facilitator, and advocate roles. Problem-solving skills must be explained and modeled. A problem such as ascertaining the status of community health, on the other hand, frequently requires fact-gatherer and analyst roles. Some problems, such as the example of infant malnutrition, require multiple roles. In that case, managing conflict among the involved health care providers demanded process skills. Collecting and interpreting the data necessary to document the problem required both interpersonal and analytical skills.

The community's history of participation in decision making is a critical factor. In a community skilled in iden-

tifying and managing its problems, the nurse may appropriately serve as technical expert or advisor. Quite different roles may be required if the community lacks problem-solving skills or has a history of unsuccessful change efforts. The nurse may have to focus on developing problem-solving capabilities or achieving one successful change so that the community becomes empowered to assume responsibility for promoting change on its own behalf.

Social Change Process

The nurse's role depends on the social change process. Not all communities are receptive to innovation. Receptivity to change is often inversely related to the extent to which a community adheres to traditional norms. Innovation is often directly related to high socioeconomic status, a perceived need for change, the presence of liberal, scientific, and democratic values, and a high level of social participation by community residents (Rogers, 1983; Rothman 1974). The innovation itself affects its acceptance. Innovations with the highest adoption rates are seen as more advantageous than other alternatives, compatible with existing values, amenable to a limited trial, easily explained or demonstrated, geographically accessible, and simple (Rogers, 1983; Rothman, 1974). For example, community residents might go to an immunization clinic rather than a private physician if the clinic is nearby and less expensive and if the physician is not always available when needed.

Innovations are also accepted more readily when the innovation is disseminated in ways compatible with the community's norms, values, and customs and when information is relayed through the appropriate communication mode. The mass media is the appropriate mode for early adopters and the face-to-face mode is appropriate for late adopters. Other factors that positively influence acceptance include the support of other communities for the change efforts, identification and use of opinion leaders, and clear, unambiguous communication about the innovation (Rogers, 1983; Rothman 1974).

Many factors shape implementation and their effects on the change process are complex and varying. Therefore, the community health nurse must be adaptable. The roles used to initiate change may differ from those used to maintain or stabilize it. The roles required to initiate, maintain, and stabilize change may vary from community to community and from one intervention to another within the same community. Thus the nurse must be skilled in a variety of implementation mechanisms.

Implementation Mechanisms

Implementation mechanisms are the vehicles, or modes, by which innovations are transferred from the planners to the units of service. The community health nurse alone is never considered an implementation mechanism, for change on behalf of the community client requires multiple implementation mechanisms. The nurse must identify and use all of them appropriately. Some important implementation mechanisms or aids include small interacting groups, lay advisors, the mass media, and health policy.

Small Interacting Groups

Small interacting groups, formal and informal, are essential implementation mechanisms. Many of the groups in the community—families, legislative bodies, health care recipients, and service providers—are discussed fully elsewhere in the text. Some of the informal groups, such as neighborhoods and social action groups, have also been discussed. The common tie among these diverse groups is their location between the community and individual levels. Because of their intermediate position, they act both to support and to constrain change efforts at the community and individual levels. They are potentially powerful because they are mediating structures (Berger and Neuhaus, 1977).

Consequently, the community health nurse needs to ascertain which groups view the proposed change as beneficial and which do not. New small groups may need to be formed to facilitate the change. Accommodations may be necessary in the innovation or in the dissemination process to increase acceptance. Initially the innovation may have to be directed to groups with a majority of early adopters (those with broad perspectives and abilities to adopt new ideas from mass media information sources) and to groups whose goals parallel those of the intervention plan (Rothman, 1974). An example of a small group initiating community-oriented change is illustrated in the Progress Notes (Figure 16-7).

Lay Advisors

Lay advisors are individuals who are influential in approving or vetoing new ideas and from whom others seek advice and information about new ideas (Rothman, 1974). They often perform a similar function to that of early adopters. Lay advisors or opinion leaders are characterized by their conformity to community norms, heavy involvement in formal social groups, specific areas of expertise, and a slightly higher social status than their followers (Rogers, 1983; Warnecke et al, 1976).

Lay advisors are helpful in community-oriented intervention. In one study, they increased breast self-examination practices among Latina women by about 40% (Lorig and Walters, 1980-1981). In another study, rural African-Americans in North Carolina were found to receive more arthritis care from lay advisors than from physicians (Salber, 1981).

Mass Media

Small interacting groups and lay advisors are particularly useful in instituting change among late adopters. But groups dominated by early adopters and lay advisors can be reached through the mass media. Mass media such as newspapers, television, and radio are impersonal and formal types of communication and are useful in providing information quickly to large numbers of people. Using the mass media is efficient because the proportion of resources expended to population covered is low and larger populations can be targeted. For example, information about teenage pregnancy can be disseminated efficiently by rock music stations.

In addition to being efficient, the mass media are effective aids in intervention. The Stanford Heart Disease Program showed that community residents subject to media-only intervention increased their knowledge about cardiovascular risk factors and improved their dietary patterns. Community residents subjected to the mass media campaign and face-to-face intervention also lowered their risk for cardiovascular disease (Maccoby et al, 1977). Similar findings have been reported from the North Karelia study in Finland (McAlister et al, 1982). A small (N = 100) pilot study conducted in North Carolina also found that mailed pamphlets were as effective as telephone calls and home visits in increasing the use of selected health services (Selby et al, 1990). An example of a program with multiple intervention mechanisms directed to family, school, and community levels was reported by Simons-Morton et al (1986). They used parent groups, school lunch modifications, and physical exercise programs to improve diet and exercise behaviors in elementary school children and the mass media, community organizations, health professional education, and lay volunteers at the school district or community level.

Health Policy

Health policy can also play a critical part in the adoption of healthful community-oriented change (Milio, 1981). The major intent of public policy in the health field is to address collective human needs, and it frequently serves to constrain individual choice for the public good. For instance, drivers have been urged for several years to wear seat belts. However, the incidence of automobile fatalities was not reduced until drivers were required to observe lowered speed limits and, in some states, to wear seat belts and use special restraining seats for children. Obviously health policy can facilitate interventions that promote community health.

Progress Notes

Name of community: *Jefferson County*

Goal: *Reduce the incidence and prevalence of infant malnutrition*

Date	Narrative, Assessment, Plan (NAP)	Budget, Time
	(Record both objective and subjective data. Interpret these data in terms of whether the objectives were achieved and whether the intervenor activities used were effective. The plan is dependent on the assessment and may include both new or revised objectives and activities.)	
2-14-92	*Objective 1, Means 4*	
	Narrative: Meeting to develop needs assessment was attended by CNP, 2 WIC personnel, and physicians from health department, neighborhood health center, and local medical society. Consensus rapidly achieved among 5 of 6 participants that goal, objectives, and means (especially Objective 1, Means 4) were appropriate. Physician representing medical society consistently objected, stating vehemently that private sector had long provided adequate medical care for area youngsters. One WIC staff member angrily questioned how physician could document "adequacy." Physician responded that federal aid created more need than disease did. He would not recommend that medical society support the effort. CNP cowered, afraid that this would jeopardise entire effort. Eventually, however, physician left, and plans were made to develop and conduct needs assessment, with or without the medical society's help.	
	Agenda: CNP to develop needs assessment tool with WIC personnel and health systems agency planner. Physicians to develop list of providers to be contacted. Neighborhood health center physician to get a place on medical society agenda and attempt to clarify our plans. WIC personnel to contact nonphysician health workers to introduce plan and develop provider list.	
	Assessment: Plans made to proceed with needs assessment and partner support essential to accomplishment of objective. Group process problematical, and CNP ineffective due to discomfort with conflict between physician and WIC staff member.	*$200, 2 hours meeting and 2 hours preparation time*
	Plans: Meeting scheduled for 2-28-92 to deal with agreed-on agenda.	
	* Before 2-28 meeting, CNP will discuss ways of better handling conflict with consultation group, collaborate in drafting needs assessment, and telephone others to determine their progess.*	
	* J. Goeppinger, RN, CHP*	

FIGURE 16-7

Progress notes: infant malnutrition.

If public policy that will encourage or even simply allow health-generating choices is to be enacted, the community health nurse must lobby actively for it. The nurse must also use small groups, lay advisors, and the mass media as aids to implementation. Most community health nurses are experienced in working with naturally-occurring small groups like the family and with lay advisors. They are less experienced in working with legislators and the mass media. Yet all resources must be used to achieve healthful change in the community client.

No matter what mechanisms are used, all implementation efforts must be documented. Evaluation is also important to determine and improve the effectiveness of community-oriented nursing practice and thereby increase our knowledge base and improve our success in competing for funds.

EVALUATING INTERVENTION FOR COMMUNITY HEALTH

Simply defined, evaluation is the appraisal of the effects of some organized activity or program. It may involve the design and conduct of evaluation research, in which social science research methods are used to determine program effectiveness, efficiency, adequacy, appropriateness, and unintended consequences. Evaluation may also involve the more elementary process of assessing progress by contrasting the objectives and the results. This section deals with the basic approach of contrasting objectives and results.

Evaluation begins in the planning phase, when goals and measurable objectives are established and goal-attaining activities are identified. After implementing intervention, only the accomplishment of objectives and the effects of intervention activities have to be assessed. The Progress Notes direct the nurse to perform such appraisals concurrently with implementation. In assessing the data recorded there, the nurse is requested to evaluate whether the objectives were achieved and whether the intervention activities used were effective. The nurse also must decide whether the costs in money and time were commensurate with the benefits. This process is depicted in the Progress Notes (Figure 16-7). Here the nurse has noted progress toward the needs assessment and difficulties encountered in handling conflict among the group members.

Such an evaluation process is oriented to community health because the intervention goals and objectives are derived from the nurse's and the community's conceptions of health. Simplistic as it appears, it is not without its problems. The lack of a control community and of adequate baseline information casts doubts on the intervention. Nursing interventions may also have diffuse and weak effects that are difficult to detect. Models for the practitioner to use in determining cost-benefit and cost-effectiveness figures are complicated and therefore not readily available. And, finally, the lay role in evaluation has never been fully accepted. Professionals have adopted partnership in assessment and implementation more readily than in evaluation. The issue of who has the power to define, judge, and institute change in professional activities is by no means resolved.

CLINICAL APPLICATION

A second example of an identified community health problem is summarized here in a step-by-step format for further clarification of how the nursing process can be used to promote community health. In this example, like the earlier example of infant malnutrition, Figure 16-1 provides an overview of the entire process.

Cigarette smoking is used here as another example of how the nursing process can be applied to the community client. Recall from the infant malnutrition example that the stages of this process include: establishment of the contract/partnership, assessment, planning, implementing interventions, and evaluating interventions. Like the infant malnutrition example used earlier in the chapter, this example follows the nursing process presented by a flow chart in Figure 16-1. Therefore, throughout this example reference will be made back to Figure 16-1.

Partnership for Community Health

Establishing the contract/partnership for community health is the first stage of the nursing process. In our example community interest in the issue of cigarette smoking in Jefferson County was stimulated by community-wide discussion of a proposed local ordinance limiting smoking in public buildings. Many questions about cigarette smoking were raised by this discussion. Some members of the community decided to pursue this issue further and their decision resulted in the formation of a partnership that included the community health nurse, community members who supported the local chapter of the American Lung Association (ALA), and the ALA regional director.

Assessing Community Health

Assessing community health is the second stage of this process. In Figure 16-1, Assess, Step 1 involves both data gathering and data generation using the community oriented health record. Table 16-2 specifies different types of status, structure, and process community health indicators that can be used for assessment. One example of status data gathered for this community health assessment is the results of a recently commissioned district-wide health study that provided vital statistics such as mortality and morbidity data for Jefferson County. Also, data were generated by talking with local church leaders, health workers, and other interested lay people about perceived community health needs. These interviews provided important information about the structural and process dimensions of this community's health. Data that are gathered and data that are generated about community health status are combined during the development of a composite data base (see Figure 16-1, Assess, Step 2).

Data interpretation (Assess, Step 3) requires examination of the composite data base in order to identify problems. The identified community health problems included: concerns about drugs in the community, a high perceived prevalence of smokers in the community, and an increased need for low-income housing. Community strengths were also identified and included such things as the presence of an established community church coalition that was interested in promoting community health.

Planning for Community Health

Once community health problems and community strengths are identified, the third state involves planning.

	Problem analysis	
Name of community: Jefferson County		
Problem statement: Suspected high prevalence of smoking in Jefferson County		

Problem correlates	Relationship of correlates to problem	Data supportive to relationships (refer to appropriate sections of data base and relevant research findings in current literature)
1. Increased risk of respiratory problems	Smokers have an increased incidence of respiratory infections.	Published findings from 1990 Behavior Risk Factor Prevalence Study of Jefferson County and multiple other research studies
2. Aggressive advertising by tobacco companies	Cigarette smoking portrayed to women as a means of self-expression and an indicator of sophistication.	Observation of local magazine, newspaper, and store advertising
3. Misconceptions about smoking	Belief that "only a few a day" isn't really smoking and therefore it won't cause any harm.	Interviews in the community with smokers and health care providers
Column 1	Column 2	Column 3

FIGURE 16-8

Problem analysis: smoking.

Problem Analysis

The first planning step is to analyze each of the identified problems (Figure 16-1, Plan, Step 1). Analysis is necessary to understand the nature of the identified problem. The results of the cigarette-smoking analysis are summarized in Figure 16-8.

Problem Prioritization

Because the community health assessment usually identifies more than one problem and community resources are limited, some means of comparison is needed to determine which identified problem is most significant to the members of the community partnership (see Figure 16-1, Plan, Step 2). Six criteria were selected as a framework for analysis before completion of the community assessment. They are listed in Figure 16-9, Column 1. After community health problems were identified from the composite data base, these criteria were applied to each identified community health problem in turn.

When these criteria were applied to the problem of suspected high prevalence of cigarette smoking in Jefferson County, criteria weights (Column 2) were established by the community partnership participants. This involves examining how important each criterion is relative to any plan of action for resolving the particular community health problem being evaluated (that is, a suspected high incidence of smoking). Determining a problem rating score (Column 4) requires that community partnership participants ask themselves questions about their ability to affect the current situation in their community regarding the specific criterion

under consideration. In this example, community motivation to resolve the problem was considered the most important criterion because any community-based effort to reduce smoking incidence will require a great deal of motivation by both the community at large and the individual smokers who are interested in quitting. Therefore the problem of cigarette smoking received a significance score of 90.

Establish Goals and Objectives (Figure 16-1, Plan, Step 3)

The high prevalence of smoking was identified as the priority problem when compared to other problems identified in the community assessment. Consequently, the next step is establishing broad goals and specific objectives, or precise statements of desired outcomes. The goal statement identified here was to "reduce the incidence and prevalence of cigarette smoking." The number of specific objectives vary from problem to problem; here seven specific objectives are listed (Figure 16-10).

Intervention activities provide specific ways to meet each of the objectives that have been established to help address the problem of high incidence of cigarette smoking. Each of the seven objectives in Figure 16-10 requires a plan. For simplicity, only the plan for Objective 6, "Identified volunteers will be instructed about enrolling people interested in smoking cessation," is presented here (Figure 16-11). See Figure 16-10, Goal and Objectives (Smoking in Jefferson County), and note that the implementation activities presented in Figure 16-11 are the means of fulfilling Objective 6.

	Problem prioritization				
Criteria	**Criteria weights (1-10)**	**Problem**	**Rating (1-10)**	**Rationale for rating**	**Problem significance (weight × rate)**
1. Community awareness of the problem	9	Suspected high prevalence of cigarette smoking in Jefferson County	9	Newspaper and radio coverage of recent city council smoking restriction ordinance	81
2. Community motivation to resolve the problem	10		9	A self-help program requires individuals who want to quit and motivated community volunteers	90
3. Nurse's ability to influence problem resolution	6		5	Local organizations have their own ideas about what to do	30
4. Ready availability of expertise relevant to problem resolution	8		9	ALA has a smoking cessation self-help booklet	72
5. Severity of consequences if problem is left unresolved	10		7	Studies document harmful effects of smoking, but many smokers believe smoking will not harm their health	70
6. Quickness with which problem resolution can be achieved	3		3	Nicotine is addictive, recidivism rate for ex-smokers is high	9
				Total	362
Column 1	**Column 2**	**Column 3**	**Column 4**	**Column 5**	**Column 6**

FIGURE 16-9

Problem prioritization: smoking.

Develop Intervention Activities (Figure 16-1, Plan, Step 4)

Figure 16-11 illustrates specific intervenor activities for Objective 6. The estimated value of each intervenor activity for the identified objective is listed in Column 2. The anticipated relative probability of implementing each intervenor activity vis-à-vis successful implementation of the identified objective is listed in Column 3. A total for each intervenor activity is obtained by multiplying the number in Column 3 by the number in Column 4.

The first intervenor activity is to identify volunteers from community organizations to support the program. It has a value of 10 because without identification and recruiting of volunteers from community organizations the goal cannot be met. Although activity is critical, the nurse can expect some organizations to decline participation and others to withdraw as the process of implementation takes place. The probability assigned is therefore 7 rather than 10.

Implementing the Plan for Community Health

The process of implementing the plan itself takes place over time (see Figure 16-1, Implement). It is guided by the results of the planning stage, using the different intervention activities identified as guidelines for reaching each specific objective. The number and complexity of each intervenor activity will vary but each activity should contribute toward the successful completion of its related specific objective.

Evaluating the Intervention for Community Health

Evaluation of the community health intervention starts while planning is taking place (see Figure 16-1, Evaluate, Steps 1 to 5). It is an ongoing part of implementation of each selected intervenor activity, and it may also include retrospective evaluation to assess how successfully each specific objective was completed. Because this assessment is an ongoing process, intervenor activities that are ineffective can be modified or changed. Objectives may be added. This might happen if the intervenor activities were ineffective or

Goals and objectives

Name of community: Jefferson County

Problem: Suspected high prevalence of cigarette smoking

Goal statement: To document the prevalence of cigarette smoking and, if appropriate, intervene to reduce the incidence and prevalence of smoking

Present date	Objectives (number and statement)	Completion date
6-92	No. 1 Data on Jefferson County examined for incidence rates and risk factor mortality data.	8-92
6-92	No. 2 An individualized smoking cessation program will be identified.	10-92
6-92	No. 3 Multiple community organizations and volunteers will be recruited for program dissemination.	2-94
6-92	No. 4 Funding for self-help booklets and local media publicity support will be sought.	1-93
6-92	No. 5 Two segments of the community identified as having a high prevalence of smokers will be targeted.	10-92
6-92	No. 6 Volunteers will be instructed about enrolling people interested in smoking cessation.	2-93
6-92	No. 7 50% of the cigarette smokers enrolled in this smoking cessation program will either quit or reduce their daily cigarette intake by 25%.	6-93
Column 1	Column 2	Column 3

FIGURE 16-10

Goals and objectives: smoking.

unworkable. Figure 16-12 provides sample progress notes for the cigarette smoking example.

SUMMARY

This chapter has described and illustrated the definition of the community client being the target of service; the key concepts of community, community health, and partnership for health; and the nursing process of assessment, planning, implementation, and evaluation to promote community health. This entire process is summarized in Figure 16-13.

Community-oriented nursing practice emphasizes the community as the nurse's client. Healthful change is sought with and for the community client. Community health is the goal of practice, and partnership is the chief means of practice.

Using the nursing process as a tool for community-oriented practice includes assessment, planning, implementation, and evaluation. Assessment of a community uses a variety of techniques, including interviews, observation, analysis of existing data, and surveys. An Assessment Guide directs this process. The planning stage of the community nursing process includes analyzing and prioritizing problems, establishing goals and objectives, and identifying implementation alternatives. Several factors affect implementation, including the nurse's chosen role and the mechanisms available for implementation. The final stage of the community-oriented nursing process is evaluation.

Plan: Implement self-help smoking cessation program

Name of community: Jefferson County

Objective number 6: Identified volunteers will be instructed about enrolling interested community residents in the self-help cessation program

Date	Intervenor activities/means	Value (1-10)	Probability (1-10)	Activity/means selected for implementation*
6-92	1. Community health-promotion coalition supplies volunteers to enroll participants.	10	7 Total 70	Large numbers of volunteers will be needed.
6-92	2. ALA provides volunteers and staff to assemble self-help information packets for distribution by volunteers.	10	9 Total 90	ALA director is interested in this project and committed her agency to implementing it.
6-92	3. CNP develops step-by-step written directions for community volunteers to use in distributing the self-help packets.	8	10 Total 80	CNP can provide expertise for this activity.
6-92	4. Community health-promotion coalition representatives identify strengths and weaknesses.	8	7 Total 56	Wide diversity among coalition members will create disagreement and require negotiation.
6-92	5. Revised directions provided to volunteers at community distribution sites.	9	9 Total 81	Written step-by-step directions will be essential for community volunteers to register program participants.
Column 1	Column 2	Column 3	Column 4	Column 5

FIGURE 16-11

Plan: implement self-help smoking cessation program.

	Progress notes	
Name of community:	Jefferson County	
Goal:	High prevalence of cigarette smoking in Jefferson County	

Date	Narrative, Assessment, Plan (NAP)	Budget, Time
	(Record both objective and subjective data. Interpret these data in terms of whether the objectives were achieved and whether the intervenor activities used were effective. The plan is dependent on the assessment and may include both new or revised objectives and activities.)	
6-5-92	Objective 1, means 2	
	Narrative: Meeting with ALA regional director to discuss the details of what will be done in assembling the self-help packets for volunteer distribution. A time line was established and a list of the needed materials was generated during the meeting. The time line for accomplishing everything is very short and the number of available ALA volunteers is small. The ALA director is convinced there will be no problems in getting things done, but the CHN is not so sure. Last minute problems? There are always last minute problems. How will they be handled and who will handle them? Television, radio, and newspaper media materials have already been developed and release dates are established now. That means the self-help packets *must* be delivered for distribution before the media announcements.	$150, 1 hour meeting, 2 hours preparation.
	Agenda: CNP will recruit additional nurses to help plan. ALA regional director will enlist help from one group of local nursing home residents to start assembling packets. CNP is worried about the short time line.	
	Plans: Meeting scheduled for 6-20-92, CNP will have detailed list of what needs to be done by the local nursing home residents. ALA regional director will enlist their help and also handle the printing of all necessary materials.	
	CNP will enlist the help of other RNs, draft a detailed list of what to do, and contact the ALA director about her progress before the meeting.	
	G. Shuster, RN, CNP	

FIGURE 16-12

Progress notes: smoking cessation.

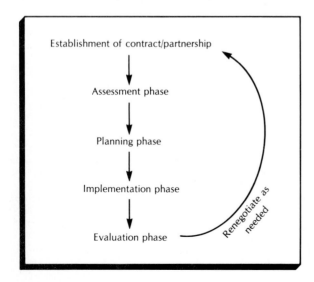

FIGURE 16-13

Summary flow sheet illustrating the nursing process with the community client.

KEY CONCEPTS

Most definitions of community include three dimensions: (1) networks of interpersonal relationships that provide friendship and support to members; (2) residence in a common locality; and (3) "solidarity, sentiments, and activities."

A community is defined as a locality-based entity, composed of systems of formal organizations reflecting societal institutions, informal groups, and aggregates that are interdependent and whose function or expressed intent is to meet a wide variety of collective needs.

A community practice setting is insufficient reason for saying practice is oriented toward the community client. When the location of the practice is in the community but the focus of the practice is the individual or family, then the nursing client remains the individual or family—not the whole community.

Community-oriented practice is targeted to the community, the population group in which healthful change is sought.

Community health as used in this chapter is defined as the meeting of collective needs through identifying problems and managing interactions within the community itself and between the community and the larger society.

Most changes aimed at improving community health involve, of necessity, partnerships among community residents and health workers from a variety of disciplines.

Assessing community health requires gathering existing data, generating missing data, and interpreting the data base.

Five methods of collecting data useful to the community health nurse are informant interviews, participant observation, secondary analysis of existing data, surveys, and windshield surveys.

Gaining entry or acceptance into the community is perhaps the biggest challenge in assessment. The community health nurse is usually an outsider and often represents an established health care system that is neither known nor trusted by community members, who may react with indifference or even active hostility.

The planning phase includes analyzing and establishing priorities among community health problems already identified, establishing goals and objectives, and identifying intervention activities that will accomplish the objectives.

Once high-priority problems are identified, broad relevant goals and objectives are developed.

The goal, generally a broad statement of desired outcome, and objectives, the precise statements of the desired outcome, are carefully selected.

Intervention activities, the means by which objectives are met, are the strategies that clarify what must be done to achieve the objectives, the ways change will be affected, and the way the problem will be interrupted.

Implementation, the third phase of the nursing process, is transforming a plan for improved community health into achievement of goals and objectives.

Simply defined, evaluation is the appraisal of the effects of some organized activity or program.

LEARNING ACTIVITIES

1. Observe an occupational health nurse, community health nurse, school nurse, family nurse practitioner, or emergency room nurse for several hours. Determine which of the nurse's activities are community-oriented and state the reasons for your judgement.

2. Using your own community as a frame of reference, develop examples illustrating the concepts of community, community client, community health, and partnership for health.

3. Read your local newspaper and identify articles illustrating the concepts of community, community client, community health, and partnership for health.

4. Using any two of the conditions of communtiy competence given in the chapter, analyze your own community briefly. Give examples of each condition.

BIBLIOGRAPHY

Anderson ET: Community focus in public health nursing: whose responsibility? Nurs Outlook 31:44-48, 1983.

Anderson E, McFarlane J, and Helton A: Community-as-client: a model for practice, Nurs Outlook 34:220-224, 1986.

Armstrong-Esther CA et al: Partnership in care, J Adv Nurs 12:735-741, 1987.

Babbie E: The practice of social research, ed 5, Belmont, Calif, 1989, Wadsworth Inc.

Berger PL and Neuhaus PJ: To empower people: the role of mediating structures in public policy, Washington, DC, 1977, American Enterprise Institute for Public Policy Research.

Blum HL: Planning for health, New York, 1974, Human Sciences Press Inc.

Bodenstein JW: The role of health professionals: Africanization in mission hospitals, Contact 21:3-10, 1974.

Bremer A: Revitalizing the district model for the delivery of prevention-focused community health nursing services, Family Comm Health 10:1-10, 1987.

Chalmers K and Kristajanson L: The theoretical basis for nursing at the community level: a comparison of three models, J Adv Nurs 14:569-574, 1989.

Chalmers K and Kristajanson L: The theoretical basis for nursing at the community level: models for community health practice. Paper presented at the 118th annual meeting of the American Public Health Association, New York City, 1990.

Cleaver VL, Ratcliff R, and Rogers B: Community health representatives: a valuable resource for providing coronary heart disease education activities for Native Americans, Health Education 20:16-20, 1989.

Combs-Orme T, Reis J, Ward LO: Effectiveness of home visits by public health nurses in maternal and child health: an empirical view, Public Health Rep 100:490-499, 1985.

Cottrell LS: The competent community. In Kaplan BH, Wilson RN, and Leighton AH, editors: Further explorations in social psychiatry, New York, 1976, Basic Books Inc, Publishers.

Dean D et al: Local health planning: a report of a collaborative process between a university and a church. Family and Community Health, 10:13-22, 1988.

Delbecq AL and Van de Ven AH: A group process model for problem identification and program planning, J Appl Behav Sci 62:467-492, 1971.

Feuerstein MT: Participatory evaluation—an appropriate technology for community health programmes, Contact 55:1-8, 1980.

Fink A et al: Consensus methods: characteristics and guidelines for use, Am J Public Health 74:979-983, 1984.

Flexner WA and Littlefield JE: Comment on alternative methods for health priority assessment, J Community Health 2:245-246, 1977.

Goeppinger J: Primary health care: an answer to the dilemmas of community nursing? Public Health Nurs 1:129-140, 1984.

Goeppinger J et al: An examination of the effective self-care education for person with arthritis. Arthritis Rheumatism, 32:706-716, 1989.

Goeppinger J, Lassiter PG, and Wilcox B: Community health is community competence, Nurs Outlook 30:464-467, 1982.

Hanchett ES: Community health assessment: a conceptual tool kit, New York, 1979, John Wiley & Sons Inc.

Hanchett ES: Nursing frameworks and community as client, Norwalk, Conn, 1988, Appleton & Lange.

Hanchett ES: Nursing models and community as client, Nurs Science Q 3:67-72, 1990.

Jamieson MK: Block nursing: practicing autonomous professional nursing in the community, Nursing and Health Care 11:250-253, 1990.

Jamieson MK: The St. Anthony Park Block Nurse Program, Am J Public Health 77:1227-1228, 1987.

Lorig K and Walters EG: Cuidaremos: the HECO approach to breast self-examination, Int Q Community Health Educ 1:125-134, 1980-1981.

Lorig K et al: The beneficial effects of the arthritis self-management course are not adequately explained by behavior changes, Arthritis Rheum 32:91-95, 1989.

Maccoby N et al: Reducing the risk of cardiovascular disease: effects of a community-based campaign on knowledge and behavior, J Community Health 3:100-114, 1977.

McAlister A et al: Theory and action for health promotion: illustrations from the North Karelia project, Am J Public Health 72:43-50, 1982.

Milio N: Promoting health through public policy, Philadelphia, 1981, FA Davis Co.

Miller MK and Stokes CS: Health status, health resources, and consolidated structural parameters: implications for public health care policy, J Health Soc Behav 19:263-279, 1978.

Mooney A and Rives NW Jr: Measures of community health status for health planning, Health Serv Res 2:129-145, 1978.

Pesznecker B and McNeil J: Collaborative practice models in community health nursing, Nurs Outlook 30:298-302, 1984.

Polit DF and Hungler BP: Observational methods. In Essentials of nursing research: methods, appraisal, utilization, Philadelphia, 1989, JB Lippincott Co.

Rogers E: Diffusion of innovations, ed 3, New York, 1983, Free Press.

Rossi PH and Freeman HE: Evaluation: a systematic approach, Beverly Hills, Calif, 1989, Sage Publications Inc.

Rothman J: Planning and organizing for social change: action principles from social science research, New York, 1974, Columbia University Press.

Rothman J and Tropman JE: Models of community organization and macro practice: their mixing and phasing. In Cox FM et al, editors: Strategies of community organization: macro practice, Intasca, Ill, 1987, FE Peacock Publishers Inc.

Ruffing-Rahal MA: Qualitative methods in community analysis, Public Health Nurs 2:130-137, 1985.

Ryan W: Blaming the victim, New York, 1976, Vintage Books.

Salber EJ: The lay advisor as community health resource, J Health Polit Policy Law 3:469-478, 1979.

Salber EJ: Where does primary health care begin? The health facilitator as a central figure in primary care, Isr J Med Sci 17:100-111, 1981.

Salber EJ, Beery WL, and Jackson JLR: The role of the health facilitator in community health education, J Community Health 2:5-20, 1976.

Schultz PR: When client mean more than one: extending the foundational concept of person, Adv Nurs Science, 10:71-86, 1987.

Scutchfield FD: Alternative methods for health priority assessment, J Community Health 1:29-38, 1975.

Selby ML et al: Public health nursing interventions to improve the use of a health service: using a pilot study to guide research, Public Health Nurs 7:3-12, 1990.

Simons-Morton BG, O'Hara NM, and Simons-Morton DG: Promoting healthful diet and exercise behaviors in communities, schools, and families. Family and Community Health 9:1-13, 1986.

Smith LS and Gentry D: Migrant farm workers' perceptions of support persons in a descriptive community survey, Public Health Nurs 4:21-28, 1987.

US Department of Health and Human Services: Consensus Conference on the Essentials of Public Health Nursing Practice and Education, Report of the Conference, September 5-7, 1984, Rockville, Md, 1985.

Warnecke RB, Mosher W, Graham S, and Montgomery EB: Health guides as influentials in central Buffalo, J Health Soc Behav 17:22-34, 1976.

Werner D: Empowerment and health, Contact 102:1-9, 1988.

Williams CA: Community health nursing: what is it? Nurs Outlook 25:250-254, 1977.

Wilson RN: Editorial note to the competent community. In Kaplan BH, Wilson RN, and Leighton A, editors: Further explorations in social psychiatry, New York, 1976, Basic Books Inc, Publishers.

World Health Organization: Community health nursing: report of a WHO expert committee, Tech Report Series No 558, Geneva, 1974, World Health Organization.

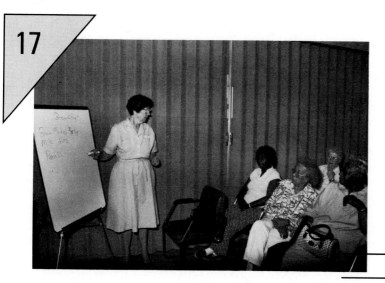

17

Working With Groups in the Community

Peggye Guess Lassiter

Group Concepts
Group Definition
Group Purpose
Cohesion
Norms
Leadership
Group Structure

Promoting Individuals' Health Through Group Work
Choosing Groups for Health Change
Stages of Group Work
Beginning Interactions
Conflict
Problem Solving for Health Change
Evaluation of Group Progress

Community Groups and their Contribution to Community Life
Identifying Community Groups
Identifying Interlinking Subsystems

Working with Groups Toward Community Health Goals

Clinical Application

Summary

OBJECTIVES

After reading this chapter, the student should be able to:

Describe member interaction and group purpose as the major elements of a group.
Describe the effect of cohesion on group effectiveness.
Identify the influence of group norms on group members.
Appreciate the usefulness of groups in promoting individual health.
Describe nursing behaviors that assist groups in promoting health for individuals.
Identify the groups constituting a community and illustrate links between them.
Describe the role of the community health nurse working with established groups toward community health goals.

KEY TERMS

cohesion	group culture	member interaction
communication structure	group purpose	norms
conflict	group structure	role structure
established groups	informal groups	selected membership groups
formal group	leadership	subsystems
group	maintenance function	task function

W orking with groups is an important skill of community nursing. Groups are an effective and powerful vehicle for initiating and implementing changes for individuals, families, organizations, and the community. Individuals naturally form groups in their home setting, and the community's health is dramatically influenced by the groups in the community. The community health nurse who works with groups must have an understanding of group concepts, practice in group work, and an appreciation of the use of group process.

All nurses have group experience. In daily practice, nurses routinely plan and implement health-focused action with clients, other nurses, and other health care workers. Nurses often participate in groups in which they are encouraged to observe their own responses to the membership and leadership. Such study and experience enrich a nurse's knowledge of group concepts and application to groups of clients, work groups, and community groups.

Additionally, groups often provide a cost-effective means of communicating instruction, making decisions, and handling issues and concerns. As discussed in Chapter 11, community health nurses often use groups to communicate health information to a number of clients who meet together once or on a regular basis, rather than repeating the information several times to individuals. During a time of decreasing resources, groups are an increasingly popular format for community health nursing intervention.

Groups have the ability to bring about changes to improve the health and well-being of individuals and communities. Groups are crucial for the development of individuals; and some individual changes for health are difficult or impossible to achieve without group support and encouragement. Individual attitudes are developed in kin and friendship groups; continued membership throughout life in other groups influences thoughts, choices, behaviors, and values. People tend to meet their social needs through association with others, and groups are a natural vehicle for meeting these needs.

Groups form for varied reasons. They may form to address a clearly stated purpose or goal, or they may form naturally as individuals are attracted to each other by shared values, interests, activities, or personal characteristics.

Community groups represent the collective interests, needs, and values of individuals; they provide a link between the individual and the larger social system. Through groups, people may express personal views and relate them to the views of others. Groups serve as communication networks and may be viewed as an organization of community parts. Identifying groups and their goals, member characteristics, and place in the community structure is an important first step toward understanding the community and assessing its health. Through community groups, nurses assist people to identify priority health needs and capabilities and to implement community changes.

GROUP CONCEPTS

The basic group concepts described in this section may be used in nursing practice to promote individual health through group work, to identify community groups and their contributions to community life, and to assist groups in working toward community health goals.

Group Definition

A *group* is a collection of interacting individuals who have a common purpose or purposes. Each member influences and is in turn influenced by every other member to some extent. The members' characteristics bring a composition to the group that in part determines the degree and kind of influence among them. Key elements in this definition of group are *member interaction* and *group purpose* (Figure 17-1).

The following examples illustrate member interaction and group purposes. Families are a unique example of community groups and the most familiar group form. Family purposes are numerous, including providing psychological support and socialization for their members. Usually, families share kinship bonds, common living space, and economic resources. Interactions are diverse and frequent because of the multiple ties between members and the particular functions delegated to families by society. Group concepts offer one study approach to family groups.

A second example is groups formed in response to particular community needs. The purpose of such community groups is to address specific problems or opportunities. For example, in one community, residents banded together to form a neighborhood association to protect their health and welfare. This neighborhood of upper middle-class homes was located in an unincorporated area. Over a period of 3 years the residents were threatened with multiple environmental hazards, including forest fire (fire hydrants had been overlooked in developing part of the area), establishment of a small airport near the homes, and construction of an interstate highway adjacent to the homes. To protect their interests, residents formed a neighborhood association and elected officers to represent their interests in a constructive manner.

Groups in the community often occur spontaneously because of mutual attraction between individuals and obvious and keenly felt personal needs. Young and single adults sharing similar desires for socialization and recreation are likely to form loosely structured groups. Through parties and other social meetings, the young adults establish new ways of behaving and relating. They select partners, test ideas and attitudes, and establish their identity within a group of people with similar developmental needs. Their unstated purpose is to test and become familiar with adult roles.

A fourth example is health-promoting groups, which are formed as individuals, meet in the community and health care settings and discover common challenges to their physical and emotional well-being. The purposes of health-promoting groups are to improve health for the members and to deal with specific threats to health. Chapters of Alcoholics Anonymous, Parents without Partners, and La Leche League illustrate health-promoting groups. Interactions between members are personally supportive and include group problem solving and education. Like other groups organized in response to community issues, health-promoting groups usually form for particular purposes, and member interactions work toward those purposes. These

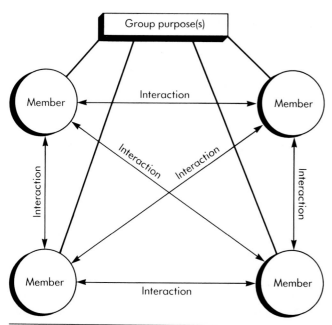

FIGURE 17-1

A group is a collection of interacting individuals who have a common purpose or purposes.

groups may be either of two types: established groups or selected membership groups. Both of these types of groups are discussed later in this chapter.

How do purpose and interaction vary in these four examples? For some groups their purpose is obvious and may be easily stated by members. This is true for groups organized to address specific community needs or health challenges. For families, social groupings, and many spontaneously formed groups, the purposes are unstated. However, the purpose for the groups can be determined by studying their activities as a group over a period of time. Highly personal and multipurpose groupings serve individual and collective needs in concrete, function-oriented ways and in subtle, less obvious ways.

Purpose and member interaction are important components of all groups, but the expression of purpose, the manner of member interaction, and the intensity of the interaction vary. Group purposes and member interactions help distinguish the group's function for its members and community.

Group Purpose

When the need for particular health changes is identified and group work is selected as the most effective intervention, a *purpose* or *goal* for a proposed group must be stated. A clear statement and presentation of this purpose are essential in establishing criteria for member selection.

Such a clear statement of purpose facilitated new group formation in a housing development in one city. The local department of social services had received numerous reports of child abuse and neglect. Routine home visits for well-child care documented high stress between parents and their offspring, and some parents requested guidance from the

community health nurse in child discipline. The community health nurse proposed a parent group to address this community need. Nurses who were involved selected the following purpose for the group: dealing with kids for child and parent satisfaction. The purpose indicated both the process—to help parents deal with kids—and the desirable outcome—satisfaction for parents and children. As potential members were approached, this statement of purpose for the group helped the individuals decide whether or not they wanted to join.

Appeals for membership in a group may be public, with all who elect to join accepted. In such situations the membership is self-selected, based on the stated group purpose. In this type of recruitment, publicity must reach those in need of particular health changes. Prospective members often wish to discuss the purpose with leaders or clarify questions concerning the purpose at the first group meeting. Their commitment to the health group is partly based on individual goals and how well the group goal satisfies their personal objectives.

Cohesion

The measure of attraction between members and to the group is called **cohesion.** This pull to each other, to the group, and to its purposes operates for an overall group valence or attraction measurement. Individuals in a highly cohesive group identify themselves as a unit, work toward common goals, are willing to endure frustration for the sake of the group, and defend the group against outside criticism. Attraction is increased when members feel accepted by others, see like qualities in each other, perceive that others like them, and believe they share similar attitudes and values (Figure 17-2). Some individual attributes that influence attraction between members include physical and interpersonal characteristics, behaviors, skills, knowledge, beliefs, and values. Members' traits that increase group cohesion and productivity include (1) congruence between personal goals and those of the group, (2) attraction to group goals, (3) attraction to other selected members, (4) distribution of leading and following skills, and (5) existence of problem-solving skills.

Functions of members that facilitate movement toward the group's purpose are termed **task functions.** Members demonstrating task-directed abilities become more attractive to the group. These traits include a cognitive ability in problem solving, access to material resources, and skills in directing. Of equal importance are abilities to provide affirmation and support for individuals in the group; these functions that help members to stay with the group and feel accepted are termed **maintenance functions.** The ability to help people resolve conflicts and ensure social and environmental comfort is also a maintenance function. Both task and maintenance functions are necessary to group progress. Naturally, those members who supply such group requirements are attractive, and an abundance of such traits within the membership tends to increase group cohesion.

Other group members' traits may decrease cohesion and productivity. These include (1) conflicts between personal and group goals, (2) lack of interest in group goals and activities, (3) poor problem-solving and communication

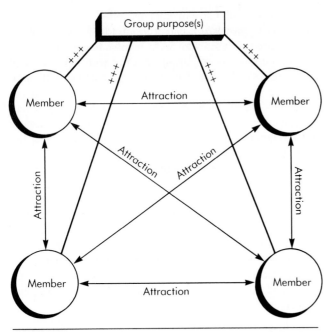

FIGURE 17-2

Cohesion is the measure of attraction between members and member attraction to group purpose(s).

abilities, (4) lack of leadership skills, (5) disagreement about types of leadership, (6) aversion to other members, and (7) behaviors and attributes that are poorly understood by others.

Commonly shared characteristics usually contribute to the group attraction for members, whereas differences tend to decrease attractiveness. Members' perceptions of differences can create marked competition and jealousy. However, differences in members' characteristics increase group cohesion if they support complementary functioning or provide contrasting viewpoints necessary for decision making. Cohesion factors are complex; multiple influences affect member attraction to each other and to the group's goal. Group productivity and member satisfaction are positively affected by high group cohesion. Two examples illustrate factors that influence group cohesion.

A community health nurse initiated and provided beginning *leadership* for a group of clients who had been treated for burns. Ten residents, all from one town, had been discharged after 3 months in the local burn unit. The stated purpose for the group was to assist members in the difficult transition from hospital to home. Each individual had been treated for extensive burns in an intensive care treatment center; each had relied heavily on health workers for physical, social, and emotional rehabilitation; and each had faced the challenge of resuming work and family roles. Individuals shared some similar experiences and hopes for the future. The individuals varied in the amount of trauma and stress experienced, and they differed widely in psychological readiness for return to ordinary daily routines. One woman was able to return quickly to her job as cashier in a large supermarket. The strength of her determination to overcome public reaction to her scars, coupled with an ability to "use

the right words" and an empathy for others, distinguished her from others in the group. These differences proved very attractive to other members, inspiring them to work toward a return to their own roles in life. Her differences were perceived as attainable by other members. The cohesion for this group was provided by the members' attraction to the common purpose of returning to successful life patterns and managing relations with others. Each member also believed that interaction with others with similar burn experiences could facilitate goal attainment. This example shows that certain member experiences, such as crises or traumas, may help individuals identify with each other and may increase member attraction.

Being different from the general population and similar to the other group members is, for some, a compelling force for membership in the group. (Others are repelled by the group because they do not wish to be identified by an aversive characteristic, such as disfigurement.) Empathy for another's pain, learned only through mutual experience, may provide each individual with a required perspective for problem solving or validation of reality. The nurse in this example helped members use common experiences and learn from their differences. The group was effective.

Differences created tension in one self-help group for victims of spouse abuse; in this group, nurses met a severe challenge stemming from the differences they presented as nonvictims. The community health nurses had been invited by professional staff to assist the group in its process toward the goal of "learning to manage: safety, health, independence." Victim members of the group felt that the nurses could not truly understand the intensely personal and devastating injury each had experienced and told the nurses so. They isolated the nurses from membership but tolerated their presence. Attraction of the group diminished, and attendance at meetings fell. Discussion of superficial issues occupied group time as the victim members avoided topics of member safety and violence in general. Differences among members decreased group cohesion; the group was not effectively addressing its goal, and members felt isolated.

In response to this deterioration, the nurses encouraged all members to describe experiences seen as threatening to self-respect in their family and work roles. The nurses revealed some of their own struggles for responsible self-direction and control. Revealing their vulnerability made the nurses more attractive to the group. The members were able to accept the nurses, whom they now saw as more similar to themselves. They promptly refocused their efforts on the purpose of the group.

Group members supported one another to assert individual rights for safety, to locate employment, to make necessary living arrangements for independence from the abuser, and to identify needs for personal interactional changes. Cohesive forces for responsible status and the clear purpose of maintaining member safety contributed to successful group work.

Members' attraction to the group depends also on the nature of the group. Factors include the group programs, size, type of organization, and position in the community. When goals are perceived clearly by individuals and group programs or when activities are believed to be effective, attraction to the group is increased.

The concept of cohesion helps to explain group productivity. Some cohesion is necessary for people to remain with a group and accomplish the set goals. Attractiveness positively influences members' motivation and commitment to work on the group task. Cohesion for groups may be increased as members better understand the experiences of others and are able to identify common ideas and reactions to various issues. Nurses facilitate this process by pointing out similarities, contrasting supportive differences, or helping members redefine differences in ways that make those dissimilarities compatible.

Norms

Norms are standards that guide, control, and regulate individuals and communities. The group **norms** represent the standards for group members' behaviors, attitudes, and even perceptions. All groups have norms and mechanisms whereby conformity is accomplished (Sampson and Marthas, 1981). Group norms serve three functions: (1) to ensure movement toward the group's purpose or tasks, (2) to maintain the group through various supports to members, and (3) to influence members' perceptions and interpretations of reality.

The task function means that certain norms keep the group focused on its task. Diversion from a steady focus is permitted only to the extent that members respect central goals and feel committed to return to them. This commitment to return to the central goals is the task norm, the strength of which determines the group's intensity in keeping to its work.

In the maintenance function, norms create group pressures to ensure affirming actions for members and to help in maintaining comfort. Individuals in groups seem most productive and at ease when their psychological and social well-being is nurtured. Maintenance behaviors include identifying the social and psychological tensions of members and taking steps to support those members at high stress points. Healthy maintenance norms may direct the group's attention to conditions such as temperature, space, and seating to ensure the physical comfort of the group during meeting times. This attention to arrangements may include meeting in places that are easily accessible and comfortable to the participants, providing refreshments, and scheduling meetings at convenient times. The group is maintained by those arrangements that minimize physical tension for members.

The third function of group norms relates to members' perceptions of reality and is of equal importance to group performance. Daily behavior is largely based on the way each aspect of life is understood. Through socialization, individuals learn how to gather information, assign meaning to that information, and react to situations in a way that satisfies needs. Decision-making and action-taking processes are influenced by the meanings ascribed to reality. Individuals need validation of their interpretations of reality and look to others to reinforce or to challenge and correct their ideas of what is real. Groups serve to examine the life situations confronting individuals. As individuals gather information, attempt to understand that information, make

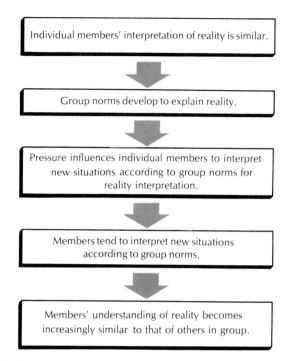

FIGURE 17-3

Influence of group reality norms on individual members.

decisions, and consider the facts and their implications, they can take responsible action, not only in relation to themselves and their group, but also for the community.

A **group culture,** or composite of the norms, develops, and these norms dictate behaviors and perceptions. It is important to know that the nurse cannot dictate them. However, the nurse can implicitly and explicitly support rules, attitudes, and behaviors, which in turn can lead to certain norms. Only when the rules, attitudes, and behaviors become part of the life of the group, independent of the nurse, are they norms.

Figure 17-3 shows that reality norms affect members, tending to pressure them to see relevant situations in the same way that other members view them. Strong normative pressure may develop to provide support for members considering change. Benne, describing the function of small groups for planned change, pointed out that individuals develop their value orientations through internalizing the norms of small groups on which they depend, notably families. "Changes in value orientations of individuals may be accomplished by seeking and finding significant membership in a small group with norms that are different in some respects from the normative orientation these individuals bring to a group" (Benne, 1976, p. 76).

To illustrate, if a group of individuals with diabetes defines an uncontrollable diet as harmful, they will direct their efforts toward influencing each other to maintain diet control. The role of the nurse in such a group would involve providing accurate information about diet and the disease process, including cause and effect relations between food intake and disease, and continually displaying a belief that health through diet control is attainable and desirable.

When members of any group have similar backgrounds,

their scope of knowledge may be limited. For example, female members in a spouse-abuse group may believe that men are exploitive and harmful based on common childhood and marriage experiences. Such a stereotyped view of men could be reinforced by members similar perceptions and might lead to continuing anger, fear of interactions with men, and a hostile or helpless approach to family affairs. Nurses or group members who have known men in loving, helpful, and collaborative ways can describe their different and positive perceptions of men, thereby adding information and challenging beliefs. Thus the group functions to influence members' perceptions and interpretations of reality. The health and condition of the individual improves as members' perceptions of reality become based on a full range of data, and cause and effect factors are understood. Nurses bring an important perspective to groups in which similar backgrounds limit the understanding and interpretation of personal concerns.

Leadership

Leadership in groups is an important and complex concept. In a group the behavior of members' that guides or directs includes all of those actions that determine and influence the group movement. Leadership behaviors and definitions are listed in the box at right. Members who have a strong influence over others are identified as leaders.

Sources of leader influence are knowledge, ability, access to needed resources, personal attractiveness, status or position in the community or organization, and ability to control sanctions for others. Leadership behaviors may be concentrated in one or a few persons, or they may be shared by many. Effective leadership is necessary for positive group functioning. Leadership is often described as patriarchal, paternal, or democratic, and each of these styles has a particular effect on members' interaction, satisfaction, and productivity. Some groups reflect a combination of leadership styles.

When one person has the final authority for group direction and movement, the leadership style is patriarchal or paternal. Patriarchal leadership may control members through rewards and threats, often keeping them in the dark about the goals and rationale behind prescribed actions. Paternal leadership wins respect from and dependence of followers by parental-like devotion to members' needs. The leader controls group movement and progress through interpersonal power. Patriarchal and paternal styles of leadership are authoritarian. These styles are effective for groups such as a disaster team, in which the immediate task accomplishment or high productivity is the goal. However, group morale and cohesiveness are typically low under these styles of leadership, and members may fail to learn how to function independently. In addition, issues of authority and control may disrupt productivity if the group members challenge the power of the leader.

A paternal style was effective in the following situation. Mary Jones, a community health nurse, called her neighbors together to alert them to the threat of drug traffic in the neighborhood. The residents agreed with Mary that several recent drug-related arrests in the area signaled a need for community concern. No one knew what to do, but all felt

---

EXAMPLES OF LEADERSHIP BEHAVIORS

Advising—introducing direction based on knowledgeable opinion.

Clarifying—checking out meanings of interaction and communication through questions and restatement.

Confronting—presenting behavior and its effects to the individual and group to challenge existing perceptions.

Evaluating—analyzing the effect or outcome of action or the worth of an idea according to some standard.

Initiating—introducing topics, beginning work, or changing the focus of a group.

Questioning—bringing about analysis of a view or views by questions that support examination.

Suggesting—proposing or bringing an idea to a group.

Summarizing—restating discussion or group action in brief form, highlighting important points.

Supporting—giving the kind of emotionally comforting feedback that helps a person or group continue ongoing actions.

---

quick action was desirable. Mary had experience in organizing people, knew of local resources, and thought that information, education, and residents' collaboration with police could substantially control the local drug-traffic problem. She organized the neighborhood group, assigned and monitored their tasks, and praised them as progress was made toward the goal of keeping the area free of drug sales.

A democratic style of leadership is characterized by a cooperative structure that promotes and supports members' functioning in all aspects of decision making and planning. Members influence each other as they explore goals, plan steps toward the goals, implement those steps, and evaluate progress.

A more common experience for nurses is illustrated in the following example. A committee of nurses for a small community health organization met weekly to improve nursing services. Tom initiated a revision of written standards. Several members of the group felt threatened by Tom's idea. They feared that their daily work would change and that a resulting evaluation using new standards would find them inferior or necessitate that they alter familiar procedures. Jane supported updating the standards. She also recognized the necessity of continuing support and affirmation of each nurse's worth on the committee. While Tom pushed the committee toward revising the standards, she often interrupted to ask members to respond and to make suggestions, noting to the group the excellent contributions. Sara provided a touch of humor whenever group tension became high. Amber provided a critical, questioning support to the decision-making process and encouraged the members to evaluate each step. In these and other ways, group members shared leadership tasks. Some served predominately to push the group toward its objective, whereas others facilitated that movement by maintaining member involvement through support. For this group, the chairperson served as convener but did not dominate in leader activities. The members accomplished the work of writing and implementing an audit for new nursing standards in a democratic leadership style.

Generally speaking, shared leadership in groups increases productivity and cohesion, resulting in friendly interactions between members. It builds appreciation for the work of leadership and inhibits power seekers. Shared leadership supports an idea of group wholeness, flexibility, and freedom.

Both members and health care workers demonstrate leadership abilities. Nurses use varied leadership styles according to their assessment of members' leadership abilities, their knowledge about how groups learn and change, their flexibility in leading behaviors, and the group's pressures for autonomy and control. Leadership is a dynamic concept. Nurses are active in all stages of group development and usually initiate and aggressively promote group establishment. They subsequently facilitate leadership development within and among members and frequently relinquish control. This encourages the members to work toward group goals to determine the pattern of leadership and the ultimate structure of the group.

Group Structure

Structure describes the particular arrangement of group parts that make up the group as a whole. *Communication structure* and *role structure* are two such descriptive frameworks. A communication structure identifies the parts according to message pathways and member participation in sending and receiving messages. Such communication structures can be identified by observing groups in action. People who are active in receiving and sending messages and who serve as channels for messages are important in the structure. These "central" individuals influence the group because of their access to and interpretive control over communication flow. Communication and role structures are interrelated.

Role structure for a group describes the expected behaviors of members in relation to each other as the group interacts. The role assumed by each group member has certain functions, or behaviors, that are displayed in the group and serve a purpose in the life of that group. Examples of roles are leader, follower, task specialist, maintenance specialist, evaluator, peacemaker, and gatekeeper (see box at right). Members' roles in the group may be described by their predominate actions. A group's role structure can be identified by observing the members' behavior as the group operates. Identification of communication patterns also helps to determine roles because people occupying particular roles characteristically use certain kinds of communication.

Group structure emerges from various member influences, including the members' understanding and support of the group purpose. Nurses assess the group structure as it relates to goal accomplishment. Many groups also consider their own structure, assess its usefulness in relation to member comfort and productivity, and then plan for a different division of tasks that is agreeable to the whole.

In the earlier example of nurses working on standards of nursing service, Tom served a role as task specialist, Jane as maintenance specialist, and Amber as evaluator. These members consistently occupied particular roles and were expected by others to maintain their behavior to serve the purposes of the group.

EXPECTED BEHAVIORS DEFINING GROUP ROLES

Leader—guides and directs group activity.
Follower—seeks and accepts the authority or direction of others.
Task Specialist—focuses or directs movement toward the main work of the group.
Maintenance Specialist—provides physical and psychological support for group members, thereby holding the group together.
Evaluator—analyzes the effect or outcome of action or the worth of ideas according to some standard.
Peacemaker—attempts to reconcile conflict between members or takes action in response to influences that disrupt the group process and threaten its existence.
Gatekeeper—controls outsiders' access to the group.

A person occupying a gatekeeper's role controls outsiders' access to the group. Gatekeepers either facilitate or block communication between outsiders and group members. Identification of those in gatekeeper's roles is crucial when established groups are used for community health. The gatekeeper usually confronts the nurse after beginning contacts are attempted. An invitation to communicate further with group members is extended only after the nurse and gatekeeper determine mutual benefits and possible risks from continued contact between the nurse and the group.

Conflicts in groups may be caused by competition for roles or member disagreement about the role ascribed to them. Struggles between members often result more from disagreement over dominance or competition for a favored position than from a conflict regarding group goals or steps in decision making. When group structures are considered from role and communication perspectives, the nurse and members of the group can more clearly understand the pressures affecting conflicting behavior and can work to resolve matters productively.

The following is an illustration of structure analysis leading to conflict resolution. A small church in a rural town initiated a project for youth recreation because driving around the countryside was the primary form of recreation for the teens. The roadway was frequently used as a speedway by the restless youth. The church enlisted the high school principal and the community health nurse to work with a project group. All supported the development of a local youth center and worked energetically toward the goal.

After 2 months of steady cooperation, many arguments began to erupt at meetings. Conflicts about the supervision of the proposed center, the site for the physical plant, and numerous smaller concerns seemed to dominate planning time. The group consisted of active, aggressive members; four of these individuals seemed to dominate the discussions and to resist argument resolution. After several frustrating meetings, the nurse asked the group to consider their roles in decision making. She suspected that the disagreements were related to members' functions in the group rather than their ideas. The nurse was supportive of each person as the roles and expectations of each member were explored. The four dominant individuals expressed personal wishes to direct the planning and displayed aggravation when these attempts were thwarted. Other members described supportive and task functions but did not seek dominance in leadership functions. The open analysis of role structure made clear to the members that arguments grew out of competition for directing roles rather than from true disagreements about the recreation project. The open discussion in this situation also resulted in an agreement to divide the project work into several task areas to be led by separate area directors. Members expressed relief that basic agreement about the purpose remained intact, and they were able to modify their role expectations to accommodate all members. They joked together about being a collection of bosses and renewed their productive work.

PROMOTING INDIVIDUALS' HEALTH THROUGH GROUP WORK

Health behavior is influenced greatly by the groups to which people belong. Individuals live within a social structure of significant others such as family members, friends, co-workers, and acquaintances. The patterns and directions of everyday activities are learned in a family, and these are later reinforced or challenged by new groups. These groups constitute the context in which values, beliefs, and attitudes are formed; individuals usually consider the responses of others in all types of decisions regarding personal welfare.

The following example illustrates the effects of a person's social network on health behavior. Mary Berton was worried about a lump she had recently discovered in her breast. She first asked her husband, Lew, to confirm its presence, which he did. He agreed that she should arrange for a diagnostic evaluation, and an appointment was arranged. Mary talked with Lew about the possible consequences of malignancy, and she noted Lew's concern for her safety. She was fearful of radical surgery and its impact on her relationship to Lew, but she did not discuss that with him. Mary telephoned two close friends from her workplace and asked them to meet her for coffee. Although they felt it was premature to fret about the lump being malignant, they discussed all they knew about treatment for breast cancer, including the trials, defeats, and successes of three mutual friends who had had surgery for breast cancer. Each of the friends had reacted differently to her own situation, and Mary's friends retold familiar details. The retelling seemed important to understanding the current situation and helping Mary sort out her feelings. She was assisted in facing the reality of risk, recognizing the need to follow through with diagnostic procedures, selecting able medical sources, and managing her emotional stress.

Mary's friends' and husband's responses to her situation influenced her assessment, decision making, and subsequent behavior. The work done by Mary and her social network in response to her health need was important. It illustrates a common mechanism among individuals and the groups to which they belong. The groups described in this example are Mary's family group, which includes Mary and Lew, and Mary's friendship group, of which those who met for coffee are a subset.

Groups supportive of individual health changes are unavailable to some people because of their social or emotional isolation. Also, existing groups sometimes work against health goals. Individuals isolated from supportive groups or hindered by their group connections may find movement toward health difficult, and they may benefit greatly through newly organized groups established for specific purposes. Isolated individuals may have low self-esteem, be mentally ill, or occupy positions of low status in their family or community. They may be disadvantaged, gifted, or deviant, or they may simply live in a rural area or be engaged in solitary work.

As community nurses increase their knowledge of group concepts, develop skills in working with varied groups, and learn to employ the power in groups for individual changes, they will become available, visible, and sought for group work.

Choosing Groups for Health Change

Individuals, groups, or organizations may initiate various group efforts for individuals' health and recruit community health nurses as expert planners and facilitators. Nurses frequently use groups to help individuals within a community after studying the overall needs of the community and its people. Such a study is based on client contacts, expressed concerns from various community spokespersons, health statistics for the area, health resources availability, and the community's general well-being. These data point to the community's strengths and critical needs. Just as other nursing interventions are based on the assessment of needs and knowledge of effective treatment, group formation is determined by the assessment of priority community needs for individual health change.

At times community health nurses work with existing groups, and at other times they form new groups. A decision about whether to work in established groups or to begin new ones is based on the clients' needs, the purpose of existing groups, and the membership ties in existing groups.

Established Groups

There are advantages to using established groups for individual health change. Membership ties already exist and the structure already in place can be used. It is not necessary to find new members because compatible individuals already form a working group. Established groups usually have operating methods that have already proved successful; an approach for a new goal is built on this history. Members are aware of each others' strengths, limitations, and preferred styles of interaction. Members' comfort levels, stemming from their experience together, facilitate their focus on the new goal.

Established groups have a strong potential for influencing members. Ties between members have been enhanced through successful group endeavors. Their bonds are usually multidimensional because of the length of time they have spent together. Such rich ties support group change efforts for individuals' health.

Before deciding to work with particular established groups, the nurse must judge whether introducing a new focus is compatible with existing group purposes. In some cases individual health goals will enhance existing group purposes, and the nurse is an important resource for bringing information for health, behavior, and group process.

How can the community nurse enter existing groups and direct their attention to individual health needs? One nurse employed by an industrial firm noted the deleterious effect of managerial stress on several individuals. They had elevated blood pressure, stomach pain, and emotional tension. The nurse learned that the employees with stress were all members of a jogging team that met weekly for conversation in addition to regular workouts. The other joggers readily accepted the offer to work together on individual stress management, recognizing that their fellow members were facing high-stress circumstances and the accompanying danger to health. High-level health had been a value shared by all team members, and although jogging was seen as an enjoyable and health-promoting activity, they had never talked about a shared purpose for improved health. In this circumstance the nurse observed a need for stress reduction, thought that the individuals at risk would be able to achieve stress reduction if supported through a group process from valued friends, and proposed that a new purpose be added to the jogging team's activities.

Selected Membership Groups

In some situations using existing groups is undesirable or impossible. The nurse then begins a selection process and brings a new group into existence. Nurses are familiar with group work in which members are selected because of their health. For instance, individuals with diabetes are brought together to consider diet management and physical care and to share in problem-solving remedies; community residents are brought together for social support and rehabilitation following treatment for mental illness; or isolated elderly persons are brought together for socialization and hot meals.

Members' attributes are an important consideration in composing a new group. Members are attracted to others from similar backgrounds, with similar experiences, and with common interests and abilities. Selecting members so that common ties or interests balance out dissimilar traits is, therefore, an important consideration.

Membership ties are influential; even in newly formed groups people bring emotional and social ties from previous and parallel group memberships. People are influenced by the interaction in the newly formed group and by their alliance with other important groups to which they belong. Memory serves to keep the norms and role expectations from one group present in a person as he or she moves from one group to another. Individual behavior is then influenced not only by the membership, purpose, attraction, norms, leadership, and structure of the group but also by those processes remembered from other valued group memberships. Consideration of the multiple influences on members helps to determine an appropriate grouping for each situation and its particular dimensions.

When the nurse is able to arrange it, the membership for *selected membership groups* should contain one or more individuals with expressive and problem-solving skills and others who are comfortable in supportive roles. Many people

demonstrate abilities in task and maintenance functions, and others have undeveloped potential for such functions. Support and training for group effectiveness within the unit build cohesion. As members perform increasingly valuable functions for the group, they become more attracted to it and more attractive to others.

The size of the group influences effectiveness; generally, eight to twelve people is considered a good number for group work focused on individual health changes. Groups of up to 25 members may be effective when their focus is on community needs, such as the group discussed previously that formed a neighborhood association. Large groups often divide and assign tasks to the smaller subgroups, with the original large groups meeting less frequently for reporting and evaluation.

Recruitment and selection among candidates for optimum group membership require judgment based on knowledge of group concepts. Selection can be facilitated by setting member criteria for specific groups. The criteria usually suggest a mixture of member traits, allowing for balance for the processes of decision making and growth.

STAGES OF GROUP WORK
Beginning Interactions

Once a group forms, work begins on the stated purpose. Early meetings require further clarification of both individual and group goals. Members with varying degrees of openness present themselves and their backgrounds. They begin to interact with each other by seeking and giving information about themselves and their circumstances and simultaneously demonstrating their capabilities in problem solving and group participation. The nurse assists by supporting ideas and feelings, inviting participation, giving information, seeking and providing clarification, and suggesting structure. The method for proceeding toward the purpose varies not only according to the nurse's skill and preference but also to the group composition and the skills brought by members.

Nurses in beginning groups should place priority on helping members interact with a degree of satisfaction. This requires close attention to maintenance tasks of attending, eliciting information, clarifying, and recognizing contributions of members. Attending includes simple responses to people, such as listening carefully to their speech and noting their mood, dress, and informal conversation as they enter the meeting. Attending behavior communicates recognition and acceptance of the person and his or her presentations to the group.

A beginning format that focuses on whatever brought each member to the group provides recognition and helps the individual acknowledge similar and different perspectives. Members may be asked to describe what each hopes to accomplish in the group and what experiences each has previously had in groups. Member-to-member exchanges are encouraged; individuals are recognized and supported as they take on leadership functions.

Even in beginning sessions of groups, some patterns of work are formulated. Members try out familiar roles and test their individual abilities. Those approaches to member support, leadership, and decision making that are comfortable and productive for the members become normative ways for the group to work. The nurse enters into such models creatively, evaluating the appropriateness of style and productivity of roles for the members and nurse. The work of the group is begun even as the goals for health change are examined carefully and are realistically accepted. During this early period, members' attractions to each other and to the group begin to develop.

Conflict

Groups at work experience *conflict.* Members have unique personalities and often disagree about many aspects of the group's work and the part that each member plays. Open discussion of differences and disagreements can promote individual and group growth. The nurse should promote such openness, making it clear that respect for each person and each person's point of view is necessary. This lays the groundwork for a group norm that supports esteem for each member during conflict and resolution.

Conflict in groups may grow from unspoken or generally unrecognized issues. These conflicts are sometimes communicated subtly in themes such as control and dependence. Often the conflict regarding status in the health group represents the concerns of members who experienced similar problems in other important groups, such as their families. For example, one person's struggle for leadership and dominance is mirrored in a similar struggle at home.

Problem Solving for Health Change

Work toward established health goals is facilitated by community health nurses through their considerable knowledge of health and health risks for individuals, groups, and communities. Problem-solving and decision-making skills and strategies for change are part of the nurse's resources for such group work.

Basic teaching is sometimes used as the first step in effecting change. Members benefit from understanding the known associations between environment, body response, wellness, and pathological states that are pertinent to the health change goal. Participation in formal learning may help members focus on the reality of the problems and ways to understand them. The potential of a group for effecting individual change is only addressed fully when members work actively and directly through discussion and other approaches to problem solving. Expectant-parent groups illustrate a type of community group in which teaching is a highly appropriate method. Participants need to understand facts concerning pregnancy, labor and delivery, self-care and infant care, parenting, and adjusting to change. They also need an opportunity to practice the skills required in anticipated tasks and to explore their attitudes and emotional responses to the anticipated family changes. Specific learning activities in the group might include demonstration and practice for baby baths and situation enactment of family activity after the baby comes home. Such experiential learning activities, which require interaction between members and involve topics highly relevant to the goal of change, are useful.

One way to consider changes for improved health is through analysis of motivating and restraining forces for individuals and groups. The group considers major factors that influence the particular change proposed for improved health. Included are the encouraging and supportive forces for change and the interfering and resistive influences that each person experiences from sources such as important individuals within the family and work and community groups. These forces are identified during group meetings when others help to plan steps for overcoming interferences and promoting facilitative factors. The group members learn from each other and the nurse to deal effectively with multiple outside influences as they relate to the individuals' desired health goals.

Describing and listing the supportive forces and resistive influences for change help people clarify the multiple factors operating in any change. The study of factor sources— whether they arise within the individual, the work group, other valued groups, or the community at large—reveals areas requiring action. Such an analysis encourages consideration of diverse influences.

Relationships within the group become increasingly important because of the shared understanding of the what, how, when, and where of health needs and changes. Normative pressures within the group keep members engaged in the work agreed on and support the progress made by each individual.

Evaluation of Group Progress

Evaluation of individual and group progress toward health goals is important. (A Guide for Evaluation of Group Effectiveness is shown in Appendix I3). Action steps toward the goal are identified early in the planning stage. These small steps may be responses to learning objectives (listed action steps designed to support facilitative forces and deal with resistive forces) or they may reflect the group's problem-solving plan. These action steps and the indicators of achievement are discussed and written in a group record. Celebration is built into the group's evaluation system to help individuals recognize and reinforce each step toward the health goal. Celebration may include concrete rewards such as special foods and drinks, or it may be the personal expression of joy and member-to-member approval. Celebration for group accomplishments marks progress, rewards members, and motivates each person for continuing work.

COMMUNITY GROUPS AND THEIR CONTRIBUTION TO COMMUNITY LIFE

An understanding of group concepts provides a (beginning) basis for identifying community groups and how they function as components of a community. Groups represent the collective interests, needs, and values of a locality. Because individuals develop, refine, and change their ideas within the context of the groups to which they belong, those groups are vital to community well-being. Groups encourage citizen participation in problem identification. They also are keys in the management of interactions within the community and between the community and larger society. Nurses are interested in the whole of the community, the components comprising it, and how interaction contributes to community competence and a comprehensive state of physical, emotional, and social well-being.

Identifying Community Groups

Community groups and their purposes and memberships are identified to describe the community. Community groups may be informal—such as social networks, friendships, and neighborhood groups—or formal—such as school, church, and business groups. *Formal groups* have a defined membership and specific purpose. They may or may not have an official place in the community's organization. In *informal groups,* the ties between members are multiple and the purposes are unwritten yet understood by members. Informal groups can be identified through interviews with key spokespersons. Information about when and why they gather is learned through interviews or observing gatherings to which the nurse is invited. Informal groups often are recognized in the news when they are distinguished for community action or service. Formal groups usually can be identified in a variety of community media. Meetings usually are announced, and business is reported publicly; members often can be identified from membership lists. The goal and mission statements are usually written and available to interested persons.

Typically, residents willingly describe the informal and formal groups in their communities after they learn the nurse's purpose for entering and studying their community. Resident informants may not identify all groups; a more complete list emerges through the study of community subsystems.

Identifying Interlinking Subsystems

Each community contains differentiated and interlinking subsystems such as family, economy, government, religion, education, health, and welfare systems. Demarcation between subsystems and the formal groupings within and links between them is determined by studying who belongs to, works with, or affiliates with particular groupings. Informal groups also function as ties within and between subsystems. Linking occurs whenever an individual belongs to two or more groups. Various communications and cooperative exchanges connect groups and contribute to community integration. Interrelatedness is built on the network of roles and status levels that exist in the various formal and informal groups in the community's social structure (Edwards and Jones, 1976).

Group norms regarding member communication and interaction with others and shared group goals influence the overall harmony and free exchange between individuals and groups in the community. Links between formal groups depend on the degree of coordination, cooperation, and competition between community subsystems. Many communities sanction cooperative links by establishing coordinating groups such as interagency councils.

The nurse considers the extent to which formal or informal groups are linked through family and friendship ties. For example, the relationships and patterns of influence existing in local extended family groups are likely to influence the many other groups to which those family members belong. For example, members of a family in one county actively participate in the board of county directors, the school board, the Protestant mission council, the youth advisory commission, and the county rescue squad. This family's conservative financial views are reflected in the conservative fiscal posture of these five separate community groups.

The nurse also notes vertical links between community groups and county, state, and national subsystems. For example, decisions of a city school board are influenced by the standards, funding, and communications from the county board of education, which is in turn influenced by the state's department of education. Ties may be clearly understood and described by local informants. Sometimes the links are informal and established through friendship or other spontaneous associations. (These informal links are usually discerned only after the nurse establishes a planning role in the community.) Vertical affiliation is always influential for groups. Links between groups and their vertical affiliates are quite strong whenever survival of the local group depends on funds or sanctions from the higher body.

Residents rank groups by characteristics such as social prestige or power in a particular area. In turn, power is associated with the hierarchies of position in the community subsystems. Those in high-level positions have greater capacities for influencing community-wide matters than those in relatively lower positions.

The community health nurse discerns goals for the community and for various groups through media reports, from community informants, and from local archives. These goals tell of resources and visions for change as perceived by the people living and working in the local community. Data may be organized according to the opinions and behaviors of the groups identified. Such information about community groups and assessment data are used with community representatives to plan desired interventions. Groups are both units of community analysis and vehicles for change.

The small group has the potential to influence and change the larger social community of which it is a part. The social system depends on groups for governing, making policy, determining community needs, taking steps to alleviate those needs, and evaluating program outcomes. The small group is a mechanism for interrelatedness between community subsystems, certain subsystems and their counterparts in the larger social structure, and factions within subsystems. Change in the composition and function of strategic small groups may produce change for the wider social system that depends on small groups for direction and guidance (Benne, 1976).

WORKING WITH GROUPS TOWARD COMMUNITY HEALTH GOALS

Community health nurses use their understanding of group principles to work with community groups to make needed health changes. The groupings appropriate for this work include both established, community-sanctioned groups and groups for which nurses select members representing diverse community sectors.

Existing community groups formed for community-wide purposes such as elected executive groups, health-planning groups, better-business clubs, women's action groups, school boards, and neighborhood councils are excellent resources for community health assessment because part of their ongoing purpose is to determine and respond to community needs. These types of groups are also excellent vehicles for community health because they are already established as part of the community structure. When a group representing one community sector is selected for community health intervention, the total community structure is studied. Data about family ties, experiences with resource centers, and lifelong contacts to other sector groups are evaluated. Groups reflect existing community values, strengths, and normative forces.

How might community health nurses help established groups to work toward community goals? The same interventions recommended for groups formed for individual health change are beneficial to community health-focused groups. Such interventions include building cohesion through clarifying goals and individual attraction to groups, building member commitment and participation, keeping the group focused on the goal, maintaining members through recognition and encouragement, maintaining member self-esteem during conflict and confrontation, analyzing forces affecting movement toward the goal, and evaluating progress. On entering established groups, nurses seek to assess the leadership, communications, and normative structures. The nurse's skills facilitate group planning, problem solving, intervention, and evaluation. The steps for community health changes parallel those of decision making and problem solving in other methodologies.

One community health nurse, Mrs. Winter, was asked to meet with a neighborhood council to help them study and "do something about" the number of homeless living on the streets. Mrs. Winter was known to residents from a local clinic, and they knew she also consulted at a shelter for the homeless in an adjacent community. When the council invited her, they stated that "our intent is to be part of the solution rather than part of the problem." Mrs. Winter accepted the invitation to visit. She learned that the neighborhood council had addressed concerns of the neighborhood for 20 years—protecting zoning guidelines, setting up a recreational program for teens, organizing an after-school program for latch-key children, and generally representing the homeowners of the area. The neighborhood was composed of low-income families who took great pride in their homes. After meeting with the council and listening to their description of the situation, Mrs. Winter agreed to help and she joined the council.

As the first step in addressing the problem, the council conducted a comprehensive problem analysis on the homeless situation. All known causes and outcomes of homeless persons on the street were identified, and the relationships between each factor and the problem were documented from literature and from the local history relative to the problem. Mrs. Winter lent her expertise in health planning and her knowledge of the homeless and health risks. She suggested negotiation between the council and the local coalition for the homeless, recognizing that planning would be most relevant if homeless individuals participated. The council was cohesive, was committed to the purpose, had developed working operations, and did not need help with group process. They made adjustments in their usual group operation to use the knowledge and health-planning skills of Mrs. Winter.

Interventions for the homeless included establishment of temporary shelter at homes on a rotating basis, provision of daily meals through the city council or churches, and joining the area coalition for the homeless. This example shows how an established, competent group addressed a new goal successfully by building on existing strengths in partnership with the community health nurse.

Community groupings, because of their interactive roles, seem to be logical and natural ways for people to work together for community health change. As the decision-making and problem-solving capabilities of community groups are strengthened, the groups become more able representatives for the whole community. Community health nurses improve the community's health by working with groups toward that goal.

CLINICAL APPLICATION

Community health assessment in a small rural county revealed a rate of chronic diseases that was much higher than the rates for the neighboring urban county and for the state as a whole. Individuals and their families received health care supervision in the local clinics and through nursing visits to them in their home. Still, the chronically ill persons were not managing their pain and mobility problems to their own satisfaction. Community health nurses set up an initial group meeting, inviting all of the persons with chronic illness in the county seat. The invitation was published in the county newspaper and all local church bulletins. Free transportation was provided by the auxiliary club at one county church. Thirty individuals came to the first meeting and indicated great dissatisfaction with their health and interest in working with the nurses on a better approach to their chronic diseases.

At the first meeting, three groups were organized, which would meet regularly for 6 weeks each. Members selected a group based on their scheduling needs and friendship ties. The nurse then met with each group to facilitate the process of setting goals and selecting a variety of group-work intervention steps toward the goal.

One group decided to review each member's individual health care plan and assist in finding needed resources, thereby encouraging members to continue their participation. Another group thought that the stress related to their chronic condition was their biggest concern. They requested a course in stress management, which a community resident taught. Group learning experiences were facilitated by the community health nurse. The third group's primary concern was that many residents with chronic disease failed to use existing health care services. Because they thought that lack of transportation was a key causative factor for underuse of services, they decided to seek transportation from members of the Ruritan Club. Because the group had strong family links to the Ruritans and because their arguments were convincing, they were able to establish a carpool at no cost to residents needing rides to health care services. Interventions were planned and implemented by resident and nurse partnerships.

Follow-up evaluation showed that individuals were more successfully managing pain and mobility; patients attributed these changes to the collective group efforts. Group meetings didn't change the rate of chronic illness; they did successfully intervene to address specific health concerns, whereas the nurse working alone or with individuals could not accomplish these interventions as effectively or as efficiently. This nursing intervention was effective for individuals and for the rural community.

SUMMARY

The concepts presented in this chapter—member interaction, group purpose, cohesion, norms, leadership, and structure—provide a basic framework for understanding group behavior. The concepts appear deceptively simple, but their application to real groups reveals their complexity for individuals wishing to influence group behavior. Although each group concept is initially considered in isolation, the combination of concepts provides a multidimensional structure for group analysis. Group behavior is complex because of the many factors influencing individual members, member interaction within the group, and the group's community environment.

The examples of group work throughout this chapter show various ways that community health nurses apply knowledge of group concepts in their assessment of individuals' and communities' needs. A group perspective of behavior is more comprehensive than one based on individual dynamics alone. Examples show that group factors affect behavior, at times influencing health risks and the needs for healthful changes; they show that group influences may facilitate or hinder health-seeking action. Community health nurses should apply group knowledge in the assessment of health and assist clients in this assessment process.

Group intervention examples show community health nursing approaches to needed healthful changes. The client group may be persons with comparable health information needs, a group of friends responsive to a sick member, a family who works together to manage a crisis, or a committee that organizes health resources and services. Nurses lead others in using established groups or selecting and recruiting new groups to address both individual and community health needs. Nurses also demonstrate these intervention and evaluation skills as they serve as members of community action groups. Such nursing group skills are based on knowledge and are developed in community practice.

The examples in the chapter describe real group situations. However, it is impossible to describe every feasible combination of elements in a "cookbook" fashion. The nurse must use creativity in applying knowledge in unique situations. A series of questions to guide the implementation of concepts should be asked. What is the problem? Who are the people involved? Are group methods the best route to accomplish the objectives with these particular people? If so, at what level should the objectives be accomplished—on an individual member or community level? Will the problem be best addressed by an established group, or should members be selected for forming a new group? What is the nursing role in establishing the new group? What strategy is suitable for entering an existing group?

Interventions are products of established knowledge, techniques, and personal attributes such as life experiences, personality, and personal style. Ability to work in a group context may vary according to all of these factors, and group members' attributes and needs as well.

Supervision or consultation assists in self-evaluation and the development of group strategies. Such feedback is essential to developing self-awareness in a group. Literature describing specific interventions with particular problems or types of groups is available (see bibliography).

Through knowledge of group behavior, skill in group practice, and appreciation of the power that groups have, community health nurses may substantially increase their impact on the health of individuals and communities. Community health nurses are challenged to use the opportunities for change through work with groups—an instrument of power for health.

KEY CONCEPTS

Working with groups is an important skill for community health nurses. Groups are an effective and powerful vehicle for initiating and implementing healthful changes.

A group is a collection of interacting individuals with a common purpose. Each member influences and is influenced by other group members to varying degrees.

Group cohesion is enhanced by commonly shared characteristics among members and diminished by differences among members.

Cohesion is the measure of attraction between members and the group. Cohesion or the lack of it affects the group's function.

Norms are standards that guide and regulate individuals and communities. These norms are unwritten and often unspoken and serve to ensure group movement to a goal, to maintain the group, and to influence group members' perceptions and interpretations of reality.

Some diversity of member backgrounds is usually a positive influence on a group.

Leadership is an important and complex group concept. Leadership is described as patriarchal, paternal, or democratic.

Group structure emerges from various member influences, including members' understanding and support of the group purpose.

Conflicts in groups may develop from competition for roles or member disagreement about the roles ascribed to them.

Health behavior is greatly influenced by the groups to which people belong and for which they value membership.

An understanding of group concepts provides a basis for identifying community groups and their goals, characteristics, and norms. Community health nurses use their understanding of group principles to work with community groups toward needed health changes.

LEARNING ACTIVITIES

1. Consider three groups of which you are a member. What is the stated purpose of each one? Are you aware of unstated but clearly understood purposes? What is the nature of member interaction in each group? How do purpose and interaction differ in the three groups?

2. Observe two working groups in session from the community, a health care agency, or a school. Notice the overall attractiveness of each group through the eyes of its members.
   a. List actions that nurses may take to assist groups in various aspects of their work, such as member selection, purpose clarification, arrangements for comfort in participation, and group problem solving.
   b. Observe a nurse working with a health promotion group. Does he or she function in the way you anticipated? What nursing behavior facilitated the group process?

3. List the areas of skill and knowledge most likely to be expected of the nurse by the community residents.

BIBLIOGRAPHY

Alexander JL: Support group for mothers. In Spradley BW, editor: Readings in community health nursing, ed 3, Boston, 1986, Little, Brown & Co.

Benne KD: The current state of planned changing in persons, groups, communities, and societies. In Bennis, WG et al, editors: The planning of change, ed 3, New York, 1976, Holt, Rinehart, & Winston,

Bennis WG et al, editors: The planning of change, ed 3, New York, 1976, Hold, Rinehart, & Winston.

Bowers JE et al: Analysis of a support group for young spinal cord-injured males, Rehabil Nurs 12(6):313-315, 322, 1987.

Budman SH et al: Cohesion, alliance and outcome in group psychotherapy, Psychiatry 52(3):339-350, 1988.

Butterfield PG: Nominal group process as an instructional method with novice community health nursing students, Public Health Nurs 5(1):12-15, 1988.

Campbell J: A survivor group for battered women, ANS 8(2):13-20, 1986.

Cecere MC: PIP (positive image program): a group approach for obese adolescents. In Spradley BW, editor: Readings in community health nursing, ed 3, Boston, 1986, Little, Brown & Co.

Chinn PL: The reality of group dynamics, ANS 8(2):vii, 1986.

Cook HL et al: A reexamination of community participation in health: lessons from three community health projects, Fam Community Health 11(2):1-15, 1988.

Cottrell LS: The computer community. In Kaplan BH, et al, editors: Further explorations in social psychiatry, New York, 1976, Basic Books.

Edwards AD and Jones D: Community and community development, The Hague, 1976, Mouton Publishers.

Fontes HC: Small group work: a strategy to promote active learning, J Nurs Educ 26(5):212-214, 1987.

Hess-Haber CA: Graduate students' use of group work with adolescents for primary prevention, J Nurs Educ 24(9):380-382, 1985.

Howlett M and Archer VE: Worker involvement in occupational health and safety. In Spradley BW, editor: Readings in community health nursing, ed 3, Boston, 1986, Little, Brown & Co.

Janosik EH and Phipps, LB: Life cycle group work in nursing, Boston, 1986, Jones & Bartlett.

Langford RW: Chronic illness: a small group approach. Rehabil Nurs 12(4):179-185, 187, 1987.

Lassiter P and Goeppinger J: Education for rural community health nursing practice, Fam Community Health 9(1):56-67, 1986.

Marley MS: The making of a group. In Spradley BW, editor: Readings in community health nursing, ed. 3, Boston, 1986, Little, Brown & Co.

McHale M: Getting the joke: interpreting humor in group therapy, J Psychosoc Nurs Ment Health Serv 27(9):24-28, 1989.

Morgan DL: Adjusting to widowhood: do social networks really make it easier? Gerontologist 29(1): 101-107, 1989.

Munger L: A hero's journal: special editor—J Assoc Pediatr Oncol Nurses 6(2):34-36, 989.

Ochoco L and Shimamoto Y: Group work with the frail ethnic elderly, Geriatr Nurs 8(4):184-187, 1987.

Sampson EE and Marthas M: Group process for the health professions, ed 2, New York, 1981, John Wiley & Sons.

Schoonover-Shoffner K: Improving work group decision-making effectiveness, J Nurs Adm 19(7):10-15, 1989.

Staples NR and Schwartz M: Anorexia nervosa support group: providing transitional support, J Psychosoc Nurs Ment Health Serv 28(2):6-10, 1990.

White EM: Conceptual basis for nursing intervention in groups. In Hall JE and Weaver BR, editors: Distributive nursing practice: a systems approach to community health, ed 2, Philadelphia, 1985, JB Lippincott.

Wiggens NC: Education and support for the newly diagnosed cardiac family: a vital link in rehabilitation, Adv Nurs 14(1):63-67, 1989.

Yalom ID: The theory and practice of group psychotherapy, New York, 1975, Basic Books.

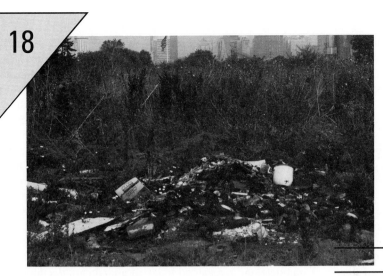

18

Environmental Health and Safety

Jeanette Lancaster

OBJECTIVES

After reading this chapter, the student should be able to:

List the major environmental health hazards and describe why and how they pose a serious threat to quality of life.

Briefly discuss the science that provides a model for looking at human and environmental interaction.

List several recent environmental hazards and discuss the health hazards associated with them.

Define environmental health and identify three routes of entry of environmental hazards.

Describe the federal agency with primary responsibility for regulating environmental health and safety.

Describe the role of the community health nurse as both a concerned citizen and a health provider in environmental health.

Plan an intervention strategy complete with an evaluation schedule to deal with one environmental issue in your community.

KEY TERMS

acid rain
air pollution
biosphere
carbon monoxide
chemical additive contamination
chlorine
chlorofluorocarbons
Clean Air Act
ecology
ecosystem
environmental health

Environmental Protection Agency (EPA)
greenhouse effect
hazard
microbiological contamination
natural radiation
nitrogen oxide
noise pollution
ozone

pesticides
radiation
radioactivity
radon
synthesis radiation
toxic wastes
vector
vector control
water pollution

F ew areas of public health policy are as riddled with ironies and setbacks as is environmental health. The health of the environment is a long-standing public health problem for which every gain seems to be met with new problems. Historically, citizens have relied on the government to ensure a safe environment; this approach is no longer effective. The complexity of the ravages and constant assaults against the environment make this a problem for everyone. Every individual, including community health nurses, must become advocates for safer environmental health.

The twentieth anniversary of Earth Day was celebrated in April 1990. This was an occasion to look back and document how the environment has changed and what measures have been taken to protect the world's most priceless resources: air, land, and water. Twenty years had passed since the passage of the Clean Air Act, yet more than 100 major cities failed to comply with the standards. In 1990 the Environmental Protection Agency (EPA) measured some of the worst and most widespread urban smog on record; the worst oil spill disaster in American history occurred when the Exxon Valdez ran aground in Alaska's Prince William Sound. Lakes and rivers were continuing to be turned into acid waterways by polluted rain. As Lewis (1990, p. 7) said, "Everything was different, but it seemed little had changed".

Stranahan (1990, p. 10) described the two decades since Earth Day 1970, saying, "Something did happen. The next two decades produced a tidal wave of new laws, scientific research and technological advances, and public awareness—all geared toward making the United States a cleaner and healthier place. But the same period has also brought discoveries of environmental problems no one dreamed of in April 1970," including acid rain, carcinogens, radon, dioxin, global warming, and places such as Love Canal, Bhopal, and Prince William Sound, which have been drastically changed by environmental disasters. Most environmentalists today agree that many of the less serious problems have been solved. What remains are those that are complex and extraordinarily difficult to resolve.

This chapter discusses briefly some milestones in the development of an environmental perspective, relates ecology to environmental health, examines key environmental hazards, and discusses the roles of the government, the community health nurse, and those in the private sector in maintaining the environment for future generations.

HISTORICAL PERSPECTIVE

Human health has always been dependent on the relationship of people to their environment. Archaeological evidence indicates that the Minoans (3000 to 1430 BC) and Myceneans (1430 to 1150 BC) built drainage systems, toilets, and water-flushing systems (Pickett and Hanlon, 1990). As people congregated in cities, problems such as those of adequate water supplies and waste removal developed. The Egyptians built flood dikes, and drainage and irrigation systems (3000 to 1500 BC), and the Romans built impressive drainage systems, gutters, and public baths.

Most of the early public health activities in the United States were concerned with poor sanitation and the prevention of exotic diseases. As early as 1647 the Massachusetts Bay Colony passed a regulation to prevent pollution of Boston Harbor. However, in the early eighteenth century when the American colonies were organizing, little progress was made in public health, including environmental health.

In the late 1700s, boards of health were established in several eastern coastal cities. Many of their early efforts dealt with environmental health concerns such as the drainage of marshes, construction of sewers, planting of trees, and the construction of walls along waterways (Pickett and Hanlon, 1990).

Environmental health in the United States was seriously questioned after 1850, following publication of the *Report of the Sanitary Commission of Massachusetts* (Rosen, 1957). This report, although largely ignored at the time of publication, is regarded today as a landmark document because of its implications for environmental health. Environmental health recommendations included the development of a systematic plan for the observation of atmospheric phenomena, for smoke prevention, and for measures to ensure pure air and water and adequate drainage, sewage, and pest control. Ironically, many of the problems identified in this classic report exist today.

The Industrial Revolution brought new hazards to people and the environment. The use of machinery and poor working conditions caused stress, physical injuries, and chemical exposures. As cities grew, knowledge of sanitation and personal hygiene were unavailable for the poor.

Conditions in mines and steel mills were terrible in the early twentieth century. In large cities, sweatshops were a constant threat to life and health for many workers. Men, women, and children worked 70 to 80 hours a week in factories. Tuberculosis was common among workers. The early 1930s brought badly needed legislation that prescribed reduced working hours for children and adults. Automated machines and improved techniques were introduced and led to mass production. Cities became overcrowded; emissions from industries and cars polluted the air; and industrial wastes from factories contaminated the air and waterways.

The number of working women greatly increased during World War II. Women began working with chemicals and gases, such as benzidine and vinyl chloride, both of which are now considered to be carcinogenic. After the war, men replaced many women in the work force, and they, too, were exposed to these carcinogenic agents.

As the demand for supplies and products increased, so did the pressures to keep costs down and production up. This led to more accidents, injuries, and deaths. As described in Chapter 41, legislation was eventually passed in 1970 that established the Occupational Safety and Health Act (OSHA) and the National Institute for Occupational Safety and Health (NIOSH).

Unfortunately, despite considerable knowledge about the relation between health and the environment, waterways continue to be polluted, the air is filled with irritating and often toxic elements, and radiation and nuclear waste continue to threaten the lives of people, animals, and plants. It seems that each attempt to make life more comfortable and pleasant through labor- and energy-saving devices and processes has led to new sources of pollution and stress.

Past models for dealing with environmental health assaults are no longer effective; what is called for is a new approach that includes all people and will require a considerable change of habits.

ECOLOGY AND ENVIRONMENTAL HEALTH

According to Last (1987, p. 131) *environmental health* is the "aspect of public health concerned with all the factors, circumstances, and conditions in the environment or surroundings of humans that can exert an influence on human health and well-being." Environmental health is intimately related to *ecology,* the study of living organisms in interaction with the environment. Ecology, then, provides a model for looking at environmental health. Ecology is concerned with the interrelations between living and nonliving things. Ecology literally means the study of organisms at home. It is concerned with both the structure and functioning of organisms; it attends to the surroundings, as well as to that which is surrounded.

Ecology is action oriented and focused on what can be rather than what has been or what is. In ecology, the term *biosphere* refers to the world of living things. The biosphere is made up of numerous ecosystems. Each *ecosystem* represents all living and nonliving parts that support a chain of life within a selected area (Wilner et al., 1978).

In each ecosystem, nature provides specific conditions essential for supporting plant and animal life. Each ecosystem is a "circle of life" comprising four principal types of components: (1) sunlight, water, oxygen, carbon dioxide, organic compounds, and other nutrients for plant growth; (2) plants, which convert carbon dioxide and water into carbohydrates; (3) consumers of the products of plants; and (4) decomposed organisms such as bacteria, fungi, and insects.

Barry Commoner's "laws of ecology" help to explain the scope of environmental health. Commoner (1971) organized an informal series of laws of ecology. The first law holds that "everything is connected to everything else"; therefore sunlight, water, oxygen, carbon dioxide, organic compounds, and all organisms are interconnected. The second law—"everything must go somewhere"—stipulates that one organism's excretion or waste is taken up by another organism as food. The third law—"nature knows best"—holds that human changes within a natural system do not always improve that system and may prove to be detrimental. The fourth law is that "there is no such thing as a free lunch." If the environment is to be preserved, anything removed from it by human effort must be replaced and anything added to it must be removed. The extent to which these laws are violated or obeyed determines the status of the environment.

In studying ecosystems it is also necessary to consider people as part of a life-support system. When people are considered a part of their environment, it is essential to consider attitudes, values, and perceptions. The behavior of people is influenced by their values and attitudes about themselves, others, and the world around them. A person's perception of reality is usually more influential in determining behavior than the reality itself.

From an ecological perspective the environment is a multifaceted system made up of biophysical and sociocultural components. The interrelations between the person and the environment are dynamic. People either try to adapt to the environment or modify their needs and desires according to the current state of the environment. Adaptation is a process, not an event. For any organism to survive, it must learn to adapt. Nothing remains fixed or constant in a living system. Living systems are in a constant state of adaptation as organisms continually accommodate to new stressors. Not all adaptations are smooth or positive in outcome. For example, people may adjust to the sound of large airplanes landing near their homes. However, if the noise overload is too great or is constant, they can experience psychotic symptoms caused by continuous sensory overload.

People often overlook the multiple interactions required to maintain a stable relation among living and nonliving parts of the environment. A classic example began in Borneo with a World Health Organization mosquito control program (Harrison et al., 1969). After a community was heavily sprayed with dichlorodiphenyltrichloroethane (DDT), the mosquitoes were controlled but roofs began to be eaten by caterpillars, which were unaffected by DDT. The spray also killed wasps that previously ate the caterpillars. The problem was complicated after indoor spraying to control houseflies. Previously, a small harmless gecko lizard ate the houseflies. However, when the lizards ate the diseased flies, the lizards became debilitated and were easily captured by their predators, the cats. As cats disappeared because of the consumption of DDT, which was passed from one animal to another in the chain, the rat population boomed, invading houses and threatening Borneo with the plague (Hanlon and Pickett, 1984). This example shows how easily, with the help of people, an ecosystem can be thrown out of balance. Throughout the remainder of this chapter, consider how each of the environmental hazards could ultimately lead to an undesirable outcome.

Not only do people contribute to the status of their environment, but they are products of that environment; therefore the environment is a determinant of health and well-being. Environmental health therefore is concerned with those forms of life, substances, forces, and conditions in the environment that may exert an influence on people's health and well-being. Environmental health considers the absence or presence of illness, health maintenance, human efficiency, and the enjoyment of life.

In the 20 years since Commoner discussed his "laws of ecology," advances in technology have done untold damage to the ecological balance in the environment. Currently, Commoner calls for a "negotiated peace" between what he calls the "technosphere" and the ecosphere (1990, p. 589). For example, we have produced algae-fouled lakes and seas by changing crop fertilization methods and have created smog by increasing the compression ratio in automobile engines, thereby creating a nitrogen oxide emission. New forms of technology, including nondevastating energy, pesticides, and methods of farming, must be developed in a worldwide effort with a view to the long-term rather than the short-term future. In the short term, many of the newer, more ecologically sound methods will be expensive, but when the cost of the environment is considered, the price is far less than the initial investment.

IDENTIFICATION OF ENVIRONMENTAL HAZARDS

Environmental problems, because of their interactive effect, cannot be considered in isolation but rather must be viewed from an ecological perspective. Community health nurses provide information to consumers and agencies about the effects of the environment and serve as advocates for a healthier environment. They must also be able to assess the risk the environment poses to health.

Environmental *hazards* can be classified as psychosocial, biological, physical, or chemical. Biological hazards include water, food, and air. Physical hazards include radiation, noise, waste disposal, vector control, and accidents. Dusts, organic and naturally occurring chemicals, molds, pulmonary irritants, and chemical pesticides constitute chemical hazards. Chapter 40 discusses selected biological, chemical, mechanical, physical, and psychosocial agents that have particular effects on the work environment.

Psychosocial Hazards

Sociological and psychological variables in the environment are more difficult to define than are biological, chemical, and physical hazards. However, any consideration of the environment must take into account hazardous psychosocial influences. Many of these hazards are described in Chapters 18, 33, and 34, which deal with community mental health, violence and human abuse, and the recognition and management of stress, respectively. To avoid redundancy, this section is somewhat brief, but this should not be interpreted as a lack of attention to the health hazards associated with the psychosocial components of the environment.

Dubos (1969) contends that mental characteristics are shaped by the environment and that genes determine only responses to stimuli. Environmental stimuli affect people from the time of conception. Survival depends on a variety of environmental stimuli, but often it is the amount and rapidity of stimuli that determine a person's ability to adapt. Although people can adapt to psychosocial stressors, they often experience stress that ultimately leads to disorders of the body and mind.

Noise, overcrowding, lack of privacy, lack of opportunity for social interaction, lack of space, boredom, excessive leisure, tedium, traffic, crowds, and feelings of estrangement from the mainstream of life can be psychosocial hazards.

Change constitutes a psychosocial hazard for nearly everyone. Both positive and negative changes require human energy for adaptation. Change, which is inevitable for most people, is more tolerable if it occurs at a reasonable rate and does not conflict with previously held values or beliefs.

Many societal changes result in potential psychosocial hazards such as increasing mechanization and automation, mobility, and dehumanization of societal institutions. People must adapt to new jobs, new homes, and new social groups, often without assistance from friends, family, or social support networks. Other psychosocial stressors and potential health hazards come from changing female and, ultimately, family roles as described in Chapters 26 and 27.

The United States has increasingly become a country of many cultures. When people holding highly divergent beliefs and attitudes live in close proximity, the potential for stress and, often, conflict arises. Chapter 6 describes key social and cultural variables affecting community health nursing.

Biological Hazards

Biological hazards include disease-producing agents that can enter the human body. They consist primarily of bacteria, viruses, and other microorganisms and parasites. For a disease to be transmitted, a host source, causative agent, and means of transmission must be present. Biological hazards are primarily concerned with the entry of disease-producing infectious agents into the body (Purdom, 1980). Common forms of invading pathogens are bacteria, fungi, and mold. They may be transmitted through water, food, or air.

Water

Throughout history, access to safe water has played an important role in people's lives. Wars have been fought and migrations have occurred so that people could gain access to water. With population growth and urbanization have come the increasing pollution of water sources and an overuse of available water, especially in the more affluent and developed countries.

Water pollution is broadly defined as the addition of a substance that changes the natural qualities of water. Substances that can pollute water and pose health hazards include waterborne viruses and bacteria, waste, heat, radioactivity, industrial pollutants, oil spills, and underground pollution from dumping. Drinking water comes either from surface sources such as lakes or streams or from underground sources. Drinking water can be contaminated in one of four ways: (1) when water is used that has never been treated with protective chemicals; (2) when deficiencies exist in the distribution system (i.e., if sewage and water lines are crossed); (3) when deficiencies exist in the treatment system; or (4) when a properly functioning system is unable to remove contaminating agents or chemicals (Blumenthal, 1985).

The most common contaminants of water are fertilizers, herbicides, fungicides, irrigation residues, detergents from homes and industry, radioactive wastes from power plants and industrial and research facilities, heavy metals, and salts. Many of these contaminants are not easily broken down and are therefore unaffected by usual water treatment methods so that they build up in water. In recent years, the damage to water from oil spills has become an increasing problem. Oil spills also kill fish and certain birds and pollute beaches.

Bacteria and viruses can enter wells by contaminated ropes, buckets handled with unclean hands, the use of contaminated water to prime pumps, or cross-connectors between water pipes and waste piping. Waterborne bacterial diseases include typhoid and paratyphoid fever, dysentery, and cholera. Waterborne viral diseases include infectious hepatitis and poliomyelitis. The pathogens responsible for these diseases are found in the intestinal and urinary tracts of infected people.

Although the Clean Water Act was passed in 1972 and has been amended several times since then to prevent the direct discharge of pollutants into navigable water, a major problem exists for rural residents because water sources serving fewer than 25 people and having less than 15 service connections are generally not monitored by water-quality agencies. This means that homes and small businesses served by wells are generally not monitored for water purity.

Not only is water pollution a problem, but also the increased consumption of water comes at a time when natural sources of water are decreasing. The average American uses 150 gallons of water daily for cooking, washing, toilet flushing, and watering. Indirect use per person is about 1840 gallons per day. Indirect use includes growing the crops people eat and feeding livestock, as well as industrial needs.

NURSING ACTIONS. Nurses must help people learn both how to conserve water and how to avoid polluted water. Some ways to conserve water include the following:

◇ Spend less time in the shower or purchase a low-flow shower head that can cut use by 75%.
◇ Turn off the water tap when brushing teeth, shaving, or scrubbing.
◇ Water the lawn early in the evening to prevent the sun from evaporating the water rapidly.

People should learn how safe their water is, whether they live in a rural area served by a well or in an urban area beset with groundwater pollution. If water is impure, residents can use bottled water for drinking or install a purifying device in their home water system. When traveling abroad where water is not routinely purified, people should be advised to avoid water and foods that cannot be cooked or peeled. No matter how clean a restaurant or home looks and how appealing the food may appear, many countries have bacteria in their water to which the residents have become immune but that can cause dysentery in visitors.

As nurses make visits in the community, they can continually assess for water pollution. Look at household or city drinking water to determine if it is discolored or has an odor or obvious particles in it. Nurses should encourage clients to report signs of impure water and to test their own water source, especially if it comes from a source not regulated by city or state guidelines for water safety. Nurses should be vigilant for any illnesses that might be associated with water used for drinking, swimming, or bathing.

Food

There are three types of environmental hazards related to food: micobiological contamination, chemical additive contamination, and suboptimal food handling.

Microbiological contamination usually results from deposits of toxins on food. There are an estimated 80 million cases of foodborne illnesses annually. The majority of the illnesses result from toxins transmitted through dairy, meat, poultry, and egg products (ADA Reports, 1990). Contaminated foods can cause salmonellosis and shigellosis; illness from *Clostridium perfringens, Vibrio organism*, and viruses; and food poisonings from *Staphylococcus organism* and *Clostridium botulinum* toxins. The most common form of parasitic food transmission is trichinosis, caused by eating undercooked pork infested with *Trichinella spiralis*. Food poisoning from microbiological contamination is caused by the transfer of an organism through food to a human victim. After the transfer, the organism grows within the person's body. Control of microbial growth depends on cooking food at the proper temperature and cooling and storing food at the correct temperature.

Chemical food additives fall into two categories: intentional additives and incidental additives. Intentional additives are deliberately used in food processing to improve or retain nutritional value, flavor, color, texture, or consistency. Many foreign products have been added to foods to make them last longer or make them more convenient to the user. The use of these additives is sanctioned by the Food and Drug Administration (FDA) under the GRAS (Generally Recognized As Safe) list. Typical GRAS additives include vitamins A_1, D_2, and D_3, carotene, ascorbic acid, and riboflavin.

Incidental additives enter and remain in food as a result of their use as pesticides or herbicides, after being added to animal food, from packaging material, or through chemical changes brought about by processing methods. Ironically, the use of pesticides and fungicides has greatly increased food production; however, these same chemicals pollute the food and the underground sources of water. The levels of additives in food are established by the FDA and must not exceed those limits.

Careless food handling, inadequate pretreatment, a contaminated environment (such as one using dirty machinery to prepare food), a high bacterial count, and poor food storage are examples of suboptimal food handling that threaten food safety and quality.

NURSING ACTIONS. Community health nurses play an active role in educating others about food hazards caused by contamination, additives, and improper handling. Nurses can explain to families the importance of properly cooking foods and the dangers associated with eating raw or undercooked eggs, meat, poultry, and fish. Many people fail to read the expiration dates on foods or to know what additives, including sugar and salt, the product contains. People on restricted diets should be taught to read carefully the contents of packages or canned foods and to take into account additives when they plan their daily diet. It is important to remember that infants, young children, pregnant women, frail elderly, and immunocompromised people are at particular risk from contaminated food (ADA Reports, 1990). The simplest way to prevent contaminants from affecting food is by the careful washing in safe water of all food.

Nurses can teach clients to keep perishable foods refrigerated, to throw away old, spoiled food, to avoid food that comes in dented or swollen cans, and to cook foods thoroughly by bringing water to a full boil if the food is unsafe when eaten raw. Nurses also have a responsibility to raise public awareness about public food establishments that are unclean and pose health risks.

Air Pollution

Air pollution has always been present in the forms of volcanic eruptions, tree and grass pollination, and swamp gas. Currently, most air pollution comes from industrial emissions. Air can contain water vapor and particulates such as dust, haze from chemical reactions, and smoke (Reist, 1985). Air is continuously circulating, and this circulation affects the extent and concentration of pollutants present.

In the broadest sense, air pollution results from the presence of foreign materials in the air and is either natural or man-made. Air pollutants are categorized as particulates (aerosols), inorganic gases, and organic gases. Although all three forms are present in the atmosphere simultaneously, gases comprise about 90% of all pollutants. A pollutant exerts its effect by either depressing or stimulating normal functioning within an organism.

Virtually all human activities bring people into contact with some form of air pollution. Five main classes of human-generated air pollution are: (1) carbon monoxide, a major part of automobile exhaust; (2) sulfur oxides, produced mostly by the combustion of coal, fuel oil, and natural gas; (3) hydrocarbons, a family of compounds containing carbon and hydrogen; (4) nitrogen oxides, mainly emitted by power plants and in transportation vehicle exhausts; and (5) particulate matter such as dust, soot, or ash.

The number of diseases and symptoms associated with air pollution is large, ranging from respiratory problems such as nose and throat irritations to bronchial asthma, emphysema, cardiovascular disease, lung cancer, and genetic mutations. It is difficult, however, to establish an unquestionable cause and effect association between the source of air pollution and the disease or symptom.

Most people in Western societies spend 16 to 17 hours per day indoors. Nonmalignant respiratory effects have been associated with exposure to indoor pollutants such as nitrogen dioxide, formaldehyde, and wood and tobacco smoke. Nitrogen dioxide results from the use of unvented gas appliances in the home (Boleij and Brunekreff, 1989). Wood smoke consists of a complex mix of suspended particles such as nitrogen dioxide, carbon monoxide, polycyclic aromatic hydrocarbons, and aldehydes. In Western societies, the effects of wood-burning stoves is small compared with the effects in developing countries, where primitive stoves and open fires are common.

In addition to indoor pollutants from wood and tobacco smoke, people breathe vapors in the kitchen, fumes from cleaning materials, particulates in cosmetics, aerosols in spray cans, fibrous particles from rugs, draperies, blankets, and clothes, and radon, which is a radioactive gas given off by home appliances. In homes and businesses, central heating and air conditioning circulate dust continuously, and deteriorating asbestos insulation can be a source of dangerous asbestos fibers in the air. Indoor-air pollutants can initiate or aggravate acute life-threatening events such as asthma attacks.

Outside, people are exposed to particles from insects, animal and human excretion, odors, gases from marshes, and dust from fields and streets. Spores, constituents of decaying plants and animals, bacteria, and viruses permeate the air throughout the year. During spring and summer, pollen adds to the number of particles that can be inhaled. The terrain also influences air pollution. For example, in a hilly region, fumes are more easily concentrated in one area, the valley.

Outdoor pollutants are rapidly increasing in countries that are expanding their industrialization. For example, many of the large Asian and South American cities are seeing a rapid growth of cars, trucks, and buses that do not have pollution-control devices. Consequently, eye irritation and upper respiratory problems are growing problems in such densely populated and increasingly polluted cities.

Three especially difficult aspects of air pollution are acid rain, depletion of the ozone layer in the atmosphere, and warming of the earth, called the "greenhouse effect."

A substance is considered acidic if it has a pH level of less than 7 and alkaline if its pH is greater than 7. Acid rain is formed primarily from two pollutants, sulfur dioxide (SO_2) and nitric oxide (NO). Lightning, soils, and oceans are natural sources of NO. Volcanos, soils, crops, and decaying vegetation are natural sources of SO_2. Cars, factories, and other industrial activities that use fossil fuels are sources of both SO_2 and NO. *Acid rain* is not just rain. Snow, sleet, fog, or even dry particles can be as acidic or more so than rain.

Once the pollutants are in the air, the lighter particles usually do not fall to the earth immediately. While aloft, they combine with water vapor, undergo chemical reactions, and eventually form sulfuric acid and nitric acids. They are often carried long distances before they fall. Acid rain affects the environment by causing abnormalities in fish and amphibian eggs and by killing algae and other organisms that fish eat. Acid rain also damages the leaves of trees and plants and is a danger to buildings and statues. Acidity and moisture react with stone to form a crust that is easily chipped off or washed away by rain, causing statues to lose their distinct features and buildings to lose a layer of stone.

In recent years, chemicals used in air conditioners have caused large holes to form in the ozone layer above Antarctica. The hole in the ozone layer over Antarctica, discovered in 1985, was about the size of the United States. At ground level, *ozone* is a major pollutant and health threat. However, in the stratosphere, it protects people by absorbing the sun's ultraviolet rays. When these rays reach Earth unfiltered, they may cause skin cancer in people and serious damage to plants and animals (Starr, 1988).

Some of the chemicals most damaging to the ozone layer are *chlorofluorocarbons* (CFCs), a family of chemicals that contains chlorine and fluorine. The most destructive are CFC 11 and 12. These chemicals are commonly used to blow bubbles into flexible foam for furniture, bedding, carpet padding, and dashboards (CFC 11). An alternative is to use spring mattresses and nonfoam furniture. Both CFC 11 and 12 are used in the rigid foam for egg cartons, coffee cups, and home insulation. Cardboard packaging can be used instead of rigid foam (Starr, 1988). It is clear that many of the current convenience items are destroying the environment. Interestingly, McDonald's was the first company in the fast-food industry to require their packaging be made of nonCFC materials. Their foam packaging is made of alternative blowing agents that will not destroy the ozone layer (McDonald's, 1990).

Protection of the ozone layer may be easier to achieve than decreasing the greenhouse warming effect that is occurring as a result of increased carbon dioxide in the air. Carbon dioxide is given off by the burning of fossil fuels—gasoline, natural gas, coal, and peat—and from deforestation (Begley, 1990). By burning these fossil fuels, "we are putting into the air more of the gases that act much like a globe of glass around the planet" (Matthews, 1990, p. 72), and that is what is called the *greenhouse effect*. Besides carbon dioxide, 39 other known gases are said to be warming the earth. The three most common are methane, produced in cattle's digestive tracts and anaerobic bacteric in rice paddies: nitrous oxides, primarily from bacteria, and CFCs.

Why should we worry about a greenhouse effect? The average temperature worldwide has increased 1° F in the last century. In just this century, the 1980s saw the 6 warmest years in recorded history. At high latitudes, winters will be shorter, wetter, and warmer; summers longer, hotter, and drier; and sea levels will rise. As a result of the earth's warming, water supplies will diminish in the western United States. Destructive droughts, such as the one in 1988 in North America, could devastate crops; storms such as hurricanes and tornadoes might become more violent; as ocean waters warm and expand and the ice on Greenland and Antarctica melts, the seas will rise onto the edge of continents, and low areas such as Bangladesh—which is already ravaged by floods and typhoons—may become submerged (Matthews, 1990).

The health consequences of global climatic changes could increase mortality, especially among older people, as a result of heat stroke. With global warming, respiratory irritants can be expected to increasingly pollute the air and cause morbidity and mortality from lung diseases such as bronchitis, bronchiectasis, asthma, and chronic obstructive pulmonary disease (Leaf, 1989). There could be a greater incidence of skin cancer and cataracts because of the lack of protection from the ultraviolet B rays from the sun.

What can be done to prevent an increase in the greenhouse effect? Actions include slowing the release of greenhouse gases by decreasing fossil-fuel use; reducing the burning of rain forests; planting more trees; and developing new forms of fuel such as nuclear power to reduce the "pouring of gases" into the atmosphere. A certain level of greenhouse effect is essential to life; otherwise, the atmosphere would be covered with ice. The solution is in the control of the effect, not its elimination (Albritton, 1990).

CONTROL. It was not until 1963, with passage of the *Clean Air Act,* that the federal government got involved in setting air pollution standards. Two types of standards were considered: (1) ambient air quality standards to apply to outside air in a town, city, or other defined region, and (2) emission standards to apply to industrial emissions. The Air Quality Act of 1967 mandated the establishment of criteria for six major pollutants: sulfur oxides, total suspended particulates, hydrocarbons, carbon monoxide, photochemical oxidants, and nitrogen oxides. The Amendments of 1970 and 1977 constituted the Clean Air Act that expired in 1981. The latest Clean Air Act was signed into effect on November 15, 1990, by President George Bush. The goal of this legislation is to cut acid rain by half, sharply reduce urban smog, and eliminate most of the toxic chemical emissions from industrial plants by the year 2000. The cost of adhering to these new regulations is expected to be $25 billion per year (Daily Progress, 1990).

NURSING ACTIONS. Just as with the detection of potential health problems resulting from food sources, community health nurses often assess environments for the presence of air pollution. Frequently the community health nurse is the one individual who recognizes the total type and amount of pollution with which clients come in contact. For example, a person working in an industry that emits noxious fumes and living in an area polluted by a different type of substance is particularly at risk for developing a pollution-related health problem. Also nurses have many opportunities to assess the hazards of air pollution in the home and to instruct families in proper ventilation, cleaning techniques, and the conservative use of pollutants.

Physical Hazards

Physical hazards can cause death, disease, or disability. Historically (and especially in the past 5 years), the effects of earthquakes, volcanic eruptions, floods, and tidal waves have been dramatic. In recent years, synthetic physical hazards have become as destructive as naturally occurring and unavoidable hazards. Among the more widespread physical hazards are radiation, noise, solid waste, insects and rodents, and accidents.

Radiation

People have always been exposed to *radiation* from the sun and from minerals in the earth. The extent and effect of natural radiation is not entirely measurable. Of the natural sources, cosmic radiation comes from the sun and other parts of earth; it is highest in areas at high altitudes. As mentioned earlier, in recent years it has become apparent that many of the gases generated on Earth, particularly fluorocarbons, are destroying the stratospheric protective layer of ozone that prevents the sun's ultraviolet radiation from reaching the earth.

Natural radiation also comes from the soil and some rocks. Radioactivity is low in most rocks, except volcanic rocks. Living in a brick or stone home adds more human exposure to radiation than living in a wooden house. In recent years the exposure to natural radon, especially in homes, has become a major concern (Loken and Loken, 1989). Radon is a radioactive gas caused by the decaying of uranium. It cannot be seen, smelled, or tasted. Radon is found in high concentrations in soils that contain uranium, granite, shale, phosphate, and pitchblende. It may also be found in soils contaminated with industrial wastes containing the byproducts of uranium or phosphate mining (Centers for Disease Control, 1986). It can enter a home through dirt floors, cracks in concrete floors and walls, floor drains, sumps, joints, and tiny cracks or pores in hollow-block walls. Radon can also enter the home through private wells and be released when the water is used. It is estimated that up to 15% of lung cancers are due to radon exposure.

The two most popular forms of radon detectors are the charcoal canister and the alpha-track detector. Both of these are available in hardware stores and can be used by the homeowner. Nurses should advise clients that their state's department of health, the EPA, and the Centers for Disease Control all publish guides about detecting radon in the home.

Uses of *synthetic radiation* include X rays and radioisotopes in clinical diagnosis and treatment; radioisotopes in industry for measuring, testing, and processing; electric power generation; lasers in science, industry, and medicine; and electronic devices at home. Medical uses account for a significant portion of all exposure to synthetic radiation. Nurses must monitor their own exposure to radiation, as well as exposure for the patient. As concern over radiation exposure has increased, equipment has become more efficient in terms of the radiation emitted. New techniques such as ultrasonography do not use x-rays and are far more safe.

The effects of radiation depend on the dose, type of radiation, and the sensitivity of various organs to the particular form of radiation. Some side effects of high levels of radiation are disruption of bone marrow, skin ulcers, decreased kidney function, pulmonary edema, and a reduced concentration of red and white blood cells and platelets. Other side effects are linked to genetic consequences, thereby placing fetuses at high risk from radiation used during pregnancy.

A growing industry is that of artificial radionuclides and compounds for use in hospitals and research establishments. Through the injection of radioisotopes into the body, organs can be scanned to detect the presence of certain diseases. Industry, biology, and agriculture use radioisotopes as tracers. These procedures pose environmental health hazards when radioactive materials are dumped with sewage into the waterways, thus affecting water life and people through the food chain and by contaminating drinking water.

The interest in nuclear energy as a source to generate electric power has increased as a result of declining oil sources. However, the meltdown of the Soviet atomic energy plant at Chernobyl in 1986 and the partial meltdown in the United States at Three Mile Island have caused the world to realize the dangers that can occur from nuclear energy. Because the effects of exposure to radiation do not always become evident for 20 years or more, the effects of these accidents are still unknown. At Chernobyl, it is estimated that over 1 million people will be affected.

NURSING ACTIONS. The community health nurse can educate clients and communities about the dangers of radiation exposure. Nurses should also encourage compliance with state or federal safety guidelines and reporting noncompliance that affects clients' health and well-being.

Noise

Noise is defined as any unwanted sound in the environment. *Noise pollution* is more prevalent in large cities, with increasingly urban areas becoming noisier. Noise pollution comes from construction activity, airplanes, diesel trucks, power mowers, radio and television sets, and people. For noise to be considered a health hazard, the level, frequency, and length of exposure must be considered. Whether noise is an environmental pollutant is subjective; some people tolerate and, in fact, enjoy high levels of noise; others are annoyed by loud noise. The effects of noise pollution range from annoyance to loss of hearing and finally mental and physical deterioration.

The magnitude or level of noise is measured in decibels (dB). The dynamic range of the ear, or the difference between the loudest and the faintest sound, is about 120 dB (Bruce, 1985). The dB scale is based on powers of 10. Each increase in 10 dB is equivalent to multiplying the intensity by 10; in other words, 30 dB is 10 times as intense as 20 dB and 40 dB is 10 times as intense as 30 dB. Generally, the danger level for hearing loss for most people is about 80 dB, and the current standard for workplace exposure is 90 dB averaged over 8 hours.

Noise can affect a person's physical and emotional well-being. Communication is disrupted by loud noise, especially in industries where people must shout over machinery to speak with each other. Physiological reactions to noise include vasoconstriction of the peripheral blood vessels, slow and deep breathing, skeletal muscle tension, and galvanic skin responses. People exposed to loud noises for a long time have increased urinary output and blood pressure. Sudden, loud noises that startle people affect their emotional well-being, as do noises that keep them awake when they desperately want to sleep.

NURSING ACTIONS. Nursing actions that can help people cope more effectively with noise pollution include wearing protective earplugs when in contact with sustained, loud noises. These ear plugs come in a variety of materials such as foam rubber or soft plastic and can be purchased in most pharmacies. Also, if loud or abrupt noises occur regularly, a dull, constant sound, such as that from a fan or clean-air filtering machines or soft music, can be used to prevent the annoyance from or startle effect of the sound.

Waste Disposal

Waste disposal has two major concerns: What should be done with the enormous amount of solid waste that is being generated, and what should be done with the toxic wastes that are being generated as a result of urbanization and advanced technological development?

Approximately two thirds of the cost of solid waste disposal comes from pickup and transfer to a collection site. Compactors can reduce cost by providing a smaller mass for collection. There are at least five reasons to more effectively manage solid wastes (Chanlett, 1985). Effective management of solid wastes can:

1. Decrease pathogen transmission
2. Reduce discarded toxic and infectious materials
3. Increase aesthetic effects of areas previously used for waste disposal
4. Recover materials and energy
5. Maintain costs

SOLID WASTE. "Each American tosses 4 pounds of stuff daily, or more than half a ton a year. As a nation, it adds up to 179.5 million tons annually—enough to fill a convoy of 10-ton garbage trucks more than 145,000 miles long" (DiChristina, 1990). Solid waste provides fertile areas for pathogen transmission as a result of its attraction for flies and rodents. Mosquitoes breed on the water accumulated in bottles, cans, and other containers in open dumps. Mosquitoes are associated with the transmission of yellow fever, dengue, or hemorrhagic fever.

The traditional method of disposing of solid wastes was to burn them in an open dump or in an incinerator. However, burning pollutes the air, and the dumps serve as breeding grounds for rats, flies, and other pests. These problems led to sanitary landfills and more efficient forms of incineration.

In sanitary landfills, waste is dumped into canyons, swamps, ravines or man-made holes and then compacted by heavy machinery and covered with dirt before rodent infestation occurs. By filling the landfill carefully, it can later be used for public and private purposes. This method has its limitations: chemicals can leak out into the soil, get into the waterways, and contaminate sources of water and the land on which crops are grown. In particular, landfills built before 1985 have been found to allow contaminants to diffuse into the ground (Science News, 1989). Most urban areas are also running out of space for landfills.

The burning of solid wastes greatly reduces the bulk of the waste needing to be disposed. However, hazards of incineration result from noise, the smell of the process, and the dust and other air pollution generated.

Essentially, two choices have existed for the disposal of waste: "burn it" or "bury it." Both methods are currently in use; however, the latter will become more difficult as the population increases and less land is available for waste disposal.

An increasingly popular goal is "transform it," and this includes composting. However, in the United States, composting has been less successful than in other countries. Basically, composting is an aerobic process whereby bacteria, especially fungi, feed on organic material. A carbon/nitrogen ratio of 30:1 is needed to provide the nitrogen for forming new protoplasm. If the pile is stirred regularly to renew its oxygen supply, it produces rich soil. Composting has been effective in many countries including Switzerland, Japan, Thailand, South Africa, Israel, West Germany, The Netherlands, England, Scotland, France, and Mexico (Chanlett, 1985).

In the future there will be new methods of solid waste disposal. Integrated waste management that includes recycling (including composting), burning, landfills, and reducing the amount of garbage generated is the likely answer (DiChristina, 1990).

TOXIC WASTES. Other wastes include *toxic materials* such as poisons, inflammables, infectious contaminants, explosives, and radionuclides (Chanlett, 1985). Hazardous materials make up about 10% of industrial waste. The most dramatic problem in recent decades related to toxic waste occurred in the 1970s at Niagara Falls, New York. A canal once used to divert water from the Niagara River to produce cheap electricity was later abandoned, then used as a toxic waste dump for a chemical company. Over time the dump was discarded, and the land was sold to the city and later developed into lots for home construction. In 1976 one of the homeowners presented the EPA with ooze from her basement containing 82 chemicals; 11 of the chemicals were associated with cancer. The health problems that have been associated with the toxic waste at Love Canal include increased birth defects, children being burned when they touched the oozing liquid in their hand, and cancer. The economic loss that occurred from the devaluation of the homes and the emotional loss from fear were high (Chanlett, 1985), but the actual loss caused by physical consequences has yet to be determined.

NURSING ACTIONS. Community health nurses should be advocates for transforming waste into usable products, for simply producing less garbage, and for moving toward an integrated system of waste management. Interestingly, 40% to 50% of landfill space is used by nondegradable paper that was labeled as degradable. Reuse is a key to decreasing garbage. For example, using cotton rather than disposable diapers, glass rather than plastic bottles, cotton or mesh rather than paper or plastic shopping bags and composting yard waste such as grass clippings and leaves and recycling metal cans, motor oil, rubber, and some types of plastics eliminate considerable garbage (DiChristina, 1990).

Insect and Rodent Control

Insect and rodent control is commonly referred to as *vector control* because of the disease-transmission potential. A *vector* is an agent that actively carries a germ to a susceptible host. Vectors are considered animate vehicles for the transmission of pathogenic organisms and include birds, beasts, bugs, and people. Vector control is most effectively carried out by modifying and regulating the environment to reduce or prevent propagation. Vectors that concern community health nurses are rodents and arthropods. The most significant rodent vectors are rats, ground squirrels, and prairie dogs because they spread the plague.

Of the arthropods, ticks are especially problematic because some carry bacteria that cause Lyme disease (Wickelgren, 1989). There was an increase in the primary Lyme-carrying tick in the northeast and upper midwest sections of the United States in the late 1980s. The transmission of the Lyme disease bacterium is one example of a complex ecosystem chain. A slender spiral-shaped bacterium, *Borrelia burgdorferi,* was first spread in the 1970s by deer ticks in Lyme, Connecticut. Forests support deer, and deer support this particular tick. People come into contact with deer, and the disease progression continues.

A different species of tick carries the disease in different parts of the country, and a variety of animals serves as host. The symptoms of Lyme disease are flu-like illness, rashes, arthritis, and neurological problems such as severe headaches and a stiff neck (Wickelgren, 1989). At present, the best way to control transmission of Lyme disease is to avoid high-risk areas such as parks and woods that are likely to be infected. An additional precaution is to wear a covering of light-colored clothes and to use insect repellent. It is important for people who spend time in wooded areas to carefully inspect themselves for ticks when they leave the woods and to remove the ticks carefully as soon as possible.

Insect and rodent control requires the cooperation of many groups, organizations, and the public. Buildings must be constructed to keep rodents from entering, kept in good repair, and maintained free of food wastes. Pest-control measures must be carefully carried out so that unsuspecting people and animals are safe.

Trapping is often used in rodent control, although it is a slow and difficult process. Poisons, although effective for rodents, do pose new hazards for people, especially children. One material, red squill, kills rodents because they cannot regurgitate it but only acts as an enteric for humans, poultry, and other animals (Wilner et al., 1978).

Mosquitos transmit yellow fever and dengue. Because mosquito "eggs hatch and the larvae and pupae develop only in quiet water and under certain conditions, mosquito control is most effectively accomplished by eliminating or modifying these waters" (Wilner et al., 1978).

Mosquito control includes draining and filling marshes and low areas, stocking larvae-eating fish, varying water levels to cause larvae and pupae to be exposed to waves and currents, spraying, improving irrigation practices, providing better drainage systems, and conducting public-education programs on control methods.

NURSING ACTIONS. Community health nurses can assist with vector control by observing the homes, schools, work sites, and other community facilities they visit to see if rubbish is adequately handled, watching for standing water around the structure, and noting if there are holes in the walls or other parts of the building that may allow rodents to enter. Once vectors are found, nurses can provide relief measures through education of clients or referral to agencies that provide control services. Nurses can also teach clients how to avoid ticks and other forms of pests.

Accidents

Accidents are a major cause of death in the United States. The major causes of accidental injury and death are carelessness or ignorance; many accidents are preventable. The most common accidents are motor vehicle accidents, falls, drownings, and fires. It is difficult to accurately report the number of annual accidental injuries because many do not require medical care and, hence, go unreported.

Injuries occur most frequently in males between the ages of 6 to 44 years. In the over-65-years age-group, women have the highest rate. As income increases, the rate of accidents decreases. Teenage boys, because of their activities and often daring and risk-taking behavior, are a high-risk category. Contact sports, motorcycling, high-speed driving, and the use of firearms increase the accident rate for this age-group.

NURSING ACTIONS. Because community health nursing emphasizes prevention and health education, it is important to review several common, preventable causes of accidents. During home visits, community health nurses should assess home safety and educate clients about reducing or eliminating actual or potential hazards.

In the home, injuries result from fires, falls, poisoning, and lacerations, abrasions, and fractures from tools or equipment. A home survey includes observation for fire hazards, combustive materials, access to matches by children, malfunctioning smoke detectors, and improper use of heaters.

Falls can be prevented by securing loose rugs or cords, removing furniture from walkways, putting rails on stairs, keeping stairs and steps free from slippery rugs, toys, and other objects, and installing a gate at the top or bottom of stairs if small children or confused adults are present. Toys and pets should be kept out of walkways, especially when elderly people whose balance may be poor live in the home.

Bathtubs and showers should have nonslip bottom surfaces or rubber mats. Handrails are useful if someone in the family has poor balance or vision problems. Sharp instruments such as razors and knives should be kept out of the reach of children. Likewise, medicine and chemicals such as bleach, cleaning materials, and liquid plumbing solutions should be safely secured. Small, inexpensive locking devices can be attached to cabinets to prevent access by small children or adults who may be confused and unaware of potential danger.

Yard and farm equipment should be used as intended and kept away from children. Tools, fertilizers, and insecticides should be safely stored. The same principles of safety used in the home should be maintained in schools, businesses, and particularly health care facilities. In addition, community health nurses can provide first aid and cardiopulmonary resuscitation (CPR) classes, encourage regular fire drills in schools and the workplace, and inform the community regularly about the location of shelters that are available during storms or disasters.

Chemical Hazards

Chemical hazards, although by no means a new hazard, are increasing annually. In addition to chemicals occurring in nature, an estimated 2 million others are currently known. Many chemicals, as discussed in Chapter 41, are found in the workplace. Others are used as food additives and in pesticides, drugs, and household materials, and others are found in industrial wastes.

In recent years one of the most controversial household products has been dioxin. In 1988, dioxin was linked to bleached paper products. Coffee filters, disposable diapers, paper towels, milk cartons, newspapers, and facial tissues are bleached products that have recently been found to contain both dioxin and its "chemical cousin" furan (Raloff, 1989). Technically, a dioxin is any of 75 structurally related chlorinated compounds. Processes creating dioxins often yield comparable levels of furans. Incinerators of municipal and hazardous wastes are major sources of these chlorinated compounds.

Three examples of chemical hazards are discussed in detail: pesticides, dusts, and pulmonary irritants.

Pesticides

Pesticides are a variety of chemical poisons used to eliminate pests and to increase annual crop production by generating healthy crops. The use of arsenic began with the ancient Greeks and is still continued. Because pesticides are so effective in reducing crop loss to insects, control of their use has been difficult, although many have been associated with ill effects on humans. Chemical pesticides vary considerably and include insecticides, fungicides, herbicides, rodenticides, arachnicides (spider killers), and nematocides (worm killers). Over the past 20 years the use of these chemical substances to destroy unwanted insect, animal, or vegetable life has increased tremendously. Spraying, dusting, baiting, drenching, dipping, and painting are used to eliminate pests. In an attempt to avoid one hazard to health, other hazards are often invited—air pollution, water pollution, and consumption of these chemicals through food products. Not all noxious material acts on the desired target. A portion of the applied chemical contaminates the air, water, soil, plant life, wildlife, and humans.

Pesticides remaining in the air are quickly diluted in large masses of air to what appears to be harmless concentrations. The "harmless concentration" in the air must be questioned, however, when concentrations of chemicals are found in migrating animals thousands of miles from its use. Pesticides settling on soil may be carried into larger bodies of water by runoff. Pesticides in water are concentrated in fish, which in turn are consumed by humans. Pesticides falling on plant surfaces may be consumed by animals or harvested with crops, or leaves may be carried away by wind or water. In any event, the pesticide is eventually consumed by people either by consumption of the crop or of animals grazing on the crop.

Some of the most well-known pesticides are DDT and aldicarb. DDT was discovered in 1874; however, its use as a pesticide did not begin until 1939. Over the years it has been proclaimed a wonder substance because of its ability to kill insects. When DDT began to be associated with cancer and also began showing up in foods, it was eventually banned by the EPA in 1973. Banning DDT did not solve the pesticide problem with regard to effects on humans.

In 1985 the pesticide aldicarb, which was sold under the name of Temik, was sprayed on watermelons that were served at a Fourth of July celebration. Over 300 people who ate the contaminated watermelons demonstrated flu-like symptoms: dizziness, nausea, perspiration, shaking, and blurred vision. Over 1 million watermelons had to be destroyed as a result of this contamination (Marshall, 1985).

Sevin (carbaryl) a frequently used pesticide around the home, is chemically related to Temik. In 1986, Sevin killed or injured thousands of people when a chemical leakage occurred in Bhopal, India. Both aldicarb and Sevin were initially regarded as clean and miraculous pest killers: now both have fallen from grace (Science, 1985).

Unfortunately pollution from pesticides knows no boundaries. A few examples illustrate the scope of the problem. Begley (1990) describes the complicated route of the pesticide toxaphene, a known carcinogen that is banned in the United States. The chemical is used in Latin America to kill grubs that eat corn roots. It seems likely that toxaphene is carried by the wind into the Great Lakes region and has been infecting the fish in Lake Superior.

In 1986, 1000 metric tons of dyes, insecticides, and mercury spilled into the Rhine River in West Germany after a fire at the Sandoz pharmaceutical company in Basel, Switzerland. The spill carried noxious waste through West Germany to the river's mouth at the North Sea in the Netherlands. That same year, radioactive particles from the Chernobyl nuclear power plant accident rained across the northern hemisphere (Begley, 1990).

Daily, pesticides and heavy metals such as mercury, cadmium, and lead run off the land into waterways from the Chesapeake Bay in the east to the Puget Sound in the west. Nearly half of the acid rain falling on eastern Canada comes from the United States, and 10% of the acid rain in the northeast comes from Canada. There has been some success in controlling acid rain. In 1979, 32 European nations, Canada, and the United States signed the Convention on Long Range Transboundary Air Pollution and pledged to reduce their 1980 emissions by 30% by 1993.

NURSING ACTIONS. How can community health nurses help clients control pests safely? The places where people are most likely to use pesticides are: (1) in the home to kill

---

NATURAL ALTERNATIVES TO THE USE OF PESTICIDES

HOME

Ants: Find the place of entry and squeeze lemon juice on the spot; leave the peel. Ants will also retreat from lines of talcum powder, chalk, damp coffee grounds, bone meal, charcoal, dust, and cayenne pepper.

Cockroaches: Plug all small cracks along baseboards, wall shelves, cupboards, pipes, sinks, and bathtubs. Borax sprinkled around an entry point controls cockroaches.

Flies: Close windows before sun comes up because sunny open windows are a favorite entry point for flies; catch flies with honey on yellow paper.

Ticks and Fleas: Wash infested pets with soap and warm water, dry thoroughly, and use this herbal rinse—2 tablespoons of rosemary in ½ pint of boiling water; steep 20 minutes, strain, cool, and spray or sponge on pet and allow to dry; do not towel; let the pet dry before going outside.

GARDEN

Organic gardening: This will require some initial costs to purchase the equipment to compost, fertilize without excess chemicals, trap insects, and naturally control disease.

LAWN

Plant well-adapted and pest-resistant grass.
Aerate the grass regularly.
Control thatch buildup.
Balance the lawn's pH level.
Water properly.

---

bugs, flies, mosquitoes, spiders, and ants; (2) in the garden to protect flowers, vegetables, trees, and plants; and (3) on lawns (Hollender, 1990).

The box above contains suggestions about natural alternatives for use in the home, garden, and lawn.

Dusts

Dusts, extremely common in the home and workplace, are composed of many different kinds of substances. The lung disease associated with dusts is called *pneumoconiosis*. One problem with dusts results from the size of the particles. Some are so small (visible only through a microscope) that they can easily enter the nasal passages and remain in the lungs. The classic example of exposure to a dust particle that is linked to cancer is exposure to asbestos. Asbestos, a fibrous mineral, has been used widely for insulation and fireproofing, in textiles, drywall compounds, cement, and thousands of other products. For years scientists knew that exposure to asbestos caused asbestosis, a severe and sometimes fatal scarring of the lungs, but it was not until the 1960s that asbestos was recognized as the cause of mesothelioma. This type of cancer is associated with the membranes that surround the lungs and line the abdominal cavity. Asbestos has also been linked with cancer of the larynx and the gastrointestinal tract. It is difficult to estimate the number of workers and consumers who have been exposed to asbestos. Increasingly, asbestos has been found in the insulation material in public buildings. Asbestos removal is necessary; however, it is expensive.

In the past many employees working with asbestos brought the fibers home on their clothes, thus exposing their families. A worker exposed to asbestos for 1 day may develop cancer in later life as a result of the exposure. The asbestos entering the nasal passages remains deposited in the lungs. It is estimated that hundreds of thousands of asbestos workers will die as a result of exposure. This estimate does not include family members or consumers who have been exposed.

Dusts in the home, school, and workplace can aggravate any respiratory problems. Special filters can be added to central heating systems to reduce the number of dust particles. Frequent dust removal from furniture by using a damp cloth also helps relieve circulatory dust.

Pulmonary Irritants

Some substances pass rapidly through the respiratory system, whereas others remain in the lungs for extended periods of time. Prolonged or continuous exposure to certain gases, vapors, and fumes can lead to chronic inflammatory or neoplastic change and lung fibrosis. Gases and vapors of low-water but high-fat solubility pass through the lungs to the blood and are carried to organ sites for which they have affinity.

The principal respiratory diseases induced by pollutants are bronchiectasis, emphysema, pulmonary fibrosis, pulmonary edema, and partial collapse of lung tissue. Although the range and list of pulmonary irritants is endless, some are particularly common and exhibit diverse effects.

Sulfur oxide has been extensively researched; its presence is an indicator of pollution because it gives off bluish-white fumes and reduces visibility. This substance is generated by burning wood, coal, and petroleum products. The degree of irritation depends on the concentration in the atmosphere and the size of the particles (Waldbott, 1978). Sulfur oxide interacts with a variety of other pollutants.

Nitrogen oxide comes primarily from automobile exhaust and almost all forms of combustion; it is a byproduct of many industries and is used in making explosives. Nitrogen oxide reacts with alkali in lung tissue, causing edema. In high concentrations, nitrogen oxide reduces the oxygen-carrying capacity of the blood by increasing the blood level of methemoglobin.

In contrast, **nitrogen dioxide** is about four times as toxic as nitrogen oxide. Insoluble in water, nitrogen dioxide passes through the trachea and bronchi into the alveoli of the lungs where it forms nitrous and nitric acid. Both are highly irritating to the mucous lining of the lungs. Both short- and long-term exposure to nitrogen dioxide increases an individual's susceptibility to infection by decreasing the ability of the lungs to clear inhaled infectious organisms.

Acute nitrogen dioxide poisoning can occur in farmers filling silos. During the early weeks when a silo is being filled, nitrogen dioxide is generated from moldy silage. Similar incidents occur in power plants in people who work with boilers and industrial gases. Symptoms of chronic poisoning range from slight irritation and burning and pain in the throat and chest to violent coughing and shortness of breath. Nitrogen dioxide interacts with tobacco smoke, causing smokers to be at higher risks for developing health problems. This gas has poor warning qualities because it smells good.

Ozone is an unstable, colorless gas found in smog and created by the interaction of hydrocarbons, nitrogen oxides, and sunlight. It is a dangerous irritant to the eyes, throat, and lungs. Because it depresses respiration and causes lung edema, ozone interferes with lung ventilation. Synthetic sources of ozone include high-voltage electrical equipment (electrical insulators; x- and u.v.–ray equipment, quartz lamps; electrostatic air cleaners). Ozone is used as a commercial bleaching compound and sterilant.

Chlorine, a common toxic gas, is frequently used in the chemical industry for preparation of organic and inorganic agents such as trichlorethylene, vinyl chloride plastics, pesticides, herbicides such as DDT, refrigerants and propellants such as fluorocarbons (Freon), detergents, and pharmaceutical agents. It is also used in the paper industry. Acute epidemics have occurred from accidents associated with the handling or emptying of liquid chlorine cylinders. A chlorine spillage can lead to congestive heart failure, pulmonary edema, and pneumonia.

Carbon monoxide is a poisonous gas produced by incomplete combustion and is particularly dangerous because it cannot be seen, smelled, or tasted by potential victims. Carbon monoxide is considered the greatest single, nonindustrial hazard. It is responsible for half of all fatal poisonings in the United States; often the engine of a running car or an open, unlighted gas burner is used in suicide. Oceans are a major source of carbon monoxide, as are automobile exhausts, cigarette smoke, and gas and coal heating systems.

Because it deprives the hemoglobin of its oxygen-carrying ability, carbon monoxide is a common asphyxiant (Waldbott, 1978). When carbon monoxide replaces oxygen in the blood, the functioning of lungs, brain, and heart is impaired. Initial symptoms range from dizziness, headaches, nausea, and general fatigue to impairment of memory and loss of muscular control (Waldbott, 1978).

COMMUNITY HEALTH NURSING AND ENVIRONMENTAL HEALTH

Community health nurses must have an understanding of the psychosocial, biological, physical, and chemical hazards affecting both men and women, elderly people, and children, as well as potential health effects on the unborn fetus. Community health nurses may be actively involved in the control of communicable diseases. Therefore nurses must be aware of the many factors that influence the spread of disease. Nurses who work in the community should be aware of the types of environmental hazards present. They must also known where to locate sources of information identifying the specific effects a hazard may have on an individual or an entire community. Nursing actions have been integrated into several previous sections of the chapter. Selected actions are discussed in the following sections.

Resources

Currently, there are many environmental health resources available. These include programs offered by universities, public health departments, medical centers, community health centers, or information obtained from federal agencies such as the EPA, OSHA, NIOSH, CDC, and the National Institutes of Health (NIH).

Voluntary agencies are excellent sources, because they are involved in health maintenance and disease prevention. The American Heart Association, the American Lung Association, the American Cancer Society, the National Association for Mental Health, and the Arthritis Foundation are some of the voluntary agencies available. These organizations have pamphlets that are excellent resource materials both for the nurse and for the consumer.

Newspapers are also excellent resources. In some cities articles that discuss the effects of environmental degradation and deterioration appear daily or weekly. Some articles address current research, whereas others discuss the role of the federal government.

Environmental Assessment

A key community health nursing role is assessment of the environment: home, school, recreational area, work site, or community as a whole. Community health nurses, especially those involved with home health care, must carefully assess the safety of the home. Electrical cords should not be hidden under throw rugs. This is especially true in situations in which elderly people might trip. Cleaning agents contain chemicals, and if not used and stored properly, these agents may be hazardous. Elderly people with poor eyesight are at risk. For example, one elderly woman mixed several cleaning agents, which led to unconsciousness and severe respiratory irritation. Improper food storage in the home has resulted in many cases of food poisoning. Children who have ingested cleaning agents or plant fertilizers are taken to emergency departments. For some, ingestion has been fatal.

Schools present many hazards. Accidents occur on playgrounds and in gyms, grandstands, and bleachers. Secondary schools have laboratories with chemicals that may cause burns to individuals or fires from explosions. Machinery in shops poses a threat. Poor lighting, littered floors, and narrow or broken stairs are other areas of concern. Improper playground equipment has caused numerous injuries to children.

In assessing the environment, community health nurses should consider the degree of potential toxicity present or proposed through an introduction of some substance or activity and should determine whether a health hazard is likely. From the perspective of physical, chemical, and biological hazards, toxicity refers to the ability of a substance to cause injury to biological tissue. The hazard associated with the substance is the likelihood that it will cause injury in a given environment or situation.

Both recognition and interaction are important. The person who drives to work in heavy traffic or walks down a busy street is exposed to carbon monoxide. This exposure may be greater than the carbon monoxide exposure in the workplace. The person who smokes a pack of cigarettes a day may be exposed to higher levels of carbon monoxide than those associated with the workplace. People who consume excess amounts of alcohol are more susceptible to the effects of carbon tetrachloride. Similarly, exposure to silica increases the susceptibility to tuberculosis. People with asthmatic conditions should not be placed in dusty work areas. Consequently, both an assessment of the individual and the environment are necessary. It is often the accumulation of several seemingly harmless pollutants that constitutes the health risk.

Community health nurses must be aware of the hazards that exist in the community. This information is gained by careful observation as the nurse travels through the community. Observations might include the presence and characteristics of trash collection sites, standing water, the quality of the air as determined by sight and smell, the level and type of noise, and the conditions of housing, including the closeness of homes to one another.

Community health nurses use the nursing process to assess the quality and safety of the environment and to plan and implement interventions. Because other health and safety providers often have greater designated responsibility for environmental control, the nursing role as health educator and advocate or catalyst for environmental change includes the assessment and reporting to the appropriate agency.

After observing potential or actual environmental hazards, nurses report them to the appropriate regulatory or intervening authority or citizen action groups. In some cities, the health department, county commission, housing authority, or other agency maintains responsibility for some aspect of environmental safety. It is important to know which local agencies handle specific environmental problems so quick and accurate referrals can be made. Frequently, citizen action groups are vital forces in instigating environmental change. The nurse alerts such groups to health hazards and works with them as they establish an intervention plan.

Education

A major nursing activity in environmental health is education of environmental health and safety to school children, health providers, fire and police personnel, and the general public. Health education includes both formal and informal teaching. Community groups must be informed about environmental issues such as pollution, vehicular safety, product safety, and the presence of or potential for additional physical, chemical, biological, and psychosocial hazards.

Nurses must often serve as catalysts to see that actions are taken. It is not always easy to persuade individuals and groups that an environmental health threat may be imminent or actually present. The nurse serves as a vital force to see that people follow through on the plans and commitments they make.

Nurses have an important role to play as informed citizens who can recommend actions that lay people can implement to save the environment. The box on p. 306 describes several useful tips for environmental protection. It is important to remember that preserving the environment will necessitate a change in old habits and some inconvenience and

WAYS TO SAVE THE ENVIRONMENT

WATER

1. Turn off water faucets while washing your face or brushing your teeth. A running faucet uses about 3 to 5 gallons of water per minute. Just wetting and rinsing teeth and using a wet cloth uses only ½ gallon of water.
2. Washing a car at home using a hose can consume 150 gallons of water compared to 5 to 10 gallons at a self-service car wash.
3. Use a low-flow shower head to reduce water use by 75%.

AIR AND PRESERVING THE OZONE LAYER

1. Avoid polystyrene foam, such as the materials that protect electronics in boxes during shipping, coolers and foam "peanuts."
2. Do not buy aerosol cans containing CFCs (Nos. 11, 12, 113, 114, or 115).

WASTE DISPOSAL

1. Use rechargeable batteries; household batteries contain mercury. When thrown out, these batteries corrode, break apart, and release mercury or cadmium into the soil.
2. Plastic shopping bags are never totally biodegradable, so use paper. Even better, bring a cloth bag when you shop.
3. Avoid flea collars for animals; use citrus oil spray instead. Run orange or grapefruit skins through a blender, and simmer in water. Cool and brush onto the animal's skin. The chemicals in flea collars can cause cancer, nerve damage, and mutations in animals and are dangerous when thrown away.
4. Use recycled oil when you change the oil in your car. It is estimated that a single quart of motor oil poured into the ground can pollute 250,000 gallons of drinking water.

HAZARDOUS HOUSEHOLD PRODUCTS

Replace toxic with nontoxic substances such as:

Air freshener	Set vinegar out in an open dish.
Drain cleaner	Use baking soda or salt followed by boiled water.
Spot remover	Apply soap to clothing spots; dishwashing detergent removes spots on rugs.
Furniture polish	Use 1 tsp lemon oil in 1 pint mineral oil.
Oven cleaner	Use baking soda, salt, and water.

For more information see Hollender, 1990; The Earth Works Group, 1989. Hollender J: How to make the world a better place, New York, 1990, William Morrow; The Earth Works Group: 50 simple things you can do to save the earth, Berkeley, Calif, 1989, Earthworks Press.

that environmental awareness actions involve some costs associated with buying newer products.

As health care professionals, nurses must objectively assess the effect of the environment on health. As new legislation is passed and old legislation amended, they must continue to ask questions, attempt to remain objective, and weigh the evidence of both sides. They must be able to comprehend the complexity of each problem and the ram-

ifications involved in possible alternatives, bearing in mind that the best approach toward solving any environmental problem is an informed one.

ROLE OF GOVERNMENT IN ENVIRONMENTAL HEALTH AND SAFETY

In the past 20 years, people have finally begun to recognize how badly they have fouled up their own "nests" with pollution. Over the years, standards for control of emission of air pollutants were established and the Environmental Protection Agency (EPA) was created.

Early local governmental efforts in the United States dealt with services such as water supply, sewage collection and deposit, refuse collection and disposal, control of rodents and pests, and regulation of housing and recreation. Some of the earliest efforts at environmental control were performed by the official health departments in Philadelphia, New York, Baltimore, and Charleston in the late 1700s. They directed activities toward community sanitation and the prevention of filth and oral disease. In some instances the specialization was extreme, with food sanitation divided into milk, meat, and food divisions. The states' health departments and other statewide environmental health and safety agencies are responsible for ensuring that all people within the state receive comprehensive services. Few if any direct services are performed at the state level, and the pattern of organization among states varies.

Political systems respond to the concerns of the public. This has certainly been evident in environmental health. In the decade following World War II, the U.S. government addressed conservation in response to public concerns about the abuse of natural resources (Rabe, 1990). The 1960s and 1970s were devoted to concerns about environmental abuses of air and water. In the late 1970s and throughout the 1980s concerns intensified about hazardous wastes, toxic substances, and some escalating and far-reaching problems such as depletion of the ozone layer and the growing "greenhouse effect."

At the national level, U.S. funding for environmental problems has historically been scarce, with regulatory authority scattered throughout the federal bureaucracy. As a result of the outcry over the degradation of the environment in the 1960s and the pressures on President Nixon, the Congress, and state legislatures, in 1970 Congress passed the National Environmental Policy Act (NEPA) to "take into account all anticipated environmental ramifications from proposed development projects supported by national government funding" (Rabe, 1990, p. 321). It also created the Council on Environmental Quality (CEQ) to assist in coordinating the environmental efforts of the government. The ***Environmental Protection Agency (EPA)*** was also established in 1970 and was to be responsible for all environmental media, including air, water, and land, and most of the major pollution problems. The agency, however, never achieved its potential as a result of political pressures from groups such as large companies that stood to lose much if the EPA enforced stringent policies. Other departments within the federal government failed to give up environmental components of their programs. At the state level, both NEPA and state versions of the EPA were established in many states. Often state and federal agencies work at cross-purposes with one another, leading to both duplication of services and omissions.

The role of the government, both federal and state, in environmental issues is likened to the ebb and flow of water. During some administrations there is concentrated attention on environmental issues; in other administrations, environmental issues are ignored or become political pawns. Many landmark pieces of legislation fail to be reauthorized or the states are unwilling or unable to fully implement the acts.

In recent years consumers have been forces to reckon with in terms of environmental health. A little known federal law called the Emergency Planning and Community Right-to-Know Act, or Title 111 of the Superfund Amendments and Reauthorization Act of 1986, gives every citizen the right to information not only about the scope of the state or national pollution problems but also how much and what kind of toxic waste is being released by factories in specific towns and neighborhoods. This Act was passed in 1986 after the Union Carbide catastrophe that killed or injured more than 200,000 people in Bhopal, India. This law requires approximately 30,000 industrial facilities to report all releases of any of the 308 chemicals officially implicated by the EPA as disturbing the environment or creating health hazards (Lawren, 1990).

CLINICAL APPLICATION

In the community health nursing course, you are required to make a home visit and assess the home for environmental hazards. You are instructed to thoroughly examine the house and the land near the house and to make a list of all potential health hazards that you observed.

You actually feel fortunate about this assignment because your assigned family is young, middle class, college educated, and lives in a small but well-maintained home. When you arrive, you are greeted by Mrs. Smith and her 18-month-old son David. You explain your assignment and ask if you can walk through the house and around the yard to determine if any health hazards exist. You really do not expect to find many hazards in this clean and attractive home.

Upon first examination, you see a three-bedroom home with a basement, built in a heavily wooded area. Being conscious of energy costs, the Smiths cook with gas and heat the house primarily with an energy-efficient wood-burning stove. To save money they also have a well-maintained vegetable garden and several small fruit trees. Upon closer inspection, you notice that there is a significant crack in the concrete in the basement. You also learn that they use a variety of pesticides to keep their garden in good condition. Soon you are surprised at the number of small safety problems that you have found. These include the following.

◊ Although the Smiths get their water from a well, they have never had it checked for pollutants.

◊ Mrs. Smith is not aware that radon gas is regularly found in the homes in her county and that the crack in the concrete could allow radon to escape into the house if the gas is present in their soil.

◊ Mrs. Smith does not know that they should use hardwoods in the stove to reduce the pollution from the smoke

generated from burning the wood. They have not been cutting their wood 6 months or more before using it and storing it in a covered area above the ground.

◊ Members of the family occasionally eat raw vegetables directly from the garden, failing to realize the importance of scrubbing all fresh fruits and vegetables thoroughly under running water to rid them of the residue from the pesticides.

◊ Inside the home you notice that there are no locks on the cabinets in the kitchen and bathroom that contain chemicals and other toxic materials; the pet food is on the floor in the kitchen, easily available for a young child to eat; none of the electrical outlets have caps on them to protect the child from sticking objects into the outlet.

Following your walk through the home with Mrs. Smith and her son, you sit down at the kitchen table and review your checklist with her. Mrs. Smith asks many questions as you describe why the hazards are potential health problems. Mrs. Smith seems embarrassed that she had not even thought of the need to cover the electrical outlets and to place locks on her cabinet doors. You find out that she has never been around young children and missed the postnatal child rearing classes offered by the local hospital, but she expresses interest in attending, even though her son is 18 months old.

Between you and Mrs. Smith, you devise the following goals and strategies to make the Smith's home a safer and healthier environment for the whole family.

◊ Within 1 week, Mrs. Smith will call the local hospital to sign up for the child-rearing program. She will purchase outlet plugs and place them throughout the house by the end of the week.

◊ Mrs. Smith will call the local health department to obtain a radon gas testing kit and have their well water tested for pollutants by the end of the week.

◊ Tonight Mrs. Smith will discuss with her husband the home health and safety checklist and explain the need to learn more about wood-burning stoves and smoke pollution in the home.

◊ Mrs. Smith will obtain a book from the local library in order to read about the use of pesticides with gardening; she will begin to scrub all fruits and vegetables immediately.

◊ To evaluate these strategies, you will make a follow-up telephone call at 2 weeks and at 4 weeks to determine the Smiths' progress in making their home safer and healthier.

This clinical application depicts the role of the community health nurse in environmental and home health. Both accurate assessment with family participation and mutual goal setting help families change their homes from hazardous to healthy and safe environments. When family members are able to identify risk factors, they often are able to develop strategies on their own. The follow-up visit or telephone call provides the family with additional guidance as needed. In addition, learning how to access and use community resources is a benefit of developing a plan that requires the family to solve their own health needs. In subsequent visits, observe and inquire about the actual changes that have been made.

SUMMARY

The challenge of maintaining individual, family, community, and worldwide environmental health and safety is tremendous. Community health nurses are in an ideal position to detect environmental hazards and to instruct individuals, families, and communities in ways to avoid or alter environmental hazards. Nurses may not always directly combat these hazards, but they do monitor, report, advise clients, and serve as action-oriented catalysts to initiate community activity. Water, air, soil, and food hazards are only a few of the potential community hazards. To implement an ecological approach, nurses must continually recognize the interaction among people and the environments in which they live. This human and environment interaction and its effect on health have been sources of concern since early recorded history. Many problems have been solved, but new and often more difficult and resistant ones continually arise. This is what makes the role of the community health nurse dynamic and exciting.

KEY CONCEPTS

Nurses play an important role in detecting environmental hazards and in developing and implementing health promotion and treatment programs.

The production and maintenance of a healthy environment will require a combination of increased legislation, vigorous enforcement of existing laws, increased cooperation by business, and greater public awareness and education. Community health nurses can make significant contributions to this process.

Ecology, the study of living organisms in interaction with the environment, provides a model for looking at environmental health.

Two contexts have been proposed for describing the human and environmental relationship. The first includes elements of the natural environment hazardous to health, such as biological agents of disease or injury. The second context consists of health hazards created by actions and maladaptations of people to their environment.

Community health nurses must have an understanding of the biological, physical, chemical, and psychosocial hazards affecting both men and women, the elderly, and children, as well as potential health effects on the unborn fetus.

A major community health nursing activity regarding environmental hazards is education.

Assessment of the client's environment is also an important community health nursing role.

The federal government has been involved in environmental legislation since the 1800s. However, the biggest nationwide effort at pollution control began in the 1960s.

The modern environment is hazardous in at least two ways: it contains noxious and stressful events and it changes so quickly that people are unable to adapt.

LEARNING ACTIVITIES

1. Read the local newspaper to gain information about major environmental hazards in a given community.

2. Describe one real or potential chain of events in a community that could have negative ecological results.

3. Review one environmental hazard that has occurred in the last 10 years and discuss three potential long-range consequences.

4. Drive through a community and identify potential disasters. You may have to assume that certain weather conditions prevail.

5. Drive through a community and identify the quality of environmental health and safety.

BIBLIOGRAPHY

ADA Reports: Food and water safety (ADA timely statement), J Am Diet Assoc 90(1):111, 1990.

Albritton DL: What we know; what we don't know, EPA J 16(2):4, 1990.

Begley S: Pollution knows no boundaries, Natl Wildlife 28:34, 1990.

Blumenthal DS: Introduction to environmental health, New York, 1985, Springer Publishing.

Boleij JS and Brunekreef B: Domestic pollution as a factor causing respiratory health effects, Chest 96(3):368S, 1989.

Bush signs Clean Air Act, Charlottesville, VA, Daily Progress, November 16, 1990.

Centers for Disease Control: A citizen's guide to radon, Richmond, VA, 1986, Virginia Department of Health, Bureau of Radiological Health.

Chanlett ET: Solid waste management. In Jarvis LL, editor: Community health nursing: keeping the public healthy, ed 2, Philadelphia, 1985, FA Davis.

Commoner B: Ending the war against earth, Nation 250(17):589, 1990.

Commoner B: The closing circle: nature, man and technology, New York, 1971, Alfred A Knopf.

DiChristina M: How we can win the war against garbage, Pop Sci 237:57, 1990.

Dubos R: The crisis of man in his environment. In Proceedings of symposium on human ecology, Pub No 1929, 1968, Department of Health, Education, and Welfare.

Hanlon JJ and Pickett GE: Public health: administration and practice, ed 8, St Louis, 1984, Mosby-Year Book, Inc.

Harrison G, Gates D, and Halling CS: Ecology: the great chain of being, Ekistics 27:161, 1969.

Hollender J: How to make the world a better place, New York, 1990, William Morrow.

Last JM: Public health and human ecology, Norwalk, Conn, 1987, Appleton & Lange.

Lawren B: How safe is your world? Natl Wildlife 28:18, 1990.

Leaf A: Potential health effects of global climatic and environmental changes, N Eng J Med 321:1577, 1989.

Lewis TA: A new day must dawn, Natl Wildlife 28:4, 1990.

Loken S and Loken T: Radon: detection and treatment, Nurse Pract 14(11):45, 1989.

Matthews S: Is our world warming?: under the sun, Natl Geo 178(4):66, 1990.

McDonald's: Ozone 8: McDonald's environmental affairs, Oak Brook, Ill, 1990, McDonald's.

Monastersky R: Global change: the scientific challenge, Sci News 135:232, 1989.

Pickett G and Hanlon HH: Public health: administration and practice, ed 9, St Louis, 1990, Mosby-Year Book, Inc.

Purdom PW, editor: Environmental health, New York, 1980, Academic Press.

Rabe B: Environmental health policy. In Pickett G and Hanlon JJ: Public health: administration and practice, ed 9, St Louis, 1990, Mosby Year-Book, Inc.

Raloff J: Dioxin: paper's trace, Sci News 135(7):104, 1989.

Reist PC: Air pollution. In Jarvis LL, editor: Community health nursing: keeping the public healthy, ed 2, Philadelphia, 1985, FA Davis.

Rosen G: A history of public health, New York, 1957, MD Publications.

Starr D: Protecting the ozone layer, Earth Sci 41(3):18, 1988.

Stranahan SQ: It's enough to make you sick, Natl Wildlife 28:8, 1990.

The Earth Works Group: 50 simple things you can do to save the earth, Berkeley, Calif, 1989, Earthworks Press.

Unexpected leakage through landfill liners, Sci News, 135(11):104, 1989.

Waldbott, GL: Health effects of environmental pollutants, ed 2, St Louis, 1978, The CV Mosby Co.

Wickelgren I: At the drop of a tick, Sci News, 135(12):184, 1989.

Wilner DM, Walkley RP, and O'Neill EJ: Introduction to public health, ed 7, New York, 1978, MacMillan Publishing.

PART FOUR

Common Community Health Problems

As the twentieth century draws to an end, common community health problems are more societal, or community based, than individual problems. The complexity of current health problems is growing. Solutions will require an integrated social and health care approach that will include preventive, therapeutic, and rehabilitative intervention. Primary prevention is the desired way to maintain community health, yet funding for prevention has never been equal to that devoted to curative practices.

Communities continue to experience significant problems as a result of communicable and frequently expensive diseases, violence against people and property, unresolved mental illnesses, abuse of substances among people of all groups, and increasing numbers of people disenfranchised from society whose personal resources are severely limited. This section presents a discussion of the most common problems currently faced by communities.

Chapter 19 discusses communicable diseases and examines prevention and treatment. Chapter 20 presents an in-depth discussion of human immunodeficiency viruses and other sexually transmitted diseases. Chapter 21 talks about the mental health needs and challenges being faced in communities in a time of increasing personal and group stress. For many, these problems are compounded by decreasing financial and other resources. Chapter 22 looks at many of society's most needy, who are vulnerable to a wide range of physical and psychosocial threats. Chapters 23 and 24 talk about substance abuse and human abuse, respectively, by looking at causes of these forms of abuse and forms of intervention.

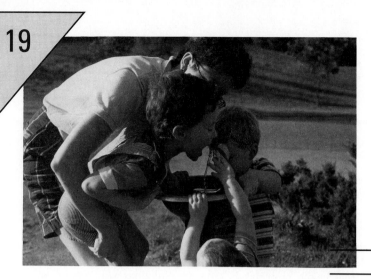

19

Communicable Diseases and Infection Control Practices

Joan G. Turner

Myra Lovvorn

OBJECTIVES

After reading this chapter, the student should be able to:

Explain the host-agent-environment triad and how these factors may interact to cause infectious disease.

Explain the process and goal of surveillance activities in infectious and communicable disease.

Discuss the impact of communicable and infectious diseases in terms of morbidity and mortality.

Explain the difference between active and passive immunity and give several examples of each.

Discuss the indications or contraindications and untoward effects of active and passive immunity.

Explain the ramifications of antibiotic-resistant organisms to community health nursing practice.

Explain the treatment for pediculosis and helminth infections.

Identify and define opportunistic infections.

Identify the hosts at risk of opportunistic infections.

Discuss prevention measures to control opportunistic infections in identified populations.

KEY TERMS

acquired immunodeficiency syndrome (AIDS)
agent
botulism
communicable disease
delta hepatitis
dosage
drug resistance
endemic
enzyme-linked immunosorbent assay (ELISA)

epidemic
haemophilus influenzae
host
immune globulin
immunization
infectivity
invasiveness
legionellosis
nationally notifiable conditions

nosocomial infections
pandemic
passive immunization
pediculosis
salmonellosis
sexually transmitted diseases
temporal patterns
vaccines
virulence

I n recent decades the impact of communicable diseases on society has been drastically reduced by the combined efforts of pharmacology, sanitary engineering, public health, medicine, and nursing. In view of the current declining mortality and rare need for hospitalization caused by communicable diseases, this still remains a significant area of concern for the community health nurse.

This chapter defines basic terminology and discusses the role of the community health nurse dealing with communicable and infectious diseases. Community health nurses must be knowledgeable about disease processes and methods of prevention and control. Informed nurses can play an important role in reducing the impact of communicable diseases in their communities.

HISTORICAL PERSPECTIVE

Communicable diseases have affected human life since earliest times. Evidence gathered by anthropologists indicates that humans who lived in the Paleolithic period (18,000 to 6000 BC) were susceptible to tapeworms, roundworms, tetanus, and gas gangrene. However, epidemics, or outbreaks involving large numbers of people were not a problem until approximately 5000 to 4000 BC. As the first large cities developed and great numbers of people lived in close proximity, the stage was set for epidemics of communicable diseases. Occasionally these epidemics came close to exterminating organized society.

Some of history's most notorious and lethal epidemics were the Black Death in Europe in 1345, smallpox among the North American Indians in 1633, dysentery during the Crusades, and the influenza pandemics of 1889 and 1918. In just a few days, an epidemic of yellow fever left Napoleon with 3000 survivors out of 25,000 troops. Such mortality figured heavily in his ultimate defeat at Waterloo (Hare, 1955).

Communicable diseases played a significant role in the death and illnesses of people during the colonial period in the United States, and they were still leading causes of death in 1900. In fact, the need to control the spread of communicable diseases stimulated the first health legislation in the United States, including the establishment of health departments in colonial America. The antibiotics of the 1940s, the vaccines of the 1950s, 1960s, and 1970s, and the general improvement in nutrition and sanitation gradually brought many of the traditional killing and crippling communicable diseases under control in the United States and other industrialized nations. Methods used to control communicable diseases in these developed nations could be applied to the developing Third World countries of Asia and Africa to protect the new world community from pandemics.

With the 1980s came acquired immunodeficiency syndrome (AIDS), which has been called one of the most complex problems of the century. AIDS has produced a virtual renaissance in worldwide concern with communicable diseases. AIDS is discussed more fully in Chapter 20. Regardless of treatment advances, community health nurses must appreciate the real and potential effects that communicable and infectious diseases currently have on society.

DEFINITIONS

To be fully knowledgeable about the problems associated with communicable diseases, some basic terms must first be defined.

Communicable disease: Illness caused by an infectious agent by transmission of that agent to an infected person, animal, or inanimate reservoir to a susceptible host (Benenson, 1990)

Infectious disease: A disease of man or animal resulting from an infection (Benenson, 1990)

Host: A human or other animal, including birds and anthropods, in which an infectious agent may enter and cause disease (Benenson, 1990)

Infectious agent: An organism (virus, rickettsiae, bacteria, fungus, protozoa, or helminth) capable of producing infection in a susceptible host (Benenson, 1990)

Agent factors: Characteristics of an agent that allow it to invade a host and cause disease

Endemic: The constant presence of an infectious agent in a given area (Benenson, 1990)

Epidemic: The occurrence of disease in a region clearly in excess of expected incidence (Benenson, 1990)

Pandemic: A worldwide outbreak of an epidemic disease phenomenon

EFFECTS OF COMMUNICABLE DISEASES ON SOCIETY

New information and changes in disease-causing organisms present a challenge for today's community health nurses to prevent the spread of communicable diseases. Knowledge of current prevention and control measures can assist the community health nurse in recognizing and treating changing communicable diseases. In addition, educating the client and the community regarding potential spread of disease is very important.

The types and causes of these diseases are not static. They constantly change and are updated by new knowledge. For instance in the past decade it was discovered that various herpesviruses caused innumerable perinatal and adult diseases previously attributed to noninfectious or nonspecific etiologic factors. Additionally, several new infectious diseases have been documented. The changing incidences of these diseases are shown in Table 19-1.

Increasingly, communicable diseases fail to respond to previously successful treatments as the result of a phenomenon known as *drug resistance* (antibiotic resistance). It has been documented in a wide range of communicable diseases such as tuberculosis, malaria, salmonellosis, and gonorrhea. When a disease becomes resistant to conventional treatment,

TABLE 19-1

Incidence of AIDS, legionellosis, toxic shock syndrome, and hepatitis B, 1982–1988

	1982	1984	1988
AIDS	—	4445	31,001
Legionellosis	654	750	1085
Toxic shock syndrome	400	482	390
Hepatitis B	22,177	26,115	23,177

other methods must be explored. Drug resistance is discussed in more detail later in this chapter.

The scope of communicable disease is changing as new information and new vaccines become available and as standard immunization schedules are modified. Information of this sort is vital to community health nursing practice.

Community health nurses must be knowledgeable about communicable diseases so that they can effectively counsel clients regarding prevention and control. They are often in a position to recognize signs and symptoms of actual or impending disease and can make referrals for diagnosis that leads to treatment and control of spread. They can monitor current vaccines to educate the public and clients regarding current time tables for vaccination.

Morbidity and Mortality

Table 19-2 shows that the total number of deaths attributed to reportable communicable diseases in the United States in 1986 was 14,576. The total figure for infectious diseases is 114,276 to 254,276 if nosocomial infections that contributed to death are counted. Deaths attributable to AIDS since 1986 would certainly inflate annual counts of deaths caused by infectious diseases. Projections made by the Society of Actuaries in 1989 estimate that, by the year 2000, AIDS deaths could be 12 to 24 times the 1988 total of 57,754 deaths (CDC, 1991). In January 1991, the death totals related to AIDS approached 100,000 thus far in the epidemic.

Tables 19-3 and 19-4 further illustrate the impact of communicable disease. Note that there is no effective active immunization for six of the seven communicable diseases with the highest incidences. The incidence of hepatitis B remains significant, despite the available immunization.

Certain communicable or infectious disease processes occur more frequently during one season of the year, as is shown in Table 19-5. Awareness of these seasonal fluctuations, known as temporal patterns, can alert the community health nurse to which disease phenomenon might be expected any given time of year.

The term *pandemic* refers to a worldwide outbreak of an epidemic disease phenomenon. Contemporary pandemics of communicable diseases have been limited essentially to influenza A types. In this century there has been the Spanish (swine) influenza pandemic (1918 to 1919), the Asian in-

TABLE 19-2
Number of deaths in the United States attributable to infectious or communicable diseases (1986)

Cause of death	Number of deaths (1983)	Number of deaths (1986)
Specific notifiable communicable disease	3592	14,576
Respiratory infections	56,771	69,700
Nosocomial infections	30,000-90,000	90,000-130,000
Total:	90,363-170,263	114,276-254,276

TABLE 19-3
Incidence of notifiable communicable diseases in the United States (1984–1988)

Disease	Number of cases reported (1984)	Number of cases reported (1988)
Gonorrhea	878,556	719,536
Chickenpox	190,894	192,857
Syphilis (all stages)	69,888	40,117
Hepatitis (all types)	52,026	56,773
Salmonellosis (excluding typhoid fever)	40,861	48,948
Tuberculosis	22,255	22,436
Shigellosis	17,371	30,617
Measles (rubeola)	2587	3396
Mumps	3021	4866
Aseptic meningitis	8326	7234
	1,283,950	1,126,780

Data from Centers for Disease Control: MMWR 38:53-59, 1989. These data do not include estimates of the common cold nor do they include pneumonia and influenza, which are not mandatorily reportable diseases.

TABLE 19-4
Deaths from specified notifiable diseases, United States (1983–1986)

Cause of death	Number of deaths (1983)	Number of deaths (1986)
Tuberculosis (all forms)	1937	1782
Hepatitis (all forms)	862	1006
Menogococcal infections	459	286
Encephalitis	164	230
Syphilis	136	80
Totals:	3558	3384

Data from Centers for Disease Control: MMWR 37:57, 1988.

TABLE 19-5
Temporal patterns in communicable or infectious diseases

Type of disease	Season of peak occurrence
Polio	Spring
Roseola infantum	Spring
Rubella	Late winter and spring
Meningococcal infections	Winter and spring
Rubeola (measles)	Late winter and early spring
Diptheria	Autumn and winter
Rocky Mountain spotted fever	Summer
Legionellosis	July through October
Reye syndrome	December through March

fluenza pandemic of 1958 to 1959, and the Hong Kong influenza pandemic of 1968 to 1969. According to the Centers for Disease Control (CDC) an excess of 40,000 deaths were attributed to influenza in U.S. epidemics from 1957 to 1986 (CDC, 1990a).

Failure to enforce the recommended schedule for communicable disease control or a break in community sanitation or water purification can result in an epidemic at any given time. An epidemic is not the only threat; communicable diseases also result in chronic disability and irreversible disease processes every year. For instance it is estimated that the occurrence of measles (rubeola), a disease that is 95% preventable by immunization, resulted in 600 cases of mental retardation and 89 deaths in the United States in 1990 (CDC, 1991).

Economic Effects

Communicable disease plays a tremendous role in the economic viability of both specific communities and the nation. The U.S. Department of Health, Education, and Welfare estimated that the total economic loss from the 1968 to 1969 Hong Kong influenza in the United States alone was $46 million (Beveridge, 1978). The cost of treating persons with AIDS was estimated to be $45.6 billion through the end of 1986 (Volberding and Abrams, 1985). In addition, acute respiratory disease (i.e., the "flu" or a "cold") is the most common human illness and the principal reason people consult a physician. Approximately 156 million workdays are lost annually at a cost of $24 billion as a result of communicable and infectious diseases (Healthy People, 1979).

Surveillance of Communicable Diseases

Trends in the occurrence of communicable diseases are monitored in the United States by the Centers for Disease Control (CDC) in Atlanta, Georgia, and on a worldwide level by the World Health Organization (WHO). The WHO monitors and reports communicable disease information in the *Weekly Epidemiological Record*. Updates can be obtained from the United Nations Building in New York City.

The CDC publishes the *Morbidity and Mortality Weekly Report (MMWR)*. These reports include weekly and cumulative totals of reported communicable diseases by geographic region and individual state. *MMWR* provides enlightening, authoritative, and up-to-date information on many facets of communicable disease occurrence, prevention, and control. Additionally, various topics of public health interest such as unusual cases of disease, communicable disease outbreaks, and environmental and occupational hazards are discussed.

Diseases are classified according to reporting requirements. Federal law requires that the occurrence of certain communicable disease be reported to the CDC by all states on weekly, monthly, and annual bases. These are classified as nationally notifiable conditions. Examples include sexually transmitted diseases, tetanus, and rabies. Other diseases may be classified as "optionally reported." States may choose to report these diseases based on their individual state health regulations. *MMWR* and the national surveillance program also monitor the occurrence of other conditions classified as nonnotifiable conditions. These communicable disease phenomena are optionally reported by state health departments and include conditions such as giardiasis, histoplasmosis, infectious mononucleosis, meningitis, Reye syndrome, strep throat, scarlet fever, toxoplasmosis, and influenza. In some instances these diseases are reported only when they are believed to be occurring in epidemic proportions. At other times a given disease is reported in a particular state because it is believed to be endemic or continuously present in the area and is therefore considered to be an ongoing public health problem. For instance, histoplasmosis is believed to be endemic to the Ohio Valley region.

TRANSMISSION OF COMMUNICABLE DISEASE

The community health nurse should have a clear understanding of how disease is transmitted to prevent and control the spread of communicable diseases. Factors that affect disease progression can be studied, and control measures can be instituted. Agent factors refer to the invading organism that causes disease in the susceptible host. Host factors are characteristics that make a host susceptible. Factors in the environment can predispose a host to invasion of the agent, rendering the community at risk of an epidemic if appropriate measures are not taken to control the spread of communicable disease.

Agent Factors

Four agent characteristics influence the transmission and severity of disease. *Infectivity* is the ability of an organism to spread rapidly from one host to another. *Invasiveness* is an agent's ability to spread within the host. *Virulence* refers to the agent's ability to produce severe disease. *Dosage* refers to the fact that multiple organisms invading the host are more apt to overwhelm the host's defenses, whereas small numbers of the same organisms are frequently suppressed or tolerated without disease occurring.

Each agent factor can exist independently of the others. For example, chicken pox virus is one of the most infectious agents, but the disease is generally self-limited. Organisms like *Treponema pallidum*, which causes syphilis, are very invasive. The organism spreads rapidly and effectively throughout the host. The influenza A virus exhibits a much more virulent characteristic than does the influenza C strain by producing a more severe disease.

Food poisoning is a good example of how the dose of the agent affects the host. For instance a host eating a hearty portion of *Salmonella* organism-infected food is more likely to get food poisoning than one who ate sparingly of the same food. Also, a mixed or multiple-agent infection often produces more serious effects than separate invasion by the various agents. For example, the onset of bacterial pneumonia, in addition to a generalized influenza syndrome, greatly increases the threat to the affected host. To prevent epidemics and severity of illness the community health nurse's focus should be to control the spread and progression of the more virulent and invasive organisms.

Host Factors

Host factors include age, heredity, and resistance to infection. In general, most disease processes produce the greatest morbidity and mortality in the very young and the very old. There are, however, some important exceptions. Many viral diseases produce much less disturbance (are less virulent) in the young. For instance, mumps are generally tolerated better by young children than middle-age adults. However, chickenpox in a newborn, although rare, is frequently life-threatening.

Heredity can genetically predispose a host to an increased risk for disease. Children born with the retinoblastoma gene have a 100,000-fold increased risk of developing retinoblastoma. Studies done on the various ABO blood types have indicated an increased risk of gastric cancer or duodenal ulcer related to the type of blood reported (Mausner and Kramer, 1985).

Resistance to infection by the host can prevent invasion of the agent when the immune system is healthy. Diet and overall well-being of the host can affect the immune system's ability to control the organism. As we have witnessed in the AIDS epidemic, a compromised immune system allows the host to develop many debilitating and fatal conditions.

Environmental Factors

Environmental factors are both social and physical. Social factors such as cultural habits or economic constraints can affect the transmission of disease. Education plays an important role in improving unhealthy social factors, such as types of food and preparation methods or wearing shoes to prevent invasion by hookworms. However, as we have seen in many Third World countries, change may be slow to occur.

Physical factors may be a direct result of the social factors in an area. Conditions caused by overcrowding, such as inadequate sewage, can pollute the environment, causing disease.

The quality and safety of any community's drinking water is usually ensured by a municipal system designed to meet community needs. Also, community building codes usually require that plumbing be designed, installed, and maintained to avoid contamination of the water supply. However, a natural disaster such as a flood can overload individual and community plumbing systems, causing sewage to mix with drinking water. Because sewage contains numerous microbiologic pathogens (such as the hepatitis B virus and *Salmonella* organisms), a community-wide epidemic could result if inhabitants consume contaminated water.

Overcrowding promotes the transmission of communicable diseases. Culture and societal circumstances both promote the overcrowding of much of the world's current population. Inner cities are often plagued with pollution, inadequate sanitation, improper food storage and preparation, and housing too poor to provide protection from the elements. The future challenge for community health nurses lies in their ability to deal with the daily physical factors while attempting to affect changes in social factors to promote a more healthy environment.

TREATMENT OF COMMUNICABLE DISEASE

The community health nurse's role in the treatment of communicable diseases is three-fold. First, prevention of disease is accomplished by immunization against specific agents and through education to prevent contact with disease-causing organisms. Second, prompt treatment of communicable disease is important to limit the disease's severity. Last, surveillance is important in the treatment of communicable diseases and to track the progression of a disease and take measures to stay one step ahead of it. In addition, from previous outbreaks, we can learn the course that certain organisms follow as they are transmitted from host to host.

Drug Resistance

Microorganisms occasionally undergo genetic mutations as a result of alterations in the enzyme production of mutant cells. Mutation may occur in a cell of a microorganism that is multiplying in a host who is being treated with an antibiotic or chemotherapeutic agent. The subsequent change occasionally alters a few cells in such a way that they are no longer susceptible to the action of the drug. These microorganisms are then said to be *antibiotic resistant*, or drug fast. The resistant cells multiply and ultimately replace sensitive cells.

The most common reason for the phenomenon of resistant organisms is overuse or abuse of antibiotics. This abuse includes excessive doses, prophylactic use in preoperative or postoperative situations or in the presence of presumed viral infections, and prescription without culture and sensitivity reports. Other examples of real or potential antibiotic abuse include the practice of adding various antibiotics to cow, pig, and poultry feed and the over-the-counter sales of antibiotics in some countries.

Antibiotic resistance has been of great concern to infection control practitioners in episodic settings for over two decades, but resistance patterns are increasingly affecting a broader range of microbiologic agents, including communicable diseases. Some of the best known and most notorious drug-resistant communicable diseases are tuberculosis and gonorrhea. *Staphylococcus aureus* and pneumococci organisms are also frequently penicillin resistant. Instances of full–drug-resistant pneumococci were reported in 1985 (CDC, 1985h). In recent years, reports of infections with methicillin-resistant *Staphylococcus aureus* (MRSA) have increased. In 1984 a documented outbreak of drug-resistant *Salmonella* organisms in four midwestern states was ultaimtely traced to consumption of meat from animals who were fed antimicrobial agents. The study done as a result of the outbreak demonstrated empirically that antimicrobial-resistant organisms of animal origin cause serious human illness. Such findings emphasize the need for more prudent use of antibiotics in both people and animals (Homberg et al., 1984).

It is difficult to accurately predict where resistant patterns will end or what the full ramifications of drug-resistant strains are for the future. Researchers must continue to develop new treatment alternatives, while government and health care providers carefully control antibiotic use.

Antibiotics may be obtained without a prescription in many countries. This is believed to account for the high rate of chloramphenicol resistance in their populations. Requiring a prescription for antibiotics would help control this problem. Antibiotics important for the treatment of human infections should be excluded from animal feeds, and as many diseases as possible should be positively identified by clinical and laboratory data before antibiotics are prescribed. Even topical gentamicin should be avoided if possible because pathogens such as *Pseudomonas aeruginosa* may acquire resistance in its presence.

The community health nurse can make a major impact on drug resistance. Assessment of home care clients for whom medicines have been prescribed will reveal any misinformation regarding drug regimens. Education is an important component of the home care management for clients and their families. Often a client will pass an antibiotic prescription to another member of the family because it worked for someone else. Also, clients often terminate antibiotic therapy before completion of the prescribed dose, which can sensitize the surviving organisms to the antibiotic and allow the strain to become resistant.

Prevention

The most effective way to prevent communicable diseases is to prepare the host's immune system to prevent invasion by the organism. Immunization has proved effective in the prevention of many diseases; however, many organisms prove difficult or impossible to immunize against.

Although immunizing agents, or vaccines, are available for about 18 disorders (see box at top right), only 7 of these vaccines are recommended for routine use. The remaining 11 diseases are sufficiently rare to preclude routine immunization, except to special high-risk individuals. These special health-status situations are discussed later in this chapter.

Types of Immunity

Immunity can be either active or passive. Passive immunity is effective almost immediately and includes transplacental, natural passive, or artificial passive immunity. Passive immunity is temporary, lasting weeks to months. Active immunity results from actual invasion of the organism that initiates an immune response in the host or from injection of killed or partial organisms into the host to initiate a similar response. Active immunity has proved to last for years, and in some cases permanent immunity is achieved. The box at bottom right lists diseases for which no immunization is available.

Inoculation of the host by one of the two routes provides passive immunity. Transplacental immunity is achieved when the mother's antibodies are passed to the fetus. The degree to which this protection prevents infection in the infant after birth varies. Artificial passive immunity can also be administered to the host after exposure to certain disease-causing organisms (see box at right). Antibodies from the same or a different species may be used. An example of antibodies from the same species is immune serum globulin (ISG), which is taken from human serum. Until human ISG was available for rabies and tetanus, serum from animals that increased the allergic reaction to the serum was used. Currently, only a few diseases require serum from animals, such as diptheria, botulism, or gas gangrene.

Active immunization is achieved by introduction of a live, killed, or partial component of the invading organism.

DISEASES FOR WHICH ACTIVE IMMUNIZATION IS AVAILABLE

Calmette-Guérin bacillus
Cholera (vaccine has only limited value)
Diphtheria
Haemophilus influenzae (type B)
Hepatitis B
Influenza
Measles (rubeola)
Meningococcal infections
Mumps
Pertussis
Plague
Pneumococcal infections
Polio
Rabies
Rubella
Tetanus
Typhoid
Yellow fever

COMMUNICABLE DISEASES FOR WHICH NO ACTIVE OR PASSIVE IMMUNIZATION IS AVAILABLE

Actinomycosis
Amebiasis caused by *Escherichia* species
Arbovirus A (all except yellow fever)
Ascariasis (roundworm infection)
Aspergillosis
Balantidiasis
Blastomycosis
Brucellosis (undulant fever)
Candidiasis (moniliasis, thrush)
Cat-bite fever
Cat-scratch disease
Chlamydiosis
Clostridium perfringens food poisoning
Coccidioidomycosis
Cryptococcosis
Echoviruses
Enterobiasis (pinworm infection)
Erythema infectiosum infection
Escherichia coli diarrhea
Gas gangrene
Genital herpes
Giardiasis
Gonoccal infections
Hemorrhagic fever
Herpes simplex virus
Histoplasmosis
Impetigo
Larva migrans
Leprosy
Leptospirosis
Listeriosis
Lymphocytic choriomeningitis
Lymphocytosis
Malaria
Molluscum contagiosum
Mononucleosis

DISEASES FOR WHICH PASSIVE IMMUNIZATION IS AVAILABLE

Viral hepatitis type A (ISG)
Measles (rubeola) (ISG)
Mumps
Rubella (ISG)
Tetanus
Varicella-zoster virus infection
Otitis media (caused by *Streptococcus pneumoniae*)

The host's immune system initiates a humoral response to the organism, recognizing the species and forming antibodies that will identify and destroy the initial and any subsequent invasion by the identified organism.

The community health nurse should realize that an artificially acquired immunity or vaccination is not without some risks to the host. Risks or side effects associated with vaccination depend on whether it has bacterial or viral antigens and if antigens are killed whole organisms or live attenuated organisms. In general, the vaccine label explains its composition.

Table 19-6 describes some side effects of administering recommended childhood immunizations and corresponding nursing actions. There are several contraindications and special circumstances for which the routine immunization administration schedule may be temporarily interrupted (Table 19-7).

Common Immunizations

DIPTHERIA, PERTUSSIS, AND TETANUS. DPT (diptheria, pertussis, and tetanus) is a common combination of vaccines used to prevent these communicable diseases. Although diptheria was once common in the United States, its current rarity is due primarily to the fact that an estimated 96% of all children entering school have received three or more doses of DPT vaccine. An immunized host is still capable of carrying *Corynebacterium diptheriae* in the nasopharynx. Therefore there is always a potential for outbreak among the unimmunized and the inadequately immunized host.

Adequate immunization is thought to protect the individual from diptheria for at least 10 years. The ages of those infected with diptheria over the last few years suggest that many American adults are not protected. Thus it is currently recommended that adults receive a combination tetanus-diptheria (Td) toxoid every 10 years. Because Td contains much less diptheria toxoid than other diptheria combinations, such as DPT, reaction to the diptheria component is much less likely to occur.

The routine use of pertussis vaccine has resulted in a substantial reduction in the incidence of and mortality from pertussis. The number of cases, however, remained fairly constant from 1979 to 1989. An average of 2529 cases and 6.5 fatalities occurred each year during that period (CDC, 1989). Moreover, several documented outbreaks in 1986 produced the largest annual total of cases since 1970. Examination of these 4195 cases revealed that 1548 of the cases occurred in children under the age of 1 year. This age

group is at greatest risk of disease morbidity and mortality. Most of those infants under 6 months of age had not received their third DPT booster and were therefore inadequately immunized (CDC, 1989).

Pertussis is often underreported because many cases are not recognized or are inaccurately diagnosed. Many microbiology laboratories do not possess the proper equipment or expertise to correctly identify *Bordetella pertussis*.

Because the incidence and severity of pertussis decreases with age and because the vaccine may cause side effects and adverse reactions (Table 19-6), routine pertussis immunization is not recommended for those over 7 years of age.

Tetanus occurs almost exclusively in unimmunized or inadequately immunized individuals. In 1984, 74 cases were reported in the United States. In 1988, 91 cases of tetanus were reported from 24 states across the country (CDC, 1989).

Of the 74 cases reported in 1984, no deaths occurred in persons under 30 years of age. Fifty-two percent of the persons over 60 years of age infected with tetanus died from the disease (CDC, 1985). Because tetanus occurs most often and most lethally in adults, the CDC has suggested that the administration of booster doses of Td toxoid at mid-decade years—that is, at 15 years of age, 25 years of age, 35 years of age, and continuing. In fact, Td toxoid is the only universally recommended immunization for individuals of all ages.

Side effects from DPT immunization. Local reactions, generally erythema and induration with or without tenderness, are common after the administration of vaccines containing diphtheria, tetanus, or pertussis antigens. These reactions occur in approximately 40% to 70% of all persons who have undergone DPT immunizations, are usually self-limited, and require no therapy. Mild systemic reactions such as fever, drowsiness, fretfulness, and anorexia occur quite frequently. Fever and other systemic symptoms are much less common after administration of preparations that do not contain pertussis vaccine (CDC 1985e).

Because severe systemic reactions such as generalized urticaria or anaphylaxis have been reported, epinephrine should be accessible during the immunization process. The exact frequency of severe events following pertussis vaccination is unknown, but some possible adverse phenomena and their reported ranges are shown as follows:

1. Collapse or shocklike state (60 to 300 per 1 million doses).
2. Persistent screaming episodes—prolonged periods of peculiar crying or screaming that cannot be controlled by comforting the infant (70 to 2000 per 1 million doses).
3. Isolated convulsions with or without fever (40 to 700 per 1 million doses).
4. Encephalopathy, with or without convulsions, and manifested by a bulging fontanel with changes in the level of consciousness or focal neurological signs; the encephalopathy may lead to permanent neurologic deficit (1.3 to 30 per 1 million doses) (CEDC, 1984a).

It is important for community health nurses to be aware of these and subsequent findings so that they can properly

TABLE 19-6
Possible side effects and nursing responsibilities of recommended childhood immunizations

Immunization	Reaction	Nursing responsibilities
Diphtheria	Fever, usually within 24-48 hours; soreness, redness, and swelling at injection site.	Instructions for DPT: Advise parents of possible side effects; may recommend prophylactic use of aspirin or acetaminophen if fever occurs following previous DPT immunization; recommend its use if fever occurs following present immunization; advise parents to notify physician immediately if any unusual side effects, such as those listed under pertussis, occur.
Tetanus	Same as for diphtheria, but may include urticaria and malaise; all may have delayed onset and last several days; lump at injection site may last for weeks or even months, but gradually disappears.	
Pertussis	Same as for tetanus, but may include loss of consciousness, convulsions, and thrombocytopenia.	
Poliovirus (TOPV)	Essentially no side effects; vaccine-associated paralysis usually occurs within 2 months of immunization.	See general comments to parents.*
Measles	Anorexia, malaise, rash, and fever may occur 7-10 days after immunization; rarely (estimated risk 1 in 1 million doses) encephalitis may occur.	Advise parents of more common side effects and use of antipyretics for fever; if a persistent high fever with other obvious signs of illness occur, have them notify physician immediately.
Mumps	Essentially no side effects other than a brief, mild fever.	See general comments to parents.*
Rubella	Mild rash that lasts 1 or 2 days within a few days after immunization; arthralgia, arthritis, or paresthesia of the hands and fingers may occur about 2 weeks after vaccination and is more frequent in older children and adults.	Advise parents of side effects, especially of time delay before joint swelling and pain; assure them that these symptoms will disappear; may recommend use of mild analgesics for pain.

Modified from Whaley LF and Wong DL: Nursing care of infants and children, ed 4, St Louis, 1991, Mosby-Year Book.
*General comment to parents regarding each immunization: The benefit of being protected by the immunization is believed to greatly outweigh the risk from the disease.

TABLE 19-7
Vaccines and toxoids indicated or specifically contraindicated for special health-status situations

Health situations	Indicated	Vaccines or toxoids contraindicated
Pregnancy	Diphtheria and tetanus toxoids (TD)	Live-virus vaccines
Immunocompromised	Influenza Pneumococcal polysaccharide	Live-virus vaccines
Splenic dysfunction, anatomic asplenia	Influenza Pneumococcal polysaccharide	
Hemodialysis	Hepatitis B (double-dose) Influenza Pneumococcal polysaccharide	
Deficiencies of factors VIII or IX	Hepatitis B	
Chronic alcoholism	Pneumococcal polysaccharide	
Diabetes and other high-risk diseases	Influenza Pneumococcal polysaccharide	

NOTE: Refer to text on specific vaccines or toxoids for details on indications, contraindications, precautions, dosages, side effects and adverse reactions, and special considerations.

counsel clients. Such findings sometimes cause generalized panic when presented in a biased fashion by the media. The community health nurse should encourage reporting of adverse reactions by parents and clients. Reports of severe or unusual reactions that seem to temporally correspond with immunization procedures should be forwarded to local or state health departments.

MEASLES (RUBEOLA), MUMPS, AND RUBELLA. Rubeola, more commonly known as measles, is often a severe disease complicated by middle ear infection or bronchopneumonia. In 1 of every 1000 cases reported, encephalitis develops, and survivors often have permanent brain damage. Infection during pregnancy leads to higher rates of premature labor, spontaneous abortion, and low birth weight infants (CDC, 1989a).

Over 14,000 cases of measles were reported for the first 4 months of 1989. This represented a substantial increase over the 1497 cases reported in all of 1983. Although reported cases of measles increased significantly, the 1989 figure is far lower than the 525,000 cases reported annually in the prevaccine era from 1950 through 1962 (CDC, 1989a).

Of the 16,819 cases of measles reported between 1985 and 1988, 42% were appropriately vaccinated and 92% occurred among persons 5 years of age and older. A third of the 16,819 cases proved to be persons for whom vaccination was indicated but who were never vaccinated.

Two major types of outbreaks have occurred in the United States, one among school-aged children and one among college students, causing the Immunization Practices Advisory Committee on Measles Prevention to issue new recommendations for vaccine administration. In addition to the single-dose vaccine given at 15 months, new recommendations suggest a second dose be given to children at the time they enter school (or preschool in high-risk populations), to students entering college, to health care personnel, to international travelers, and to individuals to control outbreak (CDC, 1989a).

Mumps is a viral disease characterized by fever, swelling, and tenderness of the salivary glands. Orchitis occurs in 20% to 30% of postpubertal males, with encephalitis reported as high as 5 per 1000 cases. Mumps infection during the first trimester of pregnancy may increase the number of spontaneous abortions with no firm evidence that it causes congenital malformations (Benenson, 1990).

Since the introduction of live mumps virus vaccine in 1967, the occurrence of reported mumps cases in the United States decreased steadily until 1987, when the number increased 150% from the previous year. Recent studies have shown that mumps can occur in highly vaccinated populations. This may account for the increase in numbers (CDC, 1989a).

The CDC recommends that the mumps vaccine be included with the measles vaccine in the form of an MMR (Measles, Mumps, Rubella) vaccine to provide additional safeguards against failures. The vaccine should be given at least 14 days before a person receives immune globulin (IG), whole blood, or other blood products containing antibodies. It should be deferred for at least 6 weeks (and preferably 3 months) after administration of these products. Furthermore,

the vaccine should not be given to persons who are immunocompromised or who have generalized malignancies.

Serologic surveys have indicated that most individuals have been infected with mumps by their twentieth birthdays. Most adults can therefore be considered immune, even if they did not have clinically recognizable mumps disease. However, persons who received killed mumps vaccine that was available from 1959 until 1978 might benefit from vaccination with the currently available live-mumps vaccine (CDC, 1984b).

Rubella, or German measles, is a febrile, viral disease with a type of scarlet-fever rash. About half of the infections occur without the rash, and encephalitis is seen more frequently in adults but rarely in children. Unlike the previous conditions, rubella causes anomalites or congenital rubella syndrome in at least 25% of infants born to mothers infected in the first trimester (Benenson, 1990).

The incidence of rubella continues to decrease. (Figure 19-1), with 225 cases reported in 1988 (CDC, 1989). Several outbreaks account for the reported cases involving university students, hospital employees, and office workers. These cases resulted in disruption of work and time lost through illness and exposed pregnant women to the disease. Several studies have shown that the rubella susceptibility rate for adolescents and young adults continues to be 10% to 20% (CDC, 1988).

The community health nurse can play an important role in the national initiative to achieve and maintain a 95% immunization level in susceptible persons, to intensify surveillance of rubella, and to promptly control outbreaks. Specific activities focus on delivery of the vaccine to women of childbearing age and increasing the awareness of the need for vaccination (CDC, 1985).

Because of the potential risk to the fetus, reasonable precautions should be taken before women of childbearing age are immunized with MMR vaccine. Precautions include drawing a titer to assess immune status, pregnancy testing before administration with exclusion of those having positive test results, counselling pregnant women about the possible risk to the fetus, and advising women to avoid becoming pregnant for 3 months after vaccination. Any woman who becomes pregnant within the specified 3 months after vaccination should be reported to the Division of Immunization, Centers for Disease Control, through the local state health department.

Children should be vaccinated after recovery from a moderate or severe febrile illness to avoid superimposing adverse effects of the vaccine and masking potentially important symptoms of a reoccurring febrile illness. The community health nurse should advise the parent or guardian to measure the child's temperature for several days after a recent febrile illness.

Hypersensitivity reactions following MMR vaccination are rarely reported; generally, only local minor reactions occur at the injection site. Persons with a history of an anaphylactic reaction to neomycin, which is found in trace amounts in the vaccine, should not be given the MMR vaccine.

The live–measles virus vaccine has not been shown to exacerbate tuberculosis as does the actual natural infection

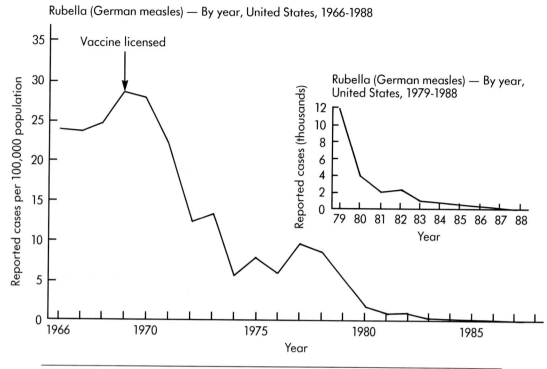

FIGURE 19-1   Rubella (German measles)—By year, United States, 1966 to 1988.

of measles. However, the measles vaccine may suppress tuberculin activity; therefore the tuberculin test should be postponed for 4 to 6 weeks (CDC, 1989a).

HAEMOPHILUS INFLUENZAE. *Haemophilus influenzae* is a leading cause of serious systemic bacterial disease in the United States. Approximately 1 in 1000 unimmunized persons under the age of 5 years develop a systemic disease caused by *H. influenzae* each year (CDC, 1985). *H. influenzae* is the most common cause of bacterial meningitis and is credited with causing 12,000 cases a year among children 5 years old or younger. Meningitis caused by *H. influenzae* has a fatality rate of 5%, and neurological sequelae are observed in approximately 25% to 35% of survivors.

Various strains of *H. influenzae* have been identified: six types (a to f) that are capsular and other strains that are noncapsular (American Academy of Pediatrics, 1988). Although influenza B accounts for only one of six known species, it causes virtually all cases of *H. influenzae* meningitis among children. Influenza B (Hib) is also responsible for other invasive diseases, including epiglottis, sepsis, cellulitis, septic arthritis, osteomyelitis, pericarditis, pneumonia, and occasionally otitis media (CDC, 1985b).

Approximately 35% to 45% of associated disease occurs among children 24 months of age or older. Children who are at high risk for *H. influenzae* infection include native Americans (Indians) and Eskimos, African-Americans, persons from low-socioeconomic backgrounds, persons with asplenia, sickle cell anemia, Hodgkin's disease, or antibody deficiency syndromes, and those under 5 years of age who attend day-care centers (CDC, 1985b).

The *Haemophilus influenzae* vaccine, consisting of purified capsular polysaccharide type b, was licensed in 1985. A conjugate vaccine using the PRP and a diptheria toxoid was licensed in 1987 for use in children 18 months of age

(American Academy of Pediatrics, 1988). It is recommended that children in high-risk groups be immunized at 18 months, and these children should receive a second dose within 18 months of the initial dose to ensure protection. All other children should be immunized at 24 months of age; it is thought that immunization at 24 months of age will protect the child from 18 to 40 months of age, without recommendation of an additional vaccination. At present, there is insufficient data on which to base recommendations for vaccination of children older than 2 years of age or adults who have never been immunized (CDC, 1985a).

Immunization Under Special Circumstances

Many vaccines have been licensed for use in special circumstances to prevent transmission of communicable disease to persons at high risk. Table 19-8 indicates health and occupational situations for which vaccines are recommended. In most instances vaccination is elective; however, some institutions have policies that require vaccination for their employees. For example, some hospitals require immunization with the hepatitis B vaccine for workers in high-risk areas.

IMMUNIZATION FOR HEPATITIS B. Hepatitis B is a virus causing anorexia, vague abdominal discomfort, nausea, and vomiting, and it can progress to jaundice. The disease may be mild, progressing to mortality with hepatic necrosis. The case fatality rate increases significantly after age 40 years (from about 1% for those hospitalized patients). A carrier state can exist without manifestation of the disease. The virus is transmitted through blood, saliva, semen, and vaginal fluids (Benenson, 1990).

The CDC estimates that hepatitis B virus (HBV) infections occurred in at least 200,000 Americans each year before hepatitis B vaccine was available; annual treatment costs were estimated at $365 million (Dowdle, 1983). Fur-

TABLE 19-8
Immunobiologics recommended for specific life situations

Indication	Immunobiologic(s)
OCCUPATION	
Hospital, laboratory, and other health care personnel	Hepatitis B Polio Influenza
Staff of institutions for the mentally retarded	Hepatitis B
Veterinarians and animal handlers	Rabies
Selected field workers	Plague
LIFESTYLES	
Homosexual males	Hepatitis B
Illicit-drug users	Hepatitis B
ENVIRONMENTAL SITUATION	
Inmates of long-term correctional facilities	Hepatitis B
Residents of institutions for the mentally retarded	Hepatitis B
TRAVEL	Measles Rubella Polio Yellow fever Hepatitis B Rabies Meningococcal polysaccharide Typhoid Cholera Plague
FOREIGN STUDENTS, IMMIGRANTS, AND REFUGEES	Measles Rubella Diphtheria Tetanus

NOTE: Refer to text on specific vaccines or toxoids for use by specific risk groups, details on indications, contraindications, precautions, dosages, side effects and adverse reactions, and special considerations.

thermore, it was estimated that, each year, at least 4000 persons would die of chronic effects of HBV infection, such as cirrhosis, acute hepatitis, and liver cancer.

An HBV vaccine was licensed in 1981; however, 26,115 cases were reported to the CDC for 1984 (CDC, 1985i). The majority of cases occurred in individuals 20 years of age or older, and 6% to 10% of affected adults became chronic carriers. The CDC estimates that the United States has between 750,000 and 1,000,000 carriers of hepatitis B. The estimated risk of acquiring HBV infection in the United States is approximately 5% for the total population, but it may reach 100% for the higher risk groups (CDC, 1984b; CDC, 1990).

Occupational, social, family, environmental, or illness-related factors may increase the risk of HBV infection. Groups at increased risk of contracting HBV include immigrants and refugees and their descendants from areas where there is a high-endemic rate for HBV, actively homosexual men, users of illicit injectable drugs, inmates of prisons (who may have a history of prior parenteral drug abuse), patients and staff in custodial institutions for the mentally retarded, classroom contacts, teachers of some deinstitutionalized carriers, household contacts and sexual partners of HBV carriers, hemodialysis clients, health care workers who have contact with blood and body fluids, inmates of long-term care or correctional facilities, and international travelers to select countries (CDC, 1985d; CDC, 1990).

To administer HBV vaccine, a series of three 1-ml doses containing 20 units/ml of HBsAg protein should be given intramuscularly in the deltoid muscle. Completion of the series of three such injections provides protective antibodies in over 90% of healthy adult recipients for at least 2 years. A course of three doses of 10 units/ml induce antibody formation in virtually all infants and children from birth to 9 years of age. The first two doses should be given 1 month apart, and the third dose should be administered 5 months after the second dose. For susceptible hemodialysis clients, three 2-ml doses should be given at the above stated schedule (CDC, 1985d; CDC, 1990).

HBV vaccine is recommended for most individuals who are members of high-risk groups. Because some areas of the world, such as eastern Asia and sub-Saharan Africa, have high endemic rates of HBV, travelers who plan to have close contact with the local population should complete the series of immunizations before leaving the United States. HBV vaccine is primarily intended for preexposure prophylaxis; however, when exposure to HBV occurs in a high-risk person with no preexposure immunization, the vaccine may be administered in combination with hepatitis B immune globulin (HBIG). When HBV vaccine and HBIG are given in combination, they provide sustained protection levels of antibody and eliminate the need for a second dose of HBIG. The series of HBV vaccine should still be completed (CDC, 1990).

Unlike live-virus vaccines such as rubella, pregnancy is not a contraindication for the use of HBV (CDC, 1990). In fact, one of the most efficient modes of HBV transmission is from the mother to the infant during birth. Because HBV in a pregnant woman may result in severe disease for the mother and chronic infection or even fulminant hepatitis in the neonate, all pregnant women should be serotested for the presence of hepatitis antibodies.

PASSIVE IMMUNIZATION FOR HEPATITIS A AND B. Hepatitis A is not associated with high mortality; however, it does cause significant morbidity. Hepatitis A is primarily transmitted by person-to-person contact, with no associated carrier state. Transmission is accomplished by poor personal hygiene, poor sanitation, and household or sexual contact. Common-source epidemics from contaminated food and water also occur. Hepatitis A has occurred at an endemic level for the past 15 years in the United States; in 1988, 28,507 cases were reported.

The passive immunization for both hepatitis A and B is by immune globulin (IG) vaccine. Immune globulin is essentially a sterile solution of antibodies from human plasma that contain anti-hepatitis A virus (anti-HAV) and anti-HBV antibodies. The only difference between IG and HBIG is that HBIG contains higher titers of antibodies to hepatitis B (CDC, 1985d; CDC, 1990).

Immune globulin should be given as soon as possible after exposure to HAV because it is much more effective very early in the incubation period. The index case (see Chapter 9) in any outbreak should be serologically tested for infection by HAV before that person receives IG. However, serologic testing of contacts for anti-HAV before giving IG is not recommended after the index case is established because the screening tests are more costly than IG vaccine and delay administration. Giving IG more than 2 weeks after exposure is not recommended. Specific recommendations for prophylaxis of HAV depend on the nature of the HAV exposure. Those recommendations are adopted from recommendations by CDC (CDC, 1990).

INFLUENZA VACCINE. Influenza is an acute viral disease of three types. Each causes symptoms of the respiratory tract of sore throat and cough, fever, headache, and myalgia. Influenza A is usually associated with widespread epidemics and pandemics. The more regional epidemics are caused by the influenza B strain, whereas influenza C has been identified in more sporadic minor outbreaks.

Influenza viruses repeatedly cause major and excess morbidity and mortality. In the years from 1957 to 1986, 19 epidemics of influenza have been associated with 10,000 or more deaths annually. In the 1984 to 1985 flu season, influenza A viruses were isolated in every state in the United States. These viruses were associated with the highest ratio of pneumonia and influenza deaths (as a percentage of total deaths) since 1976 (CDC, 1990).

The greatest impact of influenza normally occurs when new strains appear and most of the population is not immune to them. In those circumstances, pandemics occur. Only influenza A, which is generally more severe than either influenza B or C, is capable of causing pandemics.

The two groups most often and most severely affected are chronically ill persons and those over 65 years of age. Approximately 80% to 90% of deaths related to influenza and pneumonia occurred in the 65-year-old or older age group (CDC, 1990a). Because these two groups are increasing in size, the toll of influenza may increase further unless control measures are more vigorously implemented.

Several high-risk groups that would benefit from annual influenza vaccination have been identified. These groups include adults and children who have chronic disorders of the cardiovascular or pulmonary systems and who attended required regular medical checkups or underwent hospitalization during the preceding year; residents of nursing homes and other chronic-care facilities; health care personnel who have extensive contact with high-risk clients; otherwise healthy individuals who are 65 years of age and older; and adults and children with chronic metabolic diseases, renal dysfunction, anemia, immunosuppression, or asthma that required regular medical follow-up or hospitalization during the preceding year. Influenza immunization is also available for otherwise healthy children and adults who wish to reduce their chances of acquiring influenza infection.

When target or risk groups overlap for influenza and pneumococcal vaccination, both may be given simultaneously at separate anatomical sites. Although influenza vaccine should be administered annually, pneumococcal vaccine should be given only once.

The occurrence of influenza, similar to other communicable diseases, is temporal, occurring from October to February and declining in March. The vaccine should be administered from mid-October through December. If given earlier, protection may be waning when there is still widespread influenza activity. Influenza vaccine may be given to pregnant women after the first trimester. In fact, immunization during the third trimester, when it occurs from October to December, may provide antenatal protection to the mother and the fetus (CDC, 1990a).

It is necessary to obtain an adequate history before immunizing an individual for influenza. Persons who are allergic to eggs or those with acute febrile illness should not be immunized. As with any vaccine, clients should be advised of possible reactions. Reactions to influenza vaccines may be either local or systemic. Approximately one third of those immunized develop redness or induration at the injection site. Two types of systemic reactions have been reported. The first consists of fever, malaise, and myalgia. Although these reactions are infrequent, they occur most often in children and in those who have had no exposure to the particular viral antigen. The second type of systemic reaction is immediate and anaphylactic in nature. Anaphylaxis occurs very rarely and is presumed to be attributed to egg allergy (CDC, 1990a).

PNEUMOCOCCAL POLYSACCHARIDE VACCINE. Pneumococcal pneumonia is caused by *Streptococcus pneumoniae*. Of the 83 known strains, 23 capsular types cause 90% of the pneumococcal infections in the United States. As with influenza, pneumococcal pneumonia is seen in the young and very old populations.

Symptoms are usually abrupt, with fever and chills, pleural pain, dyspnea, and cough; however, the elderly may present less abrupt symptoms. Transmission is person-to-person, by direct oral contact, and by droplets. Antibiotic therapy is used as treatment for the *S. pneumoniae* infection (Benenson, 1990).

Precise data on the occurrence of pneumococcal disease in the United States is not available, partly because it is not a nationally notifiable disease. However, the annual incidence of pneumococcal pneumonia is estimated to be 68 to 260 cases per 100,000 U.S. population. The incidence of pneumococcal pneumonia increases in those over 40 years of age and shows a two-fold increase in those over 60 years of age. Mortality from pneumococcal disease is highest among individuals who develop bacteremia or meningitis, persons with underlying medical conditions, and elderly persons (CDC, 1984b). Persons at increased risk for developing severe pneumococcal disease include those with sickle cell anemia, multiple myeloma, cirrhosis, alcoholism, renal disease, splenic dysfunction, diabetes mellitus, chronic pulmonary disease, or conditions associated with immunosuppression.

Licensed in 1978, the pneumococcal polysaccharide vaccine provides protection against the various types of *Streptococcus pneumoniae* that are responsible for 87% of recent bacteremic pneumococcal disease in the United States. Most healthy adults who receive the vaccine demonstrate rises in titer that indicate immunity (CDC, 1984b).

About half of the persons given the vaccine experience mild side effects, but severe adverse effects such as anaphylactic reactions have rarely been reported. Although it is unknown how long vaccine-induced immunity lasts, booster doses are not recommended because of increased adverse reactions associated with second doses of the vaccine (CDC, 1984b).

Community health nurses often administer the vaccine to high-risk or elderly clients. Pneumococcal vaccine should be given subcutaneously, and the client or parent should be informed that mild side effects, such as low-grade fever, mild erythema, and induration at the injection site, may be experienced from about 4 hours after inoculation up to 4 days afterward. Typically, mild reactions subside within 24 hours.

MENINGOCOCCAL VACCINES. *Neisseria meningitidis* is the causative organism for meningococcal meningitis. The bacterial infection presents with abrupt onset of fever, nausea and vomiting, intense headache, and a rash. *N. meningitidis* causes both endemic and epidemic disease and is the second most common cause of bacterial meningitis in the United States. Bacterial meningitis affects between 3000 and 4000 persons each year. Case fatality rates have fallen to less than 10% with current treatment regimens, but rates rise to 20% for meningococcemia despite therapy with antimicrobial agents such as penicillin.

As noted in Table 19-5, the incidence of meningococcal disease peaks in the late winter to early spring. Incidence is highest among children, particularly those 6 to 12 months of age. Incidence steadily declines after 1 year of age. By age 5 years, the incidence among children approximates that for adults. Serogroup B, for which a vaccine is not yet available, accounts for 50% to 55% of all cases. Although serogroup A causes only a small portion of endemic meningitis disease in the United States, it is the most common cause of meningitis epidemics elsewhere in the world (CDC, 1985c). The vaccine containing group A, C, Y, and W-135 meningococcal polysaccharides was licensed and is currently the only quadrivalent vaccine used in the United States (Benenson, 1990). The serogroup A polysaccharide has been shown to induce antibody production in some children as young as 3 months of age, although a response comparable to that seen in adults is not achieved until 4 or 5 years of age. Antibodies formed after a single dose of vaccine decline markedly over the first 3 years, although the antibody decline is more rapid in infants and young children than in adults (CDC, 1985c).

Routine vaccination is not recommended because the risk of infection in the United States is low, and the serotype B is not affected by the present vaccine. However, immunization with the quadrivalent vaccine is recommended for particular high-risk groups, including individuals with terminal complement component deficiencies and those with anatomic or functional asplenia. When indicated, the vaccine can be given at the same time as other immunizations. Subsequent antibody titers are achieved within 10 to 14 days after vaccination (CDC, 1985c).

Antimicrobial chemoprophylaxis of persons in intimate contact with individuals having meningococcal disease remains the chief preventive measure in sporadic cases of *N. meningitidis* disease in the United States. Examples of "intimate contact" include household members, day-care center contacts, and anyone directly exposed to the patient's oral secretions, such as through mouth-to-mouth resuscitation or kissing (CDC, 1985c).

DISEASES OF SPECIAL CONCERN

Communicable diseases for which no vaccine is available pose a major challenge for the community health nurse. Mycobacterial infections, pediculosis, botulism, salmonellosis, legionellosis, delta hepatitis, and opportunistic infections are discussed in the following sections. Each disease is unique in spread, control measures, and treatment regimens.

Mycobacterial Infections

The incidence of infection with *Mycobacterium tuberculosis* and *Mycobacterium avium* has steadily increased in the 1980s according to the CDC (CDC, 1989c). The further spread of tuberculosis (TB) infection may increase dramatically unless appropriate measures to control the spread are taken (CDC, 1989c).

Human immunodeficiency virus (HIV)–infected individuals are at a higher risk for developing TB and, in many instances, present with TB before being diagnosed as having HIV infection. Two studies cited in the report published by the CDC in 1989 indicate that latent, subclinical TB infection may progress to clinical TB during immunosuppression caused by the HIV 1 or 2 months before HIV is discovered (CDC, 1987; CDC, 1986).

Symptoms of TB include productive cough, fever, wasting, and weight loss. Tuberculosis findings on chest radiographs associated with AIDS differ from non-AIDS patients by the presence of infiltrates found in any lung field associated with mediastinal and hilar lymphadenopathy (CDC, 1989c). Also unlike non-AIDS patients, 40% to 75% of HIV-infected patients develop extrapulmonary disease (CDC, 1989c). Diagnosis is by demonstration of acid-fast bacilli from sputum or bronchial washings. The Mantoux tuberculin skin test may be used as the initial test (CDC, 1989c).

Treatment with anti-TB chemotherapy should begin as soon as acid-fast bacilli are detected in a specimen because differential diagnosis may take several weeks. Isoniazid, rifampin, and parazinamide are administered in combination for at least 9 months and are continued for 6 months following documented culture conversion of three negative culture findings (CDC, 1989c). Compliance with the extended regimen and side effects of the medicines complicate the successful treatment of TB.

Mycobacterium avium, seen since the early 1950s, has become a major pathogen for immunosuppressed patients (Gee and Moran, 1988). Found in the blood, *Mycobacterium avium* is believed to enter the host by inhalation and ingestion of water. The organism has been cultured from blood, bone marrow, lymph nodes, and the liver of infected individuals. Damage to the tissues of an HIV-infected person presents without the classical granulomas found in non–HIV-infected patients with mycobacterial infection. As in many other opportunistic infections (which are discussed later) *Mycobacterium avium* intracellulare (MAI) is not contagious and is a reactivation of a prior exposure to *Mycobacterium avium* (Gee and Moran, 1988).

Unfortunately, symptoms of MAI are very similar to many other diseases. They include fever (usually less than 101° F), fatigue, weight loss, and bone marrow suppression. Abdominal cramps, diarrhea, and anorexia can mimic cryptosporidiosis, indicating a need for differential diagnosis.

Isolation of *Mycobacterium avium* is the only diagnostic indicator for the disease. However, cultures may take from 2 to 6 weeks to prove positive results. For this reason, when the acid-fast bacilli are identified in culture, medications should be instituted. The medical regimen is controversial and many studies using combination therapy are underway, with no single "best" treatment regimen. Treatment for MAI is, however, recommended to preserve the life of the patient. Isoniazid and ethambutol are commonly used, and clofazimine has been tested (Gee and Moran, 1988).

Tuberculosis Control and Treatment Practices

Although the number of pulmonary tuberculosis (PTB) cases reported to the CDC steadily declined throughout the last few decades, that trend has reversed since 1988. In 1990, 25,701 cases were reported, an increase of 9.4% over the 1989 figure and the largest annual increase since 1953. Further, 31 states reported increases in cases in 1990 compared with 1989.

There is some evidence that the epidemic of HIV infection may be contributing to the rise in tuberculosis cases, as large numbers of HIV infected individuals have developed PTB, and the largest increases in PTB cases have been reported among 25- to 44-year-old men, the age and sex group that also accounts for 68.4% of persons with AIDS. However, an increase in PTB has also been noted among racial and ethnic groups such as Asians/Pacific Islanders, and the reported incidence of HIV infection among these peoples is comparatively low (CDC, 1992).

When antituberculosis drugs were first introduced over 40 years ago, it was hoped that the disease would eventually be eliminated in the United States. However, control and prevention have been hampered by several factors. First, PTB is an airborne pathogen. That is, when an infected individual coughs, sings, or otherwise creates an aerosol, a nearby susceptible individual inhales organisms. A second problem is noncompliance with prescribed therapy. Most clients require a minimum of 9 months of treatment, including ongoing monitoring for drug toxicity and response to therapy. Some individuals are unwilling or unable to complete such a long course of therapy. When the drug regimen is interrupted, they may become reinfected, symptomatic, and contagious.

A third obstacle is the emergence of tuberculosis-causing organisms that are resistant to antituberculosis drugs, especially isoniazid and streptomycin. When resistance occurs, drugs and dosages must be promptly adjusted to control symptoms and prevent further transmission.

A fourth compounding factor is that an estimated 10 million persons in the United States are infected with the tubercule bacilli and thus carry a lifelong risk of developing tuberculosis. Even if all infected individuals could be identified and treated, it is still likely that tuberculosis would continue to occur.

TUBERCULIN SKIN TEST. An intracutaneous administration using 5 U of purified protein derivative tuberculin (PPD-T) or the Mantoux test should be used to identify individuals infected with tubercle bacilli. False-negative reactions may occur in 30% of persons tested with the multiple-puncture devices. As a result of the 60% false-negative result rate seen in individuals with TB and HIV infections, other indicators of disease, such as chest radiographic and bacteriologic examinations, are very important (CDC, 1990c).

The Mantoux test should be administered according to the package instructions, usually on the inner aspect of the forearm. The reading of the reaction should be done by a trained professional 24 to 72 hours after administration of the PPD-T. The test result is considered to be positive or converted if the area of reaction is 10 mm or greater for persons less than 35 years of age or 15 mm or greater in persons older than 35 years of age. Each person who has a positive test result undergo chest radiographic examination and treatment according to the findings (CDC, 1990c).

Community health nurses need to be aware of several factors that influence TB skin testing: (1) reactivity to tuberculin skin testing may be depressed or suppressed for up to 4 weeks by viral infection or live-virus vaccines such as those for measles, polio, rubella, and mumps; (2) a reactive skin test result indicates exposure to the causative agent for tuberculosis; (3) all instructions should be carefully read before skin testing and the test should be performed in the specified manner; and (4) a person who has had a known, positive tuberculin reaction should not undergo the Mantoux skin test.

Pediculosis

Pediculosis, or lice infestation, occurs worldwide. Outbreaks are common among school-aged children and institutionalized individuals. Pediculosis refers to infestations of the head or hairy parts of the body or clothing with adult lice, larvae, or nits (eggs). This leads to severe itching and excoriation of the scalp or scratch marks on the body (Benenson, 1990).

From a public health standpoint, the louse is not only a human nuisance but also transmits epidemic typhus, trench fever, and louse-borne relapsing fever (Benenson, 1980). The mode of transmission is direct contact with an infected person and indirect contact with infected personal belongings, especially clothing and head-gear. Pediculosis is communicable as long as lice remain alive and until eggs in the hair and clothing have been destroyed. Diagnosis of pediculosis is accomplished by finding either lice or nits on hairy surfaces of the body.

Pediculosis is treated with lindane (Kwell). Kwell comes as a lotion and a shampoo and contains 1% lindane as its active ingredient. Refer to the package insert for directions for use on the appropriate body surface. One application is usually curative. Some people do suffer persistent pruritus after treatment; however, retreatment should not be instituted unless living mites are seen.

Measures that can be instituted to prevent spread, aside from specific treatment, include avoiding physical contact with infected persons or their belongings or clothing and dry cleaning, laundering, in hot water (55° C or 131° F for 20 minutes), or exposing clothing and bedding to sunlight to destroy nits and lice.

Botulism

The incidence of botulism in adults in the United States is low. This is fortunate because botulism causes severe morbidity and sometimes mortality. Although botulism outbreaks are most commonly associated with consumption of improperly prepared home-canned foods, *Clostridium botulinum* can also contaminate fresh foods. Fresh foods, especially those harvested from the ground, may contain *C. botulinum*. When these foods are initially cooked and then stored at ambient temperatures for 14 to 16 hours, toxin from the spores is released, as in improperly prepared home canning.

Two key factors affect community health nursing intervention. First, clients should be taught that fresh foods can be a source of botulism poisoning. Therefore foods initially heated for serving should either be eaten hot or refrigerated and later reheated thoroughly. Second, when botulism poisoning is suspected, requests should be made for stool and serum specimens to test for butulinial toxin. Trivalent botulism antitoxin can be obtained through state health departments and administered intravenously or intramuscularly as soon as possible. Immediate admission to the hospital, preferably the intensive care unit, is necessary to monitor respiratory status because respiratory compromise is the usual cause of death (Benenson, 1990).

Salmonellosis

Salmonellosis (*Salmonella* organism-induced gastroenteritis) is a disease that is usually accompanied by nausea, abdominal pain, abdominal cramping, and diarrhea. It is believed that the 20,000 to 30,000 cases reported each year in the United States probably represents only 1% to 10% of the cases that actually occur. The overall mortality is very low (probably less than 1%), although the death rate is much higher in infants and among elderly persons (Tortora, Funke, and Case, 1982).

The normal habitat for *Salmonella* organisms is the intestinal tract of humans and some animals. Prevention of salmonellosis depends on good sanitation practices to avoid initial contamination or inoculation of food with the organism. Another practice that prevents outbreaks is refrigeration, refrigeration of foods that may be mildly inoculated with organisms prevents further growth. The severity and incubation time of the disease depend on the number of *Salmonella* organisms ingested. Poultry, eggs, and egg products have been implicated in salmonellosis outbreaks. The organisms are generally destroyed by normal cooking that heats food to an internal temperature of about 60° C (145° F). Refrigeration is useful to prevent the organisms from reproducing before cooking. *Salmonella* organisms are sometimes found in dairy cattle and raw milk, but pasteurization kills the organism.

Legionellosis

Legionnaire's disease is caused by *Legionella pneumophila*, a gram-negative bacillus. Contrary to popular belief, the outbreak that occurred in Philadelphia at the fiftieth annual convention of the American Legion in 1976 was not the first recorded outbreak. The bacillus was isolated as early as 1947, and the first well-documented outbreak of the disease occurred in 1957 (Edelstein and Meyer, 1984). However, legionellosis was recognized as a distinct clinical entity in 1976 during the outbreak. Much more is now known about legionellosis, its distribution, and clinical presentations. For instance, a nonpneumonic form of disease associated with *L. pneumophila* (Pontiac fever) has been described, and at least nine other species of the bacillus have been discovered or rediscovered.

Environmental risk factors associated with legionellosis include contaminated potable water and water fixtures and contaminated heat-exchange apparatuses in large buildings. Host risk factors include advanced age or the presence of underlying chronic cardiopulmonary disease, chronic renal failure, or diabetes mellitus. In addition, legionellosis is more common in men, in those who smoke, and in those who are immunosuppressed from either primary disease or medication(s) that affect cellular immunity. Person-to-person transmission does not occur. Transmission is by air in the environment (Edelstein and Meyer, 1984).

In 1988, 1085 cases of legionellosis were reported to the CDC. The occurrence of legionellosis is generally categorized as either community or nosocomially acquired. Whenever clusters of legionellosis appear, investigations should be undertaken to locate the reservoir. The environment must then be modified to eliminate the reservoir. The overall fatality rate is affected by drug therapy and the client's underlying disease. Death rates rise up to 80% in untreated immunosuppressed patients. Overall, the fatality rate is about 15% to 20% (Edelstein and Meyer, 1985).

The literature to date estimates that the legionellosis seen in nonhospital settings constitutes between 1% and 15% of all community-acquired pneumonias. Community health nurses should be aware that the sputum of clients with legionellosis is usually nonpurulent and watery, but it may be grossly bloody. Thick green or yellow sputum is almost never observed with legionellosis. If a sputum specimen is obtained for Gram stain only, it is unlikely that *L. pneumophila* can be identified. To diagnose legionellosis, it is necessary to submit a sputum specimen for *L. pneumophila* identification by direct immunofluorescent examination. When laboratories have the capability, urine specimens may be collected and tested for soluble antigens. Besides sputum and urine testing, blood can be drawn for serologic examination (Edelstein and Meyer, 1984).

It is important to specifically identify pneumonias caused by *L. pneumophila* so that effective treatment with erythromycin or a similar drug can be started. Additionally, the client who is treated at home should be observed for signs of respiratory failure or hypotension, which are common in legionellosis. If the client is receiving immunosuppressive agents, including corticosteroids, this therapy should be discontinued or the dosage reduced whenever possible.

Delta Hepatitis

A new form of hepatitis, delta hepatitis, has been detected in all areas of the United States and is thought to affect 200 million people worldwide. Delta hepatitis results from a virus that cannot cause infection alone. When the delta virus "piggy backs" with the hepatitis B virus, the result is an illness more severe than that caused by HBV alone (Altman, 1984).

Symptoms of delta hepatitis are more severe than are those for HBV alone but delta hepatitis is often misdiagnosed as HBV infection. Superinfections with delta hepatitis result in a more severe or chronic form of the disease and may progress to chronic hepatitis (Benenson, 1990).

Although it is known that the virus that causes delta hepatitis may be transmitted by blood transfusion or parenteral drug use, other mechanisms of spread are unclear at this time. Many cases probably go undiagnosed because there is presently no diagnostic test available. Experts agree that delta hepatitis may be avoided in large part by widespread use of HBV vaccine. However, no vaccine is available to prevent transmission of the delta virus to carriers of HBV or those already infected with HBV (Benenson, 1990).

Opportunistic Infections

In 1981 the use of the term *opportunistic infection (OI)* took on new meaning as the identification and spread of HIV was discovered. Before this time, OIs were associated with individuals who were immunosuppressed as a result of leukemias or drug suppression in conjunction with organ transplantation. As the term implies, these diseases manifest themselves whenever the opportunity arises. Many organisms invade the human body and never cause disease because of the effectiveness of the immune system. However, as the immune system becomes ineffective, various opportunistic infections occur. These organisms have become the major causes of death for HIV-infected individuals. The following conditions are some of the OIs the community health nurse must consider in the treatment of the increasing number of immunosuppressed patients.

Pneumocystis Carinii Pneumonia

Pneumocystis carinii pneumonia (PCP) was one of the first OIs identified. It continues to affect 60% to 70% of HIV-diseased patients and is the leading cause of death for AIDS patients. *P. carinii* is a protozoan that affects the lower respiratory tract of persons with immunodeficiency disorders. With the recent use of inhaled medication for prophylaxis against PCP, *P. carinii* has disseminated to other organ systems.

Symptoms are vague and slow to manifest but begin with a dry, persistent cough. The symptoms progress until shortness of breath and fever develop. The more marked these findings, the poorer is the prognosis for recovery from the infection. Diagnosis is important to effectively treat the cause of the pulmonary symptoms. Chest radiographic examinations and arterial blood gas analyses may or may not indicate disease, especially early in the disease process. Induced sputum is the most economical test; however, bronchoscopy with bronchoalveolar lavage is often necessary for definitive diagnosis.

Treatment for PCP depends on the severity of the infection. Severe cases require hospitalization and intravenous therapy of trimethoprim-sulfamethoxazole or pentamidine. This therapy has a 60% to 80% success rate. Milder cases of PCP can be effectively treated with oral trimethoprim-sulfamethoxazole, aerosolized pentamidine, dapsone plus trimethoprim, and trimetrexate. The use of steroids is controversial, and their effectiveness is under study (Landesman, et al., 1988).

Prophylactic treatment is recommended for persons at risk for PCP because 20% to 30% of all PCP patients relapse within 6 months (Gee and Moran, 1988). Trimethoprim-sulfamethoxazole has proved effective, although allergic reactions and hypersensitivity are common. Monthly or bimonthly treatments using inhaled pentamidine through a respiratory nebulizer is another effective method of prophylaxis for PCP when patients are allergic to one of the systemic drugs. However, disseminated *P. carinii* infections have been seen with the use of inhaled pentamidine alone as a result of the local effects of this treatment. More research using systemic drugs is currently underway (Landesman et al., 1988).

Cryptosporidiosis

Cryptosporidium muris is another protozoan that is checked by the normal immune system (Gee and Moran, 1988). The organism is found in the respiratory and gastrointestinal (GI) tracts of birds, reptiles, and other mammals. These serve as a potential reservoir for infection for the immunocompromised patient. When the immune system becomes ineffective, the organism causes severe watery diarrhea, affecting the small bowel and causing a malabsorption syndrome. Nausea, vomiting, anorexia, fatigue, and fever may accompany the diarrhea. These conditions compound the electrolyte disturbances and dehydration effects.

For this reason, patients may require hospitalization for supportive therapy. Drug therapy is limited to oral spiramycin. Other antiprotozal agents have proved ineffective against *C. muris* (Gee and Moran, 1988). The diagnosis should be made by ruling out bacterial causes for the chronic diarrhea. Analyses of stool specimens for ova, parasites, and white blood cells can assist with the diagnosis and should be completed before bowel biopsy (Gee and Moran, 1988). Symptoms usually persist for 30 days in a person with a healthy immune system and longer for the immunocompromised patient.

Rehydration is the only treatment to date, with cessation of immunosuppressive drugs in patients whenever possible (Benenson, 1990).

Toxoplasmosis

Toxoplasma gondii is another protozoal organism that causes disease in the immunodeficient patient. Serologic studies revealed that about 20% to 50% of adults in the United States have been infected by *T. gondii* but are protected by a normal immune system (Landesman et al., 1988). Toxoplasmosis was first seen in the 1920s as an ophthalmologic infection. However, since the onset of the AIDS epidemic, toxoplasmosis has been found in brain, skeletal, and cardiac tissues.

T. gondii are found in cats and other felines, who are the only hosts that harbor the parasite. The sexual stage of the organism's life cycle occurs in the feline intestinal tract, and oocysts are passed in the feces. Transmission occurs when other animals, birds, and rodents ingest the oocysts and are later eaten by other felines. During the tachyzoites stage, the protozoan form circulates in the blood stream causing disease. The third form of the parasite becomes encapsulated in tissue cysts, which infect tissue or muscle, and is transmitted when raw or undercooked meat is ingested (Benenson, 1990). These oocysts, which are shed in the feces, have been known to remain infectious for up to 1 year (Gee and Moran, 1988).

Manifestation of symptoms of toxoplasmosis can be gradual or abrupt, with fever and a wide range of neurological signs and symptoms. Because of the wide range of neurological symptoms, HIV dementia syndrome may be misdiagnosed. Definitive diagnosis using computerized tomographic (CT) scans of the brain with contrast-material enhancement allow for visualization of the ring-enhanced lesions. In some cases, magnetic resonance imaging (MRI) scanning or brain biopsy becomes necessary for the diagnosis of toxoplasmosis (Gee and Moran, 1988).

Sulfadiazine sodium and pyrimethamine are used in combination in the absence of sulfa allergy because both drugs readily cross the blood-brain barrier. Pancytopenia is seen, and the laboratory values must be monitored closely during treatment. Clindamycin can be administered intravenously or orally when the patient has an allergy to sulfa drugs or marked bone marrow suppression. Most patients improve with drug therapy. However, toxoplasmosis is fatal in as many as 60% of AIDS patients (Gee and Moran, 1988). Prevention of exposure to *T. gondii* is important for the HIV-infected persons. Proper handling and cooking of raw meat and disposal of cat litter boxes using gloves and masks become vital practices to protect HIV-infected persons (Landesman et al., 1988).

Candidiasis

Candidiasis, commonly known as thrush, involves the GI tract, primarily the oral mucosa. The causative organism is a fungus known as *Candida albicans,* which is commonly found in humans worldwide. As the normal flora of the host decrease, *C. albicans* increases in number, causing symptoms. When the flora is suppressed for long periods of time, the symptoms become more pronounced. *Candida* organisms may infect the oral mucosa, causing mild discomfort. Infection may involve the entire GI tract, with dysphagia, nausea, vomiting, and retrosternal pain (Gee and Moran, 1988). Colonization of the pulmonary tract and dissemination of *C. albicans* in the blood has been seen. Definitive diagnosis is important in determining the type of treatment for disseminated *candida* organism infections. Microscopic examination of the specimen reveals the pseudohyphae or budding-yeast cells (Gee and Moran, 1988).

Nystatin or Mycelex are used for esophageal or oral candidiasis in either liquid or troche form. When candidiasis has been successfully treated, prophylactic treatment using either mycelex or nystatin is beneficial to prevent any recurrence. Amphotericin B (intravenously) or ketoconazole (orally) are administered for systemic treatment of *Candida* organism infections. Liver function studies should be monitored closely during the use of these medications because of potentials for liver toxicity with amphotericin B. Diarrhea, nausea, vomiting, and adrenal suppression may also result. Amphotericin B is not appropriate for long-term use because of its toxic effects and is not appropriate for prophylactic use (Gee and Moran, 1988).

Cryptococcal Infections

Cryptococcus neoformans is a fungal organism that is commonly found in the soil and in pigeon droppings. Transmission is primarily by inhalation of organisms from the environment. Large numbers of the general population react to skin tests, indicating prior exposure to the organism. Normal immune systems are able to contain the organism. However, *C. neoformans* is able to cause disease (Gee and Moran, 1988).

C. neoformans enters the host through the lungs without clinical manifestations and is transmitted from there to the brain through the blood. The organism has an unexplained affinity for the central nervous system (CNS). If found in the blood or lung, possible CNS involvement should be investigated (Gee and Moran, 1988).

Progression of cryptococcosis symptoms is usually slow, taking from weeks to months. High fevers, headache, and malaise indicate chronic infection, and stiff neck, nausea and vomiting, photophobia, and mental status changes may present after several weeks with cryptococcal meningitis. In pulmonary cryptococcosis, symptoms include chest pain, cough, or dyspnea (Gee and Moran, 1988).

The diagnosis of cryptococcosis includes serologic antigen testing and lumbar puncture tests for antigen titer or cultures of cerebrospinal fluid for *C. neoformans;* CT and MRI scans may rule out other pathologic conditions that may cause similar symptoms. Chest radiographic examination and evaluation of bronchial secretions for the organism can indicate the diagnosis of infection. However, if these diagnostic techniques are unsuccessful, a needle biopsy may be necessary (Gee and Moran, 1988).

Amphotericin B is administered intravenously for about 6 weeks for treatment of systemic cryptococcosis. Renal function studies should be monitored carefully because of the toxic properties of amphotericin B. An oral agent called 5-flucytosine can be used in conjunction with amphotericin B to increase the effectiveness of treatment while minimizing its nephrotoxicity. Lumbar puncture tests should be repeated 2 to 3 weeks after drug therapy is completed to assess the cerebrospinal fluid for antigen titers or to culture *C. neoformans* in the fluid. Initial infections of *C. neoformans* currently have a mortality of about 17%, and the rate increases with each episode of infection (Gee and Moran, 1988).

Histoplasmosis

Histoplasma capsulatum is another fungal agent found in the soil and bird droppings. Chicken coops, bat caves, and areas where pigeons are found, especially along the Mississippi Valley area, have produced numerous cases of histoplasmosis. Approximately 70% to 90% of the people tested in this region of the United States have positive skin test results for histoplasmosis; however, because of an intact immune system, very few individuals show symptoms of disease. Similar to *C. neoformans*, *H. capsulatum* enters the host by inhalation and spreads to other organs of the body rapidly in the immunodeficient host (Gee and Moran, 1988).

The clinical symptoms resemble sepsis with a very high fever, hypotension, enlarged liver and spleen, pulmonary symptoms, and altered mental status. Serologic studies are used to identify the organism in blood or sputum cultures. Treatment for histoplasmosis is the same as for cryptococcosis. Amphotericin B is administered in much the same dose and treatment regimen (Gee and Moran, 1988).

CLINICAL APPLICATION

Community health nurses are instrumental in all facets of prevention and promotion of public health. Immunization plans are devised to protect individuals from identified communicable diseases to decrease morbity and mortality. Community health nurses are the key to implementation and success of these plans, proving again their importance in the community. The following is an actual mass immunization program planning that was reported by the CDC in 1989. Precise data on the occurrence of pneumonococcal disease in the United States is not available, partly because pneumonococcal disease is not a nationally notifiable disease. However, the pneumococcal infection is estimated to annually cause 150,000 to 570,000 cases of pneumonia, 16,000 to 55,000 cases of bacteremia, and 2600 to 6200 cases of meningitis and to contribute to or cause a total of 40,000 deaths.

Persons at increased risk for developing severe pneumococcal disease include adults with chronic diseases such as Hodgkin's disease, multiple myeloma, cirrhosis, alcoholism, renal failure, splenic dysfunction, conditions associated with immunosuppression, and most recently, otherwise healthy persons over 65 years of age.

The polysaccharide vaccine currently used contains antigen from the organisms that cause 88% of the bacteremic pneumococcal disease. The CDC (1989) estimates that, if mass immunization were accomplished for the identified risk population with 60% efficacy and 60% coverage, about 12,000 deaths from pneumococcal disease might be prevented each year.

Community health nurses can influence a patient's decision regarding vaccination. Assessment of the immuni-

zation status of risk groups and administration of the vaccine to those identified at risk helps to lower the incident of pneumococcal-related diseases. Education regarding efficacy and administration of the vaccine can also influence the public to participate in mass immunization.

California instituted a mass-immunization program in 1986 to provide protection to senior citizens and others at high risk for infection. Each autumn, as many as 500,000 citizens receive pneumococcal immunization either in conjunction with the influenza vaccination or through health department clinics. The promotion of the vaccine comes from leaflets, posters, and recommendations by staff members to the public.

During the first year of the mass-immunization project, from July 1986 through June 1987, health departments administered 41.8% of the dose inventory of pneumococcal vaccine. The departments who promoted the vaccination administered the majority of those doses given. From July 1987 through July 1989, the local health departments increased the number of vaccines administered to 69,054, or 64.1% of the total dose inventory. This reflected an 82.3% increase in just 1 year (CDC, 1989c).

Mass immunization can be used in the future when statistics indicate that the administration of effective vaccines will significantly decrease the morbidity and mortality of a disease. Another example of future uses might include the hepatitis B vaccine, for which there are significant statistics to support the use of the vaccine.

SUMMARY

Although communicable diseases are no longer the most frequent cause of morbidity and mortality, they still represent a major health problem. The natures and sometimes the names of communicable processes change over time, but they nonetheless retain a sinister ability to weaken, disable, and kill.

The effort to monitor and control communicable disease phenomena is worldwide. However, the effectiveness of larger surveillance systems depends on astute individuals on the local level who must identify individual cases and implement preventive, controlling, and maintenance strategies. Because of the practice arena involved, the community health nurse occupies a position of responsibility for all these functions. There are few other instances in which the opportunity to contribute in an interdisciplinary fashion for the common good is so operative.

KEY CONCEPTS

The vast majority of persons who succumb to communicable or contagious diseases contract them in the community and are cared for at home throughout minor illnesses or periods when th disease process can be managed on an outpatient basis.

Some infectious diseases, such as smallpox, have been completely eliminated throughout the world, and most traditional communicable diseases can be therapeutically managed so that, often, death can be prevented.

The information about types and causes of communicable diseases is not static but is constantly being changed and updated by new knowledge.

Community health nurses must be knowledgeable about communicable diseases so that they can effectively counsel patients, family, or friends about the care of potentially exposed or frankly infected persons.

Communicable disease plays a tremendous role in the economic viability of both specific communities and the nation.

Failure to enforce the recommended schedule for communicable disease control or a break in community sanitation or water purification can result in an epidemic at any given time.

Infectivity is the ability of the organism to spread rapidly from one host to another.

Invasiveness refers to the agent's ability to spread within the host.

Virulence is the ability to produce severe disease.

In general, most disease processes produce the greatest morbidity and mortality in the very young and the very old in any given population, but there are some important exceptions.

Some factors of the host's ability to ward off infection are interdependent with environmental factors such as humidity, temperature, and crowding. Other environmental factors that influence the incidence of communicable diseases are atmospheric conditions, availability of nutrients, and contamination of food and water supplies.

According to the U.S. Centers for Disease Control, social, demographic, and behavioral changes within the U.S. population during the past decade have placed an increased proportion of people at risk for sexually transmissible diseases.

LEARNING ACTIVITIES

1. Write a paper covering the stage of susceptibility of the Natural History Model on a communicable or infectious disease (student's choice, subject to faculty approval). Host, agent, and environment factors should be clearly delineated, and nursing strategies relative to primary prevention should be included.

2. Ascertain the mechanisms for reporting various types of infectious or communicable diseases in the country.

3. Instructors may plan a clinical rotation for students in local sexually transmitted disease (STD) clinics. Local and state statistics on STD should be compared with the national incidence.

4. Survey health or nursing personnel in local schools to ascertain when the last outbreak of pediculosis occurred in the community.

BIBLIOGRAPHY

Altman LK: Mysterious form of hepatitis seen as widespread threat, New York Times, August 28, 1984.

American Academy of Pediatrics: Report of the Committee on Infectious Diseases, ed 20, Evanston, IL, 1988, The Academy.

Benenson AS, editor: Control of communicable diseases in man, ed 15, Washington, DC, 1990, American Public Health Association.

Beveridge WI: Influenza: the last great plague, New York, 1978, Prodist Publishers.

Centers for Disease Control: Measles—United States, 1990, MMWR 40(22):369, 1990.

Centers for Disease Control: Genital herpes infections: United States, 1966–1979, MMWR 31:137, 1982.

Centers for Disease Control: Annual summary, MMWR 33:27, 1984.

Centers for Disease Control: Diphtheria, tetanus, and pertussis: guidelines for vaccine prophylaxis and other preventive measures, MMWR 133:392, 1984a.

Centers for Disease Control: Mumps: United States, 1983–1984, MMWR 33:533, 1984b.

Centers for Disease Control: Elimination of rubella and congenital rubella syndrome: United States, MMWR 34:65, 1985.

Centers for Disease Control: Update: milk-borne salmonellosis—Illinois, MMWR 34:215, 1985a.

Centers for Disease Control: Vaccine for prevention of Haemophilus influenzae, MMWR 34:201, 1985b.

Centers for Disease Control: Meingococcal vaccines, MMWR 34:255, 1985c.

Centers for Disease Control: Recommendations for protection against viral hepatitis, MMWR 34:315, 1985d.

Centers for Disease Control: Pertussis: Washington, 1984, MMWR 34:314, 1985e.

Centers for Disease Control: Measles on college campuses: United States, 1985, MMWR 34:445, 1985f.

Centers for Disease Control: Isolation of multiply antibiotic-resistant pneumococci: New York, MMWR 34:545, 1985g.

Centers for Disease Control: Tetracycline-resistant Neisseria gonorrhoeae: Georgia, Pennsylvania, New Hampshire, MMWR 34:356, 1985h.

Centers for Disease Control: Final 1984 reports of notifiable disease, MMWR 34:590, 1985i.

Centers for Disease Control: Tuberculosis and acquired immunodeficiency syndrome: Florida, MMWR 35:587, 1986.

Centers for Disease Control: Tuberculosis and acquired immunodeficiency syndrome: New York City, MMWR 36:785, 1987.

Centers for Disease Control: Rubella and congenital rubella syndrome: U.S., MMWR 37:178, 1988.

Centers for Disease Control: Summary of Notifiable diseases: United States, MMWR 38:29, 1989.

Centers for Disease Control: Measles prevention and recommendations of the immunization practices: Advisory Committee (ACCP), MMWR 38:1, 1989a.

Centers for Disease Control: General recommendations on immunization, MMWR 38:205, 1989b.

Centers for Disease Control: Tuberculosis and HIV infection: recommendations of the Advisory Committee for the Elimination of Tuberculosis (ACET), MMWR 38:236-238 and 243-250, 1989c.

Centers for Disease Control: Protection against viral hepatitis, MMWR 39:1, 1990.

Centers for Disease Control: Prevention and control of influenza, MMWR 39:1, 1990a.

Centers for Disease Control: Meningococcal vaccine in single-dose vials for travelers and high-risk persons, MMWR 39:763, 1990b.

Centers for Disease Control: Guidelines for preventing the transmission of tuberculosis in health-care settings, with special emphasis on HIV-related issues, MMWR 39(RR-17):1-29, 1990.

Centers for Disease Control: HIV/AIDS surveillance report, MMWR Feb. 1991, p. 1-10.

Centers for Disease Control (1992). Tuberculosis Morbidity in the United States: Final Data, 1990, *Weekly Morbidity and Mortality Report, 40*(SS-4), pp. 23-26.

Committee on Infectious Diseases, American Academy of Pediatrics: Report of the Committee on Infectious Diseases, ed 21, Elk Grove Village, IL, 1988, The Academy.

Dowdle WR: Surveillance and control of infectious diseases: progress toward the 1990 objectives, Public Health Rep 98(3):210, 1983.

Edelstein PH and Meyer RD: Legionnaires' diseases: a review, Chest 85(11):114, 1984.

Gee G and Moran TA: AIDS: concepts in nursing practice, Baltimore, MD, 1988, Williams & Wilkins.

Hare R: Pomp and pestilence, New York, 1955, Philosophical Library.

Healthy people: the Surgeon General's report on health promotion and disease prevention, DHEW Pub No (PHS) 79-55071, Washington, DC, 1979, US Department of Health, Education and Welfare.

Holmberg SD et al.: Drug-resistant *Salmonella* from animals fed anitmicrobials, N Engl J Med 311(10):617, 1984.

Landsman S et al., editors: Management of HIV disease: treatment team workshop handbook, New York, 1989, World Health Communications.

Mausner JS and Kramer S: Mausner & Bahn's epidemiology—an introductory text, Philadelphia, 1985, WB Saunders.

Society of Actuaries: US general population projected AIDS mortality rates (AIDS reference guide) Schaumberg, IL, 1990, Atlantic Information Services.

Tortora GJ, Funke BR, Case CL: Microbiology: an introduction, Menlo Park, CA, 1989, Benjamin Cummings Publishing.

Whaley LF and Wong DL: Nursing care of infants and children, ed 4, St Louis, 1991, Mosby Year–Book.

Wolberding P and Abrams D: Clinical care and research in AIDS, Hastings Center Report, pp. 16-18, August 1985.

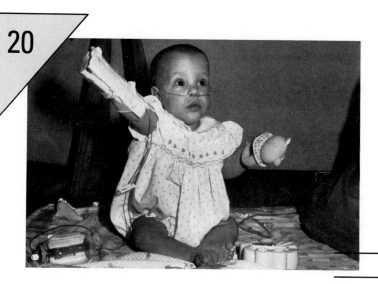

20

HIV and Other Sexually Transmitted Diseases

Patty J. Hale

OBJECTIVES

After reading this chapter, the student should be able to:

Describe the spectrum of human immunodeficiency virus infection and appropriate client education and counseling at each stage.

Describe the clinical signs of the major sexually transmitted diseases.

Identify the trends in incidence of the major sexually transmitted diseases and groups that are at greatest risk.

Identify activities that place people at risk of contracting sexually transmitted diseases.

Discuss the impact of sexually transmitted diseases in terms of morbidity and mortality at the individual and community levels.

Describe activities to prevent and control sexually transmitted diseases.

Explain the roles of community health nurses in the prevention and control of sexually transmitted disease.

KEY TERMS

acquired immunodeficiency syndrome (AIDS)
chancroid
chlamydia
epididymitis
genital herpes
genital warts
gonorrhea
HIV
HIV antibody test

HIV disease
HIV infection
HIV seronegative
HIV seropositive
HIV seroprevalence
human papillomavirus infection
incubation period
injectable drug use
nongonococcal urethritis

nonoxynol-9
partner notification
pelvic inflammatory disease
risk assessment
salpingitis
seroconversion
sexually transmitted disease
syphilis

T he scientific fields concerned with *sexually transmitted diseases* (STDs) have experienced unprecedented changes in recent years. For several decades following the development of antibiotics in the 1940s, STDs were considered to be a problem of the past. Recently, the *human immunodeficiency virus* (HIV) has been identified and other STDs, such as *gonorrhea*, have posed new challenges because of emerging antibiotic-resistant strains.

Because nearly all STDs are acquired through behaviors that can be avoided or changed, the focus of intervention has turned from cure to prevention. At the same time the infection rate is climbing, the number of people who are sexually active and use injectable drugs has risen, causing a parallel rise in the population at risk of acquiring STDs (CDC, 1991; Cates, 1987). For these reasons there is greater urgency than ever to develop effective methods to prevent and control STDs. Education and counseling to facilitate behavior changes are of primary importance and are being given new emphasis in community health nursing practice.

This chapter examines HIV infection and other significant STDs. The implications for community health nursing practice regarding disease prevention and control are reviewed.

HUMAN IMMUNODEFICIENCY VIRUS INFECTION

Human immunodeficiency virus (HIV) disease, a term used to refer to symptomatic *HIV infection* and *acquired immunodeficiency syndrome (AIDS)*, is unlike other illnesses because it affects nearly every level of society. Awareness of the political and social impact of HIV infection is growing as decisions are made about how to control its spread. The public's reaction to fears about HIV disease is complicated by the fact that this disease has commonly afflicted homosexuals and injectable drug users, two groups that have been largely scorned by society. In addition, numerous controversies have arisen over many aspects of HIV—from prevention to diagnosis and treatment. One dispute involves whether programs should be conducted to disseminate clean needles. Another involves the use of testing: Which groups should be tested and should this testing be done confidentially or anonymously?

Economic costs are growing as HIV causes premature disability and death. Ninety-five percent of those afflicted are between the ages of 20 and 59 years, resulting in disrupted families and lost creative and economic productivity at a period of life when growth is the norm. The direct cost of health care for HIV disease alone is staggering. It is of much greater concern when added to a health care system that is already unable to meet the needs of many people. Estimates of the total lifetime health care costs for an individual with HIV disease range from $65,000 to $85,000 (Hellinger, 1990; Institute of Medicine, 1988). This cost is likely to rise as new, more expensive treatments are developed and as life expectancy increases.

Pathogenesis

HIV infection is caused by a retrovirus, the human immunodeficiency virus, which was discovered in 1983. HIV causes immunologic deficiencies that leave the host susceptible to opportunistic infections and cancers. Retroviruses produce an enzyme called reverse transcriptase that tran-

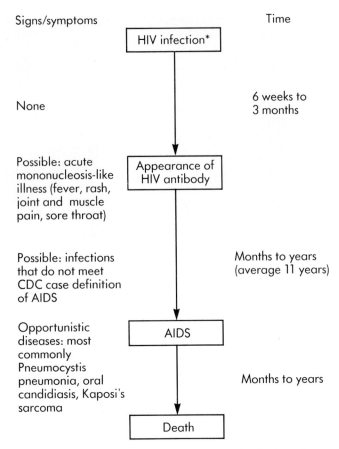

*Incubation period varies between individuals and may last from several months to several years.

FIGURE 20-1

Natural history of human immunodeficiency virus.

scribes the viral genome onto the DNA of the host cell. This results in viral replication by the infected cell.

HIV infects many cells, including the dendritic cells, endothelial cells, Langerhans' cells, lymphocytes, monocytes, and macrophages. The greatest damage is from the infection of the T4, or helper T-, lymphocyte, the cell that induces nearly every immune response. The progressive decline in numbers of T4 lymphocytes causes disruptions in immune functioning. For example, HIV adversely affects antibody production and decreases intracellular killing of pathogens following phagocytosis.

Natural History of HIV

The natural history of HIV is described in Figure 20-1. On entering the body, HIV infects cells and becomes latent for several months or years, causing no symptomatic illness. After a variable period of time—commonly from 6 weeks to 3 months—HIV antibodies appear in the blood. Although most antibodies serve a protective role, it appears that HIV antibodies do not. However, with the HIV, antibody production is significant because most tests for suspected HIV

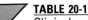

TABLE 20-1
Clinical manifestations of AIDS

Disease	Clinical signs
Candidiasis (oral or esophageal)	White patches on tongue, difficulty eating
Cryptococcal meningitis	Fever, headache, stiff neck
Pneumocystis carinii pneumonia	Shortness of breath, dry cough, fever, fatigue
Toxoplasmosis	Hemiparesis, seizures, aphasia
Cryptosporidum enteritis infection	Diarrhea, weakness
Mycobacterium tuberculosis infection	Productive, purulent cough, fatigue, weight loss
Cytomegalovirus retinitis	Visual blurring
Herpes simplex virus infection	Painful vesicles
Kaposi's sarcoma	Purple skin lesions, localized edema

infection detect the antibody presence. In some instances, however, individuals have not shown positive antibody tests for as long as 42 months following infection, but this delay is believed to be rare (Wolinsky et al., 1989). Future research will provide more information. Around 4 weeks after infection and during the time of antibody production, some individuals experience a short-term mononucleosis-like illness. This is a self-limiting illness with the symptoms of lymphadenopathy, myalgias, pharyngitis, lethargy, rash, and fever (Kessler et al., 1987).

The *incubation period* for HIV lasts from several months to many years. The average time for the development of symptoms is 11 years or longer (Lemp et al., 1990). During this long period of latency, the infected person carries and is able to transmit the virus to others.

AIDS is the last stage on the long continuum of HIV infection. AIDS is defined as a disabling or life-threatening illness caused by HIV. It is characterized by encephalopathy, wasting syndrome, or certain diseases caused by immunodeficiency in a person with laboratory evidence for HIV infection or without certain other causes of immunodeficiency (CDC, 1987). AIDS can result from damage caused by HIV, secondary cancers, or opportunistic organisms. The case definition of AIDS includes specific criteria set forth by the Centers for Disease Control (CDC). However, some symptomatic illnesses caused by HIV, such as pneumonia in injectable drug users, are not covered under this definition (CDC, 1989a).

Many of the opportunistic infections that occur are caused by microorganisms that are commonly present in healthy individuals but do not cause disease in persons with an intact immune system. These microorganisms proliferate in those with HIV infection because of a weakened immune system. Opportunistic infections may be caused by bacteria, fungi, viruses, or protozoa. The most common opportunistic diseases are *Pneumocystis carinii* pneumonia and oral candidiasis. Table 20-1 describes diseases commonly associated with AIDS and their clinical manifestations.

MODES OF HIV TRANSMISSION

HIV can be transmitted in the following ways:
(1) sexual contact, involving the exchange of body fluids, with an infected person;
(2) transfusions or other exposure to HIV-contaminated blood or blood products, organs, or semen;
(3) perinatal transmission from an infected mother to her fetus during pregnancy or delivery or to an infant when breast feeding; and
(4) sharing or reusing needles, syringes, or other equipment used to prepare injectable drugs.

Transmission

Concerns about the transmission of HIV may be expressed by clients, their families, friends, and other groups. Among many questions, the community health nurse is likely to be asked to explain the modes of transmission. Because others will look to the community health nurse for information and as a model for how to behave toward those with HIV infection, it is important to understand how transmission occurs.

HIV is not transmitted through casual contact. Family members of persons with HIV disease have shared towels, dishes, and other household equipment. Except for those who had sexual or needle-sharing contact with an infected person, none develop infection (Friedland and Klein, 1987). HIV is not transmitted by insects, coughing, sneezing, sharing office equipment, or sitting next to or eating with someone who has HIV infection. It is safe to touch, hug, or shake hands with someone who has HIV disease.

HIV transmission occurs only through exposure to blood, semen, vaginal secretions, and breast milk. Although the virus has been isolated in several other fluids including saliva, tears, cerebrospinal fluid, synovial fluid, amniotic fluid, and urine, no cases of transmission through contact with these fluids have been documented. It is believed that the low concentration of the virus in certain body fluids and the fact that some fluids do not come into contact with openings in the skin make them unlikely to be efficient modes of transmission. The most efficient transmission is believed to be through a transfusion with contaminated blood, because blood has a high concentration of the virus and it is placed directly into another's bloodstream, where many T4 lymphocytes are located. Saliva, on the other hand, has a low-viral concentration and is unlikely to gain access to the cells that HIV infects. The modes of transmission are summarized in the box above.

Screening of potential donors of blood and tissues includes the use of the *HIV antibody test* and interviews to assess for a history of high-risk activities. Blood or tissue is not used from individuals who have a history of high-risk behavior or who are *HIV seropositive* (contain antibodies of HIV in their serum). In addition to screening, coagulation factors used to treat hemophilia and other blood disorders are made even more safe through heat treatments to inactivate the virus. Such screening has significantly reduced the risk of transmission of HIV by blood products

TABLE 20-2

AIDS cases by exposure category reported through January 1991, United States

Adult and adolescent exposure category	%	Pediatric (<13 years of age) exposure category	%[a]
Male homosexual and bisexual contact	59	Hemophilia and coagulation disorder	5
Intravenous drug use (heterosexual)	22	Mother with or at risk of HIV infection	84
Intravenous drug use and male homo-sexual and bisexual contact	7	Receipt of blood transfu-sion, blood components, or tissues	9
Hemophilia and coagulation disorder	1	Undetermined	3
Heterosexual contact	5		
Blood transfusion, blood components, or tissue	2		
Other and undetermined[b]	4		

[a]The total of 101% is due to rounding errors.
[b]"Other" refers to three health-care workers who exhibited HIV seroconversion and developed AIDS after occupational exposure to HIV-infected blood. "Undetermined" refers to clients whose mode of exposure to HIV is unknown. This includes clients under investigation; clients who died, were lost to follow-up, or refused interview; and clients whose mode of exposure to HIV remains undetermined after investigation.
Adapted from Centers for Disease Control: HIV/AIDS surveillance report, Feb. 1991.

and organ donations. It is estimated that the odds of contracting HIV infection through blood transfusion are one in 153,000 per unit of blood transfused. Since the test to screen blood donors was instituted in 1985, 15 people have become seropositive after receiving contaminated blood (Cumming et al., 1989). However, because the average incubation period is 11 years, some people who received blood transfusions prior to 1985 may develop AIDS in the future.

Distribution and Trends

AIDS was first recognized in 1981 in Los Angeles. Five homosexual men were discovered to have *Pneumocystis carinii* pneumonia, a disease that occurred almost exclusively in immunosuppressed individuals. By mid-1981, Kaposi's sarcoma was diagnosed in 26 young, homosexual men in New York and San Francisco. Seven of the twenty-six also had *Pneumocystis carinii* pneumonia. From these early cases the number of diagnosed cases has grown rapidly. By 1986, 24,000 individuals were diagnosed with AIDS, and by 1990 the number had grown to 157,000.

Since the first cases in 1981, it has been recognized that the groups with the highest incidence of HIV infection are homosexual and bisexual males, injectable drug users and their sexual partners, and hemophiliacs (CDC, 1989b). Table 20-2 identifies the transmission categories for persons with AIDS. Identifying groups at highest risk allows the nurse to target prevention efforts toward these individuals.

Gender

Males represent 90% of the reported adult cases of AIDS in the United States. The rate has increased for women from 7% of the total cases in 1984 to 10% of the total cases in 1990. A majority of the adolescent and child cases are also males. This is mostly a result of hemophilia, which is a risk factor afflicting mostly males (CDC, 1989a).

Age

The largest number of reported AIDS cases (46%) is in the age group from 30 to 39 years (CDC, 1991). Eighty-eight percent of all AIDS cases are between the ages of 20 and 49 years (CDC, 1990b; CDC, 1990d). Because the incubation period is so long, the infection is likely to have occurred during adolescence and young adulthood. This period of life is characterized by experimentation with various roles and behaviors that may include *injectable drug use (IDU), sexual experimentation, and other activities that place adolescents and young adults at risk.*

Although the number of pediatric cases is a fraction of the adult cases, it is of growing concern that HIV infection in women and, consequently, neonates is increasing. AIDS ranks among the top 10 causes of death for those from 1 to 4 years old and is likely to increase (Kilbourne, Buehler, and Rogers, 1990).

Geographic Location

The geographic distribution of AIDS is uneven and clustered. Previously the disease was found mostly in identified urban areas, but increasingly it is moving into rural areas. Locations with the highest prevalence of AIDS are Florida, New York, New Jersey, California, District of Columbia, and Texas. Regionally, the Northeast section of the U.S. and some U.S. territories (Puerto Rico) reflect the highest rates (CDC, 1990a).

Race and Ethnicity

AIDS has disproportionately affected minority groups. African Americans made up 11.2% of the total U.S. population according to the 1980 census, but they represent 27.6% of those reported to have AIDS (CDC, 1990d). This overrepresentation is associated with urban residence, poverty, transmission through the use of injectable drugs, and prostitution (Aral and Homes, 1990; Moran et al., 1989).

Seroprevalence

It is estimated that there are 1 million people infected with HIV in the United States and between 5 and 10 million people infected worldwide (CDC, 1990c; WHO-ICN, 1988). AIDS is a reportable condition within the United States, but the reporting of HIV infection varies among states.

It is expected that the number of AIDS cases in the United States will increase at least through 1993. This rise is anticipated in all of the main transmission categories; homosexual and bisexual men, IDUs, heterosexuals, and children infected perinatally (CDC, 1990c). An increasing proportion of the total AIDS cases are expected to involve injectable drug users, their sexual partners, and their children.

Study of already diagnosed cases of AIDS does not necessarily reveal current HIV infection patterns because of the long interval between infection with HIV and the onset of disease. Moreover, identification of new cases of AIDS does not distinguish between those recently infected and those infected several years ago.

Studies known as *HIV seroprevalence* studies involve the screening of populations for the HIV antibody. These studies provide specific information about the number of HIV carriers and the spread of the virus within populations. Seroprevalence rates of several groups have been investigated. It has been found that 4.2% of those attending STD clinics were seropositive (Cannon et al., 1989); 15% of military recruits were seropositive (Kelley et al., 1990), and 5% to 33% of injectable drug users were seropositive (Hahn et al., 1989).

Mortality

As of 1990, 63% of all adults and 52% of all children reported to have AIDS had died (CDC, 1990d). Five years after the diagnosis of AIDS, the fatality ratio is nearly 100% (CDC, 1989a). With the use of antiretroviral therapy, such as zidovudine, the survival period has increased and is likely to continue to increase (Lemp et al. 1990).

HIV Testing

Testing for HIV infection is offered at many sites, including health departments, sexually transmitted disease clinics, family planning clinics, and freestanding HIV-counseling and HIV-testing sites. The test most commonly used is the HIV antibody test. This test does not reveal whether or not the individual has AIDS nor does it isolate the virus. It does indicate the presence of the antibody to the virus. The most commonly used form of this test is the enzyme linked immunosorbant assay (ELISA), but other tests are being developed. The ELISA was developed to screen blood and other donor products and is very effective in doing so. However, there are sometimes false-positive results, so a confirmatory test, the Western blot, is used to verify the results. False-negative results may also occur after infection before antibodies are produced. This is sometimes referred to as the window period and can last usually from 6 weeks to 3 months.

Voluntary screening programs for HIV may be either confidential or anonymous. With confidential testing, the person's name and address is obtained, but the information is considered privileged. With anonymous testing, the client is given an identification number that is attached to all records of the test results. Demographic data such as the person's sex, age, and race may be collected, but there is no record of the client's name and address. Anonymous testing is thought to increase the number of people who are willing to be tested, because many of those at risk are engaged in illegal activities. The anonymity eliminates their concern about the possibility of arrest or discrimination.

The community health nurse should recommend that persons who have engaged in high-risk behavior be tested. The following people are considered to be at risk and should be offered the HIV antibody test: those with history of STD (because STDs are transmitted through the same behavior), multiple sex partners, or IDU; those who have had sex with a prostitute; those males with a history of homosexual or bisexual activity; those who have been a sexual partner to anyone in one of these groups; and those who underwent blood transfusion between 1978 and March 1985.

If HIV infection is discovered early, the disease process can be monitored for changes, such as a decrease in the T4 lymphocyte count, that signal the need for early treatment. Antiretroviral therapy, such as zidovudine given early in the infection, may delay the onset of symptomatic illness. For these reasons, persons at high risk should be encouraged to be tested. Testing may also alleviate worry and provides an excellent opportunity for risk-reduction education.

HIV Test Counseling

An important facet of client care is counseling regarding the HIV antibody test. It is essential that the client understand that the test is not a diagnostic test for AIDS but is indicative only of HIV infection.

PRETEST COUNSELING. Special considerations should be made in pretest counseling. Exploration of what a client will do if the test is positive is important to assess their support systems. Asking clients to review how they have handled difficult situations in the past can determine how they might cope with learning they are HIV seropositive.

Information about who will have access to the test results should be given to the client. Although AIDS is reported nationally, the reporting of HIV infection varies among states. States that mandate the reporting of HIV infection differ over whether or not the client's name must accompany the report.

Because there is no cure or vaccine available, prevention of transmission of the HIV requires an assessment of the client's risk behavior and counseling on how to reduce identified risks. Sexually active individuals who have multiple partners must be encouraged to abstain, to enter a mutually monogamous relationship, or to use condoms. IDUs should be advised to enter a treatment program or discontinue drug use. If they continue to use drugs, they should be warned to not share needles, syringes, or any other drug paraphernalia.

POSTTEST COUNSELING. Persons who have a negative test result are said to be *HIV seronegative,* and they should be counseled about risk reduction activities to prevent any future transmission. It is important that the client understand that the test may not be truly negative, because it does not identify infections that may have been acquired several weeks before the test. As noted earlier, *seroconversion* takes

RESPONSIBILITIES OF PERSONS WHO ARE HIV SEROPOSITIVE

Have regular medical evaluations and follow-ups.

Do not donate blood, plasma, body organs, other tissues, or sperm.

Take precautions against exchanging body fluids during sexual activity.

Inform sexual or injectable drug-use partners of their potential exposure to HIV or arrange for notification through the health department.

Inform health care providers.

Consider the risk of perinatal transmission and follow-up with contraceptive use.

from 6 weeks to 3 months. The client must be aware of the means of viral transmission and how to avoid infection. The risk to needle-sharing partners and sexual partners of seropositive clients should be evaluated, and the client should identify ways to communicate this risk to them.

If pretest counseling was adequate, clients are likely to have contemplated the meaning of a positive test result. All clients who are antibody positive should be counseled about the need for reducing their risks and notifying partners. If the client is unwilling or hesitant to notify past partners, *partner notification*, or contact tracing, as described later in this chapter, should be done by the health department. The client should visit a primary health care provider so physical evaluation can be performed, and if indicated, antiviral or other therapies begun. The box above describes responsibilities of an individual who is HIV seropositive.

Psychosocial counseling is indicated when positive HIV test results precipitate acute anxiety, depression, or suicidal ideation. Follow-up counseling sessions and telephone calls are important to monitor the client's status. The client should be informed about available counseling services. The person should be cautioned to consider carefully who should be informed of the test results. Many individuals have told others about their HIV-seropositive status, only to experience isolation and discrimination. Plans for the future should be explored and clients should be advised to avoid stressors, drugs, and infections to maintain optimal health.

Perinatal HIV Infection

Women who are HIV infected must be aware of and consider the risk of perinatal infection. They should be counseled to prevent pregnancy. It is estimated that 30% to 40% of those women infected who become pregnant will pass the virus on to their infants (CDC, 1989c). Women who are HIV infected and asymptomatic are more likely to develop AIDS than are their nonpregnant counterparts as a result of alterations in immune-system functioning during pregnancy. Women must consider who will rear their children if they do become ill. If pregnancy occurs, the decision of whether or not to terminate it through therapeutic abortion will be influenced by the woman's personal beliefs and values, legal parameters, and the availability of health care and financial resources.

The clinical picture of pediatric HIV infection differs greatly from that of adults. The incubation period in neonates is shorter. Infected infants usually become symptomatic within the first year of life. Children also have a shorter survival period. Because 83% of children with AIDS contract the disease through maternal transmission, many die within the first 3 years of life (Grossman, 1989). HIV infection in children of seropositive mothers is difficult to detect before 1 year of age because the antibody test reflects maternal antibodies and thus even a seronegative infant may show a positive test result. Other tests, such as viral cultures, are diagnostic but are currently performed at very few laboratories. Children develop different physical signs and symptoms than adults. These include failure to thrive, diarrhea, developmental delays, and bacterial infections such as otitis media and pneumonia.

AIDS in the Community

Because AIDS is a chronic disease, afflicted individuals live and function in the community. Much of their care is provided in the home. The community health nurse must teach families and significant others about infection control and care, treatments, and other special needs. Infection control and care in the home is discussed in Section 11 of the Appendix.

Persons with AIDS have bouts of illness interspersed with periods of wellness when they are able to return to school or work. This return to normal life is of therapeutic benefit to persons with HIV disease. Policies regarding school and worksite attendance have been developed by most communities and some businesses. These policies provide direction for the community's response when an individual presents with HIV infection or AIDS. Community health nurses are frequently asked to interpret specific, local policies and thus should be familiar with them.

School Attendance

Children who are HIV infected should be allowed to attend school because the benefit of attendance far outweighs the risk of transmitting or acquiring infections. None of the cases of HIV infection in the United States are known to have been transmitted in a school setting. Decisions regarding educational and care needs should be based on an interdisciplinary team that includes the child's physician, public health personnel, and the child's parent or guardian (CDC, 1985).

Individual decisions about risk to the infected child or others should be based on the behavior, neurological development, and physical condition of the child. Attendance may be inadvisable in the presence of cases of childhood infections, such as chickenpox or measles within the school, because the immunosuppressed child is at greater risk of suffering complications. Alternative arrangements, such as home-bound instruction, might be instituted if a child is unable to control body secretions or displays biting behavior.

HIV and the Workplace

The 1974 Vocational Rehabilitation Act protects employees from termination of employment or other discriminatory action based solely on the presence of the disease.

Businesses are often unprepared and uninformed about how to deal with situations involving HIV infection (Hale, 1990). Community health nurses can assist employers by identifying the importance of sponsoring programs on HIV prevention at the workplace and acceptance of HIV-infected co-workers. Educating managers on how to deal with workers who are sick or infected is vital to reduce the risk of breach of confidentiality or wrongful actions such as termination. Revealing a worker's infection to other workers, terminating employment, or isolating an infected worker are examples of situations that have resulted in litigation between employees and employers.

Community-Based AIDS Service Organizations

As the number of individuals afflicted with AIDS increased in the 1980s, many clients' and families' needs were not addressed. Voluntary service organizations developed throughout communities to address these needs. Services that are commonly provided by these groups include client and family counseling and support groups, legal aid, personal care services, housing programs, and community education programs. Community health nurses frequently collaborate with workers in the client's home and may serve to advise community-based groups in their supportive work.

OTHER SEXUALLY TRANSMITTED DISEASES

In recent years, there has been an increase of many other STDs. These include *genital herpes, human papillomavirus infection (genital warts), chancroid,* syphilis, and antibiotic-resistant gonorrhea. The common STDs are described in Table 20-3 and are categorized by their biologic origin: those that are caused by bacteria and those caused by viruses. The bacterial infections include gonorrhea, syphilis, chlamydia, and chancroid. Most of these are curable with the use of antibiotics. The newly emerging antibiotic-resistant strains of gonorrhea are an exception.

There are no cures for STDs caused by viruses. Therefore they are frequently chronic diseases that result in years of symptom management and infection control. The viral infections include herpes simplex virus and genital warts.

Gonorrhea

Neisseria gonorrhoeae is a gram-negative intracellular diplococcus bacteria that infects the mucous membranes of the genitourinary tract, the rectum, and the pharynx. It is transmitted through genital-genital contact, oral-genital contact, and anal-genital contact.

Gonorrhea is identified as either uncomplicated or complicated. Uncomplicated gonorrhea refers to limited cervical or urethral infection. Complicated gonorrhea includes *salpingitis, epididymitis,* systemic gonococcal infection, and gonococcal meningitis. The signs and symptoms of infection in males are typically purulent and copious urethral discharge and dysuria, although it is estimated that 10% to 20% of males are asymptomatic. In females, it is thought that 25% to 80% have no symptoms, but there may be minimal vaginal discharge or dysuria (Hook and Handsfield, 1990). The asymptomatic state is dangerous because individuals who are unaware of their infection may continue to infect others, whereas those who are symptomatic usually

cease sexual activity and seek treatment. Up to 45% of those infected with gonorrhea are coinfected with *Chlamydia trachomatis.* It is therefore recommended that treatment that is effective against both organisms, such as doxycycline and ceftriaxone, be selected (CDC, 1989c).

Gonorrhea is the most common of all reported communicable disease. Groups with the highest reported incidence of gonorrhea include males; those between the ages of 15 to 24 years; urban residents (CDC, 1989d); nonwhites (Quinn, O'Reilly, Khaw, 1988; McEvoy and LeFurgy, 1988); and those with multiple sexual partners and low-socioeconomic status (Barnes and Holmes, 1984). In the years 1980 to 1988, the annual incidence ranged from 719,000 to just over 1 million cases. The CDC estimates the actual number of annual cases to be 1.5 million. The discrepancy between actual and reported cases may occur because gonorrhea is sometimes unreported by health care providers. In addition, infected clients who are asymptomatic do not seek treatment and are therefore not identified. Overall rates declined between 1980 and 1988, with greater rates within some populations. In the late 1980s, the rate of gonorrhea declined in homosexual males. This is thought to have occurred because the impact of HIV infection led to safer sexual practices in this population. However, the lack of decline in incidence within the black and teenage populations and in the number of cases of antibiotic-resistant gonorrhea is cause for concern (CDC, 1990a).

The number of antibiotic-resistant cases of gonorrhea in the United States is rising at an alarming rate, as depicted in Figure 20-2. Penicillin-resistant gonorrhea was first identified in 1976 when 15 cases were reported. By 1990, 64,972 cases were reported (Phillips, 1976; J. Blount, 1991). Although a strain of tetracycline-resistant *N. gonorrhoeae* (TRNG) has also developed, the most common antibiotic-resistant strain of gonorrhea is penicillinase-producing *N. gonorrhoeae* (PPNG). PPNG produces an enzyme called β-lactamase that renders penicillin ineffective in curing gonorrhea. The increase in PPNG infection is partially attributed to the indiscriminate or illicit use of antibiotics as a prophylactic measure by those with multiple sexual partners (Zenilman et al., 1988). To ensure proper treatment and cure, those diagnosed with infection are recommended to return for a rescreening test 1 to 2 months after completing therapy.

The development of *pelvic inflammatory disease (PID)* is a risk for women who remain asymptomatic and do not seek treatment. PID is an infection of the fallopian tubes (salpingitis) and is the most common of all complications of gonorrhea but may also result from chlamydia infection. PID can result in ectopic pregnancy and infertility as a result of fallopian-tube scarring and occlusion. It also may cause stillbirths and premature labor. It has been estimated that the cost of the complications resulting from PID is over $2.5 billion annually (Washington, Arno, and Brooks, 1986). Symptoms of PID include fever, abnormal menses, and lower abdominal pain.

Syphilis

Syphilis is caused by a member of the *Treponeme* genus of spirochetes called *Treponema pallidum.* It infects moist mu-

TABLE 20-3
Summary of sexually transmitted diseases

Disease/pathogen	Incubation	Signs and symptoms	Diagnosis	Treatment
BACTERIAL				
Chlamydia: *Chlamydia trachomatis*	3-21 days	Male: nongonococcal urethritis (NGU); painful urination and urethral discharge; epididymitis Women: none or mucopurulent cervicitis (MPC), vaginal discharge. If untreated, progresses to symptoms of pelvic inflammatory disease (PID) diffuse abdominal pain, fever, chills	Tissue culture; gram stain of endocervical or urethral discharge	Tetracycline, doxycycline, or erythromycin Partner(s) must be examined and treated
Gonorrhea: *Neisseria gonorrhoeae*	3-21 days	Male: urethritis, purulent discharge, painful urination, urinary frequency; epididymitis Female: none or symptoms of PID	Culture of discharge; gram stain of urethral discharge, endocervical, or rectal smear	Ceftriaxone and doxycycline PPNG: spectinomycin or ceftriaxone 3-7 days after completion of treatment, patient must be tested for cure; partners of the last 30-60 days should be contacted for examination and treatment
Syphilis: *Treponema pallidum*	10-90 days	Primary: usually single, painless chancre; if untreated, heals in few weeks	Visualization of pathogen on dark field microscopic examination; single painless ulcer (chancre) FTA-ABS[a] or MHA-TP[b] VDRL[c] (reactive 14 days after appearance of chancre)	Benzathine penicillin G
	6 weeks-6 months	Secondary: low-grade fever, malaise, sore throat, headache, adenopathy, and rash	Clinical signs of secondary syphilis	For those allergic to penicillin, tetracycline hydrochloride (do not administer to pregnant women, those with neurosyphilis or congenital syphilis.)
	Within 1 year of infection	Early latency: asymptomatic, infectious lesions may recur	VDRL; FTA-ABS or MHA-TP	Benzathine penicillin G
	After 1 year from date of infection	Late latency: asymptomatic; noninfectious except to fetus of pregnant women	Lumbar puncture, CSF cell count, protein level determination and VDRL	Counsel to be tested for HIV infection

Continued.

TABLE 20-3
Summary of sexually transmitted diseases – cont'd

Disease/pathogen	Incubation	Signs and symptoms	Diagnosis	Treatment
	Late Active: 2-40 years 2-30 years 10-30 years	Gummas of skin, bone, and mucous membranes, heart, liver CNS involvement: paresis, optic atrophy Cardiovascular involvement: aortic aneurysm, aortic value insufficiency		
Chancroid: *Haemophilus ducreyi*	3-7 days	Small irregular papule progressing to deep ulcer that is painful and drains pus or blood on the penis, labia, or vaginal opening; inguinal tenderness, dysuria	Visual inspection of lesion	Erythromycin or ceftriaxone Partners from past 3 weeks must be examined and treated Condom use; regular pelvic examination of prostitutes
VIRAL				
Genital warts: Human papillomavirus (HPV)	4-6 weeks most common; up to 9 months	Painless lesions near vaginal opening, anus, shaft of penis, vagina, cervix; lesions are textured, cauliflower appearance; may remain unchanged over time.	Visual inspection for lesions; papamicolaou smear; colposcopy	No cure; one third of lesions will disappear without treatment Topical podophyllin or trichloracetic acid; cryotherapy with liquid nitrogen, laser, or surgical removal Partners from past 3 months should be examined Lesions highly contagious; condoms recommended
Genital Herpes: Herpes simplex virus 2 (HSV-2)	2-20 days; average 6 days	Vesicles, painful ulcerations of penis, vagina, labia, perineum, or anus; lesions last 5-6 weeks and recurrence is common; may be asymptomatic	Presence of vesicles; viral culture (obtained only when lesions present and before have scabbed over)	No cure; acyclovir for partial control of signs and symptoms and to accelerate healing; lidocaine jelly as topical anesthetic; Papanicoalaou smear annually; sexual abstinence until 10 days after lesions heal

[a]*FTA-ABS* indicates fluorescent treponemal antibody absorption test.
[b]*MHA-TP* indicates microhemagglutination–*Treponema pallidum*.
[c]*VDRL* indicates Venereal Disease Research Laboratory test for syphilis.

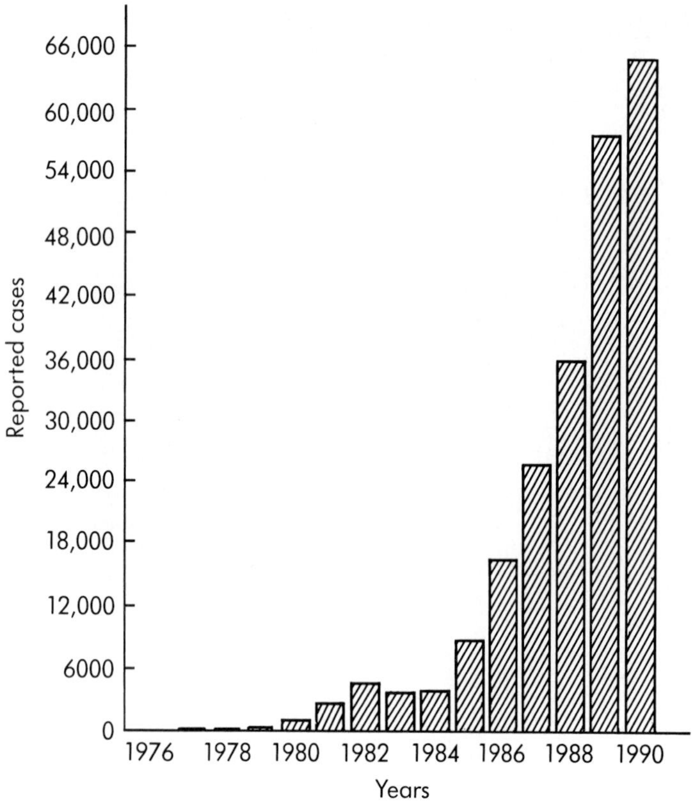

FIGURE 20-2

Total antibiotic resistant strains of gonorrhea, United States, 1976 to 1990. *(Information obtained from Centers for Disease Control, Division of HIV-STD Prevention.)*

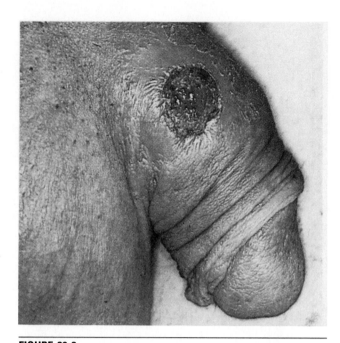

FIGURE 20-3

Primary syphilitic chancre on penile shaft. *(Reprinted with permission from Burroughs-Wellcome Company.)*

cosal or cutaneous lesions and is spread through direct contact, usually by sexual contact or from mother to the fetus in utero. In sexual transmission, microscopic breaks in the skin and mucous membranes that occur during sexual contact create a point of entry for the bacteria.

Syphilis is a reportable disease in the United States, and the number of reported cases has rapidly increased in recent years. The annual incidence rose from 27,883 in 1986 to 40,117 in 1988 (CDC, 1989d). The number of cases in 1988 was the highest in the last 40 years. The highest incidence was in males between the ages of 20 and 24 years who reside in an urban area.

Syphilis is divided into early and late stages. As defined by the U.S. Public Health Service, the early stage consists of the time period during 1 year after infection. The late stage is the time after the first year following infection. The early stage includes primary, secondary, and early latent stages; late syphilis includes late latency and tertiary syphilis. Latency may occur during the early and late phase. During this period there are no clinical signs of infection, but the person has historical or serological evidence of infection. The possibility of relapse remains.

Primary Syphilis

When acquired sexually, the bacteria produces infection in the form of a chancre at the site of entry, as shown in Figure 20-3. The lesion begins as a macule, progresses to a papula, and later ulcerates. If left untreated, this chancre persists for 3 to 6 weeks and then heals spontaneously.

Secondary Syphilis

Secondary syphilis occurs when the organism enters the lymph system and spreads throughout the body. Signs include rash, lymphadenopathy, and mucosal ulceration. Symptoms of secondary syphilis include sore throat, malaise, headaches, weight loss, variable fever, and muscle and joint pain.

Tertiary Syphilis

This phase of the illness may involve the complications of blindness, congenital damage, cardiovascular damage, or syphilitic psychoses. Another potential outcome of tertiary syphilis is the development of lesions of the bones, skin, and mucous membranes, known as gummas. Tertiary syphilis usually occurs several years after initial infection and is rare in the United States because the disease is usually cured in its early stages through the use of antibiotics. Tertiary syphilis does, however, remain a major problem in developing countries.

Congenital Syphilis

Syphilis in pregnancy and congenital syphilis are growing problems. The number of reported cases of congenital syphilis increased more than 500% in New York City from 1986 to 1988 (CDC, 1989e). Syphilis is transmitted transplacentally and if untreated can cause premature stillbirth, blindness, deafness, facial abnormalities, crippling, or death. The current treatment is penicillin. However, close follow-up is necessary because some treatment failure has occurred.

Chlamydia

Chlamydia infection results from the bacteria *Chlamydia trachomatis*. It infects the genitourinary tract and rectum of adults and causes conjunctivitis and pneumonia in neonates. Transmission occurs when mucopurulent discharge from infected sites, such as the cervix or urethra, come into contact with the mucous membranes of a noninfected person. As with gonorrhea, the infection is commonly asymptomatic in women and if left untreated can result in PID. When symptoms of chlamydial infection are present in females, they include dysuria, urinary frequency, and purulent vaginal discharge. In males the urethra is the most common site of infection, resulting in *nongonococcal urethritis (NGU)*. The symptoms of NGU are dysuria and urethral discharge. Epididymitis is a possible complication.

The incidence of chlamydial infection in the United States is currently unknown because it has only recently become a reportable disease in specific states. Based on morbidity reports from STD clinics, the CDC estimates that 3 million cases occur annually (Washington et al., 1985). Risk factors that positively correlate with chlamydial infection include young age and oral contraception use (Winter, Goldy, and Baer, 1990); multiple sexual partners (Handsfield et al., 1986; Addiss et al., 1987); and the presence of gonorrhea (Addiss et al., 1987; Winter et al., 1990). The high frequency of chlamydial infections in individuals infected with gonorrhea requires that effective treatment both for chlamydia and gonorrhea be administered when a gonorrheal infection is identified (CDC, 1989c).

Chancroid

Chancroid is caused by *Haemophilus ducreyi* and is spread from person to person through sexual contact. Chancroid is characterized by a type of ulcer lesion occurring on the penis, labia, or clitoris or at the vaginal orifice. About a week after infection, a small papule develops and soon progresses to a painful, deep ulceration, as shown in Figure 20-4. The infection spreads to the inguinal lymph nodes and causes tenderness. Usually one to two lesions occur, but there may be up to 10.

In the United States, chancroid is a less-frequent cause of genital ulcers than are herpes simplex virus 2 (HSV-2) or syphilis, but it is increasing rapidly. In 1984, 665 cases were reported in the United States, and by 1988, 5001 cases were reported (CDC, 1989d). Although it is not as common as the other reportable STDs in the United States, it is much more prevalent worldwide than gonorrhea and syphilis.

Herpes Simplex Virus 2 (Genital Herpes)

Herpesvirus is a virus that infects genital and nongenital sites. Herpes simplex virus 1 (HSV-1) primarily causes nongenital lesions such as cold sores that may appear on the lip or mouth. Herpes simplex virus 2 (HSV-2) is the primary cause of genital herpes.

There is no cure for HSV-2 infection, and consequently, it is considered a chronic disease. The virus is transmitted through direct exposure and infects the genitalia and surrounding skin. After the initial infection, the virus remains latent in the sacral nerve of the central nervous system and may reactivate periodically with or without visible vesicles.

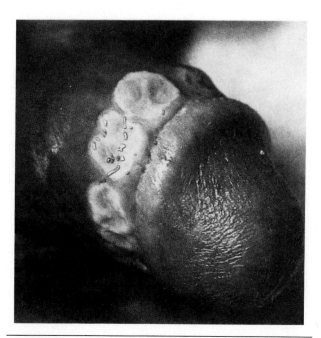

FIGURE 20-4

Chancroid: multiple, punched-out ulcers on penile shaft. *(Reprinted with permission from Burroughs-Wellcome Company.)*

Signs and symptoms of HSV-2 infection include the presence of lesions (Figure 20-5). These lesions begin as vesicles and ulcerate and crust within 1 to 4 days. Lesions may occur on the vulva, vagina, upper thighs, buttocks, and penis and have an average duration of 11 days. The vesicles can cause itching and pain and may be accompanied by dysuria or rectal pain. Although infectivity is higher with active lesions, some individuals can spread the virus even when they are asymptomatic. Approximately 50% of people experience a prodromal phase. This may include a mild, tingling sensation up to 48 hours before eruption or shooting pains in the buttocks, legs, or hips up to 5 days before eruption (Corey, 1990).

The prevalence of HSV-2 is difficult to determine because of the large proportion of subclinical cases and the difficulty in making a diagnosis. Based on one study, HSV-2 infection affects 16.4% of the U.S. population between 15 to 74 years of age, or 25 million persons (Johnson et al., 1989).

The consequences of HSV-2 are of particular concern for women and their children. HSV-2 infection is linked with the development of cervical cancer. There is also an increased risk of spontaneous abortion and risk of transmission to the newborn during vaginal delivery (Puligheddu et al., 1988). A pregnant woman who has active lesions at the time of birth should be advised to deliver by caesarean section before the rupture of amniotic membranes to avoid fetal contact with the herpetic lesions. The mortality rate for infected neonates is estimated to be as high as 60%, and neurological damage is a major complication (Benoit, 1988). The possibility of intrauterine transmission has not been eliminated because some infected neonates are born

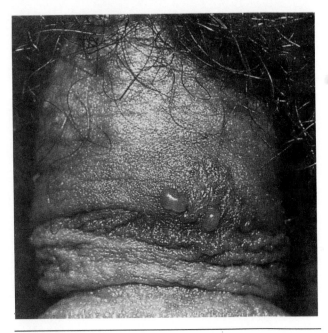

FIGURE 20-5

Herpes simplex lesions. *(Reprinted with permission from Bur-roughs-Wellcome Company.)*

to women who are asymptomatic at delivery or have had no history of genital HSV (Stone et al., 1989).

Genital Warts (Human Papillomavirus Infection)

Human papillomavirus (HPV) can infect the genitalia, anus, and mouth. Transmission of HPV occurs through direct contact with warts that result from HPV. However, HPV has been detected in semen, and exposure to the virus through body fluids is also possible. Genital warts are most commonly found on the penis and scrotum in men and the vulva, labia, vagina, and cervix in women. Figure 20-6 shows the textured surface of the lesions, sometimes described as a cauliflower appearance. The warts are usually multiple and vary between 1 and 5 mm in diameter. They may be difficult to visualize, so careful examination is required.

The prevalence of genital HPV infection is estimated to be between 10% and 20% of American women of child-bearing age, and 5% to 19% of women visiting family planning and university student health clinics (Aral and Holmes, 1990). As with genital herpes, the actual preva-lence is difficult to ascertain because it is not a reported disease and many infections are subclinical.

Complications of HPV infection are especially serious for women. The link between HPV infection and cervical cancer has been established and is estimated to be between 25% and 100% (Koutsky, Galloway, and Holmes, 1988; Reeves, Rawls, and Brinton, 1989). HPV infection is ex-acerbated in both pregnancy and old age as a result of a decrease in cell-mediated immune functioning. HPV may infect the fetus during pregnancy and can result in laryngeal papilloma. Genital warts may enlarge and become friable

during pregnancy, and therefore surgical removal may be recommended.

Because there is no cure for HPV, the goal of therapy is to eliminate the lesions. Genital warts spontaneously dis-appear over time, as do skin warts. However, because the condition is worrisome for the client and HPV may lead to the development of cervical neoplasia, treatment of the le-sions through surgical removal, cytotoxic agents, or im-munotherapies is used.

PREVENTION AND CONTROL OF SEXUALLY TRANSMITTED DISEASES

The community health nurse uses several means to prevent the spread of STDs. These include risk assessment, client education and counseling, partner notification, street out-reach, and education of community groups.

Risk Assessment

Risk assessment for STDs provides an opportunity for the community health nurse to teach about sexuality, assess the client's ability to discuss behaviors, and identify the client's needs. These assessments should not be limited to those clients presenting for care at a STD clinic. Risk assessment should be incorporated into baseline assessment data of those attending all clinics or those who receive school health, occupational health, public health, and home nursing services.

To assess the risk of acquiring STDs, the community health nurse must obtain a sexual and injectable drug-use history for clients and their partner(s). The sexual history provides information about the need for specific diagnostic tests, treatment modalities, and partner notification. It also facilitates evaluation of risk factors and is necessary for the nurse to be able to provide relevant education for the client's lifestyle.

A thorough sexual history should include information about the types of relationships, the number of sexual part-ners and encounters, and types of sexual behaviors prac-ticed. The confidential nature of the information and how it will be used should be shared with the client to establish open communication and a purposeful interaction. Most clients feel uneasy disclosing such personal information. The community health nurse can ease this discomfort by remaining supportive and open during the interview to fa-cilitate honesty about intimate activities. The community health nurse serves as a model in discussing sensitive in-formation in a candid manner by using appropriate words when discussing body parts or sexual behaviors. This en-courages the client to openly discuss sexuality during this interaction and with future partners. When discussing pre-cautions, direct and simple language should be used to de-scribe specific behaviors. Community health nurses who are uncomfortable discussing topics like sexual behavior or sex-ual orientation are likely to avoid assessing risk behaviors with the client. They will, consequently, be ineffective in identification and in assisting the client in modifying risks. It is important that community health nurses become adept at these skills to prevent and control STDs.

Because the chance of exposure decreases as the number of partners decreases, people in mutually monogamous re-lationships are at low risk for acquiring STDs. However,

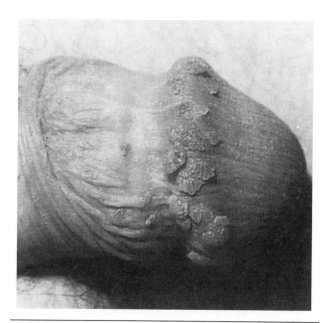

FIGURE 20-6

Genital Warts. *(Reprinted with permission from Burroughs-Well-come Company.)*

the long incubation of HIV and the subclinical phase of many STDs leads some monogamous individuals to erroneously assume that they are not at risk. Identifying the total number of sexual and IDU partners and the number of contacts with these partners provides information about the client's risk. This information can be obtained by asking, "How many sex partners do you have?" It is important to avoid assumptions about the sexual partner(s) based on the client's gender, age, race, or any other factor. Stereotypes of what people are and what they do must not prevent the community health nurse from asking questions. For example, it should not be taken for granted that if a male is homosexual he always has more than one partner.

It is important to identify whether the person has sexual contact with men, women, or both. This information is relevant to sexual practices and risk. Women who are exclusively lesbian are at low risk for acquiring STDs, but bisexual women may transmit STDs between male and female partners. In addition it is possible for men to have sexual contact with other men and not label themselves as homosexual. Therefore, risk reduction education campaigns that are aimed at homosexual males will not be heeded by this group. In such situations, the nurse can ask, "When was the last time you had sex with another male?"

Certain sexual practices are more likely to result in exposure to and transmission of STDs. Dangerous sexual activities include unprotected anal or vaginal intercourse, use of urination in the sexual encounter, oral-anal contact, and insertion of finger or fist into the rectum. These practices introduce high risks of transmission of enteric organisms or result in physical trauma during sexual encounters. The community health nurse can obtain information about sexual encounters by asking, "Can you tell me the kinds of sexual practices in which you engage? This will help to determine

what kind of problems that you may have, the type of tests we should run, and your risk." Clients who engage in genital-anal, oral-anal, or oral-genital contact will need throat and rectal cultures as well as cervical and urethral cultures.

Drug use is linked to STD transmission in several ways. Sexual enhancers, such as alcohol or other drugs, are disinhibitory and put people at risk because they can impair judgement about engaging in risky behaviors. Drugs such as crack cocaine or amyl nitrate can cause an ability to have multiple orgasms. This increases both the frequency of sexual contacts and the chances of contracting STDs. Addiction to a drug may lead to intense craving for the drug and to trading the drug for sexual behaviors. The nurse should obtain information on the type and frequency of drug use and the presence of risk behavior.

Client Education and Counseling for Preventing Sexually Transmitted Diseases

Assessments of clients' risk of acquiring STD should be done with all sexually active individuals. Based on the information obtained in the sexual history and risk assessment, the community health nurse is able to identify specific education and counseling needs of the client.

Sexual abstinence is the best way to prevent STDs. However, for many people, sexual abstinence is undesirable and information about making sexual behavior safer must be taught. Safer sexual activities include masturbation on intact skin, dry kissing, touching, fantasy, and vaginal and oral sex with a condom.

Condom Use

The use of condoms can prevent the exchange of body fluids during sexual activity. If used correctly and consistently, condoms can prevent both pregnancy and STDs. Condoms that contain lubricants with *nonoxynol-9* can inactivate HIV. Although the failure rate of condoms has been estimated to be up to 10%, most agree that condom use should be encouraged (Goldsmith, 1987). This failure rate is related to incorrect use rather than condom failure. Condoms are widely disseminated, but information about their proper use and how to communicate about initiating safer sex practices with a partner is also necessary. The community health nurse has many opportunities to teach groups and counsel individuals on both of these topics. Recommendations about condom use are included in Appendix I2 on Safer Sex Guidelines.

Condom use may be viewed as inconvenient, messy, or decreasing sensation. As a result, many sexually active individuals refrain from using them (Strader and Beaman, 1989). The community health nurse can assist clients to become more skilled in discussing safer sex through role modeling and can suggest that condom application be incorporated as part of foreplay. Table 20-4 describes common reasons for refusing to use condoms and ways clients can encourage partners to use them.

Clients should understand that it is important to know the risk behavior of their sexual partners, including a history of IDU and STDs, bisexuality, and any current symptoms. It is important to stress that, when a sexual encounter takes place, each partner is exposed to all the microorganisms of all the people that the other partner has been intimate with.

TABLE 20-4
Discussing condoms with resistant, defensive, or manipulative partners

Partner response	Rejoinder
YOU DON'T NEED IT	
"I'm on the Pill, you don't need a condom."	"I'd like to use it anyway. It protects us both from infections we may not realize we have."
"I *know* I'm clean (disease free); I haven't had sex with anyone in X months."	"Thanks for telling me. As far as I know, I'm disease free too. But I'd still like to use a condom since either of us could have an infection and not know it."
"I'm a virgin."	"I'm not. This protects us both *and* the relationship."
IT'S A TURN-OFF	
"I can't feel a thing when I wear a condom; it's like wearing a raincoat in the shower."	"I know there is some loss of it, but there's still plenty of sensations left."
"I'll lose my erection by the time I stop and put it on."	"Maybe I can help you put it on—that might give you extra sensations, too."
"By the time you put it on, I'm out of the mood."	"I know it's distracting but what we feel for each other is strong enough to help us stay in the mood."
"It destroys the romantic atmosphere."	"It doesn't have to be that way. It may be a little awkward the first time or two but that will pass."
"It's so messy and smells funny."	"Well, sex is that way. But this way we'll be safe."
"Condoms are unnatural, fake, a total turn-off."	"There's nothing great about genital infections either. Please let's try to work this out—either give the condom a try or let's look for alternatives."
ALTERNATIVES	
"What alternative do you have in mind?"	"Just petting and maybe some manual stimulation. Or we could postpone orgasm, even though I know we both want it."
MANIPULATIVE PLOYS	
"This is an insult! You seem to think I'm some sort of disease-ridden slut or gigolo."	"I didn't say or imply that. I care about us both and about our relationship. In my opinion, it's best to use a condom."
"None of my other boyfriends use a condom. A *real* man is not afraid."	"Please don't compare me to them. A real man cares about the woman he dates, himself, and their relationship."
"You didn't make Jerry use a condom when you went out with him."	"It bothers me that you and Jerry talk about me that way. If you believe everything Jerry says, I won't argue with you."
"I love you! Would I give you an infection?"	"Not intentionally, of course not. But many people don't know they're infected. I feel this is best for both of us at this time."
"Just this once."	"Once is all it takes."
"I don't have a condom with me."	"I do" or "This time, we can satisfy each other without intercourse."
"You carry a condom around with you?! You were planning to seduce me!"	"I always carry one with me because I care about myself. I made sure I had one with me tonight because I care about us both."
"I won't have sex with you if you're going to use a condom."	"Let's put it off then, until we have a chance to work out our differences" or "OK. But can we try some other things besides intercourse?"

Greico A: *Medical Aspects Hum Sex* 21:78, 1987. Reprinted with permission from *Medical Aspects of Human Sexuality* © Cahners Publishing Company. Published March 1987. All rights reserved.

Injectable Drug Use

Injectable drug use is risky because the potential for injecting pathogens exists when needles and syringes are shared. During injectable drug use, small quantities of drugs are repeatedly injected. Blood is withdrawn into the syringe and is then injected back into the user's vein. Individuals should be advised against using injectable drugs and sharing needles, syringes, or other drug paraphernalia. If needles and syringes must be shared, they should be rinsed twice with bleach, then twice with water to prevent injecting bleach.

Partner Notification

Partner notification, also known as contact tracing, is a traditional public health intervention aimed at controlling STDs. It is done by confidentially identifying and notifying exposed sexual and injectable drug-using partners of those found to have reportable STDs. These partners are counseled to seek evaluation and treatment. Partner notification programs usually occur in conjunction with reportable disease requirements and are carried out by most health departments.

Individuals diagnosed with a reportable STD are asked to provide the names and locations of their partners so that they can be informed of their exposure. The identity of the infected client who names sexual and IDU partners cannot be revealed. Maintaining confidentiality is critical with all STDs, but particularly with HIV, because antidiscrimination laws may not be in place or may be inadequate. Clients should be encouraged to notify their partners and to encourage them to seek treatment. If the client agrees to do so, suggestions on how to tell partners and how to deal with possible reactions may be explored. In some instances clients may feel more comfortable if the health department staff notifies those who are exposed. At a minimum, the health department staff contacts health care providers or clinics to verify examination of exposed partners.

The community health nurse is often involved in notifying individuals that they have been exposed to a STD and in counseling them on the reasons why evaluation and treatment are important. Literature regarding treatment, test site location and hours of operation, and risk reduction may be offered. This outreach provides an opportunity to work with those at greatest risk and provides clients with important information.

Street Outreach

Because of the illegal nature of IDU and the poverty associated by many at risk for HIV, many people at risk do not have the inclination or resources to seek health care. Opportunities for counseling on the prevention of HIV and other STDs are increased by bringing services into the neighborhoods of those at risk. Community health nurses may work with communities to establish programs of street outreach. Workers go into communities to disseminate information on safer sex, drug-treatment programs, and discontinuation of drug use or safer drug-use practices (such as cleaning equipment with bleach and water or using new needles and syringes with each injection). Some programs provide sterile needles and syringes, bleach for cleaning needles, condoms, and literature on anonymous test sites. Street outreach is often located near "shooting galleries" or "crack houses" (Liebman et al., 1990).

Education of Community Groups

The dissemination of accurate health information to large numbers of people is vital for preventing the spread of STDs. Community health nurses often provide educational sessions to community groups about HIV and other STDs. Such educational sessions are most effective in settings where groups normally meet and may include schools, businesses, or churches. When addressing groups about HIV infection, it is important to cover the number of people who are diagnosed with AIDS, the number infected, modes of transmission of the virus, how to prevent infection, common symptoms of illness, the need for a compassionate response to those afflicted, and available community resources. Teaching about other STDs can be incorporated into these presentations because the mode of transmission (sexual contact) is the same. Other information on these diseases can include the distribution, incidence, and consequences of the infection for individuals and society.

CLINICAL APPLICATION

The issues surrounding pregnancy when the mother is infected with HIV are profound and complex and require difficult life decisions. As the entire health system begins to deal with the growing number of HIV-infected women who become pregnant, community health nursing care will be increasingly directed toward providing adequate care and counseling to these women and their families.

Consider the case of Sandra Smith, a 26-year-old woman who visits the Madison County Health Department maternity clinic. Sandra is examined and found to be at 10 weeks of gestation. She is married and has been in a mutually monogamous relationship for the past 2 years. She states that she and her husband have no other children but have been saving money over the past year because they have been planning to start a family. When interviewing Sandra to gather baseline assessment data, the nurse finds that, in the past, Sandra has injected heroin and cocaine. Sandra denies current use and reports that she stopped using drugs 3 years ago, but that she did share drug paraphernalia with others. Sandra's husband, Phil, is aware of Sandra's drug use, but he has never used intravenous drugs.

The nurse evaluates Sandra's understanding of IDU as a risk behavior for HIV infection and the effect of HIV on pregnancy. Sandra is aware that sharing needles is one way that people get AIDS, but thinks that because she has not had symptoms, she is not sick; therefore she is not worried. The nurse explains the difference between symptomatic and asymptomatic HIV infection and the incubation period for HIV.

The nurse shares information about the HIV antibody test and explains some of the reasons that Sandra might choose to have the test. Specifically, the nurse reviews the effect of HIV on the fetus and the mother. She explains that transmission to the fetus is possible during the pregnancy and that if infected, the mother has a greater chance of progressing from asymptomatic infection to symptomatic HIV disease. With knowledge of her HIV antibody status, Sandra can make informed decisions about her health and her pregnancy and can decide whether she wishes to continue the pregnancy, given the risk to the infant and herself. After this discussion, the nurse and Sandra explore sources of HIV antibody testing.

The nurse evaluates Sandra's comfort in sharing the information with Phil and explores what Sandra thinks Phil's response might be. Sandra states that she thinks it throws a complication into an otherwise happy situation, but since she does not think that the test will be positive, it will not be hard to tell Phil about it. The nurse encourages that, although it is hard to imagine the possibility of a positive result, Sandra should think about it to prepare herself and her husband in case it is positive. The nurse offers to role play the situation of Sandra telling Phil about the possibility of infection, its risks, and the importance of testing for both of them.

The nurse closes the interview by stating that she realizes that they have covered a lot of information and that Sandra may have questions after she leaves; the nurse gives her a telephone number where she can be reached if she needs more information. Although it will take time for Sandra and her husband to think about the possibilities and options, it is important that they both consider returning to the clinic for an HIV antibody test at the next testing clinic so that enough time is left for the test results to return and various options to be explored early in the pregnancy. Even if Phil is not ready to have the test immediately, it is crucial for Sandra to know about her health, her ability to bear a child, and both their abilities to raise a child.

Sandra and Phil return to the health department to have the test. During pretest counseling, information is shared about the test. The implications of a positive test result, the persons or agencies to whom the results will be given, and the information that results reveal only whether one is infected and not whether one has AIDS are discussed. In the event that one or both of them have positive results, infection-control practices related to the risk factor, IDU, and implications for other routes of transmission are briefly reviewed. They are asked about how they will cope if a test result is positive and if they have thought about how they will feel. The nurse explores past crises in their lives and how they have coped with these situations that arose. They state that they have discussed the possibility of one or both of them being infected with HIV and that they feel they can handle it because it is important to find out the information.

When the Smiths return for the test results, they are counseled individually about the findings. Sandra's HIV antibody test result is positive and Phil's is negative. Information is gathered from Sandra about past IDU and sexual partners. Rather than contacting these individuals herself, she requests that health department staff contact them about possible contact with HIV.

Sandra initially reacts with a feeling of disbelief about the test results. Understanding that this is a common reaction initially, the nurse schedules a second appointment for follow-up counseling 1 week after the initial test results are given. She also gives Sandra the telephone number of the local AIDS-support group.

The need to continue prenatal care through the health department and to seek on-going care to monitor the HIV infection and the decision of whether or not to continue the pregnancy are the most immediate concerns for the couple. The nurse discusses the meaning of the test results with the Smiths and how it may affect the infant's and mother's health. The nurse evaluates whether Sandra has a primary health care provider, provides a list of providers, and stresses the importance of establishing an ongoing relationship with a primary health care provider for follow-up of the HIV

infection. She tells them that important information about Sandra's health may be identified that will help to determine her ability to carry and deliver the baby if she chooses to continue with the pregnancy. The nurse explores possibilities with Sandra and Phil about the decision regarding their ability to physically, emotionally, and financially cope with rearing a child that possibly may be ill. Family members and other potential resources are explored with the couple. The nurse telephones the Smiths the day after the test results are given to offer support and information if needed.

At the follow-up visit 1 week later, information is given regarding infection control in the home, safer sexual relations, and the need to tell health care providers or blood handlers about the HIV infection. The nurse ensures that Sandra is taking steps toward receiving prenatal care and medical care for the HIV infection. Sandra and Phil decide to continue the pregnancy and risk the chance of illness for the mother and baby. The nurse reviews information about how to maintain health and avoid stressors and contracts with Sandra to initiate home visits to provide reinforcement of adequate prenatal nutrition and teaching and to assess Sandra's physical health as the pregnancy progresses.

SUMMARY

Sexually transmitted diseases are having an increasing impact on individuals, families, and society. Not only is the number of persons infected with STDs increasing, but there is difficulty in reaching the groups most at risk to promote positive behavior changes. STDs may be subclinical in their presentation, may be expensive to diagnose, or may have no cure. Thus, STDs are a challenging health problem. Social and economic costs are expected to climb as a result of the chronic nature of some STDs and their association with some forms of cancers and neonatal morbidity and mortality.

Despite all of the difficulties associated with STDs they result mostly from behaviors that can be changed. Given this challenge, community health nurses must use skills for assessing risk and preventing and controlling STDs. Community health nurses have many opportunities in their practice to identify risks and explore ways with individuals and groups of all ages to reduce these risks. Community health nurses can influence how others respond to those infected with HIV by disseminating accurate, current information about HIV to community groups and by modeling appropriate behavior toward those infected.

KEY CONCEPTS

Nearly all sexually transmitted diseases are preventable because they are transmitted through specific, known behaviors.

Sexually transmitted diseases are one of the most serious public health problems in the United States. HIV infection has been identified as the most urgent public health problem of this century, and increases are occurring in the incidence of syphilis, drug-resistant gonococcal infection, chancroid and chlamydial infections.

Sexually transmitted diseases affect certain groups in greater numbers. Factors associated with risk include being under 25 years of age, being a member of a minority group, residing in an urban setting, being impoverished, and using crack cocaine.

The increasing incidence, morbidity, and mortality of sexually transmitted diseases documents the need for community health nurses to become actively involved in counseling about sexually transmitted disease prevention.

Aside from death, the most serious complications caused by sexually transmitted diseases are pelvic inflammatory disease, infertility, ectopic pregnancy, neonatal morbidity and mortality, and neoplasia.

Several sexually transmitted diseases, including genital warts, HIV, and genital herpes are associated with cancer.

AIDS is the most extreme stage of HIV infection. As more is learned about methods to prevent disease progression, such as antiretroviral therapy, stress reduction, and proper nutrition, more emphasis is being placed on the early recognition and management of HIV infection.

HIV testing plays an important role in early detection and treatment and provides opportunities for risk assessment and preventive counseling. However, individuals must seriously consider the psychological and social consequences of a positive test result before having the test.— Why?

Partner notification, also known as contact tracing, may be done by the infected client or by the health professional. It is done by identifying, contacting, and encouraging evaluation and treatment of sexual and injectable drug using partners.

AIDS has created an entirely new group of people needing health care. This rapidly growing population is causing strain on a health care system that is already unable to meet the needs of many.

Most of the care that is provided, both home and outpatient care, is done within the community setting, which reduces direct health care costs but increases the need for financial-support of home and community health services.

LEARNING ACTIVITIES

1. Identify the number of reported cases of AIDS and the number of reported cases of HIV infection (if reportable in your state) within your state and locale. How are the cases distributed by age, sex, geographic location, and race?

2. Identify the location(s) of HIV-testing services and whether the test results are anonymous or confidential. Describe how and to whom the results are reported.

3. Identify counseling and home care services that are available for the person with HIV infection within your community.

4. Form small groups and role play a nurse-client interaction involving a risk assessment and counseling regarding safer sex and injectable drug-use practices.

BIBLIOGRAPHY

Addiss DG et al.: Selective screening for *Chlamydia trachomatis* infection in nonurban family planning clinics in Wisconsin, Fam Plann Perspect 19(6):252, 1987.

Aral SO and Holmes KK: Epidemiology of sexual behavior and sexually transmitted diseases. In Holmes KK et al., editors: Sexually transmitted diseases, New York, 1990, McGraw Hill.

Barnes R and Holmes KK: Epidemiology of gonorrhea: current perspectives, Epidemiol Rev 6:1, 1984.

Benoit JA: Sexually transmitted diseases in pregnancy, Nurs Clin North Am 23(4):937, 1989.

Blount J: Personal communication, January 18, 1991.

Cannon RO et al.: Human immunodeficiency virus seroprevalence in persons attending STD clinics in the United States, 1985-1987, Sex Transm Dis 16(4):184.

Cates W: Epidemiology and control of sexually transmitted diseases: strategic evolution, Infect Dis Clin North Am 1(1):1, 1987.

Centers for Disease Control: Education and foster care of children infected with human t-lymphotropic virus type III/lymphadenopathy-associated virus, MMWR 34:517, 1985.

Centers for Disease Control: Revision of the CDC surveillance case definition for acquired immunodeficiency syndrome, MMWR 36(1S):3s, 1987.

Centers for Disease Control: AIDS and human immunodeficiency virus infection in the United States: 1988 update, MMWR 38(S4):1, 1989a.

Centers for Disease Control: First 100,000 cases of acquired immunodeficiency syndrome: United States, MMWR 38(32):561, 1989b.

Centers for Disease Control: 1989 sexually transmitted diseases treatment guidelines, MMWR 38(S8):1, 1989c.

Centers for Disease Control: Summary of notifiable diseases: United States—1988, MMWR 37(54):3, 1989d.

Centers for Disease Control: Congenital syphilis: New York City—1986-1988, MMWR 38(48):825, 1989e.

Centers for Disease Control: Progress toward achieving the 1990 objectives for the nation for sexually transmitted diseases, MMWR 39(4):53, 1990a.

Centers for Disease Control: Update: acquired immunodeficiency syndrome United States—1989, MMWR 39(5):81, 1990b.

Centers for Disease Control: Estimates of HIV prevalence and projected AIDS cases: summary of a workshop, MMWR 39(7):110, 1990c.

Centers for Disease Control: HIV/AIDS surveillance report, 1990.

Corey L: Genital herpes. In Holmes KK et al., editors: Sexually transmitted diseases, New York, 1990, McGraw Hill.

Cumming PD et al.: Exposure of patients to human immunodeficiency virus through the transfusion of blood components that test antibody-negative, N Engl J Med 321(14):941, 1989.

Friedland GH and Klein RS: Transmission of the human immunodeficiency virus, N Engl J Med 317(18):1125, 1987.

Goldsmith MF: Sex in the age of AIDS calls for common sense and "condom sense," JAMA 257(17):2261, 1987.

Grossman M: Pediatric AIDS. In Corless JB and Pittman-Lindeman M, editors: AIDS: principles, practices and politics, New York, 1989, Hemisphere Publishing.

Hahn RA et al.: Prevalence of HIV infection among intravenous drug users in the US, JAMA 261(18):2677, 1989.

Hale PJ: Employer response to AIDS in a low prevalence area, Fam Community Health 13(2):38, 1990.

Handsfield HH et al.: Criteria for selective screening for *Chlamydia trachomatis* infection in women attending family planning clinics, JAMA 255(13):1730, 1986.

Hellinger FJ: Updated forecasts of the costs of medical care for persons with AIDS: 1989–93, Public Health Rep 105(1):1, 1990.

Hook E and Handsfield H: Gonococcal infections in the adult. In Holmes KK et al., editors: Sexually transmitted diseases, New York, 1990, McGraw Hill.

Institute of Medicine National Academy of Sciences: Confronting AIDS: update 1988, Washington, DC, 1988, National Academy Press.

Johnson R et al.: A seroepidemiologic survey of the prevalence of herpes simplex virus type 2 infection in the United States, N Engl J Med 321(1):7, 1989.

Kelley et al.: Human immunodeficiency virus seropositivity among members of the active duty US army, 1985–1989, Am J Public Health 80(4):405, 1990.

Kessler HA et al.: Diagnosis of human immunodeficiency virus infection in seronegative homosexuals presenting with an acute viral syndrome, JAMA 258(9):1196, 1987.

Kilbourne BW, Buehler JW, and Rogers MF: AIDS as a cause of death in children, adolescents, and young adults, Am J Public Health 80(4):499, 1990.

Koutsky L, Galloway D, and Holmes K: Epidemiology of genital human papillomavirus infection, Epidemiol Rev 10:122, 1988.

Lemp GF et al.: Survival trends for patients with AIDS, JAMA 263(3):402, 1990.

Lemp GF et al.: Projects of AIDS morbidity and mortality in San Francisco. JAMA 263(11):1497, 1990.

Liebman J et al.: AIDS prevention for IV drug users and their sexual partners in Philadelphia, Am J Public Health 80(5):615, 1990.

McEvoy BF and Le Furgy WG: A 13 year longitudinal analysis of risk factors and clinic visitation patterns of patients with repeated gonorrhea, Sex Transm Dis 15(1):40, 1988.

Moran JS et al.: The impact of sexually transmitted diseases on minority populations, Public Health Rep 104(6):560, 1989.

Phillips I: Beta-lactamase producing, penicillin-resistant gonococcus, Lancet ii:656, 1976.

Puligheddu P et al.: HSV-2 and cervical intraepithelial neoplasia: cytological, histological and serological features, Clin Obstet Gynecol 15(3):88, 1988.

Quinn R, O'Reilly K, and Khaw M: Gonococcal infections in women attending the venereal disease clinic of the Nashville Davidson County Metropolitan Health Department: 1984, South Med J 81(7):851, 1988.

Reeves W, Rawls W, and Brinton L: Epidemiology of genital papillomaviruses and cervical cancer, Rev Infect Dis 11(2):426, 1989.

Stone K et al.: National surveillance for neonatal herpes simplex virus infections, Sex Transm Dis 16(3):152, 1989.

Strader MK and Beaman ML: College students' knowledge about AIDS and attitudes toward condom use, Public Health Nurs 6(2):62, 1989.

Washington AE et al.: Oral contraceptives, *Chlamydia trachomatis* infection, and pelvic inflammatory disease, JAMA 253(15):2246, 1985.

Washington AE, Arno PS, and Brooks MA: The economic cost of pelvic inflammatory disease, JAMA 255(13):1735, 1986.

Winter L, Goldy S, and Baer C: Prevalence and epidemiologic correlates of *Chlamydia trachomatis* in rural and urban populations, Sex Transm Dis 17(1):30, 1990.

Wolinsky SM et al.: Human immunodeficiency virus type 1 (HIV-1) infection a median of 18 months before a diagnostic Western blot, Ann Intern Med 111(12):961, 1989.

World Health Organization–International Council of Nurses: Guidelines for nursing management of people infected with HIV, (pamphlet), Geneva, 1988, WHO.

Zenilman J et al.: Penicillinase-producing *Neisseria gonorrhoea* in Dade County, Florida: evidence of core-group transmitters and the impact of illicit antibiotics, Sex Transm Dis 15(1):45, 1988.

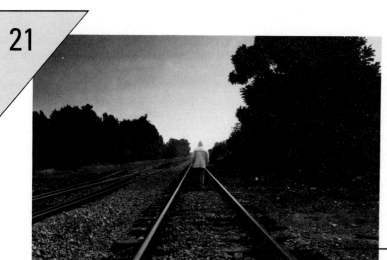

21

Community Mental Health: Problem Identification and Treatment

Diane E. Boyer

Irma Heppner

OBJECTIVES

After reading this chapter, the student should be able to:

Briefly summarize the development of community mental health as a system of care.

Discuss legislation leading to the establishment and continuation of community mental health centers.

Discuss the impact of *Action for Mental Health*.

Evaluate deinstitutionalization as a viable mechanism for caring for seriously ill psychiatric patients.

Discuss case management as a system of treatment for the seriously mentally ill patients in the community.

Explain psychosocial rehabilitation as a treatment modality in community mental health.

Identify how the consumer movement and family movement have influenced client rights and the improvement of community mental health services.

Describe the mental health nurse's role in the community support system.

Identify the needs of different high-risk populations served by the community mental health nurse.

Discuss why nurses are uniquely prepared to work in the field of community mental health.

KEY TERMS

case management
catchment area
community support system
deinstitutionalization
dual diagnosis
homelessness

International Association of Psychosocial Rehabilitation Services (IAPSRS)
least restrictive alternative
primary consumer
secondary consumer
mental illness

National Alliance for the Mentally Ill (NAMI)
National Institute for Mental Health (NIMH)
psychosocial rehabilitation
psychotropic medication
serious mentally ill

T he problems of clients with mental health needs are often complicated, resulting from the interaction of many factors, including heredity, living conditions, social and economic constraints, and family relations. People suffering from mental illness often remain in or return to the community following treatment. Therefore community health nurses must have skills both in assessing the presence of mental health problems and developing treatment plans based on the resources available in the community. The nurse must also be able to implement and evaluate these plans. To work effectively in the community mental health field, the nurse must gain knowledge in treatment modalities of mental illness including counseling techniques, medication, and psychosocial rehabilitation. The nurse must also understand how mental health services are typically organized and the history of their development. Their organization includes the community support-systems model and case management. It is also important for the community mental health nurse to understand major factors working against the advancement of community mental health on a local, state, and national level. This chapter focuses on the development of community mental health care and the evolution of the community mental health nurse. Also discussed are high-risk populations served by the community mental health nurse.

DEVELOPMENT OF COMMUNITY MENTAL HEALTH AS A SYSTEM OF CARE

Community mental health is generally implemented through comprehensive community mental health centers. It is considered the fourth revolutionary development in the field of psychiatry. The first revolution occurred in 1793 when physician Phillips Pinel removed the chains from mentally ill patients confined in Bicetre, a hospital outside Paris. The second revolution occurred with the inception of Freudian psychoanalytic treatment about 100 years after Pinel. The advancement of psychotropic drugs began the third revolution and opened the door for the birth of community mental health treatment.

Community mental health is all-encompassing, focusing on helping the individual, the family, and the community to interact in more adaptive ways so that the best adjustment possible is achieved and maintained.

Humanitarian Reform in Mental Health

Before 1840 people deemed to be mentally ill were sent to jails, asylums, or country homes. These forms of removal of afflicted people protected them from harming others and being harmed. It also provided them with food and shelter. Treatment was unheard of for what was considered an incurable affliction.

Benjamin Rush, often called the "father of American psychiatry," led the movement for humane treatment of mentally ill people. Although instrumental in introducing a humanitarian way of thinking into psychiatry, he continued to use remedies such as bloodletting, purgatives, and a torturelike device known as the "tranquilizer."

The work begun by Rush was carried on enthusiastically by a former schoolteacher, Dorothea Dix. In 1841 Dix appointed herself inspector of institutions for the mentally ill.

Traveling across the United States, she crusaded for enlightened treatment for patients. Dix insisted that each state assume the financial and caretaking responsibility for its own residents. Her exhaustive efforts on behalf of mental health led to the establishment of 32 mental hospitals in the United States. Most of the hospitals were built in rural areas to give the patients the benefit of fresh air and to keep them isolated from a society that feared them.

As the population of the United States grew, so did the number of hospitals. In 1900, however, the building of new hospitals virtually came to a halt. Existing facilities soon became overcrowded and deplorable conditions became the standard. The care of mentally ill people in the United States continued to deteriorate until Adolf Meyer took up Dix's crusade. Meyer was the first person to describe and campaign for community mental health. He proposed that a clinic for the mentally ill be established in communities so that certain population groups could be studied and treated.

The mental health movement received a major boost in 1908 from the publication of Clifford Beers' book, entitled *A Mind That Found Itself*. In this book, Beers graphically recounted his experiences as a psychiatric patient and urged reform and public education for mental health (Pickett and Hanlon, 1990). He is credited with establishing the Connecticut Society for Mental Hygiene, whose purpose was to combat ignorance about the cause and nature of mental illness. In 1909 the National Committee for Mental Hygiene was organized. This organization was a forerunner of the National Association for Mental Health.

In the following decade, 19 state mental hygiene societies in the United States and 16 societies in other nations were organized. The International Congress for Mental Hygiene was established in 1922, and in 1930 the first International Mental Hygiene Congress was held in Washington, D.C. (Pickett and Hanlon, 1990).

Governmental Involvement in Mental Health

The federal government first became involved in the financing of mental health services with the 1935 passage of the Social Security Act. This shift in responsibility from the state to the federal government was based on the notion that, if local communities could not care for their ill people, then the federal government should undertake this responsibility. The impact of World War II on community mental health was unprecedented; 875,000 of 15 million draftees, or almost 6%, were rejected from military service because of existing mental illness (Snow and Newton, 1976).

The government's role in mental health care expanded significantly after the war. In 1946 Congress enacted the National Mental Health Act, making grants available to states to develop programs outside of state hospitals. This legislation sought to apply a community health approach to the treatment of mentally ill people. In reality, individual psychotherapy based on a medical model was the primary mode of treatment used (Ramshorn, 1971). The act did establish the National Institute of Mental Health (NIMH) in 1949 and designated it as the agency responsible for mental health in the United States. Two important types of treatment facilities came into existence in the 1940s—outpatient clinics and psychiatric units in general hospitals.

The next major piece of legislation to affect mental health was the creation of the Joint Commission on Mental Health in 1955 (Snow and Newton, 1976). This commission consisted of representatives of 36 organizations and agencies chosen by the NIMH. In 1961, 5 years after its inception, the Joint Commission submitted its report to Congress. This historical document, entitled *Action for Mental Health,* emphasized the need for better training of personnel, providing early and intensive treatment for the acutely ill, and carrying out research activities. The report also recommended developing additional facilities, including units in general hospitals and clinics and programs for aftercare, rehabilitation, and mental health education (Joint Commission, 1961).

Following the publication of this report, President John F. Kennedy appointed a cabinet-level committee to review the report and make recommendations for federal action. In 1963, Kennedy made the first presidential address on behalf of the mentally ill and called for a "bold new approach" to maintain and return patients to their local community. These actions culminated in the concept of community mental health centers (Rubin, 1971).

Deinstitutionalization

In the 1960s large numbers of mentally ill people were moved out of psychiatric hospitals all over the country in an effort to improve the quality of life of the mentally ill in their home communities. It was thought that treating them in their natural environment, surrounded by their families and nonmentally ill people would help to create a more "normal" life for them. Many large hospital wards were closed, and the clients were sent to a variety of homes in the communities. Many were sent to live in adult homes, in supervised apartments, with families or relatives, and in nursing homes. Although placements were found for them, they generally lacked the supportive resources in the community to be able to function there. The result has been a decreased quality of life for many people. Many are now actually homeless, living on streets and in shelters.

One reason deinstitutionalization has not succeeded as hoped is that the community resources necessary to provide a quality life for the mentally ill in the community have not been in place. The funds have not been available to create them, and knowledge on how to care for the mentally ill in the community has been scant, at best. Meanwhile, the mentally ill still live in communities without the supports and treatments that they need. Slowly, the models and concepts are being developed to respond to this tremendous need.

Legislation for Community Mental Health

Community mental health centers became a reality on October 31, 1963, when Congress enacted Public Law 88-164, the Mental Retardation Facilities and Community Mental Health Centers Construction Act of 1963. This act sought to provide comprehensive mental health services to all residents in a specific catchment area. A catchment area is a designated service area for a community mental health center and usually consists of 75,000 to 200,000 people. Besides providing five essential services to qualify for funding, centers were encouraged to implement five additional ser-

---

ESSENTIAL AND SUPPLEMENTARY SERVICES OF COMMUNITY MENTAL HEALTH CENTERS AS SPECIFIED IN FEDERAL LEGISLATION

ESSENTIAL SERVICES

Inpatient care for patients requiring short-term hospitalization

Partial hospitalization, including day and night care

Outpatient treatment

Emergency services on a 24-hour basis

Consultation and education for members of the community

SUPPLEMENTARY SERVICES

Diagnostic services including the making of treatment recommendations

Rehabilitation services and vocational counseling

Precare and aftercare services

Training for all kinds of personnel

Research and evaluation

From Landsberg G and Hammer R: Community Ment Health J 13:63, 1977.

---

vices. Both the essential and supplementary services are listed in the box on this page.

In 1964 Congress established Public Law 89-105, providing the "seed money" concept of financing centers based on a declining formula of federal support over a 51-month period. The original legislation envisioned that funding would be provided to centers to enable them to get started, at which time federal funds would decrease as state and local funds increased. This plan did not work in many areas because state and local funds rarely increased sufficiently to take over much of the federal portion.

In 1974 the NIMH began to formally address the needs of the mentally ill in the community. The NIMH began studying the problems resulting from deinstitutionalization with the goal of developing a recommendation for community mental health services. They solicited input from a variety of sources, including consumers, family members, and mental health professionals. The result of this study was the concept of the community support system (CSS). A CSS is defined as "an organized network of caring and responsible people committed to assisting persons with long-term mental illness to meet their needs and develop their potential without being unnecessarily isolated or excluded from the community" (NIMH, 1980).

The philosophy behind the CSS concept is consistent with the thinking that began the deinstitutionalization movement. It definitely values community-based treatment and uses the hospital only for short-term evaluation and stabilization. This system emphasizes maintaining the dignity and respect of individuals, giving them the same rights and opportunities as any other citizens. It creates opportunities for individuals to grow, improve, and move towards independence in a way that is not possible with lifelong hospitalization.

In 1975 Congress overrode a presidential veto to pass the Community Mental Health Centers Amendments of 1975 (PL 94-63). These amendments provided a more stable source of funding for centers, made available distress grants, and extended the funding cycle to a maximum of 12 years. The amendments also provided grants for specialty areas, including child care, aging, court screening, care for discharged mentally ill people, transitional services, and substance abuse. These amendments have been severely criticized because of their lack of flexibility and limited responsiveness to the unique needs of individual communities (Citizens Guide, 1977).

The 1977 report of the President's Commission on Mental Health recommended strengthening the community mental health system and again extended funding. The 117 recommendations of the report were divided into eight sections: community support systems, service delivery, financing, personnel, patients' rights, research, prevention, and public understanding. The main thrust of the recommendations was to establish a new federal grant program for community mental health services that were inadequate and to increase the flexibility of communities in planning a comprehensive network of services. In general, the report called for many of the same priority areas as mentioned in the original legislation of the 1960s (President's Commission, 1978).

Following publication of the President's Commission on Mental Health report, legislation passed in 1980 emphasized the need for communities to be flexible in planning services to meet their unique needs. This legislation gave states greater authority over mental health funds and allowed for flexible and innovative program planning and development. It also emphasized prevention and the development of new approaches to meet the mental health needs of priority populations. Linkages were also supported among agencies to reduce duplication (Nation's Health, 1981).

Despite financial difficulties, the community mental health movement continued to improve services for mentally ill clients. For example, in 1985 the Robert Wood Johnson Foundation, in collaboration with the U.S. Department of Housing and Urban Development, announced a $100 million program for community-wide projects. These projects were aimed at consolidating and expanding services for the long-term mentally ill. As part of the program, the Social Security Administration (SSA) brought SSA workers into mental health settings to help grantees improve the disability determination process. The program has funded projects in eight of the 60 largest urban centers, and it has allowed for the development of community mental health authorities. It has also funded projects that provide a wide spectrum of services including health services, social services, and housing for large mentally ill populations that did not have access to these services (Mechanic, 1986).

Recently, federal law has mandated "case management" services for all individuals with serious mental illness who receive public funds. Individual states are struggling to include some version of case management in their individual mental health programs and legislation. The practical application of case management principles varies in each locality. Efforts are consistently being made to move to a case management model of community care of mentally ill individuals.

Caution from the government has not hindered the advancement of mental health public policy. In 1986 a federal law was passed entitled the Protection and Advocacy for Mentally Ill Individuals Act of 1986. It was passed because it was found that mentally ill individuals were "vulnerable to abuse and serious injury" and that they were "subject to neglect, including lack of treatment, adequate nutrition, clothing, health care, and adequate discharge planning." Furthermore, state systems varied widely and frequently were inadequate. The purposes of the Act were to ensure the protection of the rights of the mentally ill and to assist states in establishing and operating a protection and advocacy system for mentally ill individuals. It included a Bill of Rights for Mentally Ill Patients (see box on p. 355).

Consumer Involvement

Consumer empowerment is a goal of the CSS concept and has become a goal for the consumer movement (Chamberlin, 1989). The rights, wishes, and needs of primary and secondary consumers are paramount in planning and delivering services. Primary consumers are persons who are current or former recipients of mental health services. Secondary consumers include family members and other significant persons in the life of a primary consumer (Chamberlin, 1989). As in other areas of medical treatment, the consumers of the services are now recognizing their right to information about their illnesses, the options for treatment, and the side effects of treatments. They are claiming their right to have a say in decisions regarding their treatment.

Whereas this phenomenon is not particularly remarkable in society at large, it is very significant for the mentally ill individual. The passivity established in many long-term institutionalized clients, together with the deficits experienced because of the illness itself, have resulted in dysfunctional, disempowered individuals. On the other hand, consumer empowerment can mean a new sense of self-respect, hope, self-determination, and competence. Collectively, it means their voice is heard in planning, policy-making, and service-delivery areas (Chamberlin, 1989).

The consumer movement has received funding from the NIMH for consumer organizing activities. This includes the National Ex-Patient Teleconference, the National Mental Health Consumer Self-Help Clearinghouse, and the anual consumer conference, Alternatives, held in a different state each year (Chamberlin, 1989).

The National Alliance for Mental Patients (NAMP) and the National Mental Health Consumers' Association (NMHCA) are national consumer organizations that were formed in 1985. Both share the goals of promoting mutual support, empowerment, and advocacy. The International Association of Psychosocial Rehabilitation Services (IAPSRS) is made up of consumers and providers. It was organized in 1975 to promote psychosocial rehabilitation and provide a forum for the exchange of views and experiences. It holds an annual conference and has continued to gain respect in several countries because of its successful accomplishments in the field.

The goal of many consumer groups is to change the existing mental health system to be more responsive to consumers. They continue to struggle for basic civil rights, to stop unjust and oppressive treatment, to have a voice in their own treatment, and to end victimization and discrimination in such areas as housing and employment. The con-

A BILL OF RIGHTS FOR MENTALLY ILL PATIENTS

Federal law now includes a Bill of Rights for persons receiving mental health treatment services.

Title V. Section 501 of the Mental Health Systems Act, 42 U.S.C. 9501, for the first time defines in United States law a Bill of Rights for mentally ill patients.

Each State should review and revise its laws to ensure that mental patients receive the protection and services they require. A person admitted to a program or facility for the purpose of receiving mental health services should be accorded the following:

The right to treatment and services under conditions that support the person's personal liberty and restrict such liberty only as necessary to comply with treatment needs, law, and judicial orders.

The right to an individualized, written, treatment or service plan (to be developed promptly after admission), treatment based on the plan, periodic review and reassessment of needs, and appropriate revisions of the plan, including a description of services that may be needed after discharge.

The right to ongoing participation in the planning of services to be provided and in the development and periodic revision of the treatment plan, and the right to be provided with a reasonable explanation of all aspects of one's own condition and treatment.

The right to refuse treatment, except during an emergency situation, or as permitted under law in the case of a person committed by a court for treatment.

The right not to participate in experimentation in the absence of the patient's informed, voluntary, written consent; the right to appropriate protections associated with such participation; the right and opportunity to revoke such consent.

The right to freedom from restraint or seclusion, other than during an emergency situation.

The right to a humane treatment environment that affords reasonable protection from harm and appropriate privacy.

The right to confidentiality of records.

The right of access, upon request, to one's own mental health care records.

The right (in residential or inpatient care) to converse with others privately and to have access to the telephone and mails, unless denial of access is documented as necessary for treatment.

The right to be informed promptly, in appropriate language and terms, of the rights described in this section.

The right to assert grievances with respect to infringement of this Bill of Rights, including the right to have such grievances considered in a fair, timely, and impartial procedure.

The right of access to a protection service and a qualified advocate in order to understand, exercise, and protect one's rights.

The right to exercise the rights described in this section without reprisal—including reprisal in the form of denial of any appropriate, available treatment.

The right to referral, as appropriate, to other providers of mental health services upon discharge.

From Miller R and Fiddleman P: Hosp Commun Psychiatr 35(2):147, 1984.

sumer movement is also dedicated to fighting the stigma of mental illness. One such effort has been fighting the use of disempowering labels. Hence the term *chronically mentally ill* became *long-term mentally ill* and ultimately the *seriously mentally ill*.

Families of the mentally ill have also made great strides in the last two decades. No longer does one encounter the helpless, disempowered, guilt-ridden parent with no resources or supports. In the United States, families of the mentally ill have found and empowered one another. They eventually formed a nationwide organization known as the National Alliance for the Mentally Ill (NAMI), with state and local chapters throughout the country. This group evolved as a self-help and advocacy group. It has presented a major force for legislative changes on a state and national level and for programmatic changes locally.

The self-help aspect of these groups has provided a forum for family members to tell their stories and to elicit support and advice. Many families have been frustrated and helpless regarding their specific situations. The advocacy and lob-

bying aspects of these groups have provided an avenue for families to channel their energies into positive, constructive efforts to improve the lot for the mentally ill. As a result, families are becoming better equipped to press for involvement in service delivery in appropriate ways and to establish collaborative relationships with the health care providers serving their relatives (Chamberlin, 1989).

Psychosocial Rehabilitation

One important aspect of the CSS concept is psychosocial rehabilitation. The goals of rehabilitation are to build the skills and access the supports for the client to function as actively and independently as possible (Stroul, 1989). Psychosocial rehabilitation emerged as the prevailing 1980s ideology of treatment of long-term mental illness. The focus of psychosocial rehabilitation is to assure that individuals with psychiatric disabilities can perform the physical, emotional, social, and intellectual skills needed to live, learn, and work in the community with the least amount of support possible from professional care providers. Interventions derived from this framework involve teaching of necessary skills essential for strengthening and supporting present functional levels (Anthony and Lieberman, 1986). These services are provided by psychosocial rehabilitation centers, club houses, drop-in centers, a range of supported programs, and recreational programs. Both consumers and families value rehabilitative services (Anthony, 1989). This approach to treatment stands in sharp contrast to the custodial model practiced for so many years in state institutions. In contrast, rehabilitation and social supports increase self-esteem, sense of mastery, and coping ability. They decrease symptomatic behavior and enhance mental status and quality of life (Parish, 1987).

One model that has become widely accepted as a successful method of psychosocial rehabilitation for the seriously mentally ill is the *clubhouse model*. The pioneer of the clubhouse movement was Fountain House in New York City. Since begun in 1948, club houses have developed across the nation. The mentally ill are eligible to become members in an exclusive club in the community where only mentally ill are allowed membership. Club members attend functions at the club house Monday through Friday during the day and sometimes on evenings and weekends. Members work in the kitchen unit, planning and cooking the daily meal; the maintenance unit, maintaining the club house and yards; or the clerical unit, answering the phone and publishing the newsletter. There are four messages that constitute the heart and center of the club house model: membership, being expected, being wanted, and being needed (Fountain House, 1981).

Looking back over the past three decades, it is possible to see that the community mental health care movement was ushered in with many simplistic notions. On the one hand, the significance of psychoactive medication and a stable source of financial support was understood. On the other hand, the development of fundamental resources such as housing, case management, substance abuse treatment and social and vocational rehabilitation was not effectively implemented (Mechanic, 1986). In the 1990s new challenges to the mental health care system have arisen. One example is the seriously mentally ill adolescent who has grown up in an era of substance abuse, increasing crime, and the proliferation of AIDS. To address the spiraling mental health needs of communities in an era of limited resources, the mental health system is undergoing many changes. The role of the community health nurse in the mental health system continues to evolve as mental health services expand. Through education in the nursing process and relevant practical experience, the nurse can become uniquely prepared to work effectively with high-risk populations in community mental health.

Evolution of the Community Mental Health Nursing Role

The role of the community psychiatric and mental health nurse has always been important and has changed considerably over the last three decades. A number of factors have influenced and shaped this role as it has emerged as an important discipline in community mental health. Nursing as a discipline is rising to the unique opportunities and challenges presented by the seriously mentally ill in the

community. The challenge is especially great when major mental illness is coupled with substance abuse, personality disorders, or mental retardation. Limited funding and nationwide cutbacks have forced a re-prioritizing of populations who need mental health services. There is nationwide outrage at the homeless mentally ill, for example. Society feels obligated to take care of the seriously mentally ill, so more and more public dollars are being put into programs and care for them. Thus, a fair portion of this chapter deals with the nursing role as it is emerging in relation to services for the seriously mentally ill in the community.

The vast body of knowledge that has resulted from intensive research in the field has established that major mental illnesses have a physiological basis. This has created an unprecedented need for nursing expertise in the field of mental health. Deinstitutionalization essentially moved the locus of care for the seriously mentally ill from the hospital to the community. This, in turn, led to the development of the CSS concept. The CSS was demonstrated to be a successful model for caring for the mentally ill in the community and supported the belief that the community is the best location to treat the mentally ill. The family movement, the consumer movement and, with them, the emphasis on rights of the mentally ill also changed the face of community mental health. This change contributed to the evolution of the community mental health nursing role. Psychosocial rehabilitation for the mentally ill recently emerged as an important aspect of treatment in the community. This was followed by a focus on case management philosophies. These, too, have helped to shape the role of the psychiatric and mental health nurse in relation to the seriously mentally ill in the community as we know it today.

Nursing's role in relation to the many factors of care of the seriously mentally ill in the community is being defined by nurse pioneers currently in those roles. Clearly nurses' training in the biological sciences is emerging as a significant element in the understanding and treatment of the disease process, itself. Also, the nurse's observations and assessments of daily functioning is crucial to satisfactory adjustment in the community. Health and medical needs are emerging as a distinct need for the seriously mentally ill in the community. As new models and approaches to care emerge, nurses are redefining their roles and educating other disciplines regarding nurses' unique preparation and contribution. In addition to serving the seriously mentally ill, the psychiatric mental health nurse deals with many other high-risk populations in the community. These include women and children, adolescents, geriatric clients, people with AIDS, forensics clients, and the general public in crisis.

HIGH-RISK POPULATIONS SERVED BY THE COMMUNITY MENTAL HEALTH NURSE

In 1985 the National Association of State Mental Health Directors reported that nursing provided more direct–patient-care hours of service in mental health organizations than psychiatry, psychology, and social work combined (Public Health Service, 1986). In the community, nurses work with many different high-risk populations, including the homeless, seriously mentally ill, the dually diagnosed (those with both mental illness and chemical dependence), children and families, adolescents, geriatric clients, AIDS victims, forensic clients, and the general public in crisis. To work with these high-risk populations in community mental health, nurses must be educated to focus on the daily adaptation, function, comfort, health status, and quality of life of individuals, families, and communities. It is also important that the nurse have an understanding of the impact of deinstitutionalization on community mental health. A working knowledge of the community support system and case management is also vital for the community mental health nurse.

Seriously Mentally Ill Clients
Community Support Systems

The guiding principles of the community support systems (CSS) philosophy are that services should empower clients, be consumer centered, be racially and culturally appropriate, be flexible, focus on strengths, be normalized and incorporate natural supports, meet special needs, be accountable, and be coordinated (Stroul, 1989). The CSS concept includes the entire array of treatment, life-support, and rehabilitation services needed to assist persons with severe, disabling mental illness to function at optimal levels within the community. Essential components include client identification and outreach, mental health treatment, crisis response services, health and dental care, housing, income support and entitlements, peer support, family and community support, rehabilitation services, protection and advocacy, and case management (Figure 21-1). Stroul states that each community should provide these essential functions (1989). A careful look at the CSS model reveals a holistic nursing-care model. As with any other specialty in nursing, effective psychiatric mental health nursing must consider all aspects of need and must design treatment plans that include interventions to meet those needs. The psychiatric mental health nurse is perfectly suited to function in this CSS model in a number of ways.

Within the CSS, nurses still perform the important role of medication nurse—giving shots, providing medication education, observing for side effects such as tardive dyskinesia, and drawing blood samples for medication-blood level analyses. Frequently, nurses function as case managers, putting together a comprehensive care plan, including clinical treatment, psychosocial rehabilitation, and medical treatment. Nurses assists clients to find suitable housing in the community or accompany them to apply for entitlements. They work with the family and other secondary consumers, offer individual supportive counseling, and make referrals to other agencies and collaborate closely with psychiatrists to treat the disease symptoms. Nurses are directly involved in developing, coordinating, and implementing many aspects of the CSS.

One specific component of the CSS is *client identification and outreach*. Although clients are referred directly to community treatment programs on discharge from an inpatient facility, some cannot or will not come to a clinic for treatment. A comprehensive CSS must include a plan for serving these clients. This plan should include services for the homeless who are mentally ill. Locating and serving some clients may necessitate effective linkage with other com-

COMMUNITY SUPPORT SYSTEM

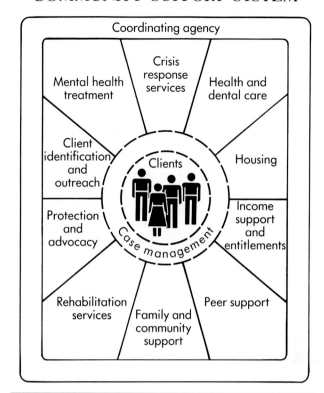

FIGURE 21-1

A client-centered comprehensive mental health system. *(From Stroul BA: Community support systems for persons with long-term mental illness: a conceptual framework, Psychosocial Rehabilitation Journal, vol 12, no 3, 1989.)*

munity groups, such as police departments or emergency rooms. This component also includes addressing transportation needs.

Another specific service component of a CSS is *mental health treatment*. It should include diagnostic evaluation and an individualized treatment plan. This plan should be used in the ongoing assessment and monitoring of the psychiatric condition. Medication management includes prescribing, ensuring the medications are available, monitoring clients to ensure maximal effectiveness and minimal side effects, and educating the client and family regarding medications. Supportive counseling and therapy is also an important factor of mental health treatment. Generally, treatment should focus on managing symptoms and medications, recognizing signs of relapse and assisting the client to cope with daily living. Mental health treatment should also include treatment programs for special problems of dual diagnosis such as mental illness and substance abuse or mental illness and mental retardation (Stroul, 1989).

The mentally ill client living in the community always functions with some degree of deficit, and the nature of most illnesses are such that there will be relapses. Therefore an effective *crisis response service* is essential to providing a CSS. The goal of this service is to assist the client to maintain or resume community functioning. As such, an effective crisis response service helps avert hospitalization, which is a major disruption in anyone's life. Crisis response services may be in the form of a hotline, a walk-in emergency center, mobile crisis outreach, crisis stabilization center, or family-based crisis homes.

Mentally ill persons have higher rates of physical illness, creating the need for services regarding *health and dental care*. Problems to be addressed in this area include locating practitioners to provide the service and paying for the service. Benefits such as Medicaid and Medicare frequently cover these services. In this component of the CSS, a nurse's background and training in medical conditions can be specifically used to develop appropriate programs.

Housing is an immediate need created by deinstitutionalization and is demonstrated graphically by the many homeless mentally ill. Decent affordable housing is essential for a mentally ill client to be able to grow, improve, and move toward independence. To offer this to each client, the community needs a variety of housing options, ranging from highly structured, supervised residences to minimally supervised independent apartments. The client's functioning level, as well as his preferences, values, and goals should be considered in determining suitable housing.

Mentally ill clients may be unable to earn money to pay for basic life necessities. Whereas these basic necessities were taken care of in the hospital, the client in the community must arrange for them. Therefore *income support and entitlements* are another essential component of a CSS. Assistance in the bureaucratic application process is generally needed.

Peer support is important in a CSS because the diagnosis of mental illness still has a stigmatizing, alienating effect. Self-help groups and other forms of peer support provide companionship, empathy, sharing, and assistance. Because peer support empowers mentally ill clients, it helps them make a more satisfactory adjustment in the community. Progress can be facilitated by drop-in centers, day programs, and encouraging consumer-run programs.

There is an increasing recognition of the need for *family and community support*. Families need to be involved appropriately, educated, provided with supportive counseling, and offered respite care. Establishing and maintaining family support groups should be encouraged. To promote genuine integration of mentally ill clients into the community, the general public, especially individuals who interact with the mentally ill, must be educated and supported.

Social and vocational *rehabilitation services* should be an integral part of a CSS. The goals are to build the client's skills to enable him to function as independently as possible. Social rehabilitation is aimed at developing daily living skills and interpersonal and leisure-time skills. Vocational rehabilitation assists the person in becoming productive and contributing to the greatest degree possible. This may involve coordination with other vocational programs and employers or developing transitional employment programs, sheltered workshops, or other forms of supported employment.

Another function of a CSS is that of *protection and advocacy*. Clients should be regularly informed of their rights and resources. They should be assisted to procure treatment in the least restrictive setting.

Case Management

Case management is the component of a CSS that coordinates all the others. It ensures that the client receives the services needed, that the various services are coordinated, and that they are modified appropriately to changing needs over time.

Various approaches in case management have been identified. The *expanded broker model* links individuals with community resources. The *personal strengths model* works to improve quality of life and achievement. The *rehabilitation model* aims at remedying deficits to overcome barriers. The *full-support model* attempts to decrease symptoms and increase functionality (Robinson, 1989).

Case managers for the seriously mentally ill have been described as "life coaches." They directly help to ensure that day-to-day activities are successfully accomplished and that individuals make choices about their own existence and are as independent as possible (Robinson, 1989).

Client identification and outreach, one component of case management, is especially important for the homeless mentally ill, drop-outs from treatment programs, and no-shows for referrals. Various strategies are being explored for successfully locating clients in need of services and ensuring that they receive support. It is becoming apparent that services must be offered in response to client's perceived needs to keep them engaged in community mental health treatment.

Both initial and ongoing *individual assessment* is essential to good case management. This ensures that services are appropriate to changing needs over time. The case manager should coordinate and assist in the development of a comprehensive *service plan* based on the client's needs and goals. This is accomplished in consultation with clinical, rehabilitation, and residential staff. Frequently, mentally ill clients require services from a variety of agencies and sources. The case manager assumes the role of a broker, *linking* the clients with requisite services. The adequacy and appropriateness of services need continual *monitoring,* followed by appropriate interventions of changes in service plans. Client *advocacy* may include accompanying a client to an appointment to help explain a problem, submitting written reports for acquisition of benefits, or presenting information at a public hearing in relation to the general needs of the mentally ill.

Crisis assistance is an essential component of a comprehensive treatment plan. Crisis services can assist the client to stabilize and readjust to community living, often averting hospitalization. If a case manager has a long-term supportive relationship with the client, he/she is in the best position to assist a client through a crisis. If this assistance cannot be provided directly, it must be arranged for by the case manager.

Homeless Seriously Mentally Ill Clients

Homeless seriously mentally ill clients represent a thorough picture of all the challenges the nurse will meet in working with high-risk populations in the community. The ubiquitous problem of homelessness is closely linked with deinstitutionalization (Mechanic, 1986). About 30% to 40% of the homeless in America are thought to be suffering from mental illness. It is claimed that the mentally ill were moved from state psychiatric institutions to ill-prepared communities, only to find themselves unable to organize their lives to secure the basics of living. Although many of these people do not present a danger to others, their quality of life has definitely not been improved by the deinstitutionalization movement.

It is necessary to consider what conditions these persons must face in the community, what needed resources are lacking, and the nature of mental illness itself. Mentally ill clients may experience poor follow-up from hospital discharge planning or may not be compliant with community treatment. Once on the street, they often stop taking prescribed medications. They may lose contact with financial and social supports (Gullberg, 1989). They are vulnerable to developing dependence on both alcohol and illicit drugs. They may begin to engage in disruptive behaviors that often lead to hospitalization or jail (Lamb and Talbott, 1986). These realities encourage the self-sustaining cycle of homelessness and the lack of appropriate care that evolves.

Community mental health nurses are uniquely prepared to provide health care services and other necessary assistance to integrate the homeless seriously mentally ill client into the community. To work effectively with clients, nurses make daily visits to their gathering places such as soup kitchens, parks, streets, bridges, and river beds (Gullberg, 1989). Nurses develop relationships by conversing with homeless people and explaining about services that are available. Other tasks of the nurse working with the homeless include completing need assessments and determining levels of functioning to develop and implement appropriate plans of care. As case manager, the nurse's interventions include both treatment planning and therapeutic involvement with each client. Initially, attention is focused on the basic needs for food, shelter, and clothing. Other services offered through case management include transportation and facilitation of additional assessments such as medical and psychiatric evaluation. If indicated, clients are referred to various programs within the community, including crisis management and hospitalization. During the full evaluation and development of a therapeutic relationship, different housing options may be considered. These include transitional placement or more permanent housing.

One of the most important and challenging responsibilities of the health care professional working with the seriously mentally ill is the establishment of a trusting relationship with clients. This requires development and maintenance of a therapeutic alliance. Developing a therapeutic alliance can be especially difficult with the homeless seriously mentally ill because they are often victimized by other homeless people and thus become unwilling to trust others (Gullberg, 1989). Their feelings of vulnerability strengthen a reluctance to share beliefs and ideas. As a result, these clients appear to be uninvolved and show little interest in professional care. It is the nurse's challenge and obligation to sensitively explore their fears and to listen to their painful experiences without withdrawing emotionally. This process is timely and requires much patience on the nurse's part. It is easy for the nurse to feel discouraged, helpless, and judgmental towards the homeless mentally ill client. The nurse must also be certain to avoid hasty offers of referrals. Responsiveness to the individual's needs and fears requires awareness of one's own prejudices and proper timing of interventions. Success of interventions with these clients depends on the professional's ability to be both enduring and insightful to sensibly personalize interventions.

Young Adult Chronic Clients

Another group of clients that present a challenge to the mental health system are those who are diagnosed with a serious mental illness by the time they become adolescents. This client has come to be known as the young adult chronic client (Pepper and Ryglewicz, 1985). The difficulty in treating these individuals and of finding suitable programs for them has heightened criticism, contributing a growing belief that deinstitutionalization has failed (Minkoff, 1987). Young adult clients with serious mental illness have enormous needs. Although unable to meet the expectations of society, they may still not choose to accept the role of patient. Mentally ill adolescents can be particularly tempted to use alcohol and drugs not only to appear more normal to their peers but also to escape into fantasy from the fear and pain caused by their mental illness. Because mental illness tends to begin in adolescence, young seriously mentally ill clients are often faced with a major conflict. They can become passive, dependent, resigned, and content with limited goals or they can choose to become adults. As adults they must become independent, risk taking, adventurous, and intimate (Lamb, 1982). They may ask for assistance and then be unwilling to cooperate with the available treatment. They struggle with a sense of failure and a low self-esteem and often lack the ambition to participate in the difficult regimen required to treat their mental illness. At a time when they are struggling for independence they feel forced into being dependent, compliant clients.

Working with young adult chronically mentally ill clients can be demanding because they are often noncompliant and critical of community mental health treatment. The nurse frequently faces frustration about feeling disregarded by clients who are quite demanding. This is an example in which peer support for the nurse is crucial to prevent burnout. To help the young adult chronic client to function optimally in the community, the community mental health nurse must understand their developmental challenges to provide accurate evaluation and effective treatment.

A holistic approach to nursing intervention for a client diagnosed with a serious mental illness works well. It is important for the nurse to examine a number of areas in addition to mental health needs. Physical health generally requires attention, as do basic life supports for food and shelter. The client's day-to-day functioning demands careful assessment, with particular attention to areas of deficits caused by the mental illness or institutionalization. Environmental factors include family interactions and support or lack of family or other close supports. The client's living arrangement and its impact on the client's well-being also must be considered. Socialization needs are often more acute than they were in the hospital. Legislative and bureaucratic decisions often directly affect the client's life and needs. Nurses can assess and intervene on each of these levels and can address the needs of the client as a whole person.

Children and Families

An array of services are available to children and families in the community mental health system. Pregnant women who may be at risk of complications during their pregnancy and who could benefit from mental health services are identified and followed until after the birth of their children. Infants who are diagnosed with developmental disabilities are also followed by the community mental health system. Some nurses specialize in infant development and work with infant-stimulation programs. As described in Chapter 32, these nurses work not only with the child but with the entire family involved with the child. Families of children with emotional problems—from early childhood through school age—are also tracked through the community mental healthy system. During adolescence, many problems may arise, including the first signs of serious mental illness and substance abuse. At this stage, treatment is focused on the client and the entire family.

Nurses may specialize in any number of the previously described areas. In addition, families in which abuse has occurred to children, spouses, or both are often served by nurses who have developed specialties in this area of need. Basic nursing knowledge includes knowledge of developmental stages and tasks, family systems, and home assessments. Nurses develop and participate in programs that include outreach as a means of preventing illness, abuse, and crisis. Their holistic approach often takes them into homes, schools, and the community at large.

The Adolescent Client

During adolescence, all young people begin to face the tasks of becoming adults. They struggle to achieve a measure of independence, to choose a vocation, to establish satisfying interpersonal relationships, and to acquire some sense of identity. Becoming an adult in the 1990s presents the adolescent with many hazards such as the threat of nuclear disaster or war, more accessible and affordable illicit drugs, more identified and potentially lethal sexually transmitted diseases, the decline of the family unit, and an economic recession. As a result, the incidence of suicide among adolescents is higher. There is a demand for an increase in mental health services available for this age group, many of the members of which are having difficulty dealing with modern society and the related challenges. Drug and AIDS education are becoming a part of the adolescent's education. Often these education programs and related counseling services are provided by community mental health nurses.

Geriatric Clients

As the percentage of elderly persons in our society increases, there is a corresponding increase in the need for mental health services available to this population. Two major illnesses that challenge the nurse are Alzheimer disease and dementia. Providing care for individuals with these illnesses is often difficult and frustrating for all involved. Other important issues that must be monitored by the community mental health nurse are that of abuse and neglect. Because the mental health needs of these individuals and their families and care givers are so intense, a specialty field of psychiatric nursing known as psychogeriatric nursing has emerged. Psychogeriatric nursing addresses interventions for developmental issues of aging, loss, loneliness, and preparation for one's own death. The development of psychogeriatric nursing comes at a crucial time because the development of federal and state mental health policies for the aged has been uncoordinated and funding for services has been sparse (Swan, Fox, and Estes, 1989).

Seriously mentally ill geriatric clients comprise one of the most underserved groups in the community mental health system. Geriatric clients in psychiatric hospitals who are ready for discharge need well-designed discharge plans that include instructions for care givers; once in the community, nurses need to develop follow-up services for these clients, including liaison work with nursing home staff and case management of the individual clients. An important issue in case management is inclusion of family members and significant others.

There is also a need for trained nurses to provide counseling and therapy to geriatric clients wherever they may be living. In nursing homes, geriatric clients and their families have needs that can be addressed through counseling with a trained psychogeriatric nurse. Some of these clients may be struggling with the loss of loved ones, loss of their home, loss of independence, anger at being placed in a nursing home, difficulty getting along with strangers, drug or alcohol abuse, and fear of what lies ahead. In many cases elderly clients who are living with family members or living independently may also be dealing with similar problems. Currently this group of clients is underserved, but with the increasing numbers of aged individuals in the population, the mental health system is being forced to examine ways to increase and improve services to these clients. Nurses involved in the field of psychogeriatrics are securing government grants to study these issues.

Clients with Acquired Immunodeficiency Syndrome

Because AIDS generates a unique series of stressors for clients and their lovers, spouses, family members, friends, and employers, it creates serious problems for everyone involved (Flaskerud, 1987). The complexity and multiplicity of problems encountered by people with AIDS and the psychological terror it causes affects every aspect of an individual's life.

Because many individuals experiencing the stressors related to AIDS are living in the community, it is crucial that community mental health nurses are trained to address the needs of these clients. The nursing interventions necessary to address the mental health needs of clients with AIDS require special attention to the psychosocial aspects of the disease, such as dealing with impending loss, judgment from others, effects on significant relationships, and participation and functioning as a community member. AIDS-related dementia is another issue that may need to be dealt with by everyone involved. Other issues that must be considered by nurses working with these clients are the stresses experienced by the lovers and families of AIDS patients and the stresses they, themselves, experience in providing care to AIDS patients. The mental health nurse may address the mental health issues related to AIDS by developing AIDS-support groups in the community.

One of the biggest challenges to the nurse working with the AIDS-infected client is that of a client's noncompliance with the practice of safe sex. The client may prefer that no acquaintances be told of the diagnosis. The nurse must understand the legal importance of strictly adhering to confidentiality policies when the most ethical action may appear to be to break confidentiality and inform sexual partners of the potential for contracting AIDS. The nurse must always confront personal preferences and judgements triggered by clients and their significant others. This may be especially challenging with a client with AIDS as issues of sexual preference and drug use may need to be explored. At times the nurse may be put in the situation of having to support a client who is struggling to accept his or her own lifestyle choices, which may differ significantly from the lifestyle of the nurse. At the same time the client may be feeling punished by the disease. It is at this point that the nurse must once again put aside preconceptions to intervene in a therapeutic way.

Forensics

The field of forensic psychiatry is expanding as more and more individuals with significant mental health needs are being dealt with in the criminal justice system. To address this problem, nurses working in community mental health serve as liaisons to the court and prison system. Issues surrounding the problem of the increasing need for mental health services in the field of forensics are complicated, but there are two evident factors that contribute to this trend. The most apparent problem is the increase in the availability, use, and profit of illicit drugs along with related legal issues. Another more subtle issue is the changing legislation around involuntary commitment and providing the least restrictive treatment alternative to seriously mentally ill clients.

As a result of the availability of highly addictive illicit drugs and the resulting sale and use of these substances, there has been an increase in the number of women and adolescents being held either in jails or on parole in the community. The problems of treating these individuals effectively within the criminal justice system are complicated by many factors such as insufficient funding for services, inadequate available preventive services—such as drug education, family planning, and counseling—and meager follow-up services once individuals are released from the judicial system. Appropriate treatment of clients is further complicated by clients who are often unwilling or (for various complex reasons) incapable of participating in the preventive and follow-up services that are available to them.

As mentioned earlier, one goal of deinstitutionalization legislation was related to the client's individual right to be provided with the least restrictive alternative of treatment. In an effort to provide patients with the greatest freedom from restrictions, major changes in commitment procedures

occurred. As a result of these changes, it became more difficult to protect patients and the community during serious psychiatric episodes. Many seriously mentally ill clients who are unsuitable for civil commitment but who are involved in law violations were then, and are now, increasingly dealt with through the criminal justice system (Mechanic, 1986). The chronically mentally ill client with a criminal history often ends up cycling through the criminal justice system as a result of the lack of extensive and conclusive research on how to best treat them in the community.

Nurses working in the field of forensics are involved in many activities for which they have not been prepared in a formal way. One challenge for the community health nurse working with forensic clients is recognizing that there are differences between the goals of correctional institutions and community mental health care systems (Niskala, 1986). The criminal justice system is designed to discipline criminal behavior and rehabilitate individuals to prevent future criminal activity. The goal of community mental health care is to help individuals with mental health needs to receive treatment in the least restrictive and most therapeutic environment. The nurse must not only work therapeutically with the client, through assessments and treatment planning and implementation, but must also understand and respect the goals of the correctional system to work most effectively with the client.

General Public in Crisis

In community mental health centers attention has changed from developing local, involuntary, care hospitals to the development of voluntary crisis options in local communities (Wilson, 1989). This change in focus and the resultant increase in crisis management options available outside of hospitals has not only increased services available to the seriously mentally during crisis episodes, but it has also increased crisis intervention services for the general public. Crisis intervention centers, crisis stabilization units, hotlines, and shelters have been established for both intervention and prevention purposes. Individuals who are depressed and potentially suicidal may choose to contact the crisis team of their local community mental health center. Crisis services are also available to those who may be dealing with chemical dependency issues or who have relatives or friends who are in need of help. Often, families who are experiencing functional emergencies will contact crisis services for assistance in resolving the emergency. During tragedies, such as earthquakes, tornadoes, train wrecks, teenage suicide, and car accidents, survivors may be overwhelmed with terror, grief, or both. Community nurses trained in crisis intervention may be called in to offer support and mental health services to those who are dealing with the shock of the tragedy. Nurses working on crisis teams within community mental health centers may be trained in critical incidence stress debriefing (CISD). This training prepares crisis workers to assit emergency staff (such as rescue-squad workers, policemen, firemen, and evacuation teams who have been involved in giving assistance during a disaster) and to deal with personal stress and other mental health issues that may arise in the aftermath of a disaster. In working with the many different types of crisis that may be experienced by the general public, nurses must be skilled in identifying those who will be served appropriately with brief interventions and those who will need longer term assistance.

CLINICAL APPLICATION

Jack is a 21-year-old unemployed white male who was referred to the Mental Health Center by his parents. Since graduation from high school, he has undergone seven psychiatric hospitalizations. During high school, he abused several different drugs, including LSD, heroine, cocaine, amphetamines, marijuana, and alcohol. The client claimed the drugs induced psychosis, for which he was hospitalized. He was given fluphenazine (Prolixin) 5 mg q hs and amantidine (Symmetrel) 2 mg q hs, and the diagnosis of atypical psychosis was made.

The client was born in a large city and was the middle of three siblings. His medical history indicated that he had hemophilia. His father was a professor in nuclear engineering; his mother was trained in social work. His older brother had graduated from college and was successful in his journalism career. His younger sister was an A student in the local university. For the previous year Jack had been staying in a halfway house in another state. He recently returned to live with his parents in one of the affluent suburbs of the city.

Following his first psychotic episode and hospitalization, Jack enrolled in a drug rehabilitation program. However, he continued his drug use and continued to have psychotic episodes. Two years before coming to the clinic he began to attend Narcotics Anonymous (NA). He became active in this group and was attending the local NA group, abstaining from illegal drugs, and taking his prescribed medication at the time he first presented at the Mental Health Center. He had had two serious suicide attempts by injecting an overdose of Tylenol into his veins.

The mental status examination revealed a neatly and casually dressed male sitting in a chair. He was cooperative, maintained good eye contact, and looked his stated age. The client stated that his mood was average/content. Affect was appropriate. The client claimed to have a good appetite, no crying spells, and had never had trouble sleeping. He denied current visual and auditory hallucinations; however, he reported three times in his life when he had heard voices that mumbled to him. There was no evidence of psychosis. The client's insight and judgment were fair.

Jack presented as someone with a history of psychotic episodes and substance abuse who was currently stable on medication and welcome at his parent's home. His nurse, as case manager, designed a comprehensive plan that included maintaining stability in regard to his psychosis; remaining free of all substance use; and ensuring follow-up for his medical problems. She arranged an appointment for him with the psychiatrist at the Mental Health Center to do an initial evaluation and made arrangements for him to be seen subsequently at regular intervals in the medication clinic. At times, she recommended minor changes be made in his medication dosages. His nurse monitored the effectiveness of the medicine and side effects. She also offered supportive counseling. Jack continued to attend NA regularly and discussed issues related to his substance abuse with the nurse. She made sure he saw a hematologist at the hospital for his hemophilia and discussed issues concerning the risk of AIDS in individual counseling.

Four months after beginning treatment, Jack overdosed on fluphenazine (Prolixin) and was rushed to the emergency room. The nurse arranged for psychiatric hospitalization and offered support to the family. She began to explore his depressive episodes in greater depth. She discussed the possibility of a bipolar disorder diagnosis with his psychiatrist. Subsequently, he was administered lithium, which resulted in less frequent and less severe depressive episodes.

Because Jack's expressed goals were to find employment, go to shcool, and begin moving towards independence, his nurse referred him to the Department of Rehabilitation Services for assistance in locating a job. He tried several part-time jobs, but eventually decided to enroll part-time in the local community college and continued living at home.

His parents were supportive, yet frustrated with Jack's lack of progress. After obtaining his permission, the nurse met with Jack's parents to discuss how to best help him and the importance of allowing him to make his own choices. She referred them to the local chapter of NAMI for support and education regarding mental illness.

She then referred Jack to a "lithium" group, consisting of eight stabilized clients receiving lithium therapy who met monthly with the psychiatrist and the nurse for support, education, and medication review. Jack attended regularly and soon developed good friendships with others in the group. The nurse maintained regular contact with Jack to evaluate the effectiveness of the plan.

SUMMARY

The "knowledge explosion" regarding mental illness, coming on the heels of the deinstitutionalization movement, has resulted in dramatic implications for the psychiatric mental health nurse in the community. As the philosophy of the community support system unfolds throughout the country, effective models for caring for the seriously mentally ill in the community are being created, consumers and families are being empowered and organized, the importance of psychosocial rehabilitation is being recognized, and case management is being required by law.

In addition to serving the seriously mentally ill, the psychiatric mental health nurse deals with many other high-risk populations in the community. Although the community mental health system has had its own special problems in developing adequate programs, it is emerging as a needed, respected institution, ripe with opportunity and challenge for the psychiatric mental health nurse.

KEY CONCEPTS

Persons with mental health problems and needs frequently are clients of the community mental health nurse.

After two decades of federal and local funding, many mental health centers have achieved their original goals of providing accessible, comprehensive mental health services at the local level. They continue to struggle with budget cuts.

The most effective treatment modality in the community for persons with serious mental illness is psychosocial rehabilitation in combination with psychotropic medication.

In recent years the deinstitutionalization of seriously mentally ill clients has dramatically altered the services provided by community mental health nurses.

Homelessness in combination with serious mental illness is one of the biggest challenges facing the community mental health nurse.

Case management includes an understanding of community mental health needs, including the special needs of the population, as well as those of the individual.

Nurses are uniquely prepared to work with the high-risk populations served in the community mental health system.

LEARNING ACTIVITIES

1. From at least two different clients, obtain all information necessary to assess their medication regime.

2. Using a community resources guide, determine what resources are available in your community for seriously mentally ill clients and their families.

3. Interview the parents of a person with a diagnosis of a serious mental illness. Determine their perceptions of community mental health services.

4. Interview seriously mentally ill consumers of mental health care in your community concerning their perceptions of community mental health services.

5. Interview community mental health nurses in your community to determine their perception of the stressors of the mentally ill and their families.

6. Evaluate the preceding three sets of interviews for consistency and contrasts in types and amounts of stress.

7. By reading your local newspaper, observing occurrences in your community, listening to the radio, and watching television, determine what potential threats to mental health exist in your community.

BIBLIOGRAPHY

Andreason NC: Diagnosis. In National Institute of Mental Health: Special report: schizophrenia, Rockville, MD, 1987, The Institute.

Anthony WA and Blanch A: Research on community support services: what have we learned? Psychosoc Rehabil J 12(3):93, 1989.

Anthony W and Lieberman P: The practices of psychiatric rehabilitation, Schizophrenia Bulletin, 12(4):542, 1986.

Brown NB: Guest editorial. Psychosoc Rehabil J 12(3):1, 1989.

Chamberlin J, Rogers JA, and Sneed CS: Consumers, families, and community support systems, Psychosoc Rehabil J 12(3):93, 1989.

Citizen's guide to the Community Mental Health Centers Amendment of 1975, Washington, DC, 1977, Government Printing Office.

Flaskerud JH: AIDS: psychosocial aspects, J Psychosoc Nurs Ment Health Serv 25(12):9, 1987.

Fountain House, Inc: Concept paper, New York, 1981, Fountain House, Inc.

Fox JC and Chamberlin J: Preparing nurses to work with the chronically mentally ill, Community Ment Health J 24(4):296, 1988.

Fox JR: Galt report. Unpublished manuscript, Department of Mental Health, Retardation and Substance Abuse, University of Virginia, Richmond, Va.

Goldstein MZ: Psychosocial issues. In National Institute of Mental Health: Special report: schizophrenia, Rockville, Md, 1987, The Institute.

Gottesman II, McGuffin P, and Farmer AE: Genetics. In National Institute of Mental Health: Special report: schizophrenia, Rockville, Md, 1987, The Institute.

Gullberg PL: A psychiatric nurse's role, J Psychosoc Nurs Ment Health Serv 27(6):9, 1989.

Hall H: The homeless: a mental health debate, Psychol Today, 25:65, 1987.

Hanlon J and Pickett G: Public health administration and practice, ed 9, St Louis, 1990, Mosby-Year Book.

Holzman PS: Psychophysiology. In National Institute of Mental Health: Special report: schizophrenia, Rockville, MD, 1987, The Institute.

Institute for Health Policy Studies: Nation's Health, Washington, DC, 1981, US Government Printing Office.

Joint Commission on Mental Illness and Health: Action for mental health, New York, 1961, Basic Books.

Lamb HR. Young adult chronic patients: the new drifters, Hosp Community Psychiatry, 33:465, 1982.

Lamb HR and Talbott JA: The homeless mentally ill: the perspective of the American Psychiatric Association, JAMA 256(4):498, 1986.

Landsberg G and Hammer R: Possible programmatic consequences of community mental health center funding arrangements: illustrations based on inpatient utilization data, Commun Mental Health J, 13:63, 1977.

Mechanic D: The challenge of chronic mental illness: a retrospective and prospective view, Hosp Community Psychiatry 37(9):891, 1986.

Mechanic D: Evolution of mental health services and areas for change, New Directions in Mental Health, 36:3, 1987.

Meltzer HY: Biological studies. In National Institute of Mental Health: Special report: schizophrenia, Rockville, MD, 1987, The Institute.

Minkoff K: Beyond deinstitutionalization: a new ideology for the postinstitutional era, Hosp Community Psychiatry 38(9):945, 1987.

National Institute of Mental Health: Announcement: community support system strategy, development and implementation grants, Rockville, MD, 1980, The Institute.

Niskala H: Competencies and skills required by nurses working in forensics, West J Nurs Res 8(4):400, 1986.

Parrish J: Community support program: vision impossible, Community Support Network News, 4:2, 1987.

Pepper B and Ryglewicz H: The developmental residence: a "missing link" for young adult chronic patients, Tie Lines 2(3):1, 1985.

Peplau H: Tomorrow's world, Nurs Time 7:29, 1987.

Peplau H: Future directions in psychiatric nursing from the perspective of history, J Psychosoc Nurs 27(2):19, 1989.

President's Commission on Mental Health: Report of the Task Panel on the Nature and Scope of the Problem. In Psychiatric mental health nursing: proceedings of two conferences on future directions, vol 2, DHHS Pub No ADM 86-1449, Washington, DC, 1978, US Government Printing Office.

Ramshorn M: The major thrust in American psychiatry: past, present, and future, Perspect Psychiatry Care 9(4):144, 1974.

Robinson GK and Bergman GT: Choices in case management: a review of current knowledge and practice for mental health programs, Contract B4 No 278-87-0026, Washington, DC, 1989, National Institute of Mental Health.

Rubin J: The community mental health movement in the United States circa 1979, Am J Psychoanal 31(1):68, 1971.

Snow D and Newton P: Task, social structure and social process in the community mental health center movement, Am Psychol 31(8):582, 1976.

Stroul BA: Introduction to the special issue: the community support systems concept, Psychosoc Rehabil J 12(3):5,

Swann JH, Fox PJ, and Estes CL: Geriatric services: community center boon or bane? Community Ment Health J 25(4):327, 1989.

Tarail M: Current and future issues in community mental health, Psychiatr Q 52(1):27, 1980.

Torrey FE: Continuous treatment teams in the care of the chronically mentally ill, Hosp Community Psychiatry 37(12):1243, 1986.

Wilson SF: Implementation of the community support system concept statewide: the Vermont experience, Psychosoc Rehabil J 12(3):27, 1989.

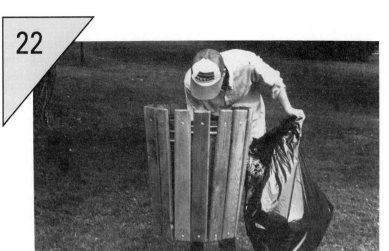

22

Vulnerable Populations in the Community

Juliann G. Sebastian

OBJECTIVES

After reading this chapter, the student should be able to:

Evaluate the usefulness and validity of a conceptual model of vulnerability.

Describe social trends that have contributed to the development of vulnerable groups in society.

Analyze the socioeconomic and age-related bases for vulnerability in selected groups including the near poor, medically indigent, homeless, runaway children, pregnant adolescents, and frail elderly and their caregivers.

Describe demographic trends in vulnerable groups.

Describe the health and social outcomes of vulnerability for selected groups.

Analyze issues in the provision of direct care to vulnerable individuals, the program planning for vulnerable groups, and the policy and health planning for these groups.

Explore political and ethical ramifications of policies relating to vulnerable groups.

KEY TERMS

anxious runaway	fluidity of poverty	social care system
basic activities of daily living	health-field concept	social darwinism
	homelessness	spend down
case management	instrumental activities of daily living	temporary homelessness
chronic homelessness		terrified runaway
comorbidity	medical indigency	throwaways
cost-sharing	medigap insurance	uncompensated care
disenfranchisement	near poor	underinsured
enabling	power	uninsured
episodic homelessness	rationing health care	vulnerability
federal poverty guidelines	rootless runaway	worthiness

N ursing has long been concerned with vulnerability, although that concept has rarely been explicitly stated or examined. For example, Florence Nightingale taught nurses to manage patients' environments in ways that would best enable patients to get well (see Chapter 1), implying that this was something that ill individuals were unable to do for themselves and that therefore they were in a vulnerable condition. Virginia Henderson's (1964) classic definition of nursing addresses the performance of those things that people are unable to do for themselves, thereby also implying the vulnerability of patients. Nurses have recently been concerned with *risk factors* for health problems and providing health services for groups at risk. Again, the idea of vulnerability is implicit. How might community health nurses more explicitly think about the concept of vulnerability?

This chapter addresses issues surrounding vulnerable population groups within the community and the role of community health nurses in meeting their health needs. The nature of vulnerability is explored, and the socioeconomic and age-related causes are analyzed. What are some variables that influence coping with vulnerability in these groups? What are some potential nursing responses to direct care issues, program planning, and policy development? These questions are addressed throughout the chapter.

CONCEPTUAL BASES OF VULNERABILITY

Vulnerability is a condition in which individuals or groups are highly susceptible to harm. In the context of community health, vulnerability is characterized by personal, social, and environmental variables (Dever et al., 1988). Health risks, limited control, disenfranchisement, victimization, disadvantaged statuses, and powerlessness are some of the major concepts that contribute to an understanding of vulnerability. The dynamic interplay between these characteristics is indicated in Figure 20-1.

Health Risk

The concept of risk is based on the natural history of disease model in which certain aspects of physiology, environment (including personal habits, social environment, and physical environment), or both make it more likely that one will develop particular health problems. An outgrowth of this concern for risk factors and high-risk groups has been increasing attention to the needs of special population groups. According to the work *Promoting Health/Preventing Disease: Year 2000 Objectives for the Nation* (Public Health Service, 1991), special population groups are defined as age groups, minority groups, or low-income groups with a greater likelihood of developing particular diseases or conditions than the population as a whole. These groups include the near poor, medically indigent, and homeless persons, runaways, pregnant adolescents, and the frail elderly and often suffer from "cumulative risks" from combinations of risk factors (Nichols, Wright, and Murphy, 1986).

Limited Control

The description of the *health-field concept* by Dever et al. (1988, p. 26) explains factors contributing to the development of vulnerability. In this model, individuals are described as having some control over their health status but not complete control. In fact, individuals comprise only one of four factors in the model, which includes biology, environment, and the health care system. According to the health-field concept, individuals share *control and responsibility* for their health status with society as a whole.

Individuals largely determine whether the behavior they engage in is health promoting or potentially health damaging. Although individuals do not control their biological heritage, they share some responsibility for the heritage they pass on to their offspring. For example, the health status of an infant reflects the prenatal health status and lifestyle of the mother. Society determines types of health services and the means of reimbursement that are available. Pregnant adolescents who live in communities with limited financial support for prenatal services find it more difficult to obtain early and continuous prenatal care. Society is also responsible for many environmental hazards. Thus the health-field concept is helpful in explaining how health status is affected by both individual factors (individual and biology) and broader societal-level factors (environment and health care system).

Certain aspects of the physical and social environment adversely affect the health status of special population groups, causing vulnerability. Many of these conditions are beyond the control of these groups and are thus the responsibility of society. For example, homeless individuals are affected both by conditions in their physical environment, such as constant mobility and exposure, and by social factors such as an overwhelming sense of disenfranchisement.

Disenfranchisement

Disenfranchisement refers to a feeling of separation from mainstream society. The individual does not have an emotional connection with any particular group or with society in general. In many ways, disenfranchisement seems to be related to the degree of deviance thought to be displayed by these groups. Productive members of society are not thought of as disenfranchised because they are fulfilling expected social roles, whether they are adolescents participating in society as students or are employed and self-sufficient adults. However, runaway adolescents are not fulfilling expected social roles and are thus disenfranchised.

Disenfranchised groups such as the homeless may essentially be "invisible" to other members of society and may be forgotten in terms of health and social planning. The frail elderly may be similarly invisible to the majority of society. Disenfranchisement suggests that vulnerable groups lack the social supports necessary to effectively manage an emotionally and physically healthy life-style.

Victimization

Dever et al. express concern (1988) that the current focus on the individual's control of many chronic health problems through life-style choices may result in *blaming the victim* for areas outside individual control. Rosner (1982) explored the social history of the concepts of *worthiness* and *truly needy* in American society and concluded that victim blaming has become part of the outlook on care for the poor and serves certain functions for society. Blaming the individual

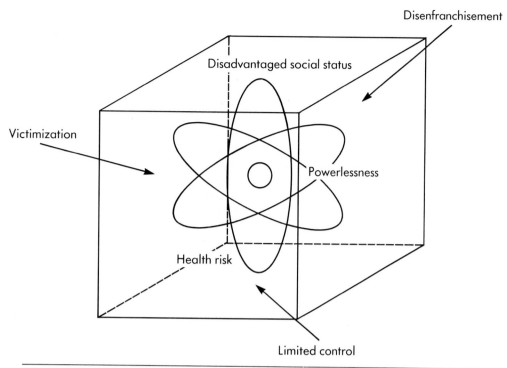

FIGURE 22-1

Dimensions of vulnerability.

may relieve society from assuming responsibility for environmental issues and issues surrounding the delivery of health services.

In the early days in the United States, public attitudes held that poverty was temporary and could be overcome. People felt a sense of responsibility to help the truly needy. The thought that poverty might be permanent opposed the developing American ideals of self-sufficiency and individual achievement.

Rosner (1982) explained that Americans eventually adopted an attitude of ambivalence toward the poor and dependent. Those who were seen as temporarily poor were considered worthy of help, whereas those for whom poverty was considered a permanent state were not considered worthy of help. The attitude that poor and dependent members of society somehow deserved their station in life justified limitations on social welfare that were actually caused by financial constraints on service availability.

Such ambivalence seems to have increased in the last decade; this time period has seen an increase in policies resulting in stringent eligibility criteria for services. This may have resulted in part from efforts to avoid paying for those who do not wish to help themselves. Also, it may have resulted partly from professional opinions regarding *enabling* behavior. The concept of enabling comes from the literature on addictions. Enabling is the behavior of people in the dependent person's environment that makes it possible for the addiction to continue and includes behavior such as covering up and "making things right."

Some professionals feel that the presence of loose eligibility criteria for health and social services enables individuals to maintain patterns of dependency. However, strict eligibility criteria are more likely during times of severely limited economic resources (Rosner, 1982). The emphasis on cost-containment has resulted in policies designed to limit those eligible for free or government-financed care, as opposed to earlier efforts to expand accessibility of services (Grau, 1987; Rosner, 1982).

As a result, victimization of vulnerable groups has included limited access to services, particularly to preventive and outpatient services. The limits to access have been both economic and social. Economically, fewer services are covered by third-party payors, and those which are covered often only provide partial payment for services, requiring individuals to pay larger amounts, themselves. Socially, many services have strict eligibility criteria that are intended to help people become self-sufficient but often have the effect of limiting services. For example, a food bank limits receipt of free food to emergency situations once every 3 months and places a limit on the total number of times a family can receive food. If the food bank is the major source of free food in the community, a frail elderly couple who regularly have to choose between paying for medication and buying groceries because they run out of money near the end of the month will probably opt to forego their medications. A choice such as this does nothing to promote their independence.

Disadvantaged Status

In many ways, vulnerable groups have limited involvement in the health planning to meet their own needs. Because these groups are primarily minorities, they are more *dis-*

advantaged than more mainstream groups because typical health planning focuses on the majority. They have far less political power than do groups that are better represented in health planning. Plans for health services are built around the needs of the majority of people. The emphasis in health planning is on areas of greatest need. Although the degree of need in a community is not always determined by the sheer number of people with a certain problem, it is an important factor.

In addition to minority status, members of vulnerable groups are often thought of as unable to credibly advocate for their own interests. For example, runaway adolescents living on the streets are not as likely to be sought out for involvement in planning clinic services for this population as are professionals. Involving community members as partners in planning (refer to Chapter 16) is one way to give vulnerable groups the opportunity to overcome a disadvantaged status.

Powerlessness

Poverty is common among vulnerable groups. Moccia and Mason stated that poverty is a *power* issue because it involves a lack of control over critical resources needed to function effectively in society (1986, p. 23). Vulnerable groups lack control over critical financial resources. In contemporary American society, money is one of the most critical resources; insufficient financial means puts individuals in dependent positions and further removes their control over choices between available options. Additionally, insufficient financial resources limit the potential power (Provan, 1980) groups may have and constrains the degree of participation they may have in making decisions that will affect them, thus limiting their potential to influence even the kinds of options that are available.

Members of vulnerable groups often lack the knowledge of resources that would help them be more effective health care participants. They may not be effective self-advocates (Riesdorph-Ostrow, 1989), either because they lack political skills or because others hold stereotyped perceptions of them. Certainly, not all vulnerable groups are poorly educated; however, many are. Education helps people make more informed choices about the degree of effort and expense they are willing to put into becoming and staying healthy (Grossman, 1972). Social networks are another important resource that may be less available to vulnerable groups. Disenfranchisement means that these groups are isolated from mainstream society and do not have strong social networks to help them increase their power base. For example, homeless individuals have very little power in part because of their lack of financial and social resources. Although some homeless individuals are well educated, they have less access to information sources like newspapers, periodicals, and public opinions simply because of their isolation, mobility, and financial problems.

CAUSES OF VULNERABILITY

Both socioeconomic and age-related factors may contribute to the development of vulnerability. The groups discussed in this chapter are all influenced by one of these factors and sometimes by both.

Socioeconomic Factors

Poverty is a primary contributing factor to vulnerability and is a growing problem in this country (Pesznecker, 1984). Poverty is a relative state. The government has a definition of poverty that is used to develop eligibility criteria for entitlement and other programs. However, many people who earn just above the government-defined poverty levels are unable to meet living expenses and are not eligible for assistance programs. Poverty causes vulnerability by making it more difficult for people to function in society. It is often difficult for a young family with an employed father in the home to obtain financial support from social services, even if the father is earning less money than the family needs. A family such as this is considered *near poor;* sometimes in these situations the family decides it would be better for them financially if the father leaves because they may become eligible for just enough financial assistance to make ends meet. In this type of situation, vulnerability results from the family's efforts to do what is necessary to manage, although it is disruptive to the family system.

People who do not have the financial resources to pay for medical care are considered *medically indigent*. They may be self-employed, lacking insurance coverage or have insufficient insurance and are therefore *underinsured*. In these situations, poverty (in its relative sense) causes vulnerability because these people are unlikely to seek preventive health care because of the expense and are more likely to suffer from consequences of preventable illnesses.

Currently, the structure of health care reimbursement policies and the mood of the country in general is based more on a *market model* than on a human service model. This type of model is thought to perpetuate inequities in service availability and accessibility. The market model of service purchase is built on the assumption that those who have the resources to purchase services are the ones entitled to those services. One assumption that some think underlies this model is that individuals unable to purchase services must somehow not be "fit" to receive services. Moccia and Mason (1986) observed that *social darwinism* is once again becoming a predominant social value in this country. Social darwinism refers to the idea of survival of the fittest in relation to social goods and services.

However, this view does not explain the extent of public monies currently spent to subsidize health care. Social darwinism also conflicts with the alternate view that at least some level of health care is a right and should be provided regardless of ability to pay. The two perspectives reflect the degree of controversy over the appropriate role of government in the provision of health and social services to vulnerable groups.

One of the problems of the market model of health care is that policies reflecting this posture reinforce a cycle nearly impossible for disenfranchised individuals and groups to break out of (Curtin, 1986). For example, groups unable to afford adequate preventive services are likely to develop more chronic diseases, thus limiting their ability to effectively work to change the status quo. Such depletion of health status limits the abilities of group members to obtain employment, seek advanced education, or accomplish other goals that may lead to improved health status.

Age-Related Causes

Vulnerable groups may share certain physiologic and developmental characteristics that predispose them to unique risks. Among these, *age* is probably the most central variable. It has long been known that clients at the extreme ends of the age continuum are less able physiologically to adapt to stressors. It seems that certain individuals are most vulnerable at particular ages as a result of the interplay between crucial developmental characteristics and socioeconomic tensions. Infants and the elderly probably account for most health care expenditures as a result of vulnerability associated with physiological immaturity (infants) or declining physiological adaptability (the elderly). Further discussion of infants can be found in Chapter 28, and general concerns surrounding care of the elderly are discussed in Chapter 31. Factors related to the vulnerability of these two groups are described in this section.

Although adolescents are not at the extremes of the age continuum, they are vulnerable to health and social problems because of the interaction between developmental characteristics such as feelings of invulnerability and high risk-taking behavior. Pregnant adolescents and runaway adolescents are two groups discussed in this chapter.

Adolescents in the United States face a high risk of pregnancy with the associated possibility of delivering low–birth-weight infants and the likelihood of interrupted education with subsequent economic hardship. Adolescent females (especially those who are under 14 years of age) are more likely to deliver low-birth-weight infants than are women in their twenties and thirties. This is probably a result of physiological variables (Yoos, 1987), although socioeconomic conditions may play an equally important role (Trussell, 1988). An inability to afford prenatal care, lack of awareness of the existence or importance of prenatal care, and a tendency to seek such care later in pregnancy than older mothers also contribute to the poor pregnancy outcomes of adolescent females.

In another example of adolescent vulnerability, family stress and dysfunction may lead to withdrawal behaviors by preteenage children and adolescents, which may manifest as running away from home, either temporarily or permanently. Runaways are more vulnerable to social, health, and economic problems than are their peers in intact families because they are confronted with the normal adolescent developmental needs for independence and identity solidification but lack the supports present in the usual environment to meet these needs. In addition to lacking supports, these children are faced with unusual and terrifying stressors that they usually do not know how to deal with effectively (Manov and Lowther, 1983).

Health-Related Causes

Another example of a common physiological variable that predisposes individuals to vulnerability is *alteration in normal physiological status*. This may result from disease processes, such as in someone with single or multiple concomitant chronic diseases. Physiological alterations may also result from accidents, injuries, or congenital problems leading to mental or physiological disability. Elderly individuals often exhibit vulnerability resulting both from age and the presence of multiple chronic illnesses. Both factors result in limitations in functional status for many elderly persons, thereby leading to vulnerability to safety hazards and to loss of independence. Disabled individuals are another example of a vulnerable group; this population group is discussed in Chapter 32.

As the exptected length of life has increased, the proportion of elderly in the population has also increased dramatically. The over-85-years age group has increased the most rapidly. Many of these people are frail, either as a result of health problems or advanced age. Most of these frail older people are living in the community and must depend on family or friends for assistance with daily living and health maintenance tasks. The stress of these new roles and altered family dynamics makes frail elderly individuals and their caregivers vulnerable to health, social, and financial problems.

SOCIOECONOMIC VULNERABILITY

A major category of vulnerability is based on socioeconomic characteristics. This includes groups that are vulnerable because of insufficient financial resources and those that may be socially disenfranchised. The groups that will be discussed here are the near poor, the medically indigent, and the homeless.

Near Poor

Poverty refers to having insufficient financial resources to meet basic living expenses. These expenses include costs of food, shelter, clothing, transportation, and medical care. Most often, poverty is thought of in terms of federal poverty guidelines. In 1987, the *federally defined poverty level* for a family of four was $10,989 or less per year (Brown, 1987). However, many people have earnings just over the federally defined poverty levels and, using these levels as the standard for poverty, are therefore barely able to make ends meet.

These groups are considered the *near poor*. Most of the near poor do not qualify for various forms of financial support and as a result are more disadvantaged in some respects than those who do meet federal poverty guidelines (Curtin, 1986). Because of the similarity in socioeconomic disadvantage experienced by those who meet federal poverty guidelines and the near poor, some characteristics of the poor are examined below. The problems the near poor have in coping with these disadvantages because they do not qualify for governmental assistance are emphasized.

Demographics

Certain groups are consistently overrepresented among the poor and presumably among the near poor. These include women, children, ethnic groups such as blacks, Hispanics, Native Americans, and Southeast Asian refugees, and many elderly persons (Pesznecker, 1984), although the economic status of the elderly as a group appears to be improving. In fact, only 12% of the elderly were considered to be below the federal poverty level in 1987, as opposed to 35% in 1959 (US News and World Report, Oct. 9, 1989). Unfortunately, more elderly are among the near poor than any other age group (Grau, 1987). In addition to recognizing the demographic characteristics of the near poor at any one point in time, it is important to recognize what Grau (1987, p. 107) has called the *"fluidity of poverty,"* which means that people may move in and out of poverty over a lifetime. Situational factors such as widowhood or illness may precipitate poverty, particularly in groups with limited resources to start with, such as the elderly.

Standards of Poverty and Eligibility for Assistance

One of the problems with current health and welfare-assistance programs is the emphasis these programs place on eligibility based on federal poverty guidelines. As described in Chapter 4, federal poverty guidelines use an *absolute standard* of poverty that does not adequately reflect inflationary pressures. If a *relative standard* of poverty were used, many more people would qualify for federal programs because this approach more accurately reflects the effects of inflation, although such an approach would considerably increase federal health and welfare expenditures.

With the current system, many people find themselves having great difficulty obtaining affordable housing, sufficient food, adequate clothing, and medical care because they do not meet federal poverty guidelines, and as a result, they do not quality for many aid programs. Yet, these individuals and families find themselves unable to consistently afford the basic necessities of a healthy, productive life and thus are considered poor, using the more general criteria of being able to sustain a certain basic standard of living. The problems the near poor have are related to "falling between the cracks" of the current health and welfare system. It has been noted that the United States has a weak "safety net . . . [which is] the system of support for people who live in or close to poverty" (Brown, 1987, p. 40), particularly in comparison with other countries.

In addition to being ineligible for health and welfare programs because of stringent poverty guidelines, many people find that, even if they are under federal poverty guidelines, they may not qualify for assistance because eligibility levels are set far below poverty levels. Benefits for those who are eligible may be very limited. For example, the federal government tightened eligibility requirements and reduced benefits available from the food-stamp program in the early to middle 1980s, with the result that ". . . nearly half of the Americans in poverty receive no food stamps. Those who do get stamps receive an average benefit of 49 cents per meal" (Brown, 1987, p. 40). Similarly, in many states, nearly one half of those who are below federal poverty guidelines do not quality for Medicaid as a result of efforts by states to best use the limited funds that are available (Grau, 1987). Although these groups are categorized as below poverty level, from the perspective of health access, they have some of the same problems as the near poor.

Effects of Poverty on Health

It has been well documented that health status is inversely correlated with socioeconomic status (Haan, Kaplan, and Camacho, 1987; Pesznecker, 1984; U.S. Department of Health, Education, and Welfare, 1979). Health status indicators such as infant mortality rates, incidence and prevalence data for chronic illnesses, and accident rates provide convincing evidence of the poor-health outcomes in low-income groups. Infant mortality is higher for the poor and for ethnic groups, which are often disadvantaged. For example, the mortality for white infants in 1985 was 9.3%, whereas for black infants it was 18.2% (National Center for Health Statistics, 1988). In addition, lower socioeconomic groups have higher maternal mortality, they have ". . . higher morbidity and mortality rates for the leading chronic disease conditions, more restricted activity days, and greater need for dental care, and they are more likely to perceive their health as 'fair' or 'poor'" (Pesznecker, 1984). Presgrove (1985) observed that Medicaid patients were more ill and had longer average lengths of stay in hospitals than did patients covered under Blue Cross insurance.

USE OF SERVICES. Health service use varies by demographic group and may account for poorer health outcomes. For example, prenatal care was begun as late as the third trimester or not at all by 4.7% of white Americans in 1985, whereas 11.5% of American Indians either had no prenatal care or began prenatal care in the third trimester (National Center for Health Statistics, 1988). The poor are less likely to use preventive services, particularly if these services result in out-of-pocket expenses. Conversely, they are more likely to use inpatient services because these are more often covered by third-party reimbursement.

ENVIRONMENTAL INFLUENCES. Low-socioeconomic groups are less likely to be able to afford a nutritious diet and are more likely to live and work in hazardous environments. Crime, poor housing, stressful employment circumstances, environmental contamination, and transportation problems are thought to contribute to the poorer health status of low-socioeconomic groups (Haan, Kaplan, and Camacho, 1987). Access to services is a frequent problem, particularly because of transportation difficulties.

Although it has often been assumed that, if the environment of low-socioeconomic groups was altered to one that was more favorable, the risk of health problems would proportionately decrease, this may not be the case. In a retrospective study of 103,072 black and white births in Chicago, Collins and David (1990) found that traditional risk factors such as maternal age, marital status, and education did not completely account for the greater risk of delivering low birth weight infants by black mothers. Even those black mothers who were affluent had a significantly higher risk of delivering low birth weight infants than the white mothers. In fact, black mothers were twice as likely as white mothers to have had a low birth weight infant, irrespective of maternal age, education, or income. The researchers concluded that more than one generation of nonpoverty may be necessary to overcome the effects of poverty.

Other research reinforces the theory that the sociophysical environment of low-socioeconomic groups (rather than lifestyle habits alone) is a source of higher morbidity and mortality (Haan, Kaplan, and Camacho, 1987). In a 9-year-study of adult residents of a low-income area in Alameda County, California, it was found that the sample group experienced higher mortality than a similar group living in a more affluent area. This result was found even when the researchers adjusted the statistical analysis to control the factors typically considered to be the major risks in lower socioeconomic groups, that is, ". . . baseline health status, race, income, employment status, access to medical care, health insurance coverage, smoking, alcohol consumption, physical activity, body mass index, sleep patterns, social isolation, marital status, depression, and personal uncertainty" (Haan, Kaplan, and Camacho, 1987, p. 989).

Findings such as these two studies support the idea that individuals do not have complete control over their health status and that a hazardous environment may have an even more insidious and long-lasting effect than once thought. The near poor seem to suffer from the same adverse environmental conditions as those who meet federal poverty guidelines and who lack the support provided by some governmental programs.

Community Health Nursing Interventions

Community health nurses can intervene in many different ways to help the near poor improve their health-management skills. Recognition of the unique life circumstances of these clients and respect for their views of their own needs is crucial to successful interventions. Attempting to impose traditional care regimens on individuals without the basic needs of food, shelter, or human relationships or without the ability to functionally manage these needs is ineffective. Communication of acceptance, creation of a trusting environment, and a willingness to begin working with clients' perceptions of their needs are particularly important aspects of the nurse-client relationship. Communication strategies should be tailored to recognize cultural variations in communication styles (Martin and Henry, 1989). In addition, impoverished clients should be involved in the determination of their treatment plans because this may help break the "we-they" dichotomy that exists between middle-class health care providers and clients from lower socioeconomic backgrounds. The following case illustrates these points.

> The Hernandez family has been coming to the Well-Baby Clinic since their first child was born 5 years ago. Mrs. Hernandez is mildly mentally retarded and, although she is concerned about her three young children, seems to need constant reinforcement of proper child-care techniques from the nurses at the clinic. Mr. Hernandez works intermittently as a farm hand and carpenter and earns just enough money that the family is over federal poverty guidelines. The family lives in a run-down apartment in the inner city. They normally have some food in the house, although it is not always very nutritious. When Mrs. Hernandez brings the children to the clinic, they are often not dressed appropriately for the weather, but they do always wear shoes, shirts, and pants. The policy in the clinic is that all clients attending the clinic receive follow-up home visits from one of the nurses to make certain that the clients understand and are able to follow the directions for the health care of their children. On a recent visit, the nurse who visits the Hernandez family observed that Mrs. Hernandez was more concerned about how she was going to get to the local food bank to get extra food supplies to tide the family over for the next several days than she was about going to the pharmacy to get the antibiotic prescribed for her 3-year-old child's strep throat. The nurse decided the most effective approach would be to help Mrs. Hernandez problem solve about how she could get to the food bank before discussing

the need for the antibiotic. In the end, Mrs. Hernandez decided to ask her sister to watch her children while she borrowed her sister's car to go to the food bank and to the pharmacy located a few blocks away.

Some have questioned whether the poor have different value systems than those who are more affluent (Martin and Henry, 1989). Such a belief may interfere with the provision of health services (Moccia and Mason, 1986). However, because ethnic groups tend to be overrepresented among the poor, it is crucial that both individual health services and health programs reflect an awareness and understanding of cultural values (Martin and Henry, 1989).

On the other hand, it may be that basic social values are not extremely different between socioeconomic groups, but that, because of varying levels of basic need fulfillment, it simply appears that the poor have different values from the more affluent. For example, the young mother who has to choose between paying the rent and buying an expensive ointment for her child's skin rash may decide to use a home remedy for the rash and save her money for the rent. She is not necessarily demonstrating a strong value for home remedies; she may simply be making a pragmatic decision about how to use her resources most effectively. Another example that is common and confounding for many health professionals is the situation encountered with the family receiving food stamps who opts to buy chips, cookies, soft drinks and other high-fat, high-caloric density, nutritionally empty foods. Decisions like this may result from the pleasure derived from consuming these foods and the limited ability to purchase other pleasurable items.

Based on these ideas, the near poor may respond optimally to the provision of basic services initially, followed by services that reflect higher needs, such as health promotion services. It is important that community health nurses assess the presence of adverse *sociophysical variables* for clients and the actual and potential impact of these variables on client health.

What nurses should do as a result of the assessment of sociophysical stressors has been the subject of some debate. Moccia and Mason (1986) observed that many nursing interventions focus on helping clients cope with their situation. They pointed out that his approach ". . . reinforces the thinking that poverty is unavoidable" (p. 20). Because they viewed poverty as involving limited control over critical resources, they recommended that nursing interventions focus both on helping clients gain power and assisting clients to cope with their situation as effectively as possible. An integrated approach to interventions might include teaching clients how to approach those in power, such as landlords and employers, with the goal of improving the social and physical environment, while helping clients learn how to improve their environments themselves. For example, the nurse might help a client determine how to most effectively negotiate with an employer over hazardous working conditions and teach the client the importance of following through with safety precautions such as using hearing-protection devices on the job.

On a broader scale, community health nurses should become involved in health and welfare policy issues and decisions affecting low-socioeconomic groups. In one community, an entire low-income area was razed to allow for construction of a multimillion dollar facility city planners felt would be good for the local economy. Nurses in the area were active in pressing for adequate housing for displaced families. Voting for legislators with an understanding of the interrelatedness of social, economic, and health issues is another example of a broad-scale community health nursing intervention.

Medical Indigency
Definition of Medical Indigency

Medical indigency refers to the inability to pay fully for one's health care either privately, through private insurance, or with forms of government insurance such as Medicare or assistance programs such as Medicaid (Milburn, 1986). Medically indigent groups include those who are *uninsured* and those who are *underinsured*. Individuals who are medically indigent may or may not be near federal poverty guidelines; this term refers specifically to the inability to pay for medical care, rather than to the ability to afford the usual necessities of life such as shelter, food, and clothing.

Uninsured Clients

Individuals may be uninsured because they are unemployed, because their employer does not offer health insurance as a benefit, because they are self-employed, because they do not qualify for government insurance or assistance programs such as Medicare and Medicaid, or because they have a preexisting health condition that makes them uninsurable (Curtin, 1986; Wilensky, 1987). Cost for uninsured individuals was less problematic before 1980. Before that time, uncompensated care was commonly handled through *cost-sharing;* costs for those who could not pay for care were simply either passed on to those who could or underwritten by hospitals and private physicians. The increases in the cost of health care and the institution of a prospective payment system in 1983 with the passage of the Tax Equity and Fiscal Responsibility Act made it prohibitive for hospitals to share costs of uncompensated care or to pass that cost on to consumers. Many private physicians are willing to provide uncompensated care, but not all are, and patients may not know which physicians are willing to do so. Also, some patients object to receiving charity care and are unwilling to seek health care under these circumstances.

It has been estimated that between 31 and 37 million Americans are uninsured at any point in time, although these figures have been subject to some debate (Dentzer, 1989; Griffith, 1987; Wilensky, 1987). This represents between 15% and 20% of the American population who are uninsured (Parker, 1989; Rooks, 1990). The number of those uninsured in this country has increased significantly from the 1970s when approximately 25 million people were estimated to be uninsured (Wilensky, 1987). As this country moved away from cost-based reimbursement of health care in the 1970s and toward increased cost consciousness and an emphasis on competitiveness in the health care marketplace, the problems of the uninsured became more visible (Wilensky, 1987). The economic recession of the early 1980s further compounded the problem as unemployment increased, individuals changed jobs, and part-time jobs and job restructuring (such as job-sharing) limited benefits for health insurance (Presgrove, 1985), resulting in greater numbers of uninsured individuals and increases in uncompensated care.

The uninsured population is not a stable population group; rather, people may be uninsured for varying lengths of time. The uninsured population can be categorized into three groups: the *nonworking uninsured,* the *working uninsured,* and the *medically uninsurable* individual (Wilensky, 1987). It is a myth to assume that the uninsured are unemployed people living in poverty. It has been estimated that approximately three fourths of the uninsured population are employed individuals and their dependents (Griffith, 1987; Wilensky, 1987). Many of these people are referred to as the *working poor,* i.e., those who barely make ends meet, but who do not qualify for assistance programs because they make just over the minimal amount of money to qualify for Medicaid. In many cases, these people fall below federal poverty guidelines but are above the level set for Medicaid eligibility by their state of residence. Another sizable portion of this population is not poor; Wilensky (1987, p. 35) observed that ". . . while 35 to 40 percent were in families who are poor, at least one-third of the uninsured were in families whose income was twice the poverty line." Consider health needs in the following example of a working uninsured individual.

> Jane is a 30-year-old woman with a graduate degree in philosophy. She has been working at an assortment of part-time jobs for the past several years because it is very difficult to find full-time jobs in her field at the present time. She has no health insurance as a result of her part-time status in each of the positions she holds. This had not really been a problem for her until recently. She normally seeks preventive gynecological care at a family planning clinic that operates on a sliding scale basis. Over the last 2 years her weight has dropped precipitously following a rigid weight loss diet and rigorous adherence to a demanding exercise regimen. In fact, she has become so preoccupied with her weight that she spends several hours each day preparing special foods and exercising. In the last several months, she has developed amenorrhea and has begun noticing hair loss. She recognizes that her behavior is not normal and has sought assistance from her physician at the family planning clinic. He has become quite concerned and told her that she is anorexic and needs inpatient treatment. However, because she has no insurance, this type of treatment is not available, unless she loses 10 to 20 more pounds, when she could be treated on an emergency basis. This is not an acceptable option to her because she knows that she would be billed for the hospitalization and she would feel a constant duty to attempt repayment. At this point, the only real choice is for her to attend a support group for women with eating disorders at the family planning clinic.

Underinsured Clients

The underinsured population are usually thought to be those who have only minimal coverage (for example, self-employed individuals) and those who have exhausted their benefits and resources by paying for catastrophic illnesses (for example, elderly people in nursing homes) (Curtin, 1986). Another example of underinsured individuals are those elderly who have Medicare but cannot afford *"Medigap"* insurance to pay for those services and supplies not covered by Medicare. *Medigap insurance* is a term used to refer to any insurance policy which covers expenses not covered by Medicare. For many impoverished elderly, Medicaid functions in this way; for those not eligible for Medicaid, severe financial hardship may result (Grau, 1987).

Health Consequences

Individuals who are uninsured or underinsured tend not to seek health services as readily as those with sufficient coverage (Wilensky, 1987). In particular, this population group is more likely to delay nonemergency services and is less likely to participate in illness prevention and health promotion programs (Presgrove, 1985). Paradoxically, this group uses emergency services more often than others.

Medicaid Coverage

The primary approach to serving uninsured women and children in this country has been through benefits provided by the Medicaid program.

ELIGIBILITY. Although Medicaid is an assistance program, rather than an insurance program, it provides for basic health services for needy and low-income people, for those who are blind and disabled, and for families with dependent children. (Refer to Chapter 4 for more information on the specific types of coverage available to Medicaid recipients). The Medicaid program is crucial to the many uninsured women and children in this country as a result of the size of this population group and the extent of their need for services. Griffith (1987, p. 90) noted that ". . . thirty-six percent of America's 9 million poor women and 30 percent of America's 5 million near-poor women of childbearing-age were completely uninsured in 1984. One-third of all poor children and 29 percent of all near-poor children under 18 were also uninsured." Although a 1989 federal law required that ". . . all states must . . . provide Medicaid coverage for pregnant women and for children up to the age of six if the family incomes are less than 133% of the federal poverty level" (Rooks, 1990), this still leaves gaps in coverage for those who just exceed the eligibility criteria. In fact, Medicaid now covers only 40% of the poor, whereas in 1975, 63% of those living in poverty were covered by Medicaid (Parker, 1989). In addition, roughly 2 million people (Parker, 1989) were cut from the Medicaid program in a Congressional effort to reduce expenses.

PROBLEMS. Why are fewer than half of the poor in this country covered by Medicaid (Griffith, 1987)? Because individual states determine the policies that apply to the disbursement of limited Medicaid funds, many people are not eligible to receive funds although they may be needy. States commonly have policies that restrict Medicaid eligibility to those who are well-below federal poverty guidelines. Some states restrict the eligibility of families with children to those in single-parent homes although the two-parent family may be below federal poverty guidelines (Griffith, 1987). These policies occur because states have only three options to manage limited funds for Medicaid: They can raise taxes, which is not politically popular; they can lower reimbursement rates for providers, which is similarly unpalatable; or

they can tighten eligibility criteria (Rooks, 1990).

An example of a program that has received a great deal of attention for the controversial way in which eligibility for Medicaid support has been revised is the Oregon Plan. The state of Oregon developed a plan that results in explicitly rationed health services based on levels of state funding. The 1989 Oregon Basic Health Services Act provides basic health services to the entire population of the state (Rooks, 1987). ". . . Its key feature is a process to rank health services according to their effectiveness and to the importance of the benefit expected to result from each service" (Rooks, 1987, p. 41). The state legislature analyzes high-priority services in light of absolute costs and cost effectiveness and determines those services the state can pay for. Those that meet both the criteria of high priority and cost effectiveness are made accessible to all people in the state. Employers are required to provide coverage for the same services for their employees (Larkin, 1990).

The plan has generated heated discussion, largely centered around issues of *rationing health care*. Proponents have observed that health care is implicitly rationed in this country at the current ime; when eligibility limits are set, essentially those who meet the criteria receive any services that are necessary, whereas those who do not meet the criteria do not receive any services. With the Oregon plan, all citizens receive a basic predetermined level of cost-effective, high-priority health services. Opponents of the plan criticize the explicit rationing of health services because the plan will not cover certain expensive services for single individuals such as transplants of various types, and the prioritization is relevant only to those who cannot afford services that others can purchase privately (Parker, 1989). In other words, some see this as further movement toward a two-tiered system of health care in this country, with one set of services available to the affluent and another set of services available to the poor. Some are concerned that, if funds run short, the list of covered services will be so short that many essential services will not be available to the poor. This plan essentially operates out of a utilitarian concept of justice with the focus on providing the "greatest good to the greatest number."

Another problem in financing health care for a vulnerable group has been that elderly individuals are largely unable to sustain the costs of extended illness and nursing home placement without impoverishment of their spouses as a result of Medicaid regulations. When an individual is placed in a nursing home, the individual must pay for that care until he or she has met the *"spend-down"* requirements of Medicaid. "Medicaid policies require that spouses be economically responsible for each other" (Grau, 1987, p. 110). Therefore spouses must deplete economic assets to pay for health care until they reach the eligibility level set by Medicaid. In this way, the spouse becomes impoverished and is likely to eventually become a Medicaid recipient as well (Grau, 1987).

One way some families have manged this is by *divestment*. In this situation, the elderly individual turns over his or her economic assets to a family member other than the spouse, thereby protecting the assets. Unfortunately, in addition to losing control over their assets, this may also place

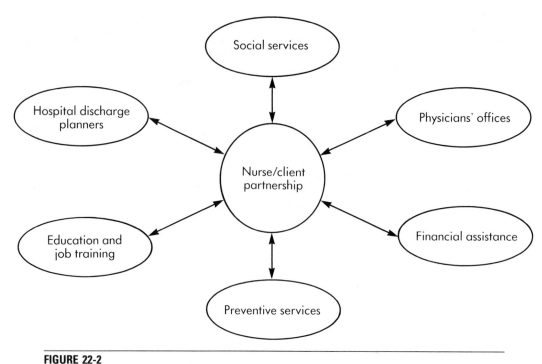

FIGURE 22-2

The community health nurse's mediating role with vulnerable populations.

some elderly individual's at a disadvantage if nursing home placement is contingent on having the economic resources to pay for the care (Grau, 1987). Recent changes in Medicaid that should help resolve this problem have resulted in allowing the spouse of a nursing home resident ". . . to keep $786 a month in income and $12,000 in assets" (U.S. News and World Report, Dec.11, 1989).

Role of the Community Health Nurse

Probably the most important aspect of the role of the community health nurse when working with medically indigent individuals, families, and groups is to help connect the client with community resources that can help supplement either their reimbursement resources or their health service needs (Figure 22-2). Often, the best way to proceed is to contact the local social services department and refer the client to a social worker for a workup for possible inclusion in a medical assistance program of some sort.

Also, the nurse should consider referring the client to community programs that can help provide the service the client needs at an affordable cost. Most communities have voluntary groups that can help fill the gaps in services that clients need. For example, one community had a medication program in which individuals with documented chronic diseases could obtain a card that entitled them to significant medication discounts at participating local pharmacies. In these cases the nurse should investigate the services before making the referral to ensure that the client is eligible for services. Then, the client should be carefully instructed on how to make the best use of the services to avoid frustration by the client or the providers. It is wise to follow up on the referral to ensure that the client has successfully obtained

the necessary services and that the intended service goals are being achieved. The nurse serves as an advisor by helping the client learn to use the system. This type of approach should help the client become more skillful in managing his or her own health care and avoid inducing dependency.

Homelessness

Homelessness is a condition with social and economic causes that affect individual and group health in very basic ways. Definitions of homelessness vary and indicate the difficulties in neatly categorizing this population group. The definition of homelessness cited in the Stewart B. McKinney Homeless Assistance Act (P.L. 100-77) of 1987 is shown in the box on p. 375. This definition implies transience and suggests that these individuals may be otherwise housed at other points in time. In fact, this impermanence results in fluctuating periods of stability and a lack of regular, sustained social relationships. The Committee on Community Health Services of the American Academy of Pediatrics noted that ". . . the U.S. General Accounting Office defines homeless individuals as those persons who lack resources and community ties necessary to provide for their own adequate shelter" (1988, p. 938). This definition underscores the role insufficient resources and social support play in homelessness.

These characteristics lead to the often mentioned "disenfranchisement" of the homeless with the associated lack of usual social supports (Baxter and Hopper, 1981; Sebastian, 1985). This disenfranchisement results in part from active efforts on the part of many homeless to avoid contact with any form of legal authority (Larew, cited in Boondas, 1985) and in part from the efforts of discouraged families and

---

HOMELESSNESS

1. An individual who lacks a fixed, regular, and adequate nighttime residence *or*
2. An individual who has a primary nighttime residence that is one of the following:
   a. A supervised or publicly operated shelter designed to provide temporary living accommodations (including welfare hotels, congregate shelters, and transitional housing for the mentally ill)
   b. An institution that provides a temporary residence for individuals intended to be institutionalized
   c. A public or private place not designed for, or ordinarily used as, a regular sleeping accommodation for human beings

From National Academy of Sciences Homelessness, health, and human needs, Washington, DC, 1988, National Academy Press.

FACTORS CONTRIBUTING TO THE DEVELOPMENT OF HOMELESSNESS

Individual health status
   Alcoholism
   Mental illness
Immediate social environment
   Unemployment
   Poverty
   Family dysfunction
   Lack of low income housing
Health and social policies
   Deinstitutionalization
   Reduction in health and welfare benefits

---

sometimes social agencies who discontinue contact with recalcitrant homeless individuals unwilling to comply with family or agency norms. In fact, some have said that the lack of social supports is the characteristic that most distinguishes the homeless from the poor (Lindsey, 1989).

Demographics

From a program-planning and policy-development perspective, it is difficult to estimate the numbers of homeless with any precision, and therefore it is difficult to precisely measure the health and social needs of this group. Recent estimates of the numbers of homeless range from 350,000 to between 3 and 4 million (Wright and Weber, 1987). Regardless of the exact number of homeless in this country, increasing numbers of persons became homeless during the 1980s (Wright and Weber, 1987; Francis, 1987).

The demographic picture of the homeless population has changed in the last decade. Recent studies have found that the "new homeless" (Wright and Weber, 1987) are far more heterogeneous than suggested by old stereotypes of the older, alcoholic white male or severely mentally ill individual. They are younger and better educated than in years past and include more women, families with children, racial and ethnic minorities, and people with neither alcohol problems or mental illness (although the mentally ill and substance abusers do continue to make up a large part of the population). In fact, minority groups are overrepresented in the homeless population.

Regional variations have been found in the demographic characteristics of the homeless (Maurin, Russell, and Memmott, 1989). For example, more two-parent families can be found in the homeless populations of the West and Southwest than in large urban areas in the East, such as New York City (Institute of Medicine, 1988). Approximately one third of the homeless are families with children, although this figure has been estimated to be much higher in some cities. Additionally, some ". . . studies show that more than half of homeless children are less than 5 years of age and are preponderantly minority children" (Committee on Community Health Services, 1988, p. 938).

The numbers of homeless families have reportedly been increasing faster than any other group of homeless in recent years. It is thought that this is largely the result of increasingly limited low-income housing and an increasing proportion of families below federal poverty guidelines (Wood, 1989). Welfare benefits are limited, and when these stresses are combined with family conflicts, marginal employment, and single parenthood, homelessness may result (Bassuk and Rubin, 1987).

Types of Homeless Individuals

Homeless individuals may be thought of as *temporarily homeless, episodically homeless,* or *chronically homeless* (Arce et al., 1983; Institute of Medicine, 1988; Splatman, 1983). An Institute of Medicine (1988) report on the homeless defined temporarily homeless individuals as those who have been ". . . displaced from their usual dwellings by natural or man-made calamities" (p. 23). Families temporarily dispossessed by disasters such as fires exemplify the temporarily homeless. The assumption is that these groups tend to have greater stability in their living conditions over longer periods of time and perhaps more sources of support.

"Episodically homeless people are those who frequently go in and out of homelessness" (Institute of Medicine, 1988, p. 23). Migrant workers or runaway youth are examples of episodically homeless. Episodically homeless families who obtain temporary shelter from friends are considered to be among the "hidden homeless" while they maintain these living arrangements.

"Chronically homeless" individuals and families are those without permanent residences for a year or more (Institute of Medicine, 1988). The differences in these groups suggest that they have different needs and that programs should be tailored with an understanding of those needs.

Factors Contributing to the Development of Homelessness

Factors that contribute to the *development of homelessness* are diverse and synergistic (see box top right). They include factors related to (1) the health status of the individual, such as alcoholism and mental illness; (2) the immediate social environment of the individual or family, such as unemployment, poverty, family dysfunction, and insufficient amounts of low-income housing; and (3) those relating to the larger social environment including broad social- and health-related policies (Francis, 1987; Wright and Weber, 1987), such as deinstitutionalization of the chronically mentally ill and reductions in benefits from health and welfare programs (Abdellah, Chamberlain, and Levine, 1986).

INDIVIDUAL HEALTH STATUS. In the past the steroeotype of the homeless was that they were largely alcoholic. Although this is changing, alcoholism can be and often is the catalyst that ultimately results in loss of home, family, friends, and job. Significant others in the alcoholic's environment may either tire of the problems resulting from alcoholism or may be counseled to avoid enabling behaviors. Either can result in the alcoholic person hitting rock bottom as a homeless and disenfranchised individual.

A large number of the homeless are mentally ill. In many cases it is thought that homelessness among this population results from inadequate community support systems for the seriously mentally ill who have been discharged from inpatient facilities in the hope of integrating them into the larger society. Often, family members find it difficult to care for seriously mentally ill members either because of the disruption they cause or because the affected individual runs away. Seriously mentally ill individuals have frequent difficulties following their medication regimens and can relapse into psychoses. Their often marginal functional status prohibits them in many cases from maintaining an independent residence, holding a job, or managing daily responsibilities such as shopping, cooking, or cleaning.

IMMEDIATE SOCIAL ENVIRONMENT. Maurin, Russell, and Memmott (1989) found that the primary reasons given for homelessness by respondents to the Utah Homeless Survey were unemployment, ". . . inability to stay with family or friends" (p. 318), and family conflict. Interestingly, one of the major reasons for homelessness was "other," which included diverse problems ranging ". . . from having been robbed to experiencing many medical problems" (p. 320). The authors observed that people with marginal resources may become homeless following a seemingly minor crisis with which they are unable to cope as a result of their limited financial, social, and emotional resources.

Becaue of the severely strained financial resources of the near poor, a seemingly small crisis such as an increase in rent or an inability to pay rent for several months may be enough to result in loss of a home. When the situation is prolonged, it is difficult to maintain a job because of the daily difficulties of managing personal hygiene and obtaining rest, thus resulting in even greater financial difficulties. A cycle of difficulties begins, which some are unable to break out of without significant assistance.

Lack of sufficient low-income housing is a major contributor to homelessness. Wright and Weber (1987) noted two factors related to this problem. Both the effect of inflation on the price of housing in recent years and an overall increase in the proportion of those in this country living at

HEALTH PROBLEMS OF THE HOMELESS
PHYSICAL HEALTH PROBLEMS
Acute: Infectious processes
Trauma
Upper respiratory tract diseases
Food poisoning
Dermatologic infestations
Chronic: Hypertension
Chronic lung disease
Peripheral vascular disease
Heart disease
Tuberculosis
Malnutrition
MENTAL HEALTH PROBLEMS
Schizophrenia
Bipolar disorders
Major depression
Substance abuse

or below federal poverty levels have contributed to a relative insufficiency of low-income housing.

In a study of homeless and housed families receiving public assistance in New York City, Weitzman (1989) found a correlation between pregnancy and recent births with homelessness. Furthermore, she found that teenage pregnancy was strongly linked with homelessness among families receiving public assistance. Additionally, the homeless women had ". . . fewer of their own children living with them . . . this finding potentially lends support to the hypothesis that the homeless 'give up' some of their children during difficult periods" (Weitzman, 1989, p. 178). She speculated that, rather than pregnancy causing homelessness, factors associated with pregnancy, such as the need for safe, sanitary housing, and policies favoring pregnant women and new mothers in emergency shelters may have influenced the findings. However, she noted that a constellation of factors, including early family dysfunction, poverty, housing conditions, and social policies, may all contribute to homelessness and the subsequent decision to seek emergency shelter.

BROAD SOCIAL ENVIRONMENT. Following the passage of the Community Mental Health Centers Act of 1963, large numbers of chronically mentally ill individiuals were deinstitutionalized in an effort to provide less restrictive care (Riesdorph-Ostrow, 1989). Such care was made possible by the development of relatively safe, effective psychoactive drugs during the 1950s. Unfortunately, although the act called for provision of appropriate community support services for this population, in many cases such services were either never developed or were inadequate. The services that currently exist are often fragmented and disorganized. It is difficult for many chronically mentally ill individuals to function effectively in such circumstances or to negotiate the bureaucratic systems often in place. In addition, some services, such as Supplemental Security Income, may not be available to those in need because one of the eligibility criteria is residency (Riesdorph-Ostrow, 1989). As a result, many homeless individuals are mentally ill, although the definition of mental illness and the actual number of those who are homeless are subjects of great dispute (Francis, 1987; Wright and Weber, 1987).

Health Problem

The primary *health problems* found among homeless populations are both physical and mental (see box at right). Among the physical problems commonly found in homeless populations are acute illnesses and injuries, including infectious processes, trauma, upper respiratory tract diseases, food poisoning, and dermatologic problems. Exaccerbations of chronic illnesses are also common, such as hypertension, chronic lung diseases, peripheral vascular disease, heart disease, tuberculosis, and malnutrition (Bowdler, 1989; Breakey, et al., 1989; Damrosch and Stasser, 1988). *Co-morbidity,* or the simultaneous existence of more than one health problem, is common. Mental health problems include major mental illnesses such as schizophrenia, bipolar disorders, major depression, and substance abuse (Breakey et al., 1989). Alcholism and drug abuse are thought to affect approximately 30% of the homeless (Bowdler, 1989). It is particularly difficult to manage co-morbidity of mental health problems. Alcohol abuse, drug abuse, and mental illness often coexist. Not only is it difficult to persuade clients to accept treatment, it is difficult to find programs that treat multiple problems (Institutes of Medicine, 1988).

Unfortunately, many common treatment approaches for these problems are unworkable for the homeless, who may not have storage space for medications and supplies and who do not follow a traditional daily schedule (Sebastian, 1985). For example, homeless diabetics have great difficulty in maintaining insulin, syringes, and blood–glucose-testing supplies and using them as instructed. Instructions to take medications with every meal are meaningless for homeless individuals who may eat whenever food is found. Another common problem is that it is extremely difficult to prevent reinfestation of homeless individuals following delousing treatments (Lindsey, 1989).

Homeless Children

Health needs of *homeless children* are related to age and life-style (See box). Health problems include scabies, lice, dermatologic problems, dental problems, chronic cardiovascular problems, neurological disorders, anemia, asthma and bronchitis, incomplete immunization status, developmental problems, behavioral and school problems, such as erratic attendance (Institute of Medicine, 1988) and failure, anxiety, and depression (Bassuk and Rubin, 1987; Committee on Community Health Services, 1988; Wood, 1989). In addition, the condition of living in shelters, with the associated transience and dislocation from friends, schools, and other social supports negatively influences the development of these children (Bassuk and Rubin, 1987; Committee on Community Health Services, 1988).

HEALTH PROBLEMS OF HOMELESS CHILDREN

PHYSICAL HEALTH PROBLEMS

    Scabies
    Lice
    Dermatologic infections
    Dental problems
    Chronic cardiovascular problems
    Neurological disorders
    Anemia
    Asthma
    Bronchitis
    Incomplete immunization status

SOCIAL AND DEVELOPMENTAL PROBLEMS

    Developmental problems
    Behavioral problems
    School-related problems
        Erratic attendance
        Failure
    Anxiety and depression

Homeless Elderly

The homeless elderly population is at the other end of the age continuum in relation to vulnerability. In a study of older men in the Bowery in New York City, Cohen et al. (1988) found a much higher incidence of physical problems among those who were homeless than among those who were at least marginally sheltered. In addition to the higher incidence of health problems, the homeless men were less likely to be receiving those benefits for which they were eligible, such as Medicaid. A primary reason given for this was the lack of an address. In general, these older men were much less likely to seek care for their health problems than their community-living counterparts. The normal developmental processes of the elderly may conflict with the homeless life-style to create an even more hazardous situation. Boondas (1985) explained that the normal phase of disengagement from society by the elderly becomes pathological for older homeless individuals who lack basic necessities such as food, clothing, and shelter while becoming socially disengaged.

Approaches to Working with the Homeless

Approaches to working with homeless populations are varied. Most authors emphasize meeting this population group in their own physical environment and accepting their perception of needs. Health and social programs are more likely to be effective if they are planned in areas frequented by the homeless, rather than in traditional settings, which may be inconvenient and less responsive to this group. Additionally, programs are most likely to be effective if they are located in close geographic proximity so that clients are not forced to walk or take public transportation to a myriad of different services. Programs may be focused on a single need, such as food, shelter, em-

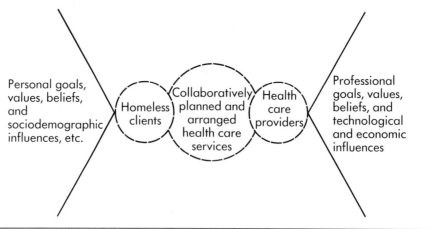

FIGURE 22-3

Framework for providing service to the homeless. *(From Nichols J, Wright LK, and Murphy JF: Framework for providing service to the homeless J Community Health 11(3):206, 1986.)*

ployment assistance, or medical care, or they may be broadly based with a rehabilitative focus designed to help the homeless become more self-sufficient, thereby reducing vulnerability.

Rehabilitation requires provision of long-term support of skills necessary for acquisition of and maintenance of jobs, homes, and social networks. Assignment of staff who have specific responsibilities for the rehabilitation program has been found to be an effective approach to inclusion of this second level of programming for the homeless (Greiff, Zipple, and McCarthy, 1987).

An example of a large scale effort to provide health care to the homeless was the Robert Wood Johnson and the Pew Memorial Trust initiative established in 1983 to fund demonstration projects in 19 cities. A study of the sites funded by the Robert Wood Johnson and the Pew Memorial Trust found that although the programs differed, seven common elements could be identified in each program. These were the use of a holistic approach toward clients, outreach, empathetic staff, a multidisciplinary approach, case management and coordination of services, provision of continuity, and a broad range of services (Institute of Medicine, 1988).

Nurses provide health care to homeless groups in soup kitchens, churches, missions, and shelters, to name a few of the many creative locations where such care is provided. Nursing care may be the only health service available or may be provided as part of a multidisciplinary program. Screening, first aid, referrals, health teaching, crisis intervention, provision of prescribed medical treatments, health monitoring, and counseling are examples of the types of care that might be provided in this situation.

Two approaches that are similar and potentially effective are case management and agency coalitions. Both recognize the importance of mediating community systems for and with the homeless client. Abdellah, Chamberlain, and Levine (1986) observed that the most important role nurses have with homeless groups may be that of mediating, or "brokering" services. This is done by assumption of a *case management* role in which a nurse coordinates all care re-

ceived by an individual, follows up on referrals, and essentially "connects" a client with the needed services, while helping the client learn the skills necessary to maximize the use of the services. The usefulness of such an approach stems from the recognition of the "multifaceted needs of homeless persons" (p. 497).

An example of a similar approach to service coordination on a broader scale was provided by Nichols, Wright, and Murphy (1986). Figure 22-3 illustrates the framework used in coordinating services for the homeless by a coalition of agencies in one city. In this framework the personal goals, values, and beliefs of health providers mesh with the goals, values, and beliefs of homeless clients through collaboratively planned and executed services. These authors described a tool used to track referrals made for homeless clients in a Southwestern city by the City Coalition for Health Care for the Homeless, funded by the Robert Wood Johnson Foundation and the Pew Memorial Trust. The tool, called the Tool for Referral Assessment of Continuity (TRAC) of health, was used to assist with intersystem coordination of referrals and service provision. Each cooperating agency had one individual responsible for following clients receiving services originating within that agency, rather than each homeless client having a specific case manager. Such a role is appropriate for community health nurses.

This approach is similar to case management, but it recognizes that, in practice, it may be difficult to arrange for homeless clients to work through one case manager. Instead, depending on the number and type of agencies serving the homeless, these individuals may initiate services in any of a number of agencies. For example, a client may initially seek care at an emergency room following a street fight or may first become known to health care workers in a soup kitchen. This tool was also used to assist with evaluation of program effectiveness because it provided information on service use and follow-up.

For most community health nurses, an acute sensitivity to the pressing and multifaceted needs of the homeless should lead to an active role in coordinating services and providing support for clients no matter what the setting. Homeless clients need specific, simple instructions and should have referrals arranged in such a way that they can easily follow through. For example, it would be unrealistic for a nurse in a primary care clinic to refer a homeless pregnant woman to a Women, Infant, and Children's (WIC) clinic to obtain food supplies when the woman has no way to store or prepare those foods. It would be far more realistic to refer her to a source of housing with transportation back to the clinic for continued prenatal care, combined with referral to a social worker who could begin to help her make plans for more permanent housing and a source of income with which to support her infant. At that time a WIC referral would be useful.

Interventions on behalf of the homeless should take place at broader levels to make changes in the basic causes of homelessness. Berne et al. (1990, p. 12) observed that ". . . most health services for the homeless are really secondary and tertiary prevention." They recommended that primary preventive measures target public policies and focus on provision of adequate education, job training, affordable housing, child care, reasonable wages, and access to preventive services. Community health nurses should take active roles in the resolution of these issues.

AGE-RELATED VULNERABILITY

Certain groups are particularly vulnerable to poor health outcomes because they are exposed to both socioeconomic stressors and age-related physiological stressors that interact synergistically. The three groups that are described in this chapter are runaway youth, pregnant adolescents, and the frail elderly and their caregivers.

Runaway Youth

Runaway youth are *episodically homeless*. In fact, running away has been described as ". . . not so much an event as a process" (Institute of Medicine, 1988, p. 14) and involves running away for progressively longer periods of time before becoming chronically homeless. Runaways have been defined as ". . . minors who leave home without permission from parents or guardians" (Englel and Lau, 1983, p. 74), although some children may be *throwaways* whose parents have forced them to leave or have abandoned them. Reasons for running away vary, although Mirkin, Raskin, and Antognini (1984) describe three groups whose running is precipitated by different family dynamics. The *rootless runaway* is reacting to a family environment that was lenient until adolescence, when unaccustomed restraints on behavior were imposed. The *anxious runaway* is fleeing a dysfunctional family and excessive responsibilities. Finally, the *terrified runaway* is escaping an abusive family environment, particularly one involving sexual abuse and incest. Family conflict and abuse are common patterns causing running away. Some have said that running away may be the healthy response to such a situation (Community Council of Greater New York, 1984; also cited in Institutes of Medicine, 1988).

The absolute number of runaways in the United States is difficult to establish. Estimates range from 1 to 2 million (Engel and Lau, 1983; Manov and Lowther, 1983), but definitive statistics are unavailable (Institutes of Medicine, 1988). In general, runaways tend to take more risks than other youths, lack acceptance of societal values, need immediate gratification, and often function as a protector of the parents' marriage and a parent of the parents (Engel and Lau, 1983; Mirkin, Raskin, and Antognini, 1984). Runaways may also serve the function of preserving a dysfunctional family because the family can focus on the problems created by the runaway, rather than on the core dysfunctions (Mirkin, Raskin, and Antognini, 1984).

Health Problems

Health problems result from the activities runaways engage in to support themselves and from their tendency to postpone health care because of fear of authorities. It is not unusual for runaways to resort to prostitution and drug dealing to support themselves. Runaways often exhibit poor general health from malnutrition, poor hygiene, and interrupted or insufficient sleep (Manov and Lowther, 1983). Anemia, infestations, and dental problems are common. Depression and self-destructive behavior, including substance abuse and suicide, are problems in this group. Sexually transmitted diseases, trauma, and pregnancy result from prostitution and sexual abuse. The sequelae from sexual activity may result in chronic problems, including ". . . rectal fissures, lesions, poor sphincter control, lacerated vaginas, foreign bodies in the anus or vagina, perforated anal and vaginal walls, [and] chronic choking from gonorrhea tonsillitis" (Manov and Lowther, 1983, p. 337).

Role of the Community Health Nurse

Establishing trust with the runaway is the critical element in provision of health services. Without a completely unjudgmental and trusting relationship, the youth is unlikely to return for future services. In addition, word will spread that the health care provider is untrustworthy, thereby further limiting the likelihood of others seeking care. Nurses should be clear about values they hold that may interfere with care for runaways. They must treat runaway clients with respect for and understanding of their chaotic life circumstances. Manov and Lowther (1983) recommend the cultivation of a sense of humor when working with this population. They also recommend development of interviewing and communication skills so that clients will clearly understand what information is confidential and what information cannot be confidential (such as suicidal or homicidal intentions). Furthermore, they suggest that nurses provide as many services as possible at one time, because the runaway may never return for follow-up. Finally, they suggest giving the runaway youth a card with names and phone numbers of community services for future use. It is helpful to include the nurse's first name and the name, address, and phone number of the clinic so the youth can call with questions following the visit.

Pregnant Adolescents

Adolescents who have children are another example of a group that has combined developmental and situational demands with limited support systems for coping with those demands.

Scope of the Problem

The adolescent pregnancy problem has been increasing in the United States with an associated increase in low birth weight infants and an infant mortality rate that is higher than that of 16 other developed countries. "Annually, more than 1.1 million teenagers (or 11% of all teenage females) in the U.S. become pregnant, resulting in approximately 700,000 live births. The majority of these mothers keep and raise their children. This means that teenagers in the United States now bear and rear about one out of every six children" (Yoos, 1987, p. 193).

In fact, according to 1980 data, the United States had higher rates of adolescent pregnancy, adolescent livebirths, and abortions than six other countries with which it was compared. The number of livebirths to parents under the age of 20 has declined over the last several decades, although the number of births to mothers between 10 and 14 years of age has nearly doubled in that period of time (U.S. Bureau of the Census, 1990). Comparisons of coital frequency and contraceptive use between adolescents in the United States and in other industrialized countries suggests that the reason for the higher rates of pregnancy, livebirths, and abortions is because American teenagers are less likely to use contraceptives and, when they do, they tend to use the less effective forms (Trussell, 1988).

Risk Factors

While adolescents in general are at risk for pregnancy, the highest risk groups are ". . . young adolescents and those from socially and economically disadvantaged backgrounds" (Panel on Adolescent Pregnancy and Child Rearing, 1987, p. 120). Certain ethnic groups may also have a higher risk of adolescent pregnancy (National Center for Health Statistics, 1987; Pletsch, 1990). Teenage boys should be considered part of the risk group, rather than assuming that this is a problem of young girls only. Adolescent pregnancy seems to be correlated with problems in the home and at school. In a study of participants in an alternative educational program for pregnant adolescents, Palmore and Shannon (1988) found that many of the subjects had attendance problems in school, had repeated grades in school, had dysfunctional family relationships, reported family violence, had mothers who themselves had experienced teenage pregnancy, and reported exposure to substance abuse.

Problems

In addition to delivering low birth weight newborns, adolescents are more likely to become toxemic and to develop pregnancy-induced hypertension and anemia. The maternal mortality for adolescents is more than twice as high as it is for mothers in their twenties (Auvenshine and Enriquez, 1990). Although it has commonly been thought that these problems are the result of age, it may be that poverty influences adverse outcomes. Insufficient prenatal care is thought to be an important influence on adolescent pregnancies (Trussell, 1988; Auvenshine and Enriquez, 1990).

Adolescents and their infants are highly vulnerable to the development of ineffective parent-child relationships as a result of the dual demands of self-development and learning parenting skills by the adolescent. The unfinished devel-

---

NATIONAL ACADEMY OF SCIENCES' GOALS OF POLICIES FOR TEENAGE PREGNANCY

1. Reduce the rate and incidence of unintended pregnancy among adolescents, especially among school-age teenagers
2. Provide alternatives to adolescent childbearing and parenting
3. Promote positive social, economic, health, and developmental outcomes for adolescent parents and their children

From Panel on Adolescent Pregnancy and Childbearing: Comment: risking the future, Family Plan Perspect 19(3):120, 1987.

---

opmental task of separation and regeneration is likely to be further interfered with by pregnancy and child rearing (Poole, 1987); that is, it is difficult for an adolescent to complete the task of emotional separation from others while simultaneously building a close and nurturing relationship with an infant. This may result in the potential for neglect (Bobak, 1987).

Economic outcomes of teenage pregnancies have long-range effects. Adolescents who have children are more likely to discontinue their education, thereby limiting future career opportunities. Adolescent girls who choose to keep their infants are more likely to raise their children alone. If they do marry, the family is ". . . likely to become dependent on public assistance and remain dependent longer than those who delay childbearing until their twenties" (Panel on Adolescent Pregnancy and Child Rearing, 1987, p. 119). Furthermore, these young people are likely to be chronically unemployed or underemployed. Children of adolescent parents are less likely to be academically successful and more likely to repeat patterns of early childbearing and higher fertility rates (Trussell, 1988).

Interventions

A 1987 National Academy of Sciences' Report on Teenage Pregnancy recommended three overall goals of policies dealing with these problems: reduction of unplanned pregnancies, provision of alternatives to teenage childbearing, and promotion of healthy outcomes for adolescent parents (see box above).

These recommendations are based on recognition of the limited use of contraceptives by sexually active teenagers and include suggestions for public financial support of contraceptive services for adolescents, for education to correct misinformation about contraceptives, and for development of school-based clinics. Comprehensive school-based clinics have been used with positive results to help adolescents deal with health problems, generally, and with reproductive problems in particular (Heller, 1988). The goal of these clinics is holistic, emphasizing improved physical and mental health of adolescents.

This approach has been controversial as a result of adolescents' status as minors. Some believe that adolescents do not need parental permission for treatment (Panel on Adolescent Pregnancy and Child Rearing, 1987). They feel that the care and counseling adolescents receive in these clinics should be confidential and should not be disclosed to the client's parents without the permission of the client because adolescents are more likely to seek services under these circumstances. Most clinics require that parents sign blanket permission forms for treatment of adolescents but are not informed when their children seek services. Others argue that parental interests, concerns, and responsibility supercede the adolescent's right to confidentiality.

The easy access to services provided by school clinics and the orientation of these clinics to adolescents have been thought to be important factors leading to their success. Confidentiality and low cost are other factors that make these clinics appealing to adolescents (Heller, 1988). Some school-based clinics are located on school property, whereas others are not but are located close by. Adolescent health clinics are most effective when they are near schools because the proximity of services alleviates transportation problems and facilitates participation in health services. The approach used in these clinics recognizes their unique concerns and developmental needs.

For example, it has been found that peer-role modeling and peer counseling are effective in increasing contraceptive use among sexually active adolescents. This method recognizes the adolescent's need to identify with a peer group. Also, adolescents are more likely to develop comfortable relationships with the nurses in the clinics because the nurses may participate in health education classes, thereby enhancing their visibility (Heller, 1988).

Staff nurses may perform the initial assessments, which is an ideal time to establish rapport with the adolescent and to begin the development of a picture of the interrelatedness between health, developmental, and social concerns of the adolescent. Nurses in these clinics have contact with adolescent males, as well as females, and should expand educational efforts to include the males (Heller, 1988). Young adolescent boys have been found to report no perceived responsibility for contraception and have less knowledge of contraception than do girls (Reis and Herz, 1987). Nurses are in roles pivotal to designing and providing health education classes, peer-support programs, and counseling for reproductive and general health matters for both boys and girls.

The recommendations also recognize that for low-income adolescents, many disincentives to delayed childbearing exist in a world in which these youths are discouraged, feel they have limited opportunities, and have few role models in situations characterized by several generations of poverty. School health nurses should understand the interactions between social and health outcomes of this vulnerable group and work with teachers and parents to provide programs that respond to these needs. Pletsch (1990) described an example of the interface between program planning and culture. She noted that in certain Hispanic cultures, adolescent females may not be highly valued and stressing delayed childbearing and higher education in family planning programs would not be very effective. However, emphasizing the economic realities in this country may be a more acceptable way to approach this dilemma.

It is unlikely that contraceptive education alone will successfully reduce the rate of adolescent pregnancy (Burke, 1987) and the associated poor social, economic, and health outcomes. Some schools have developed day-care facilities

on their campuses and others offer parenting classes in conjunction with day care. Programs such as these provide direct support to adolescent parents who wish to continue their education and who need help learning their new roles as parents, while coping with their own developmental needs.

It is important to actively try to involve the adolescent father in parenting classes and in discussions of his feelings about dealing with the new experience of parenthood (Bobak, 1987). He may not only have an active role in parenting the infant but may also be a source of support to the young mother. In turn, he may need the nurse's assistance in mobilizing his own sources of support. Community health nurses can make referrals to other programs that may help provide material or financial support to adolescent parents.

A wide variety of other programs exist to help disadvantaged adolescents gain realistic hope about the future, including programs such as Big Brothers and Big Sisters, which provide role models and adult friends for these youths. Community health nurses function both as participants in programs such as these and can become politically and socially involved to stimulate new program development.

Finally, the report by the National Academy of Sciences recommended providing for availability of abortion and adoption services, prenatal care, and family planning to reduce subsequent pregnancies during the adolescent years. Closely spaced, subsequent pregnancies tend to compound the health, social, and economic risks faced by adolescent parents (Polit and Kahn, 1986). Special educational and employment programs should be targeted to the needs of these adolescents, including supports such as child-care programs in schools. Considering the vast array of supports potentially needed by adolescent families, case management has been suggested as the most effective method of linking teenage parents to services and helping them use those services most effectively (Panel on Adolescent Pregnancy and Child Rearing, 1987).

Frail Elderly and Their Caregivers

A final example of age-related vulnerability is the growing number of frail elderly individuals attempting to avoid institutionalization and to continue living independently in the community. Together with their caregivers, they comprise a vulnerable group that has developed as a result of demographic and health-status changes.

Introduction

Frail elderly persons have fewer physiological reserves with which to respond to stressors than they once did, and many have limited social supports to help them compensate. It is well known that the majority of elderly are living in the community rather than in institutions, although many may be institutionalized at some point in their lives. The elderly depend on informal social networks, which include family, friends, and acquaintances such as postal carriers, for many sources of assistance before seeking help from formal sources (Hooyman and Kiyak, 1991). Federal policy changes in the United States during the 1980s resulted in greater emphasis on caregiving by these informal social networks. At the same time demographic changes have made it more difficult for these networks to function. Families are smaller and more mobile, with far greater numbers of employed women. These two factors alone severely limit the number of potential caregivers and their ability to provide the kinds of care and support required by many elderly persons living in the community.

Changing womens' roles have had an impact on the degree of stress and isolation felt by caregivers, who are typically women. In fact, most caregivers are not prepared for the duration and extent of caregiving needs frail elders may have (Brody, 1985). This is the first time in history that so many older people (some with serious levels of impairment) are being cared for by others for such lengthy periods of time (Hooyman and Kiyak, 1991). It is not yet known what impact other changes in family structure—such as blended families following divorce and remarriage or ". . . cohabitation by unmarried couples"—will have on support of the frail elderly population (Hooyman and Kiyak, 1991, p. 297).

Scope of the Problem

Who are the frail elderly? Although any elderly individual with multiple impairments adversely influencing functional status may be frail, the population of particular concern are the "old old." The old old are those elderly who are 85 years of age or older. This segment of the elderly population is ". . . increasing at six times the rate of the general population" (Fowles, 1985; also cited in Brown, 1988, p. 13). The old old are more likely to be poor or near poor and the majority are women without spouses (Hooyman and Kiyak, 1991). In addition to increasing limitations on physiological reserves at this age, the number of chronic illnesses of those in this age group is significantly greater than before the age of 75 years, resulting in further physiological and caregiving demands (Brown, 1988). Comorbidity of chronic conditions is a particular problem that increases with age and increases the likelihood of requiring assistance with activities of daily living (MMWR, 1989).

Caregivers are most often women and are usually spouses or children of care recipients (Bowers, 1987; Stone, Cafferata, and Sangl, 1987). Many caregivers are over 65 years of age, themselves; those who are younger are often still caring for their own dependent children (Brody, 1981). Men do provide some caregiving services, but these tend to be limited to financial assistance and other forms of less direct care; rarely are men involved in the provision of personal care (Hooyman and Kiyak, 1991).

Although some caregivers live in the same household as the older person, most do not. Caregivers may live nearby or at great distances from the older individual. In these cases the types of care may differ and may involve more emotional support and coordination of the care provided by others, such as neighbors and formal care providers.

Characteristics

Although medical problems of the very old are being managed increasingly effectively, problems persist in maintaining the *functional status* of elderly individuals living in the community. In fact, both the Surgeon General's 1979 Report on Healthy People and the Year 2000 Objectives for the Nation (U.S. Department of Health, Education, and Welfare 1979; Public Health Serivce, 1989) placed a priority on reduction of disability. In one example of this phenomenon, a visiting nurses association in Massachusetts found that the elderly clients' medical diagnoses were secondary in importance to the nursing diagnoses, which focused largely on impairments in functional status and the resulting potential for injury and deleterious impacts on family coping (Soderlind, 1989). The primary outcome of functional disability is nursing home placement (Pearlman, and Ryan-Dykes, 1986).

Factors related to nursing home placement and that describe the most vulnerable frail elderly are similar to those examined for other vulnerable groups, with the addition of risks from decreases in functional status in this group. For example, in a study of low-income community-living elderly persons in Washington state, it was found that being poor and female, ". . . using an ambulatory aid and requiring help with certain activities of daily living, such as handling money, preparing meals, walking, and dealing with transportation" (Pearlman and Ryan-Dykes, 1986) were predictors of nursing home placement. Changes in the elderly person's social and health situation also preceded institutionalization. These variables included loss of retirement pensions, decreased number of phone conversations by the elderly individual, changes in medical status, and losses in functional status (i.e., decreased ability to walk and transfer from the bed) and initiation of wheelchair use. Diminished mental status is a potent predictor of nursing home placement, although in many cases, if it is recognized early, interventions can be designed to either maintain cognitive capacities or build in supports to compensate for limitations. Mental status can be assessed using a tool such as the Mini-Mental Status Examination (Figure 22-4).

Problems of the Elderly

Changes in federal policies have resulted in greater reliance by many elderly individuals on what has been called the ". . . '*social care system*' in which continuous or intermittent ties and interchanges of assistance help older persons to maintain their psychological, social and physical integrity over time" (Cantor, 1983; also cited in Grau, 1987, p. 105). For example, the prospective payment system used for Medicare recipients emphasizes timely hospital discharge. This places greater responsibility on family and friends of frail elderly individuals to provide health monitoring, personal care, help with remembering to take medications, help with homemaking chores, and help with working with health care personnel and agencies (Truglio-Londrigan, 1986).

Frail elderly persons may need assistance managing both instrumental and basic activities of daily living (Figure 22-5). *Instrumental activities of daily living* refer to activities necessary to manage the environment, including the homemaking chores of shopping, cooking, cleaning, paying bills, and using the telephone. *Basic activities of daily living* are those tasks that involve maintenance of personal hygiene, mobility, and nutritional status, such as feeding, bathing, dressing, toileting, and transferring (Katz, 1983; Kane, Ouslander, and Abrass, 1984).

Problems of the Caregivers

Although caregivers may wish to provide home-based care for their elderly family members, some find provision of this type of care to be exhausting because they frequently

---

Mini Mental State Examination

Patient _____
Examiner _____
Date _____

"MINI MENTAL STATE"

Maximum
Score   Score

ORIENTATION

5   ( ) What is the (year) (season) (date) (day) (month)?
5   ( ) Where are we: (state) (county) (town) (hospital) (floor).

REGISTRATION

3   ( ) Name 3 objects: 1 second to say each. Then ask the patient all 3 after you have said them. Give 1 point for each correct answer. Then repeat them until he learns all 3. Count trials and record.

Trials

ATTENTION AND CALCULATION

5   ( ) Serial 7's. 1 point for each correct. Stop after 5 answers. Alternatively spell "world" backwards.

RECALL

3   ( ) Ask for the 3 objects repeated above. Give 1 point for each correct.

LANGUAGE

9   ( ) Name a pencil, and watch (2 points)
Repeat the following "No ifs, ands or buts." (1 point)

Follow a 3-stage command:

"Take a paper in your right hand, fold it in half, and put it on the floor"
(3 points)

Read and obey the following:

Close your eyes (1 point)

Write a sentence (1 point)

Copy design (1 point)

Total score

ASSESS level of consciousness along a continuum _____
Alert   Drowsy   Stupor   Coma

A

FIGURE 22-4

A, Mini-mental state examination. **B,** Instructions for administration of mini-mental state examination. *(From Folstein MF, Folstein SE, and McHugh PR: "Mini-mental state": a practical method for grading the cognitive state of patients for the clinician, J Psychiatr Res 12:189, 1975.)*

Continued.

**Instructions for Administration of
Mini Mental State Examination**

ORIENTATION

(1) Ask for the date. Then ask specifically for parts omitted, e.g., "Can you also tell me what season it is?" One point for each correct.

(2) Ask in turn "Can you tell me the name of this hospital?" (town, county, etc.). One point for each correct.

REGISTRATION

Ask the patient if you may test his memory. Then say the names of three unrelated objects, clearly and slowly, about 1 second for each. After you have said all three, ask him to repeat them. This first repetition determines his score (0-3) but keep saying them until he can repeat all three, up to six trials. If he does not eventually learn all three, recall cannot be meaningfully tested.

ATTENTION AND CALCULATION

Ask the patient to begin with 100 and count backwards by 7. Stop after five subtractions (93, 86, 79, 72, 65). Score the total number of correct answers.

If the patient cannot or will not perform this task, ask him to spell the word "world" backwards. The score is the number of letters in correct order, e.g., dlrow = 5, dlorw = 3.

RECALL

Ask the patient if he can recall the three words you previously asked him to remember. Score 0-3.

LANGUAGE

Naming: Show the patient a wrist watch and ask him what it is. Repeat for pencil. Score 0-2.

Repetition: Ask the patient to repeat the sentence after you. Allow only one trial. Score 0 or 1.

3-Stage command: Give the patient a piece of plain blank paper and repeat the command. Score 1 point for each part correctly executed.

Reading: On a blank piece of paper print the sentence "Close your eyes" in letters large enough for the patient to see clearly. Ask him to read it and do what it says. Score 1 point only if he actually closes his eyes.

Writing: Give the patient a blank piece of paper and ask him to write a sentence for you. Do not dictate a sentence, it is to be written spontaneously. It must contain a subject and verb and be sensible. Correct grammar and punctuation are not necessary.

Copying: On a clean piece of paper, draw intersecting pentagons, each side about 1 in, and ask him to copy it exactly as it is. All ten angles must be present and two must intersect to score 1 point. Tremor and rotation are ignored.

Estimate the patient's level of sensorium along a continuum, from alert on the left to coma on the right.

A score of 24 points or less suggests mental impairment, although it has been recommended that cutoff scores be lowered to 20 to 22 points for patients who have less than an eighth grade education. (From Irby JP, Schmitt FA, Gardner C, et al: Utilizing mental status examinations for cognitive screening in the elderly; strengths and limitations, Unpublished paper, Lexington Veterans' Administration Center Geriatric Evaluation Unit and University of Kentucky Medical Center, 1988.)

FIGURE 22-4, Cont'd

---

must fit caregiving duties in with other responsibilities to their spouses, their employers, and their own children (thus caregivers are sometimes called the "sandwich generation"). Elderly individuals may be reluctant to allow someone else to perform these tasks for them, leading to tension and ethical dilemmas over the degree of autonomy that the elderly person may safely maintain and the degree the elderly person desires to maintain a sense of dignity. Prior personality conflicts and tensions between the caregiver and elder may be intensified with the role reversals involved in caregiving. Beliefs about the caregiving role, the role of the elder, and the image the caregiver has of the elder seem to influence the type of caregiving strategies used and whether or not these strategies are abusive (Phillips and Rampusheski, 1986). Often, both caregivers and frail elderly feel isolated and lonely as they attempt to manage (Robinson, 1988; Ryan and Patterson, 1987).

Interventions

Community health nurses are often among the first professionals to observe subtle changes in mental status of elderly clients. This is particularly important for the

TABLE 1

Index of independence in activities of daily living

The Index of Independence in Activities of Daily Living is based on an evaluation of the functional independence or dependence of patients in bathing, dressing, going to toilet, transferring, continence, and feeding. Specific definitions of functional independence and dependence appear below the index.

A — Independent in feeding, continence, transferring, going to toilet, dressing, and bathing.
B — Independent in all but one of these functions.
C — Independent in all but bathing and one additional function.
D — Independent in all but bathing, dressing, and one additional function.
E — Independent in all but bathing, dressing, going to toilet, and one additional function.
F — Independent in all but bathing, dressing, going to toilet, transferring, and one additional function.
G — Dependent in all six functions.
Other — Dependent in at least two functions, but not classifiable as C, D, E, or F.

Independence means without supervision, direction, or active personal assistance, except as specifically noted below. This is based on actual status and not on ability. A patient who refuses to perform a function is considered as not performing the function, even though he is deemed able.

Bathing (sponge, shower, or tub)

Independent: assistance only in bathing a single part (as back or disabled extremity) or bathes self completely

Dependent: assistance in bathing more than one part of body; assistance in getting in or out of tub or does not bathe self

Dressing

Independent: gets clothes from closets and drawers; puts on clothes, outer garments, braces; manages fasteners; act of tying shoes is excluded

Dependent: does not dress self or remains partly undressed

Going to toilet

Independent: gets to toilet; gets on and off toilet; arranges clothes; cleans organs of excretion; (may manage own bedpan used at night only and may or may not be using mechanical supports)

Dependent: uses bedpan or commode or receives assistance in getting to and using toilet

Transfer

Independent: moves in and out of bed independently and moves in and out of chair independently (may or may not be using mechanical supports)

Dependent: assistance in moving in or out of bed and/or chair; does not perform one or more transfers

Continence

Independent: urination and defecation entirely self-controlled

Dependent: partial or total incontinence in urination or defecation; partial or total control by enemas, catheters, or regulated use of urinals and/or bedpans

Feeding

Independent: gets food from plate or its equivalent into mouth; (precutting of meat and preparation of food, as buttering bread, are excluded from evaluation)

Dependent: assistance in act of feeding (see above); does not eat at all or parenteral feeding

FIGURE 22-5

Katz index of independence in activities of daily living. *(From Katz S, et al.: Studies of illness in the aged. The index of ADL: a standardized measure of biological and psychosocial function. JAMA 185(12):915, American Medical Association.)*

old for whom cognitive impairment is especially prevalent (Evans DA et al., 1989). It is important to recognize early signs of decreasing mental status in order to make prompt referrals for medical care. For example, confusion may simply be an early sign of systemic infection, which can easily be corrected. If changes in mental status result from organic problems, the nurse can help family members develop strategies to keep the elder as oriented as possible. The **Mini Mental State Examination** is a quick screening tool that is useful in monitoring subtle changes in mental

status (Lindeborn, 1988; Folstein, Folstein, and McHugh, 1975) (see Appendix 1).

When initiating services with a potentially frail older person, the nurse should determine whether the individual needs help with activities of daily living. The **Katz Index of Independence in Activities of Daily Living** assessment guide is helpful in determining an elderly client's abilities to manage basic ADL's (see Appendix 2). Sometimes family or friends can provide the additional assistance the elder needs, and sometimes it is preferable to make a referral

TABLE 2
Evaluation form

Name _____ Date of evaluation _____

For each area of functioning listed below, check description that applies. (The word "assistance" means supervision, direction of personal assistance.)

Bathing—either sponge bath, tub bath, or shower

☐ | ☐ | ☐

Receives no assistance (gets in and out of tub by self if tub is usual means of bathing) | Receives assistance in bathing only one part of the body (such as back or a leg) | Receives assistance in bathing more than one part of the body (or not bathed)

Dressing—gets clothes from closets and drawers—including underclothes, outer garmetns and using fasteners (including braces if worn)

☐ | ☐ | ☐

Gets clothes and gets completely dressed without assistance | Gets clothes and gets dressed without assistance except for assistance in tying shoes | Receives assistance in getting clothes or in getting dressed, or stays partly or completely undressed

Toileting—going to the "toilet room" for bowel and urine elimination; cleaning self after elimination, and arranging clothes

☐ | ☐ | ☐

Goes to "toilet room," cleans self, and arranges clothes without assistance (may use object for support such as cane, walker, or wheelchair and may manage night bedpan or commode, emptying same in morning) | Receives assistance in going to "toilet room" or in cleansing self or in arranging clothes after elimination or in use of night bedpan or commode | Doesn't go to room termed "toilet" for the elimination process

Transfer—

☐ | ☐ | ☐

Moves in and out of bed as well as in and out of chair without assistance (may be using object for support such as cane or walker) | Moves in or out of bed or chair with assistance | Doesn't get out of bed

Continence—

☐ | ☐ | ☐

Controls urination and bowel movement completely by self | Has occasional "accidents" | Supervision helps keep urine or bowel control; catheter is used, or is incontinent

Feeding—

☐ | ☐ | ☐

Feeds self without assistance | Feeds self except for getting assistance in cutting meat or buttering bread | Receives assistance in feeding or is fed partly or completely by using tubes or intravenous fluids

FIGURE 22-5, Cont'd

for homemaker services. Most communities have these services available, although long waiting lists are often a problem. In these situations church groups or other voluntary groups may be able to fill the gap in services needed.

Caregiver strain has been found to be one of the major predictors of institutionalization (Martin et al., 1985). Robinson (1988) found that caregivers of elderly dementia victims reported significantly less perceived burden and in-

creased self-esteem and social support following a caregiver training program. This program emphasized development of social skills such as assertiveness and network-building skills. Reasoning that caregivers represent essentially " hidden populations at risk for loneliness and little social support" (p. 60), the researcher used a structured learning approach to teach caregivers how to identify potential helpers, how to request help, how to express appreciation, how to say no, and how to avoid being overwhelmed. Similar programs emphasize the support and knowledge that group participants can gain from other members of the group (Pesznecker and Zahlis, 1986; Truglio-Londrigan, 1986). Interventions such as these hold promise for decreasing the strain on caregivers and promoting positive-family functioning when caring for a frail elderly person.

It is necessary to keep clients' *life circumstances* in mind when designing programs for vulnerable groups. For example, in planning a support group for caregivers of frail elderly persons, it is important to be aware that caregivers may need someone to provide respite care for the elderly person during the caregiver's absence (Robinson, 1989). Part of the support program therefore may be inclusion of arrangements for someone else to care for the elderly person during the support-group meeting. Other successful approaches to care for frail elders and ther caregivers have included adult day-care centers, inpatient–geriatric-evaluation units, and homecare and homemaking services. Some companies are beginning to offer a new benefit called "Eldercare," in which employees caring for an older family member may receive services such as information, referrals, or group support. Case managed care is the cornerstone of provision of a coordinated package of services targeted at the elderly individual and the family.

CLINICAL APPLICATION

Use the ideas presented in this chapter to analyze the following situation. Focus on a broad range of issues, including health, social, economic, and environmental concerns. Try to think of strategies that will ultimately help to empower the client and break the cycle of vulnerability. Figure 22-2 illustrates the nurse's role as a mediator of services or case manager. This may provide ideas for the types of interventions that could be effective in helping to empower this client.

Imagine you are a nurse in a mission clinic for the homeless. Several days ago, Dorothy, a homeless 40-year-old woman who is pregnant with her fifth child, came in requesting treatment for her swollen ankles. During your *assessment* of her, Dorothy gave you a fairly complete picture of her recent health and social history. She went to the prenatal clinic at the health department once a couple of months ago. At that time she was given a couple of sample bottles of multivitamins, but she lost them. Dorothy is now on a waiting list to receive free obstetrical care but is not expecting to reach the top of the list before her due date. Her four prior pregnancies were fairly uneventful, although she mentioned that she became "toxic" with the last child. Her blood pressure today is 150/80 and she has pitting edema up to her ankles. She noted that a physician once told her that she should watch her blood pressure, but she has never taken medication for it. She is 5′ 2″ tall and weighs 170 lbs.

Dorothy commented that she normally takes chlorpromazine hydrochloride (Thorazine), but she ran out of her medicine 3 weeks ago and has not had the money to get her prescription refilled. She did not mention this medication to the physician who saw her at the prenatal clinic. She says that she has been in the local state mental hospital several times over the last few years. The usual course of events proceeding these hospitalizations is one of progressive agitation and difficulty in managing her normal responsibilities of child care, paying bills, and keeping house, resulting in tremendous stress for her and culminating in aggressive behavior and "hearing voices."

Her plans for caring for her infant are vague and include asking her unemployed boyfriend for help, although she is not able to say specifically how he will be able to help. Her four other children range in age from 16 to 23 years. None of them are with her. The two oldest live in another state; the third child lives with her biological father; and the youngest, a son, ran away several months ago following the loss of their most recent trailer. Dorothy, her boyfriend, and her teenage son had been renting a trailer, but they lost it when her boyfriend was laid off and they could no longer pay the rent. She and the boyfriend have been sleeping under a nearby bridge overpass since that time, eating fast food at a local burger emporium when they can get money and scavenging food from garbage cans when they cannot. She expresses optimism that she or her "old man" will find a room somewhere before the baby is born, but she observes that, if they don't, they can probably borrow a car to sleep in.

What other information would you want to help you assess this client's situation? What nursing diagnoses are suggested by the brief historical, physical, and social data presented here? Which of the potential diagnoses should you focus your efforts on today? Why?

Based on your *assessment,* you decide it is important to check Dorothy for proteinuria. Her urine specimen yields positive test results for protein (1 +) and negative test results for glucose. Her hands and face seem somewhat swollen, and she has a mild headache. Dorothy has become increasingly agitated as you are completing your assessment. She mentions that she is tired and wants to go to get something to eat and watch television in the guest area of the mission.

What short-term goals do you think would be most appropriate today?

At this point, your *plan* is to contact the health department and make an appointment for her to be seen within the next day or two. She agrees to this course of action, but she does not seem particularly committed to it. You further decide to help her get a nutritious meal from the kitchen and relax on a couch with her feet elevated following her lunch.

What other plans might help you handle the immediate problems Dorothy seems to have? How should you approach the long-term problems suggested in this vignette? What other agencies might be able to provide services this client needs? How should you coordinate these services? How might you function as a case manager in this situation?

Your *interventions* went fairly smoothly. Dorothy got a filling meal from the mission kitchen, although it was higher in sodium than you wanted because it consisted of a bologna and cheese sandwich, an apple, some carrot sticks and prepackaged dip, and a glass of milk. Your call to the health department resulted in an appointment later in the afternoon with the same physician who had seen Dorothy earlier. At this point, you want to find some means of transportation so Dorothy will not have to walk the 5 miles to the clinic.

What outcome criteria should you use to evaluate the effectiveness of your interventions so far? How would you evaluate the effectiveness of other interventions you may have discussed in class, but which have not been described here?

Three weeks have passed since your initial meeting with Dorothy. You had arranged for temporary housing for her through a local social service agency and provided a comfortable, but noisy, place at the mission for her to rest during the day. She hs not been able to make firm plans for housing and child care following the birth of her baby, and a social worker has been talking with her about placing the baby in a foster home until more stable arrangements can be made for the family. She has been monitored carefully by the health department's physician and was finally referred to the local community hospital where she was admitted last week for preeclampsia. In addition to the physician, she has met with a therapist through the local community mental health center for counseling and monitoring of her psychiatric condition. How would you *evaluate* the effectiveness of your interventions?

SUMMARY

Community health nurses must be sensitive to the unique combination of social, economic, and health risks that characterize vulnerable groups. Vulnerability includes cumulative risks, limited control over health behaviors, potential disenfranchisement, victimization, disadvantaged status and powerlessness. The near poor, the medically indigent, and the homeless are vulnerable primarily as a result of socioeconomic factors. Age-related factors help explain the vulnerability of runaway youth, pregnant adolescents, and the frail elderly and their caregivers.

Each of the special populations described could potentially benefit from programs using a community systems approach, including broad-based assessment, interdisciplinary planning and interventions, and assistance with referral use and follow-up. Communication and interviewing skills are particularly crucial as the nurse begins establishing a rapport with vulnerable clients. These clients need tangible forms of help that are responsive to their perceived needs, rather than to the interests of health professionals. Community health nurses must be politically active to change policies that are essentially dysfunctional for vulnerable population groups (Abdellah, Chamberlain, and Levine, 1986). Areas of policy concern for community health nurses must include social and economic health parameters.

KEY CONCEPTS

Individuals and groups may be vulnerable to social and health problems, both as a result of their own actions and the policies and decisions made at the societal level.

Vulnerability involves the concepts of health risk, limited control, disenfranchisement, victimization, disadvantaged status, and powerlessness.

Vulnerable individuals are more likely to have a low-socioeconomic status, be at either end of the age continuum, and are often from dysfunctional families.

Health outcomes of vulnerability include higher morbidity and mortality overall, including higher infant mortality and rates of low–birth weight than the population in general.

Vulnerable groups generally have lower rates of health service use than the population as a whole, particularly with regard to outpatient and preventive services.

The near poor are vulnerable because of the limited safety net in health and social services that exists in this country. This group does not qualify for existing services because their financial resources are just above those set by eligibility requirements. However, they do not have sufficient resources to be able to afford the necessary services.

Medically indigent groups are unable to pay for health services. They may be near poor, but they also may have adequate financial resources for daily needs but not for health care.

Homelessness has been increasing in this country as a result of shortage of low-income housing, increasing unemployment, restrictions in benefits from health and welfare programs, and (possibly) deinstitutionalization policies. Homeless families are the fastest growing segment of this population.

Health problems of the homeless result from inadequate nutrition, environmental hazards such as trauma and infestations, improperly treated chronic health problems, and sleep deprivation.

Runaway youths are episodically homeless. The risk of environmental hazards in this group is immense, including those precipitated by prostitution, substance abuse, and drug dealing.

Treatment of runaways must be comprehensive, recognizing that they may never return for follow-up. Creation of a trusting relationship, based on confidentiality and realism, increases the chances of follow-up.

Pregnant adolescents face immediate risks to the health of both themselves and the fetus, and long-term problems of curtailed educational achievements, chronic unemployment, poverty, long-range dependence on public assistance, unstable family relationships, and the likelihood of perpetuating a cycle of early childbearing and high-fertility rates.

Frail, community-living elderly individuals are at risk for safety and social hazards resulting from limitations in functional status, chronic health problems with high co-morbidity, and strains on caregivers.

Supports for both the elderly and their caregivers are necessary to prevent unnecessary institutionalization, further disability, and untimely death.

Clinical issues surrounding services for vulnerable groups center around recognition of needs perceived as high priority by these individuals and provision of services in areas that are convenient and both physically and emotionally comfortable.

Health and welfare policies must be designed with a clear understanding of their impact on the status of vulnerable populations and the drain on human capital when their needs are not met.

LEARNING ACTIVITIES

1. Debate with your class the nature and extent of services that you believe should be made available to the homeless. Defend your position regarding the concepts of "enabling" and "worthiness."

2. How would needs vary for families and individuals who are temporarily, episodically, or chronically homeless? Consider the time factors involved (i.e., whether assistance is needed for a short-term or long-term period). Give examples of the types of services that might be needed by a family temporarily without a home as a result of a fire. Which agencies might be helpful in resolving these needs? What services might be needed by a 14-year-old runaway girl who is earning money through prostitution and has a drug habit? What factors would the nurse need to consider in planning care for a 50-year-old chronically homeless insulin-dependent diabetic male with regular foot lesions aggravated by constant mobility? How might a nurse function as a case manager in these situations?

3. Discuss the pros and cons of expanding reimbursement for health services for the near poor. Include some analysis of the costs and benefits of expansion of service reimbursement. If possible interview someone in your community involved in developing policies for provision of indigent care.

4. Examine the pros and cons of school-based clinics for adolescents. Do you think reproductive services should be included in such clinics? What are the ethical issues involved in providing reproductive information to adolescents with or without parental consent and involvement?

5. Imagine you are a home health nurse scheduled to make three visits to the home of a 57-year-old woman who is the caregiver for her 85-year-old father who is in the end stages of Alzheimer disease. He lives with her, her husband, and their college-aged son. You are to help her learn a new and complicated medication regimen for her father. The reimburser will pay for no more than three visits. Although your supervisor is normally sympathetic to no-charge visits, your employer has a very high caseload presently, so it will not be possible to make any more than the three reimbursable visits. The caregiver tells you that she doesn't know how she can hang on any longer; the physical care required to meet her father's needs is exhausting; he doesn't recognize her and is combative much of the time; and her employer is threatening to dismiss her because of interference of the caregiving demands with her job. Her husband is complaining; her son is in need of money and the sitter, who helps with her father's care, plans to quit in a month. The woman tells you that there are times when she wishes her father were dead. What might you do to help this family?

6. Examine health statistics and demographic data in your geographic area to determine which vulnerable groups predominate in your area. Look through your phone book for examples of agencies that you think provide services to these vulnerable groups. Make appointments with key individuals in several of these agencies to discuss the nature of their target population, the types of services provided, and the reimbursement mechanisms for these services. Various class members should visit different agencies and then share their results during class. Based on your findings, identify gaps or overlaps in services provided to vulnerable groups in your community. What might be some ways to manage these gaps and overlaps to help clients receive the services they need?

BIBLIOGRAPHY

A health care debacle: lessons to learn from the retreat on the catastrophic-costs law, US News World Report 107(14):16, 1989.

Abdellah FG, Chamberlain JG, and Levine IS: Role of nurses in meeting needs of the homeless: summary of a workshop for providers, researchers, and educators, Public Health Rep 101(5):494, 1986.

Arce A et al.: A psychiatric profile of street people admitted to an emergency shelter, Hosp Community Psychiatry 34(9):812, 1983.

Bassuk E and Rubin L: Homeless children: a neglected population, Am J Orthopsychiatry 57(2):279, 1987.

Baxter E and Hopper K: Private lives/public space: homeless adults on the streets of New York City, New York, 1981, Community Service Society.

Berne AS et al.: A nursing model for addressing the health needs of homeless families, Image 22(1):8, 1990.

Bobak IM and Jensen MD: Essentials of maternity nursing, St Louis, 1987, The CV Mosby Co.

Boondas J: The despair of the homeless aged, J Gerontol Nurs 11(4):9, 1985.

Bowdler JE: Health problems of the homeless in America, Nurse Pract 14(7):44, 1989.

Breakey WR et al.: Health and mental health problems of homeless men and women in Baltimore, JAMA 262(10):1352, 1989.

Brody E: Women in the middle and family to help older people, Gerontologist 21:471, 1981.

Brody E: Parent care as a normative family stress, Gerontologist 25:19, 1985.

Brown MD: Functional assessment of the elderly, J Gerontol Nurs 14(5):13, 1988.

Burke PJ: Adolescents' motivation for sexual activity and pregnancy prevention, Issues Compr Pediatr Nurs 10:161, 1987.

Cantor M: Social care for the aged in the United States: issues and challenges, New York, 1983, The Haworth Press.

Cohen CI et al.: Survival strategies of older homeless men, Gerontologist 28(1):58, 1988.

Collins JW and David RJ: The differential effect of traditional risk factors on infant birthweight among Blacks and Whites in Chicago, Am J Public Health 80(6):679, 1990.

Committee on Community Health Services, American Academy of Pediatrics: Health needs of homeless children, Pediatrics 82(6):938, 1988.

Community Council of Greater New York: Comorbidity of chronic conditions and disability among older persons: United States—1984, MMWR 38(46):788, 1989.

Cotton P: Plan to rework catastrophic care bill triggers outrage, Med World News 30:20, 1989.

Curtin L: Throwaway people? Nurs Manage 17(12):7, 1986.

Damrosch S and Stasser J: The homeless elderly in America, J Gerontol Nurs, 14(10):26, 1988.

Dentzer S: A health-care debacle: lessons to learn from the retreat on the catastrophic-costs law, US News World Rep 107(14):16, 1989.

Dever GEA, Sciegaj M, and Wade TE: Creation of a social vulnerability index for justice in health planning, Fam Community Health 10(4):23, 1988.

Dryfoos JG: A time for new thinking about teenage pregnancy, Am J Public Health 75(1):13, 1985.

Engel NS and Lau AD: Nursing care for the adolescent urban nomad, MCN 8:74, 1983.

Evans DA et al.: Prevalence of Alzheimer's disease in a community population of older persons: higher than previously reported, JAMA 262:2551, 1989.

Folstein MF, Folstein SE, and McHugh PR: "Mini-mental state": a practical method for grading the cognitive state of patients for the clinician, J Psychiatr Res 12:189, 1975.

Fowles DG: A profile of older Americans: 1985, Washington, DC, 1985, Program Resources Department, American Association of Retired Persons and the Administration of Aging, US Department of Health and Human Services.

Francis MB: Long-term approaches to end homelessness, Public Health Nurs 4(4):230, 1987.

Grau L: Illness-engendered poverty among the elderly, Women Health 12(3/4): 103-118 1987.

Greiff I, Zipple AM, and McCarthy K: Beyond shelter: providing rehabilitation services to the homeless, Psychosoc Rehabil J 11(1):72, 1987.

Griffith H: Capitol commentary: access to health care, Nurs Econ 5(2):90, 1987.

Grossman M: On the concept of health capital and the demand for health, J Polit Econ 80:223, 1972.

Haan M, Kaplan GA, and Camacho T: Poverty and health: prospective evidence from the Alameda County study, Am J Epidemiol 125(6):989, 1987.

Hansen MM and Resick LK: Health beliefs, health care, and rural Appalachian subcultures from an ethnographic perspective, Fam Community Health 13(1):1, 1990.

Heller R: School-based clinics: impact on teenage pregnancy prevention, Pediatr Nurs 14(2):103, 1988.

Henderson V: The nature of nursing, Am J Nurs 64(8):62, 1964.

Hooyman NR and Kiyak HA: Social gerontology: a multidisciplinary perspective, Boston, 1991, Allyn & Bacon.

Iglehart JK: Medicare's new benefits: "catastrophic" health insurance. N Engl J Med 320(5):329, 1989.

Institutes of Medicine: Homelessness, health, and human needs, Washington, DC, 1988, National Academy Press.

Kane RL, Ouslander JG, and Abrass IB: Essentials of clinical geriatrics, New York, 1984, McGraw-Hill.

Katz S et al.: Studies of illness in the aged: the index of ADL—a standardized measure of biological and psychosocial function, JAMA 185(12):914, 1963.

Katz S: Assessing self-maintenance: activities of daily living, mobility, and instrumental activities of daily living, J Am Geriatr Soc 31(12):721, 1983.

Larkin H: CEO's split over Oregon Medicaid reform, Hospitals 64(2):75, 1990.

Levin P: Becoming the way we are, ed 2, Wenatchee, WA, 1985, Directed Media.

Lewis O: The culture of poverty, Sci Am 215:19, 1966.

Linderborn KM: The need to assess dementia, J Gerontol Nurs 14(1):35, 1988.

Lindsey AM: Health care for the homeless, Nurs Outlook 37(2):78, 1989.

Manov A and Lowther L: A health care approach for hard-to-reach adolescent runaways, Nurs Clin North Am 18(2):333, 1983.

Martin ME and Henry M: Cultural relativity and poverty, Public Health Nurs 6(1):28, 1989.

Martin DC et al.: Community-based geriatric assessment, J Am Geriatr Soc 33:602, 1985.

Maurin JT, Russell L, and Memmott RJ: An exploration of gender differences among the homeless, Res Nurs Health 12:315, 1989.

Mayberry RM and Lewis RF: Ten-year changes in birthweight distributions of black and white infants: South Carolina, Am J Public Health 80(6):724, 1990.

Milburn L: Medical indigency: annotated bibliography of recent research and policy documents, Nurs Econ 4(6):289, 1986.

Mirkin MP, Raskin PA, and Antognini FC: Parenting, protecting, preserving: mission of the adolescent female runaway, Fam Process 23:63, 1984.

Moccia P and Mason DJ: Poverty trends: implications for nursing, Nurs Outlook 34(1):20, 1986.

National Center for Health Statistics: Adolescent and adult history questionnaire from Hispanic health and nutrition examination survey: 1982-1984, DHHS, PHSNCHS, public use data tape documentation, tape 6521, version 2, Washington, DC, 1987, US Government Printing Office.

National Center for Health Statistics: Health United States: 1987, DHHS Pub No (PHS) 88-1232, Washington DC, 1988, US Government Printing Office.

Nichols J, Wright LK, and Murphy JF: A proposal for tracking health care for the homeless, J Community Health 11(3):204, 1986.

Palmore SU and Shannon MD: Risk factors for adolescent pregnancy in students, Pediatr Nurs 14(3):241, 1988.

Panel on Adolescent Pregnancy and Childrearing: Comment: risking the future—a symposium on the National Academy of Sciences' report on teenage pregnancy, Fam Plann Perspect 19(3):119, 1987.

Parker S: A ration of care, a measure of doubt, New Physician 38(6):23, 1989.

Pearlman RA and Ryan-Dykes M: The vulnerable elderly, J Gerontol Nurs 12(9):14, 1986.

Pepper C: Long-term care insurance: the first step towards comprehensive health insurance, Caring 8:4, 1989.

Pesznecker B: The poor: a population at risk, Public Health Nurs 4(1):237, 1984.

Pesznecker BL and Zahlis E: Establishing mutual-help groups for family-member care givers: a new role for community health nurses, Public Health Nurs 3(1):29, 1986.

Phillips LR and Rampusheski VF: Caring for the frail elderly at home: toward a theoretical explanation of the dynamics of poor quality family caregiving, ANS 8(4):62, 1986.

Pletsch PK: Hispanics: at risk for adolescent pregnancy? Public Health Nurs 7(2):105, 1990.

Polit DF and Kahn JR: Early subsequent pregnancy among economically disadvantaged teenage mothers, Am J Public Health 76(2):167, 1986.

Poole C: Adolescent pregnancy and unfinished developmental tasks of chilhood, J School Health 57(7):271, 1987.

Presgrove MV: Indigent patients: more nursing on less revenue, Nurs Manage 16(1):47-51, 1985.

Provan K: Recognizing, measuring, and interpreting the potential/enacted power distinction in organizational research, Acad Manage J 5:549, 1980.

Public Health Service: Promoting health/preventing disease: year 2000 objectives for the nation, Washington, DC, 1989, US Department of Health and Human Services.

Reis J and Herz L: Young adolescents' contraceptive knowledge and attitudes: implications for anticipatory guidance, J Pediatr Health Care 1(5):247, 1987.

Riesdorph-Ostrow W: Deinstitutionalization: a public policy perspective, J Psychosoc Nurs Ment Health Serv 27(6):4, 1989.

Robinson KM: A social skills training program for adult caregivers, Adv Nurs Sci 10(2):59, 1988.

Rooks JP: Let's admit we ration health care: then set priorities, Am J Nurs 90(6):39, 1990.

Rosner D: Health care for the "truly needy": nineteenth-century origins of the concept, Milbank Mem Fund Q 60(3):355, 1982.

Runaway and homeless youth in New York City: findings from recent research. In Leavitt RL, editor: New York, 1984. Community Council of Greater New York.

Ryan MC and Patterson J: Loneliness in the elderly, J Gerontol Nurs 13(5):6, 1987.

Sebastian JG: Homelessness: a state of vulnerability, Fam Community Health 8(3):11, 1985.

Soderlind S: Weaving a safety net, Geriatr Nurs 10(4):187, 1989.

Splatman S. Cited in Friedman E: Hospitals wrestle with the problem of homeless patients, Hospitals 57(16):97, 1983.

Stone R, Cafferata GL, and Sangl J: Caregivers of the frail elderly: a national profile, No. 15020614, Washington, DC, 1987, US Department of Health and Human Services.

Truglio-Londrigan M and Hayes RM: Carers learn to cope, Geriatr Nurs 7(6):310, 1986.

Trussell J: Teenage pregnancy in the United States, Fam Plann Perspect 20(6):262, 1988.

The short life of catastrophic care, US News World Report, 107(23):72-73, 1989.

US Bureau of the Census: Statistical abstract of the United States: 1990, ed 110, Washington, DC, 1990, US Government Printing Office.

US Department of Health, Education, and Welfare: Healthy people: the Surgeon General's report on health promotion and disease prevention, DHEW (PHS) Publication No. 79-55071, Washington DC, 1979, Government Printing Office.

Weitzman BC: Pregnancy and childbirth: risk factors for homelessness? Fam Plann Perspect 21(4):175, 1989.

Wilensky G: Viable strategies for dealing with the uninsured, Health Aff 16(2):33, 1987.

Wood D: Homeless children: their evaluation and treatment, J Pediatr Health Care 3(4):194, 1989.

Wright JD and Weber E: Homelessness and health, Washington, DC, 1987, McGraw-Hill.

Yoos L: Perspectives on adolescent parenting: effect of adolescent egocentrism on the maternal-child interaction, J Pediatr Nurs 2(3):193, 1987.

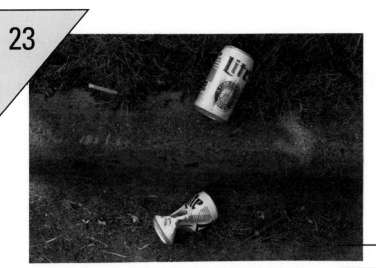

23

Substance Abuse in the Community

Mary Lynn Mathre

OBJECTIVES

After reading this chapter, the student should be able to:

Examine personal attitudes towards substance abuse to enhance therapeutic effectiveness.

Differentiate between the terms *substance use*, *abuse*, *dependence*, and *addiction*.

Discuss the differences between the major psychoactive drug categories.

Use seven drug consumer safety rules during client education to promote harm reduction from drug use.

Identify at least three groups at high risk for substance abuse.

Describe the progression of addiction and appropriate treatment modalities available.

KEY TERMS

addiction	enabling	set
Al Anon	fetal alcohol syndrome	setting
Alcoholics Anonymous	freebasing	sidestream smoke
alcoholism	mainstream smoke	substance abuse
blackout	methadone	tolerance
chemical dependency	maintenance	treatment
codependency	Narcotics Anonymous	triggers
cross-addiction	physical dependency	withdrawal
denial	polysubstance abuse	
detoxification		

S ubstance abuse is clearly a national health problem that is linked to numerous forms of morbidity and mortality. Approximately 30% to 50% of all hospital admissions are related to the effects of substance abuse (Bush, 1987; Lewis and Gordon, 1983). The substance abuser is not only at risk for personal health problems but may pose a threat to the health and safety of family members, co-workers, and other members of the community.

Substance abuse and addiction affect all ages, races, sexes, and segments of society. Community health nurses can play a significant role in the reduction of substance abuse for individuals, families, and communities.

This chapter gives a historical perspective on substance abuse. In addition, various attitudes, myths, and current social conditions are examined to differentiate the real problems from those created by lack of information and unfounded fears. Relevant terms are clearly defined to decrease the confusion caused by misuse of terms. The major drug categories are also described including information on onset and duration of action, main effects and side effects, adverse reactions, overdose effects, and nursing actions and considerations. The remainder of the chapter looks at the role of the community health nurse from a prevention point of view, including primary, secondary, and tertiary prevention of substance abuse.

UNDERSTANDING THE PROBLEM

Clearly, substance abuse and addiction to alcohol and other drugs can cause multiple health problems for individuals. Heavy tobacco, alcohol, and other drug use has been associated with many problems, including the following: neonates with low–birth weight and congenital abnormalities; accidents, homicides, and suicides; chronic diseases, such as cardiovascular diseases, cancer, and lung disease; violence, and family disruption. Factors that contribute to the substance-abuse problem include: lack of knowledge about the use of drugs; the labeling of certain drugs (alcohol, caffeine, and nicotine) as nondrugs; lack of quality control of illegal drugs; and the presence of drug laws that label certain drug users as criminals.

Community health nurses have a responsibility to seek the underlying roots of various health problems and to plan action that is realistic, nonjudgemental, holistic, and positive.

Historical Perspective

Psychoactive drug use has been endemic to virtually all cultures since the beginning of man. Often, a culture encourages the use of some drugs, while discouraging the use of others. Coffee, alcohol, and tobacco are drugs that are socially acceptable in the United States and Canada, whereas other cultures consider these drugs evil and thus prohibit their use. Conversely, marijuana, cocaine, and heroin use is not accepted in the mainstream U.S. society, but they are considered sacred and their use is encouraged in various other cultures.

Careful exploration of the history of drug acceptance and disapproval in American society will uncover strong irrational fears, prejudices, and greed as the basis of many current drug laws (Brecher, 1972; Herer, 1990; Kolb, 1956).

For example, if alcohol or tobacco were introduced today, the FDA would likely withhold approval because of the health-risk potential. Marijuana, on the other hand, was widely used at the turn of the century (tincture of cannabis) for a variety of medicinal purposes. However, as recreational use of it among blacks and Hispanics began to spread and a powerful synthetic fiber company saw marijuana (or rather, its hemp fiber) as an economic threat, laws were created to prohibit its use (Herer, 1990).

The United States' quick answer to various "drug problems" has been prohibition. During alcohol prohibition from 1920 to 1933, the United States experienced a sharp increase in violent crime and corruption among law officials secondary to the illicit market of alcohol. Distilled beverages were pushed because of the higher profit margin per bottle of liquor than wine or beer. Severe health problems were caused by the high-alcohol content in illicit moonshine.

Similar problems are occurring with current prohibition on marijuana, cocaine, and other drugs. An increase in violent crime and corruption among law officials as a result of the illicit drug market is becoming a major national problem. Stronger drugs are pushed because of their greater profits. Marijuana, (bulky and distinctly odorous) is more difficult to obtain than cocaine (compact and odorless). Crack (smokeable cocaine) is replacing cocaine because it is more addictive and yields a higher profit margin. A new drug called "Ice" (smokeable methamphetamine) is beginning to replace cocaine because it is easy to manufacture and has a longer duration of action than does cocaine. Many deaths are occurring as a result of the lack of any quality control to yield the unknown content and strength of these drugs.

Historically, confusion has existed as to whether substance abuse or addiction is a health care or criminal justice problem. Current support for legalization suggests that problems with substance abuse are health care problems and that it is the "prohibition of drugs" rather than simply the "use of drugs," which is the root of the drug problem. Newer laws are creating mandatory sentences, destroying civil liberties, and putting most resources into law enforcement rather than education and treatment (Brecher, 1972; Institute of Medicine, 1990; Trebach and Zeese, 1990).

Currently, education is beginning to address the dangers of alcohol abuse and establish guidelines for safe alcohol use. Alcohol consumers are choosing lower alcohol-content products such as beer and wine coolers rather than distilled products (Kinney and Leaton, 1991). Research shows that responsible, moderate use of alcohol can have some long-term health benefits.

As research has begun to show the extensive health risks of tobacco use, educational campaigns have been mounted to inform the public. Warnings have appeared on tobacco product labels since 1967 as a result of the Surgeon General's 1966 report on the dangers of smoking. In 1971 a ban on TV and radio cigarette advertising was imposed. Per capita cigarette consumption has fallen every year since 1973, with a decline of about 2% each year (U.S. Department of Health and Human Services, 1989).

In the 1950s and 1960s, amphetamines were widely prescribed as diet pills for women (Abadinsky, 1989). In the 1960s the benzodiazepines appeared on the market as safe

COMMON MYTHS ABOUT ALCOHOLISM AND ADDICTION AND REFUTING FACTS

MYTHS	FACTS
"An alcoholic is a skid row bum."	Less than 5% of the alcoholics fit this category.
"An alcoholic gets drunk every day."	Often, as the disease progresses, some alcoholics drink more and more on a daily basis to prevent withdrawal, but for other alcoholics their drinking pattern may be in binges, followed by periods of sobriety.
"If you teach people about drugs, they will abuse them."	It is true that people may choose to use drugs if they have knowledge about drugs; however, it is probable that people will abuse drugs if they have no knowledge about them.
"Knowledge about drugs prevents addiction."	The more a person knows about drugs does not prevent them from developing addiction. Nurses, physicians, and pharmacists have a high rate of addiction.
"Addiction is a sin or moral failing."	The disease of addiction is recognized as a health problem involving biopsychosocial factors. Persons who choose to use drugs do not do so with the intent to become addicted.

solutions to everyday stressors and were heavily marketed towards housewives. These drugs were thought to be safe and not habit forming, and the benzodiazepines were even encouraged in the treatment of alcoholism. These drugs were greatly overprescribed, and it soon became evident that they were not "a magic cure" and that many persons were having difficulties with dependence and addiction to these drugs (Weil and Rosen, 1983).

In the last decade America's "war on drugs" has escalated. Persons who use illegal drugs are arrested or put into treatment programs. This punitive approach to illicit-drug use hinders open communication between the health care professional and the drug user. Those who are abusing drugs, experiencing secondary health problems, or possibly becoming addicted may not seek help for fear of being arrested or confined.

To hope for a drug-free society is both unrealistic and probably unhealthy. Reduction of substance *abuse* and improved treatment of *addiction,* however, can be realistic goals. Community health nurses can play an important part in achieving these goals.

Attitudes and Myths

Attitudes are developed through cultural learning and personal experiences. Attitudes towards substance abuse are influenced by the way society categorizes "good" and "bad" drugs. In the United States, good drugs are over-the-counter (OTC) drugs or those prescribed by a health care provider, yet this makes them no less problematic or addictive. Also, chemicals such as alcohol, caffeine, and nicotine are given the legitimate status of "nondrugs," and their consumption is accepted as a means of enjoyment and relaxation.

Americans have come to rely heavily on prescription and OTC drugs to relieve (or mask) fear, tension, fatigue, and physical or emotional pain. Rather than learning nonmedicinal methods of coping, many people choose the "quick fix" and take pills to deal with their problems or negative feelings.

Americans also rely on drug use to enhance their social activities. Alcohol is clearly the nation's drug of choice for most social occasions, and the marketing of alcohol focuses on the enjoyment and relaxation associated with alcohol consumption. Among some wealthy groups, cocaine (intranasal) was considered the drug of choice at party gatherings during the 1970s and 1980s. For many college students and middle class adults, marijuana has been a drug to be shared among friends since the 1960s.

Addicts are often viewed as immoral, weak-willed, or irresponsible people who should try harder to help themselves. Although alcoholism was recognized as a disease by the American Medical Association in 1954 (Levine, 1984) and drug addiction was recognized as a disease some years later, the public and many health care professionals have failed to change their attitudes and accept alcoholics and addicts as ill persons in need of health care.

Community health nurses must examine their attitudes towards substance use and abuse and drug addiction before working with this health problem. To be therapeutic, the nurse must develop a trusting, nonjudgmental relationship with the client. Systematic assessment for substance abuse problems is based on awareness that there may be problems with legal drugs, as well as illegal drugs. If the nurse's attitude towards a client with a drug-abuse problem is negative or punitive, the issue may never be directly addressed or the client may be avoided. If the client senses the negative attitude of the health care provider, communication may cease and information thus withheld (Mathre, 1988). To develop a therapeutic attitude, the nurse must realize that any drug can be abused, that anyone can develop a drug addiction, and that drug addiction can be successfully treated.

Myths develop over many years, and if not questioned many attitudes may be formed based solely on fiction rather than fact. See the box above for some of the common myths and the refuting facts.

Social Conditions

Social conditions influence the use of drugs. The fast pace of life, competition at school or in the workplace, and the pressure to accumulate material possessions contribute to the daily stressors. Pharmaceutical, alcohol, and tobacco companies are continuously bombarding the public with enticing advertisements "pushing" their products as a means of feeling better, sleeping better, having more energy, or just as a "treat." People grow up believing that most of life's problems can be solved quickly and easily through the use of a drug.

For persons of a lower socioeconomic background and with minimal education or employment possibilities, many of life's opportunities may seem out of reach. For these people, psychoactive-drug use may offer a way to numb the pain or escape from their hopeless reality. These people rarely seek relief through a physician's prescription or other therapeutic measures. Instead, they rely on alcohol or illicit drugs, which are more readily available. For some, illicit-drug dealing may appear to be the only way out of the poverty-unemployment rut.

The solution of "Just Say No" is not only much too simplistic but is dangerously misleading. Indiscriminate use of "good" drugs has caused more health problems as a result of side effects, adverse reactions, drug interactions, addiction, and overdoses than has the use of "bad" drugs. The black market associated with illicit drug use puts otherwise law-abiding citizens in close contact with criminals, prevents any quality control of the drugs, increases the risk of AIDS and hepatitis caused by needle sharing, and hinders the health care professionals' accessibility to the abuser or addict.

The community health nurse is in a key position to reduce the problem of substance abuse. By approaching substance abuse as a real health problem rather than a moral or criminal problem, community health nurses can use their knowledge and skills to assist individuals, families, and the community in reducing this problem.

Definitions

The terms *drug use* and *drug abuse* have virtually lost their utility because the public and government have narrowed the term *drug* to include only illegal drugs, rather than including prescription, OTC, and legal recreational drugs. The term *substance* broadens the scope to include alcohol, tobacco, legal drugs, and even foods. The term *substance abuse* is the use of any substance that threatens a person's health or impairs their social or economic functioning. This definition is more objective and universal than the government's definition of drug abuse, which is the use of a drug without a prescription or any use of an illegal drug. Although any drug or food can be abused, the focus of this chapter is on *psychoactive drugs:* drugs that affect mood, perception, and thought.

"Drug dependence" and "drug addiction" are frequently used interchangeably, but they are not synonymous. *Drug dependence* is a state of neuroadaptation (a physiological change in the central nervous system [CNS]) caused by the regular administration of a drug in which continued use of the drug is necessary to prevent withdrawal symptoms. This happens when persons are put on an opiate such as morphine on a regular basis for pain management. To prevent withdrawal symptoms, the morphine should be gradually tapered rather than abruptly stopped.

Drug addiction is a pattern of drug abuse characterized by an overwhelming preoccupation with the use of a drug, securing its supply, and a high tendency to relapse if the drug is removed (Jaffe, 1986). Frequently, addicts are physically dependent on a drug, but there also appears to be an added psychological component that causes the intense craving and subsequent relapse. In general, anyone can develop a drug dependence caused by regular administration of drugs that alter the CNS; however, only 7% to 15% of the drug-using population will develop drug addiction. The reason some people develop drug addiction and others do not is not completely understood and continues to be an area of much research.

Alcoholism is addiction to the drug called alcohol. Alcoholism and drug addiction are recognized as illnesses under a biopsychosocial model (Donovan and Marlatt, 1988). Simply stated, the disease concept of addiction/alcoholism identifies this as a chronic and progressive disease in which a person's use of a drug(s) continues, despite problems it causes in any area of life—physical, emotional, social, economical, and spiritual.

Many theories exist on the etiological factors of addiction, and there is no consensus on specific causes. The underlying etiological factors include the belief that addiction is a disease, a moral failing, a psychological disturbance, a personality disorder, a social problem, a dysbehaviorism, or a maladaptive coping mechanism. The reality may be that different persons develop addiction in different manners. For example, some alcoholics have made statements such as, "I knew I was an alcoholic from my first drink; I drank differently than others." These people may be genetically predisposed to alcoholism and their chemical makeup is such that the disease will begin simply by consuming the drug. Others may have no family history of addiction but who suffer from great stress (chronic pain, significant losses, or abusive relationships resulting in low self-esteem) may find that drugs offer an escape from their stress. Over time, heavy use of a drug(s) to cope with their stress may develop into addiction. The biopsychosocial model provides a framework to understand addiction as the result of the interaction of multiple causes.

PSYCHOACTIVE DRUGS

Although any drug can be abused, substance abuse and addiction problems generally involve the psychoactive drugs. The psychoactive drugs are used in social and recreational settings and for personal use to self-medicate uncomfortable feelings because they are capable of changing the way a person feels. These drugs are divided into categories according to their effect on the CNS and the general feelings or experiences the drugs may induce. Often if a person cannot obtain their drug of choice, another drug from the same category may be substituted. For example, a person who cannot drink alcohol may begin using a benzodiazepine as an alternative. The box at right provides an overview of the general categories and the common drugs in each.

In addition to the specific drug being used, there are two other major factors that will influence the particular drug experience: set and setting (Zinberg, 1984). *Set* refers to the attitude of the person at the time of use, including per-

PSYCHOACTIVE DRUG CATEGORIES WITH EXAMPLES OF COMMON DRUGS

DEPRESSANTS

Alcohol
Barbiturates
   Phenobarbital
   Amobarbital (Amytal)
   Pentobarbital (Nembutal)
   Secobarbital (Seconal)
Chloral hydrate
Methaqualone (Quaaludes)
Glutethimide (Doriden)
Methyprion (Noludar)
Ethchlorvynol (Placidyl)
Minor tranquilizers
   Benzodiazepines
      Diazepam (Valium)
      Chlordiazepam (Librium)
      Lorazepam (Ativan)
      Alprazolam (Xanax)
      Oxazepam (Serax)
      Flurazepam (Dalmane)
      Temazepam (Restoril)
      Triazolam (Halcion)
   Mephrobamate (Miltown)
Opiates
   Morphine sulfate
   Heroin
   Opium
   Codeine
   Meperidine (Demerol)
   Methadone
   Porpoxyphene (Darvon)
   Hydromorphone (Dilaudid)
   Oxycodone (Percodan)

STIMULANTS

Caffeine
Cocaine
Amphetamines
   Amphetamine (Benzedrine)
   Dextramphetamine (Dexedrine)
   Methamphetamine (Methadrine)
Nicotine

MARIJUANA

Sinsemilla
Hash
Nabilone (Oral THC)

HALLUCINOGENS

LSD
Psilocybin
Mescaline
Peyote
Phencyclidine (PCP)

INHALANTS

Solvents
Amyl nitrate
Nitrous oxide

---

sonality and mood. *Setting* is the influence of the physical and social setting within which the use occurs. To understand various patterns of drug use and abuse by individuals, all three factors should be considered.

Depressants

Depressants lower the body's overall energy level, reduce sensitivity to outside stimulation and, in high doses, induce sleep. Low doses of depressants may produce a feeling of stimulation caused by initial sedation of the inhibitory centers in the brain. In general, depressants decrease heart rate, respiratory rate, muscular coordination and energy, and dull the senses. Higher doses lead to coma and, if the vital functions shut down, death. Major categories include alcohol, barbiturates, tranquilizers, and the opiates.

Alcohol

Alcohol (ethyl alcohol or ethanol) is probably the oldest and most widely used psychoactive drug in the world. Alcohol abuse ranks third, following coronary diseases and cancer, as the major cause of death in the United States. In 1988 the Surgeon General reported that 125,000 persons die each year from alcohol. At least 70% of Americans consume alcohol and, of those, approximately 10% will become alcoholic. The alcoholic's life expectancy is reduced by 15 years, and the mortality is 2 ½ times greater than that of nonalcoholics (Kinney and Leaton, 1991).

Alcohol abuse costs the country billions of dollars in lost productivity, property damage, medical expenses with alcohol-related illnesses and accidents, family disruptions, alcohol-related violence, and neglect and abuse of children. In 1984 a Harris poll reported that 38% of U.S. households were adversely affected by alcohol problems (Kinney and Leaton, 1991). The World Health Organization has estimated that, by the year 2000, alcoholism will be the world's number one health problem (Spickard, 1986).

The concentration of alcohol in the blood is determined by the concentration of alcohol in the drink, the rate of drinking, the rate of absorption (slower in the presence of food), the rate of metabolism, and a person's weight and sex. The amount of alcohol the liver can metabolize per hour is equal to about ¾ oz of whiskey, 4 oz of wine, or 12 oz of beer. Figure 23-1 shows the effects on the CNS as the blood-alcohol level (BAL) increases. However, with chronic consumption, tolerance develops and a person may reach a high BAL with minimal CNS effects.

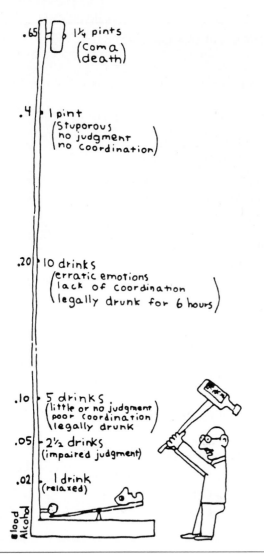

FIGURE 23-1

Blood-alcohol level and related CNS effects on a normal drinker (160-lb male) according to the number of drinks consumed in 1 hour. *Illustrated by Stuart Copans, MD, from Kinney & Leaton's* Loosening the Grip *(ed. 4), p. 33. St Louis, Mosby-Year Book, Inc. 1991.*

Chronic alcohol abuse exerts profound metabolic and physiologic effects on all of the body's organ systems. Gastrointestinal (GI) tract disturbances include inflammation of the GI tract, malabsorption, ulcers, liver problems, and cancers. Cardiovascular disturbances include cardiac arrhythmias, cardiomyopathy, hypertension, atherosclerosis, and blood dyscrasias. CNS problems include depression, sleep disturbances, memory loss, organic brain syndrome, Wernicke-Korsakoff syndrome, and alcohol withdrawal syndrome. Neuromuscular problems include myopathy and peripheral neuropathy. Males may experience testicular atrophy, sterility, impotence, or gynecomastia, and females may produce neonates with fetal alcohol syndrome (FAS). Some of the metabolic disturbances include hypokalemia, hypomagnesia, and ketoacidosis. Also, endocrine disturbances may result in pancreatitis or diabetes.

Barbiturates

Barbituric acid was discovered in 1864, and since then hundreds of derivatives have been developed. These drugs are generally known as sleeping pills or "downers." High doses help people sleep, and low doses have a calming effect.

The short-acting barbiturates are similar to alcohol in their effects and are frequently abused. These drugs are not as toxic to the body's organ systems as is alcohol; however, the tolerance that develops is much more dangerous. Tolerance to the effects on mood develop faster than the physical tolerance to the lethal dose, resulting in a greater risk of accidental overdose. When used in combination with alcohol, a synergistic reaction occurs and the risk of overdose is greatly increased.

Benzodiazepines

These drugs were introduced in the 1960s and marketed towards housewives as a cure for everyday stress. In 1985, 81 million benzodiazepine prescriptions were filled (Miller and Gold, 1989). At one time diazepam (Valium) and chlordiazepam (Librium) were marketed for the treatment of alcoholism, but it soon became apparent that these drugs produced an alcohol-like effect and that alcoholics were now also addicted to these drugs.

These drugs continue to be misprescribed for long-term therapy, rather than treating the underlying stress. The benzodiazepines have a relatively safe therapeutic index (difficult to overdose), but withdrawal can be life-threatening.

Opiates

Opiates include the natural drugs found in the opium poppy—opium, morphine, and codeine. The opiates are by far the most effective drugs for pain relief. Opioids are synthetic drugs, such as heroin (semisynthetic), meperidine, methadone, oxycodone, and propoxyphene, which mimic the effects of the natural opiates.

It is estimated that there are 500,000 heroin addicts in the United States and more than 2 million persons who use the drug occasionally (Greenstein, Resnick, and Resnick, 1984). Tolerance develops quite readily with opiates and can reach striking levels. Tolerance to one opiate extends to other opiates and thus *cross-tolerance* can occur. Physical dependence also develops quite quickly; less than 2 weeks of continuous use can cause withdrawal symptoms.

Chronic abuse of the opiates causes few physiological problems except for constipation. The negative consequences primarily result from their illegal status. Lack of quality control (varied strength and purity) often results in unexpected overdoses or secondary effects of the impurities. Unsafe methods of administration (contaminated needles) lead to local and systemic infections. The high cost on the black market leads to crime to support the addiction.

Stimulants

The primary reason for using a CNS stimulant is to feel better. Many persons consume mild stimulants on a daily basis in some form of caffeine. An increase in alertness and energy results as the stimulant causes the nerve fibers to release noradrenaline and other stimulating neurotransmit-

HOW MUCH CAFFEINE IS THERE...

	Range/mg	Average		mg
In one cup of coffee? (150 ml/5 oz)			Pepsi	41
Brewed, drip method	60-180	115	Pepsi, Diet	38
Brewed, percolator	40-170	80	Tab	47
Instant	30-120	65	Orange	0
Decaffeinated, brewed	2-5	3	Other citrus	0-54
Decaffeinated, instant	1-5	2	Gingerale, rootbeer	0
			Tonic water	0
In chocolate and cocoa?			Soda, seltzer	0
Cocoa (150 ml/5 oz)	2-20	4	Other soft drinks	0-43.2
Chocolate milk (240 ml/8 oz)	2-7	5	*In these prescription drugs?*	
Chocolate syrup (30 ml/1 oz)		4	Cafergot	100　mg
Milk chocolate (1/12 chocolate cake and frosting	1-15	6 / 15.8	Darvon	32.4
			Fiorinal	40
Dark, semi sweet chocolate (30 ml/1 oz)	5-35	20	*In these OTC stimulants?*	
			Caffedrine	200　mg
Baker's chocolate (30 ml/1 oz)		26	No Doz	100
			Tirend	100
In one cup of tea? (150 ml/5 oz)			Vivarin	200
US brands, brewed	20-90	40	*In these OTC menstrual drugs?*	
Imported brands, brewed	25-110	60	Aqua-ban	100　mg
			Aqua-ban plus	200
Instant	25-50	30	Flowaway water 100's	20
Iced (300 ml/12 oz)	67-76	70	Midol	32.4
			Odrinil	50
In a soft drink? (360 ml/12 oz)		mg	Permathone H₂Off	200
Coca-Cola		45	*In these OTC analgesics?*	
Dr. Pepper		40	Anacin, maximum strength	32　mg
Mello Yellow		40	Excedrin	65
Mountain Dew		53	Vanquish	33
Mr. Pibb		54	Cope	32
			In these OTC cold tablets?	
			Coryban D 10	30　mg
			Dristan decongestant tablet and	16.2
			Dristan A-F tablet	
			Duradyne-Forte	30
			Kolephrin	65
			Triaminicin	30

From FDA (Drug intelligence and Clin Pharm, Jan 1984); National Soft Drink Association; and Wells SJ: Am J Orthopsychiatr, July 1984.

ters. However, these drugs do not actually give the person more energy; they only make the body expend its own energy sooner and in greater quantities than it normally would.

If used carefully, stimulants may be useful and have little negative health effect. The body must be allowed time to replenish itself following use of a stimulant. There is a cost for the "high," which is the "down" state following the use of a stimulant: a feeling of sleepiness, laziness, mental fatigue, and possibly depression. Many persons abusing stimulants soon find themselves in a vicious cycle of avoiding the down feeling by taking another dose and can become physically dependent on the stimulant to function. Major stimulants include caffeine, cocaine, amphetamines, and nicotine.

Caffeine

Caffeine is the most widely used psychoactive drug in the world, with a U.S. daily per capita consumption of 211 mg (Griffiths and Woodson, 1988). Caffeine is found in coffee, tea, chocolate, soft drinks, and various medications (see box above).

Moderate doses of caffeine from 100 to 300 mg per day probably have little negative effect on health and serve to increase mental alertness. Higher doses can lead to insomnia, irritability, tremulousness, anxiety, and headaches. Regular use of high doses can lead to physical dependence. Treating afternoon headaches with analgesics containing caffeine may in reality be preventing a withdrawal symptom from the heavy morning coffee consumption.

Cocaine

Cocaine comes from the coca shrub found on the eastern slopes of the Andes and has been cultivated by the South American Indians for thousands of years. The Indians chew a mixture of the coca leaf and lime to get a mild stimulant effect similar to coffee. By 1860 cocaine was isolated from the plant as a hydrochloride salt. It could be dissolved in water and used intravenously or orally when mixed in soft drinks. By the early 1900s the common route of administration of the white powder was intranasal ("snorting").

In the 1970s, *freebasing* was introduced. This involved converting the hydrochloride salt into a more volatile substance using highly flammable substances such as ether to convert the powder to a crystal, which could then be smoked in a pipe. By the early 1980s, another form of smokeable cocaine was introduced. Cocaine was dissolved in water, mixed with baking soda, and then heated to form rocks or "crack."

Among the routes of administration, 52% is taken intranasally, 30% by inhalation, and 18% intravenously (Higgins, 1989). Surveys from the National Institute on Drug Abuse (NIDA) indicate there were 22.2 million lifetime users of cocaine in the United States in 1985 with an estimated 5.75 million current users (used within the last month). Cocaine administered by intranasal route has been a popular recreational drug among the "rich and famous," but the cheaper "crack" form has become quite popular among the lower income black population.

Persons use cocaine for the intense euphoria, increased confidence, and willingness to work for long periods. When smoking cocaine, the effects are extremely intense as the drug quickly reaches the brain through the blood vessels in the lungs.

Cocaine's interaction with dopamine seems to be the basis for the addictive patterns. The extreme euphoria is believed to be caused by cocaine's effect of dopaminergic stimulation. Chronic administration can lead to neurotransmitter depletion (especially of dopamine), which results in an extreme dysphoria characterized by apathy, sadness, and anhedonia (lack of joy). Thus a cocaine user can get caught up in a dangerous cycle of gaining an extreme high followed by an extreme low and avoiding that low by consuming more cocaine. Crack addiction develops quite rapidly and users soon make the connection between their ill health and the drug use but are frequently overwhelmed by cravings, despite a sincere desire to stop using the drug.

Crack addicts may spend $100 to $1000 per day on the drug and soon find themselves selling their possessions to pay for it. Many addicts begin dealing (selling) the drug to supplement their costly addiction. Males and females have also resorted to prostitution in exchange for the drug.

Street cocaine ranges in purity from 5% to 60% and may be cut with other drugs, such as procaine or amphetamine, or with any white powder, such as sugar or baby powder. Since 1976 there has been a 15-fold increase in emergency room visits due to abuse of the drug. Some of this increase is due to the lack of quality control; however, most is due to the use of crack (Digregorio, 1990). High doses can cause extreme agitation, hyperthermia, hallucinations, cardiac arrhythmias, convulsions, and possibly death.

Amphetamines

Amphetamines are a class of stimulants very similar to cocaine, but the effects last much longer and the drugs are much cheaper. Included in this class are amphetamine (Benzedrine), dextramethamphetamine (Dexedrine), and methamphetamine (Methedrine). Amphetamines have a chemical structure similar to adrenaline and noradrenaline and are generally used to decrease fatigue, increase mental alertness, suppress appetite, and create a sense of well-being. Amphetamines were issued to American soldiers during World War II to decrease fatigue and increase mental alertness. They are currently popular among truck drivers and college students.

These drugs are taken orally or intranasally or by smoking or injecting them. When taken intravenously, these drugs quickly induce an intense euphoric feeling (a "rush"). The user may "speed" for several days (go on a "speed run") and then fall into a deep sleep of 18 or more hours ("crash"). "Ice," a smokeable form of crystallized methamphetamine was introduced in the late 1980s as an alternative to crack because it can be easily manufactured and the effects last up to 24 hours.

The Controlled Substances Act of 1970 placed amphetamines in the schedule II category, thus greatly decreasing their availability. Other drugs containing caffeine, ephedrine, or phenylpropanolamine (singly or in combination), which are referred to as "look alikes," gained attention on the market. These chemicals are often found in OTC cold remedies as a nasal decongestant and in diet pills (e.g., Dexatrim).

Nicotine

Nicotine, the active ingredient in the tobacco plant, is one of the most toxic and addictive drugs known to man. One in six deaths in the United States are attributed to cigarettes (U.S. Department of Health and Human Services, 1989). In 1991 the Centers for Disease Control estimated 434,000 deaths per year are caused by complications of cigarette smoking. Diseases and health problems related to smoking account for an annual cost of $22 billion in health care and $43 billion in lost productivity. Cancer mortality could be reduced by approximately 25% if smoking were eliminated.

Nicotine is one of the most toxic drugs known. To protect itself, the body quickly develops tolerance to the nicotine. If a person smokes regularly, tolerance to nicotine develops within hours, compared to days with heroin or months with alcohol. Pipes and cigars are less hazardous than cigarettes because the harsher smoke discourages deep inhalation. However, pipes and cigars increase the risk of cancer of the lips, mouth, and throat.

Nicotine can also be taken in the form of chewing tobacco and snuff. Marketed as "smokeless tobacco," a wad is put in the mouth and the nicotine is absorbed sublingually. Higher doses of nicotine are delivered in the smokeless forms because the nicotine is not destroyed by heat. Nevertheless this form is less addictive because nicotine enters the bloodstream less directly.

Currently, the prevalence of cigarette smoking has dropped to 31.7% for men and 26.8% for women. Most of

TABLE 23-1 Diseases and health hazards of smoking	
Active smoking	**Passive smoking**
CANCER	
Oral cavity, pharynx, larynx, esophagus, lung, pancreas, kidney, bladder	Lung
CARDIOVASCULAR	
Aggravation of exercise-induced angina, coronary artery disease, myocardial infarction, cardiac arrhythmias, sudden cardiac death, stroke, aortic aneurysm, arteriosclerotic peripheral vascular disease, thromboangiitis obliterans (Buerger's disease)	Aggravation of exercise-induced angina, premature ventricular contractions
PULMONARY	
Impaired pulmonary function, emphysema, acute and chronic bronchitis, chronic cough, hoarseness due to vocal cord irritation	Impaired pulmonary function in adults and children, asthma attacks, pulmonary infections, bronchiolitis, decreased growth rate of lungs
PERINATAL EFFECTS OF MATERNAL SMOKING	
Increase in fetal mortality, low–birth weight, spontaneous abortion, sudden infant death syndrome, congenital abnormalities, hyperactivity in childhood, risk of cancer in later life	Low–birth weight
MISCELLANEOUS	
Peptic ulcer disease, erythrocytosis, peripheral blood leukocytosis, smoker's skin, decreased ability to taste and smell, abnormal sperm counts and evidence of chromosomal damage, decreased fertility, increased accident rate, altered drug metabolism, adverse health consequences in women taking oral contraceptives	Increased hospital admissions of infants, middle ear effusions and sinusitis in children, decreased growth rate

With permission of Milhorn, HT. American Family Physician Vol 39(3), p. 215, 1989

the decline has occurred among the better educated and white populations. However, more women are becoming new users than men and by the year 2000 it is estimated that more women will smoke than men (U.S. Department of Health and Human Services, 1989).

Smoke can be inhaled directly by the smoker (*mainstream smoke)*, or it can enter the atmosphere from the lighted end of the cigarette and be inhaled by others in the vicinity (*sidestream smoke)*. The sidestream smoke contains greater concentrations of toxic and carcinogenic compounds than mainstream smoke. Diseases and conditions associated with smoking include cancer, cardiovascular and pulmonary problems, and perinatal effects (Table 23-1).

Marijuana

Marijuana (*Cannabis sativa* or *Cannabis indica*) is the most widely used illicit drug in the United States. Estimates of regular users range from 20 to 30 million Americans and as many as 60% of those between the ages of 18 and 25 years have tried marijuana at some point in their lives (Doweiko, 1990). There is no typical marijuana user (Mathre, 1988) because use cuts across all demographic lines.

In the United States, marijuana was a popular plant growth for its fiber (hemp), seed (popular birdseed), oil, and medicinal as well as psychoactive properties. During

World War II, the hemp fiber was so valuable that farmers were required to grow marijuana to ensure a supply. Tincture of cannabis was listed in the U.S. Pharmacopoeia through 1941 for such ailments as migraines, spasticity, and dysmenorrhea and in the treatment of heroin or cocaine addiction.

The marijuana plant contains hundreds of compounds, including 61 cannabinoids, of which δ-9-tetrahydrocannabinol (THC) is the main psychoactive chemical. The leaves and buds contain most of the THC and are generally referred to as marijuana.

Compared to the other psychoactive drugs, marijuana has very little toxicity and is one of the safest therapeutic agents known to man (Randall, 1988). However, because of its illegal status, there is no quality control and a user may consume contaminated marijuana. Users enjoy a mild euphoria, relaxed feeling, and an intensity of sensory perceptions. Side effects include dry and reddened eyes, increased appetite and dry mouth, drowsiness, and mild tachycardia. Adverse reactions include anxiety, disorientation, and paranoia.

The greatest physical concern for chronic users is the possible damage to the respiratory tract. Tolerance and physical dependence can develop; however, the withdrawal symptoms are quite benign. Addiction can occur for some chronic users and is difficult to treat because the progression tends to be quite subtle.

In 1971 marijuana was placed in the schedule I category of drugs by the passage of the Controlled Substances Act and has not been available for medicinal use. Since 1972 the National Organization for the Reform of Marijuana Laws (NORML) has attempted to have marijuana removed from the Schedule I category through court action so that it may be prescribed by physicians. Together with the Alliance for Cannabis Therapeutics (ACT), their case against the Drug Enforcement Agency (DEA) was heard in 1988 and the DEA's administrative judge ruled to move marijuana from schedule I to schedule II. However, the DEA continues to protest the decision, and currently, marijuana remains in schedule I.

Hallucinogens

Also called psychedelics ("mind vision"), these drugs are capable of producing hallucinations. Many of these drugs have been used for centuries in religious ceremonies and healing rituals and by many cultures to produce euphoria and as aphrodisiacs (Doweiko, 1990). For these drugs, the user's mood, basic emotional makeup, and expectations (set), along with the immediate surroundings (setting) will have a great influence on the mental effects experienced by the user. The physical effects are more constant and produce CNS stimulation.

There are two broad chemical families of hallucinogens: the indole hallucinogens and the phenylethylamines. The indoles are related to hormones (serontonin) made in the brain by the pineal gland and include such drugs as: LSD, psilocybin, morning glory seeds, ibogaine, dimethyltryptamine (DMT), and Yage. The phenylethylamines, which closely resemble adrenalin and amphetamines, include peyote and mescaline, STP, MDA, and MDMA (Ecstasy). Phencyclidine (PCP) is in a class by itself. LSD and PCP are discussed here.

LSD

Lysergic acid diethylamide (LSD) is the most well-known drug in this category. It is a semisynthetic drug first made in 1938 from lysergic acid, a chemical in ergot, the fungus that attacks cereal grains. It is one of the most potent drugs known—as little as 25 μg in a single dose lasts 10 to 12 hours. It is administered orally in small tablets, in gelatin chips ("window panes"), or on pieces of paper soaked with the drug or stamped with ink containing LSD.

The desired effects include euphoria, a heightened sense of awareness, distorted perceptions, and synesthesia (a mixing of senses; i.e.,sounds appearing as visual images). Adverse reactions to LSD include depersonalization, hypertension, panic, and psychosis. Another adverse reaction may be a flashback, which is a recurrence of the "trip" weeks or months after the LSD has been ingested. Flashbacks can be frightening, especially because of their unpredictability, but they decrease in frequency over time.

PCP

PCP is a potent anesthetic and analgesic with CNS depressant, stimulant, and hallucinogenic properties. In the late 1960s, PCP emerged in the Haight-Ashbury district of San Francisco and was known as the "peace pill." By the early 1970s PCP accounted for 25% of the psychedelic drugs consumed in the U.S. (Giannini, 1987). PCP comes in pill or powder form and has often been sold as mescaline, psilocybin, THC, or other drugs. "Angel dust" is PCP sprinkled on a marijuana joint.

The mental effects are variable but often include a feeling of disconnection from the body and reality, apathy, disorganized thinking, a drunklike state, and distortions of time and space perception. Adverse reactions include combative behavior, inability to talk, a rigid robotic attitude, confusion, paranoid thinking, catatonia, coma, and convulsions. Unlike the other hallucinogens, addiction can develop with this drug.

Inhalants

The inhalants do not fit neatly into other categories, but include gases and solvents. The three main types of inhalants are organic solvents, volatile nitrites, and nitrous oxide. These substances are inhaled ("huffed") from bottles, aerosol cans, or soaked cloth or are put into bags or balloons to increase the concentration of the inhaled fumes and decrease the inhalation of other substances in the vapor (i.e., paint particles).

The *organic solvents* include rubber cement, model airplane glue, paint thinner, lighter fluid, varnish, spot removers, and aerosol products such as spray paint, deodorant, and hair spray. The majority of users are between the ages of 10 and 20 years. These drugs are inexpensive and easy to obtain for that age group.

The effects of inhalants are similar to those of alcohol, but they have a rapid onset and last a short time. The user initially feels stimulated as the inhibitions are depressed, then a drunklike state is experienced and possibly hallucinations.

Amyl nitrite is the most common of the *volatile nitrites* and is most often used by urban male homosexuals. It is frequently used during sexual activity to intensify the experience and prolong the orgasm. This yellow liquid is packaged in cloth-covered glass capsules that have to be popped (hence, the common name of "poppers") to release the drug for inhalation.

Often referred to as "laughing gas", *nitrous oxide* was introduced in 1776. It is widely used in dentistry and minor surgery as a tranquilizer to sedate and create an analgesic effect by changing the patient's mood and interpretation of pain. Nitrous oxide is also found in whipping cream aerosol cans ("whippets") and is released by spraying the can upside down. Dangers with administration increase when inhaling directly from pressurized tanks because the gas is very cold and can cause frostbite to the nose, lips, and vocal cords. Also, if not mixed with oxygen, the user may die from asphyxiation.

PRIMARY PREVENTION

Primary prevention for substance abuse includes (1) education about drugs and guidelines for use and (2) the promotion of healthy alternatives to drug use for recreational purposes or to cope with various stressors. Unfortunately our society has focused on certain illegal drugs of abuse rather than on the use patterns of various drugs. This has led to a dangerous belief among the general population that there are "good" (legal) drugs and "bad" (illegal) drugs. Community health nurses have a focus on health promotion and can play an important role in educating the public about drugs and healthy alternatives to indiscriminate, careless, and oftentimes dangerous drug use.

Drug Education

The problems of substance abuse extend beyond the abuse of psychoactive drugs. Currently, there are over 450,000 different drugs and drug combinations available. It has been estimated that prescription drugs are involved in almost 60% of all drug-related emergency room visits and 70% of all drug-related deaths (Weiss and Greenfield, 1986). Approximately 25% of elderly hospital admissions result from problems related to noncompliance and drug reactions (Larrat, Taubman, and Willey, 1990).

Nurses are experts in medication administration and understand the potential dangers of indiscriminate drug use and the inherent inability of drugs to "cure" all problems. The community health nurse can greatly improve the health of clients by destroying the myth of "good drug" vs. "bad drug" and by teaching that no drug is completely safe and that any drug can be abused.

An effective way to begin drug education on an individual basis is by reviewing the client's prescription medications. Because a physician has prescribed the medication, clients often presume there is little risk involved. Does the client know the name of the medication and how and where it works in the body? Does the client know the importance of taking the correct dose to get the greatest benefit yet to limit the possible side effects? Is the client aware of any untoward interactions this drug may have with other drugs being used or with food?

People need to know why they are using a medication. If it is a long-term therapy, will a tolerance develop and the safe dose no longer be effective? Could physical dependence develop, making it difficult or unsafe to abruptly discontinue the use? Some medications are necessary for people to achieve optimal health, such as insulin for a person with diabetes. Some medications are used only to mask the symptoms of an underlying problem, which is not being addressed, such as pain medications for headaches induced by stress.

We live in a world of ever-growing drug technology, and yet the public receives very little information about how to safely use this technology. People need to know what questions to ask regarding their personal drug use and should be encouraged to seek the answers to these questions before using any drug. Encouraging clients to ask questions regarding their drug use can increase their responsibility for personal health and their awareness that drugs alter their body chemistry. The box above lists seven questions that can assist clients in obtaining the essential information necessary to decrease the possible harm from unsafe medication consumption.

The community health nurse can assist in identifying the various references and community resources available to provide the necessary information. The nurse can also assist in clarifying the information. Griffith's *Complete Guide to Prescription and Non-prescription Drugs* (1989) offers in-

---

DRUG CONSUMER SAFETY GUIDELINES

1. Determine the chemical being taken.
2. Determine how and where the drug works in the body.
3. Determine the correct dosage.
4. Determine whether there will be drug interactions.
5. Determine if there are allergic reactions.
6. Determine if there will be drug tolerance.
7. Determine if the drug will produce physical dependence.

Caution: Approximately 10% of the population may suffer from the disease of addiction. For those persons, responsible use of psychoactive drugs is limited as a result of their disease. Always notify your physician of your addiction if use of psychoactive medicines is being considered in your treatment. With permission of Miller, M. Drug Consumer Safety Rules, Mosier, OR, 1985, MAMA.

---

formation regarding drug interactions between medications and other drugs (including alcohol, tobacco, marijuana, and cocaine) and other substances (food and beverages) and serves as an excellent guide for nurse, as well as for the client's personal use.

Harm reduction as a goal recognizes the reality that people consume drugs and that information about the use of drugs and risks involved is necessary for persons to make responsible decisions about their drug use. As clients learn to ask questions about their prescription medications, the nurse can encourage them to ask the same questions regarding self-administration of OTC and recreational drugs. This does not mean that nurses should encourage other drug use, but rather that the potential harm from self-medication can be reduced if the clients have the necessary information to make informed decisions about their drug use.

A common occurrence with drug users is the use of drugs from different categories used together or at different times to regulate how they feel—known as *polysubstance use or abuse*. For example, a person may drink alcohol when snorting cocaine to "take the edge off." Or a person may use barbiturates to assist with sleep after using a stimulant. Polysubstance use has the potential for causing various drug interactions. The interactions may result in additive, synergistic, or antagonistic effects. Indiscriminate polysubstance abuse may lead to serious physiological consequences and can be very complicating for the health care professional to assess and treat.

As parents learn to seek information regarding their use of medications, they begin to act as role models for their children. It can be confusing for children and adolescents to be told to "just say no" to drugs yet, at the same time, to watch their parents or drug advertisements try to "quick fix" every health complaint with a medication.

The simple "just say no" approach does not help young people for several reasons. First, children are naturally curious and drug experimentation is often a part of normal development (Shedler and Block, 1990). Second, children from dysfunctional homes often use drugs to obtain attention or to escape the intolerable environment. And finally, it does not address the powerful influence of peer pressure (Engs and Fors, 1988).

Basic drug education programs for young people should include the following areas: self-esteem, decision-making skills, assertiveness skills, stress management, recreational activities, and factual information about drugs, especially the commonly used psychoactive drugs.

Community health nurses can serve as educators or as advisors to school systems or community groups to ensure that all of these areas are addressed. Role playing can be an effective method of teaching many of these skills.

Promotion of Alternatives

Nurses are experts in health promotion. Assisting clients to achieve optimal health includes identifying interventions other than or in addition to the use of drugs whenever possible. Teaching assertiveness skills and decision-making skills helps clients increase their responsibility for their health and their awareness of various options available.

Nagging health problems such as difficulty sleeping, muscle tension, lack of energy, and mood swings are common reasons people turn to medications, especially the psychoactive drugs. The nurse can help clients understand that these medications are only masking their problems rather than solving them. Stress reduction and relaxation techniques along with a balanced life-style can address these problems more directly.

Often, stress is created by lack of balance in a person's life-style. Lack of sleep, improper diet, and lack of exercise contribute to many health complaints. Assisting clients to balance their rest, nutrition, and exercise on a daily basis can greatly reduce these complaints. The nurse can be resourceful in providing this information to various groups, assisting in the development of community recreational resources, or facilitating groups on stress reduction, relaxation, or exercise.

Lack of educational opportunities, job training, or both can contribute to socioeconomical stress and poor self-esteem, which can lead to drug use to escape the situation. Again, the community health nurse can assist clients with identifying community resources and with problem solving to address these basic needs rather than avoid them.

Frequently, recreational activities are centered around the use of drugs. Nurses can help persons increase their awareness of drug-free community activities and recreational and hobby classes that address this area.

SECONDARY PREVENTION

To identify substance abuse and plan appropriate interventions, community health nurses must assess each client on an individual basis. When drug abuse, dependence, or addiction is identified, community health nurses must assist clients to understand the connection between their drug use patterns and the negative consequences on their health, their families, and the community.

Illicit drug users are reluctant to seek related health care for fear of the consequences. By working within the community, community health nurses can reach out to those who need health care rather than wait for individuals to seek care. Developing a therapeutic relationship can increase the effectiveness of resources and interventions. Substance abusers will be more honest about their drug use patterns if the nurse can offer assistance rather than judgment.

```
┌─────────────────────────────────────────────┐
│             STAGES OF DRUG USE              │
├─────────────────────────────────────────────┤
│  1. Experimental: Drugs are used for fun    │
│     and to satisfy curiosity or to experi-  │
│     ment with feelings.                     │
│  2. Social/recreational: Drugs are used to  │
│     share a common experience with friends. │
│  3. Circumstantial/situational: Drugs are   │
│     used to help in coping with such things │
│     as moods, work, and sex.                │
│  4. Intensified: Drugs are used to escape   │
│     from problems, including emotional      │
│     problems.                               │
│  5. Compulsive: Drugs are used to maintain  │
│     a drug high or drug state.              │
└─────────────────────────────────────────────┘
```

From the National Commission on Marihuana and Drug Abuse, Drug Use in America: Problem in Perspective, Washington, DC, 1975, National Academy Press.

Identifying high-risk groups helps the community health nurse to design programs to meet their specific needs and to help mobilize community resources to meet these needs most effectively.

Assessing for Substance Abuse Problems

Assessing for substance abuse problems should be a routine part of all basic health assessments. An assessment of self-medication practices and recreational drug use should be done at the time of the "medication" history. This puts all relevant drug-use history together and aids in the assessment of drug-use patterns. When working with a client over time, periodic assessment of drug-use patterns alerts the nurse to any changes requiring intervention. To help clarify patterns of drug use, the National Commission on Marijuana and Drug Abuse (1973) described five stages of drug use (see box above).

After obtaining a medication history, follow-up questions will help to determine if any problems exist. For prescription drug use, is the client following the directions correctly? Be especially inquisitive about any prescribed psychoactive drug use: How long has the client been taking the drug? Has the client increased the dosage or frequency above the prescription?

When assessing self-medication and recreational and social drug-use patterns, the reason for use should be elicited. Some underlying health problems (i.e., pain, stress, weight or insomnia) may be alleviated by nonpharmaceutical interventions. Duration, amount, frequency, and route of administration of each drug must be explored.

The occurrence of *blackouts* should also be assessed. Blackouts are intervals of temporary memory loss during which a person remains conscious and active and may even appear sober, but later has no recollection of where he/she was and what he/she may have done or said. Blackouts are considered a "red flag" for alcoholism.

To establish the presence of a substance abuse problem, the nurse must determine if the drug use is causing any negative health consequences or problems with relationships, employment, finances, or the legal system. The box on p. 403 provides examples of questions to ask clients to determine the presence of socioeconomic problems that are often caused by substance abuse.

If a pattern of chronic, regular, and frequent use of a drug is revealed, the nurse must assess for a history of withdrawal symptoms to determine if there is physical dependence on the drug. A progression in drug-use patterns and related problems alerts the nurse to the possibility of addiction.

One of the primary symptoms of addiction is *denial*. Methods of denial include lying about use, minimizing use patterns, blaming or rationalizing, intellectualizing, changing the subject, use of anger or humor, and "going with the flow" (agreeing there is a problem, stating behavior will change, but not demonstrating any behavior changes). The nurse should suspect a problem if the client becomes defensive or exhibits other behavior indicating denial when asked about alcohol or other drug use.

Drug Testing

During the 1980s preemployment or random drug testing gained much popularity. Drug testing can be done by examining a person's urine, blood, saliva, breath (alcohol), or hair. The limitations of drug testing must be understood to yield any benefits.

When is drug testing appropriate? Drug testing as a result of documented impairment may be helpful in substantiating the cause of the impairment, thus being used as a backup rather than the primary screening method. Another time it is useful is for recovering addicts. Part of their treatment is to abstain from psychoactive drug use, therefore a urine test yielding positive results for a drug indicates a relapse.

The most common method of drug screening is urine testing. Urine testing only indicates past use of certain drugs, not intoxication. Thus persons can be identified as having used a certain drug in the recent past, but the degree of intoxication and extent of performance impairment cannot be determined with urine testing. Also, most drug-related problems in the workplace are due to alcohol, and alcohol is not identified in a urine drug screen.

To properly conduct a urine screen, the flow of urine must be closely monitored to ensure that the urine is not adulterated or that the individual does not submit a "clean" specimen that has been purchased. Drug addicts may not be able to stop use long enough to produce a clean urine on a preemployment screen; however, they have learned how to manipulate the system to "pass" the test. Because the results of these tests may greatly impact the job security of the employee, a chain of custody must be maintained to ensure that the specimen is not adulterated or mislabeled on route to the laboratory.

Most urine screens are conducted on lower technology tests because they are cheaper. When a urine specimen yields positive test results, the urine should automatically be tested by a more sensitive (and expensive) method to help reduce the possibility of false-positive results.

Blood, breath, and saliva drug tests have the benefit of indicating current use and amount. Any of these can be helpful tests to determine alcohol intoxication and are often used to substantiate suspected impairment. A serum drug screen can be very useful when overdose is suspected to determine the specific drug ingested. The testing of hair is gaining attention because the results can provide a long history of drug use patterns.

ASSESSMENT QUESTIONS TO DETERMINE SOCIOECONOMIC PROBLEMS SECONDARY TO SUBSTANCE ABUSE

1. Do your spouse, parents, or friends worry or complain about your drinking/drug taking?
2. Has a family member gone for help about your drinking/drug taking?
3. Have you neglected family obligations as a result of drinking/drug taking?
4. Have you missed work because of your drinking/drug taking?
5. Does your boss complain about your drinking/drug taking?
6. Do you drink or use drugs before or during work?
7. Have you ever been fired or quit a job as a result of drinking/drug taking?
8. Have you ever been charged with driving under the influence (DUI) or drunk in public (DIP)?
9. Have you ever had any other legal problems related to drinking/drug taking such as assault and battery, breaking and entering, or theft?
10. Have you had any accidents while intoxicated such as falls, burns, or motor vehicle accidents?
11. Have you spent your money on alcohol or other drugs instead of paying your bills (such as telephone, electricity, or rent)?

Employee-Assistance Programs

Employee assistance programs (EAPs) are gaining popularity among many work settings. These programs are set up to identify health problems among employees and offer counseling or refer to other health care providers as necessary. Early identification of and intervention for substance abuse problems are often addressed through EAPs. These programs also offer services to their employees to reduce stress and provide health care or counseling so that they may prevent substance abuse problems from developing. Nurses frequently develop and run these programs.

High-Risk Groups
Pregnant Women

During pregnancy, the fetus is at risk of negative effects from most drugs. Thus the use of any drug during pregnancy should be discouraged unless medically necessary. Surveys during the last two decades have determined that alcohol and nicotine are among the top three drugs used during pregnancy (along with iron) (Martin et al., 1988). Fetal Alcohol Syndrome (FAS) has been identified as a leading cause of mental retardation in the United States (Naegle, 1988). Negative consequences of cocaine use during pregnancy are also being observed more frequently. Table 23-2 discusses drug effects during pregnancy.

Despite the increased focus in the health care system on interventions for drug abuse, many pregnant women with drug problems do not receive the help they need. Reasons for not receiving treatment may include ignorance, poverty, lack of concern for the fetus, lack of available services, and fear of the consequences. The fear of criminal prosecution

TABLE 23-2
Drug use during pregnancy

Drug	Effect on fetus	Safe use of drug
Nicotine	Heavy smoking can lead to low–birth-weight babies, which means that the baby may have more health problems. Smoking is especially harmful during second half of pregnancy.	Should be avoided
Alcohol	Daily drinking of more than two glasses of wine or a mixed drink can cause fetal alcohol syndrome. Babies tend to exhibit low–birth weight, mental retardation, physical deformity, and behavioral problems, including hyperactivity, restlessness, and poor attention spans.	Should be avoided
Aspirin	During the last 3 months of pregnancy, frequent use may cause excessive bleeding at delivery and may prolong pregnancy and labor.	Under physician's supervision
Tranquilizers	Taken during the first 3 months of pregnancy these may cause cleft lip or palate or other congenital malformations.	Avoid if possibility of pregnancy and during early pregnancy; use only under physician's supervision
Barbiturates	Mothers who have taken large doses may have babies who are addicted. Babies may have tremors, restlessness, and irritability.	Only under physician's supervision
Amphetamines	May cause birth defects.	Only under physician's supervision
Cocaine	Shortened gestation period, premature rupture of membranes, increased incidence of abruptio placentae, low–birth weight result from its use. Immediately postpartum, cocaine seropositive neonates may have withdrawal symptoms: tremors, hypertonia, poor feeding, tachypnea, and abnormal sleep patterns.	Should be avoided

From Holland JG, Graves GR, and Martin JN: J Miss State Med Assoc 31(9):287, 1990; adapted from Deciding about drugs: a woman's choice. DHEW Pub No (ADM) 80-820, Rockville, MD, 1979, National Institute on Drug Abuse, Department of Health, Education, and Welfare.

may push addicted women further away from the health care system and cause them to conceal their drug use from medical providers and deliver their babies in out-of-hospital settings, thus further jeopardizing the pregnancy outcome (Chavkin and Kandall, 1990).

Adolescents

Studies have shown that the younger a person is when beginning intensive experimentation with drugs, the more likely dependence will develop. Heavy drug use during adolescence can interfere with normal development.

More than 90% of adolescents 18 years of age and younger have consumed alcohol, making it the most popular drug used by teenagers. Prevalence of marijuana use among adolescents ranges from 27% to 59%. It is estimated that by the twelfth grade, 20% of high school students have used stimulants, 16% cocaine, and 12% tranquilizers. These figures come from self-reporting surveys, and it is likely that actual use is considerably greater (Oetting and Beauvais, 1990).

The greatest single variable influencing substance use among adolescents is peer pressure. Decreased emphasis on religion, a low value placed on achievement, poor school performance, delinquency, and a high value placed on risk taking are other factors that are linked with adolescent substance abuse (Henderson and Anderson, 1989).

Elderly

The elderly (65 years of age and older) represent 12% of the U.S. population and consume approximately 25% of all prescribed drugs. Twenty-five percent of the elderly population consume psychoactive drugs. Factors such as slowed metabolic turnover of drugs, age-related organ changes, enhanced drug sensitivities, a tendency to use drugs over long periods of time, and a more frequent use of multiple drugs all contribute to greater negative consequences from drug use among the elderly.

The increased use of prescription drugs and alcohol by the elderly may be related to coping problems. Problems of relocation, possible loss of independence, retirement, illness, death of friends, and lower levels of achievement contribute to feelings of sadness, boredom, anxiety, and loneliness.

Two types of elderly alcoholics have been identified: (1) those who have a chronic history of alcohol abuse and (2) those whose excessive drinking is reactive to the stresses of aging. Often alcohol abuse is not identified because its effects on cognitive abilities may mimic changes associated with normal aging or degenerative brain disease. Also, depression may simply be attributed to the more frequent losses rather than the depressant effects of alcohol, and the elderly person may subsequently receive medical treatment for depression.

IV-Drug Users

In addition to the problem of addiction, intravenous (IV)-drug users are at risk for other health complications. IV administration of drugs always carries a greater risk of overdose because the drug goes directly into the bloodstream. With illicit drugs, the danger is increased because the exact dosage is unknown. In addition, the drug may be contaminated with other chemicals, which can cause negative consequences. Often IV-drug users make their own solution for IV administration and any particles present can result in complications from emboli.

The sharing of needles has been a common practice among addicts. The spread of AIDS through needle sharing has become a great public health risk. Hepatitis and other bloodborne diseases can also be transmitted through contaminated needles. Infections and abscesses may develop as a result of dirty needles or poor administration techniques.

Primarily because of the growing incidence of AIDS among IV-drug users, emphasis is being placed on reducing the transmission of this disease through contaminated needles. Abstinence is the ideal method but is unrealistic for many addicts. Therefore the nurse should provide education on use of bleach to clean needles between use and needle-exchange programs to decrease the spread of the virus. Studies indicate that the needle-exchange programs have not resulted in an increase in IV-drug abuse, but have, in fact, increased the number of people entering treatment programs (Bardsley, 1990).

Codependency and Family Involvement

The disease of drug addiction is often referred to as a family disease. People in a close relationship with the addict often develop unhealthy coping mechanisms to continue the relationship. This behavior is known as *codependency*, a companion illness in which the codependent is addicted to the addict.

Strict rules typically develop in a codependent family to maintain relationships: don't talk, don't feel, don't trust, don't lose control and don't seek help from outside the family. Codependents try to meet the addict's needs at the expense of their own. Codependency may underlie many medical complaints and emotional stress seen by health care providers such as ulcers, skin disorders, migraine headaches, chronic colds, and backaches (Zerwekh and Michaels, 1989).

When the addicted person refuses to admit the problem, the family continues to adapt to emotionally survive the stress of the addict's irrational, inconsistent, and unpredictable behavior. Members of the family consequently develop various roles that tend to be gross exaggerations of normal family roles. Members cling irrationally to these roles, even when they are no longer functional.

One of the most significant roles a family member may assume is that of an enabler. *Enabling* is the act of shielding or preventing the addict from experiencing the consequences of the addiction. As a result, the addict does not always understand the cost of the addiction and thus is "enabled" to continue to use.

Although codependency and enabling are closely related, a person does not have to be codependent to enable. Anyone can be an enabler: a police officer, a boss or co-worker, and even a drug-treatment counselor. Nurses who do not address the negative health consequences of the drug use with the addicted person are enablers.

The community health nurse can assist families to recognize the problem of addiction and help them confront the addicted member in a caring manner. Whether or not the addicted family member is agreeable to treatment, the family members should be given some guidance to the literature and services that are available to help them cope more effectively. The community health nurse can help identify treatment options, counseling assistance, financial assistance, support services, and (if necessary) legal services for the family members.

TERTIARY PREVENTION

The community health nurse is in a pivotal position to help the addict and the addict's family. The nurse's knowledge of community resources and how to mobilize them can significantly influence the quality of care clients receive.

Many alcoholics and drug addicts become lost in the health care system. If satisfactory care is not provided in one agency, the addict may give up rather than seek alternative sources of care. The community health nurse who knows the client's environment and support systems can offer guidance leading to the most effective treatment modality.

After the client has received treatment, the community health nurse can coordinate aftercare referrals and follow-up on the client's progress. The nurse can provide additional support in the home as the client and family adjust to changing roles and the stress involved with such changes. The community health nurse can support addicts who have experienced relapse by reminding them that relapses may occur, yet encouraging them and their families to continue to work towards recovery and an improved quality of life.

Detoxification

Detoxification refers to the process of clearing the drug(s) from the person's body and managing of the withdrawal symptoms. Depending on the particular drug and the degree of dependence, the time period may range from a few days to several weeks. Withdrawal symptoms vary, depending on the drug used. They may range from uncomfortable to life-threatening; therefore the setting for and management of withdrawal depends on the drug used.

Drugs such as marijuana, stimulants, and opiates may produce withdrawal symptoms that are uncomfortable, but not life-threatening. Detoxification from these drugs does not require direct medical supervision, but medical management of the withdrawal symptoms increases the comfort level. On the other hand, drugs such as alcohol and barbiturates may produce life-threatening withdrawal symptoms. These clients should be under close medical supervision during detoxification, and should receive medical management of the withdrawal symptoms to ensure a safe withdrawal. For those persons who develop delirium tremons, 15% may not survive, despite medical management; therefore close medical management should be initiated as the blood level of the drug begins to fall.

A general rule in detoxification management is to wean the person off the drug by gradually reducing the dosage and frequency of administration. Thus a chronic alcoholic could be safely detoxified by a gradual reduction in alcohol consumption. In practice, however, the switch to another drug often offers a safer withdrawal, as well as an abrupt end to the intoxication from the drug of choice. For example, chlordiazepam (Librium), is commonly used for alcohol detoxification.

Treatment for Addiction

Addiction "treatment" differs from the management of negative health consequences of chronic drug abuse, drug overdose, and withdrawal. Addiction treatment focuses on the addiction process: helping clients recognize the addiction as a chronic disease and assisting them to make life-style changes to halt the progression of that disease process. According to the disease theory, addicts are not responsible for the symptoms of their disease; they are, however, responsible for treating their disease.

Most treatment facilities are multidisciplinary because the intervention strategies require a wide range of approaches and involve interactions between the addict, family, culture, and community. Included in the strategies are medical management, education, counseling, vocational rehabilitation, stress management, and support services. In general, there are two basic approaches to addictions treatment: (1) medical management/controlled use and (2) total abstinence.

Controlled Use and Medical Management

For those addicts unwilling or unable to completely abstain from psychoactive drugs, other drugs have been used to assist the client in abstaining from their drug of choice. Until the early 1900s American physicians sometimes prescribed morphine for alcoholics because of the extensive physical damage or aggressive behavior caused by the alcohol. The alcoholic instead became addicted to morphine but would not suffer the negative physical or behavioral consequences of alcohol (Brecher, 1973).

A similar philosophy is applied today with the methadone maintenance program for treatment of heroin addiction. Methadone, when administered in moderate or high daily doses, produces a cross-tolerance to other narcotics, thereby blocking their effects and decreasing the craving for heroin. The advantages of methadone are that it is long acting, effective when administered orally, and inexpensive and has few known side effects.

The oral use of methadone offers a solution to the danger of the spread of AIDS and other bloodborne infections, which commonly occur among needle-sharing addicts. More recently, trends indicate that many IV-heroin addicts are also "shooting" (taking intravenously) cocaine; because methadone does not affect the cocaine cravings, a heroin addict on a methadone maintenance program may still continue IV-drug use.

Although not recognized as a cure for heroin (or other opiate) addiction, methadone maintenance reduces deviant behavior and introduces addicts to the health care system. This may ultimately lead to total abstinence.

For some persons, medical treatment is used to negate the high from their drug of choice or to deter use by negative interactions. Naltrexone (Trexan) can be used with opiate addiction. It is a pure opiate antagonist which blocks the effects of all opium-derived compounds. The usual dose is 50 mg orally each morning. This can help the client by preventing the psychological and physical reinforcements of opiates if a person should slip and use an opiate.

Disulfiram (Antabuse) may be prescribed for the recovering alcoholic as a deterrent to drinking. Ingesting alcohol while disulfiram is in the body produces negative health effects including blurred vision, nausea, vertigo, anxiety, and cardiovascular effects, such as hypotension, palpitations, tachycardia, and flushing of the face and neck. The reaction is believed to be caused by disulfiram's inhibition of acetaldehyde dehydrogenase—the enzyme necessary for the breakdown of acetaldehyde, a product of the metabolism of alcohol.

Clients taking disulfiram need to be educated about the risks involved and hidden sources of alcohol such as other medicines, recipes using sherry or other alcohol, flavorings, and mouthwashes. Disulfiram treatment should be considered as an adjunct to a recovery program on a limited time basis for persons who believe it will prevent them from a relapse during their initial recovery period.

Total Abstinence

Total abstinence is the recommended treatment for drug addiction. Those clients who are addicted to a particular drug (such as cocaine) are advised to abstain from the use of all psychoactive substances. The use of another drug may simply reinforce the craving for the original drug and result in relapse. More commonly, the addiction merely transfers to the replacement substance.

Treatment may be received on an inpatient or outpatient basis. In general, the more advanced the disease is, the greater the need for inpatient treatment. Inpatient treatment programs usually last 28 days, although they may range from a few weeks to 90 days. Once a person has completed detoxification, the programs provide counseling and group interaction to help the addict stay clean long enough for the body chemistry to rebalance. This is often a difficult time for recovering addicts, who may experience mood swings and difficulty sleeping and dealing with emotions.

The educational segment of the program focuses on providing information about the disease concept and how drugs affect a person physically and psychologically. Addicts are informed of the various life-style changes that they must make and learn about tools to assist them in making these changes. Discharge planning continues throughout treatment as the addicts build the support systems that they will need when they leave the controlled environment of a treatment center and come face-to-face with pressures and temptations (triggers) that may lead to relapse.

Halfway houses have been developed to ease the recovering addict back into society. These facilities provide continued support and counseling in a structured environment for persons needing long-term assistance in adjusting to a drug-free life-style. The residents are expected to secure employment and take responsibility in managing their fi-

---

SMOKING CESSATION RESOURCES AND SUPPORT GROUPS

American Academy of Family Physicians, Health Education Department B, 8880 Ward Parkway, Kansas City, MO 64114-2797

American Heart Association, 7320 Greenville Ave., Dallas, TX 75231

Health Promotion Group, Inc., PO Box 59687, Homewood, AL 35259

Warner Brothers, Attention Lorimar Home Video, 4000 Warner Blvd., Burbank, CA 91522; or phone (800) 323-5275

National Cancer Institute, Office of Cancer Communications, National Institutes of Health, Bldg. 31, Room 4B43, Bethesda, MD 20892

National Audio Visual Center, Customer Services Section, 8700 Edgeworth Dr., Capital Heights, MD 20743-3701

National Heart, Lung, and Blood Institute, Smoking Education Program, National Institutes of Health, Bldg. 31, Room 4A-18, Dept. A-1, Bethesda, MD 20892

Office on Smoking and Health, 5600 Fishers Lane, Park Bldg., Room 110, Rockville, MD 20857

Local offices/divisions

American Cancer Society (see local telephone directory)

American Heart Association (see local telephone directory)

American Lung Association (see local telephone directory)

From Milhorn, HT, American Family Physician Vol. 39(3), p. 215, 1989

FIVE STAGES IN SMOKING CESSATION

1. Precontemplation: In this stage smokers are unlikely to be responsive to direct intervention. There is little concern about the negative aspects of smoking and heavy-handed messages may increase their resistance to quitting. If pushed hard, they may seek alternative health care. A calm, factual presentation of the risks delivered in a low-key manner is the best approach.
2. Contemplation: In this stage, smokers are much more receptive to information about the health hazards of smoking. They will often ask for help.
3. Action: This is the stage of quitting tobacco use.
4. Maintenance: This is the most difficult stage, which involves continued abstinent from tobacco use.
5. Relapse: A return to smoking occurs so frequently that it must be considered part of the quitting process.

From Fisher EB et al.: Chest 93(Suppl 2):695, 1986

---

nancial obligations.

Outpatient programs are similar in the education and counseling offered, but they allow the addicts to live at home and continue to work while undergoing treatment. This method is very effective for persons in the earlier stages of addiction who feel confident that they can abstain from drug use and have established a strong support network.

Most programs incorporate family counseling and education into their programs. In addition, specific programs are being developed to address the needs of various populations such as adolescents, women during pregnancy, and health care professionals.

Recovery from addiction involves a lifelong commitment and may include periods of relapse. The addict must realize that modern medicine has not found a cure for addiction; therefore returning to drug use will ultimately reactivate the disease process.

Smoking Cessation Programs

Many resources are available on smoking cessation programs and support groups (see box above). Smoking cessation program methods vary from a gradual taper to cold turkey, but research shows that the development of a plan in collaboration with the smoker is most effective. Five stages in smoking cessation have been identified (see box above right) and awareness of these stages can assist the community health care nurse in developing an effective plan in collaboration with the individual client.

Support Groups

The development of *Alcoholics Anonymous (AA)* in 1935 began a movement that has done more for the treatment of alcoholism than the health care profession. AA groups have developed throughout the world and their success has led to the development of other support groups such as Narcotics Anonymous for narcotics addicts and Pills Anonymous for polysubstance addicts. Similar programs have been developed for process addictions such as Overeaters Anonymous and Gamblers Anonymous.

AA consists of 12 steps leading toward recovery. In the first three steps, alcoholics acknowledge the problem and make a commitment to work toward resolution. During the next four steps, they take an honest look at themselves, share the information with a special person, and begin to modify behavioral deficiencies. In the succeeding four steps, alcoholics continue self-scrutiny. Finally in the last step, they reach out to help others.

AA/NA assists addicts in developing a daily program of recovery and reinforces the recovery process. The fellowship, support, and encouragement among AA/NA members, all of whom are abstaining alcoholics or addicts, provides a vital social network for the recovering addict.

Al-Anon and Alateen are similar self-help programs for spouses, parents, children, or others involved in a painful relationship with an alcoholic (Nar-Anon is for those in relationships with addicts). Al-Anon family groups are available to anyone who has been affected by their involvement with an alcoholic. The purposes of Alateen include providing a forum for adolescents to discuss family stressors, to learn coping skills from one another, and to gain support and encouragement from knowledgeable peers.

Adult Children of Alcoholics (ACOA) groups are also available in most areas to address the recovery for adults who grew up in alcoholic homes and still carry the scars and retain dysfunctional behaviors.

CLINICAL APPLICATION

A 6-week prenatal class was developed by a community health nurse for pregnant women from an inner-city low-rent housing area. The program was designed because so many women in the area did not have the resources to get routine prenatal care and were identified as a high-risk group.

One of the classes focused on drug use during pregnancy. Following the class, Jenny, a 23-year-old single black woman in her first trimester approached the nurse. She stated that she didn't know where to begin, except that she wanted the nurse to know that she really wanted her baby, but was afraid she may have already harmed the fetus. She admitted that she had used crack on a regular basis and had been trying to quit, but had used it again over the weekend when a friend brought some by. Teary eyed, Jenny stated she didn't know where to go or who to see, but that she wanted to get help.

The nurse sat down with Jenny and continued to assess Jenny's crack and other drug-use patterns and obtained a thorough biopsychosocial history. Jenny's mother had died and her father had a history of alcoholism. There was no supportive family member nearby and her older sister's husband would not let her stay with them because she had stolen money and property from them on more than one occasion to buy crack. Jenny was not sure who the father of her baby was because she had had multiple partners in exchange for cocaine. She was currently living with friends who also used crack. She was afraid that if she returned to her environment she would not be able to stay clean.

The nurse was aware of a treatment program that was affiliated with a hospital able to take pregnant women, but realized there may be a waiting list. The nurse worked with the community services board to find housing in a homeless shelter until Jenny could get into treatment. The nurse counseled Jenny about being tested for the human immunodeficiency virus (HIV) and other sexually transmitted diseases (STDs), and on Jenny's request, blood tests were arranged through the public health department. The nurse contacted the treatment program, and Jenny was admitted a few days later into their inpatient program where she would also get prenatal care as necessary.

While in treatment, Jenny was encouraged to develop an aftercare program. Finding a place to live was of great concern. The treatment team encouraged Jenny to consider a halfway house in a nearby city that was designed for pregnant women. She would have to agree to abide by their rules, attend specific classes on child care and parenting, and attend AA and NA meetings on a daily basis. If the infant had any complications as a result of Jenny's crack use, the staff at the halfway house were prepared to assist Jenny in meeting the infant's health care needs. Jenny decided to go to the halfway house and subsequently delivered a 6-pound baby girl 1 week before her due date. The baby was healthy, and Jenny remained at the halfway house with her daughter for another 4 months.

This case study shows how a community health nurse can make a difference by identifying high-risk groups within the community and developing a plan of care to bring knowledge and care into the clients' environment. Jenny may not have been aware of the full impact her crack addiction could have on the fetus and may not have sought help so early in her pregnancy. After identifying Jenny's addiction problem, the nurse was able to mobilize community resources to find her a safe place to live, to arrange for her to be screened for possible STDs, which could require treatment, and to make an appropriate referral to a treatment program that would also offer prenatal care. Although relapse is still possible, Jenny was able to abstain from further crack or other drug use during her pregnancy and therefore decreased the possibility of permanently damaging her baby in utero.

SUMMARY

Substance abuse and addiction are significant problems in all segments of our society. The current focus of America's "war on drugs," coupled with the daily bombardment of enticing advertisements for "medicines" and "nondrugs" such as alcohol, tobacco, and caffeine have created a dangerous misconception for the public that there are "good" drugs, "bad" drugs, and "nondrugs". This has led to irresponsible, indiscriminate, and dangerous substance abuse problems with legal drugs and a negative attitude towards persons who use illegal drugs. Community health nurses have the knowledge to encourage safe drug administration and can incorporate drug consumer safety principles in routine client interactions.

Attitudes about substance abuse are of critical importance in health promotion because the way people think and feel is conveyed in nonverbal, as well as verbal messages. Attitudes toward substance abuse are most helpful to clients when they are based on the premise that people use chemicals to deal with life and that addicts are not responsible for developing the disease of addiction. People need acceptance, understanding, and commitment to help them deal constructively with their health problems.

Based on the focus of health promotion through holistic health care, community health nurses have an opportunity to significantly decrease the incidence of substance abuse and related health problems. They can provide early intervention, referrals for treatment, and follow-up health care for drug addicts. The community health nurse needs information about programs and resources in the local area. Major nursing responsibilities include teaching, assessing, providing support, encouragement, counseling, and referrals, and coordinating services.

KEY CONCEPTS

Substance abuse is a national health problem that is linked to numerous forms of morbidity and mortality.

Confusion has existed for many years about whether substance abuse is a health care problem or a criminal justice problem.

All people have attitudes about the use of drugs that influence their actions.

Social conditions such as a fast-paced life, excessive stress, and the availability of drugs influence the incidence of substance abuse.

Important terms to understand when working with individuals, groups, or communities for whom substance abuse is prevalent are: drug dependence, drug addiction, alcoholism, psychoactive drugs, depressants, stimulants, marijuana, hallucinogens, and inhalants.

Primary prevention for substance abuse includes education about drugs and guidelines for use, as well as the promotion of healthy alternatives to drug use for either recreation or to relieve stress.

Secondary prevention depends heavily on careful assessment of the client's use of drugs. Such assessment should be part of all basic health assessments.

High-risk groups include pregnant women, youth, the elderly, and intravenous-drug users.

Drug addiction is often a family, not merely an individual, problem. Codependency describes a companion illness to the addiction of one person in which the codependent member is addicted to the addict.

Community health nurses are in ideal roles to assist with tertiary prevention for both the addicted person and the family.

LEARNING ACTIVITIES

1. Read your local newspaper for 4 days and select stories that illustrate the effect of substance abuse on individuals, on families, and on the community.

2. For each of the stories in the newspaper related to substance abuse, describe preventive strategies that a community health nurse might have tried before the problem reached such a dire state.

3. Looking at your local community resources directory (or the telephone book), identify agencies that might serve as referral sources for individuals or families for whom substance abuse is a problem.

4. In groups of three to five students discuss your personal attitudes toward drinking, smoking, and drug abuse. Discuss each category of substance abuse separately. Consider the following areas: sex, age, amount, time, occasion, place where substance abuse occurs, companions, motivation, and incentives.

5. In groups of four to five students develop a list of examples, incidents, regulations, or practices in U.S. society that illustrate conflicting attitudes about drinking (for example, alcoholism is an illness yet people are arrested for public intoxication; drunken driving is illegal yet bars line many roads as do billboards advertising alcoholic beverages).

6. Attend an open AA or NA meeting and an Al-Anon meeting. Go alone if possible or with a friend who is an alcoholic or drug addict. As the members introduce themselves, give your first name and state, "I am a visitor." Plan to listen and do not attempt to take notes. Respect the anonymity of the persons present. Discuss your experiences later in a group.

BIBLIOGRAPHY

Abadinsky H: Drug abuse: an introduction, Chicago, 1989, Nelson-Hall.

Abrams RC and Alexopoulos GS: Substance abuse in the elderly: alcohol and prescription drugs, Hosp Community Psychiatry 38(12):1285, 1987.

Bardsley J. Vancouver's needle exchange program, Can J Public Health 81:39, 1990.

Bennett G, Vourakis C, and Woolf DS, editors: Substance abuse: pharmacologic, developmental, and clinical perspectives, New York, 1983, John Wiley & Sons.

Brecher EM: Licit and illicit drugs, Boston, 1972, Little, Brown & Company.

Bush B et al: Screening for alcohol abuse using the CAGE questionnaire, Am J Med 82:231, 1987.

Caroselli-Karinja M: Drug abuse and the elderly, J Psychosoc Nurs Ment Health Serv 23(6):25, 1985.

Chavkin W and Kandall SR: Between a "rock" and a hard place: perinatal drug abuse, Pediatrics 85(2):223, 1990.

Digregorio GJ: Cocaine update: abuse and ther-

apy, Am Fam Pract 41(1):247, 1990.

Donovan DM and Marlatt GA: Assessment of addictive behaviors, New York, 1988, The Guilford Press.

Doweiko HE: Concepts of chemical dependency, Pacific Grove, CA, 1990, Brooks/Cole Publishing.

Engs RC and Fors SW: Drug abuse hysteria: the challenge of keeping perspective, J School Health 58(1):26, 1988.

Estes NJ and Heinemann ME: Alcoholism: development, consequences, and interventions, ed 3, St Louis, 1986, Mosby-Year Book.

Estroff TW and Gold MS: Chronic complications of drug abuse, Psychiatr Med 3(3):267, 1987.

Fisher EB Jr et al.: Implications for the practicing physician of the psychosocial dimensions of smoking, Chest 93(suppl 2):69S, 1986.

Frezza M et al.: High blood alcohol levels in women, N Engl J Med 322(2):95, 1990.

Giannini AJ et al.: Phencyclidine and the dissociatives, Psychiatr Med 3(3):197, 1987.

Giannini AJ and Miller NS: Drug abuse: a bio-

psychiatric model, Am Fam Physician 40(5):173, 1989.

Greenstein RA, Resnick RB, and Resnick E: Methadone and naltrexone in the treatment of heroin dependence Psychiatr Clin North Am 7:671, 1984.

Griffith WH: Complete guide to prescription and nonprescription drugs, Los Angeles, 1989, The Body Press.

Griffiths RR and Woodson PP: Caffeine physical dependence: a review of human and laboratory animal studies, Psychopharmacology 94:437, 1988.

Hallal J: Are coffee, cold tablets, and chocolate innocuous or is their caffeine hazardous to your patients' health? Am J Nurs 86(4):423, 1986.

Henderson DC and Anderson SC: Adolescents and chemical dependency, Soc Work Health Care 14(1):87, 1989.

Herer J: The emperor wears no clothes, Van Nuys, CA, 1990, HEMP Publishing.

Higgins R: Cocaine abuse: what every emergency nurse should know, J Emerg Nurs 15(4):318, 1989.

Holland JG, Graves GR, and Martin JN: Cocaine: a primer for providers of perinatal care, J Miss State Med Assoc 31(9):287, 1990.

Inaba DS and Cohen WE: Uppers, downers, and all arounders, Ashland, OR, 1989, Cinemed.

Institute of Medicine: Treating drug problems, Washington, DC, 1990, National Academy Press.

Jaffe JH: Drug addiction and drug abuse. In Gilman AG, et al., editors: Goodman and Gilman's the pharmacological basis of therapeutics, ed 7, New York, 1986, MacMillan.

Kinney J and Leaton G: Loosening the grip, St Louis, 1991, Mosby-Year Book.

Kolb L: Let's stop this narcotics hysteria! The Sat Eve Post 229:194, 1956.

Krug SE: Cocaine abuse: historical, epidemiologic, and clinical prospectives for pediatricians, Adv Pediatr 36:369, 1989.

Larret EP, Taubman AH, Willey C: Compliance-related problems in the ambulatory population, Am Pharm NS30(2):18, 1990.

Levine HG: The alcohol problem in America: from temperance to alcoholism, Br J Addict 79:109, 1984.

Lewis DC and Gordon AJ: Alcohol and the general hospital: the Roger Williams Interventions Program, Bull N Y Acad Med 59:181, 1983.

Martin JN et al. Pregnancy-associated substance abuse and addiction: current concepts and management, J Miss State Med Assoc 29(12):369, 1988.

Mathre ML: A survey on disclosure of marijuana use to health care professionals, J Psychoactive drugs 20(1):117, 1988.

Mikuriya TH and Aldrich MR: Cannabis 1988: old drug, new dangers—the potency question, J Psychoactive Drugs 20(1):47, 1988.

Milhorn HT: Nicotine dependence, Am Fam Physician 39(3):214, 1989.

Miller M: Drug consumer safety rules, Mosier, OR, 1985, MAMA.

Miller NS and Gold MS: Identification and treatment of benzodiazepine abuse, Am Fam Physician 40(4):175, 1989.

Mulry JT: Codependency: a family addiction, Am Fam Physician 35(4):215, 1987.

Oei S: Fetal arrhythmia caused by excessive intake of caffeine by pregnant women, Br Med J 298:568, 1989.

Oetting ER and Beauvais F: Adolescent drug use: findings of national and local surveys, J Consult Clin Psychol 58(4):385, 1990.

National Commission on Marijuana and Drug Abuse: Drug use in America: problem in perspective, Washington, DC, 1973, US Government Printing Office.

Naegle MA: Substance abuse among women: prevalence, patterns, and treatment issues, Issues Ment Health Nurs 9:127, 1988.

Randall RC, editor: Marijuana, medicine & the law, Washington, DC, 1988, Galen Press.

Schottenfeld RS: Drug and alcohol testing in the workplace; objectives, pitfalls, and guidelines, Am J Drug Alcohol Abuse 15(4):413, 1989.

Shedler J and Block J: Adolescent drug use and psychological health, Am Psychol 45(5):612.

Slade J: The tobacco epidemic: lessons from history, J Psychoactive Drugs 21(3):281, 1989.

Spickard A Jr: Alcoholism: the missed diagnosis, South Med J 79:1489, 1986.

Tongue E and Turner D: Treatment options in responding to drug misuse problems, Bull Narc 40(1):3, 1988.

Trebach AS and Zeese KB: Drug prohibition and the conscience of nations. Washington, DC, 1990, The Drug Policy Foundation.

U.S. Department of Health and Human Services: Preventing alcohol-related birth defects, Alcohol Health Res World 10(1):4, 1985.

U.S. Department of Health and Human Services: Reducing the health consequences of smoking: 25 years of progress—a report of the Surgeon General, Washington, DC, 1989, US Government Printing Office.

U.S. Prevention Services Task Force: Screening for alcohol and other drug abuse, Am Fam Physician 40(1):137, 1989.

Vener AM and Krupka LR: Over-the-counter drug advertising in gender oriented popular magazines, J Drug Educ 16(4):367, 1986.

Washton AM: Nonpharmacologic treatment of cocaine abuse, Psychiatric clinics of North America, 9(6):563, 1989.

Washton AM: Cocaine addiction: treatment, recovery, and relapse prevention, New York, 1989, WW Norton.

Weil A and Rosen W: Chocolate to morphine: understanding mind-active drugs, Boston, 1983, Houghton Mifflin.

Weiss KJ and Greenfield DP: Prescription drug abuse, Psychiatr Clin North Am 9:475, 1986.

Westermeyer J: The pursuit of intoxication: our 100 century-old romance with psychoactive substances, Am J Drug Alcohol Abuse 14(2):175, 1988.

Zerwekh J and Michaels B: Co-dependency: assessment and referral, Nurs Clin North Am 24(1):109, 1989.

Zinberg NE: Drug, set, and setting: the basis for controlled intoxicant use, New Haven, 1984, Yale University Press.

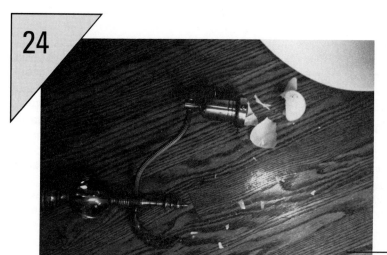

24

Violence and Human Abuse

Jacquelyn Campbell

Jeanette Lancaster

OBJECTIVES

After reading this chapter, the student should be able to:

Discuss the scope of the problem of violence in American communities.

Describe at least three factors existing in most communities that influence violence and human abuse.

Identify at least three types of common community facilities that can help mitigate violence.

Identify typically noticed indicators of child abuse.

Define the four general types of child abuse: neglect, physical abuse, emotional abuse, and sexual abuse.

Discuss abuse of the elderly as a growing community health problem.

Evaluate the role that community health nurses can assume with rape victims.

Identify primary preventive nursing interventions for community violence.

Describe the different responses that a nurse would expect to see in a battered woman from the beginning of the abuse until after the relationship has ended.

Discuss the principles of nursing intervention with violent families.

KEY TERMS

battered child syndrome	empowerment	secondary prevention
crises	helplessness	sense of cohesiveness
developmental disabilities	hostility	sense of confusion
	incest	sexual abuse
elder abuse	physical abuse	spouse abuse
emotional abuse	powerlessness	survivors
	primary prevention	therapeutic intervention

T he word "violence" comes from the Latin *violare,* meaning to violate, injure, or rape. Indeed, violence is a violation, resulting in emotional ramifications in addition to physical injuries. American society is unfortunately quite violent by most measures. Statistics indicate that the United States has the fifth highest homicide rate in the world (Rosenberg and Mercy, 1985). Newspaper headlines and television reports are rife with news of violence. Although considerable progress has been made in decreasing rates of death from all other causes since 1940, the risk of homicide in the United States is actually increasing (Farley, 1986). The violence in our streets and in our homes threatens the health and well-being of our entire population.

It is not clear from research if violence stems from an innate aggressive drive or is primarily learned behavior. However, it *is* clear that all human beings have the capability for violence. It is also clear that some entire societies are basically nonviolent (Counts, Brown, and Campbell, 1991). Therefore it is important to understand under what conditions aggression and violence are exacerbated and, conversely, what keeps them in check and promotes nonviolent conflict resolution. From a community health standpoint, nurses should be interested in these forces at a family, aggregate, and community level.

Violence is a community health nursing concern. Significant mortality and morbidity results from violence, and extensive violence within a community is distressing to all of its inhabitants. Communities across the United States are voicing anger and fear about rising crime and violence rates. Former Surgeon General C. Everett Koop stressed that violence was to be considered one of the most important public health problems facing the nation. The Surgeon General's *Workshop on Violence and Public Health Report* (1986) points out that medical, nursing, psychology, and social service professionals have been slow in developing a response to violence that is integral to their daily professional lives. As a result, the estimated 4 million victims of violence annually may not receive the best care possible. In addition, the extent of their pain that could have been avoided by community health prevention efforts is unknown.

This chapter examines violence as a community problem and discusses how the community health nurse can help families, groups, and the community cope with and reduce violence and human abuse. Community health nurses have access to clients in a wide variety of settings, including in the home. They are in key positions to detect and intervene in community and family violence. It is important that nurses have an understanding of community-level influences on all types of violence as a beginning point for addressing this important problem.

SOCIAL AND COMMUNITY FACTORS INFLUENCING VIOLENCE

Numerous variables within a community can support or minimize violence. Changing social conditions, multiple demands on people, economic conditions, and institutions that make up a given society or community influence the level of violence and human abuse. The following discussion of selected contemporary social conditions provides a basis for understanding factors that influence violent behavior.

Work

Productive and paid work is an expectation in mainstream American society, especially for men. Work can be fulfilling and thus can contribute to a sense of well-being, but it can also be frustrating and unfulfilling, contributing to stress that may lead to aggression and violence. Unemployment is also associated with violence both within and outside the home.

When jobs are repetitive, boring, and lacking in stimulation, frustration mounts. Some work environments discourage creativity and reward conformity and "following the rules." In many work settings people try to get ahead regardless of the cost to others. Workers often go home feeling physically and psychologically drained. They may have worked at a back-breaking pace all day only to be yelled at by the boss for what seemed like a trivial oversight. It is hard to separate feelings generated at work from those in the home environment.

For example, a father arrives home feeling tired, angry, and generally inadequate because of a series of reprimands from his boss. Soon after he sits down, his 4-year old son runs through the house pretending to fly a wooden airplane. After about three loud trips past his father, who keeps shouting for the child to be quiet and go outside, the airplane hits the father in the head. This provides a fertile setting for striking out in frustration and anger.

In times of economic constraints, people are often afraid to give up even those jobs that are frustrating or boring or that create great stress. Their family needs necessitate that they keep the hated job. They feel trapped and may resent those who are dependent on them. This frustration and resentment may lead to violence.

Unemployment also often precipitates aggressive outbursts. The inability to secure or maintain a job may lead to feelings of inadequacy, guilt, boredom, dissatisfaction, and frustration. Unemployment does not fit the image of the ideal man in American society, and these men are more likely to commit violence both within and outside the family (Hotaling and Sugarman, 1986).

Young, minority males have the highest rates of unemployment in the United States, ranging close to 50%. This group also has the highest rate of violence. They are described as young men living in a world of oppression, with lack of opportunity and enormous anger as a "subculture of exasperation." It must be understood that the norms developed by this group are a response to being pushed out of mainstream society and of being on the receiving end of the fallout of policies that ignore their dilemmas and give them no stake in mainstream America. Most analyses conclude that the differential rates of violence between African-Americans and European-Americans in this country has more to do with economic realities, such as poverty, unemployment, and overcrowding, than with race (Hawkins, 1986; Straus and Gelles, 1990).

Education

In recent years schools have assumed many responsibilities traditionally assigned to the family. Schools teach sexual development, discipline children, and often serve as a place to "dump" children who have no other place to go. Large

ing with these families. Nurses have a "duty to warn" family members of the possibility of homicide when severe abuse is present, just as they warn of the hazards of smoking (Campbell, 1986). Other nursing care issues are discussed further in the section on family violence.

Assault

The death toll from violence is indeed staggering. Yet, the physical injuries and emotional costs of violence are equally important issues in terms of the acute health care system and both public health nursing and home health care. There are at least 100 nonfatal assaults for each homicide that occurs in the United States (Public Health Service, 1990). In 1986 there were 1842 assaults resulting in injury per 100,000 persons. Sometimes the difference between a homicide and an assault is only the response time and quality of emergency transport and treatment facilities. Whatever community measures are used to address homicide are also useful to combat assault. In addition, nurses find that assaulted persons are often seen in home health care situations with such long-term health problems as head injuries, spinal cord injuries, and stomas from abdominal gunshot wounds. In addition to physical care, nurses must also address the emotional trauma resulting from a violent attack.

Rape

Currently, rape is one of the most underreported yet fastest growing forms of human abuse in the United States. Rape is the one category of violent crime that continued to increase during the 1980s. In 1986 there were 120 rapes per 100,000 (Public Health Service, 1990). Because many rapes are not reported as a result of fear of retaliation or stigma or a feeling of guilt about having somehow provoked the attack, the actual incidence is many times higher than reported. In spite of still prevailing myths to the contrary, the majority of rapes are perpetrated by someone known to the victim, and "date rape" is an instance of traumatic violence that often goes unrecognized by both the health care and criminal justice systems. We are also beginning to recognize that rape often happens to men, especially boys and young men. Although we need much more research in that area, beginning studies suggest that the emotional trauma to a male rape victim is at least as serious as that for a woman.

For reported rapes, cities constitute higher risk areas than do rural settings, and the hours between 8 PM and 2 AM, weekends, and the summer are the most critical times. In about one half of rapes the victim and the offender meet on the street, whereas in the other cases the rapist either gains entry to the victim's home or somehow entices or forces the victim to accompany him.

Prevention of rape, as in other forms of human abuse, requires a broad-based community focus for educating both the community as a whole and key groups such as police, health care providers, educators, and social workers. Research has shown connections between rape rates and community-level variables such as community approval and legitimization of violence (for instance, violent network television viewing and permitting corporal punishment in schools), which underscores the need for community-level intervention (Baron, Straus, and Jaffee, 1988).

Attitudes

The first priority is to change attitudes about rape and about victims. Rape is a crime of violence, *not* a crime of passion. The underlying issues are hostility, power, and control rather than sexual desire. The defining issue is lack of consent of the victim. When a woman or man refuses *any* sexual activity, that refusal means "no." People have the right to change their mind, even when they seemed initially acquiescent. Pressure in the form of physical contact, threats, or deliberate inducement of drug or alcohol intoxication is a violation of the law. There must also be an end to the myths that women say "no" to sex when they really mean "yes" and that the victims of rape are culpable because of the way they dress or act.

Pornography

There is persuasive evidence that viewing pornographic material depicting violence against women within the context of sex is correlated with aggressive and sexual behavior (Sommers and Check, 1987). More research is needed in this area before definitive public policy recommendations can be made concerning laws governing pornography. However, there is enough evidence to recommend keeping violent pornography illegal, especially for minors. Prevention also involves providing information to women about self-protection, including self-defense procedures, avoiding high-risk locations, and safeguarding one's home against unwanted entry.

The Victim

Victims can be hit, kicked, stabbed, and severely beaten. It is the violence that most traumatizes the victim—because of the fear for her life and her helplessness, lack of control, and vulnerability.

People react to rape differently, depending on their personality, past experiences and background, and support received after the trauma. Some victims cry, shout, or discuss the experience. Others withdraw and fear discussing the attack. During the immediate as well as the follow-up stages, victims need to talk about what happened and to express their feelings and fears in a nonjudgmental atmosphere. Therefore nonjudgmental listening is an essential nursing measure.

In any psychological trauma, the right to privacy and confidentiality is of the utmost importance. Victims should not be expected to answer questions in an area where others can hear them. Nurses are responsible for providing continuous care once the victim enters the health care system. This includes monitoring the actions of other workers who may be less sensitive to the psychological needs of the victim (Dietz, 1978).

In several states nurses perform the physical examination in the emergency department to gather evidence (such as hair samples and skin fragments beneath the victim's fingernails) for criminal prosecution (Lenehan, Bowie, and Ruksnaitis, 1983). This is an important intervention mode because physicians are often impatient with the time required for this procedure and nurses can take advantage of this opportunity to provide therapeutic communication. Nurses can be trained to conduct the examination easily, and their evidence is credible and effective in resultant court proceedings (Dinitto, Martin, and Byington, 1987). Community health nurses can lobby for changes in hospital policies and state laws to make this strategy a reality in all states.

Rape is a situational crisis for which advance preparation is rarely possible. Therefore nursing efforts are directed toward helping victims maximize their ability to cope with the stress and disruption of their lives caused by the attack. Counseling focuses on the crisis and the concomitant fears, feelings, and issues involved. The goal is to help the victim use problem-solving skills to develop ways to regroup personal forces.

Many rape victims need follow-up mental health services to help them cope with the long-term effects of the crisis. They may be hesitant to ask for help or to follow through on these services; therefore community health nurses must not only make appropriate referrals but must also take the initiative by calling the victim to check on her and remind her of appointments. Rape victims need support, encouragement, and acceptance from those with whom they come in contact (Burgess and Holstrum, 1979).

Suicide

Suicide is the third leading cause of death for young people age 15 to 24 years and the tenth leading cause of death overall, with white males and American Indians at greatest risk. There are approximately 11.6 suicides per 100,000 people in the United States (Public Health Service, 1990). The incidence of suicide increases with age, reaching a high of 40 per 100,000 among persons over 75 years of age. Yet attempts at suicide are most common in adolescents and college students (Hanlon and Pickett, 1984).

The leading factors associated with suicide attempts are listed by Hanlon and Pickett (1984) as broken homes or frequent moves during childhood, marital disharmony, emotional immaturity, cruelty to children, and jealousy bordering on the pathological. The abuse-prone family is likely to exhibit one or more of these factors. Among adolescents the incidence of actual suicide also is alarming. According to the National Institute of Mental Health, more than 6000 adolescents kill themselves each year. This figure means that, every 90 minutes, an adolescent commits suicide and that, every day, 1000 more will attempt it (Oliphant, 1986).

Males commit suicide three times more frequently than females, although females attempt suicide more often. The number one risk factor for actual and attempted suicide in adult women is wife abuse (Stark and Flitcraft, 1985). Suicide is four times more frequent among whites than among blacks. Affluent and educated people have higher rates of suicide than do the economically and educationally disadvantaged (Hanlon and Pickett, 1984).

Nursing care must focus on family members and friends of suicide victims. *Survivors* often feel angry toward the dead person yet frequently turn the anger inward. Likewise, survivors frequently question their own liability for the death. The impact of suicide can affect family, friends, co-workers, and the community. Survivors may have difficulty dealing with their feelings toward the dead person. They may have difficulty concentrating and may limit their social activities because it is often difficult for both survivors and

their friends to talk about the suicide. Community health nursing intervention can help survivors cope with the trauma of the loss and may include referral to a counselor or support groups.

FAMILY VIOLENCE AND ABUSE

Family violence is also responsible for significant injury and death. Reported child abuse increased during the 1980s, a decade that also witnessed more attention to wife abuse and the beginning of documentation of elder abuse (Public Health Service, 1990). The most recent random-sample family-violence survey indicates that at least 10.5 million Americans are severely assaulted by a family member each year; however, this survey excluded elder abuse (Strauss and Gelles, 1990). Although no national survey of elder abuse has been conducted, estimates of the number of elders abused by a relative per year range from 1 to 2.5 million (Pillemer and Finkelhor, 1986). These rates of family violence suggest that at least 10% of all American families are violent and that community health nurses should be actively intervening in abuse or potential abuse situations in more than 10% of their cases.

Family violence can include sexual and emotional abuse, as well as physical violence. These three forms tend to occur together as part of a system of coercive control. Generally, violence within families is perpetrated by the most powerful against the least powerful. Thus approximately 90% of all "spouse abuse" is directed primarily toward wives (although they may physically fight back), whereas approximately 7% to 8% is mutual violence, and 2% to 3% is husband abuse (Campbell and Humphreys, 1984).

Recognizing the battered child or spouse in the emergency room is relatively simple after the fact. Unfortunately, by the time medical care is sought, serious physical and emotional damage may have been done. Community health nurses are in a key position to predict and deal with abusive tendencies. By understanding factors contributing to the development of abusive behaviors, nurses can identify abuse-prone families.

Development of Abusive Patterns

Factors that characterize people who become involved in family violence include upbringing, living conditions, and increased stress. Understanding how these factors influence the development of abusive behavior can help the nurse deal with abusive families.

Upbringing

Of all the factors that characterize the background of abusers, the most predictably present is previous exposure to some form of violence (Straus and Gelles, 1990). As children, abusers were often beaten themselves or witnessed the beating of siblings or a parent. Children raised in this fashion may abhor the use of violence, but they have had no experience with other models of family relationships.

Repeated research has demonstrated that even what is considered "normal" physical punishment of children is associated with future abuse of both children and spouses (Straus and Gelles, 1990). Childhood physical punishment teaches children to use violent conflict resolution as an adult. A child may learn to associate love with violence because parents are usually the first persons to hit a child. The child can come to believe that those who love him also are those who hit him. The moral rightness of hitting other family members thus may be established when physical punishment is used to train children. This type of experience predisposes children ultimately to use violence with their own children.

People who become abusers may also learn parenting skills from dysfunctional role models. Their parents may have set unrealistic goals, and when the children failed to perform accordingly, they were criticized, demeaned, punished, and denied affection. These children may have been told how to act, what to do, and how to feel, thereby discouraging the development of autonomy, problem-solving skills, and creativity (Scharer, 1979). Children raised in this fashion grow up feeling unloved and worthless. They may want a child of their own so that they will feel assured of someone's love.

To protect themselves from feelings of worthlessness and fear of rejection, abused children form a protective shell and grow increasingly hostile and distrustful of others. The behavior of potential abusers reflects a low tolerance for frustration, emotional instability, and the onset of aggressive feelings with minimal provocation. Because of their emotional insecurity, they often depend on a child or spouse to meet their needs so that they may be valued and feel secure. When their needs are not met by others, they become overly critical. Critical, resentful behavior and unrealistic expectations of others leads to a vicious cycle. The more critical these people become, the more they are rejected and alienated from others. Abusive individuals tend to perceive that the target of their hostility is "out to get them." These distorted perceptions can be detected when parents talk about an infant crying or keeping them up at night "on purpose."

Increased Stress

A perceived or actual crisis may precede an abusive incident. Because crisis reinforces feelings of inadequacy and low self-esteem, it is often a number of events occurring in a short time that precipitates abusive patterns. Factors such as unemployment, strains in the marriage, or an unplanned pregnancy may set off violence.

The daily hassles associated with raising young children, especially in an economically strained household, intensify an already stressed atmosphere for which an unexpected and difficult event provides a catalyst for violence. Research by Straus and Gelles (1990) showed associations between stressful life events, poverty, and the number of small children with family violence.

Crowded living conditions may also precipitate abuse. The presence of numerous people in a small space tends to heighten tensions and to reduce privacy. Tempers flare because of the constant stimulation from others.

Social isolation is associated with abuse in families (Straus and Gelles, 1990). Such isolation reduces social support, decreasing a family's ability to deal with stressors. The problem may be intensified if a violent family member tries to keep the family isolated to escape detection. Therefore when a family misses clinic or home visit appointments, community health nurses need to keep in mind that abuse may be present. Community health nurses can encourage involvement in community activities and can help neighbors reach out to neighbors to help prevent abuse.

Frequent moves disrupt social support systems, are associated with an overall increased stress level, and tend to isolate people, at least briefly. Mobility can have serious negative impact for the abuse-prone family. These families do not readily seek out new relationships, leaving only the family to turn to for support. Resources may be unfamiliar or inaccessible to them. Because frequent moving may be both a risk factor for abuse and a sign of an abusive family trying to avoid detection, community health nurses should assess such families carefully for abuse.

Types of Family Violence

It is important to realize that the various forms of family violence and violence outside the home frequently occur together. When nurses detect child abuse, they should also suspect other forms of family violence. When elderly parents report that their (now adult) child was abused or has a history of violence toward others, the nurse should recognize the potential for elder abuse. Physical abuse of women is frequently accompanied by sexual abuse both inside and outside of marital relationships. Severe wife abusers are likely to have a history of other acts of violence. Families who are extremely verbally aggressive in conflict resolution (e.g., using name calling, belittling, screaming, and yelling) are more likely to be physically abusive. Although the various forms of family violence are discussed separately, they should not be thought of as totally separate phenomena.

No member of the family is guaranteed immunity from abuse and neglect. Spouse abuse, child abuse, abuse of the elderly, serious violence among siblings, and mutual abuse by members all occur. Although these examples are not inclusive, they demonstrate the scope of family violence.

Child Abuse

A recent national survey projected that nearly 1.5 million children and adolescents are subjected to abusive physical violence each year (Straus and Gelles, 1990). This is probably a conservative figure, since only the most severe cases are reported. Child maltreatment was rarely discussed in medical literature until Henry Kempe et al. published their classic article in 1962, which coined the term *battered child syndrome*.

Kempe and his associates (1962) were highly successful in generating public and professional concern over child maltreatment. Their work led to the passage in 1974 of the Child Abuse Prevention and Treatment Act, which mandated reporting by professionals of child maltreatment.

The presence of child abuse signifies ineffective family functioning. Abusive parents who recognize their problem are often reluctant to seek assistance because of the stigma attached to being considered a child abuser.

Children are frequent victims of abuse because they are small and relatively powerless in the family hierarchy. In many families only one child is abused. Parents may identify with this particular child and be particularly critical of that child's behavior. In some cases the child may have certain qualities, such as looking like a relative, being handicapped, or being particularly bright and capable, that provoke the parent.

BEHAVIORAL INDICATORS OF POTENTIALLY ABUSIVE PARENTS

The following characteristics in couples expecting a child constitute warning signs of actual or potential abuse.

1. Denial of the reality of the pregnancy, as evidenced by a refusal to talk about the impending birth or to think of a name for the child
2. An obvious concern or fear that the baby will not meet some predetermined standard: sex, hair color, temperament, or resemblance to family members
3. Failure to follow through on the desire for or seeking of an abortion
4. An initial decision to place the child for adoption and a change of mind
5. Rejection of the mother by the father of the baby
6. Family experiencing stress and numerous crises so that the birth of a child may be the "straw that broke the camel's back"
7. Initial and unresolved negative feelings about having a child
8. Lack of support for the new parents
9. Isolation from friends, neighbors, or family
10. Parental evidence of poor impulse control or fear of losing control
11. Contradictory history
12. Appearance of detachment
13. Appearance of misusing drugs or alcohol
14. Shopping for hospitals or health care providers
15. Unrealistic expectations of the child
16. Abuse of mother by father

Abusive parents tend to be very controlling of their children's behavior and insensitive to their needs (Houck and King, 1989). They often have unrealistic expectations of the child's developmental abilities. The nurse must not only teach them what is "normal" but may also attend to their underlying emotional needs. The box above lists some of the behavioral indicators of potentially abusive parents. These parents often experience pain and poor emotional stability. They are in need of intervention as much as their children.

FOSTER CARE. When child abuse is discovered, the child is often placed in a foster home. Unfortunately, there is not enough good foster care for all abused children, and many foster care situations are also abusive. Abused children generally want to return to their parents, and the goal of most agencies is to keep natural families together as long as it is safe for the child. Many times the community health nurse's role involves helping to monitor a family in which a formerly abused child has been returned after a time in foster care. Keen judgment and close collaboration with social services is necessary in these situations. The nurse must ensure the safety of the child, while working *with* the parents in an empathetic way. The nurse's goal is to enhance their parenting skills, not to be viewed as yet another "watchdog."

Another point to keep in mind about abusive parents is that the wish to replace a child who has been removed by the courts because of abuse is a normal response to the grief of losing a child. Rather than regarding another pregnancy as a sign of continued poor judgment or pathological be-

havior, the pregnancy can be perceived by community health nursing as an opportunity for intensive intervention to prevent the abuse of the expected child. Generally, the parents are equally eager to avoid further problems if enlisted as partners in the project.

INDICATORS OF CHILD ABUSE. It is essential that community health nurses recognize the physical and behavioral indicators of abuse and neglect. The box at right summarizes indicators of physical abuse, physical neglect, sexual abuse, and emotional maltreatment. Child abuse ranges from violent physical attacks to passive neglect. Violence such as beating, burning, kicking, or shaking may often result in severe physical injury. Passive neglect may result in insidious malnutrition or other problems. Abuse is not limited to physical maltreatment but includes emotional abuse such as yelling at or continually demeaning and criticizing the child.

EMOTIONAL ABUSE. Extreme debasement of feelings may result in the child feeling inadequate, inept, uncared for, and worthless. Victims of emotional abuse learn to hide their feelings to avoid incurring additional scorn. They may act out by performing poorly in school, becoming truant, and being hostile and aggressive.

Physical symptoms of physical, sexual, or emotional stress may include hyperactivity, withdrawal, overeating, dermatologic problems, vague physical complaints, stuttering, enuresis (bladder incontinence), and encoporesis (bowel incontinence). Ironically, bedwetting is often a trigger for further abuse, which makes for a particularly vicious cycle. When a child displays physical symptoms without clear physiological origin, ruling out the possibility of abuse should be part of the community health nurse's assessment process.

CHILD NEGLECT. Child neglect in general can be divided into two categories: physical and emotional. Physical neglect is defined as failure to provide adequate food, proper clothing, shelter, hygiene, or necessary medical care (Campbell and Humphreys, 1984). Physical neglect is most often associated with extreme poverty.

In contrast, emotional neglect is the omission of basic nurturing, acceptance, and caring essential for healthy personal development. These children are largely ignored or in many cases are treated as nonpersons. Such neglect usually affects the development of self-esteem. It is difficult for a neglected child to feel a great deal of self-worth because the parents have not demonstrated that they value the child.

Neglect is much more difficult to assess and evaluate than abuse because it is more subtle and may go unnoticed. Astute observations of children, their homes, and the way in which they relate to their caregivers can provide clues of neglect.

SEXUAL ABUSE. Child abuse also includes sexual abuse. Approximately one of every four female children and one in ten males in this country will be subject to some form of sexual abuse by the time they reach age 18 years. This abuse ranges from unwanted sexual touching to intercourse. The majority of childhood sexual abuse is perpetrated by someone known to the child. Between one half and one third of all sexual abuse involves a family member (Russell, 1982; Covington, 1989).

INDICATORS OF ACTUAL OR POTENTIAL ABUSE

1. An unexplained injury
   a. Skin: burns, old or recent scars, ecchymosis, soft tissue swelling, human bites
   b. Fractures: recent or ones that have healed
   c. Subdural hematomas
   d. Trauma to genitals
   e. Whiplash (caused by shaking small children)
2. Dehydration or malnourishment without obvious cause
3. Provision of inappropriate food or drugs (alcohol, tobacco, medication prescribed for someone else, foods not appropriate for the child's age)
4. Evidence of general poor care: poor hygiene, dirty clothes, unkempt hair, dirty nails
5. Unusually fearful of nurse and others
6. Considered to be a "bad" child
7. Inappropriately dressed for the season or weather conditions
8. Reports or shows evidence of sexual abuse
9. Injuries not mentioned in history
10. Seems to need to take care of the parent and speak for the parent

---

Research has shown that many of the characteristics of physically abusive and sexually abusive parents, such as unhappiness, loneliness and rigidity, are shared by both groups (Milner and Robertson, 1990). However, sexually abusive parents report fewer family problems and a more positive view of the child than do physically abusive parents.

It is estimated that at least 1 girl in 100 is abused sexually by her father or stepfather (Brunngraber, 1986). Russell's (1982) regional survey suggests that stepfathers are far more frequently the perpetrator, but that the resultant feelings of betrayal and anguish are usually similar. Many cases of parental incest go unreported because victims fear punishment, abandonment, rejection, or family disruption if they acknowledge the problem.

Incest is not limited to "backwoods" people but occurs in all races, religious groups, and socioeconomic classes. Incest is receiving greater attention because of mandatory reporting laws; yet, all too often its incidence remains a family secret.

Because nurses, particularly community health nurses, are often involved in helping women deal with the aftermath of incest, it is crucial to understand the typical patterns and the long-term implications. The daughter involved in paternal incest is about 11 years of age at the onset and is often the oldest or only daughter. The father seldom uses physical force. He most likely relies on threats, bribes, intimidation, or misrepresentation of moral standards or exploits the daughter's need for human affection (Brunngraber, 1986).

Nurses must be aware of the incidence, signs and symptoms, and psychological and physical trauma of incest. An extensive review of research (Rew, 1989) identified clusters of affective symptoms, including low self-esteem, depression, and intrusive imagery. Somatic symptoms include headaches, eating and sleeping disorders, menstrual prob-

lems, and gastrointestinal distress. Other symptoms include difficulties in social situations, especially in forming and maintaining close relationships with men, and behavioral symptoms such as substance abuse and sexual dysfunction.

Adolescents may display inappropriate sexual activity or truancy, or may run away from home. Running away is usually considered a sign of delinquency, but community health nurses should be alert to the possibility that an adolescent who runs away is displaying a healthy response to a violent family situation. Therefore assessment should include an inquiry about sexual and physical abuse at home and appropriate intervention.

In their impressive review of the literature on child maltreatment effects, Houck and King (1989) stress that the effects of any kind of child maltreatment can be lessened if the child has a nonoffending parent, another relative, or an adult outside the family to provide stable, ongoing support and emotional nurturance.

Abuse of Female Partners

Although women do abuse men, by far the greatest proportion of what is often discussed as "spouse abuse" or "domestic violence" is actually wife abuse. At least 1.8 million women are battered by their husbands each year in the United States (Straus and Gelles, 1990). Neither the term *wife abuse* nor *spouse abuse* take into account violence in dating or cohabiting relationships. Spousal or partner violence can be used as a more inclusive term to refer to all kinds of violence between partners, and all adults should be assessed for violence in their primary intimate relationships (Goldberg and Tomalanovich, 1984). However, abuse of female partners has the most serious community health ramifications because of the greater prevalence, the greater potential for homicide (Campbell, 1990), the effects on the children in the household, and the more serious long-term emotional and physical consequences.

Victims of child abuse and individuals who witnessed their mothers being battered are at risk of using violence toward an intimate partner, whether one is male or female (Straus and Gelles, 1990). However, using evidence of a violent childhood to identify women at risk of abuse is less useful. Much evidence now suggests that abuse cannot be predicted based on characteristics of the individual woman. It is the violent background of an abusive male, combined with his tendencies to be possessive, controlling, and extremely jealous, that is most predictive of abuse. Substance abuse is also associated with battering, although it cannot be said to "cause" the violence.

SIGNS OF ABUSE. Battered women often have bruises and lacerations of the face, head, and trunk of the body. Attacks are often carefully inflicted on parts of the body that can easily be disguised by clothing. This pattern of proximal location of injuries (breasts, abdomen, upper thighs, and back) rather than distal is extremely characteristic of abuse (Campbell and Sheridan, 1989). When a woman has a black eye or bruises about the mouth, the nurse should ask, "Who hit you?," rather than, "What happened to you?" The latter implies that the nurse is not knowledgeable or not comfortable with violence, and this may prompt the woman to fabricate a more acceptable cause of her injury.

Once abused, women tend to exhibit low self-esteem and depression (Campbell, 1989). They exhibit significantly more physical symptoms of stress than women in troubled relationships and also frequently complain of chronic pain. Both of these symptoms may be related to repeated injuries, as well as to the intense stress of a violent relationship (Campbell, 1989; Goldberg and Tomlanovich, 1985).

ABUSE AS A PROCESS. Research by both Landenburger (1989) and Campbell (1991) suggests that there is a process of response to battering over time wherein the woman's emotional and behavioral reactions change. At first there is a great need to minimize the seriousness of the situation. The violence usually starts with a slight shove in the middle of a heated argument. All couples fight, and if there is any physical aggression, both the man and women tend to blame the incident on something external, like a particularly stressful day at work or drinking too much. The male partner usually apologizes for the incident, and as with any problem in a relationship, the couple tries various strategies to improve the situation. Although marital counseling may be useful at this very early stage, it is generally contraindicated because of the risk to the woman's safety. Unfortunately, abuse tends to escalate in frequency and severity over time, and the man's remorse tends to lessen (Walker, 1984).

Because women have often been taught to take responsibility for the success of a relationship, they usually go through a period where they tend to change their behavior to end the violence. They may even blame themselves for infuriating their spouse. Women who blame themselves for provoking the abuse are more likely to have low self-esteem and be depressed than those who do not blame themselves. The majority of battered women do not blame themselves for provoking the abuse, and any self-blame tends to decrease over time (Campbell, 1989; Frieze, 1983). Women find that no matter what they do, the violence continues. During this period the woman tends to try to hide the violence because of the stigma attached. She tries to placate her spouse and feels she is losing her sense of self (Landenburger, 1989; Ulrich, 1989). Women are also typically very concerned about their children. An abused woman worries about the well-being of her children if she leaves and about their safety if she stays (Lichtenstein, 1981).

Some abuse escalates to the point that the woman is kept in terror, similar to a prisoner of war (Okun, 1986). She is constantly subjected to emotional degradation, absolute financial dependency, sadistic physical and sexual violence, and control of all her activities. She is in terror that her partner will try to kill her, her children, or both if she attempts to leave. This fear is, in fact, often justified. Clinically, she may be suffering from learned helplessness, traumatic stress syndrome, or both and will need intensive therapy. She may kill herself or her abuser to escape because she sees no other way out (Walker, 1984). A nurse encountering an abusive situation such as this needs to be fairly directive in arranging for the safety of the woman and her children. She will need an order of protection, a legal document specifically designed to keep the woman's abuser away from her. She will also need help in getting to a safe place, such as a wife abuse shelter. At the very least, the women must design a carefully thought out plan for escape and arrange for a neighbor or an adolescent child to call the police when there is another violent episode.

The more frequently encountered battered woman is one who has tried several times to leave. She will eventually successfully do so or otherwise manage to end the violence (Campbell, 1991; Okun, 1986). Each attempt to leave is a gathering of resources, a trial of her children's ability to survive without a father, and a testing of her partner's promises to reform. When and if it becomes clear that he is not going to change and she has the emotional support and the financial resources to do so, she will end the relationship. Often this will involve using a shelter for abused women or individual advocacy and support groups (Bowker, 1983).

An alternative to ending the relationship is the male partner's attendance at programs for batterers. These programs have been shown to be most effective if they are court mandated and if the man's underlying values about women are addressed, as well as his violence (Dutton, 1988; Gondolf and Hanneken, 1987). Abused women need affirmation, support, reassurances of the normalcy of their responses, accurate information about shelters and legal resources, and brainstorming about possible solutions. These needs can be met by other women in similar situations and professionals such as nurses (Campbell, 1986). They should not be pushed into actions they are not ready to take.

After the abuse has ended, a period of recovery ensues. This includes a normal grief response for the relationship that has ended and a search for meaning in the experience (Landenburger, 1989). Thus a formerly battered woman who is feeling depressed and lonely after the relationship has ended is exhibiting a normal response for which support is needed.

SEXUAL ABUSE. Because 40% to 45% of battered women are also sexually abused (Campbell, 1989), the nurse must carefully assess for this form of violence in women in ongoing relationships. In fact, between 10% and 14% of all American women have been raped within a marriage. This sexual abuse is not always accompanied by physical abuse (Finkelhor and Yllo, 1985; Russell, 1982).

The notion that men have a right to force their wives to have sex comes from traditional English law that stated that a woman gave irrevocable and perpetual consent to her husband on marriage to have sex whenever and however he wanted. This legal tradition was reflected in the laws of 47 states in the United States as recently as 1980 as a marital rape exemption. In other words, a man could not be charged with rape if the victim was his wife. By 1990 only 10 states still retained this provision, but the fact that it is still legal for a man to rape his wife in any state is alarming. Serious physical and emotional damage has been documented from marital rape (Campbell, 1989; Campbell and Alford, 1989). There is also an alarming incidence of date rape, the dynamics of which may parallel marital rape.

To assess for sexual assault, the question of "Have you ever been forced into sex you did not wish to participate in?" should be used in all nursing assessments. This will allow for the ascertainment of marital rape, date rape, or rape of a male.

ABUSE DURING PREGNANCY. Battering during pregnancy has serious implications for the health of both women and their children. Approximately 12% of all pregnant women are physically battered during their pregnancy. These women are at risk for spontaneous abortions, premature delivery, and low–birth-weight infants (Helton, McFarlane, and Anderson, 1987; Bullock and McFarlane, 1989). Their infants will also be at high risk of child abuse after they are born. An additional 13% of pregnant women were battered before pregnancy, which was the most important risk factor for abuse during pregnancy (Helton, 1986).

Generally, the same dynamics of coercive control are operating when a woman is battered during pregnancy. The largest group of one sample of 76 battered women were subject to the same abuse whether or not they were pregnant. About 20% escaped abuse during pregnancy, although they were abused after the baby was born. Another 20% indicated that their perception of the reason for the abuse during pregnancy was that their partner was jealous of the baby (Campbell, Bullock, and Oliver, 1991).

Abuse of the Elderly

Elder abuse is a form of family violence that is only recently being documented and explored. A national random-sample survey of elder abuse has not been conducted so the exact incidence is unknown. Estimates of elders being abused and neglected range from 1% to 10%.

As with other forms of human abuse, elder maltreatment includes emotional, sexual, and physical abuse. Other forms of elder abuse include emotional and physical neglect, financial abuse, and violation of rights (Sengstock and Barrett, 1984).

TYPES OF ELDER ABUSE. The elderly are neglected when others fail to provide adequate food, clothing, shelter, and physical care and to meet physiological, emotional, and safety needs.

Roughness in handling elderly people can lead to bruises and bleeding into bodily tissues because of the fragility of their skin and vascular systems. It is often difficult to determine if the injuries of the elderly result from abuse, falls, or other natural causes. Careful assessment both through observation and discussion assists in determining the cause of injuries. Other ways in which the elderly are physically abused occur when caregivers impose unrealistic toileting demands and when the special needs and previous living patterns of the elderly person are ignored.

The elderly are also abused with regard to nutrition. They may be given food that they cannot chew or swallow or that is contraindicated because of dietary restrictions. Caregivers may overlook food preferences or social or cultural beliefs and patterns about food. Elderly people may become undernourished if they can neither prepare their own food nor eat the food that is prepared for them.

Caregivers occasionally give elderly people medication to induce confusion or drowsiness so that they will be less troublesome, will need less care, or will allow others to gain control of their financial and personal resources. Once medicated, the elderly have few ways to act in their own behalf.

The most common form of psychological abuse is rejection or simply ignoring elderly people. This kind of treatment conveys that they are worthless and useless to others.

INDICATORS OF POTENTIAL OR ACTUAL ELDER ABUSE

Unexplained or repeated injury
Fear of the care giver
Untreated sores or other skin injuries, such as decubitus ulcers, excoriated perineum, burns
Overall poor care (e.g., unclean, given inappropriate food)
Withdrawal and passivity
Periods of time when elderly person is unsupervised
Failure to seek appropriate medical care
Contractures resulting from immobility or restraint
Unwillingness or inability of caregiver to meet elderly person's needs
Improper home repair
Unsafe home situation (e.g., poor heating, ventilation, dangerous clutter)

Modified from Phillips LR: J Adv Nurs 8:379, 1983; and Ferguson D and Beck C: Geriatr Nurs 4:301, 1983.

The elderly may subsequently regress and become increasingly dependent on others, who tend to resent the imposition and demands on their time and life-styles. The pattern becomes cyclical: The more regressed the person becomes, the greater the dependence. Furthermore, the elderly people's past accomplishments and present abilities are not consistently acknowledged, causing them to feel even less capable. Indicators of actual or potential elder abuse are listed in the box above.

PRECIPITATING FACTORS FOR ELDER ABUSE. Caregivers abuse elderly people for a variety of reasons. The elderly family member may impose a physical, emotional, or financial burden on the caregiver, leading to frustration and resentment. The abuser may be reversing earlier family patterns, whereby the abuser was previously abused by the elderly person (Elder Abuse, 1980).

Many tend to think of abused elders as dependent on others for their care. Recent research, however, indicates that, at least for those subject to physical violence, the abused elder is not significantly more likely to be physically ill than control groups (Phillips, 1983; Pillemer and Finkelhor, 1988). In fact, the one random-sample survey study to date suggests that the abuser is more likely to be financially dependent on the elder than vice versa. The single most important risk factor was that the abuser had a history of violence (Pillemer and Finkelhor, 1988). In addition, a significant proportion of female abused elders are battered women who have become old. Thus, although it is important to assess for elder abuse when the elderly person is in need of care from family members, *all* elderly persons should be assessed for abuse.

A subgroup particularly vulnerable to abuse are the confused and frail elderly. Large numbers of frail elderly people, many with serious physical or mental impairments, live in the community and are cared for by their families. Living with and providing care to a confused elderly person is a difficult, round-the-clock task, which often exhausts family members. Family stress increases as members must work harder to fulfill their other responsibilities in addition to the needs of the elderly person.

PREVENTION STRATEGIES. Fulmer (1989) suggests the following prevention strategies for communities: (1) develop new ways to provide assistance to caregiving families, including helping them with decisions about discontinuing caregiving at home; (2) publicize existing supports for caregiving families; and (3) involve all community organizations in developing new supports and training, such as Neighborhood Watch programs for families with elderly persons. In addition, community health nurses must help families who are contemplating taking care of an elder at home to fully evaluate that decision and prepare for the stressors that will be involved. A plan for regular respite care for the elderly person is absolutely necessary.

Elderly people need to retain as much autonomy and decision-making ability as possible. Community health nurses have multiple avenues for detecting abuse among the elderly and have skills and responsibility for discovering abuse, giving treatment, and making referrals. Many families who care for elderly members exhaust their resources and coping ability. Community health nurses can assist in finding new sources of support and aid.

COMMUNITY HEALTH NURSING INTERVENTION
Primary Prevention

To prevent violence and human abuse, a community approach is essential. First, the community can take a stand against violence and make sure their elected officials and the local media are clear that nonviolence is a priority in their area. In their roles as community advocates, nurses can help with this process. In the legislative arena, laws are needed to outlaw physical punishment in schools and marital rape. State laws are needed to enforce mandatory arrest for wife abusers, which has been shown to decrease repeat offenses (Humphreys and Humphreys, 1985; Sherman and Berk, 1984).

Cultural analysis of family violence suggests that strong community sanctions against violence in the home are effective in keeping abuse levels low (Counts, Brown, and Campbell, 1991; Levinson, 1989). Neighbors keeping an eye out and working together to address problems in other families is not an invasion of privacy but a sign of community cohesiveness. Nurses need to work with advocate groups to make sure police deal with assault within marriage as swiftly, surely, and severely as assault between strangers (Carmody and Williams, 1987). Nurses can encourage others to interfere when they see children beaten in a grocery store, notice that an elderly person is not being properly cared for, see a neighborhood bully beat up his classmates, or hear a neighbor hitting his wife.

Secondly, persons can take measures to reduce their vulnerability to violence by improving the physical security of their homes and learning personal defense measures. Community health nurses can encourage people to keep windows and doors locked, trim shrubs around their homes, and keep lights on during high-crime periods. Many neighborhoods organize crime watch programs post signs to the effect, in addition to signs indicating that certain homes will assist children who need help; these homes are identified by the

sign of a hand, usually posted in a window. Other neighbors informally agree to monitor one another's property and safety. Also, many law enforcement agencies evaluate homes for security and teach individual or neighborhood safety programs. Individuals install home security systems, participate in personal defense programs such as judo or karate, and purchase firearms for their protection.

Unfortunately, handguns are far more likely to kill family members than intruders (Kellermann, 1986). Accidental firearm death is a leading cause of death for young children, and handguns kept in the home are unfortunately easy to use in moments of extreme anger with other family members or extreme depression. The majority of homicides between family members and most suicides involve a handgun. All community health nursing assessments should include a question about guns kept in the home, and the family should be made aware of the risk that a handgun holds for family members. If the family feels that keeping a gun is necessary, safety measures should be taught, such as keeping the gun unloaded and in a locked compartment, keeping the ammunition separate from the gun and also locked away, and instructing children about the dangers of firearms. Lobbying for handgun-control laws is a primary prevention effort that would significantly decrease the rate of death and serious injury caused by handguns in this country.

Assessment for Risk Factors

Identification of risk factors is an important part of primary prevention. Although abuse cannot be predicted with certainty, a variety of factors tend to influence the onset and support the continuation of abusive patterns. Community health nurses are in an excellent position to identify potential victims of abuse because these nurses see clients in a wide variety of settings.

Factors to include in an assessment of an individual or family's potential for violence are categorized by Logan and Dawkins (1986, p. 743) as illustrated in Figure 24-1.

The nurse must also be able to identify "red-flag" anti-social behaviors that might lead to abusive patterns. According to Klingbeil (1986), high-risk categories of behavior include the following:

1. Psychiatric diagnosis such as depression
2. Pattern of substance abuse
3. Loss and grief after death of a loved one
4. Isolation
5. Lack of support system
6. Homelessness
7. Previous history of assaultive or suicidal behavior
8. Chronic unemployment
9. Presence or use of weapons; previous arrests
10. History of runaways
11. Single-car auto accidents
12. Psychosomatic complaints

Individual and Family Strategies for Primary Prevention

Primary prevention of abuse includes strengthening individuals and families so they can cope more effectively with multiple life stressors and demands and reducing the destructive elements in the community that support and en-

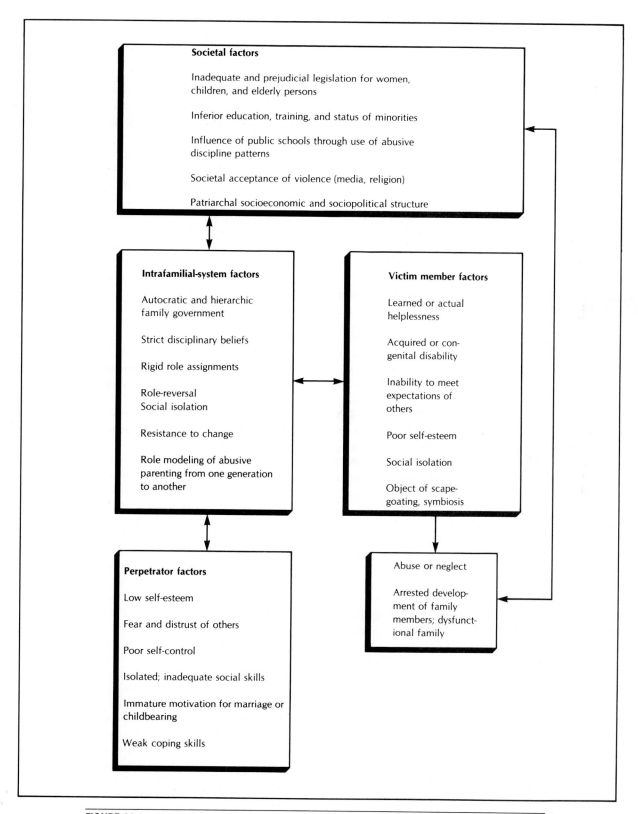

FIGURE 24-1

Factors to include when assessing an individual or family's potential for violence.

courage the use of human violence. In their work in schools, community groups, employee groups, day-care centers, and other community institutions, nurses can foster healthy developmental patterns and identify signs of potential abuse.

Many clinicians believe that providing support and psychological enrichment to at-risk individuals and families prevents the onset of health disruption. For example, community health nurses have varied opportunities to strengthen and even teach parenting abilities. Basic skills such as diapering, feeding, quieting, and even holding and rocking a baby can be the focus of a class or home or clinic visit. Parents also need to learn acceptable and workable ways to discipline children so that limits are maintained without causing the child emotional or physical harm.

Mutual support groups are valuable for new parents, families with special children, or abused people themselves. Such groups have variable formats and can provide information, support, and encouragement. Nurses can help begin such groups or can actually serve as group leaders. Chapter 17 describes the role of the community health nurse in working with community groups.

Secondary Prevention

When abuse occurs, community health nurses can initiate measures to reduce or terminate further abuse. As discussed in Chapter 35, both developmental and situational *crises* present opportunities for abusive situations to develop. The occurrence of violence represents a family crisis and should be handled using the crisis intervention strategies presented in Chapter 35.

Nursing intervention is directed toward helping participants discuss the problem and seek alternatives for dealing with the tension that led to the abusive situation. Injured persons must be temporarily or permanently placed in a safe location. Secondary preventive measures are most useful when potential abusers recognize their tendency to be abusive and seek help. For children, there is often a need for 24-hour child protection services or caregivers who can take care of the child until the acute family or individual crisis has been resolved. Respite care is extremely important in families with frail elders. Telephone crisis lines can be used to provide immediate emergency assistance to families.

There is now a 24-hour national hotline for abused women to call for help in finding a local shelter or to just talk about the violence. The number is 1-800-333-SAFE.

Effective *communication* with abusive families is important. Typically, these families are not eager to discuss their problems. Many members of such families are embarrassed to be involved in an abusive situation. Often considerable guilt is involved. Effective communication must be preceded by an attitude of acceptance. It is often difficult for nurses to value the worth of an individual who willfully abuses another. The behavior, not the person, must be condemned. The nurse must radiate caring, acceptance, understanding, compassion, and a nonjudgmental attitude.

Additionally, families do not always know how to have fun. Nurses can assess how much recreation is integrated into the family's life-style. Through community assessment, the nurse will know what resources and facilities are available and how much they cost. Families may need counseling about the value of recreation and play in reducing tension and appropriately channelling aggressive impulses.

Tertiary Prevention: Therapeutic Intervention with Abusive Families

It is extremely difficult to form a trusting relationship with abusive families, but the community health nurse is often in a key position to act as case manager, coordinating the other agencies and activities involved. Principles of giving care to families who are experiencing violence include the following: (1) intolerance for violence, (2) respect and caring for all family members, (3) safety as the first priority, (4) absolute honesty, and (5) empowerment. Nurses must clearly indicate that any further violence, degradation, and exploitation of family members will not be tolerated, but that all family members are respected, valued human beings. However, everyone must understand that the safety of every family member is the first priority.

Abusers often fear they will be condemned for their actions, so it is often difficult to make and maintain contact with abusive families. Although community health nurses convey an attitude of caring and concern for them, families may doubt the sincerity of this concern. They may avoid being home at the scheduled visit time out of fear of the consequences of the visit or an inability to believe that anyone really wants to help them. If the victim is a child, parents may fear that the nurse will try to remove the child.

Nurses are mandatory reporters of child abuse, even when only suspected, in all states. They are also mandatory reporters of elder abuse and other physically and cognitively dependent adults in most states. The mandatory reporting laws also protect reporters from legal action on cases that are never substantiated. Even so, physicians and nurses are sometimes reluctant to report abuse. They may be more willing to report abuse in a poor family than in a middle-class one or may be afraid that an elderly person or child is better off at home than in a nursing home or foster home. Referral to protective service agencies should be viewed as enlisting another source of help, rather than an automatic step toward removal of the victim or criminal justice action. This same attitude can be communicated to families so that reporting is done *with* families rather than without their knowledge and prior input. Absolute honesty about what will be reported to officials, what the family can expect, what the nurse is entering into records, and what the nurse is feeling is essential.

To further empower the family, the nurse needs to recognize and capitalize on the violent family's strengths, as well as to assess and deal with their problems. The nurse must use a nurse-family partnership rather than a paternalistic or authoritarian approach. The family is generally capable of generating many of their own solutions, which will be much more culturally appropriate and individualized than those the nurse may generate. Victims of direct attack need information about their options and resources and reassurance that abuse is unfortunately rather common and that they are not alone in their dilemma. They also need reassurance that their responses are normal and that they do not deserve to be abused. Continued support for their decisions must be coupled with nursing actions to ensure their safety.

Nursing Actions

The community health nurse can meet the families' therapeutic needs in a variety of ways. Besides referral to appropriate community agencies, nurses can act as role models for the family. During clinic and home visits, nurses can demonstrate constructive adult-child interactions. Nurses often teach mothers child-care skills such as proper feeding, calming a fretful child, effective discipline, and constructive communication.

Nurses can demonstrate good communication skills and discipline by teaching both parents and children in a calm, respectful, and informative manner. Caregivers, especially those caring for children, handicapped people, or the elderly, may need to learn age-appropriate expectations. It is unreasonable to expect a 14-month-old infant to be able to differentiate between what is right and wrong. Children at this age do not deliberately annoy caregivers by breaking delicate pieces of china. Likewise, a person with poor sphincter control does not willingly soil clothes or bedding.

Role modeling can be used with abuse victims of all ages. When providing nursing care to abused spouses or to the elderly, nurses can demonstrate communication skills, conflict resolution, and skill training. For example, adult children often become abusive toward their parents when they become frustrated and taxed in their abilities to care for the elderly person. During home visits, nurses can demonstrate ways to physically and psychologically care for family members. The nurse can work with caregivers to help them develop approaches that are acceptable to the individual elderly person. Assessment, creativity, and critical thinking help the nurse, family, and client devise ways together of meeting client and family needs, without causing undue stress and frustration.

The emotional investment and sheer drain of energy required to effectively work with abusers and victims of abuse cannot be disregarded. Abusers present difficult clinical challenges because of their reluctance to seek help or to remain actively involved in the helping process.

Referral is an important component of tertiary prevention. Community health nurses should know about available community resources for abuse victims and perpetrators. If attitudes and resources are inadequate, it is often helpful to work with local radio and television stations and newspapers to provide information about the nature and extent of human abuse as a community health problem. This also helps to acquaint people with available services and resources. Frequently, people fail to seek services early in an abusive situation because they simply do not know what is available to them. Ideally, a program or planned emphasis for abused people begins with a needs assessment to identify potential clients and to determine how to effectively serve this group. Community health nurses serve as catalysts for getting programs started and as a major source of public education.

CLINICAL APPLICATION

Mrs. Smith, a 75-year-old bedridden woman, consistently became rude and combative when her daughter, Mary, attempted to bathe her and change her clothes each morning. During a home visit, Mary told the nurse, Mrs. Jones, that she had gotten so frustrated with her mother on the previous morning that she had hit her. Mary felt terrible about her behavior. She stressed that her mother's incontinence made it essential that she be kept clean; her clothes had to be changed every day for her own safety and physical well-being.

Mrs Jones, in taking Mrs. Smith's vital signs and examining her skin turgor, engaged her in a conversation. She learned that Mrs. Smith felt stiff and seemed to have more joint pain from her arthritis in the mornings. By late afternoon, her joints were more flexible and less painful. Nurse, daughter, and client discussed their options and decided that Mary would wash only her mother's anal area in the morning and put clean pads under her if indicated. Total hygienic care would be done in the late afternoon.

Mrs. Jones demonstrated to Mary alternative ways to move, turn, and wash her mother to minimize the strain on her arthritic joints and to incorporate some effective exercise into the bath. They also decided that, on two mornings a week, a home health care aide would be employed to stay with Mrs. Smith. Mary could then do family shopping and errands and participate in activities in which she had previously been involved.

Nursing intervention was based on the principles introduced earlier. The nurse listened carefully to the pain and anguish the daughter felt about hitting her mother. She conveyed a nonjudgmental attitude and helped the daughter and mother explore ways in which both of their needs could be more effectively met. She provided information and resources to allow the daughter some respite from constant caretaking and a way to continue her own activities. The nurse also taught her ways to improve her mother's physical care. Mrs. Jones will need to monitor the situation carefully for any further signs of abuse. Any further instance of violence must be discussed with the daughter and immediately reported. In a subsequent visit, the nurse evaluated the effectiveness of her teaching and learned that Mary and her mother were working much more cooperatively on Mrs. Smith's care.

SUMMARY

The potential for human abuse and neglect in individuals and families is acquired over many years and stems from a multitude of factors, including societal influences, family history, behavioral characteristics of both the abuser and the abused, and a number of specific precipitating events. Community violence is also influenced by many factors, such as unemployment, dysfunctional community interactions, and lack of cultural activities. Increasing attention is being focused on these problems as people seek to establish a safe environment in which to live and work. Because of the stigma attached to the occurrence of human violence, reporting mechanisms have been inadequate. Yet, the occurrence of violence and abuse is significant and is, in fact, increasing in the face of rapidly changing events and social conditions.

Community health nurses may play a key role in the prevention, early detection, and prompt intervention of abuse. Addressing abuse and violence at all three levels of prevention is a task of critical importance for community health nurses.

KEY CONCEPTS

Violence and human abuse are not new phenomena, but they have increasingly become community health concerns.

Communities throughout the United States are voicing anger and frustration about increasing levels of violence.

The community health nurse is in a position to evaluate and intervene in incidents of community and family violence; to intervene effectively, the community health nurse must understand the dynamics of violence and human abuse.

Factors influencing social and community violence include changing social conditions, economic conditions, population density, community facilities, and institutions within a community, such as organized religion, education, the mass communication media, and work.

The potential for violence against individuals or against oneself is directly related to the level of violence in the community. Identification and correction of factors affecting the level of violence in the community constitute one way of reducing violence against family members and other individuals.

Violence and abuse of family members can happen to any family member: spouse, elderly person, child, or developmentally disabled person.

People who abuse family members are often persons who were themselves abused and who react poorly to real or perceived crises. Other factors that characterize the abuser are the way the person was raised and the unique character of that person.

Child abuse can be physical, emotional, or sexual. Incest is a common and particularly destructive form of child abuse.

Spouse abuse is usually wife abuse. It involves physical, emotional, and frequently, sexual abuse within a context of coercive control. It usually increases in severity and frequency and can escalate to homicide of either partner.

Community health nurses are in an excellent position to identify potential victims of family abuse because they see clients in a variety of settings, such as schools, businesses, homes, and clinics. Treatment of family abuse includes primary, secondary, and tertiary prevention and therapeutic intervention.

LEARNING ACTIVITIES

1. For 1 week keep a log or diary related to violence.
   a. Make a note of each time you feel as though you are losing your temper. Consider what it might take to cause you to react in a violent way.
   b. Think back; when was the last time you had a violent outburst? What precipitated it? What were your thoughts? What were your feelings? How might you have handled the situation or those feelings without reacting in a violent way?
   c. During this same week make note of the episodes of violent behaviors you observe. For example, do parents hit children in the supermarket? What seems to precipitate such outbursts? What alternatives might exist for reacting in a less violent way?

2. If you learned, after a careful assessment of your community, that family violence is a significant community health problem, what plan of action might you take to intervene? Remember

that the goal is to promote health; outline a plan of action with objectives, time tables, implementation strategies, and evaluation plans for intervening in family violence in your community.

3. Complete a partial community assessment to determine the actual incidence and types of violence in your community.

4. What resources are available in your community for victims of violence? Interview a person who works in an agency that seeks to aid victims of violence. What is the role of the agency? Do its services seem adequate? Who is eligible? Is there a waiting list? What is the fee scale?

5. Cut out all stories about violence in your local newspaper every day for 2 weeks. Notice the patterns. Is the majority of the violence perpetrated by strangers or family members? How are the victims portrayed? What kind of families are involved? What kinds of stories and families get front page treatment rather than a few lines in the back of the paper?

BIBLIOGRAPHY

Baron LS, Straus MA, and Jaffee D: Legitimate violence, violent attitudes, and rape: a test of the cultural spillover theory, Ann NY Acad Sci 528:80, 1988.

Bowker LH: Beating wife-beating, Lexington, MA, 1983, Lexington Books.

Bruhn J and Fuentes R: Child abuse: a societal paradox, Unpublished data, 1981.

Brunngraber BS: Father-daughter incest: immediate and long-term effects of sexual abuse, ANS 8(4):15, 1986.

Bullock L and McFarlane J: Higher prevalence of low birthweight infants born to battered women, Am J Nurs 89(9):1153, 1989.

Burgess A and Holmstrum L: Rape: crisis and recovery, Bowie, MD, 1979, Brady.

Campbell JC: Nursing assessment for risk of homicide with battered women, Adv Nurs Sci 8(4):36, 1986.

Campbell JC: A test of two explanatory models of women's responses to battering, Nurs Res 38(1):18, 1989.

Campbell JC. In Sampselle CM, editor: Violence against women: nursing research, education, and practice issues, Washington, DC, 1991, Hemisphere Publishing.

Campbell JC: Women's responses to battering over time, Unpublished manuscript, 1991.

Campbell JC: "If I can't have you, no one can": homicide in intimate relationships. In Radford J and Russell DEH, editors: Femicide: the politics of woman killing, Boston, MA, 1991, Twayne Publishers.

Campbell JC: Women's responses to sexual abuse in intimate relationships, Health Care Women Int 10:335, 1989.

Campbell JC and Alford P: The dark consequences of marital rape, Am J Nurs 89:946, 1989.

Campbell JC, Bullock L, and Oliver C: Women's perception of why they are beaten during pregnancy, Unpublished manuscript, 1991.

Campbell JC and Humphreys J: Nursing care of victims of family violence, Reston, VA, 1984, Reston Publishing.

Campbell JC and Sheridan DJ: Clinical articles emergency nursing interventions with battered women, J Emerg Nurs 15(1):12, 1989.

Carmody DC and Williams KR: Wife assault and the perceptions of sanctions, Violence Victims 2(1):25, 1987.

Counts D, Brown J, and Campbell J: Sanctions and Sanctuary, Boulder CO, 1991, Westview Press.

Covington CH: Incest: the psychological problem and the biological contradiction, Issues Ment Health Nurs 10:69, 1989.

Dietz P: Social factors in rapist behavior, In Roda R, editor: Clinical aspects of the rapist, New York, 1978, Grune & Stratton.

Dinitto DM et al.: Nurses conduct the rape kit examination, Response 10(2):10, 1987.

Dutton DG: The domestic assault of women, Newton, MA, 1988, Allyn & Bacon.

Elder abuse, Washington DC, 1980, National Clearing House on Aging.

Farley R: Homicide trends in the United States. In Hawkins DF, editor: Homicide among black Americans, Lanham, MD, 1986, University Press of America.

Finkelhor D and Yllo K: License to rape: sexual abuse of wives, New York, 1985, The Free Press.

Frieze IR: Investigating the causes and consequences of marital rape, J Women Culture Soc 8(3):532, 1983.

Fulmer T: Mistreatment of elders, assessment, diagnosis, and intervention, Nurs Clin North Am 24(3):707, 1989.

Gelles R and Conte J: Domestic violence and sexual abuse of children: a review of research in the eighties, J Marriage Fam 52(4):1045, 1990.

Goldberg WG and Tomlanovich MC: Domestic violence victims in the emergency department, JAMA 25(1):3259, 1984.

Gondolf EW and Hanneken J: The gender warrior: reformed batterers on abuse, treatment, and change, J Fam Violence 2(2):177, 1987.

Hanlon J and Pickett G: Public health: administration and practice, ed 8, St Louis, 1984, Mosby-Year Book.

Hawkins DF: Black homicide: The adequacy of existing research for devising prevention strategies, In Hawkins DF, editor: Homicide among black Americans, Lanham, MD, 1986, University Press of America.

Helton AS, McFarlane J, and Anderson ET: Battered and pregnant: a prevalence study, Am J Public Health 77(10):1337, 1987.

Helton AS: Battering during pregnancy, Am J Nurs 86(8):910, 1986.

Hotaling GT and Sugarman DD: An analysis of risk markers in husband to wife violence: The current state of knowledge. Violence Victims 1(2):101, 1986.

Houck GM and King MC: Child maltreatment: family characteristics and developmental consequences, Issues Ment Health Nurs 10:193, 1989.

Humphreys J and Humphreys WO: Mandatory arrest: a means of primary and secondary prevention of abuse of female partners, Victimology 10:267, 1985.

Kempe CH et al.: The battered child syndrome, JAMA 181:17, 1962.

Kellermann AL and Reay DT: Protection or peril?, an analysis of firearm-related deaths in the home, N Engl J Med 314(24):1557, 1986.

Klingbeil K: Interpersonal violence: a comprehensive model in a hospital setting—from policy to program. In the Surgeon General's workshop on violence and public health report, DHHS Pub No HRS-D-MC 86-1, Washington DC, 1986, Health Resources and Services Administration, U.S. Public Health Service, U.S. Department of Health and Human Services.

Landenburger K: A process of entrapment in and recovery from an abusive relationship, Issues Ment Health Nurs 10:209, 1989.

Lenehan G, Bowie S, and Ruksnaitis N: Rape victim protocol and chart for use in emergency department, J Emerg Nurs 9:83, 1983.

Levinson D: Family violence in cross-cultural perspective, Newbury Park, CA, 1989, Sage Publications.

Lichtenstein VR: The battered woman: guidelines for effective nursing intervention, Issues Ment Health Nurs 3:237, 1981.

Logan BB and Dawkins CE: Family-centered nursing in the community, Menlo Park, CA, 1986, Addison-Wesley Publishing.

Mercy JA and O'Carroll PW: New directions in violence prediction: the public health arena, Violence Victims 3(4):285, 1988.

Milner JS and Robertson KR: Comparison of physical child abusers, intrafamilial sexual child abusers, and child neglecters, J Interpersonal Violence 5(1):37, 1990.

O'Carroll PW and Mercy JA: Regional variation in homicide rates: why is the West so violent? Violence Victims, 4(1):17, 1986.

Okun LE: Woman abuse: facts replacing myths, Albany, 1986, State University of New York Press.

Oliphant C, editor: Health scene, Pendleton, OR, 1986, Pendleton, Community Hospital.

Phillips LR: Abuse/neglect of the frail elderly at home: an exploration of theoretical relationships, J Adv Nurs 8:379, 1983.

Pillemer K and Finkelhor D: The prevalence of elder abuse: a random sample survey, Gerontologist, 28:51, 1988.

Prince J: A systems approach to spouse abuse. In Lancaster J: Community mental health nursing: an ecological perspective, St Louis, 1980, Mosby-Year Book.

Public Health Service: Promoting health/preventing disease: year 2000 objectives for the nation, Washington, 1990, U.S. Department of Health and Human Services.

Rew L: Childhood sexual exploitation: long-term effects among a group of nursing students, Issues Ment Health Nurs 10:181, 1989.

Roesch R: Violent families, Parents 59:74, 1984.

Rosenberg ML and Mercy JA: Homicide and assaultive violence. In Violence as a public health problem, Atlanta, GA, 1985, U.S. Public Health Service.

Russell D: Rape in marriage, New York, 1982, MacMillan.

Scharer K: Nursing therapy with abusive and neglectful families, J Psychiatr Nurs 17(9):12, 1979.

Sengstock MC and Barrett S: Elder abuse. In Campbell J and Humphreys J, editors: Nursing care of victims of family violence, Reston, VA, 1984, Reston Publishing.

Sherman L and Berk R: The specific deterrent effects of arrest for domestic assault, Am Sociol Rev 49:261, 1984.

Sommers EK and Check J: An empirical investigation of the role of pornography in the verbal and physical abuse of women, Violence Victims, 2:189, 1987.

Stark E and Flitcraft A: Spouse abuse. In Surgeon General: Workshop on violence and public health source book, Atlanta, GA, 1985, U.S. Public Health Service.

Straus MA and Gelles RJ: Physical violence in American families: risk factors and adaptions to violence in 8,145 families, New Brunswick, NJ 1990, Transaction.

Surgeon General: Workshop on violence and public health report, DHHS Pub No HRS-D-MC 86-1, Washington, DC, 1986, Health Resources and Services Administration, U.S. Public Health Service, U.S. Department of Health and Human Services.

Ulrich YC: Cross-cultural perspective on violence against women, Response Victimiz Women Child 12(1):21, 1989.

Walker LE: The battered woman syndrome, New York, 1984, Springer.

PART FIVE

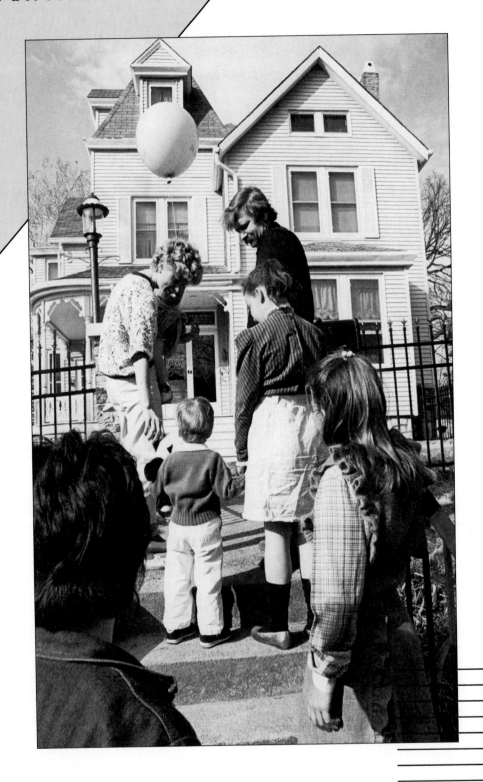

The Individual and Family as Client: A Developmental Approach

T he family is a major influence on the individual's concept of health and illness. It is within the family that the individual's sense of self-esteem and personal competence is developed. The action taken by or for the person with a health problem depends on this sense of self-worth and the family's definition of illness. The environmental, social, cultural and economic factors, as well as the resources of the community to meet health needs, influence the family's health risks and reaction to health. The goals of the nation for the year 2000 name the individual as the primary target for changing the overall health of the nation. Through family support the individual may develop the responsibility to participate in activities that will lead to a healthier life-style.

Major health problems of individuals can be identified and related to their developmental phase. This factor becomes evident when age-specific morbidity data are reviewed. The community health nurse has the opportunity to influence the actions and reactions to health of all individuals of the community from birth through senescence. The community health nurse may influence the health of neonates and infants by introducing healthy parenting bahaviors, risk factor appraisal, and interventions at this stage of life. Likewise, the community health/school health nurse is in a position to introduce illness prevention and health promotion activities to the school-age and adolescent populations. Appropriate influences during these developmental stages have the potential for changing the future outlook for the nation's health.

Young and middle-aged adults are faced with many life changes and challenges that they may find rewarding or demanding. Previous lifestyles and increases in stress from social, environmental, and economic constraints often result in risk for major health problems during this life stage.

The community health nurse's primary function with persons of all ages should be to promote quality and quantity of life. As the elderly population continues to grow, the health care delivery system and nursing must address and plan strategies to cope with increasing longevity, chronic health problems, and technological advances, as well as twenty-first century economic, social, and health issues.

Chapters 25 through 27 explore family development, the nursing process applied to family health, the health of individuals in the family system, and family health promotion issues. Chapters 28 through 31 explore the major developmental tasks, health needs, risk factors, and issues for individuals from birth through senescence. Chapter 32 focuses attention on needs of a very special population, the developmentally disabled. Community health nursing interventions must be refined to assist this group in meeting their health care needs.

25

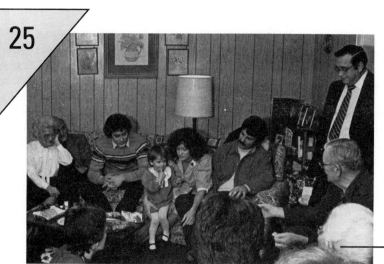

Family Development

Rosemary Johnson

OBJECTIVES

After reading this chapter, the student should be able to:

Analyze various approaches to defining the family.

Discuss the various types of family and household structures.

Identify family demographic trends that have implications for community health nursing practice.

Identify and discuss family adult roles.

Identify and discuss the functions common to most families.

Identify and discuss family health functions and tasks.

Analyze the family development conceptual approach to studying families.

Discuss the developmental tasks involved in the processes of separation and divorce.

Discuss the application of the developmental framework to community nursing practice with adoptive, single parent, remarried, and vulnerable families.

KEY TERMS

adoption	family life cycle	role sharing
cohabitation	family structure	separation
developmental task	household	sibling
divorce	marriage	single parent
family	nuclear family	stepfamily
family demography	primary relationship	stepparent
family development	remarriage	transition
family function	role	

The family, as society's most significant unit of social behavior, has been experiencing considerable changes. These changes have affected the family's development in relation to structure, functions, and interactions, both within the family and within the community. Demographic and socioeconomic changes, which had their beginnings in the late 1700s, have continued throughout the twentieth century, resulting in considerable consequences for families in the United States. Demographic trends that have had an impact on the family are related to age at time of first marriage; fertility patterns and birth rates; increases in singlehood, divorce, and remarriage; larger numbers of children experiencing family divorce or living with a never-married parent; and a growing elderly population.

Although there are general societal and familial expectations about family roles and functions, trends in marriage and the family influence the types of roles found in families, the enactment of those roles, and the functions carried out by the family. Each family tends to modify family roles and role behaviors in relation to the family structure and in relation to forces internal and external to the family unit. All families, regardless of their structure, have certain functions that are performed to maintain the integrity of the family unit and to meet the family's needs, individual family members' needs, and society's expectations.

CONCEPTUAL FRAMEWORKS
Developmental Theory

A conceptual framework is essential for guiding the community health nurse in the process of assisting families in their health-promoting efforts. One framework generated for studying families, which has been used in conjunction with other conceptual approaches, is the developmental framework. Developmental theory focuses on common general features of family life and provides a longitudinal view of the *family life cycle*. The family developmental framework identifies points in a family's development where changes occur in the status and roles of family members. Increasingly, variation in family structure such as single-parent families, remarried families, and vulnerable families are being studied from the developmental perspective.

The family development framework contributes to the community health nurse's understanding of families at different points in their life cycle. A major strength of this approach is that it provides a basis for forecasting what a family will be experiencing at any period in the family's life cycle, for example, role transitions and family constellation changes.

The developmental approach can be used successfully in practice with a variety of family structures, but the nurse must recognize that in every family there are individual and family developmental tasks to be accomplished that are peculiar to that particular family. Implicit in this approach is the need to be aware of the internal and external environmental forces (psychosocial, cultural, etc.) that influence the family's development.

Knowledge about family life stages and the accompanying tasks gives the community health nurse a focus for family assessment, planning, intervention, and evaluation. Assessing the family's developmental stage and its performance of the tasks appropriate for that stage provides the nurse with guidelines for analyzing the family's development and health-promotion needs. Anticipatory guidance can be implemented to prepare the family to cope with predictable role and position changes. The developmental approach also identifies periods in the family life cycle when problems may emerge because of limited or strained personal, emotional, and financial resources. Consequently, the family may need to be made aware of available support resources in the extended family or in the community.

Although anticipating what to expect is helpful when working with families, the nurse must recognize that not all families move through the family life cycle in the same way because of the variations among families. The nurse still can predict important things about the overall pattern of a family's developmental activities by knowing (1) where the family is in its developmental history and life cycle; (2) the number, age, and way in which family members in the household are related; and (3) the family's ethnic, religious, and socioeconomic characteristics.

Systems Framework

Systems theory was introduced by von Bertalanffy over 50 years ago as a method of thinking about the order of the environment. This framework has been applied to families. In systems theory families are described as units comprised of members whose interactional patterns become the focus of attention. The family is viewed as a whole, with boundaries that are affected by and permeated by the external environment. The family as an organizational structure is a subsystem of the community and of society. Interaction of family members is directed toward maintaining homeostasis through a feedback mechanism of input from members and from the external environment, throughput, and output from members to the external environment. Feedback may be positive or negative, and it affects the control or adaptation of the family to its environment.

Application of this framework helps the community health nurse to understand family interaction patterns, family norms and expectations, effectiveness of interaction patterns, decision-making processes, family adaptation to individual needs, family expectations of its members, and family adaption to the community. The following situation, illustrated in Figure 25–1, provides an example of how systems theory is applied to families in interaction with families and communities.

Hypothetically, assume that numerous cultural systems decide that the values of peace and general human welfare take priority over war and full domestic employment, and that there is a resulting national policy that the manufacturing of armed services aircraft will cease. Some communities would experience a loss of income and possible out-migration of engineers and skilled workers. Likewise, the families of aerospace engineers previously employed by such aircraft industries would experience economic and emotional stress. They also might experience possible role realignment or changes if, for example, the spouse had to seek employment or a child had to drop out of college. Additional changes might be the loss of health insurance and other benefits. Consequences for the individual engineer

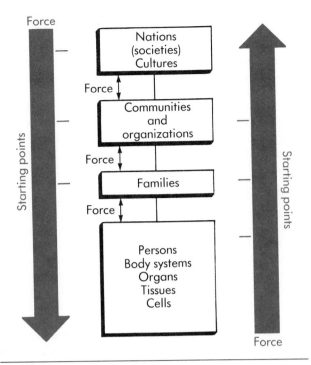

FIGURE 25-1

Family health and community health: a systems perspective. *(Modified from Blum, H.L.: Expanding health care horizons, Oakland Calif, 1976, Third Party Associates, Inc.)*

could be the loss of self-esteem, the need to learn new skills, and the need to adjust to changing lifestyles.

The final outcome for one or more family members could be the development of digressive social behaviors or stress-related illnesses. At this point, the spread of disequilibrium upward through the hierarchy of systems might be observed, as the behaviors of individual family members begin to affect the health status and coping behavior of the family. The family's ability or inability to cope adequately and to adjust with or without consequential family disorganization has obvious consequences for the community. Family disorganization places demands on the community's health and human services resources and reduces the availability of productive, contributing family members in the community. Multiple families experiencing states of disorganization eventually would affect the general health status of the community.

Interactional Framework

The interactional approach focuses on the family as a unit of interacting personalities and examines the symbolic communication processes by which family members relate to one another. Within the family each member occupies a position or positions to which a number of roles are assigned. Family members define their role expectations in each situation through their perceptions of the role demands. Family members judge their own behavior by assessing and interpreting the actions of others toward them. The responses of others in the family serve to challenge or reinforce the family members' perceptions of the norms or of role expectations (Schoaneveldt, 1967).

Central to the interactional approach is the process of role taking. Every role exists in relation to some other role, and interaction represents a dynamic process of testing perceptions about each other's roles. Through family interaction, the result of the testing process is stabilization or modification of roles. The ability to predict other family members' expectations for one's role enables each member to have some knowledge of how to react in the role. It also indicates how other members will react to the performance in the role.

Assessment of the family within an interactional framework would emphasize (1) family functioning relative to interaction between and among family members; for example, the messages communicated about family role expectations such as the socialization of children, and (2) family communication patterns relative to messages sent about health and illness behaviors appropriate for different roles such as differing behaviors appropriate for the child versus the father.

Structural-Functional Framework

Within the structural-functional framework, the family is viewed as a social system with members who have specific roles and functions. General assumptions in the structural-functional approach include the following (Eshelman, 1974):

1. The family is a social system with functional requirements.
2. The family is a small group possessing certain generic features common to all small groups.
3. The family as a social system accomplishes functions that serve both the individual and society.

Studying the family from a structural-functional perspective also includes analyzing the family as a system with boundaries that regulate input from and output to the environment. The boundaries facilitate or interfere with adaptation. The family as a social system consists of individuals organized into a single unit so that change in any family member inevitably results in changes in the entire family system (Friedman, 1986).

The structural-functional approach provides a framework for assessing family structure and functions such as the socialization process of family members for roles and behaviors necessary for living and interacting in society; the socialization process for family members in relation to cultural and social norms; values, rights, and privileges assigned to family roles; enactment of family roles; focus of authority and decision making in the family; development of coping behaviors; development of family subsystems; and communication patterns. Other examples of the structural-functional approach include the family health estate, the interrelationship between family and individual health, and the relationship between family health and community health.

DEFINING THE FAMILY

Traditionally, the family has been defined in relation to the *nuclear family* (mother, father, and young children) in which the original parents remained together throughout the family life cycle. Thus the traditional family pattern is characterized as a "legal, lifelong, sexually exclusive marriage between one man and one woman, with children, where the male is primary provider and ultimate authority'' (Macklin, 1987, p. 317).

There are six major premises related to the traditional monogamous family: (1) romantic love forms the basis for a successful marriage; (2) sexual activity should be confined to marital relationships; (3) a person should have only one partner of the opposite sex; (4) masculine and feminine sex roles should be clearly defined; (5) children should be raised in a nuclear family setting; (6) the nuclear family is the most effective unit for family living and social functioning (Gutknecht et al, 1983).

The traditional nuclear family, as a continuing unit with original parents, is no longer the predominant family structure in American society. The family as an intact social unit has become more transient. This transient nature has resulted in changes in family structure, membership goals, and in some instances, the family's reason for being. A consequence of family changes and the emergence of other family forms has been the increased difficulty in defining the family. The way the family is defined determines to some extent how the family's functions and roles in society are described.

The following definitions show several ways in which families are defined today. A family is defined as:

1. Two or more individuals who reside in the same household; who can identify some common emotional bond; and who are interrelated by performing some social tasks in common, for example, socialization of children (Baranowski & Nader, 1985, p. 54).
2. A group that engages in socially sanctioned, enduring, and exclusive relationships that are based on marriage, descent, adoption, or mutual definition, as in common-law marriage (Yorburg, 1983, p. 45).
3. Composed of people (two or more) who are emotionally involved (perceived reciprocal obligation, sense of commonness, sharing of certain obligations, coupled with caring and commitment) with one another and live in close geographical proximity (Friedman, 1986, p. 8).
4. A group of two or more persons related by birth, marriage, or adoption and residing together in a household (National Center for Health Statistics, 1990a).

Some family theorists have openly challenged attempts to define families formally because of the many exceptions and variabilities. One approach is to conceptualize the family as a primary relationship. This approach is considered particularly useful for community health nursing practice. The *primary relationship* consists of at least two persons interacting in continuing fashion within an immediate situation as well as within a larger environment (Scanzoni et al., 1989, p. 43). The primary relationship approach includes legal marriages, two natural-parent families, and other family structures.

Definitions of the family range from viewing the family as having a single, exclusive structure to perceiving the family as a household unit representing various types of family structures. A broad definition of the family is needed in community health nursing because community health nurses work with families that represent both traditional and less traditional family structures. Developing a definition of the family for research purposes is even more problematic, especially in relation to family membership, family behavior, family goals, and family life. The following definition represents the author's perspective on the family; the *family* is represented by two or more individuals, belonging to the same or different kinship groups, who are involved in a continuous living arrangement, usually residing in the same household, experiencing common emotional bonds, and sharing certain obligations toward each other and toward others.

FAMILY STRUCTURES

The social significance of the family has been founded in its mediating function between society and individual family members. The family has the dual responsibility of meeting the needs of family members and at the same time meeting the needs of the society with which it is associated. Social expectations for family members in the form of obligations and responsibilities, are modified by the family to fit the needs and abilities of its members. The family, in turn, prepares and assists family members to meet societal responsibilities and obligations. Some recent trends affecting marriage and the family are becoming quite well established, while others remain tenuous.

Traditional and Other Family Structures

Each family, regardless of its structural system, has the potential for serving societal needs in one way or another. In addition all families tend to be similar in attempting to provide for family needs, including the need to exchange affection; to provide reasonable stability; to provide financial resources for food, clothing, and shelter; to offer educational opportunities, and to make health services available and accessible.

Families that the community health nurse works with represent a variety of structures and living arrangements. The community health nurse is responsible for assisting the family to promote its health, to meet family health needs, and to cope with health problems within the context of the existing family structure and lifestyle. Thus community health nurses must be knowledgeable about family structures, functions, processes, and roles. In addition they must be aware of and must understand their own values and attitudes pertaining to the family and varying family lifestyles.

Family structure refers to the characteristics (gender, age, number) of the individual members who comprise the family unit. More specifically, the structure of a family represents the positions occupied by the individuals who are engaged in regular, recurring interactions and relationships within that family unit (Yorburg, 1983). Many people envision a family structure in which they will be married, have children, live in a single-family household, prefer heterosexuality, and desire permanence and sexual exclusivity. However, increasing numbers of people are choosing other family lifestyles at some point in their lives. As social norms have become more tolerant of a range and variety of choices in relation to managing one's life, there is no longer a general consensus that the traditional nuclear family model is the

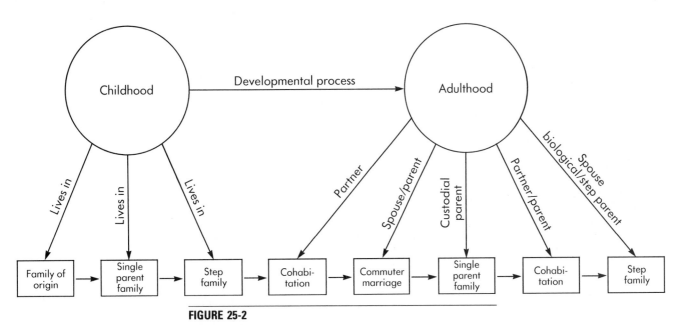

FIGURE 25-2

Family career of an individual.

only "right" model. As a consequence, there is a growing pluralism in family and household types. There is also an increasing awareness that there is more variation within particular family structures than among them. For example, the single-mother headed household may be represented by the unmarried, teenaged mother with an infant (unplanned pregnancy); the divorced mother with one or more children; or the single, career-oriented woman in her late 30s who elects to have a baby and remain single.

Thus far, attention has focused on the changing family structure, but what about the family career of the individual? It is possible that an individual may participate in a number of family life-course experiences or trajectories over a lifetime (Fig. 25-2). For example, a child may spend the early, formative years in the family of origin (mother, father, sibling); experience some years in a single-parent family because the parents divorce; and participate in a stepfamily relationship when the single parent (of custody) remarries. This same child as an adult may experience a variable conjugal career. As an adult, the individual may cohabitate while completing a desired education, marry and have a commuter-type marriage while developing a career, divorce and become the custodial parent, eventually cohabitate with another partner, and finally marry another partner who also has children.

Although variations of the traditional nuclear family have existed throughout history, the increase of variant family structures is becoming more recognized and pronounced. There are many reasons that an increasing number of families diverge from the traditional family structure. A typology of family and household structures is presented on p. 436. *Household* is defined as a single dwelling (apartment or house) occupied by an individual or a group of two or more individuals (related or unrelated). Thus two or more individuals residing in the same dwelling may be defined as a family unit by some or as a household unit by others.

Over time the community health nurse will work with many families representing various structures and living arrangements. For example, one type of family living arrangement may be found among dual career families in which spouses maintain separate residences for the purpose of pursuing their individual careers. Families experiencing *commuter marriages* may need assistance in reducing stresses associated with spousal separation, temporary or long-term parental absences, and financial management associated with maintaining two households.

Some couples deliberately elect not to have children *(voluntary childlessness)*. They may tend to associate few advantages with parenthood, and view greater couple intimacy as a more satisfying relationship. Voluntary childlessness has implications for social policy. Childlessness is perceived as noncompliance with the dominant social norm prescribing children. Thus, a social policy is needed which will increase the public's awareness of choice as well as enhance freedom of choice (Houseknecht, 1982).

Singlehood may be voluntary or involuntary, and permanent or temporary. Included in the group of singles are single parents, both women and men. The status of single parent may be due to divorce, or due to conception or adoption outside of marriage. Adults pursuing the singlehood track may need health education related to nutrition, emotional and sexual well-being, budgeting, preparation for retirement and old age, and other "living alone skills." Single parents may need assistance with parenting skills; and

FAMILY AND HOUSEHOLD STRUCTURES

Married family
Traditional nuclear family
Dual-career family
    Spouses reside in same household
    Commuter marriage
Husband/father away family
Stepfamily
    Stepmother family
    Stepfather family
Adoptive family
Foster family
Voluntary childlessness

Single parent family
Never married
    voluntary singlehood (with children—biological or adopted)
    involuntary singlehood (with children)
Formerly married
    widow (with children)
    divorced (with children)
        custodial parent
        joint custody of children
        binuclear family

Multi-adult household (with/without children)
Cohabitating couple
Communes
Affiliated family
Extended family
New extended family
Home sharing individuals
Same sex partners
Fictive kin

if employed, access to evening and weekend home visits, clinics, and group classes.

The placement of a child in another family setting, the *foster home,* may be for an unknown period of time. The foster care population is represented by children from economically deprived backgrounds (usually single parent, female headed households), children experiencing emotional and physical disabilities or abuse, and teenagers having conflictual relationships with their parents or difficulties with other authority figures (Eastman, 1982). The foster parent(s) may need guidance regarding: parenting skills appropriate to the individual child's needs, assisting the child to adjust to a new home and family environment, and providing appropriate health care.

Same sex partner households may or may not include children. Many same sex partners have been in a heterosexual marriage at one time or another, and have children from that marriage. In addition, some same sex (homosexual) partners elect to have a baby through natural means, artificial insemination, or adoption (Macklin, 1987). These families may need assistance with parenting skills, health guidance, and helping the child to cope with social attitudes about same sex partner households.

Voluntary *group living* is predicted to become an increasingly viable option for older adults. It is one solution for providing companionship and care for the elderly as health and income decline. In "share-a-home" arrangements, older persons pool their resources, share household and care responsibilities, and possibly employ a manager. In the *affiliated family* older nonkin are integrated into a younger family unit. The *fictive kin* family structure is common to low-income and minority cultures. Non-kin members of various ages are incorporated into the family structure for various economic and social reasons. Much of the work with these types of families can be conducted on a group basis.

Trends In The Family Life Cycle

During the preindustrial European period, the family was functional, patriarchal, and community dependent. Marriage was founded on rational and economic grounds, and there was little affection between family members. The affectionate, private, male-dominated nuclear family developed with industrialization. This nuclear family was a social and emotional unit. The permanent, exclusive affectionate bond between the spouses formed the foundation for the family. Today, families tend to be partial to the individualized, open, equal value pattern where independence, close emotional ties with persons outside the family, and individual interests are emphasized. The family continues to evolve, maintaining many of its traditional functions and structures while adapting to changing economic circumstances and social ideologies (Macklin, 1987).

The historical study of families in the early settlements in the United States finds that most of the family structures currently in existence were present then. The difference is the numbers found in each of the structures: the nuclear intact household, single-parent family, blended family, extended family, three-generational family, dual-job family, and other structures. Prospects for families for the twenty-first century are numerous. New family structures that currently are experimental will emerge as everyday "natural" families; for example, families in which the members are not related by blood or marriage, but who provide the services, caring, love, intimacy, and interaction needed by all persons to experience a quality life. These family structures will bring together people from different generations as well as persons of similar ages. The baby-boom cohort, with a history of low fertility rates, will find few relatives available in the years 2010 to 2020 when they reach late adulthood. New "like" families will be needed in increasing numbers to provide home-like environments and care (Sussman, 1987).

Other trends and prospects are:

1. The continued presence and existence of multiple family structures will result in changes in federal regulations related to a family's qualifications for service programs.
2. Court decisions will continue to accept broader definitions of the family than current traditional and legal definitions.
3. Middle-aged adults may find themselves "squeezed" between the prolonged dependency of adult children

remaining in the home of origin for longer periods of time and elderly parents and/or grandparents entering into their homes on a somewhat permanent basis.

4. People will move from one type of household to another more frequently than in the past.
5. People will have more complicated family histories and complicated kinship relationships resulting from divorce and remarriage.
6. Women will continue to bear most of the costs associated with technological and family changes.
7. There will be an increase in the number of women socialized to be career- or work-oriented in adulthood, particularly for personal reasons.
8. Redefinition of family roles toward equity will continue even though attempts have been made to maintain traditional roles.
9. An important function of the family will continue to be providing for individual life transitions.
10. The primary relationship between parents and children will continue to be the most enduring of family relationships (Macklin, 1987; Settles, 1987; Sussman, 1987).

FAMILY DEMOGRAPHY

Family demography is the study of the structure of families and households and the events that alter the structure (Teachman, Polonko and Scanzoni, 1987). Changes in family and household structures can be explained by the events that alter status or position within the structure. For example, the position of being a married parent is changed by the divorce process, and the family structure is altered to one of a single, divorced parent with children.

An important use of family demography is forecasting such as planning for the number of houses, types of housing, and sizes of residences needed in the future. Such forecasts become increasingly important as family and household structures change. To account for the variations in the number, timing, and sequencing of family-related events, various social, economic, and demographic influences must be examined. The following is a brief summary of the demographic changes that must be considered in working with family units.

Marriage

Presently over 90% of Americans marry, but it is predicted that by the year 2000 this percentage may drop to 85% (Macklin, 1987). In 1987 marriages declined for the third consecutive year, and the total was lower than any year since 1980. Although the total first marriage rates rose in 1987, the total remarriages declined for both men and women (National Center for Health Statistics, 1990a).

The marriage rates for divorced men and women were higher than the rates for their single and widowed counterparts. Factors associated with age differentials at the time of marriage are education, labor force participation, income, and premarital fertility. Educational and occupational aspirations tend to influence the postponement of marriage, while dating or early heterosexual involvement and sexual experimentation may lead to early marriages for both males and females. Many early marriages are accompanied by a premarital pregnancy, although willingness to have an abortion or to experience a premarital birth may delay marriage (Teachman et al., 1987).

Cohabitation

From 1970 to 1987 the number of unmarried heterosexual couples sharing the same household rose considerably, with the greatest increase occurring in the middle-age group. There were considerably more widowed women than widowed men who were cohabitating.

Singles

In 1987, 22% of the population 18 years of age and over was single. Since 1970 there has been a steady increase in the number of men and women who are single. It has been predicted that 8% to 9% of the adults in their 20s will experience a lifetime of singlehood. Also, there is an increased likelihood that an individual may be single several times in a lifetime: before marriage, after divorce, after remarriage and divorce, and after death of a spouse (Macklin, 1987).

An interesting phenomenon is the number of young single adults who remain in their parent's home or return to their home of origin after a period of absence. More males than females were in this type of living arrangement (United States Bureau of the Census, 1989, p. 49).

Divorce

Between 1970 and 1987 the ratio of the population 18 years of age and older undergoing divorce increased over 100%. In 1987 the median length of a marriage for a divorcing couple was 7 years (National Center for Health Statistics, 1990b). Approximately one third of the divorces occurred before the fourth year of marriage. Some of the factors associated with marital disruption are: less than a high school education, a premarital birth or premarital pregnancy, marrying during the teen years or in the early 20s, and husband's frequent unemployment (Teachman et al., 1987).

Remarriage

More than 75% of people who divorce remarry. In 1987 the marriage rate for divorced women was 37% higher than the rate for single women marrying, and 14 times higher than the rate for widows remarrying. The marriage rate for divorced men was 137% higher than the rate for single men and more than four times the rate for widowers. One half of the divorced and widowed men remarried within 2.2 years of the date their last marriage ended. The median interval of remarriage for divorced women was 2.5 years, and 4.6 years for widows (National Center for Health Statistics, 1990b). Studies support the fact that there is greater diversity in remarriage experiences than in first marriages; for example, men and women in remarriages tend to differ in age by a greater margin than do men and women in first marriages (Furstenberg and Spainer, 1984).

Children of Divorces

Each year in the United States, more than 1 million couples divorce, and more than 1 million children are affected. Nearly 10 million children under the age of 18 years lived with a biological parent and a stepparent or with two parents who were remarried. Seventy percent of these children lived with their biological mother and stepfather, and 30% lived with both natural parents (born after mother remarried). Nearly one half of all the children from maritally disrupted families have not seen one of their biological parents, usually the father, in the previous 5 years. Only one child in six whose parents were separated or divorced saw the outside biological parent about once a week (Furstenberg and Spanier, 1984).

One-Parent Families

In 1987 there were over 10 million single-parent, female-headed households with children, and approximately 2 million single-parent, male-headed households (United States Bureau of the Census, 1989). It has been predicted that by the age of 17, 70% of the white children born in 1980 will have spent at least some time with only one parent. The same prediction has been made for 94% of African-American children (Espenshade, 1987).

Children in Poverty

The federal poverty income guidelines for 1989 range from $5980 for one person to $20,260 for a family of eight, exclusive of Alaska and Hawaii, which have higher ranges. The poverty level income for a family unit of two is $8020, for three $10,060, and for four $12,100. For families of a larger size, $2040 should be added for each additional family member (Social Security Bulletin, 1989). These guidelines are important because they determine whether a child or family is eligible for community services such as women-infants-children (WIC) programs and Medicaid.

In 1970 almost 15% of children under 18 years of age lived in families with incomes below the poverty level. That percent increased to 20% in 1987. In 1987, 7.1 million children living in poverty were in female-headed families with no husband present (United States Bureau of the Census, 1989, pp. 453, 454). Fifty percent of single-mother households fall below the poverty level (Hanson, 1985).

Working Women

Women presently make up a large proportion of the work force. Sixty-one percent of the households consisting of married couples with children have two wage earners in the family. Seventy percent of the working mothers hold full-time jobs (Family Service of America, 1987). Thus there has been a steady increase across all marital statuses, from 1970 to 1988, in the number of women with children who are in the work force.

Elderly

In 1920 less than 5% of the population in the United States was 65 years of age or older. Presently, older people represent 12% of the population, and it is predicted that by the year 2050 the proportion will be 24% to 35%. The majority of these persons will be women. The living conditions for older women are quite different than for older men. There are more elderly women than men, almost twice as many men as women live with a spouse, and there are over three times as many widows as widowers. In addition a much higher proportion of elderly women live alone, as compared with men, and more than twice as many women as men live below the poverty level.

It should be pointed out that it is very important for community health nurses to keep themselves informed and up-to-date regarding demographic trends. Such knowledge is very important so that nurses can identify high-risk populations such as the large number of children living in poverty, children of working mothers who care for themselves, and elderly women living alone. There are implications for planning health care services for groups such as the elderly, children living in poverty, and unmarried mothers; developing community resources for adequate child care and numerous counseling services; and becoming politically active in relation to the appropriate allocation of scarce funds and resources for health services needed by a growing, diverse population.

FAMILY ROLES AND FUNCTIONS

Implicit in the study of the family are the concepts of roles and functions. The current trends in marriage and the family influence the types of roles found in families, the enactment of those roles, and the functions carried out by the family. The nurse working with families must be knowledgeable about family roles and functions and their modifying factors.

Family Roles

In every family the members hold a recognized position or status; for example, husband, wife, son, or daughter. Each family member usually occupies several positions simultaneously (husband, worker, grandfather, etc.). Individuals are guided by *roles* that are "expectations of behavior, obligations, and rights that are associated with a given position in a family or social group" (Duvall and Miller, 1985, p. 77). Individuals acquire the knowledge and develop the skills, attitudes, and competence to function in a given position through the process of socialization. Unfortunately, an individual may be thrust into a position without adequate preparation for the associated roles; for example, the young teenager who becomes a mother.

No two individuals occupying the same position will enact their role exactly the same way, although societal expectations ensure some similarities. The extent of one's commitment to or conflict about a role is affected by the socialization process. Social and cultural factors that influence role fulfillment include rates of social change, ambiguities, contradictions, modifications, and alternatives in prevailing role definitions (Yorburg, 1983). For example, the women's movement has caused some men to experience difficulties in defining their roles, while some women assume a defensive posture regarding their role as full-time homemaker.

Social class, race/ethnicity, and age/generation have significant implications for role conception and performance. Among the poor in society, a married woman with a husband present usually has few rights but has demanding domestic and economic obligations to the family. The upper class wife usually has a great deal of freedom, and serves as the manager for employed assistants who provide domestic services. Among urban, professional families, the wife may be pursuing her own career full time, sharing authority with her husband, and delegating some of the homemaking and

TABLE 25-1
Life cycle sibling role behavior

Pre-schoolers	Handling competition for parents' attention
	Handling grievances toward each other resulting from parental differential treatment
School-aged siblings	Developing an affectional sibling structure
	Engage in role-making with siblings
	Functioning as discipline to siblings
	Developing power patterns within sibling subsystem
	Gender role socialization
Adolescent siblings	Learning from each other how to relate to peers of opposite gender
	Reminder to younger siblings that adolescent tasks can be mastered
	Supply younger siblings with current information on content of adolescent tasks
	Advisor and confidant to siblings
	Provide support and understanding that can ease parent-adolescent conflicts
	Serve as mediator within family and also between family and broader community
Adult siblings	Maintain sibling contacts through obligatory parental contacts
	Maintain sibling bond
	Performing kinkeeping functions after death of parents
Elderly siblings	Reestablish sibling relationships (if necessary)
	Provide comfort and support

Modified from Aldous J: Family careers: developmental change in families. New York, 1978, John Wiley & Sons.

child-rearing responsibilities to others. Generally, married full-time working women still perform most of the household and child care activities with varying amounts of assistance from their husbands. In addition to societal and cultural expectations about the behavior of family members, each family also has expectations. These expectations may or may not be congruent with those of society. Each family tends to modify family roles and role behaviors in relation to the family structure, and to forces internal and external to the family unit.

Family Adult Roles

The enactment of family adult roles, and the behaviors associated with them, will vary. The following describes typical family adult roles (Nye, 1976):

1. Child socialization: Child socialization encompasses the processes and activities in the family that contribute to the development of the child's social and mental capacities.
2. Child care: Child care involves provision of physical and emotional care to the child for the purpose of developing a healthy individual.
3. Provider role: The role of provider includes the production of goods and services needed by the family or the obtaining of them through the exchange of goods and services.
4. Housekeeper role: The housekeeper role involves preparing and maintaining the goods and services for the family's use. This role also includes services in the home that contribute to the pleasure and comfort of the family members.
5. Kinship role: The kinship role includes the maintenance of contact with kin and, in addition, implies assistance during periods of crisis.
6. Sexual roles: Sexual roles require mutual participation of both partners, with the implicit assumption that

both partners enjoy the sexual relations.
7. Therapeutic role: The therapeutic role entails assisting the family member to cope with problems and providing emotional support, as well as handling intra-family problems.
8. Recreational role: The recreational role involves providing for family recreation and aspects of relaxation, entertainment, and personal development.

Although husbands and wives participate in the family adult roles in different ways and to a different extent, there are some couples who are subscribing to the new values of equality at work and at home. *Role sharing* as been defined as "both partners having equal claims to the bread winning role and equal responsibilities for the care of the home and children, including the obligations to contribute equally or equitably to the family expenses" (Smith and Reid, 1986, p. 6).

Sibling Roles

Siblings are both instigators of socialization in the family and recipients of the socialization process. They contribute to one another's (sibling) identity formation by serving as defenders and protectors of each other, interpreting the outside world, teaching others about equity, building coalitions, bargaining, negotiating, and mutually regulating each other's behavior. Siblings also provide direct services to each other by serving as a buffer between a sibling and the parents and by providing resources such as lending money and other material goods. As a subgroup within the family, siblings assist in establishing and maintaining family norms and contribute to the development of the family's culture (Thinger-Tallman, 1987). Aldous (1978) has examined sibling role behavior from a life cycle perspective (Table 25-1). The life cycle approach identifies sibling roles starting with preschool-aged siblings and concluding with elderly siblings.

The preceding adult and sibling roles are reviewed as formal family roles. In addition to formal family roles there are also informal family roles such as scapegoat, placater or pleaser, martyr or sacrificer, encourager, blamer or know-it-all, follower, or initiator of change.

Family Functions

All families have certain functions that are performed to maintain the integrity of the family unit and to meet the family unit's needs, the individual family member's needs, and society's expectations. Duvall and Miller (1985, pp. 8, 9) identified six family functions that are generally applicable to all types of family structures:

1. Generating affection: Affection is generated between spouses, between parents and children, and among members of the generations.
2. Providing personal security and acceptance: The family provides a home base with a stability that allows the family members to develop naturally in their own way at their own pace.
3. Giving satisfaction and a sense of purpose: In the family setting the family members enjoy life with each other through satisfying activities.
4. Ensuring continuity of companionship: In most cases family associations that provide sympathetic companionship and encouragement can be expected to endure.
5. Providing social placement and socialization: The family serves as the transmitter of culture from one generation to the next and prepares family members for their place in the social hierarchy.
6. Imposing controls and a sense of what is right: Within the family, members first learn the rules, rights, obligations, and responsibilities characteristic of human societies.

Family Health Functions

In addition to the above, a basic family function is to protect the health of the family members and to provide supportive, nurturing care during periods of illness. The family is the primary social system within which the individual develops, is nurtured and becomes socialized, and it is where personal growth and autonomy are fostered. The family contributes to the health of individual family members by supporting the biophysical and psychosocial development of the members. It is within the family unit that members develop their concept of health and establish their health habits. The family as a social unit develops a system of values, beliefs, and attitudes about health and illness that are imparted to and demonstrated through the health-illness behaviors of the family members (family health estate). The family also functions as the primary intermediary for transmitting health-related cultural traits to the next generation. It is through the family that family members learn the beliefs and practices of the larger society concerning health and illness (Johnson, 1987).

The way in which the family carries out its health-care responsibilities, and the ability of the family to do so, will be influenced by factors such as the family's structure, division of labor, socioeconomic status, and ethnicity.

FAMILY HEALTH FUNCTIONS AND TASKS

- Provision of adequate food, shelter, and clothing
- Maintenance of health-supporting physical home environment
- Maintenance of health-supporting psychosocial home environment
- Provision of resources for maintenance of personal hygiene
- Provision for meeting spiritual needs
- Health education
- Health promotion (nutrition, exercise, etc.)
- Health-illness decision making
- Recognition of developmental disruptions
- Recognition of health disruptions
- Seeking health care
- Seeking illness care
- Seeking dental care
- First aid
- Supervision of medications (prescribed and over the counter)
- Illness care (short-term and long-term)
- Rehabilitation care
- Involvement with community's health

The list of health-related functions and tasks in the box is applicable to most families, but the extent to which these functions and tasks will be observed for every family will vary in accordance with the aforementioned family characteristics. The community health nurse supports the family in its ability to perform health-related tasks, contributes by assisting the family in strengthening its resources for carrying out these responsibilities, and intervenes more directly as necessitated by the family situation.

FAMILY DEVELOPMENT THEORY

Family development refers to the process of progressive structural differentiation and transformation over time. This includes the acquisition and discarding of roles by family members as they seek to meet changing requirements for survival and adapt to recurring life stresses as a family (Hill and Mattessich, 1979). Family development theory focuses on common, general features of family life through a longitudinal view of the family life cycle (FLC). It assumes that there are successive phases and patterns that occur within the experience of family living over the years. Family development theory divides family life over time into a series of stages or phases that are qualitatively and quantitatively different from the preceding and succeeding stages. This assumes that there is a high degree of interdependence among the family members. As a consequence of this interdependence, families change each time members are added to or subtracted from the family (Duvall and Miller, 1985; Friedmann, 1986). These changes, referred to as critical transition points, also result in changes in the status and roles of family members. The family operates through roles that shift and alter during the course of the family's life. The healthy family performs all roles appropriately accord-

TABLE 25-2
Family developmental tasks

Family stages	Developmental tasks
Beginning family	Establishing a marriage Relating to kin network Family planning
Early childbearing family	Stabilizing the family unit Reconciling family members' conflicting developmental tasks Facilitating developmental needs of mother, father, and infant
Family with pre-school children	Nurturing and socializing children Maintaining a stable marriage
Family with school-aged children	Socializing children Promoting school achievement Maintaining satisfactory marital relationship
Family with teenager(s)	Balancing teenage freedom and responsibility Maintaining open parent-child communication Maintaining a stable marital relationship Building a foundation for future family stages
Launching family	Releasing children as young adults Readjusting the marriage Assisting aging parents
Middle-aged family	Strengthening the marital relationship Sustaining relationships with parents and children Providing a healthy environment Cultivating leisure-time activities
Aging family	Adjusting to retirement Maintaining satisfactory living arrangement Adjusting to reduced income Adjusting to health problems Adjusting to death of spouse

Modified from Friedman M, Family nursing: theory and assessment, New York, Appleton-Century-Crofts, 1986, pp. 59-73.

ing to family member's ages, competencies, and needs during the family life cycle.

Family development is unique as a framework for studying families. The FLC dimension provides the basis for the study of families over time, emphasizes family member's and families' developmental tasks at every stage of development, identifies family stresses at critical developmental periods, and recognizes the need for services and programs for families throughout their family life cycles (Duvall, 1988).

The family development framework, as originally formulated, focuses essentially on the life cycle of the nuclear family from the wedding, to the birth of children, to the death of the surviving spouse. In recent decades it has become apparent that not everyone fits into this normative family life cycle pattern. As stated by Duvall and Miller (1985), "Families express their individuality in the distinctive ways in which they proceed through the universal life cycle. Each family history has its own unique design" (p. 21).

At all times during the course of the family's development, there is an interrelationship among individual, family system, and intergenerational development. There are four kinds of action in the family's developmental history: movement of family members through their own unique life cycle; interaction of these life cycles; developmental movement of this interacting family system through the FLC; and the

interweaving of intergenerational FLCs (e.g., young parent in a family of procreation who is, at the same time, an adult child in a family of origin).

Family Development Frameworks

As originally conceived, the FLC, also referred to as the family career, consisted of stages related to the child's entry into and exit from the family. Events related to the child's stages in the family were considered to be transitional points for the family because role relationships among family members were significantly altered by those events (Fig. 25-2).

Duvall and Miller (1985, p. 26) categorized the family life cycle into eight stages: (1) married couple without children, (2) childbearing family in which the oldest child is 30 months of age, (3) family with preschool children (oldest 2 1/2 to 6 years of age), (4) family with school-aged children (oldest 6 to 13 years), (5) family with teenagers (oldest 13 to 20 years), (6) family launching young adults (time from first and last child leaving home), (7) middle-aged parents (residing alone to retirement), and (8) aging family members (retirement to death of both spouses). These are summarized in Table 25-2.

Assumptions of the family developmental framework can be summarized as followed (Aldous, 1978, p. 15):

1. Families develop and change over time in similar and consistent ways.

TABLE 25-3
Family life cycle stage transitions

Transition points	Issues
Commitment (late courtship, wedding, honeymoon, parenthood)	Moving away from family of origin Developing lifetime commitment to new family
Developing new parent roles	Shift from spouse to parent (within conjugal and extended families) Role transitions for numerous family members
Accepting new personality	Accept normal dependency of newborn Allow development of new individual personality (as child passes from infancy to childhood)
Introducing child to institutions outside the family	Dealing with individual's adjustment to establishing independent relationships with school, church, etc.
Accepting adolescence	Developing a sexual identity for adolescent and individual integration into peer group culture
Experimenting with independence	Lessening of ties with family of origin Allow adult strivings to emerge
Preparations to launch	Acceptance of independent adult role of first child
Letting go/facing each other again	Let go of children and face each other as spouses alone again Children leave parents to themselves Development of new roles: grandparents, parents
Accepting retirement and/or old age	New lifestyle excluding career plans, goals, and responsibilities Plan for caring for older and younger generations

Modified from Barnhill LR and Longo D: Fixation and regression in the family life cycle, Fam Proc 17(4):469-478, 1978.

2. Humans initiate actions as they mature and interact with others as well as reacting to environmental pressures.
3. The family and family members must perform certain time-specific tasks set by themselves, and they must perform tasks determined by culture and society.
4. Families tend to have a beginning and an end.

Since the early work of the family development theorists in the 1940s, considerable research and conceptualization regarding family development has continued. Over the past decade, increasing concern has been expressed about the need to minimize the emphasis placed on the FLC stages and to increase the focus on the transitional process from one stage to another. Family development includes two interrelated types of change: 1) change in the role content of family positions, essentially because of changes in age norms for those positions (e.g., moving from parent of infant, to parent of adolescent, to parent of adult children), and change in interactional patterns in the family (e.g., changes in spousal interactions when a couple become parents) (Olson & Lavee, 1989).

Barnhill and Longo (1978) formulated the key principles of the transition points for various FLC stages. The next step in this formulation, yet to be accomplished, is to identify key issues in the transitions (Table 25-3). Although it is readily apparent that this approach to transitions in the FLC focuses essentially on the entrance and exit of children in the family, it is possible that this type of model could be used to develop transitional formulations for different family structures.

Family Developmental Tasks

A *family developmental task* is defined as a "growth responsibility that arises at a certain stage in the life of a family, the successful achievement of which leads to present satisfaction, approval, and success with later tasks." Failure in completing the tasks can lead to family unhappiness, societal disapproval, and difficulty with later developmental tasks (Duvall and Miller, 1985, p. 61). Tasks are considered accomplished if the family's biological needs are met, societal obligations are fulfilled, and the family's own values and aspirations are satisfied. The developmental tasks basic to most families, such as physical maintenance and socialization of family members, tend to be congruent with the family functions discussed previously. Although specific family developmental tasks were identified for each FLC stage, many tasks are common to several stages. Examples include: providing adequate housing, facilities, and equipment; meeting family expenses; sharing responsibilities for household management and child care; maintaining mutually satisfying intimate family communications; relating to relatives; community participation; maintaining family morale; and developing mature roles within the family (Duvall and Miller, 1985). Examples of family developmental tasks by stage appear in Table 25-2. Some of the developmental tasks are more relevant for intact families (mother, father, children residing together) than for some other types of family structures.

The achievement of family developmental tasks at each family stage is interrelated with the accomplishment of developmental tasks by individual family members (see Chapters 28 through 31). Achievement of family developmental tasks assist the individual members to accomplish their tasks. This in turn enables the family to complete its task(s). In addition individual family members must accomplish many of their individual developmental tasks to be able to fulfill their family roles adequately (Aldous, 1978; Duvall and Miller, 1985; Havighurst, 1974; Stevenson, 1977).

The following example illustrates the interrelationship of the tasks and also demonstrates the complex nature of the family at this stage of its development. When an adolescent becomes pregnant, in addition to working on the developmental tasks common to adolescence, she is confronted with the developmental tasks associated with pregnancy. Pregnancy-associated developmental tasks are: (1) development of an emotional attachment to the fetus during the first trimester; (2) differentiation of the self and the fetus during the third trimester; (3) acceptance and resolution of the relationship with the pregnant woman's mother; and (4) resolution of dependency issues in relation to the woman's mother and husband/partner (if present). Successful accomplishment of these tasks should contribute to the development of a coherent sense of oneself as a person and as a parent. Thus the adolescent is confronted with a double set of developmental tasks that are not necessarily compatible. The adolescent also is confronted with premature entry into the parental role and possible premature exit from the educational role.

The tasks of the other family members become more complex because certain roles shift as a result of the pregnancy. The parents may become grandparents prematurely, and the siblings become aunts and uncles. If the adolescent decides to keep the baby and remain in the family of origin, the family unit size and composition will change.

The family development approach assists community health nurses in understanding and anticipating clinical problems in the family as well as identifying family strengths. The framework can serve as a guide in assessing the family's developmental stage, the extent to which the family is fulfilling the tasks associated with the respective stage, the family's developmental history, and the availability of resources essential for performing the developmental tasks. One example of the application of the family development framework to community health nursing intervention is its appropriateness for use in anticipatory guidance. Family members can be assisted by preparing them to cope with FLC role transitions and by making them aware of supporting community resources. For example, the early childbearing family may experience stress from the arrival of a new baby. The community health nurse can plan to share with the parents changes that they should expect in their lives and schedules (i.e., sleep, rest, feeding schedule, emotions, new demands on time). A community resource that the nurse could refer them to is a parenting group.

In summary, developmental theory as a framework assists the community health nurse to:

1. Keep the family in focus throughout its life cycle.
2. See family members in interaction with one another.
3. Observe the ways in which family members and the family unit influence each other.
4. Recognize what a given family is experiencing at a particular time.
5. Identify critical periods of growth and development for both the individual family members and the family.
6. Recognize the commonalities and variations among the life cycles of families.
7. Respect the way in which culture and families influence each other.

8. Forecast what a family will be experiencing at any period of its life cycle (Duvall and Miller, 1985, p. 16).

DEVELOPMENTAL THEORY AND NONTRADITIONAL FAMILY STRUCTURES

Increasingly the life course of many families is not following the typical life cycle of the nuclear family. Greater numbers of families are demonstrating variations in childbearing and childrearing patterns, frequency in marital disruption before widowhood, and in reconstituting family structures. The developmental framework helps to understand these family life changes. These family changes result in developmental crises that must be resolved for families to continue to function normally.

Adoptive Family

Adoptive parents, like their nonadoptive counterparts, must adapt to the increased personal and interpersonal strains that accompany parenthood. In addition there are other developmental transitional issues and stresses that adoptive parents encounter; examples of these are described in Table 25-4. Although there are numerous stresses associated with the transition to adoptive parenthood, there are also protective factors related to the transition.

Adoptive families need ongoing services to help them cope with adoptive issues in general. They also may need assistance with parenting skills that are specific to their needs as adoptive parents. Finally, family life education programs should be made available to explain the similarities and differences between adoptive and biological parenthood at various stages in the family's and child's life cycle (Di Guilio, 1987).

Separation

Separation is one set of transitions in the total process of moving from family organization in marriage to family reorganization in divorce and remarriage. Not all separations end in divorce. Major developmental role transitions in the family system occur in separation, divorce, and remarriage. At these times, families experience adjustment, restructuring, and consolidation. In the adjustment phase families attempt to handle their stresses by avoidance, elimination, or assimilation (incorporating the stress into the existing family structure in a way that reduces stress). The restructuring phase consists of families establishing new patterns of interaction that recognize that the marital relationship no longer is present. During the consolidation phase, new role patterns are incorporated into new family structures, resulting in a testing of members to see how they fit into the family structure and to see how a family fits into the community (see box). During this dynamic adjustment and adaptation process, the family and family members pursue strategies designed to regain or maintain the themes they value in family life (Ahrons and Rodgers, 1987). It should be kept in mind that adults of all ages experience separation.

Divorce

Divorce is an event that moves individuals from a condition of being legally married to a state of being legally divorced. The divorce experience begins before the actual divorce, its

TABLE 25-4
Transition to adoptive parenthood

Developmental issues	Stresses
No role models	Difficulty developing realistic expectations about the transition to adoptive parenthood
	Preparation for parenting tends to be based on experiences with own parents
Timing of transition to role	Uncertainty about the transition to parenthood—may be anywhere from a few months to 6 to 7 years
	Absence of usual pregnancy cues makes it difficult for others to alter perceptions and expectations of couple becoming parents
In-depth evaluation process	Proving their worthiness to be parents
	Process perceived as intrusive and anxiety arousing
Timing of adoption placement	Extent of attachment bonds between child and biological or foster parents
Biological risk associated with adoption	Background of child (genetic, parents' behavior, prenatal/birth complications)
Telling child about adoption	Makes explicit that adoptive parents are not biological parents
	Introduces image of natural parents into adoptive family system
	Threatens exclusiveness of relationship between adoptive parent and child

Modified from Brodzinsky DM and Huffman L. Transition to adoptive parenthood. Marr & Fam Rev 12(3-4):267-86, 1988; and DiGuillo JF. Assuming the adoptive parent role. Soc Casework 68(9):561-6, 1987.

DEVELOPMENTAL TRANSITION PHASES OF SEPARATION

Preseparation
Gradual emotional separation
Continue to enact public/social roles
Avoid exposing state of relationship to the public
Initiator usually experiences guilt
Assentor usually experiences anger

Early Separation
State of emotional and social anomie
Emotional ambivalence (feelings vacillate)
Ambiguity of separation itself
Status of family undefined

Midseparation
Emotional distress still felt
Faced with a deficit in structure (two separate households)
Realignment of family member relationships
Conflict between meeting own needs and childrens' needs
Convert anxieties into "other-directed" anger
Restructure tasks to meet children's health and nutritional needs (may require outside support)
Try to form a coparenting relationship
Seek support from friends, relatives, etc.

Late Separation
Old patterns replaced by new ones: family reorganization
Trial and error period for meeting needs
Power struggles of the marriage become more exaggerated
Reassessment of economic condition of family and friendships
Create a sense of family for all family members

Modified from Ahrons CR and Rodgers RH. Divorced families: a multidisciplinary developmental view, New York, 1987, W.W. Norton Company.

DEVELOPMENTAL TASKS FOR SINGLE-MOTHER FAMILIES	
Establishment of the single-parent family	Developing new patterns of power, communication, and affection Altering child-rearing patterns Developing new social networks Fulfilling physical maintenance tasks Coping with disrupted intimacy and sexual aspects of the marital relationship
Woman continuing, instituting, or reinstituting an occupational career	Developing new family physical maintenance arrangements Restructuring relationships with younger children Emphasizing affectional relationship with children Maintaining morale of children Providing children with needed extra nurturance Reestablishing self-esteem (mother) through outside involvement

Modified from Aldous J: Family careers: developmental changes in families, New York, 1978, John Wiley & Sons.

effects extend into the future, and each family member is affected by it. Divorce is viewed as a developmental crisis and necessitates focusing on the normal family patterns resulting from the crisis. It is possible that defining divorce as a societal institution in the United States is at hand, even though sociocultural norms are ill-defined for divorce at the present time. The directions taken by families regarding divorce are related to their history, the current family situation, and family members' desired goals for the future (Ahrons and Rodgers, 1987).

Some of the post divorce developmental tasks are a continuation of the tasks initiated during the separation transition phases. Additional tasks are handling the legal problems of the divorce and interpreting the meaning of the divorce to other family members, extended family, and friends (Duvall and Miller, 1985).

Single-Parent Family

The three most common family patterns in the United States at the present time are nuclear, single-parent, and remarried families. This discussion of single-parent families will focus essentially on the separated or divorced female as head of the household because that family structure continues to predominate for divorced single-parent families.

Aldous (1978) identified six developmental stages for single female-parent families (i.e., divorced women): establishment of the single-parent family; the woman continuing, instituting, or reinstituting her occupational career; the family with adolescents; the family with young adults; the woman in middle years; and the woman's retirement from her career and/or assuming responsibilities for parents. The box depicts some of the developmental tasks associated with the first two stages of the single-parent family. Many of the tasks related to the last four stages tend to be comparable to the tasks that have been identified for most families, with the exception of tasks related to the spouse.

Many of the family tasks delineated for the single mother family would apply to the single father family also. While the single mother may have to learn about and assume re-

sponsibility for tasks around the home that the husband formerly carried out (e.g., home repairs, yard work), similarly, the single father may face some of the same problems, especially problems related to child care (e.g., child's nutritional and health care needs).

The community health nurse working with the single-parent family will need to be prepared to assist the parent and children with developmental tasks through the provision of professional support, anticipatory guidance and problem solving, and the development of support systems and social networks. One of the major problems for single-parent families is task overload. This problem is very apparent in the single mother family with young children because the major task of raising children becomes the responsibility of one parent rather than two parents. A problem for the children is not only the absence from the home of one of the parents, but the perceived loss of both parents if the mother seeks employment outside the home at the same time that the divorce is occurring.

Remarried Family

There are several synonyms for the term remarried family: merging, blended, restructured, reconstituted, synergistic, and stepfamily. The terms remarried family and stepfamily will be used interchangeably in this section because of the selected developmental issues that will be discussed.

At the present time, there is no widely accepted, concrete model of behavioral stages related to how a remarried family, with children involved, should function normally. Stepfamilies as well as community health nurses tend to develop their ideas about the expected family roles on models of the biological nuclear family. In remarriages family members need to develop a concept of family that is acceptable to the spouses and to the stepfamily (Keshet, 1988). Stepfamilies, like some adoptive families, find children and adults, once strangers, becoming instant relatives without the shared experience of developing their parent-child relationship over time. In remarried families that include children, many habitualized family behaviors may no longer apply.

TABLE 25-5
Remarried family formation: developmental issues

Steps	Prerequisite attitude	Developmental issues
1. Entering the new relationship	Recovery from loss of first marriage (adequate "emotional divorce")	Recommitment to marriage and to forming a family with readiness to deal with the complexity and ambiguity
2. Conceptualizing and planning new marriage and family	Accepting one's own fears and those of new spouse and children about remarriage and forming a stepfamily Accepting need for time and patience for adjustment to complexity and ambiguity of: 1. Multiple new roles 2. Boundaries: space, time, membership, and authority 3. Affective issues: guilt, loyalty conflicts, desire for mutuality, unresolved past hurts	a. Work on openness in the new relationships to avoid pseudomutuality b. Plan for maintenance of cooperative coparental relationships with exspouses c. Plan to help children deal with fears, loyalty conflicts, and membership in two systems d. Realignment of relationships with extended family to include new spouse and children e. Plan maintenance of connections for children with extended family of exspouses
3. Remarriage and reconstitution of family	Final resolution of attachment to previous spouse and ideal of "intact" family Acceptance of a different model of family with permeable boundaries	a. Restructuring family boundaries to allow for inclusion of new spouse/stepparent b. Realignment of relationships throughout subsystems to permit interweaving of several systems c. Making room for relationships of all children with biological (noncustodial) parents, grandparents, and other extended family d. Sharing memories and histories to enhance stepfamily integration

From Carter E and McGoldrick M, editors: The family life cycle: a framework for family therapy, New York, 1980, Gardner Press, Inc., p. 19. Copyright 1980 by Gardner Press.

TABLE 25-6
Stepfamily developmental tasks

Stages	Tasks
1. Setting goals	Develop desired long-term goals for the family structure based on the needs of all the family members (focus on satisfactions to be gained in the stepfamily) Explore possible roles for the stepparent in relation to the stepchildren (the stepparent may or may not work toward a parental role)
2. Parental limit-setting	Biological parent (in stepfamily) in charge of setting and enforcing limits for biological child Stepparent sets limits in accordance with biological parents' rules In the family where both spouses have children, the couple will need to accept the existence of different rules for different children
3. Stepparent bonding	Create periods of time free from limit-setting, for stepparent nurturing of the stepchild for the purpose of allowing stepparent-child bonding appropriate to the age of the child
4. Blending family rules	Stepfamily develops own new rules and traditions Negotiate regarding the stepparent parental role (if there is to be one—this begins only after the initial bonding phase completed) Disagreement regarding rules resolved by the biological parent Biological parent accommodates the stepparent regarding rules to the extent that the stepparent contributes positively to the child's development
5. Stepfamily's relations in the binuclear family	Stepparent supports the child's relationship with the same sex parent in the other household Differentiate between the two binuclear households

Modified from Mills D: A model for stepfamily development, Fam Rels 33:365, 1984.

As a result, these families must solve problems unknown to other types of families. Some of the major structural elements associated with the stepfamily are (Visher and Visher, 1979):

1. Permeability of the family's boundaries—shifting boundaries and membership.
2. Presence of family members with interpersonal bonds associated with another previous family constellation.
3. Presence of at least two individuals who experienced the rupturing of spousal and/or parent-child bonds.
4. Possible presence of another natural parent with power outside the stepfamily boundary.
5. New relationships that are more difficult to negotiate because they do not develop slowly as in the early stages of the nuclear family life cycle—they possibly begin in the school age or adolescent period.
6. The rapid engagement of family members in instant multiple roles.

Table 25-5 provides a format for conceptualizing the development of a remarried family. The developmental steps in the formation of the remarried family build on the successful resolution of the developmental issues involved in the divorce process.

A model for stepfamily development constructed by Mills (1984) could be used as a guide by the community health nurse in assessing, guiding, and evaluating the family's task accomplishments relevant to the stepfamily cycle. An adequate model for the stepfamily should stress the ways in which the stepfamily functions that are unique to that type of family structure. For example, the model should focus on the development tasks appropriate for the stepparent-stepchild relationship while taking into account that this relationship will differ with different children. The stepparent eventually may be able to develop a parental role with a young stepchild but may never fully achieve the parental role with a teenager. This may be because of the lack of a common family history (for the stepparent and teenager) over most of the teenager's life and also the teenager's needs in relation to the developmental task of seeking more autonomy from the family. General characteristics of the model are: (1) both spouses, working as a pair, should assume conscious executive control of the family; (2) with the cooperation of the biological parent, the stepparent can select from a variety of possible roles (e.g., friend, parent) the role most appropriate for the stepparent-stepchild relationship; and (3) the stepfamily will need to select the family structure that best satisfies the individual needs of all its members. This structure may change considerably over time.

The developmental stages and tasks in the Mills model are presented in Table 25-6. The developmental tasks are implemented sequentially so that each task can build on the process initiated in the preceding stages. All of the tasks should continue throughout the stepfamily development process.

Certain themes emerge when considering the stepfamily structure: (1) there are no clearly delineated sociocultural norms for enactment of family roles in the stepfamily; (2) there are identifiable developmental tasks for the remarried family; (3) the boundaries of the stepfamily are permeable and sometimes changing as family members (i.e., children) move in and out of the family; (4) most of the concerns related to the stepfamily center around the stepparent-stepchild relationship; (5) the individuals in the remarried family engage in instant multiple roles and relationships; and (6) this family type experiences its own unique FLC.

VULNERABLE FAMILIES—AN ANALYSIS

In every community health nurse's case load there are one or more families who have experienced generational poverty as well as multiple problems of a physiological, psychological, and/or social nature. This is the family (to be referred to as a vulnerable family) that has never experienced financial stability; has been a long-time client of public agencies; has experienced frequent, if not continuous, states of disorganization; and whose life cycle represents an endless succession of crises. The family members of the vulnerable family usually possess deep-seated assumptions about themselves as related to the broader society: (1) they are not needed or wanted; (2) they really have no right to exist; (3) there is nothing they can do; and (4) they are being destroyed by society itself (Colon, 1980). The adults may develop a conviction that regardless of what they do to get a job or try to keep it, their efforts are useless. For this reason, they may view illegal options as the only opportunity for economic gains, and consequently they may develop a pervasive sense of impotence, rage, and despair. The important struggle is for survival.

There are certain factors related to the vulnerable family that the community health nurse should remember when preparing to work with the family: (1) the family should be viewed across a three-generational time frame that includes members of the immediate family and the extended family; (2) the vulnerable family is subject to more abrupt loss of membership through such events as desertion, death, imprisonment; and (3) the vulnerable family seems to have less calendar time in which to experience the various developmental stages. The shortened duration of the family life cycle frequently results in: (1) inadequate time to achieve the developmental tasks of each family life stage, (2) more blurring of the boundaries of the life stages of this family, and (3) difficulty with the subsequent stages because the previous developmental tasks have not been resolved. The community health nurse can assume that the vulnerable family has developed a variant family structure for the purpose of surviving and carrying out essential functions.

If the community health nurse adopts a developmental framework to guide the nursing process with the vulnerable family, it is important to know that a three-stage family life cycle framework probably will be the most appropriate. The three stages are: (1) the unattached young adult (includes late adolescence), (2) the family with children, and (3) the family in later life (Colon, 1980). The following discussion focuses on these three stages.

It generally is assumed for most young adults that the major developmental tasks for the unattached young adult are to develop an identity, make a commitment to work/career and marriage, and gradually to disengage from the family. By contrast, the adolescent (i.e., young adult) in the vulnerable family may not grow away from the family gradually but may be forced to leave the family and become independent. Another possibility may be that the adolescent/young adult will remain with the family as a source of income. This phenomenon of being forced to leave home prematurely may occur with children as young as 10 to 11 years of age. Another developmental problem for the young adult is that without viable work options it is difficult to make a commitment to work. This is particularly important for the young adult male who may infrequently have observed adult males functioning in a stable work role. Because of limited job opportunities and limited opportunities to see an adult male functioning in a stable parental role, the young adult male may function as a transient participant in heterosexual relationships.

The young adult female tends to perceive her role as a mother and develops her identity with that role. When two young adults do get married or decide to live together for a period of time, the relationship generally is unstable. There have been few models representative of a stable married couple, except those on television, and these are difficult for the young adults to identify with. As the couple moves into another stage of the family life cycle (family with children), the arrival of children coupled with unemployment results in additional problems for the family. The family may receive outside public assistance, with the result that the father becomes more peripheral to the family. Another pattern that may develop is that the parents remain primarily identified with their adolescent peer groups and avoid the adult parenting roles. By way of contrast, if the adult has not had an opportunity to develop an identity through the satisfactory fulfillment of the child and/or adolescent roles and developmental tasks, the individual may view the parental role as a source of identity.

Within the vulnerable family, one of the children may emerge as a surrogate parent to help with the siblings. In addition the school-age children may not receive adequate attention from the mother and/or father, resulting in the inadequate development of cognitive, affective, and communication skills that would enable them to benefit adequately from their learning experiences in the school system. As more children are born over a longer period of time, the child-rearing stage tends to be protracted. As a result, the older children frequently are discharged to their peer groups. That is, they turn to their peer groups for needs fulfillment because their parents are too busy caring for younger siblings to give them the needed attention.

During the life cycle stage of the vulnerable family in later life, the forward progress of the generational process may come to a standstill or may break down, especially if the household is three-generational. The adult daughter's mother may make the grandchild one of her children, the adult daughter remains a daughter instead of a mother, and family roles become very confused. The family system becomes a system for survival and homeostasis and not for change and growth. The death of the grandmother can have a devastating effect on the family both emotionally and developmentally. It is at this time that the oldest daughter, who was unable to become a mother in terms of fulfilling the role, may be able to move into that role now because

of the death of her mother. Thus the new mother role occupant begins to repeat the life cycle of the vulnerable family.

The community health nurse can combine theories about the family system's development, family roles, functions, and interactions with knowledge about vulnerable families. The emerging framework should generate a working plan that will guide the assessment of the family, assist the involvement of the family in the planning process, and provide direction for the intervention strategies and evaluation.

The community health nurse should realize that the family members may distrust professionals because of past experiences with public agencies. The nurse also should make clear to the family the kind and extent of assistance that can be expected from the nurse and the agency. It is very important that the nurse retain a flexible perspective on the family and avoid viewing the family within a middle-class family developmental model of structure, roles, and functions. The community health nurse can view the nursing process with the vulnerable family as a socializing experience for the family members in which they participate in problem solving and informed decision making, identify their strengths and resources, plan their care, and evaluate the outcomes of their health care efforts.

CLINICAL APPLICATION

Nancy approached her community health nursing experience knowing that her caseload would include families in the community. As she reviewed her assignment, she discovered that the five families with whom she would be working included a nuclear family of mother, father, and two school-aged children; a single mother with a toddler; and a stepfamily with mother, stepfather, stepgrandmothers, and two teenaged siblings, one from each prior marriage.

Nancy first *assessed* the families' development. She found that all families were meeting the appropriate tasks for each development stage except the single mother. Nancy assessed the demographics of this family and found that Mrs. Rodgers' income was lowered as a result of her divorce; she was having difficulty fulfilling the physical maintenance tasks of rent, food, and day care for her child. This was affecting her ability to show affection toward the child. Mrs. Rodgers and her child were now among the families whose life events had placed them in poverty.

As Nancy *planned* her care for Mrs. Rodgers, she considered providing anticipatory guidance regarding Mrs. Rodgers' developmental tasks and her needs to be able to meet her tasks. Nancy also considered providing guidance to Mrs. Rodgers about her toddler's tasks and the toddler's need for affection from the mother to successfully survive this life crisis. Nancy sought out community resources available to help Mrs. Rodgers and discovered that she was eligible for rent subsidy, day care subsidy, and food stamps through social services. Mrs. Rodgers also was eligible to receive a Medicaid card for preventive and illness care services for herself and her child. Nancy also discovered a single-parent self-help group to refer Mrs. Rodgers to for needed emotional support.

Nancy knew that her role in *implementing* the plan would include advocating for Mrs. Rodgers with the community resources and serving as educator, facilitator, and supporter in guiding her through this crisis. Nancy planned to include Mrs. Rodgers in establishing goals for resolving this developmental crisis and the transition to family stability.

During each visit Nancy *evaluated* Mrs. Rodgers' progress toward meeting her individual and family developmental tasks, her compliance with the interventions, and progress toward mutually agreed upon goals.

SUMMARY

Community health nurses need to increase their understanding of the process by which individuals become involved in their particular family/household structures and the factors affecting the successful or problematic transition from one structure to another. Traditional family development theory, which assumes that persons progress through identifiable stages of courtship, marriage, childbearing, and retirement is being revised. The alternative family/household structures reviewed in this chapter may be viewed as evolving modifications of the family structure in families' continual process of adaptation to changing societal conditions.

Knowledge of family theory and appropriate conceptual frameworks will assist community health nurses in applying the nursing process to families and developing a knowledge base about family health. Family development is one framework used to study families. This approach emphasizes how families change over time and focuses on interactions and relationships among family members.

This chapter examined issues relevant to family development. It discussed the developmental conceptual framework from a general perspective and in relation to various family structures. The family life cycle was examined in relation to family demography and in relation to trends in marriages and families. Other concepts related to the developmental framework presented were family structure, roles, and functions.

The reader is encouraged to draw from the many chapters in the text that have direct application to the study of the family. Especially relevant are the chapters focusing on family health (chapters 26 and 27), and the chapters emphasizing individual developmental stages (chapters 28 through 31).

KEY CONCEPTS

Family development is one theoretical framework used to study families. This approach emphasizes how families change over time and focuses on interactions and relationships among family members.

Demographic trends affecting the family's structure and development are age at time of first marriage; fertility patterns and birth rates; increase in the number of individuals engaging in singlehood, divorce, and remarriage; increase in the number of dependent children experiencing divorce in the family or living with a never-married parent; and an increase in the number of elderly.

Implicit in the developmental approach to the study of family are the concepts of family roles and functions. Knowledge in these areas is essential to adequately assess the family and to effectively plan, intervene, and evaluate care with the family.

A family developmental task is a responsibility for growth that arises at a certain stage in the life cycle of a family. Successful accomplishment of the task leads to satisfaction, approval, and success with future tasks.

Mills' model for stepfamily development can be used to help assess, guide, and evaluate the stepfamily's task accomplishment.

The family's culture affects the enactment of family roles, the timing of developmental tasks, and the meaning attached to the different stages of the family life cycle.

The family developmental framework identifies points in a family's development at which changes occur in family members' status and roles.

Increasingly, variations in family structure, such as single parent families, remarried families, and vulnerable families, are being studied from the developmental perspective.

LEARNING ACTIVITIES

1. Select six or more health professionals and other human service workers and ask them to define a family. The health professionals should include community health nurses and physicians, and the human service workers should represent social workers, teachers, and others. Analyze the responses for commonalities and differences.

2. Form small groups and discuss the implications of family demography and demographic trends for community health nursing.

3. Develop a typology of the different family structures and household arrangements representative of the community. This information may be available from various sources such as the health department, schools, and other social and welfare agencies, and census data.

4. Interview several individuals who represent different family structures and family living arrangements. Ask them to define a family and to identify their family roles and functions. Analyze the responses for commonalities and differences. Analyze the implications of your survey and your knowledge about family structures for community health nursing. (If there are several persons carrying out this activity, pool all responses and proceed with the analysis.)

5. Select several families representing first marriages and remarriages who have more than one child in the family. The children in the families should be old enough to talk about their relationships with their siblings. Ask each of the children about their relationship with their brother(s) and/or sister(s). The discussion should include the children's ideas about how their siblings help them, how they help their siblings, and their perceptions about sibling difficulties. Analyze the responses for commonalities and differences regarding age and gender of the respondents and sibling relationships (biological sibling, stepsibling, halfsibling).

6. As a group project, each student/community health nurse should select several families and interview the family, as a unit, about: a) their perceptions of their health-related functions and tasks, b) their health promotion behaviors, and c) their values and attitudes about health promotion. The families selected should represent different ethnic/racial and socioeconomic backgrounds.

7. Form five discussion groups and discuss the use of the developmental approach as a guide for the nursing process used by the community health nurses in working with the a) nuclear family, b) adoptive family, c) single-parent family, d) remarried family, and e) vulnerable family. Each group should select one family type to discuss. As a group, analyze the similarities and variations in the application of the developmental framework to the nursing process with each family.

8. As a group, discuss your attitudes about working with the different family/household types discussed in the chapter.

BIBLIOGRAPHY

Ahrons CR and Rodgers RH: Divorced families: a multidisciplinary developmental view, New York, 1987, W.W. Norton Company.

Aldous J: Family careers: developmental change in families, New York, 1978, John Wiley & Sons.

Atwater L: Long-term cohabitation without a legal ceremony is equally valid and desirable. In Feldman H and Feldman M, editors: Current controversies in marriage and family, Beverly Hills, 1985, Sage Publications, pp. 243-52.

Baranowski T and Nader P: Family health behavior. In Turk D and Kerns R, editors: Health, illness, and families, New York, 1985, John Wiley & Sons, pp. 1-22.

Barnhill LR and Longo D: Fixation and regression in the family life cycle, Fam Proc 17:469-78, 1978.

Bertalanffy, Lvon: General systems theory, New York, 1968, George Braziller.

Blum HL: Expanding health care horizons: from a general systems concept of health to a national health policy, Oakland, 1976, Third Party Associates, Inc.

Bozett FW: Gay men as fathers. In Hanson SM and Bozett FW, editors: Dimensions of fatherhood, Beverly Hills, 1985, Sage Publications, pp. 327-52.

Brodzinsky DM and Huffman L: Transition to adoptive parenthood, Marr Fam Rev 12:267-86, 1988.

Butler EW and Meints J: Notes on nontemporary singles. In Gutknicht RB, Butler EW, Criswell L, and Meints J, editors: Family, self, and society: Emerging issues, alternatives, and interventions, Lanham, Md, 1983, University Press of America, Inc., pp. 363-369.

Carter E and McGoldrick M: The family life cycle and family therapy: an overview. In Carter E and McGoldrick M, editors, The family life cycle: a framework for family therapy, New York, 1980, Gardner Press, Inc, pp. 3-20.

Clements I and Robert F: Family health: a theoretical approach to nursing care, New York, 1983, John Wiley & Sons.

Colon F: The family life cycle of the multiproblem poor family. In Carter E and McGoldrick M, editors: The family life cycle: a framework for family therapy, New York, 1980, Gardner Press, Inc., pp. 343-81.

Crane PT: Processes surrounding the decision to remain permanently voluntarily childless. In Gutknecht DB, Butler EW, Criswell L, and Meints J, editors: Family, self, and society: emerging issues, alternatives, and interventions, Lanham, Md, 1983, University Press of America, Inc., pp. 383-92.

Demick J and Wapner S: Open and closed adoption: a developmental conceptualization, Fam Proc 27:229-49, 1988.

Di Giulio JF: Assuming the adoptive parent role, Soc Casework, 68:561-6, 1987.

Duvall EM: Family development's first forty years, Fam Rel 37:127-34, 1988.

Duvall E and Miller B: Marriage and family development, ed 6, New York, 1985, Harper & Row, Publishers.

Eastman KS: Foster parenthood: a nonnormative parenting arrangement, Marr Fam Rev, 5:95-120, 1982.

Eschleman JR: The family: an introduction, Boston, 1974, Allyn & Bacon, Inc.

Espenshade, TJ: Marital careers of American women: a cohort life table analysis. In Bongaarts J, Burch TK, and Wachter KW, editors: Family demography: methods and their application, New York, 1987, Oxford University Presss, pp. 150-67.

Family Service of America: The state of families, Milwaukee, Wisc, 1987, Family Service of America.

Friedman MM: Family nursing: theory and assessment, Norwalk, Conn, 1986, Appleton-Century-Crofts.

Furstenberg FF, and Spanier GB: Recycling the family: remarriage after divorce, Beverly Hills, 1984, Sage Publications.

Gerstel N and Gross HE: Commuter marriages: a review, Marr Fam Rev 5:71-93, 1982.

Gutknecht DB, Butler EW, Criswell L, and Meints J: Alternative life styles: implications for family, self, and society. In Gutknecht DB, Butler EW, Criswell L, and Meints J, editors: Family, self, and society: emerging issues, alternatives, and interventions, Lanham, Md, 1983, University Press of America, Inc., pp. 315-8.

Hanson SMH: Single custodial fathers. In Hanson SMH and Bozett FW, editors: Dimensions of fatherhood, Beverly Hills, 1985, Sage Publications, pp. 369-92.

Havighurst R: Developmental task and education, ed. 3, New York, 1974, David McKay Company, Inc.

Houseknecht SK: Voluntary childlessness in the 1980's: a significant increase? Marr Fam Rev 5:51-69, 1982.

Hill R and Mattessich P: Family development theory and life span development. In Baltes P and Brim O, editors: Life span development and behavior, vol 2, New York, 1979, Academic Press, pp. 161-204.

Ihinger-Tallman: Member adjustment in single-parent families: theory building, Family Relations Journal of Applied Family and Child Studies, 35(1):215-221, 1986.

Johnson R: Family developmental theories. In Stanhope M and Lancaster J, editors: Community health nursing: process and practices for promoting health, St. Louis, 1987, The CV Mosby Co.

Jorgensen SR: The American family of the future: what choices will we have? In Gutnecht DB, Butler EW, Criswell L, and Meints J, editors: Family, self, and society: emerging issues, alternatives, and interventions, Lanham, Md, 1983, University Press of America, Inc., pp. 227-45.

Keshet JK: The remarried couple: stresses and successes. In Beer WR, editor: Relative strangers: studies of stepfamily processes, Totowa, NJ, 1988, Rowman & Littlefield Publishers, pp. 29-53.

Keyfitz N: Form and substance in family demography. In Bongaarts J, Burch TK, and Wachter KW, editors: Family demography: methods and their application, New York, 1987, Oxford University Press, pp. 3-16.

Macklin ED: Nontraditional family forms. In Sussman MB and Steinmetz SK, editors: Handbook of marriage and the family, New York, 1987, Plenum Press, pp. 317-45.

Marciano TD: Homosexual marriages and parenthood should not be allowed. In Feldman H and Feldman M, editors: Current controversies in marriage and family, Beverly Hills, 1985, Sage Publications, pp. 293-302.

Mills D: A model for stepfamily development, Fam Rel, 33:365-72, 1984.

National Center for Health Statistics: Advance report of final natality statistics, 1987, U.S. Department of Health and Human Services, 38(Suppl 3):1989a.

National Center for Health Statistics: Children of divorce. DHHS Pub No (PHS) 89-1924. Hyattsville, Md, 1989b, U.S. Department of Health and Human Services.

National Center for Health Statistics: Advance report of final marriage statistics, 1987, Mo Vital Stat Rep 38(suppl 12), Washington, DC, 1987, US Department of Health and Human Services.

National Center for Health Statistics: Advance report of final divorce statistics, 1987, Mo Vital Stat Rep 38(12), Supplement 2, Washington, DC, 1990b US Department of Health and Human Services.

National Center for Health Statistics (1990c): Births, marriages, divorces, and deaths for 1989, Mo Vit Stat Rep. 38(12), Washington, DC, 1990c, US Department of Health and Human Services.

Nye FJ: Role structure and analysis of the family. Beverly Hills, 1976, Sage Publications, Inc.

Olson DH and Lavee Y: Family systems and family stress: a family life cycle perspective. In Kreppner K and Lerner RM, editors, Family systems and life span development, Hillsdale, NJ, 1989, Lawrence Erlbaum Associates, Publishers.

Parrot A and Ellis MJ: Homosexuals should be allowed to marry and have children. In Feldman H and Feldman M: Current controversies in marriage and family, Beverly Hills, 1985, Sage Publications, pp. 303-11.

Pitkin JR and Masnick GS: The relationship between heads and non-heads in the household population: an extension of the headship rate method. In Bongaarts J, Burch TK, and Wachter KW, editors: Family demography: methods and their application, New York, 1987, Oxford University Press, pp. 309-26.

Renvoize J: Going solo: single mothers by choice. Boston, 1985, Routledge & Kegan Publishers.

Rexroat C and Shehan C: The family life cycle and spouses time in housework, J Marr Fam 49:737-50, 1987.

Scanzoni J, Polonko K, Teachman J, and Thompson L: The sexual bond: rethinking families and close relationships. Newbury Park, CA, 1989, Sage Publications, Inc.

Schuaneveldt JD: The interactional framework in the study of the family. In Nye FI and Berardo FM, editors: Emerging conceptual frameworks in family analysis, New York, 1967, Macmillan Publishing Co., Inc.

Settles BH: A perspective on tomorrow's families. In Sussman MB and Steinmetz SK, editors: Handbook of marriage and the family, New York, 1987, Plenum Press, pp. 157-80.

Shapiro ER: Individual change and family development: individualization as a family process. In Falicov CJ, editor: Family transitions: continuity and change over the life cycle, New York, 1988, Guilford Press, pp. 159-80.

Shostak AB: Singlehood. In Sussman MB and Steinmetz SK, editors: Handbook of marriage and the family, New York, 1987, Plenum Press, pp. 355-67.

Smith AD and Reid WJ: Role-sharing marriage, New York, 1986, Columbia University Press.

Social Security Bulletin: Federal poverty guidelines 1989, vol 52, no 3, Washington, DC, 1989, Social Security Administration.

Social Security Bulletin: SSI: Social Security Supplemental

Stevenson J: Issues and crises during middlescence, New York, 1977, Appleton-Century-Crofts.

Sussman MB: From the catbird seat: observations on marriage and the family. In Sussman MB and Steinmetz SK, editors: Handbook of marriage and the family, New York, 1987, Plenum Press, pp. XXXI-XLII.

Teachman JD, Polonko KA, and Scanzoni, J: Demography of the family. In Sussman MB and Steinmetz SK, editors: Handbook of marriage and the family, New York, 1987, Plenum Press, pp. 3-36.

United States Bureau of the Census: Household and family characteristics: March 1985, Current Population Report Series P-20, No. 411, Washington DC, 1986, U.S. Department of Commerce.

United States Bureau of the Census: Statistical abstract of the United States 1989, ed 109, Washington, DC, 1989, U.S. Department of Commerce.

Valentine D: The experience of pregnancy: a developmental process, Fam Rels 31:243-8, 1982.

Visher E and Visher J: Stepfamilies: a guide to working with stepparents and stepchildren, New York, 1979, Brunner/Mazel Publishers.

Watkins SC, Menken JA, and Bongaarts J: Demographic foundations of family change, Am Soc Rev 52:346-58, 1987.

Willekens F: The marital status life table. In Bongaarts J, Burch TK, and Watcher KW, editors: Family demography: methods and their application. New York, 1987, Oxford University Press, pp. 126-49.

Yorburg B: Families and societies: survival or extinction? New York, 1983, Columbia University Press.

THE NURSING PROCESS APPLIED TO FAMILY HEALTH PROMOTION

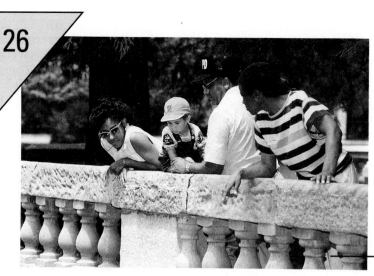

Julia W. Balzer

OBJECTIVES

After reading this chapter, the student should be able to:

Discuss family functioning as a continuum from functional to dysfunctional.

Discuss unrealistic beliefs about marriage and family life that can influence successful family functioning.

Identify family dynamics that may affect how work in the family is accomplished.

Explain the application of the nursing process—assessing, planning, implementing, and evaluating—to family health promotion.

Examine the role of humor and spirituality in working with families.

Apply the nursing process to families experiencing childbearing loss.

KEY TERMS

barriers to change	functional family	problem prioritization
blaming	humor	rescue fantasy
computing	leveling	scapegoat
distracting	multiproblem family	spirituality
dysfunctional family	nursing strategies	systems theory
failed expectations	placating	triangulation
family dynamics		

NOTE: Excerpts from this chapter were contributed by Rosemary Johnson in the first edition of this text.

T his chapter provides information about family assessment and the use of the nursing process as a problem-solving approach to promote family health. The definition of a family includes a variety of traditional and nontraditional family forms. References to the development of a family by the marriage of a couple, a traditional family form, are used in this chapter to simplify the discussion of unmet expectations that influence a family's success. A clinical application section on promoting health in a family experiencing childbearing loss is included.

FAMILY ASSESSMENT

In theory, family functioning exists on a continuum from the highly *functional family* to the severely *dysfunctional family.* In reality, every family has strengths and weaknesses.

Otto provides criteria for assessing family strengths, "those factors or forces that contribute to family unity and solidarity and that foster the development of the potentials inherent within the family" (Otto, 1963, p. 88). This framework has been useful for community health nurses in family assessment and planning family health care programs. The nurses and the family work together to identify and develop its strengths and use them in family problem solving (Otto, 1973)(see box below).

The Family as a System

The application of social systems theory to the family unit demonstrates the complexity of family functioning. Some critics of nursing education contend that there is heavy emphasis on the wellness and illness of the individual within nursing curricula, with minimal attention given to the family.

Systems theory teaches the nurse to be aware that the health status of any one family member affects that of all the other members. The general health practices of the entire family, based on their values, attitudes, and beliefs about

wellness and illness, in turn affect the health status of each individual. Some nurses approach the study of families with some degree of ethnocentricity, assuming that because they were part of a family they already understand all there is to know about families. (Chapter 25 offers several approaches to the systematic study of families to assist in the development of a family approach.)

The family does not survive alone; it interacts with its environment, society. Its functioning depends on what is happening in society. A family assessment model useful in clinical practice, and one that illustrates the application of systems theory, is shown in Figure 26-1. The outer circle represents family components for assessment. The inner circles represent family members with the same components. A stressor is an event that could potentially upset the homeostasis, or balance, of the family's ability to cope with life's problems. The five components to be assessed provide information about whether the event is causing a crisis state that would require assistance from outside the family to restore equilibrium.

Aguilera and Messick (1990) suggest three balancing factors that must be assessed to determine whether a crisis state exists: whether the person has a realistic perception of the event, whether the person has adequate coping skills, and whether an adequate support system exists. The family as a whole, for example, may be coping adequately with its tasks in the face of acute illness of one of its members, but one family member may be identified as needing additional support.

Family Dynamics

Family dynamics influences the work of the family, that is, its ability to complete its functions and tasks. From research on families and through family therapy, much information about family dynamics has been generated. An understanding of these dynamics assists the community health nurse in both collection and interpretation of data for family assessment. Figure 26-1 is an example.

Functional versus Dysfunctional Families

Identification of weaknesses in family functioning is important because they affect the family's ability to promote health. Minuchin and his colleagues (1975) theorized that certain family factors are related to the disease process in children. They studied diabetes mellitus, asthma, and anorexia nervosa. Characteristics such as overprotectiveness, rigidity, poor conflict resolution skills, and involvement of a child in conflict between parents were found to be more prevalent in "psychosomatic families." The overprotectiveness adversely affects individual family members' sense of competence and autonomy. This inhibits a sense of personal control and participation in problem solving, which the nurse seeks to encourage in health promotion.

In contrast, Pratt (1976) suggests that certain types of families have structural or undetermined patterns that are associated with coping with illness without major disruption. She calls these "energized families," characterized by frequent intrafamily communication, community ties, promotion of autonomy, creative problem solving using family strengths and goals, and flexibility in role changes in the family (Turk and Kerns, 1985). The nurse builds on family

---

CRITERIA FOR ASSESSING FAMILY'S STRENGTHS

The ability to provide for the physical, emotional, and spiritual needs of a family

The ability to be sensitive to the needs of the family members

The ability to communicate effectively

The ability to provide support, security, and encouragement

The ability to initiate and maintain growth-producing relationships and experiences within and without the family

The capacity to maintain and create constructive and responsible community relationships in the neighborhood, the school, town, local and state governments

The ability to grow with and through children

The ability to perform family roles flexibly

An ability for self-help and the ability to accept help when appropriate

Mutual respect for the individuality of family members

The ability to use a crisis experience or seemingly injurious experience as a means of growth

A concern for family unity, loyalty, and interfamily cooperation

Adapted from Otto HE: Fam Process 2:333, 1963.

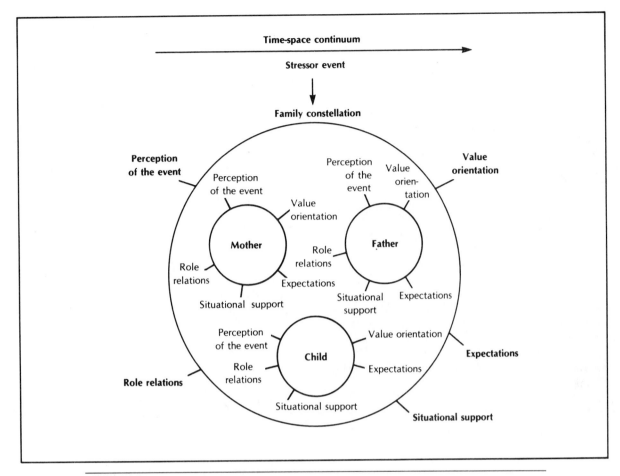

FIGURE 26-1

A model for assessment and crisis intervention with families. (Used with permission. From Oehrtman, S.E.: Assessment and crisis intervention: a model for the family, In Hall, J. E., and Weaver, B. R., editors: Nursing of families in crisis, Philadelphia, 1974, J.B. Lippincott Co.)

assessment skills (discussed later in this chapter) and evaluates problems, strengths, and resources in a variety of areas of assessment. The nurse assists the family to accomplish developmental family tasks that are unmet and assesses which family health functions and tasks are being met and which need to be supplemented to assist in health promotion. The concept of a "normal" family that has been presented in the media adds to confusion for children in the face of the reality of high divorce rates. One preadolescent whose parents share custody struggled with the notion of two homes and two parents who were seeking new definitions of self during their midlife years. Although the child was receiving counseling to assist with coping and was functioning in school and athletics, he lamented all of the changes in his life and longed for "normal" parents and a "normal" family. His mother told him, "As sad as it may seem, I think we may be a normal family these days." Assistance may be needed because family life is not always what the family expects.

Failed Expectations

When family life is not smooth and members are not healthy and happy, the family experiences *failed expectations,* which arise from myths about marriage, the faulty notion

that life must be fair, and the belief that the family members will always be healthy.

Myths About Marriage

Relationships in families are complex. In a marriage, for a nurse to listen to one spouse's point of view without consideration of the other's is to disregard the interaction patterns that may reveal how the family system works. It is impossible to quantitatively measure a healthy marriage. It is helpful, however, to consider some of the false assumptions with which marital systems are begun that lead to the family's inability to perform its functions and tasks. Lederer and Jackson (1968) identified seven false assumptions, discussed below in the box, which they call the "mirage" of marriage.

Myths in a family can serve as that family's reality. Family members may not have information about how people in other, perhaps healthier, families relate. Children may assume that it is their role to mediate in parental conflict. This can drain needed energy from the child's own quest for autonomy and independence. A child may assume that open expression of anger or disagreement is bad. This can prevent the child from developing problem-solving skills in which alternative behaviors are considered.

FALSE ASSUMPTIONS ABOUT MARRIAGE

1. **It is assumed that people get married because they love each other.** Many partners get together for reasons such as the sexual excitement of courtship, societal pressures, loneliness, a desire to better themselves, or neurotic needs to continue a pattern of relating that may be unhappy but familiar and thus comfortable.

2. **Most married people love each other.** Partners may feel they are trying to make a marriage work while actually they are acting destructively in the name of love. A wife may love to cook and see this as a way to define what a good wife, mother, and woman she is. The family members are becoming overweight. Although they may try to limit what they eat, in doing so they feel guilty and rejecting of the wife and mother who provides large quantities of rich food as a sign of love.

3. **"Romantic" love is essential for a satisfactory marriage.** Our culture worships romantic love and fosters the notion that a marriage must sparkle to be successful. Such beliefs contribute to divorce as a substitute for the work, compromise, and problem solving that is necessary to sustain any relationship.

4. **There are inherent differences between attitudes and behaviors of men and women that cause most marital difficulties.** Men and women have been socialized into different roles, and when traditional roles are challenged, the marriage may suffer. Flexibility is a keynote of a successful marriage. Roles may need to be alternated, depending on the current lifestyle, and roles may need to be merged in times of illness.

5. **Having children automatically improves a problematic marriage.** The attention a child demands for its well-being may serve to take the focus temporarily off a troubled dyadic relationship but, at best, problems may be postponed. Couples may project their hopes on their children to live the perfect lives they themselves were unable to achieve, thus unrealistic life expectations are transmitted to the future generation.

6. **Loneliness will be cured by marriage.** Often two people whose social skills are minimal marry and expect the other to bring satisfaction in the social arena. Each blames the other for bringing inadequacies to the marriage. Such couples seem to be chronically unhappy and socially isolated.

7. **If one spouse expresses open anger toward the other, a poor marriage exists.** It is impossible for there to be agreement at all times in a relationship. When conflict arises, one spouse may need to act in opposition to the other to meet personal needs and then work through the conflict. Consistent agreement is unusual. It is likely in such a relationship that one spouse is quietly giving in to the other and will eventually feel justified at getting even.

Interpreting Life

A family may have the unrealistic expectation that life is and must always be fair; in fact, life is difficult. Even if a person does all the right things, crises occur. Peck (1978), a psychiatrist, writes that once a person accepts this, life is no longer difficult. Peck offers four tools for dealing with the pain of life's problems:

1. Delay of gratification
2. Acceptance of responsibility
3. Dedication to truth
4. Balancing

Some families are able to continue to function in the face of catastrophe without denial of the reality of life's difficulty. In practice, this means one is able to put personal preferences aside, accept responsibility for the task of problem solving and hard work, face life changes, work through denial, and retain a sense of perspective and balance to life.

An example of a family who has been able to use these tools is a family whose 30-year-old son, John, was receiving the services of a home health-care agency. This son was brain damaged as the result of an assault 7 years earlier. As a result of the brain damage, John was blind, confined to a wheelchair most of the time, and had limited intellectual ability and a very short attention span. John continued to live with his parents because his wife had sought a divorce. When discussing the family's situation, John's father advised that one must give up the bitterness. This bitterness is a sign of a family being unable to move beyond the insistence that life has to be fair, that the catastrophe is undeserved and unacceptable.

John's family accepted the fact that life presents unexpected problems. Coping skills included the ability to rely on religious faith, support from friends, continued involvement with community activities, and budgeting for the son's financial resources received from litigation. John's siblings are prepared to accept responsibility for his care when his parents are no longer able. John's parents look forward to retirement, when they will be able to offer John more environmental stimulation. They are adding ramps and a deck to their home to increase John's mobility.

This family was able to use the tools Peck described to face an unexpected difficulty, ". . . common people, made uncommon by hardship . . ." (Dotson, 1985, p. 37).

Another expectation unlikely to be fulfilled is that all the family members will be healthy. People do not usually plan to be sick and dismiss thoughts of accidents, thinking that such things only happen to other people. Consider a couple who has saved money and planned for an early retirement in which they would travel. The husband is then fatally injured in an auto accident caused by an intoxicated driver. Unrealistic expectations of freedom from disease and catastrophe seem irrational and ridiculous to the experienced nurse; however, people embrace and operate on false assumptions and myths such as these.

Altered Family Communication Styles Under Stress

The family experiences stress when failed expectations occur, and this stress can alter the members' communication styles. Patterns have emerged from systematic study of families (Satir, 1972). Four problematic communication styles are *blaming, placating, computing,* and *distracting;* a healthy style is termed *leveling.*

Blaming

For some people, a serious threat to self-esteem arises when something goes wrong. A simplistic example is a man who sees himself as thoroughly organized and responsible yet forgets a dental appointment. This view of himself, which he holds as an important part of being a competent person, is threatened. At some level he says to himself "This is awful. If I have forgotten this appointment I cannot be organized and responsible. I can't have made a mistake, It must be someone else's fault." As the pressure mounts, he reacts, almost automatically, by blaming. He accuses his wife of not reminding him and moves into blaming behavior, acting and speaking in an accusatory manner.

This same blaming behavior may be seen when a family who cannot accept the failure of chemotherapy in the treatment of a family member with cancer accuses the nurse for somehow being at fault. A nurse who does not understand these dynamics may react defensively, deny blame, or retreat from the family, leaving them isolated with their pain. A more helpful response from the nurse is to acknowledge how difficult the situation is and reaffirm willingness to continue to work with the family. Further experience teaches the nurse that time and patience are often the only possible interventions. The most carefully phrased therapeutic responses of empathy cannot stop the patient from dying.

When persons continue to blame, it protects them from the anxiety that always accompanies change. In the first example, the change needed is in organizational skills. The person may note appointments on a calendar and check it daily or may need to understand and accept that everyone makes mistakes. An appointment can be rescheduled. In the second example, the change needed is in the expectation that life will provide happiness and health for all family members. The family needs to be supported while accepting the terminal illness of the family member.

Placating

Some people have such low self-esteem that it seems natural for them to accept blame even for situations in which they could not possibly be at fault. A placator moves automatically to accept the blame. The placator seeks reinforcement of the view of self as worthless or useless. Consider the wife of the man who missed the appointment. Suppose the wife does not make dental appointments for the husband and keeps no record of them. It is unreasonable that she would accept blame. It would be more helpful to help the husband figure out how he could prevent the problem from recurring.

Placating behavior also may be seen when a child is injured in a bicycle accident. A mother who placates might blame herself for allowing the child to ride a bicycle. A father who tends to blame under stress might reinforce the mother's guilt. The mother may become more overprotective instead of teaching the child safety rules and the expectation that life will present problems with which the child must cope. At this time, the nurse might intervene to focus on problem solving about specifics such as how the child will attend school with a leg cast. The nurse understands that communication patterns under stress become familiar ways of coping and are difficult to change.

Computing

Some people think than expressing feelings is a sign of weakness. It is more important to appear in control during times of stress. There is an overwhelming fear of not being able to control one's life. The person who relies on computing may talk coldly, use big words, and appear rigid and tense. Consider a woman whose husband returns home after hospitalization for treatment of serious heart disease. She focuses on prescribed treatment of the disease, asks questions focused on medical issues, but never seems to express any emotion. An inexperienced nurse might conclude that this woman does not have any feeling for her husband, that she is denying the seriousness of the disease, or perhaps that she is functioning out of a sense of duty rather than love. Observation of communication patterns within the family might reveal that one way the woman copes with stress is to control her responses and thus insulate herself from the overwhelming fears that her husband may die, that she might be left alone, and that she might have to face her complete lack of ability to control life.

Distracting

Some people seem easily overwhelmed in the face of stress. A distractor is someone whose behavioral response to a situation seems irrelevant, completely unrelated to the situation at hand. Consider a woman whose breast biopsy reveals that she has a malignancy. A distractor might offer to fix coffee for the nurse or pick lint off her sweater. This person is so unable to focus on the event or its effect on herself or others that she shuts all of it off from her immediate attention. Her conversation may be tangential and her movements actually distracting to the nurse. A nurse might intervene by speaking slowly, calling the woman by name, attempting eye contact, and acknowledging how difficult it must be to hear this information. High levels of anxiety decrease this person's ability to hear and remember details. Knowing this, the nurse can gently reintroduce the subject and spend time with this woman and her family as she attempts to focus her attention on the issue at hand.

Leveling

A healthy communication style under stress is leveling. The goal in communication between family members is for members to be able to say what they feel and believe. No feeling is bad. Feelings are amoral, neither good nor bad; they simply exist. It is no worse to experience anger, sadness, or boredom than it is to experience happiness or elation. The nurse looks for ways to help family members speak for themselves and not through another member. The nurse helps family members to ask each other for what they need and not to expect that a loved one automatically knows what will offer comfort or expect the others to "mind-read." The nurse models this through personal assertive communication with the family.

The Triangle

Triangulation is an important concept in understanding the communication between family members. How a family communicates affects the work of the family, its ability to cope with problems, and its ability to promote health among its members (Bowen, 1971).

Whenever two people form a relationship, the issues of closeness and personal need conflict. How much closeness is enough? How much closeness is too much? A couple trying to live together in the same environment is composed of two different people with different personal preferences. To compromise and make changes to live harmoniously takes energy and causes anxiety. Change produces anxiety because people are fearful of losing something valuable of themselves. Sometimes, rather than dealing with the anxiety that comes when conflict resolution is needed, a third person; two or more persons such as parents or in-laws; an object, such as a pet or boat; or an issue, such as work or alcoholism, will be used.

If a person can turn to or focus on a person, an object, or an issue, there is less need for change. For example, a wife remains silent when she disagrees with her husband but turns to her mother to berate her husband. A husband begins working later and later even though it is not necessary and apologizes for never being home with his wife with whom he is in current conflict over future career plans. A mother and father continue to have children they cannot afford financially or emotionally and live in constant chaos without any time to work on their own troubled marriage. The mother, the job, and the children have been brought in to serve as the third point of a triangle, to take the attention and focus away from working on the conflict normally experienced in a dyad. This tension-reducing mechanism prevents people from working on relationship issues and problem solving needed to promote family health.

Family members may attempt to involve the nurse in triangulation. The wife of a patient with heart disease may complain to the nurse about her husband's dependency on her and her inability to participate in any activities outside the home. For the nurse to accept this as the complete picture and to intervene with the husband strictly on the data given by the wife is to ignore the complexity of a family system and the concept of triangulation. When the wife complains to the nurse, she feels better, is less anxious, and is less motivated to work out the relationship with the husband. The nurse might listen initially and then redirect the wife to discuss this with the husband, and the nurse might be with her while she discusses it. The nurse will consider the information given by the wife when offering client education to the husband about his increasing level of activity. The nurse might initiate a discussion of his concern, knowing that change in the role of any family member affects the roles and lives of all other family members. The nurse must not assume the responsibility to "fix" the relationship between the husband and wife.

The Scapegoat

Failed expectations in families often produce further problems. What if family members are unhappy and life is not smooth? Some people come to believe that someone must be at fault. Blame can become pervasive in a family and can be focused on one member. In some families one member is unconsciously chosen as the *scapegoat,* the focus of all family difficulties. It is as if everyone believed that if only this one member were not ill, everything else would proceed smoothly, and everyone in the family would live

happily ever after. This dynamic may operate in families in which mental illness exists and the family wants an agency or healthcare worker to "do something" or remove the family member. A less severe example is a family in which an elderly woman lived most of her later years with her daughter, son-in-law, and their children. Whenever anything was misplaced or lost, everyone complained "Well, Grandma took it" or "Grandma is always giving our things away." The elderly woman began to have transient ischemic attacks, finally a stroke, and was placed in a nursing home. Then whenever the family misplaced or lost things, they learned it was not Grandma's fault.

Family dynamics can affect the nurse's ability to collect data and the family's ability to resolve problems. Recognition of communication patterns under stress enables the nurse to assist family members in better problem solving. The nurse can avoid siding with one family member when information about the nature of triangles is applied to family communication. Families that attempt to focus all family problems on one member may be using that member as a scapegoat and may require assistance from a mental health resource.

COMMUNITY HEALTH NURSING PROCESS WITH FAMILIES

The implementation of the nursing process is the foundation of nursing practice. Basic information about its application is found throughout this text and others. How the nurse uses the nursing process to promote health in families and how this is different from work with individual clients are the issues discussed in this chapter.

The family is more complex than the nurse will ever be permitted to see. Nurses work with data from family assessment in addition to data from individual assessment; this makes the process more complicated. Nurses continue to add data and change plans as a more complex view of the family begins to emerge. Nurses also recognize the effect of family dynamics not only on family life but also on how data are analyzed. Nurses reexamine their own values when confronted with lifestyles and value systems that may be unfamiliar or at least easier to minimize in the hospital or clinic setting, the nurse's "turf." It is important to remember that information about health promotion can only be made available to the family; the task of health promotion belongs to the family and can only be facilitated by the nurse (See Appendix C-4 on Lifestyle Assessment).

Assessment
Initiating Contact

Before contacting the family, the nurse clarifies with the referral source the purpose of the contact. The nurse is not a member of the family, and the contact, often involving intimate family business, may be considered an invasion of privacy if it is not clear to the family why the nurse is involved.

Data Collection

An example of a family assessment tool can be found in Appendix B3, Family Health Assessment Guide. The boxed material contains a helpful summary of the assessment cat-

FAMILY HEALTH ASSESSMENT SUMMARY TO ORGANIZE DATA COLLECTION

Consider in each category 1. Family problems/stresses
                                          2. Family strengths
                                          3. Family resources
Family composition: socioeconomic information
Family environment: residence, neighborhood, community
Family structure: roles, division of labor, authority and power, values
Family processes: communication patterns, decision making, problem solving
Family functions: physical, emotional, social
Family coping: conflict, life changes, support systems, life satisfaction
Family health behavior: health history, health status, activities of daily living, risk behaviors, health beliefs, self-care, health care resources, community health nursing service (attitudes and expectations)

egories and three issues to assess in each category used; family problems/stresses, family strengths, and family resources.

The nurse begins the family assessment by stating the initial reason for contact with the family, the identified client, and the client's health problem. Haley (1978, p. 9), a family therapist, noted that "If therapy is to end properly, it must begin properly—by negotiating a solvable problem." Trainees in family work will function "more effectively using a concrete, problem-oriented framework" (Weber, 1985, p. 358). Family assessment initially focuses on how family functioning will affect the progress of the client and how the client's health problem will affect other members, their roles and functioning, and the total family's functioning. Working with the family, the nurse can collect data that may lead to the identification of other health problems and identify areas for family health promotion. (See Chapters 25 to 27 and Appendix C, Health Risk Appraisal Forms.) Table 26-1 presents family-specific risk factors and related health problems in each stage of family development. This information gives the nurse clues to potential problems throughout the life cycle.

Johnson (1984) suggests several approaches for the collection of family data: the interview, the questionnaire, and the participant-observer method. The nurse can use a structured interview in which specific questions are asked from a prepared list. This technique is useful for short-answer factual data. A nonstructured interview allows for elaboration and open-ended questions but requires skill in keeping the interview focused on appropriate content. A typical question might be "What kinds of things do you do in your family to protect your health?"

Questionnaires may be useful to collect data from family members who are not available for interviews. The Lifestyle Assessment Questionnaire in Appendix C1 is an example of a self-report questionnaire. Attention must be paid to the reading abilities of the family members asked to provide data by this method.

The participant-observer method allows the nurse to col-

lect data about family dynamics and problem-solving skills. Cross (1986) provides a lengthy clinical example of verbatim data collection and its analysis. Additional sources of information include contacts with older human service personnel working with the family (Johnson, 1984).

Nurses might look over a list of areas of concern before contacting the family to help focus thinking during the meeting. They can review developmental tasks appropriate for each age level and observe for evidence of them (see Chapters 28-32 and Appendix A, Individual Assessment Tools) and the tasks and functions appropriate for the current stage of family life development. It is helpful to make anecdotal notes immediately after the meeting. Initially it is difficult to juggle so many concepts at once, but as nurses gain personal and professional experience, they become more comfortable and familiar with the signs and symptoms of the various stages of family life development and are better able to interpret the current stage of the client family.

Planning
Individualized Plans

It is important to remember that the family has its own agenda for how the nurse will be of use. The family or some of its members may prefer to focus solely on the original reason for contact. In these families, the nurse assists the family to meet the identified need. The nurse builds trust and, through assessment and education, identifies some mutually agreed-on problem to pursue.

Another family or one of its members may be struggling with a more urgent concern, such as needing money to pay their heating bill in a severe winter. The nurse may assist the family with the identified problem by helping the family to contact the appropriate community resource. After this need is met, the family may be ready to return to the problem for which the nursing contact was initiated.

Another family may identify the nurse as a much needed resource and greet the nurse with eager questions. In this case the nurse is challenged to provide assistance and grows professionally with the family as they learn together new ways to promote health.

Community health nurses are often faced with multiproblem families, and because of this, it is easy to forget that most families deal with their problems and rely on the problem-solving skills they have learned from other family members. Nurses learn from these families in their practices and use this knowledge to help other families cope. A newspaper article (Holland, 1986) describing health problems in a subdivision illustrates the difficulties of working with multiproblem families and some of the environmental hazards that hinder health promotion and limit interventions by community health nurses. This community had no indoor plumbing, no indoor source of water, no paved roads, no central heat, and no regular pick-up of garbage. At the time the subdivision was built, no zoning laws existed to regulate the area's development. These poor conditions resulted in unusually high rates of intestinal parasites and stomach problems in the residents.

Residents had been frustrated with attempts to get assistance. The article reported that a government grant had been promised to remedy some of the community problems. The

TABLE 26-1
Family-specific risk factors and related health problems

Stage	Risk factors	Health problems
Couple and child-bearing family	Lack of knowledge concerning family planning Teenage marriage Lack of knowledge concerning sexual and marital roles and adjustments Lack of prenatal care Inadequate nutrition Underweight or overweight Poor food habits Smoking, alcohol, and drug abuse Unmarried status First pregnancy before age 16 or after age 35 History of hypertension and infections during pregnancy Rubella, syphillis, gonorrhea, and autoimmune deficiency syndrome (AIDS) Genetic factors present Low socioeconomic status Lack of safety in the home	Premature pregnancies Unsuccessful marriage Low-birth weight infant Birth defects Birth injuries Accidents Sudden infant deaths
Family with school-aged children	Home unsafe Home not stimulating Working parents with inappropriate use of resources for child care Poverty environment Abuse and/or neglect of children Generational pattern of using social agencies as way of life Multiple, closely spaced children Low family self-esteem Child or children used as scapegoat for parental frustration Repeated infections, accidents, and hospitalizations Parents immature, dependent, and unable to handle responsibility Unrecognized or unattended health problems Strong beliefs about physical punishment for obedience Toxic substances unprotected in the home Poor nutrition (overeating or undereating)	Birth defects Behavior disturbances Speech and vision problems Communicable diseases Dental caries School problems Learning disabilities Cancer
Family with adolescents	Racial and ethnic family origin Lifestyle and behavior patterns leading to chronic disease Lack of problem-solving skills Family values of aggressiveness and competition Socioeconomic factors contributing to peer relationships Family values rigid and inflexible Daredevil risk-taking attitudes Denial behavior Conflicts between parents and children Pressure to live up to family expectations	Violent deaths and injuries Alcohol and drug abuse Unwanted pregnancy Sexually transmissible diseases Suicide
Family with middle-aged adults	Hypertension Smoking High-cholesterol diet Diabetes Overweight Physical inactivity Personality patterns related to stress Genetic predisposition Use of oral contraceptives Sex, race, and other hereditary factors Geographic area, age, and occupational deficiencies Habits (diet with low fiber, pickling, charcoal use, broiling) Alcohol and smoking Exposure to certain substances (sunlight, radiation, water or air pollution) Social class Residence	Cardiovascular disease, principally coronary artery disease and cerebrovascular accident (stroke) Cancer Accidents Homicide Suicide Abnormal fetus Mental illness

Adapted from Healthy people: The Surgeon General's report on health promotion and disease prevention, Health and Human Services Pub. No. 79-55071, Washington, DC, 1982, US Government Printing Office.
From McCarthy, N.C.: Health promotion and the family. In Edelman, C., and Mandle, C.L., editors: Health promotion throughout the lifespan, ed. 2, St. Louis, 1990, The C.V. Mosby Co.

TABLE 26-1
Family-specific risk factors and related health problems—cont'd

Stage	Risk factors	Health problems

Family with older adults	Depression
	Gingivitis
	Age
	Drug interactions
	Depression
	Metabolic disorders
	Pituitary malfunctions
	Hypercalcemia
	Cushing's syndrome
	Chronic illness
		Periodontal disease and
		    loss of teeth
		Mental confusion
		Reduced vision
		Hearing impairment
		Hypertension
		Acute illness
		Infectious diseases
		Influenza
		Pneumonia
		Injuries such as burns
		    and falls
		Depression

	Retirement Loss of spouse Reduced income Poor nutrition Lack of exercise Past environments and lifestyle Lack of preparation for death	Death without dignity

residents were skeptical and remained "locked in a living time warp, a community of numbing poverty and neglect . . ." (Holland, 1986, p. A-12).

Community health nurses conducted a study to provide documentation of internal parasites in preschool and school-aged children living in the community. Nurses checked these children regularly and treated them for whipworms and round worms. They identified sources of contamination of water by sewage and concluded that the lack of adequate sanitation contributed to high-risk pregnancies.

Families in this community struggled unsuccessfully to meet the lowest level of needs. Interventions focused on Maslow's hierarchy of self-actualization would have been inappropriate. The community health nurse had to meet these families where they were and support their community's efforts to make progress.

Prioritizing Problems

As the nurse reviews data collected about the family, it is helpful to identify problems, strengths, and resources in each area of assessment (see box on p. 459 and Family Problem-Solving Guide, Appendix B4, for details).

When a list of problems is developed, the nurse can simplify *problem prioritization* by using predetermined criteria, such as the following:

1. Family awareness of the problem
2. Family motivation to resolve or better manage the problem
3. Nurse's ability to influence problem solution
4. Availability of family or community resources to solve the problem
5. Severity of the consequences if the problem is unresolved
6. Quickness with which resolution can be achieved

Chapter 16 describes a method for rating and ranking the problems that are identified.

For example, a nurse may be working with the family of a child who will be needing insulin injections. The nurse's assessment is that the mother works during the hours the injections are needed and is limited intellectually. The mother's sister lives in the home and is willing and able to give the injections. For these reasons, the nurse, with agreement from the mother, instructs the aunt. Short-term goals focus on the aunt's being able to give the injection. This goal is evaluated by a return demonstration. Also, the family needs information about the administration of the medication, its importance, and possible reactions to the medication before the members can work on the long-term goals of accepting information about the possibility of long-range complications of the illness. The nurse supports the family in its use of various family members for resources. An older sibling of the child tells the aunt and nurse that a friend of his also has diabetes. He contributes that this child's mother said "Pow!" to distract the child when the needle was inserted. The aunt was able to use this suggestion, and the nurse helped the aunt to add this step into the steps for giving the injection.

The nurse works with the family in an ongoing process to implement strategies to promote health. It remains the family's choice as to its desire to work on the problems identified, with or without nursing intervention.

The nurse and the family may disagree about what are health problems that need resolution. For example, cigarette smoking presents a high-risk situation to individual health and to nonsmokers in the environment with the smoker, but smoking may be seen by the client as a much needed coping device to deal with anxiety.

Rescue Fantasies

The nurse must remember who owns the problem and beware of rescue fantasies. A *rescue fantasy* is a well-intentioned intervention by a helping person who unwittingly attempts to take over the person's problems to solve them for the client. For the nurse, a sign to indicate that rescue fantasies are in operation is feeling an unnecessary sense of urgency about the individual's or family's work on a certain problem. The nurse may become attached to a specific intervention similar to a personal course of action in such a situation and may be unable to stop insisting on a course of action, even when it becomes obvious that the family will not pursue it. An essential quality for a community health nurse is self-awareness, an understanding of personal strengths and limitations (see the box for a list of other qualities). All nurses need to be able to seek supervision, a problem-solving and perspective process, when a relationship with a client becomes too intense or too clouded for the nurse to analyze alone.

Consider a nurse who had made a personal decision to have an abortion when faced with an unplanned pregnancy. The nurse makes the assessment that the client, an unmarried, pregnant teenager, is not physically, emotionally, or financially prepared to parent a child. The nurse becomes attached to this young woman and envisions a different life for her, a better life. She finds herself wanting to advise the girl to have an abortion. The nurse seeks supervision from another community health nurse who helps the nurse recognize that the final decision must be made by the client, her family, and the baby's father.

PERSPECTIVE FOR THE CAREGIVER AND THE CLIENT

Seasoned community health nurses recognize two concepts that assist caregivers and clients experiencing increasing complexities in their lives. These are humor and spiritually.

Humor

Humor is an attitude that assists in facing the incongruities of life. (Robinson, 1977). Humor can assist nurses in preventing burnout while facing difficult issues. It can assist clients and their families in coping with illness and adversities. Robinson lists five purposes of humor in nursing:

1. To establish warm interpersonal relationships
2. To relieve anxiety, stress, and tension
3. To release anger, hostility, and aggression
4. To avoid or deny feelings that are too painful and stressful at the time
5. To facilitate the process of learning

These apply to clients and to nurses.

Three criteria for the appropriate use of humor in nursing have been identified. (Leiber, 1986). Questions nurses should ask for evaluation of a humorous intervention are:

1. Is the content in good taste? Does it make light of self rather than others? Is it nonoffensive? Avoid racist or sexist humor.
2. Is this the right time? In an emergency, people want prompt professional care and might interpret humor as insensitive. Humor may be more useful in assisting the client to adjust to chronic illness.
3. Is the person receptive? Some people see humor as an interruption in the serious business of life. Some see it as a sinful waste of time. It is important to respect individual differences and watch for cues that humor is useful to the client.

A playful attitude, positive thinking, and hope are useful skills to nurses. A sense of humor helps nurses to keep their perspective and take the work seriously, but take themselves lightly (Paulson, 1989). One nurse humorist provided community health nurses with bottles of bubbles to blow for comic relief when the paper work demands exceed the allotted time (Balzer, 1990). Another nurse shared a story of the rooster that chased the nurse outside the client's home. The client informed the nurse that it was an "attack" rooster. That story resurfaced in the office in tough times. Victor Borge said, "Laughter is the shortest distance between two people."

For some families humor is a natural coping device. Nurses can build on this survival skill. A nurse-clown working for a hospice related a story of an elderly man whose illness slowed him physically. The nurse bought him a button that he wore regularly with pride. The button featured a turtle with the words, "I may be slow, but I won the race." This humanized his symptoms and fostered their working relationship.

A bitter wit or tough cynicism can provide a protective distance for a client and is sometimes used by survivors of child sexual abuse (Bass and Davis, 1988), but it also can give clues to areas for further exploration. A note of caution: Some people use humor to deny serious problems in their lives. As with any use of denial it can minimize a problem that needs assessment. It is useful to listen to what the patient takes lightly. An offhand, joking comment might indicate a concern that needs further exploration.

ESSENTIAL QUALITIES FOR THE COMMUNITY HEALTH NURSE TO PROMOTE HEALTH IN FAMILIES

Holistic approach: looks for ways to promote wellness
Family centered approach: looks for how illness of one member affects all others
Nonjudgmental: recognizes that one may never have all the facts that affect another's actions
Accepting of different value system
Self-awareness: continues to increase understanding of personal weaknesses and strengths
Comfortable in nonstructured environment: is able to work with distractions
Forgiving of self and client when perfection is not possible
Sensitive, with sense of timing, awareness of another's pain
Flexible: if one tactic fails, tries another
Tolerant of the emotions of everyday life
Confident in skills
Independent in nursing judgments
Self-starter
Able to terminate a relationship
Assertive
Able to manage personal stress
Meets personal needs outside of work setting
Common sense

Spirituality

Spirituality is a way of life, centered in a human connection with a higher power (Arnold, 1989). A clear understanding of personal spirituality can assist the caregiver and the client. When nurses confront illness and social conditions that test the foundation of their personal belief systems, adverse stress reactions can erupt spontaneously. Arnold calls this erosion of the spirit. She suggests that burnout is an existential crisis of meaning in which nurses' deepest beliefs are in doubt. When a religious framework provides only rules and regulations and does not address situations that seem unfair, meaningless, and without solutions, nurses may flounder. To come to a personal spirituality that includes a belief in a higher purpose is to be able to seek meaning in the incomprehensible circumstances of pain and suffering.

Nurses' comfort with spirituality can assist clients in their life journeys. Again nurses should look for cues that the client is receptive to such discussion, but the nurse may open the conversation with questions about what provides strength and support. One hospital chaplain who works with oncology patients refers to the "ministry of listening." The intimate nature of the care given by nurses and aides often elicits clients deep concerns and fears in their search for meaning in illness. Quinn (1989) notes that some clients who may never be cured may be healed and cites an example of a frail elderly woman who finds a profound sense of peace in an ever-deepening spirituality in spite of increasing infirmity. Within each life crisis there is a problem and a lesson to be learned. Nurses help the client to move the focus from what is negative about the situation to what is to be learned—the lesson—the more positive aspect of the event.

IMPLEMENTATION OF INTERVENTIONS

Peitze (1984) suggests that family nursing care focus on transitions into parenthood, adulthood, loss from death or disability, and illness from the acute to chronic to rehabilitative stages. She describes nursing care as a bridge for the family that provides assistance with problem-solving, coping behaviors, and evaluation of health outcomes. The family is encouraged to see itself as competent to cope with the present and future. Peitze (1984, p. 235) delineates concrete nursing interventions:

1. Discussing behaviors and conversation of family members that demonstrate functional and dysfunctional areas of coping
2. Providing direct care to meet physical and emotional needs
3. Providing education and educational materials
4. Identifying appropriate resources (e.g., agencies, people, supplies, support groups)
5. Providing compassionate support throughout the nurse-patient, nurse-family relationship
6. Clarifying ways family members can and do contribute to individual and family health

Table 26-2 provides examples of interventions for health promotion and disease prevention through each stage of family development.

Barriers to Change

Transition in families means change. Change brings anxiety as the family deals with unknowns. The nurse assists the family in problem identification and prioritization, but *barriers to change* in behavior may exist that affect the family's move toward problem resolution.

The family may not understand a need for change in behavior. The family may habitually use defense mechanisms such as denial, repression, or rationalization to lessen the threat of change. Although these defenses help the client handle anxiety, they may impede the change process. The nurse can gradually decrease the client's anxiety by providing information about the disease process and ways to cope with it, thus making it possible for the client to give up the initial defense against anxiety.

A *multiproblem family* may feel powerless to control what happens to it and to effect change based on past life experiences. The nurse helps the family set small, attainable goals and focuses on successes to build the client's view of self as someone who can become more healthy.

The family may value the very behavior the nurse targets for change. For example, the family may be used to serving steak as frequently as possible as a symbol of their prosperity and ability to provide for members. If red meat is to be limited in the father's diet to promote health, the family may be reluctant to give it up.

The client may have unrealistic expectations of life and may not believe that serious illness could strike the family. The nurse helps the family cope with the diagnosis of disease in gradual steps and, if necessary, links the family to an appropriate support group (Cobb-McMahon, Williams, and Davis, 1984).

Nursing Strategies

Three *nursing strategies* summarize the community health nurse's use of the nursing process to help the family move toward wellness. (1) *The nurse functions as a health educator* to provide education to assist the family to see how its behavior affects the health of family members. Haggarty (1977, p. 276) states "One's life-style, including patterns of eating, exercise, drinking, coping with stress, and use of tobacco and drugs, together with environmental hazards, are the major known modifiable causes of illnesses in America today."

Based on epidemiological analysis, it is widely believed that the best chance for health promotion lies in decreasing self-destructive habits and increasing sound health practices (McKeown, 1976).

As a health educator, the nurse interprets health information and creates opportunities for the family to participate in health education and related activities (Breckon, Harvey, and Lancaster, 1985). For example, hospitals, competing for the health dollar in this time of change in reimbursement systems, offer health screenings in readily accessible areas such as shopping malls. Hospitals also offer health education classes such as clinics to help stop smoking. Often these are offered at a nominal fee or at no charge to attract future purchases of health care.

(2) *The nurse functions as a problem solver.* As the nurse and family formulate a plan for problem resolution, the nurse

TABLE 26-2

Nurse's role in health promotion and disease prevention through stages of family development

Stage	Nursing role	Stage	Nursing role
Couple	Counselor on sexual and marital role adjustment Teacher and counselor in family planning Teacher of parenting skills Coordinator for genetic counseling Facilitator in interpersonal relationships	Family with adolescents	Teacher of risk factors to health Teacher in problem-solving issues regarding alcohol, smoking, diet, and exercise Facilitator of interpersonal skills with teenagers and parents Direct supporter, counselor, or referrer to mental health resources
Childbearing family	Monitor of prenatal care and referrer for problems of pregnancy Counselor on prenatal nutrition Counselor on prenatal maternal habits Supporter of amniocentesis Counselor on breast-feeding Coordinator with pediatric services Supervisor of immunizations Referrer to social services		Counselor on family planning Referrer for sexually transmittable disease Participant in community organizations on disease control
Family with preschool and school-aged children	Monitor of early childhood development; referrer when indicated Teacher in first-aid and emergency measures Coordinator with pediatric services Supervisor of immunizations Counselor on nutrition and exercise Teacher in problem-solving issues regarding health habits Participant in community organizations for environmental control Teacher of dental care hygiene Counselor on environmental safety in the home Facilitator in interpersonal relationships	Family with young or middle-aged adults	Teacher in problem-solving issues regarding lifestyle and habits Participant in community organizations for environmental control Case finder in the home and community Screener for hypertension, Pap smear, breast examination, cancer signs, mental health, and dental care Counselor on menopausal transition for husband and wife Facilitator in interpersonal relationships among family members
		Family with older adults	Referrer for work and social activity, nutritional programs, homemakers' services, and so on Monitor of exercise, nutrition, preventive services, and medications Supervisor of immunization Counselor on safety in the home

From McCarthy, N.C.: Health promotion and the family. In Edelman, C., and Mandle, C.L., editors: Health promotion throughout the life span, ed. 2. St. Louis, 1990, The C.V. Mosby Co.

suggests possible solutions. This includes asking the client whether such a problem has occurred in the past and, if so, what solutions were used then. (3) *The nurse functions as a resource-linker.* As the nurse assists the family to identify problems, strengths, and resources in each area of assessment, appropriate information is shared about community resources that may not be known to the family. The nurse demonstrates the process of approaching agencies by writing down a phone number and the name of a contact person when possible. With time, the nurse's personal knowledge of community resources grows. It is helpful to carry a community resource book or an address book in which notations

can be added about specific services and helpful contact people. It is also useful to help the family learn how to call a number of agencies, if necessary, to find an appropriate resource.

The support group movement provides community resources for approximately 350 types of health and lifestyle problems. An estimated 15 million people belong to a half million support groups in the United States (Boberg and Hedrick, 1986). Referrals can be made to groups offering support for such conditions as Alzheimer's disease, arthritis, premenstrual syndrome, ostomy, diabetes, impotence, mental illness, and learning disabilities.

Evaluation

The nurse and family use mutually agreed on goals to evaluate the success of nursing intervention. The evaluation that occurs throughout the implementation phase is called *formative* evaluation; *summative* evaluation occurs when the nurse and the family decide whether the relationship needs to continue or should be terminated (see Family Health Care Plan in Appendix B1).

The nurse cannot expect family members to do comprehensive planning and evaluation at each visit. It is important for the nurse to end each visit by clarifying goals for the next meeting, summarizing progress already made, and obtaining input to formulate future goals. Strategies to consider in evaluation when the established plan is not working are the following:

1. Seek information about what prevented follow-through with the plan. Is there a family crisis? Is there a problem with resources such as money or transportation?
2. Review the family's understanding of what they had agreed to do and what the nurse had agreed to do.
3. Determine whether the problem is a priority with the family at this time.
4. Provide further client education about the problem as appropriate.
5. Ask yourself: Am I operating from a personal value system? Am I aware of a sense of personal urgency about this plan or anger with the family that might indicate rescue fantasies? Discuss these issues with nurse supervisors.
6. Reformulate the plan, if appropriate, incorporating the new data.

Three of the assumptions and beliefs about community health nursing set forth by the American Nurses' Association (1980) summarize the focus of the nursing process with the family (see Chapter 8 for the entire list):

Belief 5: Prevention of illness is essential to promote health.

Belief 7: The client is the only constant member of the health care team.

Belief 8: Individuals within a community are ultimately responsible for their own health and must be encouraged and taught to be active participants in their own health care.

CLINICAL APPLICATION

Childbearing loss is a significant family health problem. In the United States almost one of three women who conceive loses the baby to perinatal death. Perinatal death includes deaths within the first year from an unknown cause (e.g., sudden infant death syndrome); deaths within the first 6 months of life from a known cause or neonatal death; stillbirth; and prenatal deaths from miscarriage or spontaneous abortion (Knapp and Peppers, 1980).

Schiff (1977) notes that when two people marry, they seem to believe they become joined together as one. This idea is shattered with the death of a child. Each person must mourn as an individual. Perhaps this brings to consciousness each person's mortality and essential aloneness.

Information from the nurse and from other sources of support assist the family that experiences childbearing loss in coping with its grief. Literature written by families who have successfully coped with a childbirth loss can provide further information about interventions by the nurse. Some families will benefit from bibliotherapy, recommendation of books for the family to read. *When Bad Things Happen to Good People* (Kushner, 1981) and *Man's Search for Meaning* (Frank, 1963) conclude that although a person cannot always control things that happen in life, a person can control what one makes of the event, one's response. Berezin (1982) cites an extensive list of books to help children with the grief process.

How can nurses assist in family health promotion with the family experiencing a childbearing loss? Nurses can function as health educators, problem solvers, and resource links. Nurses can function as health educators with the mother, the father, and with other children and family members to help them understand the grief process.

The nurse can help the mother understand that the grief she experiences is normal and that, although there may be no solution, life cannot remain unchanged. One normal behavior of bereavement that may require reassurance is searching. The mourner, although realizing that the hope is irrational, may peer into baby strollers looking for the dead baby (Berezin, 1982).

Nurses can intervene to encourage the mother to allow herself the privilege to grieve in her own way and to be protective of her time. The mother needs to let friends and relatives know when she needs to be alone. Some people will hesitate to approach her, not wanting to interrupt the grief or will feel paralyzed for fear of saying or doing the wrong thing. The mother can be encouraged to make the first contact, if necessary, to get the assistance she needs.

The nurse can suggest that the mother look beyond the husband's facade of strength to see his hurt. One useful way of handling hurt feelings or a missed communication is for one family member to ask the other "Can we start over?" When the hurt or angry member is able, they wipe the slate clean, effectively saying they love each other enough to forgive imperfections. If one member is not quite ready to begin again, this person can indicate this and take a cooling-off time before beginning again. Physical contact such as hugging is helpful for adults and children when the words do not come out smoothly. Not every problem can be worked out, and "agreeing to disagree" on some issues clears the air. Members in healthy families do not always agree or see things the same way; that is acceptable.

The nurse can help the father by sanctioning his need to express his feelings. Crying is helpful but not easy; it may be more "manly" to be comfortable with himself than to play the expected role.

The nurse may need to initiate the discussion of how the parents are helping the other children deal with death. Some families use natural occurrences, such as the death of a pet, to explain death as a natural, although painful, part of the life cycle. Hugging and the parents allowing themselves to cry in front of the children are helpful. Children need to know that life has good and bad experiences that can be shared with others (Berezin, 1982). Furman (1978) notes that how successful parents are in helping their children deal with their bereavement may be an accurate measurement of their own coping success. Prolonged affected behavior and school problems of the children may be indicators that a referral to a mental health resource may be needed.

Rituals of mourning may serve to bring the family together. Difficult days for the family may be Mother's Day, Father's Day, Christmas, or the due date or birthdate of the baby (Berezin, 1982). Memories awaken the grief. On such occasions, a family visit to the cemetery, or, if there is no grave, a memorial service, or asking the minister to remember the family may be helpful (Berezin, 1982). A donation can be made to a favorite charity in the child's name.

Nurses can anticipate problems in such areas as lack of attention to the marital relationship. The nurse can suggest that the couple plan some time together, even if it is only an hour or two. Children can be helped to understand the parents' need for privacy by explaining to them that children grow from the parents' love. When parents take time to strengthen their love and work on their problems, the children benefit.

The nurse may identify a couple's fear of sexual intimacy at this time. Encouraging the couple to focus on caring aspects of their relationship is appropriate. Backrubs, massage, and physical closeness by mutual commitment of the spouses can substitute for intercourse for a while. When the couple is ready to resume intercourse, they may choose to use added contraceptive methods as extra protection against a pregnancy feared at this time. The idea of another pregnancy when the grief is yet unresolved, can make sexual intimacy a dreaded experience. The passage of time offers much comfort in the grief process (Panuthos and Romeo, 1984).

Reminders about proper nutrition and exercise at this time may be helpful. In one case, the father of a stillborn child reported that when he returned to a regular physical workout, it gave him more time to focus on his feelings about the death of his daughter (Panuthos and Romeo, 1984). The nurse can address the issue of exhaustion in both parents. Physical exhaustion may be magnified by sleep disturbances. The nurse can suggest that the parents try music or other brief relaxation techniques to aid sleep (see Chapter 36). Slow deep breaths and focusing on a simple word such as "calm" can be useful. It may be helpful to instruct the parents to try to visualize a familiar tranquil scene such as woods, a stream, or a beach. The nurse can encourage the person to bring to mind the sights, sounds, smells, and textures of this place. Children can also use this technique by focusing on a happy place.

Nurses can function as a link to resources by making referrals to appropriate support groups. The family gains support and finds meaning in its own experience by sharing their experience and helping others. The family's healthy resolution of grief requires mutual support and flexibility with work, social, and home schedules. Sensitive treatment by caregivers can assist family members to emerge as stronger people. Unhealthy resolution can lead to separation or divorce, psychosomatic illness, or prolonged emotional disturbance (Berezin, 1982).

Life experience is a valuable teacher. Nurses can look to literature written by parents who have survived childbirth loss to find concrete, practical suggestions for families.

Four beliefs that aid in coping and resolution of childbearing losses are offered in *Ended Beginnings*, a book written for parents by parents (Panuthos and Romeo, 1984, p. 121). They suggest that parents need beliefs in the following:

1. The drive toward psychological and physical health
2. Goodness within the human condition
3. Inner wisdom as the ultimate guide
4. The ability to accomplish healing

Emphasis on holistic care and self-care points to the importance of a family's taking responsibility for its own healing in bereavement, with assistance from helping resources. Naisbitt (1982) describes these changing attitudes, people learning to make personal decisions about health care, as a major trend in America. Opinions differ as to the statistical significance of attitude and positive thinking on health promotion, but experience in nurse-client relationships over time points to an enhanced sense of well-being, mastery, and hope in the family in which strengths rather than weaknesses are emphasized.

Health promotion in any aspect of the family is an ongoing process. Healthy grief resolution does not proceed in clear-cut stages as texts may portray but rather follows its own timetable. The effect of resolution of grief on the family's physical and emotional well-being can be profound. The nurse's intervention with clients may produce personal growth for family members of which they may never become aware. For the nurse to communicate trust in the family's strengths and not place a value judgment on the family's progress, the nurse must be involved in relationships and activities outside the nurse-client relationship that confirm the nurse's value as a person.

SUMMARY

The role of the community health nurse in health promotion in families is unique. The nurse has a view of family life to which few professionals have access. The nursing process is used as an organizing framework with which to assist family members to a higher level of functioning.

Community health nurses must be able to assess the family as a unit, in addition to assessing individuals who comprise the family system. Systems theory and developmental theories assist nurses to assess the health status of the family unit and of each family member. As nurses apply the nursing process to family health promotion, family strengths and weaknesses become apparent. Family dynamics influence the work of the family and its ability to complete its functions and roles. Application of Otto's criteria for assessing family strengths assists nurses in helping families to identify and develop their strengths and use them in family problem solving. Nurses help families to identify weaknesses that may be affecting their ability to promote health.

Often persons develop myths about marriage and family life that prevent them from coping with real life events such as illness or loss. Peck provides four tools to assist the family in dealing with life events.

During stressful events, family communication patterns may be altered. Four patterns of altered communication are blaming, placating, computing, and distracting.

In some instances families may be able to use the healthy communication style of leveling in stressful situations. However, if the family is unable to communicate effectively, triangulation may occur. The nurse must be aware of this occurrence and avoid becoming involved in triangulation. The nurse also must be aware of scapegoating of one family member by others. These communication patterns can affect the nurse's ability to collect data and the family's ability to resolve problems.

In planning and implementing strategies to promote family health, nurses function as problem solvers, resource links, and health educators. Nurses must avoid attempting to rescue families from their problems by imposing their own values and solutions on the problems of the family. Evaluation of the family's problem resolution and nurses' strategies for intervention occur throughout nurses' contact with families and at the point of terminating the relationship.

Nurses often see families without masks and defenses shown to the outside world. They grow with families through experiences with illness and wellness. Intimate moments demonstrate that the family has as much to teach the nurse as the nurse has to teach the family. Family expectations are not always fulfilled. Often nurses assist families in coping with failed expectations.

Families are complex, and family assessment is a complicated and never completed task. Some families will reveal more of themselves than others. It is a special privilege and a credit to the nurse's skills and genuineness when the family invites the nurse to take a glimpse at its work as a family.

KEY CONCEPTS

In theory, family functioning exists on a continuum from the highly functional to the severely dysfunctional family.

The application of social systems theory to the family unit demonstrates the complexity of family functioning. Systems theory teaches the nurse to be aware that the health status of any one family member affects the health of all other family members.

Family dynamics influence the work of the family and its ability to complete its functions and tasks.

When family life is not smooth and family members are not healthy and happy, the family experiences failed expectations. Failed expectations arise from myths about marriage, the faulty notion that life is or ought to be fair, and the belief that family members will always be healthy.

The family experiences stress as a result of failed expectations, and this stress can alter communication styles. Problematic communication styles are blaming, placating, computing, and distracting; a healthy style is leveling.

Triangulation, a tension-reducing mechanism to take the focus away from working on a conflict, is an important concept in understanding the communication between family members. Unconsciously, in some families, one member is chosen as the scapegoat, the focus of all family difficulties.

The nursing process provides the concrete problem-solving approach necessary to assist the family in its work to promote health.

Three strategies that summarize the community health nurse's use of the nursing process in working with the family are nurse as health educator, problem solver, and resource linker.

LEARNING ACTIVITIES

1. Using Otto's criteria for assessment of family strengths, discuss your own family's strengths and weaknesses in meeting the tasks of the family.

2. Assume the role of participant-observer at your next family gathering, perhaps at a holiday. Identify communication patterns that you or other family members may demonstrate under stress.

3. Select a family in your clinical practice caseload. Using Table 26-2, identify the stage in family life development for the selected family and discuss which risk factors are of concern in this family.

4. Select a family in your caseload and identify nursing roles appropriate for health promotion and disease prevention in this family using Table 26-1 for ideas.

5. Interview nurses in your clinical setting to collect examples of humor used by the caretaker for helping the client to cope.

6. Discuss with nurses in your clinical setting attitudes or belief systems that help them maintain their perspective and help them find meaning in their work.

BIBLIOGRAPHY

Aguilera D and Messick J: Crisis intervention theory and methodology, ed. 4, St. Louis, 1990, Times Mirror/Mosby College Publishing.

American Nurses' Association: A conceptual model of community health nursing, Kansas City, 1980, The Association.

Arnold E: Burnout as a spiritual issue: rediscovering meaning in nursing practice. In Carson VB: Spiritual dimensions of nursing practice. Philadelphia, 1989, WB Saunders, 320-353.

Aslen SP: Coping with family crisis: intervention with sudden infant death syndrome. Fam Rel 29:584-590, 1980.

Balzer JW: Survive and thrive . . . more than stress management. Workshop for the Visiting Nurses' Association, Jacksonville, Florida, 1990.

Bass E and Davis L: The courage to heal: a guide for women survivors of child sexual abuse. New York, 1988, Harper & Row Publishers.

Benfield DG, Leib SA, and Vollman JH: Grief response of parents to neonatal death and parent participation in deciding care, Pediatrics 62:171, 1978.

Berezin N: After a loss in pregnancy: help for families affected by a miscarriage, a stillbirth, or the loss of a newborn, New York, 1982, Simon & Schuster.

Bettelheim B: The uses of enchantment: the meaning and importance of fairy tales, New York, 1977, Alfred A. Knopf.

Boberg JT and Hedrick HL, editors: Support groups: potential roles for health professionals, Allied Health Educator Newsletter 17:1, Jan. 1986.

Bowen M: Family and family group psychotherapy. In Kaplan HI and Sadock BJ, editors: Comprehensive group psychotherapy, Baltimore, 1971, The Williams & Wilkins Co.

Breckon DJ, Harvey JR, and Lancaster RB: Health educator, Rockville, MD, 1985, Aspen Publications.

Carson VB: Spiritual dimensions of nursing practice. Philadelphia, 1989, W.B. Saunders Co.

Cherryholmes LG: The qualities of a home health care nurse. In Stuart-Siddell S, editor: Home health care nursing: administrative and clinical perspectives, Rockville, MD, 1986, Aspen Publications.

Clemen SA, Eigsti DG, and McGuire SL: Comprehensive family and community health nursing, ed 2, New York, 1987, McGraw-Hill Book Co.

Cobb-McMahon BA, Williams DD, and Davis JH: Changing health behavior of community health clients, J Community Health Nursing 1(1):27-31, 1984.

Cross JR: Nursing process of the family client. In Griffin-Kenney JW and Christensen PJ, editors: Nursing process: application of theories, frameworks, and models, St. Louis, 1986, The CV Mosby Co.

Crowley C, et al: Innovations in family and community health: incorporating home health care into the baccalaureate nursing program, Community and Family Health 2:81, Aug. 1985.

Dossey B, Issue Editor: Spirituality and Healing. Holistic Nurs Prac 3:(3): May 1989.

Dotson B: In pursuit of the American dream, New York, 1985, Atheneum Press.

Dowling C: The Cinderella complex: women's hidden fear of independence, New York, 1981, Summit Books.

Edelman C, and Mandle CL: Health promotion throughout the lifespan, ed. 2 St. Louis, 1990, Times Mirror/Mosby College Publishing.

Elkins CP: Community health nursing: skills and strategies, Bowie, MD, 1984, R.J. Brady.

Flynn JB and Griffin PA: Health promotion in acute care setting, Nurs Clin North Am 19(2):239, June 1984.

Frank VE: Man's search for meaning, New York, 1963, Washington Square Press.

Friedman MM: Family nursing theory and assessment, New York, 1981, Appleton-Century-Crofts.

Furman EP: The death of a newborn: care of the parents, Birth Family J 5:4, Winter 1978.

Haggarty RJ: Changing life-styles to improve health, Prev Med 6:276, 1977.

Haley J: Problem-solving therapy, San Francisco, 1978, Jossey-Bass.

Hall JE and Weaver BR: Distributive nursing practice: systems approach to community health, Philadelphia, 1985, J.B. Lippincott Co.

Hall JE and Weaver BR: Nursing of families in crisis, Philadelphia, 1974, J.B. Lippincott Co.

Havelock R: Training for change agents, Ann Arbor, Mich, 1972, University of Michigan Press.

Healthy People: The Surgeon General's report on health promotion and disease prevention, DHEW Pub. No. (PHS) 79-55071. Washington, D.C., 1979. Department of Health, Education and Welfare.

Holland N: Health hazard is home for Page's people. The Florida Times-Union, Jacksonville Journal, Jan 12, 1986.

Holmes TH and Rahe RH: The social readjustment rating scale, J Psychosom Res II:213-218, 1967.

Johnson J and Parsons M: Symposia on health promotion, Nurs Clin North Am 19(2), June 1984.

Johnson R: Promoting the health of families in the community. In Stanhope M and Lancaster J, editors: Community health nursing: process and practice for promoting health, St. Louis, 1984, The CV Mosby Co.

Johnson SH: High-risk parenting: nursing assessment and strategies for the family at risk, Philadelphia, 1979, JB Lippincott Co.

Kastenbaum R: The child's understanding of death: how does it develop? In Grollman EA, editor: Explaining death to children, Boston, 1967, Beacon Press.

Knapp RJ and Peppers LG: Doctor-patient relationships in fetal/infant encounters, J Med Educ 54:775-780, 1979.

Kohnke MF: The nurse as advocate, Am J Nurse 80(II):2038-2040, 1980.

Kolbenschlag M: Kiss sleeping beauty goodbye: breaking the spell of feminine myths and models, Garden City, New York, 1979, Doubleday & Co., Inc.

Klaus M and Kennell J: Maternal-infant bonding, St. Louis, 1976, The CV Mosby Co.

Kushner HS: When bad things happen to good people, New York, 1981, Avon Books.

Lederer WJ and Jackson DD: The mirages of marriage, New York, 1968, WW Norton & Co.

Leiber D: Laughter and humor in critical care. Dims Crit Care Nursing 5(3):162-170. May-June 1986.

Lewis CS: A grief observed, New York, 1961, The Seabury Press.

MacVicar MG and Archbold P: A framework for family assessment in chronic illness, Nurse Forum XV(2):180-195, 1976.

McCarthy NC: Health promotion in the family. In Edelman C and Mandle CL, editors: Health promotion throughout the lifespan, St. Louis, 1986, The CV Mosby Co.

McCormick MC, Shapiro S, and Starfield B: High-risk young mothers: infant mortality and morbidity in four areas in the United States, 1973-1978, Am J Public Health 74(1):18-23, 1984.

McKeown T: The modern rise of population, New York, 1976, Academic Press, Inc.

Miller JR and Janosik EH: Family-focused care, New York, 1980, McGraw-Hill Book Co.

Minuchin S, et al: A conceptual model of psychosomatic illness in children, Arch Gen Psychiatry 32:1031-1038, 1975.

Mundinger M: Home care controversy: too little, too late, too costly, Rockville, MD, 1983, Aspen Publications.

Murray RB and Zentner JP: Nursing concepts for health promotion, Englewood Cliffs, NJ, 1979, Prentice-Hall, Inc.

Naisbitt J: Megatrends, New York, 1982, Warner Books.

Nelson EC, Keller AM, and Zubkoff M: Incentives for health promotion: the government's role. In Ng L and Davis D, editors: Strategies for public health, New York, 1981, Van Nostrand Reinhold.

Northman JE: Human service program design and the family, Family Community Health 1(2):17-25, July 1978.

Oehrtman SE: Assessment and crisis intervention: a model for the family. In Hall JE and Weaver BR, editors: Nursing of families in crisis, Philadelphia, 1974, JB Lippincott Co.

Otto HE: A framework for assessing family strengths. In Reinhardt AM and Quinn MD, editors: Family centered community nursing: a sociocultural framework, vol 1, St. Louis, 1972, The CV Mosby Co.

Otto HE: Criteria for assessing family strengths, Fam Process 2:329, Sept 1963.

Panuthos C and Romeo C: Ended beginnings: healing childbearing losses, Boston, 1984, Bergin & Garvey Publishers, Inc.

Parkes CM: Bereavement: studies of grief in adult life, New York, 1972, International Universities Press, Inc.

Paulson TL: Making humor work: take your job seriously and yourself lightly. Los Altos, Calif, 1989, Crisp Publications, Inc.

Peck MS: The road less traveled, New York, 1978, Simon & Schuster.

Peitze CF: Health promotion in the well family, Nurs Clin North Am 19(2):229, June 1984.

Pratt L: Family structure and effective health behavior: the energized family, Boston, 1976, Houghton-Mifflin Co.

Quinn JF: On healing, wholeness, and the haelan effect. Nursing and Health Care. 10:(10):553-556, Dec 1989.

Robinson VM: Humor and the Health Professions, Thorofare, NJ, 1977, Charles B. Slack Company.

Rhodes S and Wilson J: Surviving family life, New York, 1981, GP Putnam's Sons.

Satir V: Peoplemaking, Palo Alto, Calif, 1972, Science and Behavior Books, Inc.

Schiff HS: The bereaved parent, Middlesex, England, 1977, Harmondsworthy Penguin Books.

Spradley BW: Community health nursing: concepts and practice, Boston, 1985, Little, Brown & Co.

Spradley BW: Readings in community health nursing, Boston, 1982, Little, Brown & Co.

Sullivan HS: Conceptions of modern psychiatry, New York, 1953, WW Norton & Co.

Turk DC and Kerns RD, editors: Health, illness and families: a life-span perspective, New York, 1985, John Wiley & Sons, Inc.

Von Bertalanffy L: General systems theory, New York, 1968, George Brazillers.

Weber T, McKeever JE, and McDaniel SH: A beginner's guide to the problem-oriented first family interview. Fam Process 24:357, Sept. 1985.

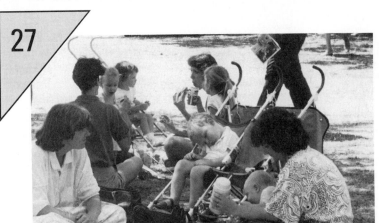

27

Issues in Family Health Promotion

Carol J. Loveland-Cherry

Concepts in Family Health Promotion
Defining Family Health
Defining the Focus of Family Health Promotion

Modalities for Promoting Family Health
Family Home Visits
Contracting in Family Health Promotion
Enabling and Empowering Families
Community Resources

Clinical Application

Summary

OBJECTIVES

After reading this chapter, the student should be able to:

Identify factors that interfere with or serve as barriers to implementing a family health promotion focus in community health nursing.

Analyze the interrelationship between individual health, family health, and community health.

Explain the relevance of knowledge about family structures, roles, and functions for the family-focused community health nursing process.

Analyze the various approaches to defining and conceptualizing family health.

Identify and analyze the factors related to family health promotion.

Analyze the relevance of conceptual frameworks (family) for the family focused community health nursing process.

Explain the application of the nursing process (assessing, planning, implementing, evaluating) to family health promotion.

KEY TERMS

adaptive model	family health	postvisit phase
clinical model	health paradigm	previsit phase
contracting	home visits	role-performance
empowerment	in-home phase	model
eudaimonistic model	pathogenic paradigm	termination phase

W orking with families is a complex task that is both rewarding and frustrating. As a major client system for community health nursing, the family is important in promoting the health of individuals and populations. The family system is a basic unit within which health behavior, including health values, health habits, and health risk perceptions, are developed, organized, and performed (Baranowski & Nader, 1985a; Doherty and McCubbin, 1985; Duffy, 1988; Litman, 1974; Mauksch, 1974; Pratt, 1976). The interrelationship between health, health behavior, and the family "is a highly dynamic one in which each may have a dramatic effect on the other" (Litman, 1974, p. 495).

Knowledge of family structure and functioning, family theory, nursing theory, and models of health behavior are fundamental to implement the nursing process with families in the community.* However, community health nurses need to recognize important issues that influence family health promotion. Issues related to family health promotion originate from three major sources: the family system itself; the health care system (which includes the discipline and profession of nursing); and the social, political, and economic environment within which the family exists.

This chapter examines issues related to family health promotion and presents some approaches to enhance community health nursing intervention with families. The focus is on a systems perspective within a developmental framework.

CONCEPTS IN FAMILY HEALTH PROMOTION

Community health nursing advocates the promotion of family health. A closer examination of the components of this goal prompts questions for the nurse to consider in working toward this goal.

Traditionally, community health nursing has been viewed as an integration/synthesis of "public health, the humanities, the social and behavioral sciences, epidemiology, and nursing science" (ANA Standards, 1986, p.2). Effective understanding of health promotion in families requires an integration of concepts and theories derived from these areas.

Within the last decade, the characteristics of the concepts of health, health protection (prevention), and health promotion as they relate to individuals have been clarified (see Chapters 2 and 8). The definition of these terms in relation to families has occurred more slowly and less clearly. Health protection has been defined as being "directed toward decreasing the probability of specific illnesses of dysfunctions in individuals, families, and communities, including active protection against unnecessary stressors" (Pender, 1987, p. 4). Thus, for a family with a history of cardiac disease, nursing interventions directed toward health protection may focus on assisting the family to pattern their eating, exercise, and stress management behaviors. Health promotion has been defined as being "directed toward increasing the level of well being and actualizing the health potential of individuals, families, communities, and society" (Pender, 1987, p. 4). A nursing intervention emphasizing health promotion may be directed toward meeting a family identified goal of

establishing an appropriate exercise program to enhance family interaction and cohesion. Historically, community health nursing has been concerned with health protection and health promotion (see Chapters 1 and 2). This chapter considers both of these issues and recognizes the distinction between the two. To promote family health, nurses must understand the dimensions of family health.

Defining Family Health

Historically, practice in community health nursing has been characterized as using a *pathogenic paradigm* (Laffrey, Loveland-Cherry, and Winkler, 1986). Within this model, health is viewed as freedom from disease, and health behavior includes behaviors related to preventing or curing disease. Human beings are viewed from a machine-like model, composed of parts that may or may not function effectively. The recipient of health services is viewed as a patient, a person who is relatively passive, dependent, and accepting of treatment by an expert practitioner, in this instance the community health nurse. Interventions are disease-specific. Examples of intervention include immunization programs, screening programs, and teaching behaviors designed to prevent specific diseases (for example, dietary practices related to preventing heart disease). The emphasis is on increasing clients' compliance with professionally prescribed regimens.

Within the *health paradigm* (Laffrey, Loveland-Cherry, and Winkler, 1986), human beings are viewed as organismic beings characterized by wholeness, the ability to initiate action, the potential for growth, and both qualitative and quantitative change. Relationships between health professionals and clients focus on interactive processes to assess the health situation and to promote higher levels of health. Health is viewed as a dynamic process defined by individuals within their own values and cultures. Community health nursing interventions in this model emphasize the importance of exploring with clients what health means to them and where it falls in their value system.

To identify the goals in working with families to promote health, community health nurses should be aware of which of these two perspectives is more appropriate in the specific situation. If the critical issue is an immediate response for a family in a crisis situation, the family may, in its best interest, give up its control and power of choice to health professionals for the immediate period. However, a different approach is proposed to be more effective in working with families to reach desired levels of health. In this approach the values, desires, and capabilities of the client are not only acknowledged but are also promoted in the process of seeking health.

Family theorists refer to healthy families but generally do not define *family health*. Based on the various family theoretical perspectives (see Chapters 8, 25, and 26), definitions of healthy families can be derived within the guidelines of any of the frameworks. For example, within a structural-functional framework, family health can be defined as the continuing ability to meet defined functions in interaction with other social, political, economic, and health systems. From the perspective of the developmental framework, family health can be defined as possessing the abilities and

*See chapters 8, 9, 22, 23, 25-29, 31-34.

resources to accomplish family developmental tasks.

Although most existing theoretical models originally were directed toward individuals, recent work has attempted to apply them to families (Chin, 1985; Clements and Roberts, 1983; Frey, 1989; Hanson, 1984; Johnston, 1987; King, 1983; Rogers, 1983; Tadych, 1985; Taylor, 1989; Whall, 1987). The extension of Orem's self-care model (1985, 1991) can define family health as a state of wholeness or integrity of the family, its parts, and its modes of functioning. The health of a family could be assessed in terms of its ability to exercise its essential self-care or dependent-care capabilities (Tadych, 1985). More specifically, family health is reflected in its abilities to meet strategic functions, including socializing family members as self-care and dependent-care agents, acknowledging therapeutic self-care demands of family members, identifying strategies to meet therapeutic self-care demands, obtaining and managing required resources to meet self-care demands (e.g., money, food, shelter), and integrating self-care and dependent-care activities into family patterns (Taylor, 1989, p. 135-136).

Within Roy's model (1984), family health can be considered as both the state and process of becoming an integrated and whole system. Because promoting adaptation should lead to health in this model, assessment focuses on dimensions of adaptation on two levels. First-level assessment is an evaluation of the family's current adaptive and ineffective behavior within the four adaptive modes of physiological function, self-concept, role function, and interdependence. Hanson (1984) has identified guidelines for each of these areas (see box). Second-level assessment emphasizes identification of focal, contextual, and residual stimuli contributing to any behaviors that were identified in the first-level assessment. Focal stimuli are those events immediately confronting the family that require a response (e.g., the birth of a new infant). Contextual stimuli are all other events existing in the situation that influence the family's behavior (e.g., the father's loss of his job). Residual stimuli are other factors that may affect behavior but cannot be validated systematically (e.g., attitudes about the parenting role).

Another dimension of family health can be identified by using JL Smith (1983a) four models of health: *clinical model, role-performance model, adaptive model,* and *eudaimonistic model* (Table 27-1).

The following clinical example applies these models to one family's situation.

The Russell family consists of Mr. and Mrs. Russell, 6-year-old Ann, 4-year-old Jim, and 1-month-old Karen. Karen was born prematurely and spent 3 weeks in a neonatal intensive care unit (NICU). The community health nurse has been working with the family after they were referred by the staff of the NICU, who said that the parents expressed concern about caring for such a small infant and about her future health.

The focus in a *clinical model* approach might be to identify realistic perceptions of health risks for Karen and to teach the parents how to recognize and deal with symptoms of distress. Assessment would include determining Mr. and Mrs. Russell's perceptions and knowledge of premature infants, identifying the family's health care resources, and

---

FAMILY ASSESSMENT BASED ON ROY'S ADAPTATION MODEL

PHYSIOLOGICAL MODE

Physical maintenance of members—food, clothing, shelter

Allocation of resources for health care needs—emergency care, medical care, dental care, preventive care

Allocation of space and equipment—rest, exercise, aloneness, togetherness

Provision of a safe environment

Provision for cleanliness and sanitation

Accessibility to goods and services

SELF-CONCEPT MODE

Solidarity of the family

Social integration of the family into the community

Understanding that the family provides to its members

Companionship that the family provides to its members

Moral-ethical values of the family

Future and present orientation of the family

Provision for sexual identity for family members

Family support for its members in conflicts with family or community

ROLE FUNCTION MODE

Decision-making processes

Clarity of roles

Flexibility of roles and tolerance for change

Division of responsibility

Clarity of communication

INTERDEPENDENCE MODE

Family interaction with neighbors and political, social, educational, health, and religious systems

Support systems

Significant others for family

---

recognizing their concerns about caring for a premature infant.

Assessment in the *role-performance model* would include exploring with the family their feelings about their abilities and resources to accomplish developmental tasks. This family is in the developmental stage of families with preschool children, based on the age of the oldest child. Developmental tasks for families in this stage include:

1. Supplying adequate space, facilities, and equipment for the expanding family.

2. Meeting predictable and unexpected costs of family life with small children.

3. Sharing responsibility for household management and care within the young family.

4. Maintaining mutually satisfying intimate communication in the family.

5. Rearing children already present and planning future family size.

6. Relating to relatives on both sides of the family in creative ways.

7. Tapping resources outside the family in the wider community.

TABLE 27-1
Smith's four models of health

Model	View of health	Assessment	Nursing goals
Clinical	*Individual* The absence of disease *Family* The absence of disease or dysfunction	Includes family health/illness history; family's definition of health and illness; family's value of health; family's knowledge of health promotion and illness prevention/treatment; family practices related to nutrition, sleep/rest, exercise, and recreation; use of alcohol, tobacco, drugs; family processes for determining illness and whether and how professional care will be sought.	To promote family's physical, mental, and social health; to provide comfort to the family; to prevent deterioration of family system
Role-Performance	*Individual* Effective performance of roles *Family* Effective meeting of family functions and developmental tasks	Includes family's current developmental stage/history; family's role structure; socialization patterns; resources for meeting functions and developmental tasks; family's perceptions of family functioning	To promote effective performance of family functions; to promote achievement of developmental tasks; to assist in identifying and mobilizing support systems and resources
Adaptive	*Individual* Condition of the whole person engaged in effective interaction with physical/social environment *Family* Condition of the whole family engaged in effective interaction with physical/social environment; family/environment fit	Includes the identification of family coping patterns, social networks, and support systems; family's perceptions of their environment; family's flexibility in altering behaviors, rules, roles, and perceptions when needed	To promote the family's adaptation and health-directed patterning with the environment
Eudaimonistic	*Individual* Complete development of individual's potential for general well-being and self-realization *Family* Development of family's well-being and maximum potential	Includes family's values and goals; family interaction patterns; family patterns of recreation and relaxation; family cohesion; family promotion of autonomy	To clarify family's values; to assist in identifying and prioritizing family's goals; to assist family in implementing plans to meet goals

Modified from Smith, JA: The idea of health: implications for the nursing professional, New York, 1983, Teachers College Press, Columbia University.

8. Maintaining morale in the face of life's changes and dilemmas (Duvall and Miller, 1985, p. 199).

Based on the assessment, the nurse can assist the family in identifying areas of strength and areas where external resources may be necessary.

Assessment in *adaptive model* would focus on identifying with the family the kinds of changes that have occurred since Karen's birth and the different or new demands that have resulted. The nurse would work with the family members to help them adapt to having a new family member and to repattern their lives to deal with the increased and different demands of having a premature infant. By pointing out the knowledge and skills that the family already has and the ways to adapt them to the changes in the family system, the nurse builds on family competencies. Another potential intervention would be to identify parent support groups in the community.

In the *eudaimonistic model*, the nurse could work with the family in reassessing family goals and ways to meet them. The addition of a family member indicates assessment of family values and goals such as socialization and education of children, family recreation, and patterns of interaction. At some point it might be appropriate to inform the family about how they could offer support to other families in similar circumstances.

Families' Perceptions

From the perspective of the *health paradigm,* another less prevalent approach to identifying dimensions of family health is to examine families' perceptions of their health. As part of a larger study of families and health behavior (Loveland-Cherry, 1982), parents and children were asked to rate their families' health on a six-point scale and to describe what they thought of when asked about family health. Characteristics of family health identified by children and parents included participation in health behaviors (eating healthy foods, getting enough rest, and exercising regularly); absence of illness (very little sickness, healthy bodies, and mental health); a feeling of well-being (high energy levels, enthusiastic living, a happy home, support, mutual respect, and love; having fun together; having regular health care; and ability to function in usual roles. Knowing what the family identifies as being healthy directs the nurse in working with the family to identify and reach health promotion goals.

Defining the Focus of Family Health Promotion
Promoting Family Members' Health

An important question for the community health nurse is the emphasis for the client unit, that is, whether the focus is on an individual family member or on the family unit. Nursing interventions may focus on promoting the health of individual family members in interaction with the family environment. In this instance the goal, whether from a pathogenic or health paradigm, is to promote the health of the individual by working with the family system unit. The basis for this approach is determined by the relationships between specific family characteristics and health and health-related behavior of family members (Duffy, 1988). Parenting styles characterized by a high degree of autonomy and support for the child, active participation in the community, health-training efforts by parents, flexible division of tasks, an egalitarian power structure, family cohesiveness, and promotion of autonomy of family members are positively related to parents' and children's health beliefs and behaviors (Loveland-Cherry, 1984, 1986; Pratt, 1976). These findings support the view that individuals' competency in managing their lives is a basis for participation in health-promoting behaviors (Loveland-Cherry, 1982; Petze, 1984; Pratt, 1973, 1976). The importance of the family as the primary environment for learning values and behavior and for reinforcing positive behaviors is critical in planning strategies for family health promotion (Duffy, 1988).

Most models for understanding health behavior, and the interventions based on these models, have been developed for individuals or for special population groups. A number of the critical variables* in the models are developed and learned within the family environment. Therefore there has been a renewed interest in designing family interventions

to promote health behavior. Some initial success of a project "encouraging family members to support each other's attempt to alter their diet and exercise patterns" has been reported by Baranowski, Nader, Dunn, and Vanderpool (1982). The intervention used tangible (provision of time and supplies, cooking meals, etc.) and emotional social support by families to promote dietary and exercise change in family members. The results indicate that promoting social support for change encourages changes in diet but not in exercise. Additionally, it was found that families need assistance in learning how to provide support to promote changes in health behavior.

Other programs have focused on promoting cardiovascular health through family intervention programs in the community (Glueck, Laskorszewski, Rao, et al., 1985; Matarazzo, Connor, Fey, et al., 1982). The benefits of family interventions for health promotion has long been advocated (Mauksch, 1974) and is now documented (Simons-Morton, O'Hara, and Simons-Morton, 1986; Baranowski and Nader, 1985b).

Promoting Family System Health

In contrast to working with the family system to promote individuals' health, the focus of nursing service can be the health promotion of the family system internally and in interaction with social, political, economic, educational, physical, and health systems. The goal is to promote the health of the family system. Areas for assessment may not differ markedly in either focus; the emphasis is on how the family system interacts as a whole and its ability to interact with other systems. The community health nurse often functions as a facilitator between the family and other systems. For example, community health nurses function as the link between schools and families in identifying health-related needs of families and assisting schools to design programs related to health (see Chapters 38 and 40).

MODALITIES FOR PROMOTING FAMILY HEALTH
Family Home Visits

Community health nurses work with families in different settings, including clinics, schools, support groups, offices, and the family home. An important aspect of community health nursing's role in promoting the health of populations has been the tradition of providing services to individual families in their homes.

Purposes

Home visits give a more accurate assessment of the family structure and behavior in the natural environment. Home visits also provide opportunities to observe the home environment and to identify barriers and supports for reaching family health promotion goals. The nurse can work with the client first hand to adapt interventions to meet realistic resources. Meeting the family on its home ground also may

---

Variables include cognitive-perceptual factors (importance of health, definition of health, perceived self-efficacy, or one's ability to successfully perform behaviors) (Pender, 1987); perceived barriers (factors such as insufficient time that would decrease the likelihood of performing an activity) (Becker, Haefner, Kasl, et

al., 1977; Pender, 1987); and generalized resistance resources (a set of repeated life experiences that exhibit consistency, opportunities to influence outcomes, and involvement in managing life events) (Antonovsky, 1979, 1987).

contribute to the family's sense of control and active participation in meeting its health needs. Most research has focused on the maternal-child population (Barkauskas, 1983, 1987; Combs-Orme, Reis, and Ward, 1985; Hall, 1980; Larson, 1980; Lowe, 1973; McNeil and Holland, 1972; Olds, Henderson, Chamberlin, and Tatelbaum, 1986; Siegel, Bauman, Schaefer, et al., 1980; United States General Accounting Office, 1990) (see Chapter 42).

A home visit may be more than just an alternative setting for service; it may be an intervention modality. If the home visit is to be valuable and effective, careful and systematic planning must occur. Mayers (1973) cautions that the process of home visits may become more a patterned response set, or ritual, than a vital exchange with productive outcomes.

Advantages and Disadvantages

Recently, the effectiveness of providing large portions of health promotion services with home visits has been reexamined by agencies, including health departments and visiting nurse associations. Barkauskas (1983) identified the following advantages and disadvantages of home visits. Advantages include convenience for the client; client control of the setting; the best option for clients unwilling or unable to travel; and a natural, relaxed environment for the discussion of concerns and needs. Costs were the major disadvantage identified by Barkauskas; the costs of previsit preparation, travel to and from the home, time spent with one client, and postvisit activities such as paperwork, making referrals, consulting, and collaborating with others about client care are high. In a study comparing teaching new mothers in groups and home visits, the group approach was more effective in terms of knowledge, and cost was approximately one third that of home visits (McNeil and Holland, 1972). The Government Accounting Office (1990), based on a review of eight home-visiting programs for at-risk families, concluded that the programs can have short- and long-term benefits for the health and well-being of families. Although potential to reduce costly interventions was documented, the report noted limited comparisons of the cost effectiveness of home visits with other intervention modalities. Many agencies have explored alternative methods of providing service to families, particularly group interventions (see Chapter 17). The important issue is determining which families would most benefit from home visits and how home visits can most effectively be structured and scheduled. With increasing demands for home health care, the home visit is again becoming a prominent mode for delivery of nursing services.

Process

The components of a home visit are summarized in Table 27-2. The sections that follow provide more information on these components.

INITIATION OF A HOME VISIT. Usually a home visit is initiated as the result of a referral from a health or social agency. However, a family may request services, or the nurse may initiate the home visit as a result of case-finding activities. Subsequent home visits should be based on need and mutual agreement between the nurse and the family. Regardless of

TABLE 27-2
Phases and activities of a home visit

Phase	Activity
I Initiation phase	Clarify source of referral for visit
	Clarify purpose for home visit
	Share information on reason and purpose for home visit with family
II Previsit phase	Initiate contact with family
	Establish shared perception of purpose with family
	Determine family's willingness for home visit
	Review referral and/or family record
III In-home phase	Introduction of self and professional identity
	Establish nurse-client relationship
	Implement nursing process
IV Termination phase	Review visit with family
	Plan for future visits
V Postvisit phase	Record visit
	Plan for next visit

the impetus for making a home visit, it is essential that the nurse be clear about the purpose for the visit and that the nurse's perception or understanding be shared with the family.

PREVISIT PHASE. The previsit phase has several components. First, if at all possible, the family should be contacted before the home visit. A telephone call to the family to introduce oneself, to identify the reason for the contact, and to schedule the home visit is highly desirable. Leavitt (1982) suggests that a first telephone contact should be brief, with an outside limit of 15 minutes. The nurse should give name and professional identity, for example: "This is Karen Smith. I'm a community health nurse from the Middle County Health Department." The family should be informed of how they came to the attention of the community health nurse, for example, a referral or a contact from observations or records in the school setting. If a referral has been received, it is important and useful to ascertain whether or not the family is aware of the referral. This will establish a perspective of valuing the client's input and involvement in care. Next, a brief summary of the nurse's knowledge and information allows the family to know the extent of the nurse's information about the family. The nurse might say "I understand that your baby was discharged from the hospital yesterday and that you requested some assistance with caring for the child at home." A visit should be scheduled for as soon as possible and as soon as is appropriate for both the nurse and the family. Letting the family know agency hours that are available for visits, the approximate length of the visit, and the purpose of the visit are helpful to the family in determining when to set the visit. Although the length of the visit may vary, depending on circumstances, approximately 45 minutes is usual (Kallins, 1967).

If possible, the visit should be arranged so that as many

of the family members as possible will be available for the entire visit. It is also important for the nurse to tell the client about any fee for the intial visit and subsequent visits and potential methods of payment. The telephone call can terminate with a review by the nurse of the time, place, and purpose for the visit and a means for the family to contact the nurse in case they need to verify or change the time for the visit or to ask questions they may not have asked during the initial phone call. If the family does not have a telephone, another method for setting up the visits can be used. The most obvious is dropping a note at the family home or sending a letter or postcard informing the family of when and why the home visit will occur, with a means for the family to contact the nurse if necessary.

Of course, the possibility always exists that the family may refuse to agree to a home visit. Less experienced nurses or students may interpret this as a personal rejection when it is not. Families regulate when and which outsiders are allowed to enter into their territory (Kantor and Lehr, 1977). The nurse needs to explore the reasons for the refusal; there may be a misunderstanding about the reason for the visit or there may be a lack of information about services. If the nurse determines that either the situation has been resolved or services have been obtained from another source, and if the family understands services available and how to contact the agency if desired, the contact may be terminated as requested. However, the nurse should leave open the possibility of future contact. There are instances when legal obligations, for example follow-up of certain communicable diseases, mandates that the nurse persist in requesting a home visit.

Before visiting the family, it can be useful for the nurse to review the referral or, if it is not the first visit, the family record. If there is a time lapse between the contact and the visit, a brief telephone call to confirm the time often avoids a visit when the family is not at home.

IN-HOME PHASE. The actual visit to the home affords the nurse the opportunity to assess the family's neighborhood. An issue that may arise either in approaching the family home or once the family has opened the door to the nurse is that of personal safety. Nurses need to examine their own fears and objective threats to determine whether safety is indeed an issue. Certain precautions can be taken in known high-risk situations. Agencies may provide escorts for nurses or have them visit in pairs; readily identifiable uniforms may be required; a sign-out process indicating timing and location of home visits may be used routinely. The nurse needs to use caution; if a reasonable question about the safety of making the visit exists, the visit should not be made.

"Pride, the ethic of self-sufficiency, territoriality, and privacy" are issues for nurses making home visits with families (Leavitt, 1982, p. 288). The nurse needs to be aware that families may feel that they are being "checked-up on," are seen as being inadequate or dysfunctional, or that their privacy is being invaded. Nursing services, especially those from health departments, have been identified by the public as being "public services" for needy families or those with insufficient funds to pay for care. These potential areas of concern underline the needs for sensitivity by the nurse, the need for clarity in information regarding the reason for visits, and the need to establish collaborative, trusting relationships with the family.

The changing nature of the American family can make it difficult to schedule visits during what have been traditional agency hours. The number of working single-parent or dual wage-earner two-parent families is increasing, which means that families are busy, with many more demands on their time. Even if one parent is at home during the usual work day, the ideal is to work with the entire family unit. This often is not possible because of conflict between agency hours and school or work schedules. It may be possible to schedule a visit at the beginning or end of a day to meet with working or school-aged members. In some parts of the country agencies are reconsidering traditional hours and Monday through Friday visits.

Families may not be able to control interruptions during the visit. Telephones ring, pets join in the visit, people come and go, televisions are left on. The nurse can ask that for a limited time televisions be turned off or other disruptive activities be limited (Leavitt, 1982). Families may be so used to the background noises and routine activities that they do not recognize them as being potentially disruptive.

The actual home visit includes several components. Once at the family home, the nurse needs to again provide personal identification and professional affiliation. This is part of the introductory phase. Then there should be a brief social period to allow the client to assess the nurse and to establish rapport (Leahy, Cobb, and Jones, 1982).

The major portion of the home visit is concerned with establishing the relationship and implementing the nursing process. Assessment, intervention, and evaluation are ongoing. It is important that the nurse be realistic about what can be accomplished in a home visit. In some situations, one visit may be all that is possible or appropriate. In this instance needs and resources for meeting needs are explored with the family and a determination is made whether further services are desired or indicated. If the latter is the case and the current agency is not appropriate, the nurse can assist the family to identify other services available in the community and help in initiating any referrals. Although it is not unusual to have only one home visit with a family, often multiple visits are made (Guilino and LaMonica, 1986). The frequency and intensity of home visits vary not only with the needs of the family but also with eligibility for services and agency policies and priorities. It is realistic to expect at least the beginning of building a relationship and initial assessment to occur during a first visit.

TERMINATION PHASE. When the purpose of the visit has been accomplished, the nurse reviews with the family what has occurred and been accomplished. This provides the client the opportunity to recognize what has been done and provides a basis for planning any further home visits. Ideally, termination of the visit and, ultimately, of service begins at the first contact, with the goal or purpose being defined. Frequently, nurses are not sure of the reason for the visit; consequently, the visit is compromised and either aimlessly comes to a close or ends abruptly. If communication has been clear to this point, the family and nurse can now plan for future visits, specifically, the next visit. Planning for future visits is part of another issue: setting goals and planning service. Contracting is a constructive approach to working with clients and is receiving increasing attention by health professionals. The purpose and components of contracting with clients will be discussed in the next section.

POSTVISIT PHASE. Even though the nurse has now concluded the home visit and left the client's home, responsibility for the visit is not complete until the interaction has been recorded. (see Chapter 13 for a discussion of the purposes of record keeping). Agencies may or may not organize their records by families; that is, the basic record may be a "family" folder or a record with all members included in one record, or each family member receiving services may have a separate record, with family members' records cross-referenced. In reality the concept of a family-focused record often breaks down. History and background usually are given to some extent for the family, but often the focus shifts to individual health histories and, consequently, nursing diagnoses, goals, and interventions that are directed toward individual family members rather than the family unit. Record systems and formats will vary from agency to agency. The nurse needs to become familiar with the particular system used in the agency. All systems should include the following elements: a data base, nursing diagnoses and problem list; a plan, including specific goals; actual actions and interventions; and evaluation. These are the basic elements needed for legal and clinical purposes. The format may consist of narrative, flow sheets, POMR, SOAP, or a combination of formats. It is important that recorded information be current, dated, and signed.

Using theoretical frameworks appropriate to working with families give direction to the family centered nursing process. For example, a nursing diagnosis of "ineffective mothering skill related to lack of knowledge of normal growth and development" is an individual-focused nursing diagnosis. "Inability for family to accomplish stage-appropriate task of providing safe environment for preschooler related to lack of knowledge and resources" is a family focused nursing diagnosis based on knowledge of the developmental approach to families. To provide family centered nursing care, diagnoses, goals, and interventions need to be family focused. At times the need also will exist to present information for a specific family member. However, the emphasis should be on the individual as a member of, and within the context of, the family.

Contracting in Family Health Promotion

Increasingly, health professionals look at working with clients in a more interactive, collaborative style. This approach is consistent with a more knowledgeable public and the recent self-care movement. *Contracting,* which is an agreement between two or more parties, involves a shift in responsibility and control to a shared effort by client and professional versus that of the professional alone. The ANA Standards of Community Health Nursing Practice (1986) explicitly state the rights of clients to participate actively in planning their own health care and designate that "in partnership with the family and individual" the community health nurse collects, interprets, and analyzes data; formulates and validates diagnoses; formulates plans and implements interventions; and evaluates process and revision of the plan. This active involvement of the client is reflected in several of the existing nursing models, particularly those of Rogers (1970), King (1981), and Orem (1991). Contracting is one strategy aimed at promoting a collaborative working relationship, in this instance, one specifically focused on health promotion.

Contracting is a way of formally involving the family in the nursing process and explaining their roles. Some nurses are reluctant to use the term *contracting* but discuss it in terms of mutual goal setting. Some of this reluctance may be because of the potential legal ramifications of a contract, whether formal or informal. There may be concern about possible liability in terms of services agreed on versus those delivered or received or attainment of agreed on outcomes. In some cases, the connection of the term *contracting* with compliance model may be contrary to a philosophy of an interactive partnership between nurse and client.

Thus, an important issue that needs to be considered is the purpose and/or philosophy that underlies the nurse's use of contracting with families. A large body of literature addresses the "noncompliant" client or family. Edel identifies the concept of compliance as applying to relationships between "those who have power and those over whom they exercise it" (Edel, 1985, p. 183). These relationships are described as vertical, with one party dominating the other. This approach contradicts the collaborative relationship. If contracting is viewed only as another approach to increase compliance, the basic premises of the concept are violated. Contracting addresses the issue of control by the client versus control by the professional (Boehm, 1989; Hayes and Davis, 1980).

Purposes

The purpose of contracting is to enhance and support the clients' active role in health care by defining clients' and professionals' roles to accomplish health-related goals (Herje, 1980). Sloan and Schommer (1975) differentiate between a legal contract and a nursing contract. The former is defined as a written, binding agreement and the latter as a working agreement that is continuously renegotiable and may or may not be written. A nursing contract may be either a contingency or noncontingency one (Boehm, 1989). A contingency contract states a specific reward for the client after completion of the client's portion of the contract; a noncontingency contract does not specify rewards. The implied rewards are the positive consequences of reaching the goals specified in the contract.

In the instance of family health promotion, it is essential that the contract be made with all responsible and appropriate members of the family. Involving only one individual is invalid if the goal is family health promotion, which requires a total family system effort. Scheduling a visit with all family members present may require extra effort; if meeting with the entire family is not possible, each family member can review a contract, give input, and sign it. This allows for active participation by all family members without the necessity of finding a time when everyone involved can be present.

TABLE 27-3
Phases and activities in contracting

Phase	Activity
I Beginning Phase:	Mutual data collection and exploration of needs and problems
	Mutual establishment of goals
	Mutual exploration of resources
	Mutual development of a plan
II Working Phase:	Mutual devision of responsibilities
	Mutual setting of time limits
	Mutual implementation of plan
	Mutual evaluation and renegotiation
III Termination Phase:	Mutual termination of contract

The Process of Contracting: Phases and Activities

Contracting is a learned skill on the part of both the nurse and the family. All parties involved need to know the purpose and process of contracting. Leavitt (1982) identifies three general phases: beginning, working, and termination. The three phases can be further specified into seven sets of activities. The phases and activities are summarized in Table 27-3, and an example of a contract is included in Appendix B2.

The first activity involves both the family and the nurse in data collection and analysis of the data. An important aspect of this step is obtaining the family's perspective of the situation and its needs and problems. The nurse can present his or her observations and validate them with the family and also gain the family's view. Leavitt (1982) suggests that the initial contract be based on the most obvious and/or concrete of the family's needs; more subtle problems can be added as the family and nurse build their working relationship.

It is important that goals be mutually set and be realistic. A pitfall for nurses and clients who are new to contracting is to set overly ambitious goals. The nurse should recognize that there may be discrepancies between professional priorities and those of the client and determine whether negotiation is required. Because contracting is a process characterized by renegotiation, the goals are not static.

Throughout the process, the nurse and family need to continually learn and recognize what each can contribute to meeting health needs. This exploration of resources allows both parties to be aware of their own and others' strengths and requires a review of the nurse's skills and knowledge, family support system, and community resources.

Developing a plan to meet the goals involves specifying activities, prioritizing goals, and selecting a starting point. Next the nurse and the family need to decide who will be responsible for which activities. Structuring time limits involves deciding on a deadline for accomplishing or evaluating progress toward accomplishing a goal and the frequency of contacts. At the agreed on time, the nurse and family together evaluate the progress to date in both process and outcome. Based on the evaluation, the contract can be modified, renegotiated, or terminated.

Advantages and Disadvantages of Contracting

Contracting takes time and effort and may require the family and nurse to reorient their roles. Increased control on the part of the family also means increased responsibility. Some nurses may have difficulty relinquishing the role of the controlling expert professional. Contracts will not always be successful, and contracting is neither appropriate nor possible in some cases. Some clients do not want to have this kind of involvement; they prefer to defer to the "authority" of the professional. Included in this group are individuals with minimal cognitive skills, those who are involved in an emergency situation, those who are unwilling to be more active in their care, and those who do not see control or authority for health concerns within their domain (Herje, 1980). Some of these clients may learn to contract; some never will.

The use of the nursing process does not necessarily provide an active role for the family as a client; it assumes that needs exist based on professional judgment and that changes can and should be made within the family unit. Contracting is one alternative approach that depends on the value of input from the nurse and family, competency of the family, responsibility on the part of the family, and the dynamic nature of the process that not only allows for but also requires continual renegotiation. Although it may not be appropriate in all situations or with all families, contracting can give direction and structure to health promotion in families.

Enabling and Empowering Families

Help-giving interventions do not always have positive outcomes for clients. If families do not perceive a situation as a problem or need, offers of help may cause resentment. Help giving may also have negative consequences if there is not a match between what is expected and what is offered. Nurses' failure to recognize families' competencies and to define an active role for families can lead to dependency and lack of growth for families. This can be frustrating for both the nurse and the family. For families to become active participants, they need to feel a sense of personal competence as well as "a desire for and, willingness to take action in, the public domain" (Zimmerman and Rappaport, 1988, p. 746). Recently, approaches for assisting individuals and families to assume an active role in their health promotion have focused on empowerment (Dunst and Trivette, 1987; Hegar and Hunzeker, 1988; Pinderhughes, 1983; Rappaport, 1987). Definitions of empowerment reflect three characteristics of the family seeking help: (1) access and control over needed resources, (2) decision-making and problem-solving abilities, and (3) acquisition of instrumental behavior needed to interact effectively with others to obtain resources (Dunst and Trivette, 1987, p. 445). The last characteristic refers to the fact that families may need to learn how to identify sources of help, how to contact agencies, how to ask critical questions, and how to negotiate with agencies to have family needs met. These characteristics generally reflect a process by which people (individuals, families, organizations, or communities) "gain mastery over their affairs" (Rappaport, 1987, p. 122).

Empowerment requires a viewpoint that often conflicts

with the perspective of many helping professions, including nursing, in which the underlying assumption is one of a partnership between the professional and the client versus one in which the professional is dominant. First, families are assumed to either be competent or to be capable of becoming competent. This implies that the professional is not an unchallengeable authority who is in control. Second, an environment that creates opportunities for competencies to be used is necessary. Finally, families need to identify that their actions result in behavior change. Dunst and Trivette (1987) propose that different models of helping result in very different outcomes. The compensatory model, which recognizes the clients' responsibility for the need/problem and emphasizes clients' responsibility for solving their problems, is proposed to lead to clients acquiring behaviors that increase independence and autonomy and a sense of self-efficacy resulting in enhanced well-being. This model has the potential to guide interventions that are empowering to families.

Specifically, a community health nursing intervention that incorporates the principles of empowerment identified by Dunst and Trivette (1987) would be directed toward the building of nurse-family partnerships that emphasize health promotion. The nurse's approach to the family should be positive and focused on competencies rather than on problems or deficits. The interventions need to be consistent with family cultural norms and the family's perception of their problem. Rather than making decisions for the family, the nurse would support the family in primary decision-making and bolster their self-esteem by recognizing and using family strengths and support networks. Interventions promoting family behaviors that increase family competency and decrease the need for outside help, resulting in families seeing themselves as being actively responsible for bringing about desired changes. The goal of an empowering approach is to create a partnership between the nurse and the family characterized by cooperation and shared responsibility.

Community Resources

Families have varied and complex needs and problems. The community health nurse often mobilizes resources to effectively and appropriately meet family health promotion needs. Although specific resources vary from community to community, general types can be identified. A number of governmental resources such as Medicare, Medicaid, Aid to Families with Dependent Children, Supplementary Security Income, Food Stamps, and Women, Infants, Children (WIC) are available in most communities. These programs primarily provide support for basic needs (e.g., illness/health care, nutritional needs, and funds for housing and clothing) and funds are based on meeting of eligibility criteria.

In addition to governmental agencies providing health-related services to families, most communities have voluntary (nongovernmental) programs. Local chapters of organizations such as the American Cancer Society, the American Heart Association, the American Lung Association, and Muscular Dystrophy Association provide educational and support services and some direct services to individuals and families. These agencies provide primary prevention

and health promotion services as well as screening programs and assistance once the disease or condition is diagnosed. Local social service agencies such as Catholic Social Services provide direct services such as counseling to families. Other voluntary organizations provide direct service (e.g., shelters for the homeless or battered individuals, substance abuse counseling and treatment, Meals on Wheels, transportation, clothing, food, and furniture).

Health resources in the community may be proprietary, voluntary, or public (see Chapter 2). In addition to private health care providers, community health nurses should be aware of voluntary and public clinics, screening programs, and health promotion programs.

Identifying resources in a community requires time and effort. One obvious and valuable source is the telephone book. Community service organizations such as the Chamber of Commerce and the local health department often publish community resource listings. Regardless of how the resource is identified, the community health nurse must be familiar with the type of service offered and any requirements or costs involved. If this information is not available, the community health nurse can contact the resource (see Chapter 39 for more discussion of available community resources).

Locating and using these systems often requires skills and patience that many families lack. Community health nurses work with families to identify community resources and as a client advocate in assisting families to learn to use resources. This may involve sharing information with families, rehearsing with families what questions to ask, preparing required materials, making the initial contact, and arranging transportation. Finally, the appropriateness and effectiveness of resources should be evaluated with families after referrals.

CLINICAL APPLICATION

The initial referral for community health nursing service to a family provides limited information, and the situation that develops may be much more complex than anticipated. The following example, based on an actual case, illustrates the issues and approaches outlined in this chapter.

A referral was received at the Middle County Health Department indicating that Amy Cress, age 16 years, had been referred by the school counselor at the local high school for prenatal supervision. Amy was 4 months pregnant, in apparently good health, in the tenth grade, and living at home with her mother, stepfather, and younger sister. The family lived in a rural area outside a small farming community. The father of the baby also lived in the community and continued to see Amy on a regular basis. The referral information provided the community health nurse with a beginning, but limited, assessment of the family situation. A home visit would allow for a more extensive assessment of the family within the four models of health: clinical, role-performance, adaptive, and eudaimonistic.

The community health nurse phoned the home to make an appointment for a home visit. Amy's mother answered the phone and indicated that Amy was at school during the day. The nurse introduced herself and explained that the counselor at the high school had talked with Amy about the possibility of having a community health nurse from the health department help her to learn more about her pregnancy, labor and delivery, and caring for a new infant. Amy's mother sounded both relieved and enthusiastic about having the nurse visit. Although Amy was in school during the day, she could arrange to be at home so that the nurse could meet her at the end of the agency working day. An appointment was made for later in the week to meet with Amy and her mother. At this point, the initiation and previsit phases of the home visit process were completed by the nurse.

At the first home visit, it became apparent that Amy and her mother were interested in continuing community health nursing service. During her visit with Amy and her mother, the nurse added to her assessment by exploring with them what they saw as problems and concerns. This is consistent with an approach focused on empowerment. Amy and her mother identified a number of questions and concerns. How could Amy finish her education and care for a child? What would labor and delivery be like? How could Amy and her boyfriend avoid unplanned pregnancies in the future? How could the family members be supportive and yet have their own needs met? To extend the assessment to the entire family system, a second visit was scheduled to include Amy's boyfriend and stepfather.

During the second visit, additional areas related to clinical health of family, in terms of acute or chronic conditions, were assessed. Because it was apparent that there was a potential conflict between individual and family development needs that had implications for the adaptive processes of the family, time was spent identifying both family needs and individual needs and how best to meet these needs. A contract was negotiated to continue visiting with Amy, but the visits would occur at school during a study period. The focus would be on prenatal teaching on the nurse's part, with Amy agreeing to attend a group for pregnant students offered at the school. Visits were also arranged with Amy's mother to discuss her concerns. These approaches reflected acknowledgement of the family's abilities to be actively and competently involved in resolving problems they had identified.

Over time, the contract was modified and expanded to include well-child supervision during the year following the birth of a healthy baby boy. During this time, Amy's maternal grandfather, who had been recently widowed, became ill and was unable to live alone. The grandfather moved into the family home and the family became a four-generation unit. Amy's mother discussed a number of conflicts about her commitment to caring for her father, assisting with the care of her grandson until Amy finished school and could make other arrangements, having time for her other daughter, and continuing to develop her relationship with her husband in a fairly new marriage (she had been widowed 3 years earlier). Although the focus of nursing assessment and intervention continued to be on increasing the skills and resources of the family, the contract was evaluated to determine both effectiveness and needs for revision to meet the changing needs of the family. The contract was modified

to include working with Amy's mother to renew her child care skills, providing health supervision for the grandfather, and identifying a schedule for the family that allowed time for the mother and stepfather to have some time alone. The complexity of the family's needs meant that the contract was frequently modified and that not all plans worked. Amy's mother eventually indicated that alternative care was needed for the grandfather and, based on options identified by the nurse and the mother, an adult foster home was located and a placement made. Conflict arose between Amy's and her boyfriends' individual developmental needs as adolescents and family developmental tasks to be accomplished. Plans and responsibilities had to be renegotiated. With much effort, some pain, and a great deal of commitment to one another, family members moved to a pattern described by Smith LA (1983) as role-sharing in incorporating the adolescent mother and child into the household. Successful completion of developmental tasks of confirming the pregnancy to the family, committing to a new system, redefining relationships, and role-sharing characterized the evolution of this family. The family has yet to deal with whether or not Amy and her son will continue to live in the family home when she finishes the beautician training she enrolled in after high school. Amy's mother has indicated a desire to have Amy, her son, and the baby's father live separately, with or without marriage.

This family situation is not an unusual one and reflects many of the problems and needs of contemporary families. The skills required of the community health nurse are many and varied. Knowledge of family structure, function, developmental tasks, family support systems, health promotion over the life span, and community resources have been essential in working with this family.

SUMMARY

Promoting health in families is a complex process that requires an understanding of family theory, health promotion, changing family structure, and forces that affect families. This chapter presented an overview of the implications of changing family and health systems for family health promotion.

Although community health nurses come in contact with families in a variety of settings, the home visit continues to be a major modality for providing service to families. The purposes and advantages and disadvantages of home visits were reviewed.

The concept of contracting families formalizes and effectively implements the nursing process in family health promotion. Three phases and specific activities provide guidelines for implementing this strategy.

Empowering families was proposed as an approach that can be integrated with home visits and contracting to enhance family competency and active participation in health promotion. Working with families to promote the health of family systems, family members, and ultimately populations will continue to be an important aspect of community health nursing.

KEY CONCEPTS

The importance of the family as a major client system for community health nursing in promoting the health of individuals and populations is well-documented; the family system is a basic unit within which health behavior, including health values, health habits, and health risk perceptions are developed, organized, and performed.

Knowledge of family structure and functioning, family theory, nursing theory, and models of health behavior are fundamental to implementing the nursing process with families in the community. However, community health nurses need to recognize important issues that influence family health promotion. Issues related to family health promotion originate from three major sources: the family system itself; the health care system, which includes the discipline and profession of nursing; and the social, political, and economic environment within which the family exists.

From the perspective of the health paradigm, another less prevalent approach to identifying dimensions of family health is to examine families' perceptions of their health.

An important question for the community health nurse to consider in working with families is the emphasis on the client unit; that is, whether the focus is on an individual family member or on the family unit.

In contrast to working with the family system to promote individuals' health, the focus of nursing service can be the health promotion of the family system both internally and in interaction with social, political, economic, educational, physical, and health systems.

An important aspect of community health nursing's role in promoting the health of populations has been the tradition of providing services to individual families in their homes.

Home visits afford the opportunity to gain a more accurate assessment of the family structure and behavior in the natural environment. Home visits also provide opportunities to make observations of the home environment and to identify both barriers and supports for reaching family health promotion goals.

Increasingly, health professionals have come to look toward working with clients in a more interactive, collaborative style.

Contracting, which is an agreement between two or more parties, involves a shift in responsibility and control to a shared effort by client and professional versus that of the professional alone.

The purpose of contracting is to enhance and support the client's active role in health care by defining who will do what to accomplish health-related goals.

Families have varied and complex needs and problems. The community health nurse often mobilizes a number of resources to effectively and appropriately meet family health promotion needs.

LEARNING ACTIVITIES

1. Select one or more agencies in which community health nurses work and examine the agency's and community health nursing's philosophies and objectives with emphasis on individual care, family care, illness care, health promotion, and prevention.

2. Form small groups and discuss approaches that can be used by community health nurses for integrating family health promotion and prevention activities into existing health services.

3. Identify three community health problems in your community and discuss the implications of these problems for the health of families. Identify three health problems common to families in your community and discuss the implications of the problems for the health and/or health care resources of the community.

4. Select three to four families (hypothetically or from actual situations) representative of different ethnic and socioeconomic backgrounds. Compare the similarities and differences in their health promotion behaviors. How are their health promotion behaviors related to the factors of motivation, perceptions, values, and attitudes?

BIBLIOGRAPHY

Antonovosky A: Health, stress, and coping, San Francisco, 1979, Jossey-Bass.

Antonovosky A: Unraveling the mystery of health: how people manage stress and stay well, San Francisco, 1987, Jossey-Bass.

American Nurses' Association: Council of Community Health Nurses: standards of community health nursing practice, Kansas City, 1986, American Nurses' Association.

Baranowski T and Nader PR: Family health behavior. In Turk DC and Kerns RD, editors:

Health, illness, and families: a life-span perspective, New York, 1985a, John Wiley & Sons.

Baranowski T and Nader PR: Family involvement in health behavior change program, New York, 1985b, John Wiley & Sons.

Baranowski T, Nader PR, Dunn K, and Vanderpool NA: Family self-help: promoting changes in health behavior, Journal of Communication 32(3):161-72, 1982.

Barkauskas VH: Effectiveness of public health nurse home visits to primarous mothers and their

infants, Am J Public Health 73(5):573-80, 1983.

Becker MH, Haefner DP, Kasl SV, et al: Selected psychosocial models and correlates of individual health-related behaviors, Med Care 15:27-46, 1977.

Berg CL and Helgeson D: That first home visit, Journal of Community Health Nursing 1(3):207-15, 1984.

Boehm F: Patient contracting. In Fitzpatrick JJ, Taunton RL, and Benoliel JQ, editors: Annual review of Nursing Research, vol 7, 143-153,

New York, 1989, Springer.

Bomar PJ, editor: Nurses and family health promotion: concepts, assessment, and interventions, Baltimore, Md, 1989, Williams & Wilkins.

Chin S: Can self-care theory be applied to families? In Riehl-Sisca J, editor: The science and art of self-care (pp 56-62), Norwalk, Conn, 1985, Appleton-Century-Crofts.

Clements LW and Roberts FB, editors: Family health: a theoretical approach to nursing care, New York, 1983, John Wiley & Sons, Inc.

Combs-Orme T, Reis J and Ward LD: Effectiveness of home visits by public health nurses in maternal and child health: an emperical review, Public Health Rep 100(5):490-9, 1985.

Doherty WJ and McCubbin HI: Family and health care: an emerging arena of theory, research, and clinical intervention, Family Relations Journal, 34:1, 5-11, 1985.

Duffy ME: Health promotion in the family: current findings and directives for nursing research, J of Advanced Nursing 13:109-117, 1988.

Dunst CJ and Trivette CM: Enabling and empowering families: conceptual and intervention issues, School Psychology Review 16(4):443-56, 1987.

Duvall EM and Miller BC: Marriage and family development, ed 6, New York, 1985, Harper & Row, Publishers, Inc.

Edel MK: Noncompliance: an appropriate nursing diagnosis? Nurs Outlook 33(4):183-5, 1985.

Frey MA: Social support and health: a theoretical formulation derived from King's conceptual framework, Nursing Science Quarterly 2(3):138-48, 1989.

Gillis C, Highley BL, Roberts BM, and Martinson IM, editors: Toward a science of family nursing, Menlo Park, Calif, 1989, Addison-Wesley Publishing.

Gluek CJ, Laskorszewski PM, Rao DC, et al: Familial aggregation of coronary risk factors. In Coonan W and Bristow D, editors: Complications in coronary health disease, Philadelphia, 1985, JB Lippincott.

Guilino C and LaMonica G: Public health nursing: a study of role implementation, Public Health Nurs 3(2):80-91, 1986.

Hall LA: Effect of teaching on primiparas' perception of their newborn, Nurs Res 29:317-21, 1980.

Hanson J: The family. In Roy C, editor: Introduction to nursing: an adaptation model, ed 2, (pp 519-33), Engelwood Cliffs, NJ, 1984, Prentice-Hall.

Hanson SMH: Healthy single parent families, Family Relations 35(1):125-32, 1986.

Hayes WS and Davis LL: What is a health care contract? Health Values: Achieving High Level Wellness, 4(2):82-9, 1980.

Hegar RL and Hunzeker JM: Moving toward empowerment-based practice in public child welfare, Social Work 33:499-502, November-December, 1988.

Helgeson DM and Berg CL: Contracting: a method of health promotion, Journal of Community Health Nursing 2(4):199-207, 1985.

Herje PA: Hows and whys of patient contracting, Nurse Educator 5(1):30-4, 1980.

Johnston RL: Approaching family intervention through Roger's conceptual model. In Whall AL, editor: Family therapy theory for nursing: four approaches (pp 11-32), Norwalk, Conn, 1987, Appleton-Century-Crofts.

Kallins EL: The textbook of public health nursing, St Louis, 1967, CV Mosby Co.

Kantor D and Lehr W: Inside the family, San Francisco, 1977, Jossey-Bass.

King IM: A theory for nursing: systems, concepts, process, New York, 1981, John Wiley & Sons.

King IM: King's theory of nursing. In Clements IW and Roberts FB, editors: Family health: a theoretical approach to nursing (pp 177-88), New York, 1983, John Wiley & Sons.

Laffrey SC, Loveland-Cherry CJ, and Winkler SJ: Health behavior: evolution of two paradigms, Public Health Nurs 3(2):92-100, 1986.

Larson CP: Efficacy of prenatal and postpartum visits on child health and development, Pediatrics 66:183-90, 1980.

Leahy KM, Cobb MM, and Jones MC: Public health nursing ed 3, New York, 1982, McGraw-Hill, Inc.

Leavitt MB: Families at risk: primary prevention in nursing practice, Boston, 1982, Little, Brown & Co.

Litman TJ: The family as a basic unit in health and medical care: a social behavioral overview, Soc Sci Med 8:495-519, 1974.

Loveland-Cherry CJ: Family system patterns of cohesiveness and autonomy: relationship to family members' health behavior, Dissertation Abstracts Intern 43(11B):35-7, 1982.

Loveland-Cherry CJ: Family system patterns of autonomy and cohesiveness: relationship to family members' health behavior, Nursing Res 33(1):51-2, 1984.

Loveland-Cherry CJ: Personal health practices in single parent and two parent families, Family Relations Journal 35(1):133-139, 1986.

Lowe ML: Effectiveness of teaching as measured by compliance with medical recommendations, Nursing Res 19:59-63, 1973.

McCubbin H and Patterson J: Family adaptation in crisis. In McCubbin H, Cauble A, and Patterson J, editors: Family stress coping and social support (pp 26-47), Springfield, Ill, 1982, Charles C. Thomas.

McNeil HJ and Holland SS: A comparative study of public health nurse teaching in groups and in home visits, Am J Public Health 62(12):1629-37, 1972.

Matarazzo JD, Connor WE, Fey SG, et al: Behavioral cardiology with emphasis on the family heart study: fertile ground for psychological and biomedical research. In Millon T, Green CJ, and Meagher RB editors: Handbook of health care psychology, New York, 1982, Plenum Press.

Mauksch HO: A social science basis for conceptualizing family health, Soc Sci Med 8:521-8, 1974.

Mayers M: Home visit—Ritual or therapy? Nurs Outlook 21(5):328-31, 1973.

Olds DL, Henderson CR Jr, Tatelbaum R, Chamberlain R: Improving the life-course development of socially disadvantaged mothers: a randomized trial of nurse home visitation, Am J Public Health 78(11):1436-1445, 1988.

Olson DH, Sprenkle DH, and Russell C: Circumplex model of marital and family systems. I. cohesion and adaptability dimensions, family type, and clinical applications, Fam Process 18:3-28, 1979.

Orem DE: The self-care deficit theory of nursing: a general theory. In Clements IW and Roberts FB, editors: Family health: a theoretical approach to nursing care (pp 205-217), New York, 1983, John Wiley & Sons.

Orem DE: Nursing concepts of practice, ed 3, New York, 1985, McGraw-Hill Book Co.

Orem DE: Nursing: concepts of practice, ed 4, New York, 1991, McGraw-Hill Book Co.

Pender NJ: Health promotion in nursing practice, ed 2, Norwalk, Conn, 1987, Appleton & Lange.

Pesznecker BL and Zahlis E: Establishing mutual help groups for family-member care givers: a new role for community health nurses, Public Health Nurs 3(1):29-37, 1986.

Petze CF: Health promotion for the well family, Nurs Clin North Am 19(2):229-37, 1984.

Pinderhughes EB: Empowerment for clients and for ourselves. Social Casework: The Journal of Contemporary Social Work 64:331-8, 1983.

Pratt L: Child rearing methods and children's health behavior, J Health Soc Behav 14:16-9, 1973.

Pratt L: Family structure and effective health behavior, Boston, 1976, Houghton Mifflin Co.

Rappaport J: Terms of empowerment/exemplars of prevention: toward a theory for community psychology, Am J Community Psychol 15(2):121-48, 1987.

Rink LT, editor: Outcome measures in home care, vol: Research, New York, 1987, National League of Nursing.

Rogers M: An introduction to the theoretical basis of nursing, Philadelphia, 1970, F.A. Davis Co.

Rogers ME: Science of unitry human being: a paradigm for nursing. In Clements IW and Roberts FB, editors: Family health: a theoretical approach to nursing care (pp 219-28), New York, 1983, John Wiley & Sons.

Roy C: Introduction to nursing: an adaptation model, ed 2, Englewood Cliffs, NJ, 1984, Prentice Hall, Inc.

Siegel E, Bauman KE, Schaefer ES, et al: Hospital and home support during infancy: impact on maternal attachment, child abuse and neglect, and health care utilization, Pediatrics 66:183-90, 1980.

Simons-Morton DG, O'Hara NM, and Simons-Morton DG: Promoting healthful diet and exercise behaviors in communities, schools, and families, Family and Community Health 9(3):1-13, 1986.

Sloan MR and Schommer BT: The process of contracting in community nursing. In Spradley BW, editor: Contemporary community nursing, Boston, 1975, Little, Brown and Co.

Smith JA: The idea of health, implication for the nursing professional, New York, 1983, Teachers College Press, Columbia University.

Smith LA: A conceptual model of families incorporating an adolescent mother and child into the household, Advances in Nursing Science 6(1):45-60, 1983.

Tadych R: Nursing in multiperson units: the family. In Riehl-Sisca J, editor: The science and art of self-care (pp 49-55), Norwalk, Conn, 1985, Appleton-Century-Crofts.

Taylor SG: An interpretation of family within Orem's general theory of nursing, Nursing Science Quarterly 2(3):131-7, 1989.

United States General Accounting Office: Home visiting: a promising early intervention strategy for at-risk families. (GAO/HRD-90-83). Washington, DC, 1990, United States General Accounting Office.

Whall AL: Family therapy theory for nursing: four approaches, Norwalk, Conn, 1987, Appleton-Century-Crofts.

Zimmerman MA and Rappaport J: Citizen participation, perceived control, and psychological empowerment, Am J Community Psychol 16(5):725-50, 1988.

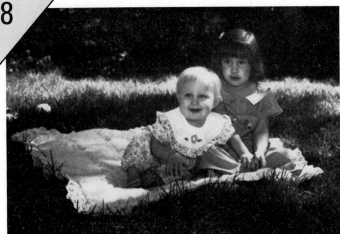

28

The First Through Sixth Years of Life

Nancy Dickenson-Hazard

OBJECTIVES

After reading this chapter, the student should be able to:

Identify and discuss significant factors in the prenatal environment that influence neonatal health.

Describe the characteristic elements of physical and psychosocial growth and development in the first 5 years of life.

Identify and discuss major factors affecting growth and development and the nurse's role in relation to these factors.

Identify and discuss major causes of death and illness in the child from birth through 5 years of age.

Discuss appropriate nursing assessment tools for the child from birth through 5 years of age.

Identify the role of the community health nurse and discuss appropriate nursing interventions that promote and maintain the health of infants, toddlers, and preschoolers.

KEY TERMS

attachment

child abuse and neglect

congenital anomaly

critical periods

child care

diet assessment

family assessment

fetal assessment

group parent education

growth spurts

heredity

homeless children

immaturity and prematurity

immunizations

infectious diseases

malnutrition

mastery

neonatal assessment

nutrition

pediatric acquired immunodeficiency syndrome (AIDS)

play

sepsis

sudden infant death syndrome (SIDS)

technology-dependent child

temperament

working mother

C hildren are one third of our population and all of our future . . . their health is our foundation. Because children must learn health practices, the opportunity to teach health promotion and maintenance is greater for children than for any other population group.

Childhood is the period of life when most behaviors are learned, and parents are the primary teachers of acceptable behavior. The community health nurse can influence this learning process by helping parents and children learn methods that promote positive health behaviors.

This chapter provides information on the assessment of child health within the community for the child from birth through age 5 years. The content includes age-specific growth, development, major health problems, and the tools and techniques of health promotion activities.

PRENATAL ENVIRONMENT

Assessing the quality of the atmosphere in which a fetus grows is the first step in ensuring a healthy childhood. The community health nurse makes this assessment in a variety of settings. Being aware of the prenatal factors that promote wellness facilitates the nurse's assessment.

Before Conception

At the moment of conception, some aspects of wellness are determined. Genetic and chromosomal abnormalities, blood group incompatibilities, and maternal age and state of health influence fetal health before and at the time of conception. Up to 10% of all births in the United States involve birth defects, the majority of which are inherited (Wegman, 1990). Although preventing genetic defects is the primary objective when advising parents at risk, facilitating parental knowledge about the disorder becomes a priority once conception has occurred. Nursing assessment and referral are essential elements in the complex process of genetic counseling.

Fetal Assessment and Parent Education

Fetal assessment evaluates the fetus's physical environment and the physical and psychosocial environment of the mother. Nurses can better assess fetal health by using their knowledge of and data from modern technologies that detect these difficulties (sonography, amniocentesis, and mechanical fetal monitoring). Being aware of the indicators of high-risk parents (i.e., adolescent, single, unplanned pregnancy, history of mental illness, substance abuse, or child abuse, previous pregnancy or child loss, no permanent living plan, or a high number of children born close together) assists the nurse in the fetal assessment. Further nursing interventions should include information sharing, explanations, reassurance, and assistance for parents in balancing family stresses and support (Miller, 1986).

Contributing to a slow decline in the overall infant mortality in the past 5 years is the lack of improvement in the rate of timely receipt of prenatal care (Wegman, 1990; National Commission to Prevent Infant Mortality, 1988). The role of the community health nurse is to educate and counsel prospective parents by implementing existing prenatal programs, identifying pregnant mothers at risk, developing adequate prenatal follow-up and referral systems, and promoting universal access to prenatal health care.

Nursing activities that promote maternal and fetal health after conception include the following:

Complete data collection mechanism, including pregnancy, maternal health, and family history

Physical assessment and appropriate laboratory studies

Plan of care in collaboration with parents-to-be, focusing on their physical and psychosocial needs, including readiness and ability to parent

As the pregnancy progresses, education about the neonate and parenting must begin and monitoring of maternal and fetal physical health must continue. The pediatric prenatal visit is an effective health promotion activity in which ex-

---

▷ **TABLE 28-1**
  Assessing the neonate

Assessment	Activity	Nursing implications
Apgar scoring	Observation and scoring of newborn appearance, pulse, grimace, activity, respiration	Identifies deviations for underlying problem
Gestational age	Record number of weeks in utero; indicators of physical maturity	Influences management of well-infant care Infuences nutrition, education, infant development, assessment, care education, referral
Physiological changes	Observe norms of: Average birth weight: 7 lbs 8 oz (3400 g) with 5-7 oz weekly gain by 1 mo Average birth length: 19½ in (49 cm) with ½ to 1 in monthly gain Average heart circumference: 12 in (33 cm) with 1.5 cm monthly gain	Periodic monitoring of weight, height, heart and chest circumference, vital signs Influences well-infant care management, particularly nutritional and growth development assessment
Reflex activity	Observe and assess for absence, asymmetry, or abnormal persistence (see Appendix K3)	Identifies and refers for deviations Influences anticipatory guidance
Sensory function	Observe and assess for response to tactile, auditory, and taste stimulation, visual acuity	Identifies and refers for deviations Influences anticipatory guidance
Normal variations	Observe and assess for normal variations and minor abnormalities (see Appendix J1)	Identifies and refers for deviations Provides anticipatory guidance for parents

pectant parents, with the nurse's help, can lay the groundwork for positive influences on the child's health. The optimal time for the prenatal assessment is at 33 to 37 weeks of gestation—before parents begin to focus on delivery (Miller, 1986).

PHYSICAL GROWTH AND DEVELOPMENT

Human growth and development are orderly, predictable processes that begin with the embryo and continue until death. Growth is the quantitative or measurable aspects of the individual's size, whereas development is the qualitative or observable aspects of progressive changes in the individual. The progression through the definite phases of growth and development are influenced by hereditary and environmental factors. The nurse must be cognizant of these factors and the overall process when assessing the measurable and observable aspects. In addition, individual variations in progression through the process must be considered.

Neonates

The period of life from birth to 1 month of age is commonly referred to as the neonatal period. During this phase of life the newborn's functioning and behavior are mostly reflexive. Stabilization of major body functions is the primary task of the neonate and occurs in a definite sequence of physiological events in the first hours of life.

Physiological stabilization is affected by birth and rapid growth of the neonate. These physiological changes are evidenced through the monitoring of vital signs. Community health nurses should be proficient in measuring vital signs and growth and need to be aware of the subtle changes that occur in these indicators during the neonatal and infancy periods to make an accurate assessment of the newborn's physiological functioning. (See a basic text in pediatric nursing for a review of vital sign values.)

The physical examination of the newborn is one of the most important tools for assessing neonatal health. With the trend toward early discharge after delivery (within 24 to 48 hours), the community health nurse frequently conducts a *neonatal assessment*. Using the data obtained from a physical examination provides the nurse with an opportunity to implement preventive health activities (Table 28-1).

Danger Signs

Although most newborns adjust to functioning outside the uterine environment without incident, the possibility of neonatal difficulty exists. The nurse should therefore be alert to the danger signs indicating a need for referral and management when assessing the newborn (Chow, et al., 1984). These danger signs are presented in the box below.

Family Adaptation to the Neonate

The birth of a child creates changes for family members. Assessment of how the family is adapting becomes an essential part of the nursing process and should focus on parenting skills, the ability of parents to assume new roles and responsibilities, sibling reaction and behavior, and changes in the marital and parent-children relationships. Communication patterns, the reorganization of daily family functioning and distribution of labor, the availability of resources outside the family, changes in extended family and friend relationships, and family adjustments should also be evaluated. Nursing interventions may include actions such as encouraging parents to go out by themselves, to set aside time alone with older children, and to ask a grandparent or friend to babysit. Referring parents for financial assistance or other government-sponsored child health programs and assisting them in planning their daily activities are other interventions.

Infants

Infancy extends from 1 month to 1 year. During this time major physical growth occurs. Generally, infants double their birth weight by 6 months and triple it by 12 months of age. By the end of the first year an infant has grown between 10 and 12 inches in length.

Although infant deaths have declined, the rate of decline has slowed. However, the black to white race ratio has been

---

DANGER SIGNS IN THE NEWBORN

A positive family history for major disease or illness	Full, bulging fontanel
Gestational or delivery complications	Small head size
Abnormal positioning of neonate	Convulsions, twitching, excessive irritability
Congenital malformations	Lethargy
Rapid or difficult respirations	Fever or hypothermia
Rapid, slow, or irregular pulse rate	Paralysis
Abnormal cry	Jaundice
Unusual cough	Pallor
Cyanosis	Petechiae
Sweating	Behavior or appearance change
Vomiting of bile	Excess salivation
Delayed or inadequate voiding	Diarrhea
Bleeding, specifically noting cord and circumcision	No meconium passage in first 48 hours
Single umbilical artery	Cord odor or exudate

Adapted from Chow MP, et al.: Handbook of pediatric primary care, ed 2, New York, 1984, J Wiley & Sons, pp. 262; and Behrman RE and Vaughan VC, editors: Nelson textbook of pediatrics, ed 13, Philadelphia, 1987, WB Saunders, pp. 373.

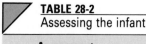

TABLE 28-2
Assessing the infant

Assessment	Activity	Nursing implications
Physiological stability	Monitor vital signs on routine basis	Influences anticipatory guidance Refers or continues to monitor vital signs if deviant
Sleep patterns	Obtain history of patterns, comparing with normal of 16 hr with short alert (7-10 min) span for newborn; 10 hr at night, with 2-3-hr day naps at 3 mo; 12 hr at night, with 1-2-hr day naps at 12 mo	Influences anticipatory guidance for promoting sleep patterns compatible with family life and for stimulating infant development
Elimination patterns	Observe and obtain history of patterns, comparing with normal of first meconium stools by 48 hr of life; one to three stools if breast fed, four to six if formula fed by 3 mo; six to eight wet diapers per day	Influences anticipatory guidance of parents for infant care Early identification of elimination problems
Feeding patterns	Observe and obtain history of feeding patterns and techniques, comparing with normal of on-demand feeding as newborn; every 3-4 hr by 3 mo; three to five times a day by 6 mo, with solid food introduction; three meals a day and snack with self-feeding and cup use at 12 mo (see Appendix J4)	Early identification and intervention for feed-difficulties Influences nutritional and feeding guidance
Neuromotor development	Observe and obtain history relevant to normal cephalocaudal progression from reflexive to purposeful and voluntary (see Appendix K7)	Early identification and management of developmental problems Influences anticipatory guidance on stimulation of development

increasing. It becomes the role of the community health nurse to identify and intervene in the situations where infants are at risk, including infants who are of low–birth weight, are premature, have congenital anomalies or chronic illnesses, have adolescent mothers, and are from low-socioeconomic backgrounds.

Nursing interventions during infancy include close monitoring of growth and development, frequent contact to assess physical and psychosocial health, and close follow-up for compliance with the nursing care plan. Particular attention should be paid to the assessment of feeding, sleeping, and elimination patterns and neuromotor development (see Table 28-2).

Growth Spurts

Physical growth in the first year is evidenced by periods of time called *growth spurts*. During these spurts, patterns of infant behavior change. Physiological functioning and subsequent metabolic requirements increase in response to the growing body's demand for increased energy through calories. The infant alters feeding patterns by increasing both the amount and the frequency of feeding. Sleeping patterns change; some infants requiring more sleep, but others may have interrupted or fretful sleep as a result of hunger. Elimination is also affected and generally decreases in frequency. However, if feeding needs are overmet, elimination patterns may increase or remain the same.

Growth spurts are most frequent and noticeable by parents in the first 6 to 8 months of life but occur periodically until adolescence. The first evident spurt occurs approximately at 6 weeks of age, and growth spurts may recur every 6 to 8 weeks until approximately 6 months of age. The behavioral changes usually last 4 to 7 days. For parents who have not been prepared to expect this normal growth occurrence, the changes in the infant's behavior can be stressful. Nurses can prevent this potential stress for parents and infants by providing (1) early anticipatory guidance and education regarding the origin and course of growth spurts, (2) counseling on how to manage them, and (3) support and reassurance when they do occur.

Toddlers and Preschool Children

The toddler years are the second and third years of life. The preschool years encompass ages 3 to 5 years. During these years growth rates decelerate and stabilize, and increased physical abilities permit an expanded exploration of the environment, both within and without the family unit.

The role of the community health nurse in the health care of this age group is continued health promotion. Nursing interventions should focus on continued growth monitoring through height, weight, vital signs, and blood pressure recording; continued assessment of feeding and sleeping patterns and neuromotor development; and initiation of dental and orthopedic assessments (Table 28-3). The community health nurse can perform these assessments during annual health maintenance visits, in the clinic or home setting, or during clinic screenings from data obtained from an interval history during the health visit.

TABLE 28-3
Assessing toddler and preschool children

Assessment	Activity	Nursing implications
Physical growth	Monitor growth, comparing with normal of annual weight gain of 5 lbs; height increases of 3-4 in annually after year 3 and up to 5 in in year 2 (see Appendix K1)	Early identification of deviant growth patterns Provides anticipatory guidance regarding normal growth patterns
Skeletal development	Observe and monitor closure of anterior fontanelle around 18 mo; normal progression from bowlegs (12-18 mo) to knock-knees (18-24 mo) to correction (see Appendix K5)	Initiates orthopedic screening Identifies deviant skeletal problems Provides anticipatory guidance and reassurance regarding normal variations
Dental growth	Inspect number and condition of teeth, comparing to normal of first tooth eruption by 6 mo; 20 primary teeth by 2 yr; addition of molars between ages 3-8 yr; loss of first primary tooth at age 5-6 yr. Initiate first dental rinses and visit by 3 yr and use of sealants and fluorides (systemic or topical)	Provides for parent and child education regarding early preventive dental care Identifies early dental problems
Sleep patterns	Obtain history on sleep requirements, comparing to normal of 8-12 night hr by 3 yr; afternoon nap until 3 yr; and establishment of bedtime routine	Provides anticipatory guidance regarding routine and common problems Early identification of deviant sleep behaviors
Feeding patterns	Obtain dietary history, focusing on distribution of calories and recommended energy intake (see Table 28-4); development of feeding skills; food preferences and food jags common at these ages (see Appendix J4)	Provides nutritional guidance Early identification of eating problems
Motor skills	Observe gross and fine skills; screen motor development by use of tools and history (see Appendix K7)	Provides anticipatory guidance on development and safety Identifies motor development difficulties

TABLE 28-4
Distribution of calories, water, and energy requirements for all age groups

Age	Protein (%)	Fat (%)	Carbohydrate (%)	Total water requirement in 24 hr (ml)	Energy needs
Low–birth weight infants	10-11	40-50	35-45	200-250	110-150 kcal/kg/day
Normal full-term infants	6-8	30-35	45-55	750 at 3 mo to 1200 at 12 mo	115 kcal/kg/day
Toddlers and preschoolers	10-12	30-45	40-50	1350 at 2 yr to 1800 at 4 yr	900-1800 kcal at 2-3 yr 1300-2300 kcal at 4-6 yr
School-age children and adolescents	10-15	30-45	35-55	2000 school-age child 2500 adolescent	1650-3300 kcal 2100-3900 kcal for males; 1500-3000 kcal for females
Adolescent athletes	10-15	25-35	50-60	2700	2000-4000 kcal

PSYCHOSOCIAL DEVELOPMENT

A child's growth process includes not only physical development but also emotional and social development. Variables that influence the child's psychosocial growth include interpersonal and cognitive characteristics and personality and temperament differences. Social and cultural variables include family structure, familial attitudes, beliefs, and economic status.

The individuality of a child's progression through the developmental phases is also influenced by the concept known as *critical periods of development.* A critical period is a specific span of time during which the environment has its greatest impact on a child's development. The nature of stimuli provided by the environment varies among children. A child's developmental progression depends on the timing and degree of environmental stimuli and his or her readiness to be stimulated by the environment. Nurses need to recognize the psychological, cognitive, social, and cultural variables that influence the child's psychosocial growth while considering normal individual differences.

Infants

Much of the foundation for psychosocial competency is built during the first year of life. The newborn enters the world dependent on others for meeting his or her needs. If basic needs are met through a close, warm, comforting relationship, a sense of trust develops. If needs are not met or are only met sporadically, a sense of mistrust develops because a child is never certain that needs will be met. The caretaker-infant relationship therefore becomes an important factor in the infant's development of a sense of trust. The quality of this relationship has a direct impact on the infant's sense of well-being, as influenced by the behavioral consistency and motivation of the caretaker. The synchronization of maternal and infant responses is termed *bonding,* or *attachment.* The interaction and attachment between mother and infant are influenced by many variables, including maternal and infant characteristics and environmental factors, such as housing conditions and sleeping arrangements, the mother's cultural and pregnancy experiences, the infant's appearance and responsiveness, and the family's financial and psychosocial support resources. Nurses can facilitate the attachment by assessing the influence these factors have on the process and intervening with support and guidance when appropriate.

The presence and development of a paternal-infant attachment and a parental unit-infant bond are additional variables influencing psychosocial growth. When appropriate, the nurse can facilitate these bonds by encouraging the father's participation in the infant's care, providing early opportunities for paternal bonding, teaching parenting skills, and providing support and empathy. In addition, nurses should teach parents how to stimulate the infant's visual, sensory, and tactile environment, thereby promoting psychosocial development. (Appendix J3 provides age-appropriate stimulation suggestions that can be used in the first year.)

Knowledge and assessment of developmental milestones are also important aspects of the nurse's role in promoting infant development. An appropriate focus when assessing psychosocial and cognitive development centers on an infant's social and language behaviors. Characteristic behaviors are reviewed in Appendixes A3 and K7.

Toddlers

During the second through third years of life, the individuality of a child becomes more apparent, as evidenced by their willingness to explore and separate from their mothers. Psychosocial development is enhanced by improved physical prowess, a developing sense of autonomy, and an expanding communicative ability.

Communication skills include those that are both expressive (active participation in the communication process) and receptive (their behavior responses to the language of their worlds). Development of these skills is important to intellectual and psychosocial development. The nurse should assess each child for appropriate language skills (see Table 26-5, Appendix K4 and Appendix K6). In addition, the developing sense of self (autonomy) should be assessed and promoted through nursing recommendations, such as parents' reading to the child, providing time for outdoor play,

TABLE 28-5	
Language development stages	
Age	**Development**
0-2 mo	Coos; small throaty sounds
2-6 mo	Babbles; single vowel and consonant sounds
8-9 mo	First word, usually imitated
9-10 mo	Comprehends simple commands
12 mo	Says two or three words with meaning
18 mo	Height of unintelligible jargon; imitates animal sounds
2 yr	Uses two- or three-word phrases; has about 300-word vocabulary
3 yr	Uses four- or five-word sentences; has 900-word vocabulary; uses plurals, pronouns, prepositions
4-5 yr	Has 500- to 2100-word vocabulary; uses correct grammatic form and complete sentences

allowing the child to help with household chores, and being concrete and concise with the child.

Providing counseling about toilet training is another way the nurse helps parents promote autonomy in their child. Educating parents about appropriate timing and techniques of toilet training facilitates success. Success for the child means a feeling of accomplishment and independence.

Play is an integral part of a child's life. It is a means to achieve developmental tasks and learn. Play contributes to a child's development in all spheres. The physical activity of play contributes to improving coordination; the explorative activity contributes to reality orientation; and the experimental activity of play contributes to self-awareness and emotional expression. Because play is a child's work, it is important for nurses to be knowledgeable about its characteristics and ways to stimulate play. Concrete, practical suggestions from nurses to parents can promote healthy, productive play. Principles useful in assisting parents to promote play are as:

- ◊ Opportunities for play that are appropriate for the child's age should be provided.
- ◊ The expense of a toy is not necessarily an indicator that it will promote development. Common household items such as plastic cartons provide as much stimulation as an expensive set of stackable cubes.
- ◊ Parents need to play with their child.
- ◊ Parents need to be aware of the child's responses to play—that is, when to stimulate and when to rest.
- ◊ Play should be pleasurable.
- ◊ Toys should be safe, durable, and suitable to the child's developmental abilities.
- ◊ Toys should promote the child's own creativity and resourcefulness and not be excessive, confusing, or overwhelming.

In addition, nurses can assist parents in directing play and selecting toys by suggesting readings and providing information appropriate to child's age and safety needs.

Preschoolers

During the preschool years, children rush to accomplish new skills, tasks, and capabilities in the expanded world of home, school, and neighborhood. They begin to assert themselves and their personalities in a world away from home. This expansion occurs comfortably when some degree of self-control is mastered. At this age, all aspects of development, (social, emotional, physical, and cognitive) must begin to come together for the child to function effectively. As the preschooler moves away from egocentric to perceptual and intuitive behaviors, his increasing use of language to express himself, rather than acting out, becomes more apparent in play and interactions. As community health nurses conduct developmental assessments of children at this age, they must consider the basic skills with which the preschooler should be equipped, including achieving fine and gross motor milestones and appropriate social behaviors and language skills (see Appendix K7).

In addition, the nurse should initiate a discussion with parents about school and the child's ability to play with peers, offering suggestions about how to select a preschool and what toys and types of play are appropriate for a child of this age.

Cognitively, the preschool child is progressing from egocentricity to prelogical thinking. In the clinical situation, the community health nurse demonstrates awareness of this ability by involving the child in what is being done. For example, the nurse might allow the child to examine a doll, performing the activities performed on the child (e.g., the nurse listens to the child's heart while the child listens to the doll's heart).

FACTORS AFFECTING GROWTH AND DEVELOPMENT

Human growth and development are continuous processes that are complex yet predictable. Although the exact age for accomplishing the specific tasks of each stage varies from child to child, a chronology of events does exist. The individual pace of a child through the developmental stages is set by a variety of factors.

Mastery

Of primary importance in developmental progression is the successful mastery of the tasks and achievement of milestones of the preceding state (Erikson, 1963). Because development is a sequential process, a child must successfully complete, in an individual style, the particular task of the specific developmental stage. For example, a 15-month-old child cannot run without first walking. Similarly, a 2-year-old child cannot separate easily from mother, unless the child has come to trust her. Although a child never completely finishes all the developmental tasks in a given stage, some degree of mastery and comfort must be achieved before proceeding successfully to the next stage (i.e., a child continues to learn to trust other people throughout life but must have developed a basic trust of mother to separate and expand into the world). As tasks are mastered, the child develops a cadre of physical and psychosocial skills that are used to expand the learning opportunities in the environment. For example, the toddler, having learned to climb, will push a chair to the countertop to reach a cookie. Once

TABLE 28-6 Temperament and personality characteristics	
Temperament	**Characteristic**
Easy	Positive mood
	Regular body functions
	Low to moderate intensity of reaction
	Adaptability to new situations
Slow-to-warm up	Low activity level
	Tendency to withdraw on first exposure to new stimuli
	Slow adaptability
	Somewhat negative mood
	Low intensity of reaction to situations
Difficult	Irregular body functions
	Intensity in reactions
	Withdrawal from new stimuli
	Slow adaptation
	Negative mood

Adapted from Chess S and Thomas A: Dynamics of individual development. In Levine MD, Carey WB, Crocker AC, and Gross RT, editors: Developmental behavioral pediatrics. Philadelphia, 1983, WB Saunders, p 158.

climbing is mastered in the home, the toddler will then use this skill at the playground, where climbing up the slide will be attempted.

By the end of the preschool years, this process of continual mastery, experience, and expansion results in a repertoire of effective behaviors, which incorporate all skill spheres. Although a distinct individual person exists in the child as an infant, this individual becomes more apparent by the end of the fifth year as a result of this integration process.

Heredity

The nurse must also be aware of the results of an individual's genetic makeup. Physical characteristics and diseases are inherited, as are some aspects of the individual's behavioral temperament (Chess and Thomas, 1983). Therefore the nurse should assess these genetic forces through an evaluation and history of the genetic makeup of several generations.

Temperament

Children differ in personality temperament. *Temperament*, defined as an individual's behavior style, is usually one of the following three types: easy, slow to warm, and difficult (Chess and Thomas, 1983). Characteristics are shown in Table 28-6. Children have been found to demonstrate temperamental characteristics in the first weeks of life. Although the environment can influence a child's behavior, the basic temperament is unique to each child.

Health and Living Environment

Children's states of health affect not only their responsiveness in the developmental process, but also the responsiveness of others to them. Similarly, conditions affecting health, such as adequacy of nutrition, sleep, rest, and exercise influence the child's development. For example, the infant who does not sleep well at night and has become a picky eater may be unable to meet the developmental task of sociability because of being tired and possibly poorly nourished.

Characteristics of the physical environment also play an important part in this process. These factors include adequacy of housing, socioeconomic status, and geographic location and resulting seasonal and climatic variations.

Family, Peers, and Life Experiences

The family's central purposes are the protection and promotion of its members. Of importance early in the child's life are the nature and adequacy of the bond developed between family members, particularly between parent and child. The quality of the parent-child relationship has been found to affect the child's development.

Second to the family in influencing development are a child's peers. Through and with a peer group, a child learns about self, others, and society, accomplishing a wide variety of developmental tasks.

Dealing with and learning through family and peers provides the child with experiences that enable progress developmentally. By applying what has been learned to new situations, the child can use experience to recognize and master further developmental tasks.

Additional nurturing influences that affect development include the child's ordinal position (oldest, youngest, or middle child), presence and sex of siblings, sex of the child, family structure and societal attitudes, and expectations and culture as interpreted within the child's home.

Working Mothers

In 1990 approximately 60% of mothers with children under 5 years of age were employed outside the home and required alternate child care. This represented 10 million children for whom care arrangements must be made (Balk and Christoffel, 1988). The primary motive for mothers working outside the home is financial need.

Because of this increasing trend toward working mothers, family functioning has changed (e.g., chores and day-to-day parenting must be shared), and many parents experience conflicting emotions (such as guilt at leaving their children in someone else's care, yet relief at having the additional income). However, the child's need for day care remains. In some working families, parents share the child-care needs by rearranging work schedules; in others, parents make arrangements in the community (e.g., day-care centers, day care by relatives, or home care by a nonrelative) (American Academy of Pediatrics, 1987). For the single working mother, child care and household management became greater challenges since these responsibilities are not shared with a spouse.

The community health nurse can facilitate the family's decision making and adjustment to the mother's return to work and selection of day care at several points in the process. Initially the nurse can assist the parent(s) in identifying the need for both parents to work and possible alternatives. For example, part-time work by one spouse may be sufficient to meet financial need or work in the home by one parent may be an alternative.

Once the decision has been made, nurses should assist parents in identifying child-care alternatives, such as care in the home; day-care centers or homes; nursery schools; play schools or groups; and kindergarten. The nurse should advise parents to consider (1) the philosophy, attitude, and emotional tone expressed by the primary caretaker; (2) the physical environment and its safety, appeal and diversity, materials and equipment, and access or proximity to parents; (3) other participants in the setting, their health, their response to caretaker and environment, and their ages and developmental levels. In addition, it is wise to counsel parents to visit and observe the care setting before final selection and to periodically evaluate the setting and its effects and influence on the child. Other factors parents should consider are the licensing and accreditation status of the facility, the amount of parental involvement allowed, the program curriculum (if applicable), and the educational qualifications of the administration and staff (Balk and Christoffel, 1988; Wong, 1986).

The community health nurse can be instrumental in developing policies at the community level that will positively affect day care. Advocating requirements for up-to-date immunizations for all children and staff, special care provisions for sick children, and sanitary codes are appropriate nursing actions. Nurses can also implement education for day-care staff to prevent the spread of infectious disease. This education should include an explanation of how diseases are transmitted, appropriate infection control principles, and guidelines for managing a child with an infectious disease (Lopez et al., 1988). Advocating separate care areas for sick children or making recommendations to employers for parental leave to care for sick children is also appropriate because of the high incidence of viral-illness communicability among day-care participants (Aronson and Gilsdorf, 1986; Waldo et al., 1988).

Finally, nurses can facilitate parental coping and adjustment to the working-mother family situation. Appropriate nursing intervention should focus on reallocating chores and responsibilities to include all family members and assisting parents to identify feelings (such as inadequacy, guilt, anger, resentment, relief, and freedom) about their return to work and the influence these feelings and behaviors have on the child's attitude toward this change. Nurses can assist the family to identify stresses created by the change that may produce tension and can help all family members develop adequate coping behaviors.

COMMON CAUSES OF MORBIDITY AND MORTALITY
Infants

Major strides have been made over the past 5 years to improve the safety of life for infants. The provisional infant mortality for the United States in 1990 is a record low 9.7 infant deaths per 1000 live births. This reduction is partly attributable to improved nutrition, housing, and prenatal, obstetrical, and pediatric care. However, the lower rates for neonates are most influenced by technology, and there has been little progress in dealing with the effects of this technology in infancy. Low–birth weight, lack of universal access to prenatal care, and the racial and ethnic components of infant mortality remain unaddressed. Nearly twice as many black infants die before their first birthday than do white infants. Similarly, infants from low-income homes and certain regional areas and infants of certain ethnic backgrounds demonstrate higher morbidity and mortality (Wegman, 1990).

Infant mortality in other developed countries has also declined over the past 5 years. However, 20 countries report lower rates than the United States. The results of collaborative research among several of these countries and the United States demonstrate that their lower rates are attributable to early high-quality prenatal care (Wegman, 1990).

The primary threats to infant health and survival are low–birth-weight associated illness, congenital anomalies with associated problems, and sudden infant death syndrome (SIDS). The incidence of short gestation and low–birth weight is the most influential factor in infant mortality. Low–birth weight caused by many prenatal conditions, such as poor prenatal care, poor nutrition, and poor maternal health. These factors contribute to many perinatal conditions (e.g., bronchopulmonary dysplasia, respiratory distress syndrome, drug withdrawal, and developmental delay). Congenital anomalies and their secondary effects are the second leading cause of death, followed by SIDS (Wegman, 1990). Before the mid–1980s, congenital anomalies were the leading cause of death, followed by SIDS and low–birth weight. This change in the order of occurrence reflects the increase in early recognition through prenatal screening and intervention for infants at risk of congenital anomalies, along with a decrease in prenatal care for mothers at risk of delivering low–birth-weight infants (National Commission to Prevent Infant Mortality, 1988).

Immaturity and Prematurity

In approximately 6.9% of all livebirths, the newborns weigh less than 5.5 lb (2500 g). Low–birth-weight survivors are twice as likely to suffer one or more handicaps, such as cerebral palsy, chronic lung problems, epilepsy, delayed speech, blindness, deafness, and mental retardation (Na-

---

FACTORS DISPOSING MOTHERS TO DELIVERING PREMATURE INFANTS

Chronic hypertensive disease
Toxemia
Placenta previa
Abruptio placentae
Cervical incompetence
Low-socioeconomic status, including poor nutrition, chronic infection, fatigue, and generally poor personal and environmental hygiene
Absence of prenatal care
Multiple pregnancies
History of previous premature delivery
Age (highest incidence under age 20 years)
Order of birth (highest incidence in first pregnancies)
Maternal infections
Maternal addictions

Adapted from Chow MP, et al.: Handbook of pediatric primary care, ed 2, New York, 1984, John Wiley & Sons; and Whaley LF and Wong D: Nursing care of infants and children, ed 4, St Louis, 1991, Mosby–Year Book.

---

tional Commission to Prevent Infant Mortality, 1988). Factors disposing infants to preterm delivery and immaturity, such as absence of prenatal care and low-socioeconomic status of the mother, should be assessed through history taking by the community health nurse (see box below). Early interventions include referral for prenatal care, frequent follow-up on compliance with care management, education that addresses diet and health maintenance during pregnancy, and education about the specific high-risk factors. After birth, many preterm, low–birth-weight infants require at-home technological care. This care may include a tracheostomy, a ventilator, suctioning equipment, oxygen, or parenteral nutrition. These infants are also at risk for developmental delay and neurological, mental, and physical problems (Rice and Feeg, 1985). This predisposition requires the community health nurse to implement early developmental screening, nutritional education, and infant stimulation teaching. The community health nurse is responsible for the coordination of care for these high-risk infants, including assessment, management, referral, and follow-up.

Definition of Prematurity

In general, high-risk infants are classified according to size, gestational age, and predominant pathophysiological problems (Whaley and Wong, 1991). Classification as premature is based on gestational age. The premature or preterm infant is one born before the end of 37 weeks of gestation, regardless of birth weight. The infant who is born prematurely is generally immature gestationally and of low–birth-weight. Low–birth-weight infants (less than 2500 g, regardless of gestational age) are classified as follows (Dubowitz et al., 1970):

◊ Appropriately grown for gestational age (AGA): infants whose rates of intrauterine growth are normal at birth but who are small because they are born before the end of week 37
◊ Small for gestational age (SGA): infants whose rates of intrauterine growth are slow but who are born at or near term (38 to 41 weeks)
◊ Small for gestational age *and* premature: infants whose rate of intrauterine growth is retarded and who are delivered before 37 weeks

Classification according to fetal outcome is associated with the state of maturity of the infant and involves chemical disturbances and the consequences of immature organ and systems functioning (Whaley and Wong, 1991).

NURSING ROLE. Follow-up care of premature infants is the primary management. A plan of care is directed toward preventing the health problems associated with immaturity and facilitating the family's coping by providing support and anticipatory guidance to the parents concerning the physical and psychosocial development of the infant. Community health nurses can implement such a plan of care through home and clinic contacts, while providing the necessary element of continuity of care.

The low–birth weight or preterm infant requires a special plan for nutrition. Basically, these infants require increased calories, protein, vitamins, and minerals for growth (see Table 28-4). Although able to absorb protein and carbohydrates efficiently, preterm infants absorb fat poorly and readily lose fat-soluble vitamins and calcium through fecal fat loss. Also, iron stores are depleted much earlier than in full-term infants, and stores of vitamin E and folic acid are deficient in the first 3 months of life (AAP Committee on Nutrition, 1985).

Because of these nutritional deficiencies and added requirements, the feeding of a low–birth weight infant must be managed very closely. This infant requires approximately 110 to 150 calories/kg/day with supplementation of vitamins A, C, D, and B group. Calcium needs to be supplemented, as does iron. Additional vitamin E and folic acid are required in the first 3 months of life.

Hints, such as offering small frequent feedings (2 to 3 oz every 2 to 3 hours), bubbling frequently, resting the infant at signs of tiring, and holding the infant's head above stomach level are all appropriate suggestions.

Although a premature infant requires more frequent follow-up visits, the preventive pediatric care does not differ significantly from that of a full-term infant. However, during the follow-up care of a preterm infant or the infant who has experienced complications or prolonged illness, extra attention in certain areas of physical and developmental assessment is required. Table 28-7 provides an appropriate plan of care for such infants.

Parents of high-risk infants also require nursing care. Appropriate instruction on the care of their infant must be provided with frequent follow-up to evaluate parent ability to implement the care. Providing emotional support is also important and may be obtained through support groups, identifying family resources, and frequent contacts with the community health nurse.

Throughout screening and follow-up, the community health nurse should maintain a positive attitude based on the knowledge that, although potentials for delay and health problems are present, *equally present is the potential for normal outcomes.*

Congenital Anomalies

A *congenital anomaly* is any deviant organ or part existing before or at birth in an abnormal form, structure, or location but not necessarily detected at birth (Behrman et al., 1987). Congenital anomalies involving the cardiovascular, circulatory, and nervous systems pose the greatest mortality threats; congenital anomalies of other major organ systems may also occur. (See a basic pediatric nursing text for a review of the major organ system anomalies and their accompanying signs and symptoms.) Other types of congenital anomalies include genetic disorders (e.g., Down's syndrome, sickle cell anemia, or cystic fibrosis) and those related to exposure of the fetus to toxic agents during pregnancy (e.g., maternal rubella, exposure to radiation and chemicals, or maternal alcohol or drug abuse).

Sudden Infant Death Syndrome

Sudden infant death syndrome (SIDS) is the sudden death of any infant or young child that is unexpected by the history and in which a thorough postmortem examination fails to demonstrate an adequate cause of death. It is responsible for approximately 5000 deaths per year in infants from ages 1 week to 1 year (Wegman, 1989). It occurs most often between 2 and 4 months of age and is uncommon before 1

TABLE 28-7

Nursing implications in follow-up care for premature infants

Nursing goal	Nursing implication
Prevent neurologic-al function impairment	Scheduling frequent follow-up visits (initially 1 to 2 times a week, advancing to once a month when a normal pattern of growth is identified)
	Complete physical and neurological assessment at each visit
	Referral as appropriate
Promote physical growth and prevent functional impairment	Monitoring of height, weight, and head circumference at each visit
	Nutritional monitoring and education; use of supplemental nutrients and calories to ensure adequate nutrition; suggested techniques for feeding
	Education regarding skin care because of maceration proneness
	Education regarding maintenance of thermal environment
	Education regarding proneness to and avoidance of infections
	Education regarding infant need for rest and gentle handling
	Referral as approriate, especially early dental assessment and hearing and ophthalmological examinations
Promote maximum development	Routine developmental screening
	Education regarding sensory stimulation
	Promotion of maternal-infant and paternal-infant bonds
	Promotion of normal newborn experiences and avoidance of overprotection
	Referral as appropriate, especially to community resource support groups

Adapted from Korones SB: High risk newborn infants, ed 4, St Louis, 1986, Mosby–Year Book; and Foster R, Hunsberger M, and Anderson J: Family centered care of children and adolescents, ed 2, Philadelphia, 1989, WB Saunders.

month and after 8 months.

The clinical picture presented by the family of a SIDS victim is relatively unremarkable. Most infants die at home, during the night while sleeping, without difficulty, and unobserved. Parents often discover their infant lying lifeless in the crib, often in a state of disarray, with blood-stained fluid in the nose and mouth.

Infants at Risk for SIDS

SIDS occurs more frequently in males, low–birth weight infants, twins, low socioeconomic groups, neonates with low Apgar scores, and infants with central nervous system disturbances. It often occurs during normal sleep periods and happens during times of the year when the incidence of upper respiratory illnesses is increased. Other at-risk infants include the "near-miss" infant who periodically ceases breathing but restarts with stimulation and the infant with true infantile apnea, who ceases breathing for at least 20 seconds and experiences bradycardia, cyanosis and pallor (American Academy of Pediatrics, 1985; Bernbaum, 1989).

The incidence of SIDS in siblings of infants who have died from SIDS is unclear. Some studies report an increased occurrence (Brooks, 1982), whereas others do not (Peterson et al., 1986).

NURSING ROLE. Currently, no reliable screening tool exists for identifying infants at risk of SIDS. The community health nurse can be a valuable resource for the family, particularly if home apnea monitoring is instituted. Appropriate nursing interventions may include parent teaching about SIDS, monitoring, and CPR; coordinating discharge planning between home and hospital; and assisting the family in securing appropriate equipment and financial resources. Assisting the family in preparing the home environment, helping the family identify changes in life-style and how to cope with them and assisting the family in identifying support groups and follow-up care are other necessary interventions (Davis and Sweeney, 1989).

If the infant dies, the parents and family require tremendous support. The nurse is in a position to provide this through the therapeutic relationship. Interventions need to be made at the time of death, as well as after the cause of death has been confirmed (see box at right).The family should be contacted at home within 5 to 7 days after the death. During this and subsequent visits, the nurse should focus on providing empathetic support and assisting the family in coping, progressing through the grief process, and dealing with siblings and relatives.

Community health nurses should be involved in the implementation of the management plan for parents and siblings of SIDS victims. This involvement requires familiarity with support groups (such as the National Sudden Infant Death Foundation or Council of Guilds for Infant Survival) and current information (available through Sudden Infant Death Syndrome Clearinghouse).

Sepsis

Neonates are particularly susceptible to sepsis and other infectious diseases. Community health nurses should be aware of the symptoms to facilitate early recognition and assessment.

The occurrence of the following symptoms should prompt the nurse to provide appropriate intervention:

Full anterior fontanel that lacks normal pulsations

Hypothermia

Continued lethargy or anorexia

Persistent apneic spells or seizures

Feeding poorly with a weak suck

Persistent diarrhea, vomiting, or spitting up

Jaundice and liver enlargement between days 4 and 8 of life

Petechiae, shrill cry, or abdominal distension

Preventive measures aimed at reducing the incidence and spread of the agents of septicemia can be implemented by the nurse. Community health nurses can initiate prevention

---

NURSING INTERVENTIONS IN SIDS MANAGEMENT

RECOMMENDED MANAGEMENT* AT THE TIME OF SIDS DEATH

◇ Performance of autopsies on all infants dying suddenly and unexpectedly

◇ Prompt notification of the results of that autopsy to the parents

◇ Use of the term *sudden infant death syndrome* on the death certificate

◇ Follow-up information and counseling for all families provided by a knowledgeable health professional

APPROPRIATE MANAGEMENT WITHIN 1 WEEK OF INFANT'S DEATH INCLUDES A HOME VISIT WITH THE FOLLOWING OBJECTIVES FOR CARE:

◇ Provide emotional support during the grieving period

◇ Listen empathetically

◇ Provide information on SIDS to the family members as they are ready for it

◇ Anticipate normal grief reactions, and reassure parents that their reactions are normal

◇ Answer all questions asked by parents, and give printed material on SIDS

◇ Assist parents in dealing with siblings and relatives

◇ Put parents in touch with parent groups and the National Foundation of Sudden Infant Death

◇ Support the whole family during the pregnancy and infancy period of a subsequent child

◇ Refer parents for psychiatric help if abnormal reactions exist and persist

INDICATIONS FOR REFERRAL

◇ Parent(s) shows no emotion

◇ Parent(s) overintellectualizes (e.g., is obsessed with scientific details)

◇ Parent(s) persistently denies the infant's death

◇ Continuing inability of parent(s) to resume previous responsibilities and level of functioning

*Recommended by National Foundation of Sudden Infant Death (NFSID) from Mile M, editor: Mental health aspects of SID: Report of a conference sponsored by NFSID and National Institute for Mental Health, Kansas City, July 30, 1975, U.S. Department of Health, Education, and Welfare. Adapted from Chow MP et al.: Handbook of pediatric primary care, ed 2, New York, 1984, John Wiley & Sons, p. 1181; and Buschbacher VI and Delcampo RL: J Pediatr Health Care 1:85, 1987.

---

through parental and family education in hygiene techniques. Potential environmental sources of the bacteria can be identified, and the client can be referred for treatment.

The nurse has a responsibility to support the parents of an infant who develops sepsis or other major infection. Particular attention to the disruption in the parent-child relationship is needed if hospitalization occurs. The nurse should identify measures that facilitate attachment and parental involvement in the care of the infant. The community health nurse can be most instrumental in a successful resolution by acting as a client advocate and supporter.

Acquired Immunodeficiency Syndrome

The majority of pediatric acquired immunodeficiency syndrome (AIDS) cases occur when certain maternal risk factors are present. These include maternal or paternal intravenous drug use, maternal promiscuity, a diagnosis of maternal AIDS, and Haitian or central African origin. Most children with AIDS are infected in utero or during birth (Brady, 1987; Williams, 1989).

Infants who have positive test results for human immunodeficiency virus (HIV) commonly present with failure to thrive, recurrent infections, including otitis media, pneumonia and septicemia, persistent oral candidiasis and chronic diarrhea. In addition, hepatosplenomegaly, lymphadenopathy and encephalopathy frequently occur. Children with AIDS are more susceptible to pyogenic bacterial infections but are less likely to develop malignancies than are adults with AIDS (Brady, 1987).

The nursing management of infants with AIDS for the community health nurse involves assessment for high-risk maternal factors, early recognition of potential signs and symptoms, and coordination of home care. Home care of the child with AIDS should focus on maintaining physical and psychosocial well-being. Basis aspects of care should include nutritional support, pulmonary toileting and support and consistent, thorough oral and personal hygiene. Other needed measures include pharmacological interventions, infection control, appropriate developmental and educational activities, individual and family support or counseling, patient and family education, and support for reintegration into the community (Berry, 1988; Williams, 1989). A system assessment and care plan for the child with AIDS is included in Appendix J13.

Toddlers and Preschoolers

Currently, children over the age of 1 year are enjoying better health than ever before. The death rate for these children has fallen to 34 per 100,000 population. Most of these deaths are attributable to accidents and associated injuries and infectious disease.

Accidents

Although the death rate from motor vehicle accidents has declined approximately 20% in the past few years, the rate for other accidents has decreased by two thirds. In descending order of incidence, the most common causes of fatal injuries in toddlers and preschoolers are motor vehicle accidents, drowning, burns, poisoning, choking, and falls. Segments of this population most at risk are boys, who demonstrate an annual death rate higher than girls, and blacks, who demonstrate an overall higher mortality (Wegman, 1990).

Practice of age-appropriate safety measures can significantly reduce and prevent most accidents. Nursing, with its emphasis on health promotion and supervision, can have a significant impact on accident prevention. The counseling and education of parents on the developmental abilities and related safety measures needed to provide an accident-free environment are responsibilities that nursing must meet when delivering well-child care. Environmental assessment tools, such as the Safety Evaluation Program, can be used by the community health nurse in evaluating home safety and in advocating and referring community safety programs, such as KISS (Kids in Safety Seats). Appendix J6 provides information on age-appropriate accident prevention.

Community health nurses have the opportunity to implement accident prevention education in the home, clinic, and school. They should counsel parents during well-child visits and in group settings on accident-prevention issues such as auto restraints, plugging electrical outlets, toy safety, poisonous plants, household products, and medication safety. A reduced number of accident-related deaths and injuries can result from organized education programs from community health nurses.

Infectious Diseases

Infection remains the primary cause of both illness and restricted activity in children ages 1 to 5 years. Although resistance to many causative agents of infectious diseases is developing in children these ages, exposure and subsequent immunity are incomplete and the infant, toddler, and preschool child are frequently plagued with these diseases. The community health nurse frequently encounters infants and children with infectious diseases. Assisting parents through education to recognize and provide responsible symptomatic management can prevent further complications (Table 28-8). In addition, facilitating client knowledge in the prevention of infectious disease spread is well within the community health nurse's role. Health promotional activities that need to be stressed include adequate nutrition, avoidance of sources of infection or ill persons, use of responsible hygiene measures, and early intervention if symptoms occur.

MAJOR HEALTH PROBLEMS

During the process of physical and emotional maturation, a child passes through many stages. Each presents risks to the child's health and well-being. Nurses should provide anticipatory guidance and, when indicated, assist parents with the management of these problems.

Neonates and Infants

Major health problems during the neonatal period include the phenomenon of jaundice and regulation of body temperature. In infants the health problems of major concern include upper respiratory tract infections, *Chlamydia* organism infections, otitis media, allergies, gastrointestinal illnesses, and malnutrition. These problems are summarized and the community health nurse's role is defined in Table 28-9 (also see Appendix J7).

Toddlers and Preschoolers

Although the major health problems of infants have significant incidence rates in the 2- to 6- year-old group, the toddler and preschool groups are also at risk of developing additional illnesses, viral illnesses, and exanthems. Viruses are the most common cause of infectious disease in children. Of particular significance are the incidences of viral hepatitis, influenza, roseola, and varicella. Appendix J7 reviews their presentation and nursing management and the features of other common infectious diseases. The role of the nurse

TABLE 28-8
General measures for symptoms of infectious disease

Symptom	Measure
Fever	Antipyretic medication
	Monitoring temperature
	Liberal fluid intake
	Avoiding chilling
	Reducing environmental temperature
	Light clothing
	Cool compresses to forehead
Upper respiratory tract symptoms	Liberal fluid intake
	Cool-mist vaporizers
	Decongestants as appropriate
	Warm gargles, saline-solution mouth and throat irrigations, cool liquids, and soft foods for sore throat as appropriate to age
	Petrolatum jelly to protect the skin around the nares
	Cough preparations generally ineffective and contraindicated in infants and young children
	Prevention of infection spread
Generalized aching and malaise	Rest and limited physical activity
	Warm baths
	Body massage
	Cold compresses for headache
	Analgesic medication
Anorexia	Small, frequent feedings of favorite foods and liquids
	Relaxed attitude about oral intake; forcing foods and fluids is usually counterproductive
	Appealing food appearance
Rash	Proper hygiene with limited bathing, using no or mild soap
	Cool baths, local applications of calamine lotion, and mild anesthetic ointments or systemic antihistamines to relieve pruritus
	Fingernail care, including frequent cutting and cleaning, to reduce effects of scratching; gloves or mittens may be used at night on younger children
	Saline mouthwashes if mucous membranes are involved
	Loose fitting clothes of nonirritating fabric (i.e., cotton)
	Avoiding overheated and high-humidity environments

is to implement preventive measures that may be directed toward primary prevention (reducing the incidence of the problem for the child) or secondary prevention (reducing the incidence of secondary complications). The major health problems of toddlers and preschoolers and the community health nurse's role in caring for clients with these problems are summarized in Table 28-9.

SOCIAL PROBLEMS AFFECTING INFANTS AND YOUNG CHILDREN

Child abuse or neglect and homelessness are two social problems that significantly affect children's health. The role of the community health nurse in regard to these problems is to implement nursing interventions focused on prevention, early recognition, management, and close follow-up.

Child Abuse and Neglect

The epidemic of child abuse is a recently discovered and unfortunate phenomenon. Although the actual number of cases of child abuse and neglect is unknown because of difficulties in identification and reporting, it is estimated that approximately 2 million children in the United States are reported as abused or neglected and that 1 out of 10 children is sexually abused (Anderson, 1987; Castiglia, 1990; Wong, 1987). Children under the age of 3 years are

the most frequent victims, and women are the most frequent abusers, although men abuse more severely and are more often involved in sexual assault. All races and socioeconomic groups are involved, but statistics indicate a higher incidence in lower socioeconomic classes (Anderson, 1987). Most perpetrators are known to the child victim (Ryan, 1984).

The psychodynamics involved in an abusive situation are characterized by the following factors:

⋄ A crisis precipitating the occurrence, preceded by multiple frustrations, problems, and an inability to cope
⋄ Socially isolated parents and children
⋄ A premeditated injury
⋄ Parents who were abused as children, who lack support systems, and who display a lack of trust
⋄ A child who has been "labeled" as different by the parent, possibly as a result of unplanned pregnancy, illness, or prematurity

Prevention is the primary goal in regard to child abuse (Ryan, 1984). Nurses have a responsibility to identify potentially abusive situations and to implement risk screening prenatally, postnatally, and periodically throughout well-child care (see Appendix J9). If a family at risk is identified, additional supportive measures need to be implemented in the interest of prevention.

TABLE 28-9
Health problems of children—birth through 5 years

Problem	Primary age affected	Nursing intervention
Allergies	Infancy (food allergies) Preschool and school-age (environmental allergens)	Obtain detailed food and environment allergy history Assess current symptoms Manage current symptoms (Table 28-8) Initiate diet control or allergy proofing as indicated (Appendix J2) Provide appropriate counseling, focusing on allergen source
Chlamydia trachomatis infection	Neonates and infants	Initiate screening of pregnant women for *Chlamydia trachomatis* infection Assure medical prophylaxis for infant at birth Promote prevention through prenatal care Assess compliance and follow-up of maternal and infant medical regimen Initiate measures to prevent infection spread
Child care epidemics of respiratory tract infections, *Haemophilus influenzae* type B disease, hepatitis, diarrheal disease, cytomegalovirus infection	Toddlers and preschoolers	Teach appropriate handwashing techniques, emphasizing frequency Instruct in proper disposal of soiled clothes and diapers Instruct in proper cleansing of changing areas Stress staff assignment to small groups that do not cross age groups Encourage proper kitchen cleaning and meal preparation by staff members other than those who change diapers Instruct in toy cleaning Advocate an exclusion policy for febrile or diarrheal children Recognize and assess initial symptoms Promote appropriate immunizations for prevention
Gastroesophageal reflex (GER)	Infants	Closely monitor growth and weight Counsel parents about feeding techniques (i.e., small, frequent, thickened with cereal; frequent burping) Educate parents about positioning after feeding (i.e., head elevated 30 degrees) Assist parents to devise a head-elevated bed and instruct in safety
Hyperbilirubinemia	Neonates	Provide adequate hydration Educate parents in safe implementation of phototherapy if appropriate Educate and counsel parents about progression of disease and signs to watch for Ensure follow-up
Lead poisoning	Toddlers and preschoolers	Assess environment for potential sources of lead Obtain detailed history of exposure Identify children at high risk (i.e., inner city, live in old building, black, history of pica) Assess for subtle signs of lead poisoning (i.e., abdominal pain, constipation, and vomiting) Screen children at risk for elevated lead levels Implement education in community and schools

Continued.

TABLE 28-9
Health problems of children—birth through 5 years—cont'd

Problem	Primary age affected	Nursing intervention
Malnutrition	Infants and toddlers	Initiate dietary assessment and history (Appendix A4) Identify children at risk Implement thorough nutritional education program for parents at each stage of infant development Provide information about food program resources in community Provide vitamin and mineral supplementation as indicated Monitor growth closely Implement follow-up
Otitis media, including serious and suppurative	Infants, toddlers, and pre-schoolers	Provide education on symptom management (i.e., fever, discomfort, drainage) (Table 28-8) Educate parents on preventive measures (i.e., feed in up-right position, use Valsalva maneuver or blowing games) Assess environment and eliminate allergens, including tobacco smoke Monitor medical regimen Monitor and assess development, hearing, and speech Emphasize and monitor follow-up care
Physiological jaundice	Neonates	Assess for signs Monitor progression of jaundice Educate parents in normal progression and signs of worsening Educate and reassure parents regarding benign nature of process Ensure adequate hydration Ensure follow-up
Temperature control	Neonates	Educate parents in maintaining environmental temperature Counsel parents regarding external warmth by using blankets and covering infant's head Assess infant for circulatory adequacy
Upper respiratory tract infections including respiratory syncytial virus (RSV), crup, larynogotracheobronchitis (LTB)	Infants, toddlers, and pre-schoolers	Promote prevention through adequate nutrition, rest, hygiene, and immunization Assess environment for allergens and irritants Educate parents regarding symptom management (Table 28-8) Assess severity of symtoms Implement measure to prevent infection spread Monitor medical regimen Implement close follow-up
Vomiting and diarrhea (see Appendix J7)	Infants, toddlers, and pre-schoolers	Differentiate vomiting and regurgitation in infants Assess frequency and character of diarrhea Assess possible causes through history, including of diet Assess for dehydration Counsel and educate parents in monitoring and managing symptoms Implement medical regimen, including dietary modifications Assess dietary compliance Monitor weight Prevent spread if infectious process Prevent skin breakdown Implement oral care Closely monitor and follow-up

Managing a situation of child abuse is difficult and requires a multidisciplinary approach. Nurses can be an integral part of this team by offering support to the parents and the child, teaching parents how to nurture and parent, and investigating community services available to the family. Both the child and the parents will require health care interventions. The goal of management is directed toward the protection of the child, support and rehabilitation of parents, and return of the child to the home when deemed safe. In addition, it is mandatory that all cases of suspected abuse and neglect in the United States be reported to the appropriate authorities. Although this responsibility is generally the physicians, nurses are also legally obligated to report abuse or neglect. Although failure to report suspected cases can result in prosecution, reporters of such cases are immune from court action for civil liability under the Child Abuse Prevention and Treatment Act. Generally, child abuse or neglect is reported to local or state government child protection agencies. Abused children usually are temporarily removed from the home until the family situation restabilizes and the parents have demonstrated both a willingness to continue care and a positive caring attitude toward their child.

Follow-up is essential in any case involving child abuse or neglect. Nurses can contribute in this follow-up by assisting parents to deal with the frustrations of parenthood, teaching parenting approaches, providing support and encouragement, and facilitating the identification and use of community resources. The community health nurse ideally can ensure that families are receiving adequate support and care through home visits and assessments. Appropriate community services may include the following (Chow et al., 1984):

Crisis hotlines
Parents Anonymous
Single parents' groups
Lay community organizations
Crisis nurseries or child care centers
Day care centers
Parent education groups
Health visitor groups
National Center for Missing and Exploited Children

Homelessness

Children do not escape the epidemic of homelessness. The number of homeless children nationwide is estimated to be between 100,000 to 750,000. More than 50% of these children are under the age of 5 years, and the infant mortality among homeless children has been reported to be as high as 24 per 1000 live births in some major cities (Shulsinger, 1990). These children have special problems and needs that can be addressed by nursing. Four primary areas of need are not being met for homeless children: health care, nutrition, education, and developmental opportunities (Shulsinger, 1990; Wood, 1987).

Access to routine health care for homeless children is minimal. Many children have not been immunized or have had sporadic immunizations. A majority need dental care and experience recurrent infectious and communicable diseases. These children are at risk of malnutrition and asso-

---

RESPONSIBILITIES OF THE OUTREACH TEAM

COMMUNITY HEALTH NURSE

◇ Develop and maintain trusting relationship with families
◇ Follow up acutely ill family members
    Review medicines and treatment plans
    Facilitate referrals and follow-up on referrals
    Provide feedback to health care teams
◇ Perform field assessments and triage to clinic
◇ Provide health education and disease prevention
◇ Continue assessment and follow-up for child abuse and neglect in high-risk families

COMMUTY WORKER

◇ Develop and maintain trusting relationship with families
◇ Help family set priorities and develop goals to meet them (e.g., find housing, resolve relationship problems, drug rehabilitation, find job)
◇ Assist families in progress toward meeting goals
◇ Provide family advocacy with public agencies (welfare, WIC, housing authority, etc.)
◇ Provide family advocacy with health agencies

From Wood D: *Pediatr Health Care* 3:198, 1989.

---

ciated illnesses because the number and assurance of nutritionally sound, regular meals is minimal. Educationally, homeless children are disadvantaged. The transient nature of their existence makes it difficult for them to attend school. Furthermore, these children have few opportunities to develop psychosocially. In shelters, a play space and materials are frequently nonexistent. Many homeless preschool-age children demonstrate one or more developmental delays. School-age children have school and behavior problems, with many being overtly depressed (Shulsinger, 1990; Wood, 1987).

The community health nurse is in a unique position to assist in meeting these needs by using outreach programs. These programs take health care services to the homeless and involve health care professionals and the community (see box above). In addition, preventive health care (including immunizations, tuberculosis testing, and physical examinations), developmental assessment, school placement, history of current and past problems, family and behavioral assessment, and screening tests (anemia, vision, hearing, and laboratory) should be developed into a care plan protocol for homeless children.

HOME CARE OF TECHNOLOGY-DEPENDENT CHILDREN

Advances in health care and technology have made it possible for many chronically ill, high-risk and technology-dependent children to be cared for at home. The goals of home care should be to support the family and the child through the process of normalizing life, to minimize disruption created by the illness, and to foster growth and development (Andrews and Nielson, 1988; Whaley and Wong, 1991). The community health nurse has the opportunity to achieve these goals by organizing services.

TABLE 28-10
Common childhood behaviors

Age (yr)	Behaviors
1	Sucks thumb, smears stools, shakes bed, bangs and rocks, and masturbates
2	As above; has temper tantrums, tears books or wallpaper, tears bed apart, removes clothes, runs around, and has many demands before sleep
2½	Above behavior to a lesser degree; stutters and has disruptive aggressive attacks such as hitting and biting
3	Less of the above behaviors
3½	Again an increase in some of the above behaviors; spits, picks nose, bites fingernails, and whines
4	Runs away, kicks, spits, bites nails, grimaces, calls names, boasts, brags, uses silly language, has nightmares and fears, needs to urinate in moments of emotional distress, has "belly" pains and may vomit
5	A decrease in some behaviors, blinks eyes, shakes head, clears throat, and sniffles
5½ to 6	All the above behaviors and increased clumsiness
7	Tries to control behaviors and may have headaches
8	Picks at fingers, cries with fatigue, and makes faces
9	Stamps feet, fiddles, drops and breaks things, picks at self, growls, and mutters

From Chow MP et al.: Handbook of pediatric primary care, ed 2, New York, 1984, John Wiley & Sons, p. 383.

Home care for high–technology–dependent children requires a multidisciplinary approach that begins with discharge planning before release from the acute care setting. The community health nurse needs to be involved in the assessment of home and environment before discharge. This assessment should include factors related to the physical environment; caretaker ability to perform the technical aspects of home care; and the availability of respite, support, and financial services.

The specific nursing care needs of the child, both physical and developmental, must be identified, and nursing interventions must be planned accordingly. This plan of care should also extend to family members, who will require regular support and guidance.

COMMON PARENTAL CONCERNS OR PROBLEMS

A common problem might be defined as a child's behavior which causes parents to be concerned. Frequently, parents have behavioral expectations in regard to some physical or psychosocial aspects of their child's growth or development. When the infant or child does not demonstrate the expected behaviors, parents often respond in an emotional, anxious, or insecure manner. The child then reacts to the parents' response, creating additional stress. For example, the mother of a 1-month-old infant expects the baby to feed every 4 hours and sleep through the night. When the infant wants to eat every 2 hours and is up three times a night, the mother becomes concerned, anxious, and may be insecure about her mothering abilities. This response subsequently affects her ability to be relaxed and motherly toward her infant, and the infant responds by being more demanding. Table 28-10 outlines common childhood behaviors that normally occur yet may create parental concern.

Many factors contribute to the occurrence of common problems. Significant variables include the following:

Parental expectations of a child's behavior and of their own behavior as parents, which are frequently unrealistic

Lack of parenting experience and knowledge

Emotional impact of becoming a parent

Age, sex, and temperament of the child as it affects the parents and family

Too much concern and emphasis on the part of parents toward common problems

The most frequently identified common concerns or problems of infancy include colic, feeding, sleeping and elimination patterns and behaviors, crying, gas, hiccups, teething, spoiling, weaning, and stranger or separation anxiety. Appendix J5 describes these problems and appropriate anticipatory guidance and management.

Specific behavioral habits of toddlers and preschoolers that evoke parental concern may include biting, hitting, masturbation, sleep and eating disturbances, negativism, temper tantrums, toilet training, discipline, and limit setting.

Nurses must educate parents about the normalcy of the behaviors and assist them in identifying effective coping behaviors, and identify appropriate approaches to handling the child and the behavior and provide support and reassurance to the parents. Appendix J8 provides information pertinent to the nursing assessment and management of these common problems.

TOOLS FOR ASSESSMENT

The nursing process involves the assessment, diagnosis, planning, implementation, and evaluation of the health needs of a client and family. An accurate assessment through data collection is the basis for any further plan of intervention. The tools and techniques used for assessment vary, depending on the child's age. However, basic methods provide nursing with a uniform and reliable approach to assessment of an individual child's health needs, as well as those of the family and community.

History

The history and subsequent assessment of the child and family begin at the moment of contact through observation. This technique of data collection provides information about the child's physical, psychosocial, developmental, and interactional growth. A more formal interview should be directed toward gathering data relative to the immediate health status. Traditional information gathered in an initial pediatric health history is reviewed in Appendix A2.

Physical Examination

Data collected from the physical assessment verifies information collected from observation and the history interview. For example, the nurse may observe that a 6-year-old child is limping; the history reveals the child complained of pain in the right ankle after falling off of a bicycle 1 day earlier. The physical examination verifies these data through findings of edema, bruising, and limited range of motion. Similarly, data collected during a health maintenance visit can verify the observation and history that a child is in good health.

Approaches in conducting a physical examination for a pediatric client are most important and must be adapted to the child's age and developmental level. Suggested approaches and sequence of conducting the physical examination are summarized in Appendix A3.

Health Assessment

Combining the components of history taking and physical assessment with the assessment of physical and psychosocial growth and development pertinent to a specific age results in a total health assessment. This includes the monitoring of growth and development by measuring height, weight, and (for infants) head circumference, monitoring vital signs, (and for children over 3 years of age) blood pressure, and screening for health problems with particular attention to dental, vision, hearing, and speech development. In pediatric patients, health assessments are generally implemented at specific time intervals. In the first 6 years of life, health assessment visits for the normally developing child are generally recommended at ages 2 to 4 weeks; ages 2, 4, 6, 9 or 12, 15, 18, and 24 months; and annually until age 6 years. Outlines for the content of these health visits are included in Appendix A3. Appendix K contains information on additional tools for screening growth and development and for health problems.

Psychosocial Development

The most useful tools available to nurses are those designed to assess psychosocial skills, developmental skills, or both. Children generally follow similar patterns of development. Subsequently, developmental standards have been established based on studies of the age levels at which the average child masters various motor, language, adaptive, and social behaviors. The Waechter Developmental Guides provide comprehensive summaries of growth and development during infancy and should be a component of the essential knowledge base for nurses involved in pediatric care (Appendix K7).

Developmental and psychosocial screening tests are designed to assess how an individual child is developing compared to the average standard. These tests are a means for determining the need for intervention and perhaps more comprehensive evaluation. Screening tests used most frequently in pediatrics are selected primarily for their ease of administration, economic feasibility, and accuracy and reliability of results. Interpretation of their results requires recognition of the range of normalcy, individual variations, and the variables present in the test situations.

Screening tools that are particularly useful to the community health nurse include the Denver Developmental Screening Test–Revised (DDST-R), the Revised Denver Prescreening Developmental Questionnaire (R-DPDQ), the Carey Infant Temperament Scale (CITS), the Home Observation for Measurement of Environment (HOME), the Denver Articulation Screening Examination (DASE), and the Preschool Readiness Experimental Screening Scale (PRESS). (Frankenburg et al. 1971; Carey, 1972; Bradley and Caldwell, 1988; Rogers and Rogers, 1972).

The DDST-R was developed to screen children from birth to 6 years of age. The Denver II is a major revision and restandardization of the DDST which includes an age scale similar to the American Academy of Pediatrics' schedule for health supervision. In addition to the items on the DDST-R, the Denver II has 36% more language items, speech, intelligibility, and a place to rate the child's behavior. The community health nurse can use it one time or for periodic screening and assessment of personal, social, fine motor, adaptive, language, and gross motor development. Results of the screening will facilitate the planning of nursing interventions to promote growth and development or to identify potential problems that need further evaluation.

The R-DPDQ is especially useful for the community health nurse because it can be easily administered during clinic or home visits and is designed to identify children ages 3 months to 6 years who require more thorough screening and intervention. The CITS also helps the nurse plan well-child care and anticipatory guidance by providing a profile of infant temperament, including parent information on patterns of sleep, feeding, and elimination and stimuli response.

The HOME (see Appendix B6) is a unique behavior and interaction inventory that assesses the quality and quantity of social, emotional, and cognitive factors available to the child from birth to 6 years of age. The community health nurse can use this tool to assess environmental adequacy for development and to initiate intervention. The PRESS helps the nurse to assess a child's overall readiness to attend kindergarten and the individual maturational level of children ages 4 to 5 years. It is useful for planning interventions for the child who needs assistance with preparation or adjustment strategies.

Family Assessment Tools

The focus of the community health nurse should be family-centered care. Although obstacles such as lack of time, professional and organizational support, and knowledge about family assessment make family-centered care difficult, family assessment remains important because the success of nursing interventions depends on the family's ability and resources to implement the care. Family assessment is particularly important in pediatric health care because chil-

TABLE 28-11
Content outline for group of parents of infants

Session	Topic and content
First	Introduction and getting to know each other Sharing the birth experience Sharing feelings about early parenting Answer immediate questions and concerns. Overview of basics of infant care: such as bathing, diapering, holding, and dressing
Second	Getting to know your infant Discussion of normals: feeding, sleeping, elimination, and activity patterns Review of feeding techniques Discussion of techniques to facilitate adjustment and realignment and redistribution of family tasks and responsibilities
Third	Your infant as a person Discussion of temperament and evolving behavior patterns Discussion about infant stimulation and promotion of development
Fourth	Nutritional and safety issues Discussion of changing infant nutritional needs over first year Discussion of safety needs as related to infant development
Fifth	Caring for a sick infant Discussion of common acute illnesses Review of symptoms and when to seek intervention Home management of symptoms, including temperature monitoring
Sixth	The working mother Selecting and making arrangements for child care Discussion of alternatives Discussion of feelings

dren rely on their families for health activities (Speer and Sachs, 1985).

Family assessment tools must be understandable, easily administered and scored, reliable, valid, and appropriate for most families (Speer and Sachs, 1985). Appendix B7 provides an evaluation summary of family assessment tools that the community health nurse may find useful.

HEALTH PROMOTION ACTIVITIES

The successful promotion of health is evident in a person when he or she is able to identify and accept realities, adjust to changes in the environment, maintain a wholesome attitude toward self and life, and assume responsibility for managing his or her own health as appropriate for age and development. For the pediatric client, health promotion must involve the family. As primary caretakers, the child's family must also be motivated to assume health promotion responsibilities.

The role of nursing is to facilitate and support individuals and their families in endeavors for health. Nurses can assist family members to use their own resources in identifying health needs and assuming responsibility for their own care.

Nurses can assist parents in learning and adapting health promotion behaviors that positively affect the health of their children. Increasing parent competence and confidence in providing self-care includes teaching parents to prevent illnesses, to assist with illness recovery, and to cope with the effects of illness (Sirles, 1988). Education to promote health must be implemented at every nurse-client encounter.

The community health nurse can assist families to promote the well-being of infants and children in a variety of ways and settings. Health assessment visits should focus on promoting health-oriented behaviors in the parent and child. Parent education and anticipatory guidance from nurses are two means of promoting such behaviors, in addition to emphasis on preventive health measures, particularly safety and accident prevention (see Appendix J6). The nursing management plan for health maintenance activity also needs to include the child. For example, even at the age of 2 to 3 years, children can be taught and encouraged to brush their teeth, thereby promoting dental health. Finally, the use of screening tools is particularly important. Age-appropriate tools are discussed earlier in this chapter and in Appendixes A3 and K.

Group Education and Home Intervention

Group health education is a popular, effective, and time efficient means of health promotion. Parenting groups often focus on a specific age, developmental stage, or health problem. Table 28-11 illustrates an overview of course content for a group of parents of infants and Table 28-12 presents an overview for a parenting class for parents of toddlers. However, before program development, as discussed in Chapter 12, nurses must assess the learning needs of clients and avoid duplication of current classes or health education resources already available in the community. (See Chapters 11 and 12 for a detailed discussion of program planning for health education.)

Community Resources

Promoting the health of children largely depends on the use of available community resources. To identify resources for a specific area or region, nurses should consider the following potential services or interest groups:

Children's services centers or clinics
Well-child clinics
Woman-infant-child programs
Immunization clinics
Communicable disease clinics
Crippled children's services
Child abuse centers or councils
School health programs
Project Grow
Head Start
Parents Anonymous
Youth services bureaus
Crisis or hotlines for parents, children, or both
Parent discussion groups
Adult education groups on aspects of parenting (e.g., infant care, coping)
Child development classes
Infant/child stimulation classes

TABLE 28-12
Content outline for group of parents of toddlers

Session	Topic and content
First	Introduction and getting to know each other
	Discussion of developmental theories and tasks of age group
	Review of mastery, investigation, testing, and manipulating
Second	An age of activity: in or out of control
	Discussion about toddler behaviors: temper tantrums, negativism, jealousy, sibling rivalry, ritualism, separation behaviors, regression
Third	Approaches to toddler behaviors
	Discussion about limit setting and discipline
Fourth	Changing physically and learning to control body functions
	Discussion about toilet training, sleeping, eating, and self-comforting behaviors and patterns
	Discussion about how to handle safety considerations
Fifth	The necessity of play and learning sex role
	Discussion of learning through play
	Review of ideas about toys, television, playmates, play groups, and nursery school
	Discussion of sex role identification and factors influencing this
Sixth	Speech and learning to express self
	Discussion of timetable, reinforcement, nonverbal activities

TABLE 28-13
Current American Academy of Pediatrics immunization schedule

Age	Immunization(s)
2 mo	DTP, TOPV, HbOC*
4 mo	DTP, TOPV, HbOC
6 mo	DTP, HbOC
15 mo	MMR¶, HbCV
15-18 mo	DTP†, TOPV†
4-7 yr	DTP, TOPV
12 yr	MMR‡
q 10 yr	dT

Adapted from American Academy of Pediatrics: Report of the Committee on Infectious Diseases, ed 22, Elk Grove Village, IL, 1991, The Academy.
DTP indicates diphtheria-tetanus-pertussis; *TOPV*, trivalent oral polio vaccine; *HbOC, Haemophilus influenzae* type b conjugate vaccine (diphtheria CRM$_{197}$ protein conjugate; HibTITER); *MMR*, measles-mumps-rubella; *HbCV*, Hib conjugate vaccine (ProHIBIT, Pedvax HIB, HibTITER); *dT*, diphtheria-tetanus.
*In October 1990, HbOC (HibTITER) was approved by the FDA for infants starting at 2 mo of age. Other Hib conjugate vaccines have submitted applications.
†Both be given at 15 mo of age and simultaneously with MMR and HbCV; DTP should be given 6-12 mos. after third dose.
‡Some states require this dose at 4-6 yr of age.
¶May be given at 12 months in areas with recurrent measles transmission.

Immunizations

Immunity is defined as the body's resistance to the effects of harmful agents. The protection of immunity can be received through active or passive means. (See Chapter 19 for a discussion of active or passive immunity.)

Active artificial immunization is initiated for infants and children to protect them against the once common and dangerous infectious diseases such as measles, mumps, rubella, tetanus, diphtheria, pertussis, and *Haemophilus influenzae* infection. The neonate enjoys a relatively short period (first few weeks to 2 months) of natural passive immunity as a result of placental transfer of maternal antibodies. However, this protection is temporary and is only against those diseases for which the mother has developed sufficient antibodies. Young infants are then at risk of infection because their immune systems are poorly developed and immature.

Active immunization is conferred through two basic types of agents—toxoids and vaccines. Antibody production for tetanus and diphtheria is stimulated through the use of a toxoid, a bacterial toxin that has been heated or chemically treated to decrease the virulence but not the antibody-producing ability. The use of vaccines, a suspension of attenuated or killed microorganisms, provides an active immunity response for pertussis (a killed bacteria), measles, mumps, rubella, polio (i.e., Sabin and Salk vaccines, attenuated and killed viruses, respectively), and *Haemophilus influenzae*. Appendix D2 and Table 28-13 provide information regarding the basic immunization agents and their administration schedule in pediatrics.

In normal infants the immune system is capable of re-

Prepared childbirth and classes or groups on raising children

Local community advocate groups (e.g., single parents, working mothers, nursing mothers)

Day care nurseries

Government-sponsored programs have played a major role in child health. Although many maternal-child health programs have suffered or been discontinued as a result of recent federal budget cuts, the following programs are cost-effective and continue to be funded (Select Committee on Children, Youth and Families, 1986):

Special supplement food program for women, infants, and children (WIC)

Prenatal care

Medicaid

Childhood immunizations

Preschool education

Compensatory education

Education for all handicapped children

Youth employment and training

The community health nurse has a responsibility to use these program resources for clients, as well as to become knowledgeable and active in legislative processes directed toward child health.

TABLE 28-14
Recommended immunization schedules for children not immunized in first year of life

Recommended time/age	Immunizations*	Comments
YOUNGER THAN 7 YEARS		
First visit	DTP, OPV, MMR	MMR if child ≥15 mo old; tuberculin testing may be done at the same visit
	HbCV†	For children aged 15-59 mo, can be given simultaneously with DTP and other vaccines (at separate sites)‡
Interval after first visit:		
2 mo	DTP, OPV, (HbCV)	Second dose of HbCV is indicated only in childlren whose first dose was received when younger than 15 mo
4 mo	DTP	Third dose of OPV is not indicated in the U.S. but is desirable in other geographic areas where polio is endemic
10-16 mo	DTP, OPV	OPV is not given if third dose was given earlier
4-6 yr (at or before school entry)	DTP, OPV	DTP is not necessary if the fourth dose was given after the fourth birthday; OPV is not necessary if third dose was given after the fourth birthday
11-12 yr	MMR	At entry to middle school or junior high
10 yr later	Td	Repeat every 10 yr throughout life
7 YEARS AND OLDER§,¶		
First visit	Td, OPV, MMR	
Interval after first visit:		
2 mo	Td, OPV	
8-14 mo	Td, OPV	
11-12 yr	MMR	At entry to middle school or junior high
10 yr later	Td	Repeat every 10 yr throughout life

*Abbreviations are explained in the footnote‡ to Table 2.
†If child is younger than 15 mo, only one HbCV (HbOC), as of October 1990, is approved for use (see *Haemophilus influenzae* infections, page 227).
‡The initial three doses of DTP can be given at 1- to 2-month intervals; hence, for the child in whom immunization is initiated at age 15 months or older, one visit could be eliminated by giving DTP, OPV, and MMR at the first visit; DTP and HbCV at the second visit (1 month later); and DTP and OPV at the third visit (2 months after the first visit). Subsequent doses of DTP and OPV 10 to 16 months after the first visit are still indicated. HbCV, MMR, DTP, and OPV can be given simultaneously at separate sites if failure of the patient to return for future immunizations is a concern.
§If person is ≥18 years old, routine poliovirus vaccination is not indicated in the U.S.
¶Minimal interval between doses of MMR is 1 month.
From American Academy of Pediatrics: Report of the Committee on Infectious Disease, ed. 22, Elk Grove Village, Il. 1991, The Academy, p. 18.

sponding with adequate antibody production by 2 months of age. This is generally the recommended age to begin artificial immunizations.

The interval between immunizations is important to the immunity response. After the first injection, antibodies are produced slowly and in small concentrations (primary response). However, the antibody-producing mechanism has been altered in response to this first injection. Therefore, subsequent injections with the same antigen are recognized by the body and antibodies are produced much faster and in higher concentration (secondary response). Because of this secondary response, once an initial immunization series has been started, *it does not need to be restarted if interrupted, regardless of the length of time elapsed.* Once the initial series is completed, boosters are required at the appropriate time intervals to maintain an adequate concentration level of antibodies.

Occasionally, children are encountered who have received no immunizations. The recommended immunization schedule for these children is listed in Table 28-14. How-

ever, if compliance with this schedule and follow-up care are doubtful, it is valid to simultaneously administer diphtheria, tetanus, pertussis (DTP) (or tetanus, diphtheria (Td) if the child is over 7 years of age), the trivalent oral polio virus vaccine (TOPV), measles, mumps and rubella (MMR), a *Haemophilus influenzae* conjugated vaccine, and tuberculin test (PPD [Mantoux]).

Three conjugated vaccines are currently licensed for use in the United States to induce antibody production to *H. influenzae* in children younger than 2 years of age (ProHibiT, HibTITER, Pedvax HIB). Current recommendations are to immunize with HibTITER (HbOC) at 2, 4, and 6 months of age, concurrent with DTP (but at a different site). Infants who are 7 to 11 months of age and who have not received HbOC need two doses 2 months apart. If the child is between 12 and 14 months of age, one dose should be given. All children should receive a booster at 15 months of age with any of the *H. influenzae* conjugate vaccines (HbCV).

Recent outbreaks of measles have prompted a reassessment of measles immunization. Although the current age for routine initial immunization with MMR remains 15 months, a second booster dose is recommended at 12 years of age by the American Academy of Pediatrics. Some states, however, recommend and require this second dose at 4 to 6 years of age.

Contraindications

Contraindications for the administration of immunizations are relatively few. Vaccines should not be administered to children with acute febrile illness or to those who have had severe reactions to the previous dose. Minor illnesses or infections are not contraindications for administration. Specific circumstances for nonadministration of a particular agent are listed in Appendix D2. In addition, the community health nurse needs to be aware of religious and cultural barriers that may prevent immunization. Finally, those with the following conditions are not routinely immunized and require medical consultation before the agent is administered, especially the live virus vaccines: pregnant women, persons with a generalized malignancy, those on immunosuppressive therapy or with immunodeficiency disease, persons with marked sensitivity to eggs or chicken, or persons who have had recent immune serum globulin or plasma or blood administration, (a wait of 3 months is advised).

Parent Education

Parental preparation and education regarding the immunization program, what responses or reactions to expect, and how to manage these common reactions is essential to the program's success. Although much discussion has occurred over these issues, parents should be informed of the risks and benefits of each immunizing agent, in addition to the common side effects. It should be stressed that the benefits generally outweigh the risks. Appendix D2 discusses potential reactions to specific immunizations and appropriate treatment measures that parents can institute to minimize discomfort.

Nutrition

One of the most important components of maintaining a child's health is the promotion of good nutrition and dietary habits. The quality and quantity of nutrition influence the growth and development of a child and the first 5 years of life are most important in developing sound eating habits. The nurse's role involves the use of a sound knowledge base to assist parents in providing adequate nutrition for the child (see Chapter 34).

Factors Influencing Nutrition

As with every aspect of human behavior, nutritional habits are influenced by a wide range of variables, which are derived from families as well as the child. Although some habits may be changed, others have to be accepted and incorporated when implementing a sound nutrition program. Among the parental factors most influential are ethnic, racial, cultural, and socioeconomic variables. How and what parents eat and their attitudes toward nutrition are invariably passed on to their child. The child also brings individual variables to the nutritional situation (i.e., a slow eater, a picky eater, periods of disinterest, development of prefer-

ences, presence of food allergy, and alterations in eating patterns during periods of growth).

No one diet is effective for all children or even for one age group. Nurses must accept and be knowledgeable about individual styles, methods, and approaches to child nutrition to assist parents in providing the appropriate nutrients for their child.

Infants

TYPES OF INFANT FEEDING. Supplying essential nutrients to an infant is done primarily through breast-feeding, bottle-feeding, or both. The method of feeding is a choice that must be made by parents with guidance and without pressure. The advantages and disadvantages of both methods should be discussed with parents prenatally, and the differences between the basic forms of milk should be reviewed. In addition, parents should also be aware of the need for vitamin and mineral supplementation as well as current recommendations on infant nutrition methods.

Breast milk is recommended by many health professionals as the preferred method of feeding an infant in the first 6 months of life. Recent studies document the nutritional efficacy and soundness of breast-feeding. However, some supplementation is necessary. For the infant who is solely breast-fed, the following need to be supplemented (AAP Committee on Nutrition, 1985; Pipes, 1989):

1. Vitamin D: Although breast milk contains adequate amounts of vitamins A and B complex, there is an inadequate amount of vitamin D to meet the 400 IU/day RDA. Additionally, vitamin C in human milk is adequate, provided that the maternal diet contains sufficient vitamin C.
2. Iron supplementation: The normal birth weight infant has sufficient iron stores until 4 to 6 months of age, at which time body stores must be supplied. Breast milk contains adequate amounts of absorbable iron to meet requirements. An infant who is exclusively breast-fed does not require exogenous sources of iron unless breast-feeding is discontinued before 6 months. Use of iron-fortified cereals and formula is recommended in this circumstance.
3. Fluoride: Breast milk contains inadequate amounts of fluoride, and supplementation in combination with other vitamins or alone is recommended.

Milks other than human milk have been used successfully for infant feeding. Commercially prepared formulas are most popular because they are convenient, contain standard ingredients, and are fortified with vitamins and minerals, negating the need for supplements. However, a formula prepared at home with evaporated or condensed milk or use of forms of cow's milk requires supplementation, generally of vitamins A, D, and C, fluoride, and iron (AAP Committee on Nutrition, 1985). Additionally, skim, lowfat, or 2% milk is not recommended for infants under 1 year of age because of insufficient fat and caloric contents.

In addition to providing nutritional facts, nurses must be prepared to instruct, encourage, reassure, and support parents in the feeding method of their choice. For breast-feeding, teaching topics include comfortable positioning, appropriate techniques, feeding frequency, the let-down reflex, care of breasts, and length of feedings. In addition, assessing the mother's feelings about nursing her infant and providing support and encouragement, the presence or absence of paternal and family support, and providing support and encouragement are important to success.

For bottle-feeding, parents require instruction regarding preparation and care of the equipment and formula, positioning of the person feeding as well as the infant and bottle, and the factors of frequency, length, and feelings about the method of feeding.

INTRODUCTION OF SOLID FOODS. Infants receiving breast milk or formula with the appropriate supplementation do not require additional foods before 4 to 6 months of age. There are no nutritional, developmental, or psychological advantages to starting infants on solids before this time and from a developmental perspective, infants are not physically able to handle solid food consumption until 5 to 6 months of age. However, the trend toward early introduction of solids does exist, and it will not be changed easily. Nurses can make a significant contribution to the nutritional adequacy of infants and children primarily through parental education and support. This requires being up-to-date on current nutritional findings and also being accepting of parents who, for a variety of reasons, wish to introduce early solids.

In addition to developmental considerations, the nurse should counsel parents regarding the nutritional value of solid foods. Generally solid baby foods are high in carbohydrates, moderate in protein, and low in fat, whereas human milk or formula is high in fat and carbohydrates and lower in protein. When infants are fed solids and also switched to whole, 2%, or low-fat cow's milk, the diet becomes excessively high in protein, sodium, and other solutes. Because the infant cannot excrete these large solutes efficiently without using large amounts of body fluid, this type of diet is hazardous for the infant.

Parents should be aware of the diversity of composition and nutritional quality of commercially prepared infant foods. Reading labels carefully is important. Parents also need to know that the cost per unit of calories is considerably higher for commercially prepared foods than for formula. In addition, the incidence of constipation in infants is greater when solid food intake is high, and the introduction of solids too early may possibly lead to overfeeding and later overeating. Finally, a greater possibility of food allergy exists for infants when solids are introduced too early because the foreign proteins in foods become antigens because of insufficient IgA production until after the age of 6 months.

Once parents have made the decision to start solid foods, nurses can assist them in developing a program for introducing appropriate foods in sensible amounts and in the best sequence. For example, it is not nutritionally sound to give an infant eggs as the first solid food, primarily because of difficulties in digesting and a high incidence of allergy to the egg protein. Dry cereal fortified with iron is a more appropriate starter food because of the ease of digestion and iron fortification (at a time when newborn iron reserves are low).

Guidelines for feeding infants from birth to 1 year are given in Appendix J4. Appendix J5 provides suggestions for anticipatory guidance for common feeding problems.

Toddlers and Preschoolers

As a child progresses through the toddler and preschool years, nutritional status and eating are affected by a decreasing physical growth rate, motor maturity, and cognitive and personality factors. Children learn to feed themselves and demonstrate food preferences and individual eating habits, thereby exerting an influence over their nutritional status. In assisting parents to maintain nutritional adequacy for their toddler or preschooler, the folling suggestions can be made:

Offer a balanced diet that meets recommended daily allowances for age, incorporating food preferences and variety.

Offer food several times a day (i.e., five to six times as opposed to three regular meals).

Limit milk intake to 16 ounces a day to avoid a filling up on milk instead of eating solids.

Offer suggested amounts of food as listed in Appendix J4.

Emphasize favorites that are nutritional and are easy to handle.

Continue to avoid nuts, bony fish, and popcorn because of risk of aspiration.

Generally, vitamin and iron supplements are not required. However, during periods when appetite and intake decrease, temporary use is appropriate. During such periods, nutritionally sound foods (especially those high in iron and low in sugar) should be offered more frequently.

Diet Assessment

One of the most useful tools for nutritional assessment is a diet or nutritional history from parents. This provides information regarding the adequacy of the diet and facilitates identification of parental concerns. Such an assessment should take place at every well-child visit, and the data obtained should be used in conjunction with current nutritional information to educate and guide parents in providing a well-balanced diet for their infant or child (Appendix A4).

Since toddlers and preschoolers can be unpredictable about the quantity as well as the quality of what they eat, periodic assessment is especially important for this age group to determine nutritional adequacy. Factors specific to these age groups that require consideration in the nurse's assessment and management include the need for (1) increased caloric intake; (2) 10% to 15% protein, 50% carbohydrate, and 35% fat caloric distribution; and (3) increased water intake (see Chapter 34).

CLINICAL APPLICATION

Rose Kendall is a 2-day-old white female referred to the health department for a postnatal nursing follow-up visit. Review of the prenatal and birth history reveals that Rose's mother is 23 years of age, gravida III, and para III, received routine prenatal care through the health department clinic, and experienced no health problems during this pregnancy. Labor was 6 hours long, followed by an uncomplicated posterior presentation and vaginal delivery with an epidural anesthetic at 40 weeks of gestation. The Apgar scores at 1 and 5 minutes were 9/8. Birth weight and length were 6 lbs 4 oz and 19 3/4 inches, respectively. Rose experienced no problems at birth and was discharged at 48 hours at a weight of 6 lbs 10 oz with her mother, who is breast-feeding her.

Anne Howard, the community health nurse, visits the home when Rose is 6 days old. Her *assessment* reveals that Rose lives in a two bedroom, sparsely furnished apartment that is gas heated and has functional utilities. Rose's mother is divorced and her two siblings, Janet (age 5 years) and George (age 3 years) live with them. The apartment is on a bus line, and Rose's maternal grandparents live several miles away and are accessible by bus. Rose's mother will be returning to her secretarial job in 4 weeks and has no arrangements for child care because the previous babysitter has moved.

Further assessment by Ms. Howard reveals that Rose is nursing four to five times a day, weighs 6 lbs 1 oz, has normal elimination patterns, exhibits satisfactory suck and grasp reflexes, and regards her mother's face when awake. Rose's mother voices concern that Rose sleeps more than her other two children did at this age, is difficult to wake for feedings, and frequently falls asleep after nursing on only one side. Ms. Howard notes that Rose's skin had a yellow hue.

In *planning* Rose's nursing care, Ms. Howard establishes the nursing diagnoses of altered nutrition resulting from potential of inadequate amount and frequency; altered physiological status caused by potential of jaundice associated with breast-feeding; altered growth as a result of a potential weight loss of greater than 10% of birth weight; and altered parenting and family life resulting from a single mother returning to work. In implementing her plan of care, Ms. Howard carried out the following nursing interventions.

Initially, she made arrangements for Mrs. Kendall to bring Rose to the health department clinic. Rose's bilirubin level was 8.3 mg/dL and her weight was 6 lbs. Ms. Howard encouraged Mrs. Kendall to continue breast-feeding and to avoid supplementation and reassured her about the benign nature of breast milk jaundice. She discussed breast-feeding techniques and encouraged Mrs. Kendall to awaken and feed Rose every 2 to 3 hours during day and evening hours. Rose and her mother returned to the clinic 1 week later. Her bilirubin level was 10 mg/dL and her weight was 6 lbs 5 oz. Ms. Howard reinforced the need to continue the frequent breast-feedings. At 3 weeks of age, Rose weighed 6 lbs 10 oz and her bilirubin was 12.5 mg/dL. Ms. Howard noted yellowing of Rose's sclera. Ms. Howard reassured Mrs. Kendall that Rose's weight gain was satisfactory and explained that the continuing rise in the bilirubin level was normal for breast milk jaundice and recommended increasing Rose's exposure to sunlight. Ms. Howard also discussed child care with Mrs. Kendall because she was planning to return to work the following week. Ms. Howard encouraged Mrs. Kendall to seek child care within the family, possibly with the maternal grandmother or aunt she had mentioned. She also discussed ways to continue breast-feeding after she returned to work and made arrangements for Mrs. Kendall to secure a breast pump from a loaner program. Mrs. Kendall brought Rose to the clinic when she was 4 weeks old. Her

weight was 6 lbs 15 oz and her bilirubin level was 8.9 mg/dL. Ms. Howard noted that the yellow appearance of Rose's scleral and skin was diminishing. Outcomes of Ms. Howard's nursing were evaluated at this 4 week visit and arrangements for further follow-up visits were made.

Outcomes of Ms. Howard's nursing *interventions* included Rose's return to her birth weight with continued weight gain; continuation of breast-feeding through the jaundiced period; beginning resolution of jaundiced appearance; securing a breast pump to facilitate continuation of breast-feeding once Mrs. Kendall returned to work; and assistance in making arrangements for child care. A follow-up visit was scheduled for 2 weeks later to further *evaluate* Rose's continued weight gain, her bilirubin level, and child care arrangements.

SUMMARY

The promotion of child health provides society with an opportunity to be a well society. The community health nurse has a unique opportunity to work with parents and children to promote positive childhood behaviors that will lead to a healthy adulthood.

At the moment of conception, some aspects of wellness are determined. Once conception has occurred, fetal growth depends on the intrauterine environment. Fetal assessment and the assessment of the mother's physical and psychosocial environment assists the community health nurse in providing interventions that will help families prepare for the baby's first year of life. Prenatal visits help the nurse lay the groundwork for positive influences on the child's health and the parents' adjustment to the child.

Assessment of physical, emotional, and social growth and development and the physical examination are important techniques the nurse can use to evaluate the health of the neonate infant, toddler, and preschooler, to predict current and future health problems, and to implement early preventive activities to ensure optimal health. Factors that affect growth and development are successful mastery of tasks and milestones of each developmental stage, heredity, temperament, health and living environment, family, peers, life experiences, and the ability of the family to cope when both parents work.

Growth and development of the toddler and the preschooler are further affected by expansion of life experiences and integration of the personality.

Although major strides have been made in the past 5 years to improve the safety of life for infants, significant problems still exist. The first year of life is the most hazardous period (until age 65 years). The primary threats to infant health and survival are low–birth weight, congenital anomalies with associated problems, and sudden infant death syndrome. The major causes of mortality of these age groups are accidents and injuries; infections are responsible for most of the morbidity. Child abuse or neglect is a phenomenon of growing concern in the United States and is becoming a major contributor to morbidity and mortality in toddlers and preschoolers.

The basic tools and techniques for assessing health problems of toddlers and preschoolers include monitoring physical growth and phychosocial development. There are many tools available to assist the nurse in identifying problems requiring intervention. Community resources are an integral part of the nurse's techniques for helping families to resolve the problems of toddlers and preschooler.

Prevention is the primary goal of the nurse in regard to accidents, infectious disease, and child abuse. Anticipatory guidance, health teaching, and counseling are appropriate community health nursing interventions that assist families in making the child's first year of life healthy and happy.

KEY CONCEPTS

Children are one third of our population and all of our future. Their health is our foundation.

Human growth and development are orderly, predictable processes that begin with the embryo and continue until death. The phases of growth and development are influenced by many hereditary and environmental influences, such as the parent-child relationship and the living environment.

The growth process includes not only physical development but also emotional and social development.

Physical and physiological growth is slower in toddlers than in infants and continues at a still slower rate during the preschool years.

One of the most important components of maintaining a child's health is the promotion of good nutrition and dietary habits. The nurse's role involves encouraging and assisting parents in providing adequate nutrition for their child.

Major health problems during the neonatal period include jaundice and problems in the regulation of body temperature.

The primary threats to infant health and survival are low–birth weight (immaturity), congenital anomalies with associated problems, and sudden infant death syndrome (SIDS). For the family of infants at risk of SIDS, the community health nurse can be a valuable resource.

Major health problems of infants are upper respiratory tract infections (URIs), otitis media, allergies, gastrointestinal illnesses, annd malnutrition.

The largest percentage of pediatric aids victims results from maternal high-risk factors.

Major health problems of toddlers and preschoolers include viral illnesses, infectious diseases in day care centers, lead poisoning, and child abuse and neglect. Viral illnesses are the most common infectious diseases in children.

Accidents are the most preventable cause of morbidity and mortality in infants and children.

Homeless children have four areas of need: access to health care, education, nutrition and developmental stimulation.

The assessment tools most useful to the nurse are those designed to assess psychosocial skills, developmental skills, or both.

The community health nurse can help families promote infant, toddler, and preschooler well-being in a variety of ways and settings, including health assessments, physical and psychological screening, diet assessment, and parent groups and parent education.

LEARNING ACTIVITIES

1. Develop a plan of immunization for a 2-month old infant who has never been immunized and a 12-month old infant who has received one DTP and OPV.

2. Administer the DDST-R to the mother of a 4-month-old infant. Then develop a plan of anticipatory guidance.

3. Conduct a diet history, and then develop a diet plan for a 6-month-old infant who is currently being breast-fed.

4. Develop a plan of nursing care for the family and premature infant, the family who has experienced a SIDS death, and the family and a technology-dependent infant.

5. Administer the press to a 4-year-old child.

6. Observe a group of toddlers *or* preschool children interacting (at a day care center, a nursery, or a nursery school). Then complete the following, based on your observations of four children:

OBSERVATIONS

Age	Level of play
_____	_____
_____	_____
_____	_____
Fine motor activity	Gross motor activity
_____	_____
_____	_____
Social activity observed	Language observed
_____	_____
_____	_____
_____	_____

BIBLIOGRAPHY

American Academy of Pediatrics, Committee on Early Childhood, Adoption and Dependent Care: Health in day care: a manual for health professions, Elk Grove Village, 1987, The Academy.

American Academy of Pediatrics: Committee on Nutrition, Pediatric Nutrition handbook, ed 2, Elkgrove Village, 1985, The Academy.

American Academy of Pediatrics: Report of the Committee on Infectious Diseases, ed 22, Elk Grove Village, 1991, The Academy.

American Academy of Pediatrics, Task Force on Prolonged Infantile Apnea: Prolonged infantile apnea, Pediatrics 76:129, 1985.

Anderson CL: Assessing parenting potential for child abuse risk, Pediatr Nurs 13:323, 1987.

Andrews M and Nielson DW: Technology dependent children in the home, Pediatr Nurs 14:111, 1988.

Apgar V: The newborn (Apgar) scoring system, Pediatr Clin North Am 13:645, 1966.

Aquilina SS: Gastroesophageal reflux: problem or nuisance?, J Pediatr Health Care 1:233, 1987.

Aronson SS and Gilsdorf JR: Preventive management of infectious diseases in day-care, Pediatr Rev 7:259, 1986.

Balk SJ and Christoffel KK: Advising the working mother, Contemp Pediatr 5:56, 1988.

Barnard MU et al.: Handbook of comprehensive pediatric nursing, New York, 1981, McGraw-Hill Book Co.

Behrman RE and Vaughan VC, editors: Nelson textbook of pediatrics, ed 13, Philadelphia, 1987, WB Saunders.

Bernbaum JC et al: Preterm infant care after hospital discharge, Pediatr Rev 10:195, 1989.

Berry, RK: Home care of the child with AIDS, Pediatr Nurs 14:341, 1988.

Bierman, CW and Pearlman DC, editors: Allergic diseases of infancy, childhood and adolescense, ed 2, Philadelphia, 1988, WB Saunders.

Bowlby J: Attachment and loss, vol 1, Attachment, New York, 1969, Basic Books.

Bradley, RH and Caldwell BM: Using the HOME inventory to assess family environment, Pediatr Nurs 14:97, 1988.

Brady M: AIDS in children, J Pediatr Health Care, 1:214, 1987.

Brown MS and Murphy MA: Ambulatory pediatrics for nurses, ed 2, New York, 1981, McGraw-Hill Book Co.

Bunch WH: Common deformities of the lower limb, Pediatr Nurs 518, 1979.

Buschbacher VI and Delcampo RL: parents response to sudden infant death syndrome, J Pediatr Health Care 1:85, 1987.

Caffey J: The whiplash shaken infant: manual shaking by the extremities with whiplash induced intracranial and intraocular bleedings, link with residual permanent brain damage and mental retardation, Pediatrics 54:396, 1974.

Caldwell B: Home observations for measurement of the environment, Little Rock, 1976, University of Arkansas Center for Child Development and Education.

Caplan F and Caplan T: The power of play, New York, 1973, Anchor Press.

Castiglia PT: Sexual abuse of children, J Pediatr Health Care 4:91 1990.

Center for Disease Control: Recommendations of the immunization practices advisory committee, MMWR 36:11, 1989.

Chess S and Thomas A: Dynamics of individual behavioral development. In Levine MD, Carey WB, Crocker AC, and Gross RT, editors: Developmental behavioral pediatrics, Philadelphia, 1983, WB Saunders.

Chow MP et al.: Handbook of pediatric primary care, ed 2, New York, 1984, John Wiley & Sons.

Davis N, Sweeney LB: Infantile apnea monitoring and SIDS, J Pediatr Health Care 3:67, 1989.

Drumwright AF: Denver Articulation Screening Examination: scoring and interpretation instruction, Denver, 1971, University of Colorado Medical Center.

Dubowitz L, Dubowitz V, and Goldberg C: Clinical assessment of gestational age in the newborn infant, J Pediatr 77:1, 1970.

Dudek B: Counseling in sudden infant death syndrome and other childhood deaths, Pediatr Rev 7:168, 1985.

Duvall E: Marriage and family development, Philadelphia, 1977, JB Lippincott.

Erikson E: Childhood and society, New York, 1963, Jeffrey Norton Publishers.

Food and Nutrition Board, National Research Council: Recommended dietary allowances, ed 9, Washington, DC, 1980, National Academy of Sciences.

Foster R, Hunsberger M., and Anderson J: Family centered care of children and adolescents, Philadelphia, ed 2, 1989, WB Saunders.

Frankenburg WK et al.: Validation of key Denver Developmental Screening Test items: a preliminary study, J Pediatr 112:560, 1988.

Frankenburg WK., Goldstein, AD., and Camp BW: The revised Denver Developmental Screening Test: its accuracy as a screening instrument, J Pediatr 79:988, 1971.

Giebink GS: Progress in understanding the pathophysiology of otitis media, Pediatr Rev 11:133, 1989.

Goldberg R: Identifying speech and language delays in children, Pediatr Nurs 10:252, 1984.

Hall JG: When a child is born with congenital anomalies, Contemp Pediatr 5:78, 1988.

Heiser CA: Home phototherapy, Pediatr Nurs 13:425, 1987.

Hoekelman RA: Pediatric primary care, St. Louis, 1987, Mosby-Year Book.

Kempe, CH and Helfer R: Helping the battered child and his family, Philadelphia, 1972, JB Lippincot.

Kempe CH and Hopkins J: The public health nurse's role in the prevention of child abuse and neglect, Public Health Curriculum 15:1, 1975.

Klaus MH and Kennell JH: Maternal-infant bonding, ed 2, St Louis, 1982, Mosby-Year Book.

Korones SB: High-risk newborn infants, ed 4, St Louis, 1986, Mosby-Year Book.

Kronmiller JE and Nirsch RF: Preventive dentistry for children, Pediatr Nurs 11:446, 1985.

Krugman S, Ward R, and Katz SL: Infectious diseases of children, ed 8, St Louis, 1985, Mosby-Year Book.

Lavengood TDN: Involuntary smoking: children in crisis, Pediatr Nurs 14:93, 1988.

Lenneberg EH: Biological foundations of language, New York, 1967, John Wiley & Sons.

Lombardino LJ: Evaluating communicative behaviors in infancy, J Pediatr Health Care 1:240, 1987.

Lopez J, Diliberto J, and McGuekin M: Infection control in day care centers: present and future need, Am J Infect Control 16:26, 1988.

Maier H: Three theories of child development, New York, 1969, Harper & Row, Publishers.

Miles M, editor: Mental health aspects of SIDS: Report of conference sponsored by the National Foundation for Sudden Infant Death and the National Institute of Mental Health—Kansas City, July 30, 1975, Washington, DC, 1975, U.S. Department of Health, Education, and Welfare.

Miller SJ: Prenatal nursing assessment of the expectant family, Nurs Pract 11:40, 1986.

Mohler SE: Passive smoking: a danger to children's health, J Pediatr Health Care 1:298, 1987.

National Commission to Prevent Infant Mortality: Death before life: the tragedy of infant mortality, Washington, DC, 1988, The Commission.

Osborn LM: Management of neonatal jaundice, Nurs Pract 11:41, 1986.

Parten M: Social participation among preschool children, J Abnorm Soc Psychol 4:242, 1932.

Rettig PJ: Infections due to Chlamydia trachomatis from infancy to adolescence, Pediatr Infect Dis 5:559, 1987.

Rice BK and Feeg VD: First year developmental outcomes for multiple risk premature infants, Pediatr Nurs 11:30, 1985.

Rogers WB Jr and Rogers RA: A new simplified preschool readiness experimental scale (PRESS), Clin Pediatr 11:558, 1972.

Rose BS: Phototherapy: all wrapped up? Pediatr Nurs 16:57, 1990.

Rudner N: Children with elevated lead levels, J Pediatr Health Care 4:46, 1988.

Ryan MT: Identifying the sexually abused child, Pediatr Nurs 10:419, 1972.

Scipien GM et al.: Pediatric nursing care, St Louis, 1990, Mosby-Year Book.

Select Committee on Children, Youth, and Families, 99th Congress, 1st session: Opportunities for success: cost effectiveness programs for children, Washington, DC, 1986, U.S. Government Printing Office.

Shulsinger E: Needs of sheltered homeless children, J Pediatr Health Care 4:136, 1990.

Sirles AT: Self care education, J Pediatr Health Care 2:135, 1988.

Smith DP: Common day care diseases: patterns and prevention, Pediatr Nurs 12:175, 1985.

Speer JJ and Sachs B: Selecting the appropriate family assessment tool, Pediatr Nurs 11:349, 1985.

Suskind RM and Varma RN: Assessment of nutritional status of children, Pediatr in Rev 5:195, 1984.

Tomlinson PS: Father involvement with first-born infants: interpersonal and situational factors, Pediatr Nurs 13:101, 1987.

Tuttle JI: Adolescent pregnancy: factoring in the father of the baby, J Pediatr Health Care 2:240, 1988.

Waldo E, Dashefsky B, Byers C, Guerra N, and Taylor F: Frequency and severity of infections in day care, J Pediatr 112:540, 1988.

Wegman ME: Annual summary of vital statistics: 1989, Pediatrics 86:835, 1990.

Weiser MA and Castiglia, PT: Assessing early father-infant attachment MCN 9:104 1984.

Whaley LF and Wong, DL: Effective communication strategies for pediatric practice, Pediatr Nurs 11:429, 1985.

Whaley LF and Wong DL: Nursing care of infants and children, ed 4, St Louis, 1991, Mosby-Year Book.

Williams JK: Screening for genetic disorders, J Pediatr Health Care 3:115, 1989.

Wood D: Homeless children, J Pediatr Health Care 3:194, 1989.

Wong D and Whaley LF: Clinical manual of pediatric nursing, ed 3, St Louis, 1990, Mosby-Year Book.

Wong, DL: False allegations of child abuse: the other side of the tragedy, Pediatr Nurs 13:329, 1987.

Wong DL: Helping parents select day care, Pediatr Nurs 12:181, 1986.

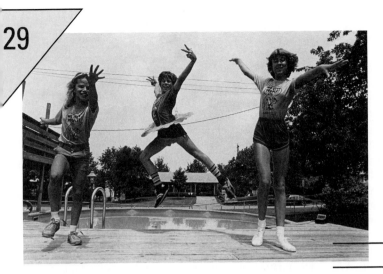

29

School-Age Children And Adolescents

Nancy Dickenson-Hazard

OBJECTIVES

After reading this chapter, the student should be able to:

Identify significant physical and psychosocial developmental factors characteristic of school-age and adolescent clients.

Define nursing activities that promote the health of school-age and adolescent clients.

Identify factors that influence the growth, development, and health of school-age children and adolescents.

Identify common causes of morbidity and mortality in school-age children and adolescents.

Identify significant health problems of school-age children and adolescents and the role of the community health nurse in alleviating them.

Discuss assessment tools appropriate for school-age children and adolescents.

Define the role of the community health nurse in the promotion of health for school-age children and adolescents in the home, school, or clinic.

KEY TERMS

accidents and injuries
adolescence
adolescent mother
asthma
cancer
child self-care
contraceptive education
dyslexia
hyperactivity

kyphosis
learning difficulties
lordosis
minimal brain dysfunction
nutrition
puberty
school adjustment
school conference

school-based health promotion
scoliosis
sexually transmitted diseases
substance abuse
suicide
teen pregnancy
vegetarian child
vitamin and mineral supplementation

B oth the school-age child and the adolescent live in rapidly expanding worlds. The experiences confronting them are diverse and complex. Although the health of this nation's children and adolescents is better than ever, school-age and adolescent persons are confronted with health problems more complex than those of preceding generations. School and societal influences create many problems for children in these age groups. Nurses in community health settings can educate school-age children and adolescents about these problems and the influence on health. These educational encounters may occur in the school, clinic, or home. Through these encounters the community health nurse can assist children and adolescents to learn behaviors that will help them become healthy adults.

This chapter focuses on the health assessment, health maintenance, and health promotion activities pertinent to the school-age child and the adolescent. The physical and psychosocial aspects of health are reviewed, as are significant factors that can positively or negatively influence health behavior.

PHYSICAL GROWTH AND DEVELOPMENT

The child from 6 to 12 years of age experiences steady physical growth, neuromuscular refinement, and rapid expansion of cognitive and social skills. During this phase of life, physical and psychosocial mastery of the expanding environment is the primary task. The period of life from 13 to 18 years is characterized by a steady progression of physiological changes. These physical changes, coupled with the emotional, psychological, and social adaptations of adolescence, require the young person to develop coping mechanisms that will be carried throughout life.

School-Age Children

Physical growth is slow and steady in school-age children. Boys are generally taller and heavier than girls until approximately age 9 to 10 years, when girls begin to grow more rapidly in height and weight. The preadolescent growth spurt usually occurs between 9 and 14 years for girls and between 12 and 16 years for boys.

Overall body appearance changes occur during this time as a result of skeletal growth. Lordotic posture is replaced by erect posture. Dental growth is evidenced by the shedding and eruption of teeth, whereas patterns of eating and sleeping are relatively stable. Neuromuscular skills, sensory organ development, and cognitive skills are refined and expanded. Sexual growth begins, as evidenced by the appearance of inital secondary sex characteristics. Nutritional needs increase toward the end of this period as prepubertal growth increases appetite and caloric and water requirement (see Appendix J4).

Monitoring of height, weight, vital signs, and blood pressure continue to be essential to the community health nurse's assessment. Observation of dental and skeletal growth is also important. Discussing a diet that promotes optimal growth and dental health is appropriate because the school-age child now has increased cognitive and development abilities and can assume a more active role in health promotion. Anticipatory guidance for preparing the school-age child for the physical and psychosocial changes of puberty should also be initiated by the nurse. (See Appendix K8 for other aspects of development health promotion that require the nurse's assessment).

Adolescents

Physical growth during adolescence is accelerated, with the majority of growth occurring over a 2- to 3-year span. For girls, this growth spurt normally begins at approximately 9½ years of age, peaks at 12 years of age, and stops by 14 years of age. The height spurt for boys begins at approximately 10½ years of age, peaks at 14 years of age, and ends at 16 years of age. Growth follows the same pattern for both sexes, beginning with leg lengthening, followed by widening of thighs, broadening of shoulders, and trunk growth. Skeletal mass doubles during adolescence, resulting in significant weight gains.

The process of sexual maturation that occurs during puberty involves rapid sexual growth following a specific sequence of events (see a basic pediatric text for a detailed discussion of sexual development). Both primary (necessary for reproduction) and secondary (differentiate gender) sex characteristics develop for completion of puberty according to the person's individual maturation rate.

The community health nurse needs to continue growth monitoring through height, weight, vital sign, and blood pressure measurements. Determination of the stage of sexual development, evaluation of normal progression, identification of any abnormalities of development, and counseling and education of adolescents in regard to the changes created by their sexual development are other essential nursing activities. Tanner staging is the most widely used tool for assessing sexual development. (See Tanner [1962] or a basic pediatric nursing textbook for a detailed discussion.)

Community health nurses also need to continue to monitor immunization and nutritional status. An additional booster for tetanus and diphtheria is indicated for children 14 to 16 years of age. A diet history provides the nurse with information about nutritional adequacy. Particular attention must be paid to the adolescent's diet because calorie and nutritional requirements increase. The community health nurse should assist the adolescent to implement a diet plan that incorporates these increased requirements and the individual's food preferences) Appendixes D2, A4 and J4).

PSYCHOSOCIAL DEVELOPMENT

From the ages of 6 to 12 years children expand their social and cognitive spheres. They learn to contribute, collaborate, and work cooperatively to become productive members of a peer group. Developing cognition permits them to differentiate, categorize, problem solve, and understand causality. Between the ages of 13 and 18 years, cognitive abilities improve to allow the use of abstract logic, deductive reasoning, and hypotheses construction. This process of formal thinking enables adolescents to establish their own identity and make decisions about life-styles and vocations. Appendixes J11 and K8 provide an overview of the psychosocial development of the school-age child and the adolescent.

School-Age Children

During school-age years, children are working toward developing a sense of industry, by using their expanding cognitive skills of reasoning and realism. Being able to differentiate, categorize, solve problems, and conceptualize allows the child to achieve social, cognitive, and physical competencies.

The community health nurse assesses this growth through history taking and observation. By knowing the typical behaviors for a specific age group, the community health nurse can assess the individual child's psychosocial health. For example, knowing that the average 10-year-old child can follow rules, participates in cooperative projects, has hobbies or distinct interests, and has a group of special friends would alert the nurse to a child who has few friends, plays alone at recess, does not follow rules, and does not appear to have any special interests. Knowledge of developmental norms can also assist the community health nurse in promoting psychosocial growth. For example, the nurse might encourage a shy child to participate in organized sports or encourage the parents of a child who is attending a new school to invite schoolmates to play after school. These nursing interventions encourage group and peer activity, which is important for the child's developing social skills.

School-age children who develop confidence in themselves and function well within societal rules are better equipped to handle the turmoil of adolescence. The nurse can positively influence this adjustment by exploring feelings of inferiority that result from their immature physical and cognitive abilities. The nurse should assist them in developing positive coping behaviors for the pressures of school, home, and friends. For example, the school nurse can hold discussion sessions on how to say no to drugs, sex, and alcohol.

Adolescents

Adolescents are trying to establish their identities while continuing to expand their concrete and abstract logical abilities. Often these two areas of development collide. For example, most adolescents are aware of the dangers of drinking and driving, yet go along with it because of their need to be a part of the peer group. The role of the nurse is to help adolescents to recognize these inconsistencies and to direct their energies toward positive health behaviors. The community health nurse can help students establish a chapter of SADD (Students Against Driving Drunk) or develop a community program that distributes information on safe driving tips at local grocery stores.

Community health nurses also need to motivate and involve adolescents in decisions about health behaviors through education. Knowledge about health facts and risks can help adolescents choose positive health behaviors. The community health nurse should educate and counsel during health visits in the school setting and during home visits. Special adolescent screening and health assessment clinics and special group health education classes in the school or clinic are frequently used by community health nurses. They often conduct scoliosis screening in schools, classes on birth control alternatives in the clinic, or health education classes in either setting on skin care, diet, and nutrition.

Additionally, the community health nurse should promote adolescent psychosocial health through education programs for parents of adolescents. These sessions can provide a forum for parents to discuss problems they are encountering—for example, dealing with the influence of peers, the argumentative teenager, sexual development, and the apparently irresponsible adolescent—or focus on topics of special interest, such as recognizing drug use in the adolescent, communicating with the adolescent, or assisting the adolescent in decision making.

For both adolescent and school-age clients, the community health nurse can make use of their children's increasing cognitive abilities. The nurse can rely on the school-age child or adolescent as historian and verify facts with parents as indicated. In addition, nurses should explain any physical assessment techniques to clients of these ages and involve them directly in their plans of care.

FACTORS INFLUENCING GROWTH AND DEVELOPMENT

As the child continues to grow and develop throughout the school-age and adolescent years, exposure to a multitude of new factors influences progression through these stages. As for the earlier years, growth and development are affected by the degree of success or failure a child has had in mastering the tasks of preceding stages. However, unlike earlier years, a child is now equipped with more complex cognitive, physical, and social skills, but faces more complex tasks. In addition, the degree of difficulty a child or adolescent experiences in accomplishing these more complex tasks influences resultant developmental abilities and skills.

Role of Peers

Of singular importance to growth and development at this stage is the role of peers. With the exception of family, a child or adolescent's peer group exerts the greatest influence on development. Peers permit the individual to try out and even fail in new skills, to validate thoughts, feelings, and concepts, and to receive acceptance and support as a unique person. Conversely, a peer group can place demands and pressure on the individual to conform that create feelings of being uncomfortable or even inferior. The balanced effect of this peer influence can be positive at times, negative at others, and almost always lasting.

Role of Family

As the child's world expands outside of the home, the family influence changes. Parents are no longer viewed as the ultimate, all-knowing authority. The child, and particularly the adolescent, learns that parents are human; they make mistakes and do not have all the answers. Frequently, parental values and ideas are questioned and differences and conflicts arise. Despite these confrontations, however, the child still needs parental love and support. Parental guidance, knowledge, and experiences continue to serve as resources for verification of their own fast-developing repertoire of behaviors. Parental values, ideas, and expectations help adolescents to develop their own. Although adolescents may diverge or digress from parental points of view, the influence remains and eventually affects decisions and behaviors (Sutterley and Donnelly, 1981).

Physical Well-Being

The state of their health and nutrition affects children's abilities to grow and develop. Optimal mastery of skills and

---

TABLE 29-1

Historical data for screening for childhood malignancies

	Family history	Review of systems
Leukemia	Relates syndromes or diseases (e.g., Down's syndrome, immunodeficiency disease) Carcinogen exposure (e.g., radiation, immunosuppressive drugs)	Signs of anemia: pallor, excessive tiredness, decreased exercise tolerance Bleeding tendencies: excessive bleeding, nosebleeds, petechiae Recurrent infections—local or systemic
Central nervous system disorders	Congenital spine or skull defects Presence of CNS-related disorders (e.g., neurofibromas, tuberous sclerosis)	Signs of CNS dysfunction: headaches; visual problems (e.g., diplopia); nystagmus; decreased acuity; ataxia; vomiting without nausea and on waking; palsies and paresis
Wilms' tumor	Associated congenital anomalies (e.g., hemihypertrophy, hypospadias, cryptorchism, renal masses)	Signs of gastrointestinal tract dysfunction: abdominal pain, distension or enlargement, diarrhea, anorexia Signs of urinary tract dysfunction: hematuria General signs: fever, lethargy

Modified from Wolf WJ and Bancroft B: Pediatr Nurs 5:43, 1980; Hockenberry MJ et al: Pediatr Nurs 16:239, 1990.

---

tasks occurs when the individual is healthy. Deficiencies in nutrition and problems with health alter an individual's sense of wellness and perceptions of self. Functioning at a diminished capacity creates difficulties in accomplishing complex tasks. Therefore promotion and maintenance of health and nutrition become important components in the normal developmental progression.

COMMON CAUSES OF MORBIDITY AND MORTALITY

Although the health of school-age children and adolescents has improved over the past 10 years, the slowness of the decline in mortality continues to be of major concern. Injury-related deaths are the predominant cause of mortality in school-age children, followed by cancer and birth defects. Violent death and accidents account for the majority of deaths in adolescence with three fourths of all deaths attributable to motor vehicle accidents, homicide, or suicide (Wilson, 1989). In addition, deaths of children younger than 15 years of age as a result of immunodeficiency virus (HIV) have increased more than 70% (Wegman, 1989).

Accidents and Injuries

Motor vehicle accidents are responsible for more than 13% of all childhood deaths in ages 1 through 4 years and 21% of all deaths for ages 5 through 14 years. Alcohol consumption has been implicated in many adolescent fatalities, which also accounts for this population having the highest number of motor vehicle accidents (Wegman, 1989; Wilson, 1989).

Bicycles, swings, and skateboard injuries account for the most accidental injuries among school-age children. For the preadolescent and the adolescent, injuries from contact sports such as football and basketball are also primary causes of injury. Furthermore, drowning accounts for a large proportion of deaths in the school-age and adolescent population. These accidental causes of death and injury require the attention of all health care professionals if the health of children is to improve.

Community health nurses should intervene to prevent accidents, primarily through education. Because prevention of accidents requires changes in behavior on the part of parents and children, incorporation of safety education and accident prevention is necessary in each contact community health nurses have with their clients. Educational efforts must be directed toward and involve the child or adolescent, the parents, the family, and the community. For example, water safety needs to be emphasized to parents and children in areas where water sports or pools are highly used and sports personnel and teachers need to be educated about the immediate management and transport of an injured athlete. Discussing bicycle safety with school-age children and automobile driving and passenger safety with adolescents should be an additional educational focus of the community health nurse. Reinforcement of this safety education can be carried out during the health maintenance visit, in collaboration with the school, and through group health education seminars and workshops. Additional appropriate safety education is discussed in Appendix J6.

Cancer

Children who are age 1 to 14 years are frequent victims of cancer, with leukemia being the most frequent childhood malignancy. The incidence of testicular cancer is particularly significant for adolescent males, making the testicular self-examination a priority educational focus for this age and gender group.

Screening for cancer through history and physical assessment is an important aspect of the nurse's role. Table 29-1 presents historical data indicative of childhood malignancies, which require immediate referral.

Suicide

The number of suicides in the preadolescent and adolescent age group has nearly doubled in the past 5 years. Children with poor social adjustment or psychiatric or family problems (see box) are at increased risk (Wilson, 1989). Nurses

---

CHARACTERISTICS OF ADOLESCENTS AND FAMILIES AT RISK OF SOCIAL PROBLEMS

ADOLESCENT BEHAVIORS

Insecure
Poor self-concept or feeling inadequate
Severe mood changes
School problems
Antisocial behavior
Substance abuse
Decreased verbal communication
Sleep disturbances
Prolonged grief reaction following divorce, death, or severing
    of a romance
Communication problems at home
"Loner"
Friends of questionable reputation
Premature "growing up"
Social, emotional, or attention deficits
Cognitive development disability

Depression
Hedonistic philosophy

FAMILY SITUATION

Divorce
Death of one parent
Frequent family relocation
Insufficient parental guidance
Frequent absences of one parent
Drug or alcohol abuse
Stepparent
Poor relationships between family members
Mental illness
Economic deprivation
Faulty communication patterns
Emotional, physical, or sexual abuse

---

have a responsibility to be cognizant of behaviors that are considered danger signs (see box) and to implement immediate intervention.

Nursing assessment and intervention directed toward the depressed or suicidal child are needed in the community, in the school, and in the ambulatory care setting. Nurses, particularly those in the school and community settings, are potentially the first persons the suicidal adolescent encounters. Frequently, a physical complaint is the initial factor precipitating an encounter between the nurse and the adolescent. Masked in the physical complaint is the major problem or concern that is promoting suicidal thoughts. Nurses facilitate the identification of such a troubled teenager by being observant of adolescent behaviors, by encouraging adolescents to discuss their feelings, and by being an available source of support (Child et al., 1980; Nelms and Brady, 1980; Valente and Saunders, 1987).

In addition, family assessment and involvement in nursing interventions are critical. The family's role in exacerbating or alleviating the depressed child's symptoms must be explored through history and interview. Assisting family members to cope with the child's behavior and feelings, helping them solve dysfunctional family relationships, and educating the family to be a support for the child are important nursing tasks.

Community resources are also essential to prevention. Crisis intervention centers and telephone hot lines provide professional help and resource referral. Educational programs directed toward the variables that create problems for adolescents facilitate early identification and provide a support group. Such programs should involve adolescents in both participation and planning.

MAJOR HEALTH PROBLEMS OF SCHOOL-AGE CHILDREN AND ADOLESCENTS

Common causes of morbidity for the school-age child and adolescent are physical and psychosocial in origin. Of primary significance to the school-age population are the prob-

---

BEHAVIORAL DANGER SIGNS

1. Giving away prized possessions.
2. Becoming increasingly isolated.
3. Recent loss, especially a parent, boyfriend, or girlfriend.
4. Statements such as, "No one cares about me. It would be better for everyone if I were dead." "How many aspirins do you have to take to kill yourself?"
5. A sudden elevation of mood following a depression. This could be misconstrued to mean improvement when actually the teenager may be experiencing a sense of relief that the decision to die has been made.

From Hart NA and Prophit SP: Pediatr Nurs 5:22, 1979.

---

lems of asthma, school adjustment, including phobia and learning difficulties, and abnormal spinal curvatures. The social and physical problems of substance abuse, sexually transmitted diseases, and pregnancy confront the adolescent. Other health problems—such as bacterial and parasitic infections, acne, eating disorders, menstrual and behavioral disorders—increase in incidence during school-age and adolescent years. (See Appendix J7 and J10 for an overview of these health problems.) The nurse's responsibility is to provide intervention to resolve problems and to reinforce preventive measures that will abate recurrence.

Asthma

One in 12 school-age children are affected by asthma, which creates physical and psychological problems affecting the child's health, growth, school performance, and social interactions.

Nursing interventions for the child with asthma begin with assessment and prompt intervention during acute episodes. Education regarding self-care at home and at school should be a priority. Such counseling should include information about prevention of acute attacks through environmental control and avoidance of infection; appropriate exercise, diet and hydration; compliance and understanding of drug therapy and regular follow-up.

School Adjustment

Starting school creates a situation that will require adjustment on the part of the child and parent, because both parent and child must now "let go" of some degree of security and comfort to allow the child to develop as an individual. Children must learn to cope with new challenges presented by school and peers, and parents must allow their children to make decisions, accept responsibility, and learn from both positive and negative life experiences. Parents and children will need support and guidance to successfully adjust to the school experience.

Nurses can promote adjustment to school by assisting individuals to identify potential stresses and by collaborating with parent, child, and teacher to prevent or minimize reactions. Primary areas of intervention include assisting parents to allow the freedom necessary for their child's development, assisting the child to cope with the social and cognitive demands of the school setting, and assisting teachers in dealing with problem or crisis situations involving children and parents.

A problem unique to the school adjustment situation is school phobia, the persistent and abnormal fear of going to school. The cause of this school anxiety behavior may be related to circumstances at home, at school, or both. Frequently identified factors include pressure to achieve, stressful relationships at school, fear of leaving home, and recent occurrence of a traumatic event associated with death, loss, or abandonment.

Nursing interventions include supporting the child and family throughout the problem identification and school reentry process; assisting child and family to follow the management plan; assisting the child to develop coping behaviors that will positively affect self-concept and esteem; assisting parents and child to identify other potential support or professional services; and facilitating interaction and relationships between child, parents and school. Additional nursing actions include prevention of school phobia. Encouraging parents to discuss school and its routines and to visit the school with the child before entry to help allay fears. Parental involvement in school-related activities, such as field trips, also helps the child adjust. Encouraging independence early in the child's life further facilitates school adjustment, preventing potential school phobia.

Learning Difficulties

Approximately 10% to 30% of all school-age children experience some degree of learning difficulty in school. The causes are complex, multifaceted, and often unidentifiable. In addition, many types of problems are frequently lumped under the labels of learning disability, minimal brain dysfunction (MBD), or attention deficit disorder (ADD). Table 29-2 identifies the more common problems associated with learning difficulties and their probable causes and appropriate interventions.

Nursing activities involve assessment and management of the problem. Participation in the early identification, observation, and data collection is a nursing responsibility, as is ensuring appropriate referral and follow-up. Coordinating the activities of all disciplines involved in the evaluation and management frequently is the nurse's role. In addition, the nurse can best explain the problem to the parents and child and provide the support and encouragement needed for a successful outcome.

Abnormal Spinal Curvatures

Abnormalities of the spinal curvature are most frequently detected during the adolescent growth spurt between the ages of 10 and 15 (Chow et al., 1984). Of particular concern are the incidences of kyphosis, lordosis, and scoliosis. Kyphosis is an exaggerated convex curve in the thoracic region resulting in a hump or hunchback appearance. Lordosis is an exaggerated concave curve in the lumbar region of the spine, resulting in a swayback appearance. Because both kyphosis and lordosis are related to poor posture, nursing actions indicated should focus on assisting adolescents to develop an exercise program and learn proper sitting and standing. To achieve maximal success, a detailed explanation of the problem and its cause should precede development of a program. Incorporating activities of interest to the individual teenager further facilitates compliance and success.

Scoliosis is an S-shaped lateral curvature of the spine with rotation of vertical bodies which occurs most frequently in adolescent girls. Immediate referral is indicated upon recognition of scoliosis. Treatment is aimed toward prevention of increasing deformity and may include use of a Milwaukee brace, traction, and surgery.

The community health nurse's role lies in the early recognition of scoliosis and the provision of resources and support during the diagnosis, treatment, and follow-up stages. Early detection and implementation of a plan of care are essential to prevent the secondary complications of lung pathological conditions and future back ailments. Thus screening for scoliosis is a necessary component of health assessment for school-age children and adolescents. Siblings of clients diagnosed with scoliosis particularly need screening because of the potential genetic etiological factor. Screening procedures are easily implemented in the school setting, in special clinics, or in the home. The procedure for screening requires complete exposure of back, chest, and hips and is based on observing the child when walking, standing erect, and bending forward (see Appendix K5).

Because the child generally returns home during treatment, the community health nurse becomes responsible for facilitating the adjustment necessary to ensure a normal life. Specific areas of intervention are indicated, particularly in the self-care of and adaptation to selected treatment methods. Table 29-3 provides guidelines by which an effective plan of nursing care can be implemented.

Substance Abuse

The use of alcohol and drugs has been increasing among adolescents over the past 10 years, and beyond the experimentation phase, adolescents are also increasing the frequency and regularity of use of tobacco, marijuana, and stimulants.

TABLE 29-2

Learning difficulties

Health problem definition	Etiology	Clinical signs	Interventions
ATTENTION DEFICIT DISORDER WITH HYPERACTIVITY (ADDH)			
A behavior disorder with characteristic clinical manifestations resulting in non–goal-directed activity in inappropriate amounts	Most common of minimal brain dysfunction disorders, occurring more frequently in boys than girls Appears to involve a delay in the maturation of cerebral inhibitory function Dietary factors may be a contributing factor	Demonstration of characteristic behaviors of increased motor activity, short attention span, poor concentration, emotionally labile, easily distracted, prone to mood swings, and temper outbursts May be accompanied by learning difficulties and "soft" neurological signs	Medical management may include the following: Use of stimulant drugs (Ritalin and Dexedrine), which stimulate release of norepinephrine, thus producing a calming effect Salicylate-free diet that eliminates all artificial colors and flavors and salicylates Nursing interventions may include facilitating provision of the following (also see interventions for MBD): Structured external stimuli environment at home and school Special education classes Outlets for family feelings of frustration, inadequacy, guilt, tension, stress Avoidance of labeling child Support and encouragement
DYSLEXIA			
Inability to read printed symbols or understand oral symbols (materials)	May be primary dyslexia, which is usually familial and may be due to weakness of learning process or immaturity of brain May be developmental dyslexia resulting from cerebral dysfunction About 15% of children have reading skill difficulty, and of these, 3% are due to primary or developmental dyslexia; developmental dyslexia is more frequent in boys than girls	Demonstrates ability to hear and understand statement but cannot read Usually average or above-average intelligence Demonstrates difficulty distinguishing similar letters (*b* and *d*): may reverse letters when reading (*saw* for *was*); sees letter upside down or mirror image	Measures include the following (also see nursing interventions for MBD and ADDH: Early identification through screening at health assessment visits Assistance with reading instruction School and family working together Use of repetition and reinforcement Positive, relaxed home and school environment Provision of informal learning at home Games to improve reading and hand-eye coordination Avoidance of negative reinforcement; praise and reassurance for child

Continued.

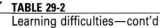

TABLE 29-2
Learning difficulties—cont'd

Health problem definition	Etiology	Clinical signs	Interventions
MINIMAL BRAIN DYSFUNCTION (MBD)			

Descriptive term for a child of average intelligence who has difficulty learning; a disorder in understanding or using language or adapting behavior	Associated with possible minimal insult to the central nervous system
	May result from infection, injury, chronic lead poisoning, or the slow maturation of brain function
		Normal or above average intelligence
		May appear as learning, motor coordination, speech, or auditory difficulty or combination of these
		Of children affected, 50% demonstrate "soft signs": they have short attention spans and mild speech impairment and are clumsy, impulsive, awkward, talkative, destructive, distractable, hyperactive, and socially immature
			Management plan is provided by team and designed for individual child
			Appropriate nursing interventions may include the following:
			  Administering screening tests
			  Assisting parents to be consistent and to design a workable day-to-day schedule
			  Supporting family when evaluating and venting their feelings
			  Assisting parents to design a schedule that keeps frustrations and obstacles at a minimum
			  Assisting parents to identify ways to positively reinforce desirable behaviors of child
			  Teaching parents to keep directions and tasks simple
			  Assisting parents to work with school, physician, and other therapists to implement plan
			  Assisting family to identify useful community resources

The cause of increased substance experimentation and use is not definitive. As with other socially related problems, many factors contribute to this behavioral expression, including the need for peer acceptance or approval, succumbing to peer pressure, curiosity, availability of substances, poor self-concept, a deteriorated parent-child relationship, and boredom.

The physical and psychological effects of substance use are highly variable and differ among individuals. However, chronic use that leads to dependence and addiction can create devastating effects such as change of life-style to accommodate drug need, malnutrition, emotional stress, and alienation from family and friends.

Much substance abuse can be prevented, but assisting adolescents to stop or avoid misuse is not easy. Prevention requires a change in social acceptability, as well as individual acceptability. Strategies for intervention differ, and nurses have a vital role in these preventive efforts. Appropriate interventions include the following:

Educational programs on substance abuse for adolescents emphasizing their decision-making capabilities

Educational programs for parents in preventing abuse or recognizing early symptoms

Early identification and referral of adolescents with a substance abuse problem

Provision of support and acting as a role model

Assistance for adolescents in identifying stressors in their lives and in developing appropriate coping strategies

Use of youth organizations (such as 4-H and Scouts) and media to reinforce substance abuse education

Provision of community programs about substance abuse

Community involvement in establishing a drug-free youth

Sexually Transmitted Diseases

Sexually transmitted diseases have become the leading type of communicable disease in our nation. Gonorrhea, syphilis, and genital herpes simplex account for an estimated 10 to 12 million cases of veneral disease per year and *Chlamydia trachomatis* is now recognized to be responsible for more episodes of sexually transmitted disease than any other organism (Brown, 1989; Marks and Fisher, 1987). Similarly,

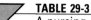

TABLE 29-3
A nursing approach to scoliosis

Areas of intervention	Nursing interventions
Client knowledge and understanding	Discuss normal anatomy and function of spine Define problem as it relates to client and discuss causes of scoliosis Discuss potential management methods in relation to how problem will be treated Discuss management method for individual client and why chosen and the purpose Discuss management course: what will occur, when, how long, how often Provide opportunity for questions; second visit may facilitate this
Client self-care	*Devices* Discuss application of device to be worn and assess its fit Discuss skin care and plan for personal hygiene Review care and cleaning of device Discuss comfortable clothing to wear Review appropriate exercise and diet Discuss management of activities Discuss recognition and prevention of potential problems Request return demonstration of appropriate activities Assess environment for hazards and discuss safety precautions *Casting* Discuss cast application and drying techniques Review care of cast Discuss skin care and personal hygiene Review safety, diet, and elimination factors Discuss impact of immobilization Review management of activities Discuss recognition and prevention of potential problems, including cast syndrome Discuss cast removal, care, and appearance (of skin) after removal
Client psychological well-being	Discuss feelings about management plan (fear, anxiety, lack of control, rejection) Discuss impact on body image and self-esteem Discuss peer and family acceptance and relationships Discuss interaction with general public Discuss ways of dressing that disguise cast or device Discuss ways to explain cast or device to others
Family support	Discuss preceding client factors with family Emphasize self-care activities Encourage understanding Discuss family feelings, perceptions, and attitudes Discuss changes in household routines and physical environment Discuss financial responsibilities

the transmission of trichomoniasis and *Candida albicans,* which most frequently creates vaginal infection, has become a widespread health problem. Condylomata acuminatum (venereal warts) is the most common external lesion seen and is the most common of viral origin. The increased incidence of acquired immunodeficiency syndrome (AIDS) among adolescents is also a major health concern (See Chapter 20 for a complete discussion of AIDS).

Nurses have a vital responsibility in the prevention, identification, and encouragement of prompt treatment of the venereal diseases. Appropriate nursing interventions can be carried out effectively in group or individual counseling sessions, need to be presented in a nonjudgmental manner, and should facilitate adolescent knowledge and understanding about their sexuality. Nursing activities include the following:

Sex education (written information)

Venereal disease education (written information)

Screening of at-risk groups

Identification and treatment of infected persons and their contacts

Teaching of preventive practices such as using a condom, washing well after sexual contact, urinating after intercourse, improving personal hygiene, and avoiding contact with persons known to be infected

Early education about AIDS, its transmission, incidence, and prevention

Pregnancy

Childbearing during adolescence is a high-risk experience for both mother and infant. More than 1 million teenage girls become pregnant annually, and over 30,000 of these pregnant adolescents are under 15 years of age. Approximately one half of these pregnancies are terminated, the remaining half ending in livebirths (Tyrer, et al., 1989; Wildey, 1987).

Maternal morbidity and mortality are higher for adolescent mothers, as is infant mortality. There is a higher incidence of noncompliance with prenatal care on the part of pregnant adolescents, leading to a higher rate of complications during the prenatal and neonatal periods. However, if adolescents receive early and comprehensive care they are at no greater medical risk than are adult mothers (Wildey, 1987).

The nurse can assist the pregnant teenager in many ways. The initial nursing assessment should focus on identifying the adolescent's feeling about being pregnant; her feelings about options (i.e., termination versus continuation); her support persons and role model; and her short-term goals (e.g., medical care, school continuation, and relationships with baby's father, her family, and peers). A nonjudgmental and supportive attitude is essential during the assessment and management phases. The pregnancy of an adolescent affects many people, as well as society in general. Handling the implications of the effects of her pregnancy is frequently difficult for the adolescent. Hence the goals of nursing interventions should be short term and directed at definition of the most appropriate way for the individual adolescent to handle the pregnancy. Appropriate nursing activities include the following:

Providing and facilitating early prenatal care

Providing pregnancy counseling, explaining fully the teenager's choices in regard to termination or continuation

Assisting the teenager to identify support persons in the family or among friends

Providing support and encouragement

Making appropriate referrals for medical care and school placement

Assisting the teenager to manage her altered life-style

Providing appropriate health education

Assisting the family to deal with and provide support to the pregnant teenager and the father

Assisting the teenage father to identify his role during and after the pregnancy

Assisting the family, pregnant adolescent, and teenage father to express their feelings about the pregnancy

Conduct close follow-up to nursing care plan

Assisting pregnant teenager to complete her education and working with the school to achieve this

The Adolescent Mother

The adolescent who decides to keep her infant poses a unique challenge for nurses (currently more than half of all adolescent mothers are raising their children alone [Wildey, 1987]). The adolescent's adjustment to parenthood relies heavily on being prepared, informed, and supported. Nurses need to be aware that adolescents are continuing to deal with their own developmental tasks in addition to the pregnancy and parenthood. Conflict between her own developmental needs and the pregnancy, and later her infant's needs, is common. The pregnant adolescent frequently discovers she is in a role that requires maturity and decision making but is unable to deal with these responsibilities. Nurses can assist teenage mothers to coordinate their roles and responsibilities and to set priorities. Appropriate nursing interventions may include the following:

Assisting teenager and family or father in distributing responsibilities of child care

Assisting teenager to identify and use support persons and groups

Providing education about infant behavior and physical care

Facilitating use of appropriate health care for teenage mother and infant

Facilitating attachment and bonding

Making referrals as appropriate, identifying appropriate resources (babysitters, living arrangements)

Assisting teenager to identify and meet goals (e.g., return to work or school)

Assisting teenager to use family planning

Facilitating expression of feelings about infant, motherhood, her family, and the infant's father

Acting as an emotional support person and source of reassurance

Contraceptive Education

Parents and adolescents need to be informed about methods of contraception. Whether this information is sought out by the adolescent or the parent or offered by the nurse, all methods require discussion, emphasizing effectiveness and appropriateness of use for the individual. In addition, education regarding sexuality is an important precursor to contraceptive education. Nurses can provide this education, focusing on (1) the physical and emotional sexuality of adolescents and their options for expression; (2) their attitude regarding sexual activity; (3) their awareness of the potential consequences of sexual activity (e.g., pregnancy, venereal disease, emotional distress); and (4) their available resource or support persons or groups should problems arise. The nurse can also assist parents to (1) recognize and deal with the present-day realities of increased sexual activity among adolescents; (2) express their feelings about sex positively to their teenagers; (3) handle sex education and discuss sexual issues at home; (4) be a positive role model; and (5) identify support and resources if a problem arises.

Follow-up of teenagers using contraceptive methods is imperative. The nurse must assess the teenager's understanding, use, and response and the efficacy of the method chosen. Follow-up visits are also a time for the adolescent to voice questions or concerns about contraception and sexuality and to receive support and encouragement. An educational tool for methods of contraception is presented in Appendix J12.

ASSESSMENT TOOLS

Once school age or adolescence is reached, the nursing process does not change significantly from that used for early childhood. However, variations in tools and techniques are indicated for the older child. These variations occur because the school-age child and the adolescent have the ability to participate more actively in all aspects of health assessment.

The child can be the primary informant or historian. The older the child becomes, the greater the degree of detail and accuracy (Gorman, 1980). Focusing on the school-age child and adolescent as the primary informant facilitates the therapeutic relationship by promoting the nurse's trust and confidence in the child's ability. This technique assists children and adolescents in taking responsibility for their health care and provides an opportunity for expression of concerns or feelings about their own health, growth, and development. If the nurse is concerned about the accuracy of the historical data, particularly in regard to early events, unsure dates, or an identified problem, validation by the parent is indicated. This verification should be done with the child or adolescent's knowledge and is best handled in a separate interview.

Health Assessment

A complete health assessment combines health history, physical assessment, and the monitoring of physical and psychological growth and development. The history is a long-term cumulative data base. The amount and type of historical information obtained depend on the purpose of the visit and the expressed concerns of the client and parents. A complete health history should be obtained in the initial visit. Supplementary information to be obtained for the adolescent in addition to the general history is summarized in the box at right.

The techniques of physical assessment vary little for the school-age child and the adolescent. Explaining each portion of the examination is most important for individuals of these age groups because concern about body functioning, changes, and normalcy is usual (see Appendix A3). In addition, explaining the what and why of the examination technique, including the results of specific parts of the examination, is useful in promoting confidence and trust.

Appropriate laboratory studies, assessment of sexual age, and screening for diseases such as tuberculosis and scoliosis are also important components of the health assessment. Based on these data, further activities that promote health can be implemented as needed for the individual child or adolescent. Once the child has reached school age, the frequency of health assessment visits is usually extended to every 2 years, unless the health status of the client warrants more frequent assessment. The general content of these visits is discussed in Appendix A3.

Setting for Adolescent Health Visit

Community health nurses must also consider the setting and tone of a healthy assessment visit for the adolescent client. Most adolescents experience some degree of discomfort in coming to a pediatric clinic. The added factor of being accompanied by parents, who possibly wish to discuss issues of concern to them, warrants special consideration. The following measures are useful in facilitating the adolescent health maintenance visit (Marks and Fisher, 1987).

Schedule adolescent appointments on days different from

SUPPLEMENTARY HEALTH HISTORY DATA PERTINENT TO THE ADOLESCENT

1. Past history
   Use of diethylstilbestrol in mother's pregnancy
2. Social history
   Behavior—as related to school, home, parents, siblings, and peers
   Parent's and adolescent's concerns regarding above behavior
   Smoking, substance usage
3. School history
   Grade, name of school, method of getting to school
   Performance in school
   Favorite, best, more difficult courses
   Attitude about school
   Goals for schoolwork
   Concerns or difficulties related to school
4. Extracurricular activities
   Work
   Social
   Hobbies
   Sports and other activities
5. Peer relationships
   Number of friends
   Relationship with siblings
   Dating activity
   Perception of social self
   Concerns regarding preceding points
6. Sexuality
   Information about sexuality (e.g., physiological)
   Sexual activity
   Knowledge of contraceptive methods
   Knowledge of venereal disease symptoms, prevention, treatment
   Concerns and attitudes regarding sexuality and sexual self
   Worries about body: height, weight, development of sex characteristics, skin problems
7. Review of systems and particular focus on general health as described by client
   Skin: acne
   Dietary history
   HEENT*: headaches, squint, hearing difficulty
   Dentition: last dental visit
   Heart: palpations
   Lungs: shortness of breath
   Gastrointestinal: abdominal pain, weight gain or loss
   Genitourinary: discharges, enuresis, dysuria, urinary tract infection
   Musculoskeletal: joint or back pain
   Neurological: emotional stress, fainting, dizzy spells
   Menstruation: age of onset, regularity, frequency, duration, last menstrual period, dysmenorrhea, premenstrual tension, attitude, feelings and beliefs regarding menses

*HEENT indicates head, eyes, ears, nose, and throat.

baby or younger-child appointments

Provide age-appropriate reading materials in waiting area, which focus on adolescent-related problems

Ask adolescent to complete any previsit history or information forms

Interview the adolescent first and then parents, unless adolescent expresses desire for parent to be present

Explain procedure for present and future visits in detail

Direct interview to adolescent; be interested in and develop a trusting relationship with adolescent

Reassure adolescent that information shared is confidential (exception being when behavior is dangerous to self or others)

Conduct interview in friendly, concerned manner

When providing health care services to the adolescent, nurses must also be aware of the constitutional rights of minors, including the right to self-consent. All states have legislation pertinent to the aspects of obtaining health care without parental permission. Because state statutes vary, nurses need to be familiar with those within their own jurisdictions. It is important to know the age at which minors can seek health care on their own and the types of health care services that can be offered.

Family Assessment

The health of a child largely depends on the family's health and ability to cope. Comprehensive nursing implies implementing the nursing process for the family as well as the individual client. Use of assessment tools such as the Family Coping Index, the Family Coping Estimate, the Family Apgar test, and the Family Function Index (FFI) define nursing plans to make them more effective. These tools assess family dynamics and abilities to adapt and grow when faced with health problems. Appendix B7 describes family assessment tools that are useful to the community health nurse.

School Conference

A major part of the older child's or adolescent's world consists of the time spent at school. Experiences, attitudes, and values encountered at school affect psychosocial development. For this reason, communication between the community health nurse and the child's teacher and the school nurse is essential in monitoring psychosocial development.

The communication nurses establish with the school can be initiated in several ways: (1) between the nurse in the community and the nurse in the school, the child's teacher, or both; (2) between the nurse in the school and the teacher; and (3) between the nurse (in the community or the school), the teacher, the parent, and the child.

The dialogue established between nurse, teacher, and child can be focused in the following directions:

A. The adjustment to school can be facilitated by:
   1. Providing support for teachers and intervening in crisis situations
   2. Providing support for parents and offering guidance and a means of participation in child's education and adjustment to school through preschool conferences, parent-teacher-nurse conferences throughout school year, involvement with parent-teacher groups (PTO)
   3. Providing support for child and assisting to identify peer group, appropriate after-school activities, and means of coping with new situation of school

B. Preventive health measures can be provided by:
   1. Screening for physical and emotional health problems (such as vision, hearing, and scoliosis screening, conversational conferences about how school is going)
   2. Conducting health education classes geared to specific age group (such as how to care for teeth, taking care of a cold, sex education, STD education)

C. Assistance can be offered in managing identified problems, both physical and emotional, such as:
   1. Cooperating with a prescribed medication regimen
   2. Facilitating a behavior modification plan
   3. Facilitating special dietary needs or requirements

For the school conference to be productive, the nurse must facilitate (1) mutual identification of health goals or problems brought to or created by the setting, (2) collaboration of all parties involved to meet goals or resolve problems, and (3) periodic follow-up to ensure that health is maintained.

Once a child has entered the school system, nursing action can facilitate adjustment to and advancement through the educational process. To do so, the nursing process must be applied to many environments, including home, school, and peer groups. The nurse must have the knowledge and skill to assess the multiple factors of these environments that influence a child's growth and development. It is the nurse's responsibility therefore to intervene, coordinate, and facilitate a positive, healthy outcome for the child.

HEALTH PROMOTION ACTIVITIES
Health Assessment

Nurses continue to implement activities to promote health throughout the school-age and adolescent years. As discussed earlier in this chapter, the health assessment visit remains a focal point for nursing intervention. Developing and implementing a health plan need to be a collaborative effort involving the child or adolescent, parents, and the school. The specific screening techniques and tools for assessment have been previously discussed. *The most important are screening of hearing, vision, dentition; assessment of sex characteristics (Tanner staging), nutrition, and school and social adjustment; screening for scoliosis, tuberculosis; assessment of common problems, venereal disease, birth control, need and learning disabilities.*

School-age children and adolescents should be encouraged to assume responsibility for their own health (Daniel, 1977). This approach requires close follow-up to ensure that health goals are being met.

The focus of anticipatory guidance is prevention of health problems. See Appendixes A, B, D, J, and K for examples of appropriate anticipatory guidance tools. Preventive health counseling should focus on nutrition, safety, school, peers, identified or at-risk health problems, sexuality (including venereal disease and birth control), family and sibling relationships, and coping strategies.

Group Health Education and Child-Focused Education

Promoting health in the group education setting is an effective technique. The principles for development of health maintenance classes can be applied to classes focusing on school-age and adolescent persons. An additional technique, which is useful and specific to these age groups, is to solicit participation of the child or adolescent in outlining the content of such courses. As interest evolves, participation can be increased to presentation of material in collaboration with the community health nurse. In some instances, adolescents may indicate interest in helping with educational classes for younger children. The primary objective, regardless of the technique, is to involve the participants and to encourage self-care responsibilities.

The setting for health education classes varies. However, use of the school setting promotes greater participation. In addition, incorporating health education into the school's curriculum is a challenge nurses should undertake. Such health programs could be a required component of the curriculum or be made available during student "free periods." The topics for such programs should be of interest to the participants and focus on a special interest group or an identified problem. Potential topics include sex education, participation in sports, self-care, coping as a teenager, the importance of friends, and the health risks of smoking.

Parent-Focused Education

Parents also need educational programs. Focusing on topics from a parental perspective may facilitate more effective parenting skills. For example, classes in how to cope with teenage crises, how to talk to a child about sex, or how to communicate with teenagers offer parents an opprtunity to learn new skills that promote both their relationships with their children and the children's health. A similar approach can be applied to teachers by offering seminars that focus on problems or concerns they may be experiencing (e.g., how to handle an inattentive child or how to promote a positive relationship with students).

Home Intervention

Home intervention is generally based on an individual's or family's health needs. Intervention at the time of a crisis is obviously indicated, but intervention before a crisis, with the goal of promoting health and preventing a crisis, is a significant contribution community health nurses can make. Assessing the home situation and environment is the nurse's responsibility. By assisting the family and child to identify and resolve problems within the home, nurses promote individual, family, and community health. A home that maintains health and relies on its resources is engaging in self-care and promoting wellness, both of which are nursing goals.

Immunizations

The process of acquiring immunity continues into the school-age and adolescent years. Nurses assist parents and children in following the recommended immunization schedule through education and counseling, record maintenance, and referral to appropriate resources or agencies for receipt of vaccines. Nurses have the further responsibilities of being knowledgeable about state legal requirements for immunizations before school entry and of advising parents and children under their care about the implications of these regulations. See Appendix D2 for specific immunization information.

Nutrition
School-Age Children

Healthy school-age children are in a period of slow and steady growth, and their nutritional needs are relatively stable. The caloric intake requirement for this age group decreases slightly as do protein and water requirements. Snacks are most likely to be the primary source of nutrients for the school-age child, and the older the child becomes, the more nutrition is obtained outside the home (Pipes, 1989). Therefore the continued promotion of good eating habits and nutritious snacks is an essential part of the health maintenance visit. Additionally, implementation of a nutrition education program is indicated for the school setting.

Although the school-age period is generally a time of few nutritional problems, the need for continued nutritional assessment is important. The diet history continues to be a useful tool, one that will involve children in their own assessment and promotion of sound eating habits (see Appendix A4). The nurse's responsibility is to ensure that previously established healthy eating patterns are maintained and that children with deviant patterns are assisted to recognize them and to change (See Chapter 33).

Adolescents

The preadolescent and adolescent years are a time of increased growth that is accompanied by increases in appetite and nutritional requirements. Caloric and protein requirements increase for boys ages 11 to 18 years. Girls have an increased protein need but a decreased caloric need during the same age span. In addition, the iron needed by the adolescent nearly doubles that needed by adults, and iodine, calcium, niacin, and thiamine requirements also increase (Pipes, 1989).

Adolescent nutritional needs are influenced not only by the physical alterations that are occurring but also by the psychosocial adjustments. Teenagers are generally free to eat when and where they choose. It is a time when eating habits acquired from the family are dropped, snacking outside the home is a major source of nutrition, and fad foods and diets are prominent (Torre, 1977).

The factors of accelerated growth and poor eating habits make the adolescent at risk of poor nutritional health. Adolescents have been found to demonstrate the most unsatisfactory nutritional status of all age groups. Deficiencies in iron, vitamins A and C, calcium, riboflavin, and thiamin are most common.

Nurses have a responsibility to intervene and initiate activities that promote improved nutritional status. Such activities include the following (see also Chapter 34):

Provision of informational material on good nutrition in group or individual encounters

TABLE 29-4
Daily food guide for adolescents

Food group	Servings
Milk and milk products	4
Meats	3
Fruits and vegetables	4
Vitamin A source	1
Vitamin C source	1
Breads and cereals	4

From Tackett JJ and Hunsberger M, editors: Family centered care of children and adolescents, Philadelphia, 1981, WB Saunders, p. 1244.

TABLE 29-5
Clinical signs indicative of nutritional deficiencies

	Clinical signs
General appearance	Lethargy, excessive or inadequate body fat, muscle wasting
Skin	Dryness, flakiness, scaling, roughness (follicular hyperkeratosis), pallor
Mouth	Angular fissures, redness at corners of mouth (cheilosis); redness, swelling, or atrophic papillae on tongue; red, swollen, or bleeding gums
Teeth	Severe caries
Eyes	Pale conjunctivae
Nails	Spoon-shaped, brittle, or ridged
Hair	Dull, easily plucked

Adapted from Foster R, Hunsberger M, Anderson J, editors: Family centered care of children and adolescents, ed 2, Philadelphia, 1989, WB Saunders.

Diet assessment using a comprehensive diet history or a 24-hour diet diary

Educational activities that focus on:

Effects of fad foods and fad diets

Supplying of "at risk" nutrients and their sources

Provision of a daily food guide (Table 29-4)

Suggested snacks and "on the run" foods that supply essential nutrients

Relationship of good nutritional habits to healthy appearance

Assessment for signs of nutritional deficiencies (Table 29-5)

Supplementation

VITAMINS. Adequate amounts of vitamins and minerals are necessary for the nutritional health of people of any age. Without these essential nutrients, physical and psychosocial health may be compromised. There is much controversy over the question of whether or not to routinely supplement the diet with vitamins and minerals. Of particular concern is the recent fad of taking megadoses (very large doses) of vitamins and minerals to ensure health.

The decision to supplement a child's or adolescent's diet with vitamins or minerals should be based on (1) the nutritional adequacy of the diet for age and growth requirements as verified by diet assessment and (2) a clinically based nutritional deficiency identified through laboratory studies and physical examination (Chow, et al., 1984).

FLUORIDE. An adequate fluoride supply is essential for dental health. Fluoride sources include treated drinking water, topical application, and oral tablets and rinses. Nurses should assess whether adequate fluoride sources are available and should assist the client to secure a source if current supply is inadequate.

Special Nutritional Situations

ATHLETIC CHILD. The child or adolescent who is engaged in athletic activities will require additional nursing assessment and intervention. For individuals involved in strenuous activities, at least 2300 to 5000 calories per day is required. Optimal distribution of calories is considered to be 10% to 15% protein, 25% to 35% fat, and 50% to 65% carbohydrate. Increases in vitamins, minerals, and water and salt

also may be indicated (AAP, 1989). Nurses should be aware of the potential need for added nutritional supplements for athletic children and should implement appropriate dietary assessment and management to meet these increased needs.

VEGETARIAN CHILD. The child or adolescent who follows a vegetarian diet requires special nursing assessment and management. Knowledge of the type of vegetarian diet followed is essential. Generally these types are (1) lactoovovegetarian, a diet of vegetables supplemented by milk, eggs, and cheese; (2) lactovegetarian, a vegetable diet with only milk and cheese added; and (3) pure vegetarian, the diet of a vegan, which excludes all foods of animal origin.

Vegetarian diets can provide the essential nutrients for the growth and development of children. Diets of these types need to be based on sound nutritional principles, and the nurse who is assessing and counseling a vegetarian should be aware of the following points (Williams, 1975):

Protein sources need to be varied to ensure adequate amounts of essential amino acids.

Amino acids in one food can supplement those in another food.

A variety of vitamin C and folacin sources must be included.

A diet that excludes all animal food is deficient in vitamin B_{12}; supplementation is essential if eggs, cheese, or milk are not used.

Adequate iodine can be obtained by using iodized salt.

Adequate vitamins and minerals are supplied if protein, vegetables, and fruit are adequate.

Nurse's role. Sound nutritional counseling includes teaching that a vegetarian diet that includes some animal foods is nutritionally adequate if well planned. Vegans, who observe pure vegetarian diets, require vitamin B_{12} supplementation. Providing sample menus for the vegetarian dieter is often helpful in promoting sound nutritional habits.

Additional Activities

Bibliographies directed toward specific concerns, problems, or age groups are useful tools. Printed materials on a diversity of topics are available from governmental agencies, special interest groups, and pharmaceutical companies. Community health nurses have a responsibility to direct their clients to these resources. Many community groups provide needed services, including the following:

Mental health hot lines
Drug abuse centers
Planned Parenthood centers
STD clinics
Alcoholics Anonymous
Community recreation centers
Child and youth organizations
Youth athletic clubs

Nurses have the knowledge, skills, and resources to have an impact on the status of child health. The challenge lies in realizing their full potential.

CLINICAL APPLICATION

Billy Thoms, an 11-year-old boy, has been referred for nursing follow-up care for a fractured right femur, sustained in a bicycle accident. His leg was casted in a full-leg, plaster cast. Orders include keeping cast elevated for 18 hours and no weight bearing for 72 hours. Jane Holmes, RN, makes a home visit 12 hours after casting.

Ms. Holmes' assessment included a circulatory check to the casted extremity, which revealed that Billy's toes were slightly swollen and cool to the touch but blanched well. The skin around the cast rim was irritated, chafed, and reddened. Billy told Ms. Holmes that he is having minimal pain except when he walks on it, which he had to do to go to the bathroom this morning. When asked about using his crutches, keeping his cast elevated and limiting weight bearing, Billy says he just gets around the best he can because both his parents work days and he has to take care of himself. His mother has left food prepared for him and the bathroom in their two bedroom, one floor house is at the end of a long hallway. Billy's two older siblings, age 12 and 14 are at school all day but will be able to help him when they get home.

Ms. Holmes plans her care based on the following nursing diagnoses: self-care deficit resulting from being left alone to manage care; impaired physical mobility caused by casting and weight bearing limit; potential for injury and tissue damage because of casting and irritation to skin; and diversional activities and development impairment as a result of lack of stimuli and missing school.

In implementing her care plan, Ms. Holmes teaches Billy how to use his crutches and has him practice. She reinforces the need not to bear weight for 72 hours and explains why. She tells Billy he must use his crutches whenever he gets up. She moves Billy to the living room from his back bedroom so that he is closer to the kitchen. There is a television and she puts some of his favorite books and toys within his reach. Ms. Holmes elevates Billy's casted leg and instructs him in the importance of keeping it elevated. She also petals the edges of the cast, cleans the exposed skin and covers his exposed foot. She teaches Billy how to check his toes for circulation and discusses other aspects of cast care, such as keeping it dry, touching it as little as possible until it is dry to prevent indentation, and not putting any objects down the cast. Ms. Holmes then contacts Billy's mother at work and explains her plan of care to her. She leaves written instructions for Billy and his parents. Ms. Holmes also contacts Billy's school and makes arrangements to have his homework sent home with his sister.

Later in the day, Ms. Holmes calls the Thoms house and learns from Billy's 14-year-old sister that Billy has been using his crutches, avoiding weight bearing, and maintaining elevation. She says his foot is warm to touch and pink in color but still swollen. Ms. Holmes makes arrangements to check on Billy the following day.

In evaluating her care 72 hours after casting, Ms. Holmes finds Billy's cast has dried evenly, the circulatory checks to his casted extremity are normal, and the exposed extremity swelling is subsiding. Billy is able to manuver well on the crutches, is weight bearing slightly without discomfort, and plans to return to school the following day. Billy's parents have made arrangements for a follow-up orthopedic visit in 1 week to evaluate the healing progression.

SUMMARY

Both the school-age child and the adolescent live in rapidly expanding worlds. The period of life from 6 to 12 years is characterized by steady physical growth, neuromuscular refinement, and rapid expansion of cognitive and social skills. Between the ages of 13 and 20 years, a person leaves childhood and becomes an adult. This period of life is characterized by a steady progression of physiological changes. These changes and the emotional, psychological, and social adaptations to them push the adolescent to learn to develop coping mechanisms that will be carried throughout life.

Growth and development throughout these stages are influenced by the degree of success or failure a child has had in mastering the tasks of preceding stages. Developing self-esteem and identifying life-style values are important accomplishments during the school-age and adolescent developmental phases.

The community health nurse can play a significant role in promoting the health of school-age children and adolescents through physical and health assessment, risk analysis, screening, anticipatory guidance, health teaching, and counseling children and their parents.

KEY CONCEPTS

Although the health of school-age children and adolescents in the United States is better than ever, these age groups are confronted with health problems more complex than those of previous generations.

Nurses in community health settings can educate school-age children and adolescents regarding health problems and their subsequent influence on future health.

Helping children develop self-esteem and identify lifestyle values is the basis of anticipatory guidance.

The physical, emotional, social, and psychological adaptations of adolescence push the young person to learn and develop coping mechanisms that will be carried throughout life.

Although the health of children in the United States is better now than 10 years ago, the slowness of

the decline in mortality remains a concern. A major contributor to this slow decline is the fact that 50% of all deaths result from accidents.

The significant health problems affecting school-age children are asthma, learning and school difficulties, and abnormal spinal curvatures.

Substance abuse, STDs and pregnancy remain significant health problems for adolescents.

Violent deaths and accidents account for the majority of deaths among adolescents and young adults.

The health assessment visit, using the health history and physical assessment components that focus on individuals and their potential health risks and stressors, remains a focal point for nursing intervention during the preadolescent and adolescent years.

LEARNING ACTIVITIES

1. Develop and implement a program on bicycle safety for 8- to 10-year-old children through the local school.

2. Construct a presentation illustrating the various methods of birth control available to adolescents.

3. Develop a nursing care plan for a 16-year-old girl who has learned she is pregnant.

4. Observe behaviors relating to the first day of school at the local school or bus stop. Note and record the "parting" behaviors of 5- to 6-year-old children and their parents. Return and make the same observation 2 weeks later and compare.

BIBLIOGRAPHY

American Academy of Pediatrics: Report of the Committee on Infectious Diseases, ed 22, Elk Grove Village, IL, 1991, The Academy.

American Academy of Pediatrics: Sports medicine: health care for young adults, ed 2, Elk Grove Village, IL, 1989, The Academy.

American Dental Association: Your child's teeth, Chicago, 1971, The Association.

Anderson B: The patient with scoliosis: Carole, a girl treated with bracing, Am J Nurs 79:1592, 1979.

Atton AV and Tunnessen WW: Acne update: help your patients help themselves, Contemp Pediatr 5:18, 1988.

Behrman RE and Vaughan VC, editors: Nelson textbook of pediatrics, ed 13, Philadelphia, 1987, WB Saunders.

Bernstein AC: Six stages of understanding how children learn about sex and birth, Psychol Today 1:31, 1976.

Boyle MP, Koff E, and Guidas LJ: Assessment and management of anorexia nervosa, Matern Child Nurs 6:412, 1981.

Brosnan J and Fond K: School phobia: the student anxiety syndrome, Pediatr Nurs 6:9, 1980.

Brown HP: Recognizing STDs in adolescents, Contemp Pediatr 6:17, 1989.

Castiglia PT: Anorexia nervosa, J Pediatr Health Care 3:105, 1989.

Child AA, Murphy CM and Rhyne MC: Depression in children: reasons and risks, Pediatr Nurs 6:9, 1980.

Chow MP et al.: Handbook of pediatric primary care, ed 2, New York, 1984, John Wiley & Sons.

Committee on Adolescence, Group for the Advancement of Psychiatry: Normal adolescence, New York, 1968, Charles Scribner's Sons.

Dunn B: Common orthopedic problems of children, Pediatr Nurs 1:7, 1975.

Erikson E: Childhood and society, New York, 1963, WW Norton & Co.

Foster R, Hunsberger M, and Anderson J: Family centered care of children and adolescents, ed 2, Philadelphia, 1989 WB Saunders.

Freeman RB and Henrich J: Community health nursing practice, ed 2, Philadelphia, 1987, WB Saunders.

Gemberling CL: An adolescent gynecologic examination: an overview J Pediatr Health Care 1:141, 1987.

Gorman G: The school age child as historian, Pediatr Nurs 6:39, 1980.

Hart NA and Prophit SP: Adolescent suicide, Pediatr Nurs 5:22, 1979.

Havinghurst R: Developmental tasks and education, New York, 1972, David McKay Co.

Health: United States and prevention profile, DHHS Pub No (PHS) 84-1232, Hyattsville, MD, 1986, U.S. Department of Health and Human Services, Public Health Service.

Hockenberry MJ, Coody DK, and Bennett BS: Childhood cancers: incidence, etiology, diagnosis and treatment, Pediatr Nurs 16:239, 1990.

Hoffman AD, editor: Adolescent medicine, Menlo Park, CA, 1983, Addison-Wesley Publishing Co.

Keenan T: School based adolescent health care programs, Pediatr Nurs 12:365, 1986.

Keller OL: Bulimia: primary care approach and intervention, Nurs Pract 11:42, 1986.

Khoiny FE: Adolescent dysmenorrhea, J Pediatr Health Care 2:29, 1988.

Krugman S and Katz SL: Infectious diseases of children, ed 8, St Louis, 1985, Mosby Year Book.

Laige J: The school aged child and his family. In Hymovich D and Barnard M, editors: Family health care: developmental and situational crises, New York, 1978, McGraw-Hill Book Co.

Lauernsen N: Recognition and treatment of menstrual syndrome, Nurs Pract 10:11, 1985.

McClellan MA: On their own: latchkey children, Pediatr Nurs 10:198, 1984.

Maheady DC: Reye Syndrome: review & update, J Pediatr Health Care 3:246, 1989.

Maran JN and Crispell KA: Lyme disease: an elusive diagnosis, J Pediatr Health Care 3:60, 1989.

Marks A: Health screening of the adolescent, Pediatr Nurs 4:37, 1978.

Marks A and Fisher M: Health assessment and screening during adolescence, Pediatrics 80(suppl):140, 1987.

Nelms BC and Brady MA: Assessment and intervention: the depressed school-age child, Pediatr Nurs 6:15, 1980.

Novotny J: Adolescents, acne and the side effects of accutane, Pediatr Nurs 15:247, 1989.

Paparone P: The summer scourge of Lyme Disease, Am J Nurs 90:44, 1990.

Pipes PL: Nutrition in infancy and childhood, ed 4, St Louis, 1989, Mosby–Year Book.

Rice MA and Kibee PE: Review: identifying the adolescent substance abuser, Matern Child Nurs J 8:139, 1983.

Rigg CA: Homosexuality in adolescence, Pediatr Ann 11:826, 1982.

Rogers M: Early identification and intervention with children with learning problems, Pediatr Nurs 2:21, 1976.

Sapala S and Strokosch G: Adolescent sexuality: use of a questionnaire for health teaching and counseling, Pediatr Nurs 7:133, 1985.

Schwartz RH, Cohen PR, and Bair GO: Identifying and coping with a drug using adolescent,

Pediatr Rev 7:33, 1985.

Smilkstein G: The family APGAR: a proposal for a family function test and its use by physicians, J Fam Pract 6:1231, 1978.

Smith N: Sports medicine, Pedatr Nurs 5:39, 1979.

Stone AC: Facing up to acne, Pediatr Nurs 8:229, 1982.

Sutterley D and Donnelly G: Perspectives in human development: nursing throughout the life cycle, ed 2, Philadelphia, 1981, J B Lippincott.

Tanner JM: Growth at adolescence, Oxford, 1962, Blackwell Scientific Publications.

Torre CT: Nutritional needs of adolescents, MCN 2:105, 1977.

Tyrer LB, Rothbart B, and Anderson K: What every teen should know about contraceptives, Contemp Pediatr 6:68, 1989.

Valente SM and Saunders JM: High school suicide prevention programs, Pediatr Nurs 13:108, 1987.

Wegman ME: Annual summary of vital statistics, Pediatrics 84:943, 1989.

Wegman ME: Annual summary of vital statistics, Pediatrics 86:835, 1990.

Whaley LF and Wong D: Nursing care of infants and children, ed 4, St Louis, 1991, Mosby–Year Book.

Wildey LS: Diagnosis and initial management of the pregnant adolescent, J Pediatr Health Care 1:60, 1987.

Williams ER: Making vegetarian diets nutritious, Am J Nurs 75:2168, 1975.

Wilson MH: Preventing injury in the middle years, Contemp Pediatr 6:20, 1989.

Wolf WJ and Bancroft B: Early detection of childhood malignancies, Pediatr Nurs 5:43, 1980.

Zahr LK, Connolly M, Page DR: Assessment and management of the child with asthma, Pediatr Nurs 15:109, 1989.

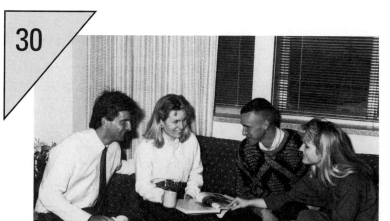

30

Young and Middle-Age Adults

Patricia L. Starck

Geneva W. Morris

Psychosocial Development
Middlescence

Factors Influencing Growth and Development
Health
Self-Care
Environmental Influences
Personal and Family Life-Styles
Promoting Changes in Life-Style
Coping with Conflict and Stress
Confronting Suffering and Death

Common Causes of Morbidity and Mortality in Young Adults

Common Causes of Morbidity and Mortality in Middle-Age Adults
Heart Disease
Cancer
Diabetes
Periodontal Disease

Work-Related Issues
Second Careers: Becoming a
Student Again

Physically Disabled Adults
Definition of Terms
Civil Rights for the Disabled
Prevention
Impact of Disability
The Family with a Disabled
Member
Careers for Disabled Adults
Community and National
Significance
Physical, Psychosocial, and
Spiritual Rehabilitation

Clinical Application

Summary

OBJECTIVES

After reading this chapter, the student should be able to:

Differentiate the psychosocial tasks of young and middle-age adults.

Discuss the major health problems of young adults—the causative factors and significant impact on individuals, families, and society.

Discuss the major health problems of middle-age adults and the risk factors and incidence.

Analyze the role of stress in health and disease as it relates to life-style.

Compare and contrast the terms *impairment, disability,* and *handicap.*

KEY TERMS

aging process	impairment	personal health profiles
burnout	logotherapy	psychosocial
cancer	middlescence	immunization
dereflection	osteoporosis	self-transcendence
disability	periodontitis	socratic dialogue
handicap		spiritual rehabilitation

The period in life categorized as young and middle adulthood is demanding and rewarding. Much is expected of the adult, who must support others on either end of the age continuum. Social role expectations of adults may result in stoicism about or suppression of their own needs while they take care of the young, cope with difficulties of adolescent offspring, and care for elderly parents. Like the middle-income strata of society, the young or middle-age adult may be considered the backbone of society—being responsible, accountable, and expected to take care of themselves, as well as others.

In the health care literature, young and middle-age adults are neglected. Other age groups are well isolated for study and even have identifying labels such as fetus, newborns, infant, toddlers, early childhood, adolescents, preteens, geriatric, and elderly. No such identifying terms exist for adult stages.

Age is used as the criterion for defining adulthood in our society. However, chronological age, maturity, and developmental tasks may vary. For the purposes of this chapter, adults are categorized as young adults (ages 20 to 35 years) and middle-age adults (ages 36 to 64 years), recognizing that the dividing line is blurred. Indeed, adults may move back and forth between the young adult and the middle-age adult lifestyles when establishing a marriage, home, and family; reentering single life; establishing a second marriage, home, and a family; and in developing a first and, later, a second career.

This chapter examines ways community health nurses can assist young and middle adults to meet health needs. Physical development and psychosocial developmental tasks are discussed, including the tasks and responsibilities characteristic of this group, the changes in biological functions and structures, and the concomitant psychosocial changes. Factors influencing progression through this stage of life, including health status, resources in rural or urban settings, and life-styles are explored, as are common causes of morbidity and mortality for young and middle-age adults. The nursing role implied by the major health problems is discussed; the discussion includes tools for assessment and strategies for implementation. This chapter also discusses health promotion from physical, psychosocial, and spiritual perspectives. Because a major task for the young and middle-age adult is career productivity, this chapter discusses careers and stress in the workplace and considers the special needs of the disabled adult. Exercises to be used by the reader to cope with health needs of this age group are also included.

PSYCHOSOCIAL DEVELOPMENT

Adults progress through successive phases of stabilization and consolidation, followed by change and growth in the pursuit of new goals and in the confrontation of life crises.

Adulthood is a time of caring for others—children and parents. Caring for children presents challenges that vary with each stage of development of the child. A growing number of single parents face child rearing without partners. Reversal of the caring role (parent or child) often requires difficult decision making about a parent's welfare. Deciding on nursing home care vs. living alone or with the primary

family group may require professional consultation.

The primary burden of income production rests with the young and middle adult. Level of income, which determines living standards, security, and satisfaction, is often considered a measure of success. Adults feel pressure to achieve in a competitive world. During these years, an individual devotes considerable time, often in excess of the traditional 40 hours per week, to economic success.

Adults also feel pressure to fulfill societal responsibilities. Because community progress depends on adult leadership, much emphasis is placed on this generation's contribution to posterity.

The community health nurse may encounter individuals who are struggling with psychosocial tasks appropriate to the stages of development or individuals who have failed to achieve normal goals. In either case, frustration affects the individual and the family system, creating barriers to achieving optimal health.

Middlescence

Middlescence is defined as the intermediate stage of life between young adulthood and old age and is marked by physical, psychological, and social changes. During middle age, life events that have been predictable may change, and this new unpredictability often initiates a crisis.

Conflicting feelings and states of being characterize midlife crises—with individuals experiencing paradoxical emotions; feeling wise yet confused; and seeming to be independent yet being dependent. This painful life dilemma is accompanied by anxiety, depression, anger, restlessness, and even physical symptoms.

FACTORS INFLUENCING GROWTH AND DEVELOPMENT

Factors that influence the growth and development of the adult include health status, a sense of responsibility for self-care, resources in rural and urban settings, and life-style. The consummation of adult growth and development is achieving fulfillment through meaning and purpose in life.

Health

Health for the adult is the balanced state of well-being resulting from the successful interaction of body, mind, and spirit. Community health nurses need to implement interventions that prevent health disruptions, promote high-level wellness, provide care and curative services for illnesses, and provide rehabilitation for chronic disabling conditions.

Self-Care

Assisting adults to reach their optimal level of functioning is a basic goal of community health nurses. If adults cannot or will not assume responsibility for their care and become active participants in the process, community health nurses will have difficulty in helping them to achieve an optimal level of functioning. Nurses need to encourage adults to be responsible for self-care. A contract between the nurse and client that makes the characteristics of self-care explicit is a possible solution to this problem (Helgeson, 1985).

A 50-year-old man, a retired military officer, has had essential hypertension for 3 years. He is not employed and spends his days at home. He is working on several projects, such as repairing a fishing boat, but he paces his day as he likes. His wife is a 38-year-old professional career woman who sometimes is annoyed that he is not working or "making any worthwhile contribution to society." In discussing his health with the nurse, the wife reveals that she suspects that he lies on the sofa all afternoon watching soap operas. He does not get any physical exercise. She puts his medicine on a dish for him every day, but is not convinced that he actually takes it. She prepares a healthy lunch for him each day before she leaves for the office, but frequently finds evidence that he has eaten salty foods while she is away. He also smokes one pack of cigarettes per day, which annoys his wife. She tells the nurse that she is at the end of her rope in trying to take care of his health.

A conference with the client reveals that he feels his wife nags him all the time. He says that all he wants is to be left alone. He feels that she treats him like a naughty child and that he deserves to live his life the way he chooses. The nurse also learns that the previous nurse assigned to this client spent considerable time in teaching health to the client and his wife. She found that both comprehended information well, but that the client's attitude was one of indifference.

Who is responsible for the client's health? The thesis of this chapter is that each adult is responsible for his or her own health. The wife in this case has been behaving as if her husband's health were her responsibility. Many people who are nurturers, such as mothers, wives, and even nurses, fail to motivate a client to assume self-responsibility. After a discusssion with the nurse, the wife had the following conversation with her husband:

> I realize that I have been nagging you about your diet, exercise, and medications. I also know that you are the one who is responsible for your health, and the choices are yours. From now on I won't constantly hover over you. I'll be glad to do whatever you need to help you carry out your plan.

The wife stopped putting out his medicine or preparing his lunch, although she did make certain plenty of nutritious foods were available. Remarkably, there was a change in the client's behavior. He purchased two exercise bicycles and began to comply with his diet and medication regimens.

The impact of self-care on the traditional health care delivery system is significant, with a shift toward client education as adults become more active in administering care. The key to intervention for the community health nurse is based on understanding and modifying factors such as cultural beliefs and practices, costs, accessibility, and previous experiences to determine the likelihood of behavioral changes. Health teaching involves changing attitudes and values and educating.

Communicate Attitude of Responsibility for Self

Community health nurses should not say: "You shouldn't eat sweets on a diabetic diet." Such a message presumes a superior-inferior position. It says that the nurse knows what is best—"I can tell you what you should do." It also creates guilt in the client who eats sweets despite knowing the dangers. A better response is: "What do you (or can you) do about your craving for sweets, which adversely affects your diabetic condition? Are there things you can do to control your desire for sweets?"

Teach Health Information

The young and middle-age adult years are a critical time for the development of behaviors and attitudes that have lasting effects on an individual's health. Teaching health information is of critical importance. Certain segments of the population enter into these years faced with the challenge of adjusting to a chronic disease such as diabetes mellitus, whereas others are developing a health profile that may put them at risk of problems in the future.

Teaching is not telling; giving accurate information does not ensure compliance. Client teaching should begin with assessment; it is important to find out what the client already knows so that time and patience are not wasted. For example, a nursing student assigned to assist with discharge planning for a client recovering from a myocardial infarction set a priority goal of emphasizing the need for a gradual return to work. The night before the assignment she prepared a simplistic drawing of the heart. She used the diagram to explain to the client how his heart would be affected by overwork. Near the end of her teaching session she asked "By the way, what do you do?" He replied, "I'm a cardiologist."

After assessment of the knowledge level of the learner, community health nurses should set objectives based on mutual goals. Learning activities are designed according to the content and learning style best suited to the client. Evaluation must follow a teaching and learning session. Retention of learned material should not be taken for granted. Often, reinforcement of the learning is also necessary.

Use Positive Reinforcement of Effective Health Behaviors

Good health has its own rewards—such as vim, vigor, and vitality. However, the first few days or weeks of losing weight may not bring such a feeling of exhilaration. Community health nurses must support clients who comply with healthy behaviors, and they also need to accept those who lapse back into unhealthy actions. In the latter case, the nurse can tell the client that it is not unusual to have occasional relapses. Many contracts for establishing healthy behaviors allow for 1 to 2 "free" days per week in which jogging, for example, can be omitted. Clients should reward themselves, for instance, by going to a movie to celebrate a week of adherence to a new diet.

Health risk appraisal (discussed in Chapter 33) is a useful technique in monitoring health status. The most effective means of promoting health and preventing disease is to have a comprehensive understanding of the disease process. Community health nurses must be able to anticipate and predict consequences of poor health practices. For example, community health nurses should be able to predict complications of uncontrolled diabetes, such as a limb amputation, and thus encourage preventive measures in the young adult who is presently healthy but has a history of diabetes, tends to eat foods high in carbohydrates, and has a sedentary lifestyle.

When healthy adults with particular genetic, dietary, and life-style antecedents become aware of the predictable nature of disease conditions, self-care can be practiced with more vigor. *Personal health profiles* may be useful in health counseling.

Environmental Influences

Adult health status and opportunities for growth and development are interlinked with environmental influences and resources of the individual, family, and community. A community assessment identifies both environmental health stressors and services available within the community. Health stressors differ according to the type of community (e.g., industrial focus).

Although many different living conditions exist, rural vs. urban settings are easily distinguished. Rural areas are defined by the United States Census Bureau as those with less than 2500 people and in open country. By this definition, about 27% of the United States population lives in a rural area. The criterion for an urban area is presence of a city with 50,000 or more people (Cordes, 1985).

The number of young and middle-age adults living in rural areas is declining, and there is a disproportionate number of people below the poverty scale in rural communities (Patton, 1989). Living in poverty increases health problems caused by poor nutrition, inadequate housing, reduced access to services, and the inability to purchase insurance. The nurse often faces greater obstacles in mobilizing resources for poor, uninsured rural clients as the availability of local, state, and federal funds for public health services decrease. Therefore the nurse in the rural area is more likely to encounter clients with chronic, long-term conditions such as hypertension, coronary heart disease, stomach and duodenum ulcers, hernias, hypertensive heart disease, gall bladder disease, and emphysema (Cordes, 1985).

Falck (1985) advocated a socioecological model to motivate change for rural health care problems. The model consists of the following:

1. Environmental determinants such as transportation and water supply
2. Social role determinants such as community leaders and nurturers
3. Group membership such as in family and ethnic groups
4. Constitutional determinates such as genetic and biological factors

To be effective, nurses must gain the trust of clients and structure the care plan according to client priorities. Only then can nurses introduce health improvement ideas that have not been previously valued by the client population. Increasingly, professionals are learning to blend medical care with folk practices for greater compliance. If clients engage in certain health rituals that do not harm them, nurses can choose to be accepting—as long as the clients also improve other health practices.

Community health nurses should also promote linkage systems between rural and urban areas to provide comprehensive, accessible care for rural citizens.

Personal and Family Life-Styles

Life-style, perhaps the greatest influence on health status, involves the practice of health habits and a philosophy of life. Individual and family life-styles vary according to resources, values, traditions, and family members. Each family has its particular sources of stressors, and each adopts coping styles to maintain balance. The roles played by each member and the extent to which the tasks of family living are accomplished also influence the amount of stress present.

Changing American life-styles alter traditional divisions of labor, rules, and values of the family and are a source of stress. Couples are having fewer children and having them later in life. Adults marry, divorce, and remarry through the age of 70 years and even beyond. Both women and men leave jobs and reenter school and work, often adopting second careers. Family structures change as adults rear children in one- or two-parent families.

Promoting Changes in Life-Style

Life-style changes result from reassessing goals, changing values, and making commitments to a new life pattern. These changes can be triggered suddenly through crisis or can develop slowly. An individual's significant others are often catalysts in the adoption of new life patterns. Nurses and other health professionals can also serve as facilitators of changed attitudes.

When attempting to motivate clients to change their life-style, community health nurses should first assess clients' and their families present life-styles, using assessment forms (such as the ones in Appendix C1) to determine if a life-style change is indicated. Community health nurses can often use the circuitous method of communication effectively. For example, a 19-year-old man injured in an automobile accident while speeding suffered a C7 spinal cord injury. After discharge from the rehabilitation center with instructions to follow a well-defined plan of care, the man was visited by the community health nurse who found the following problems:

1. He had been fasting to lose weight.
2. His fluid intake was poor.
3. He decided to drop out of college.
4. He hoped to get married at the end of the year.

While discussing his fasting, the client stated that he was getting too big for his clothes, and the wheelchair was feeling tight. In an attempt to lose weight rapidly, he discounted the risk of protein depletion that could result in skin breakdown and other problems. Although aware of the need for fluids, he said he hated to ask others to get him a drink. He was apathetic about school and yet hung on to the illusion that life would go on as planned when he married his childhood sweetheart. Because he was struggling with the psychosocial task of becoming independent of parental control, the nurse decided against using "teaching and preaching scare tactics" and instead told him about a client with similar problems who had made positive plans to resolve them. She gave him the other client's telephone number and encouraged them to converse about mutual concerns.

Community health nurses can also use a logotherapeutic approach (see later section) in working with clients who appear apathetic or otherwise lack the motivation to modify their life-styles to enhance their state of health. The aim of logotherapy is self-transcendence, or getting outside oneself to help others. Self-transcendence involves focusing on others, as compared with self-actualization, or focusing on developing and actualizing potential within oneself. As a result of focusing on a cause other than self, one finds fulfillment and motivation. The key to logotherapy is attitude change. The nurse may be innovative in techniques to modify attitudes. Various intellectual exercises, such as analyzing parables, can stimulate discussion that guides the client to a broader view of a fate that cannot be changed.

Coping with Conflict and Stress

Stress for the adult often results from time pressures—the urgency to get many things done in a limited amount of time. Anything and anybody who interferes with this speeding pace causes frustration, conflict, and consequently stress. Community health nurses can help clients assess how they spend time and then evaluate whether other activities would more appropriately meet their personal goals. One way to manage stress is to immunize the body, both physically and emotionally, from stressors that are known and preventable.

Psychosocial immunization may buffer the adult against stressors to be expected at this time in the life cycle. Anticipatory guidance (i.e., helping the adult to know what to expect from different phases of life) may be helpful. Often an old friend or mentor eases the way. For example, a 27-year-old single parent of a 10-year-old boy becomes friends with a neighbor, the mother of a 15-year-old boy who has a motorcycle and wants very much to receive a car by his sixteenth birthday. The friendship between the two women helps the first woman to anticipate what she will face in a few short years as the parent of a teenager. The neighbor helps by telling the woman about parenting techniques she found helpful when her son was 10 years old.

Confronting Suffering and Death

Frankl (1959) espoused the theory of logotherapy to help clients find meaning and purpose in life. He maintained that suffering is a common, natural condition and can be a growth experience by which individuals learn valuable lessons about life. Clients need to find meaning in suffering to cope effectively.

Strategies the nurse could use include the following logotherapeutic techniques:

1. Dereflection: Directing the focus away from the problem and toward assets and abilities (e.g., not focusing on paralyzed legs but rather on strong upper arms).
2. Paradoxical intention: Exaggerating and wishing for the opposite; using humor. This action diffuses the problem.
3. Socratic dialogue: Engaging in thought-provoking conversation with the client. For example, an elderly man who has been depressed since his wife's death is asked what would have happened if he had died before his wife. He recounts how unfortunate this would have been; she would have been afraid to live alone and she had no experience managing money. The client is reminded that he has spared his wife this suffering by living past her (Frankl, 1959).

COMMON CAUSES OF MORBIDITY AND MORTALITY IN YOUNG ADULTS

Morbidity and mortality indicators for young adults offer guidance to the community health nurse in planning strategies for this aggregate population. For young adults, major threats to health include: (1) violent death and injury involving motor vehicle accidents, suicides, and homicides; (2) alcohol and substance abuse; (3) unwanted pregnancies; and (4) sexually transmitted diseases. Life-styles and behavior patterns that affect health are often established during young adulthood. Health education programs with a community-wide audience should be geared toward avoiding risks, practicing safety precautions, emphasizing the dangers of consuming alcohol and driving, and promoting the use of seat belts and motorcycle helmets.

Community health nurses need to be involved in vehicles for social change, including public policy, to prevent suicides. A number of current policies and attitudes have been identified by Papalia and Oles (1989) as contributing to the problem, including the availability of guns. Advocating gun control and organizing suicide hot lines are two effective interventions.

The nurse should be well aware of family planning options within the community in order to educate clients about primary prevention of pregnancy and to make referrals to appropriate primary care agencies that are in keeping with the clients' values and beliefs regarding contraception. The nurse should also monitor public policy regarding allocation of dollars for comprehensive family planning for public health programs, which primarily serve indigent populations.

Knowledge of primary and secondary preventive resources for sexually transmitted disease is essential for nurses caring for adult clients. A nonjudgmental attitude is necessary to achieve the desired compliance in treatment and follow-up of contacts. Information about acquired immunodeficiency syndrome (AIDS) and other sexually transmitted diseases is presented in Chapter 20.

COMMON CAUSES OF MORBIDITY AND MORTALITY IN MIDDLE-AGE ADULTS

Common causes of morbidity and mortality in middle-age adults are heart disease, strokes, cancer, diabetes, alcohol and substance abuse, mental health problems, and periodontal disease. See chapters 21 and 23 for discussions of mental health and substance abuse.

Heart Disease

Community health nurses need to assess clients' risk factors for heart disease and strokes, such as hypercholesterolemia, hypertension, and cigarette smoking. Community screening for cholesterol levels and programs for hypertensive clients—including exercise, smoking cessation, and stress reduction programs—are effective community nursing interventions.

Cancer

Providing care to adults with cancer who are living at home presents many challenges for the community health nurse. Such care includes (1) providing physical care, (2) teaching and counseling, and (3) giving emotional support to the client and family.

Physical care may include colostomy care, dressing changes, or medication administration. With earlier hospital discharge, more patients are receiving antineoplastic chemotherapy at home. Often, analgesia is self-administered through a pump device known as patient controlled analgesia (PCA). These infusion pumps and venous access lines must be maintained. The nurse must practice safety precautions and teach the patient and family to observe those same precautions.

Diabetes

Diabetes affects 11 million persons in the United States, and an estimated 5 million of these have not yet been diagnosed. It is the seventh leading cause of death and a significant risk factor for the development of blindness, coronary artery disease, congestive heart failure, and cerebrovascular and renal disease (U.S. Preventive Services Task Force, 1989). About 90% of all diabetics are classified as having non–insulin-dependent diabetes mellitus (NIDDM), or type II. This form generally occurs in adults and becomes increasingly common after the age of 40 years. Factors associated with the development of NIDDM include family history, obesity, and a history of gestational diabetes; NIDDM is also more common in blacks, Hispanics, and Native Americans. The remaining 10% of diabetics are described as having insulin-dependent diabetes mellitus (IDDM), or type I. This disease process is characterized by an acute onset in childhood or adolescence.

The period of young and middle adulthood is a critical time for both of these groups, and the role of the community health nurse is central. For the insulin-dependent diabetic, life-style changes and health promotive behaviors developed during these years will have a great effect on the client's future health status. For the potential non–insulin-dependent diabetic client, identification and screening for risk factors, combined with education and life-style changes, can delay or possibly avert the onset of the disease process. The community health nurse also must be aware of the needs of a third high-risk group of young adults. Pregnant women without diabetes may develop gestational diabetes. Usually detected around 24 to 28 weeks of gestation, this form of diabetes is a limited condition that affects approximately 3% of all pregnancies. If left undetected and untreated, it can result in serious maternal and neonatal complications such as preeclampsia and microsomia.

The community health nurse functions at all levels of prevention and can impact client health through identification, screening, referral, and education of high-risk clients. The Diabetes Advisory Board (1987) has issued recommendations for the content of patient education programs that can be used as a guide in planning a nursing intervention. The education plan consists of the general facts and description of the disease process, including the concepts of nutrition, diet planning, exercise, and medications. The plan also stresses the importance of involving the client and family in the teaching. The diagnosis of diabetes will affect not only the individual client but all family members who care for or depend on that person. It is an important nursing goal to assist the client and family with the psychological adjustment to the diagnosis and chronic management required with diabetes.

Other areas of the teaching plan include defining the states of hypoglycemia and hyperglycemia and instructing

on the appropriate actions for each. In addition, the client and family need to fully understand the possibly acute and long-term conditions and the self-care activities necessary to maintain good health, such as proper foot, skin, and oral care. Finally, having diabetes changes the way in which the client interacts with the health care delivery system. The community health nurse needs to give the client information on their rights and responsibilities as patients and on ways to identify and gain access to resources in the community.

Despite the prevalence of diabetes in the United States, much misinformation exists. The community health nurse is in the best position to affect the client's long-term health status by intervening during the young and middle-age adult years with education, counseling, and support.

Periodontal Disease

The community health nurse should be aware that periodontitis is the leading cause of tooth loss after the age of 35 years. A careful assessment of the gums for gingivitis should be routine for the adult client. The nurse should also be involved with client and community dental education programs to heighten awareness of the problem and its prevention. Clients should be made aware of the importance of plaque control through regular brushing, flossing, and using commercial antiplaque dental hygiene products. Adults should be taught the importance of regular dental check-ups even when much of their dental budget may be allocated for orthodontics for teenage children.

WORK-RELATED ISSUES

One of the primary tasks of young and middle-age adults is engaging in purposeful, productive work. An individual's career, whether domestic or a highly challenging executive position, can affect health negatively or positively. The role of the nurse often involves counseling and referral for counseling regarding job problems or goals for second careers. Job-related problems can be physical, presenting a hazard to health, or psychosocial, creating a feeling of disparity between job and worker.

Second Careers: Becoming a Student Again

Many middle-age adults and even some young adults struggle with career identity and satisfaction and decide to pursue another career. People often want to explore new experiences; many yearn for what they wish they had become. This yearning often leads to midlife career changes, many of which require further education.

The adult population seeking college education is very heterogenous (Swift, et al., 1987). Some adults return to school to develop their personal and professional goals. Others require an education for very practical reasons. For example, a woman is suddenly divorced or widowed and has children but no job skills. This woman is very vulnerable and seeks advancement through education. She may be isolated within the community and need assistance and counseling in many aspects of her life —from ways to fix the plumbing to ways to enroll in a vocational or academic program. Without financial and emotional support, this woman cannot hope to achieve the goals she sets. The community health nurse must be able to assist her to locate needed services and establish a network of support. Nurses should also promote employer programs such as a shorter work week, flexible hours, and child care programs to provide adults with time to pursue both a career and other developmental tasks. Leaves of absence in the middle years (planned by employers) foster health and productivity.

PHYSICALLY DISABLED ADULTS

Approximately 35 million Americans are physically disabled to some degree, making this group the largest minority in the United States. Eleven million disabled individuals are under the age of 45 years, with an additional 11 million between the ages of 45 and 64 (Lambert and Lambert, 1987).

Definition of Terms

Several terms are used, often interchangeably, to describe the disability state, and various definitions may be found in the literature, including ones with a positive focus, such as "physically challenged." For purposes of discussion, the following terms are used:

Impairment: a disturbance in structure or function resulting from anatomical, physiological, or psychological abnormalities. For example, a person may have impairment of flexion and extension in the right arm.

Disability: the degree of observable and measurable physical or mental impairment. For example, a person may have a 50% disability of the right arm.

Handicap: the total adjustment to disability necessitated by an impairment or disability that limits or prevents functioning at a normal or usual level. For example, a person may be handicapped in writing, driving a car, and playing tennis because of the disability of the right arm.

People may have a high degree of disability and be minimally handicapped, such as those with quadriplegia who own their own businesses, drive specially equipped vans, and maintain active family roles. Conversely, some clients with little disability may exhibit profound limitations in satisfying life patterns. In either case, clients have disabilities, but they should not be labeled according to their disabling condition. The nurse's role is to capitalize on the individual's abilities and minimize and compensate for the disabilities. The nurse should also promote the rehabilitation process for optimal achievement of potential. Rehabilitation is the process by which individuals, their families, or both strive for the attainment and maintenance of the maximum level of need satisfaction.

A disability may be classified as congenital or acquired, visible or invisible, and stable or progressive. Regardless of the classification or the extent of the disability, individuals are entitled to equal rights for family, work, social, and sex role responsibilities. They have a right to educational opportunities, health care services, and dignity and respect from others.

Civil Rights for the Disabled

The Americans with Disabilities Act (ADA) of 1990 prohibited discrimination on the basis of disability and protected the basic civil rights of disabled citizens, greatly expanding opportunities for full participation in all aspects of society. The Act is the first major legislation for the disabled since the Rehabilitation Act of 1973. Although the 1973 legislation prohibited discrimination in any federally funded endeavor, the ADA of 1990 extends those prohibitions to the private sector in a series of progressive steps over the next few years. The Act prohibits discrimination in restaurants, theaters, public transportation, hotels, stores, and public services. Furthermore, employers are prohibited against rejecting applicants because they are disabled. The goals of the nation with regard to persons with disabilities were defined to ensure equality of opportunity, full participation, independent living, and economic self-sufficiency.

The ADA of 1990 defines a disabled person as anyone with a physical or mental impairment that substantially limits one or more of the major life activities. The bill contains five titles: 1. Employment, II. Public Services, III. Public Accommodations and Services Operated By Private Entities, IV. Telecommunications, and V. Miscellaneous Provisions. The provisions of these titles are summarized in Table 30-1. Implementation dates have been established that are judged to be reasonable and feasible and vary from immediately to up to 30 years for changes in major facilities.

Persons who are currently engaging in illegal use of drugs are *not* covered by this Act. However, those covered include (1) an individual who has completed a supervised drug rehabilitation program and is no longer engaging in illegal use of drugs; (2) an individual who is participating in a supervised rehabilitation program; and (3) an individual who is erroneously regarded as engaging in such use.

Prevention

If a large group of young healthy students were asked to indicate who had a history of diabetes in their families, many would respond positively. Of that group, some may develop diabetes and eventually have a leg amputated or suffer total blindness. Prevention and primary health care in the community is important to minimize disabling conditions and should be approached with vigor. Life-styles can be modified to promote health and decrease the possibility of impairment.

Impact of Disability

The community health nurse is challenged when assisting a family with a member who has a newly acquired disability. Many rehabilitation agencies discharge clients when they have mastered the physical skills of daily living. Yet, total adjustment for the individual and family involves much more.

Lipkin and Williams (1987) described the following stages of reaction to illness and disability: shock and numbness; denial; anger, bargaining; and acceptance and accommodation. These stages may overlap, and clients may skip or regress to certain stages. The community health nurse may determine the client is in a particular stage after discharge from an acute care institution, but mourning and depression may follow, with the client regressing to an earlier stage. The client may express feelings of helplessness, hopelessness, and sadness. Withdrawal is characterized by avoidance of social contacts, increased isolation, increased

TABLE 30-1
Summary of provisions of the Americans With Disabilities Act of 1990

Title	Provisions
I. Employment	◇ Cannot discriminate in job application procedures, hiring, advancement, discharge, compensation, job training, or other privileges. ◇ Must make reasonable accommodations for disabled.
II. Public Services A. Public Transportation	◇ All fixed route systems, demand responsive vehicles, paratransit facilities, and rapid and light rail systems shall provide services for disabled persons.
B. Public Transportation by Intercity and Commuter Rail	◇ All single or bilevel coach cars, dining cars, sleeping cars, lounge cars, and food service cars, as well as the station—including passenger platforms, designated waiting areas, ticketing areas, restrooms, and concession areas—must be accessible.
III. Public Accommodations and Services Operated by Private Entities	◇ Goods, services, facilities, privileges, advantages, and accommodations in an integrated setting shall be provided by anyone who owns, leases, or operates a place of public accommodation, including hotels, motels, restaurants, bars, motion picture houses, theatres, concert halls, stadiums, convention centers, lecture halls, bakeries, grocery stores, clothing stores, hardware stores, shopping centers, laundromats, dry-cleaners, banks, barber shops, beauty shops, travel services, shoe repair services, funeral parlors, gas stations, offices of accountants or lawyers, pharmacies, insurance offices, professional offices of health care providers, hospitals, terminals, depots, museums, libraries, galleries, parks, zoos, amusement parks, nurseries, elementary, secondary, undergraduate, graduate, or postgraduate schools, day care centers, senior citizen centers, homeless shelters, food banks, adoption agencies, or other social service agencies, gymnasiums, health spas, bowling alleys, and golf courses. ◇ Private clubs and religious organizations are exempt. ◇ Examinations or courses related to applications, licensing, certification, or credentialing for secondary or postsecondary education, professional, or trade purposes shall be accessible.
IV. Telecommunications	◇ Relay services for hearing and/or speech impaired persons shall be offered 24 hours per day at equivalent costs. ◇ Closed captioning is required for any federal public service announcement.
V. Miscellaneous	◇ It is unlawful to retaliate, coerce, intimidate, threaten, or interfere with any individual related to this act. ◇ A study shall be conducted on the ability of individuals with disabilities to enjoy the National Wilderness Preservation System. ◇ Not covered in the definition of disabled are individuals such as transvestites, homosexuals, bisexuals, pedophiles, exhibitionists, voyeurs, compulsive gamblers, kleptomaniacs, and pyromaniacs.

sleeping, fantasizing, and a general apathetic attitude. A client who is angry, hostile, or aggressive can be particularly enigmatic to the family and the nurse. Fixing blame is often the focus of the client's thoughts and actions. Clients may be abusive, argumentative, and even violent.

Logotherapy may be useful in helping the client find meaning in the suffering experience, as illustrated in the following example:

> Milly was injured by a gunshot at age 15 years during a domestic quarrel between her parents. The injury left her arms and legs completely paralyzed. She spent her day watching soap operas on television. While responding to the nursing history, Milly expressed surprise when the nurse asked what she did for others. Milly stated that she could not feed herself, bathe herself, write, sew, or even hold a telephone. Using dereflection, (deemphasizing the identified problem or deliberately focusing on something other than the problem), the nurse helped Milly to focus on her abilities—she had a bright mind with retentive and concentration skills, a melodious voice, and lively, expressive eyes. Over the course of the nurse-client interaction, Milly learned

to type with a mouthstick and wrote letters of comfort to church members who were experiencing sorrow. She began putting her inspirational messages on tape for the church library. Later she volunteered for 4 hours per week of telephone counseling.

The impact of an acquired disability on the individual varies, based on many factors. According to Maslow (1970), all people strive to meet their needs to obtain some degree of satisfaction and fulfillment. The Needs Satisfaction Scale found in Appendix A may serve as a useful tool in assessing a client's current need satisfaction level.

The Family with a Disabled Member

Often health workers focus their entire attention on the individual client and fail to see the needs of the family, particularly the client's caregiver. Disability of one family member can have a significant impact on the entire family. As the costs of institutional care continue to spiral, many families are providing care at home for members with a disability.

With these responsibilities, family members become subject to stressors that can affect their health. They may have added roles and expanded or modified patterns and lifestyles. The crisis of an injury or the shock of a diagnosis of chronic illness can greatly upset the family equilibrium.

The community health nurse must be aware of the impact of the disability on the family system. The beginning point for assessment and planning for family needs is during the initial crisis stage when most clients are hospitalized. To cope, the family needs to achieve several goals (Grieco and Kowalski, 1987):

1. They must become physically independent in the home.
2. They must become competent in applying the prescribed therapeutic regimen.
3. They must attain adequate knowledge of the disabled member's health condition.
4. They must be able to apply the principles of general hygiene to the circumstances of the homebound client.
5. They must have a positive attitude toward providing health care.
6. The care-giving individual of the family must be emotionally competent.
7. They must have a stable living pattern.
8. The physical environment must be adequate for the patient's home care needs.
9. When difficulties arise, a source of help to be used as a "safety valve" must be identified.
10. Community resources must be available to support these needs.

Family members show grief reactions just as the client does and need to maintain hope and to restore a balance to family life. Concerns expressed by family members include finances, work, housing, transportation, family activities, sexual activities, social relationships, and coping with the problems (functional and emotional) caused by the disability. Open communication between the disabled person and other family members is crucial to a healthy family pattern. Maintaining contact with the extended family through telephone conversations or letter writing is also helpful in providing an emotional support system.

The community health nurse needs to assess the family's patterns for tension management and conflict resolution (e.g., sudden outbursts, passive aggression, and psychosomatic ailments) and to assist the family in using health coping techniques. Referral for more intensive professional help may be appropriate in some cases. Environmental stimulation and social interaction are necessary for caretakers and family members as well as clients.

The community health nurse should evaluate the client's functional ability and family health, which is complicated by the added responsibilities of caring for a member with a disability. The nurse must recognize the effects on the major caretaker and others of providing long-term physical and emotional care. Respite care provides services intermittently to the family or caregiver to relieve them of the responsibilities associated with caring for a chronically ill or disabled person (Clemen-Stone et al., 1987). The long-term effects of unrelieved stress and frustration of needs can cause a breakdown of the caretaker.

Miss A. had never been married, lives with her parents, and assists with the family business. When her father died, she took on complete responsibilities for providing for herself and her mother. She worked long, hard hours at the store and then assisted her aging mother with the house and yard work. When Mrs. A. had a stroke, her daughter took care of her at home in a devoted manner. As Mrs. A.'s condition worsened, Miss A. found herself staying up at night yet continuing to put in a full day at the store. Mrs. A. become cranky and more demanding. She was incontinent and frequently called for help during the night. Although the doctor urged Miss A. to get help to supplement the daytime nurse, she declined, preferring to take care of her mother herself during the evening and night hours. Friends offered to relieve Miss A. for a weekend and urged her to take a relaxing trip, but she maintained her vigil. One day, to the surprise and consternation of relatives, Miss A. lost all control, had her mother placed in a nursing home, and said she never wanted to see her again. At the nursing home Mrs. A. made some degree of progress, and the staff attempted to plan a visit home. However, Miss A. still refused to associate with her mother and had all the locks on the doors changed to ensure that she could not return home. The mother eventually died in the nursing home. The daughter retired from the family business and became a virtual recluse.

Careers for Disabled Adults

Recent legislation has facilitated acceptance of the disabled adult into the work force. The community health nurse can be a source of support to a newly employed disabled adult who often faces many barriers, not the least of which are the attitudes of management, fellow workers, and the public. The nurse should be aware that, by law, handicapped adults who apply for job training, college, or basic adult education must be considered on the basis of their work or past academic records, not their disability.

Community and National Significance

Disability influences resources and emphasizes needs for services, including inpatient and outpatient services, emergency care services, housing, and transportation. The current philosophy of mainstreaming and integrating individuals who have disabilities into society rather than isolating them in a protective environment requires planning, and the community health nurse should be actively involved.

A community may need a variety of modules to provide housing options for its residents. The Housing and Urban Development Act of 1965 provides funds to assist handicapped individuals to obtain adequate housing through rent subsidies. This act also allows a group of handicapped people to categorize themselves as a family so that they can qualify for low-income housing.

Community health nurses should be interested in how well local health services and other aspects of the community consider the needs of individuals who are disabled. For example, do emergency medical technicians receive training on how to handle the needs of a blind person who is injured and may become emotionally hypersensitive? Do restaurants provide braille menus? Do waitresses address family members of a blind person and ask, "What would he like to order?" Are churches accessible to the disabled, or do the churches prefer a ministry to "shut-ins"? Are local government buildings accessible to the disabled?

Rehabilitation following disability is as costly to the nation as providing for special needs such as transportation or housing. However, such services may allow a disabled person and the caretaker to return to work. Thus the worker is contributing to the tax base instead of being dependent on government services. Rehabilitation contributes to the economic welfare of the nation and serves to facilitate humanitarianism.

Physical, Psychosocial, and Spiritual Rehabilitation

In a holistic approach to the rehabilitation process, attention must be given to all component parts of human existence. Specialized centers offer a variety of services to meet these needs. Clients are usually discharged from institutions when they master certain physical tasks. The community health nurse monitors treatment plans to maintain physical achievements. Often a client who has learned to work with an artificial limb goes home and hangs it in the closet; therefore, nurses must constantly encourage physical conditioning. Other nursing care focuses on promoting the continued health of nonpathological structures. For example, a client with diabetes who has had one leg amputated for gangrene should be taught to exercise all efforts to keep the other leg healthy.

People with a disability need psychosocial restoration as part of the broad perspective of rehabilitation. The achievement of self-care and mobility does not guarantee reintegration and social functioning. The community health nurse must be innovative in individual cases to promote psychosocial restoration. Encouraging self-transcendence helps clients to focus on others. For example, a man who has been injured in a deliberate attempt on his life and who is left with an ileostomy and spinal cord injury, necessitating the use of a wheel chair, can find meaning in volunteering in the recreational program in a nursing home. In meeting the needs of others, his own psychosocial health improves.

All humans have a spiritual (not synonymous with religious) dimension. The dynamic power of the human spirit can be harnessed to restore the disabled person to satisfaction and fulfillment. Logotherapeutic counseling can assist disabled persons to find meaning in their circumstances and unique purpose in life, with satisfying roles to fulfill. Life's task becomes one of finding an answer for the question, "Now that I am in this situation, what will I do with my life?"

CLINICAL APPLICATION

The following clinical situation provides an opportunity for the student to apply his or her knowledge to a typical case involving the needs and health problems of young and middle-age adults. The nursing process is used as a framework for making clinical decisions.

Mrs. Rosa Garcia is a slightly overweight 48-year-old Hispanic woman who attends the Riverview Community Center diabetic clinic. Her diabetes has been controlled with NPH insulin (30 units) for the past 5 years. She explains that recently she has experienced occasional chest tightness and shortness of breath. She is employed as a domestic worker and has noticed symptoms expecially after climbing stairs. After a thorough examination by the multidisciplinary team at the center, Mrs. Garcia is placed on nitroglycerine (1/150 g prn) for angina. She is referred to the nurse for planning community-based chronic care with an emphasis on health maintenance, decreasing cardiovascular risks, and preventing complications of diabetes mellitus.

Other members of the Garcia household include Jose, the husband, a 52-year-old construction worker who is currently unemployed because of the depressed housing market. He has been abusing alcohol in the past 3 months, which coincides with his length of unemployment. He is depressed, and the nurse suspects his drinking bouts sometimes lead to abusive behavior toward his wife and children. The Garcia children are: Maria, age 15, Jimenez, age 17, and Anna, age 18 years. They are all in high school: each has an after-school job and is making minimum wage.

1. Based on the information, what additional assessment data should be collected about the family members and household during the first home visit?
2. Identify the developmental tasks characteristic of middle-age adults in this situation.
3. An understanding of Hispanic cultural values and lifestyles will be necessary to analyze the assessment data. Describe the common values and traditions of Hispanics who are first generation Mexican-Americans.

After the first home visit, the nurse identifies several problems within the Garcia household. Mrs. Garcia works 10 hours per day, including house cleaning from 8 AM to 12 PM and managing a laundromat from 12 PM to 6 PM. In addition, she rises early to prepare breakfast for the family and to make lunches for the children. When she returns in the evening, she prepares dinner and cleans her own house. Saturdays are usually spent doing the family laundry and baking for the week. Sundays are spent at various church activities. In the past, Sundays were reserved for family outings, but now the children prefer activities with friends their own age. There is evidence that all three children are sexually active, and Mrs. Garcia is worried that Jimenez occasionally experiments with drugs.

Mr. Garcia spends most of his days out of the house, hoping to locate work and drinking. He gets very upset at the suggestion that he is drinking too much. His physical health appears good, but he has not had a thorough physical examination since he started working for the construction company 10 years ago. He is collecting unemployment insurance, but voices shame about it. His parents live in the neighborhood. His father has had a stroke but is doing well at home, where he is cared for by Jose's mother. They are both retired and have a modest but adequate income.

1. What is the nursing diagnosis?
2. What factors must be considered in developing a family plan of care?
3. What are the alternatives for modifying Mrs. Garcia's workload and energy expenditure?
4. Develop a 3-month, 6-month, and 12-month plan for

the Garcia family that demonstrates a gradual change to desired goals.

5. What are the teaching and learning needs of the Garcia family?

One evening, after a particularly stressful day, Mrs. Garcia becomes extremely dyspneic and must be hospitalized. Her complaints of chest tightness and shortness of breath subside with adequate care. Her diabetes is slightly out of control, but with several days of rest and proper diet, it is once more in balance. During the hospitalization, a number of family problems are made known to Mrs. Garcia: Jimenez is addicted to cocaine and has been skipping school for the past 6 weeks; Maria is pregnant and the father of the baby wants to marry her; Mr. Garcia has been in an automobile wreck and was arrested for driving under the influence of alcohol.

1. In coordinating discharge planning with the hospital, what priorities should be set for follow-up care?

2. What stress-reducing interventions might be useful as Mrs. Garcia faces domestic problems?

3. How might a logotherapeutic approach to intervening with the family crises be implemented?

Six months after the Garcia family became part of the caseload of the community health nurse, Mrs. Garcia's diabetic and cardiovascular conditions are stabilized. Her work schedule has been reduced to 8 hours per day with no heavy cleaning. Jimenez has entered a residential drug treatment program, where he has developed an interest in the electronics trade. Maria's pregnancy is without complications, and she is conscientious about keeping clinic appointments. She and the baby's father still want to marry but no plans have been made. Anna has entered a nursing program and is progressing satisfactorily. Unfortunately, Mr. Garcia has still not found work, continues to drink and has recently manifested hypertension.

1. What are the criteria to evaluate the progress, or lack of progress, toward health goals by this family?

2. What are the continued health risks for members of the family?

3. Based on the achievements and continued problems for each family member, what are the priorities for future plans?

SUMMARY

The major health problems of young and middle-age adults are largely the result of life-style behaviors that are influenced by specific developmental tasks. Individuals in this age group experience much stress and pressure from social role expectations to meet not only their own needs but the needs of others who are dependent on them. The adult years reflect growth and change in the pursuit of new life goals and in coping with life crises.

Assuming responsibility for self-care is the adult health task. Each person needs to exert a planned effort at maintaining optimum health, which includes exercise, nutrition, rest, sleep, play, and a healthy mental outlook on life.

Within each age category, special subgroups, such as single adults, require the specialized attention of community health nurses. The morbidity and mortality rates of young and middle-age adults give direction for the community health nurse. Suicide, homicide, and accidents are serious concerns for young adults. The nurse must assess and analyze the pressures and frustrations that lead to such consequences if this major health problem is to be resolved. Positive mental health services are needed in a community so that families can present their problems to professionals and learn to cope with crises. Sexually transmittable diseases are also a major health problem of young adults.

Morbidity and mortality factors for the middle-age adult include heart disease and stroke, cancer, alcohol and substance abuse, mental health problems, and periodontal diseases. Although singular cause-and-effect factors cannot be demonstrated, various health practices, including the avoidance of known risk factors, can contribute to disease prevention and health promotion. The community health nurse must work as a partner with the adult to reduce the risk of disease development and to promote a healthy life-style.

Community health nurses assess the impact of a physical disability on an individual, family, or community. Technology has eliminated many barriers to the disabled adult's ability to function in the larger society, and the ADA of 1990 will further expand opportunities for this group's full participation in society. As the community health nurse uses this technology and coordinates community resources, attention must be given to what is often the greatest barrier—the public's attitude toward the disabled person.

Health problems of young and middle-age adults relate to work, family, and community. Although major health hazards are reflected in morbidity and mortality statistics, community health nurses must be aware of potential problems from the emerging trends of a changing society. Anticipating new health problems requires an analysis of the life-styles and values of the adult population.

KEY CONCEPTS

Like the middle-income segment of society, young and middle-age adults may be considered the backbone of society.

Young adults are those between the ages of 20 and 35 years; middle-age adults are those between the ages of 36 and 64 years. However, adults may move forward and backward among young-adult and middle-adult life-styles.

Adults progress through successive phases of stabilization and consolidation and then change and grow while pursuing new goals and confronting life crises.

Factors that influence growth and development of the adult include health status, a sense of responsibility for self-care, available health resources, and lifestyle.

Health for the adult is the balanced state of well-being resulting from the harmonious interaction of body, mind, and spirit.

The status of adult health and opportunities for growth and development are interlinked with environmental influences and the resources of the individual, family, and community.

The middle years are crossroads in the adult developmental process, and transition is as critical as it was in adolescense.

For young adults, major health threats include violent death or injury, alcohol and substance abuse, unwanted pregnancies, and sexually transmissible diseases.

Motor vehicle accidents are the leading cause of death in young adults age 15 to 24 years.

Common causes of morbidity and mortality in middle-age adults are heart disease and stroke, cancer, alcohol and substance abuse, mental health problems, and periodontal disease.

Heart disease accounts for over 33% of deaths among middle-age adults.

The major health problems of young and middle-age adults are largely the result of life-style behaviors that are influenced by specific developmental tasks.

Approximately 35 million Americans are physically disabled to some degree; 55% of persons age 17 to 44 years have at least one chronic illness. Opportunities for persons with disabilities to participate fully in society are increasing.

LEARNING ACTIVITIES

1. Conduct an individual assessment on 10 adults. Half of these adults should be between the ages of 20 and 35 years, and the remaining five should be between the ages of 36 and 64 years. Compare the psychosocial tasks performed by members of each group as reported on their personal health assessments.
2. Interview at least six single adults. Include males and females in the group and compare the psychosocial tasks mentioned in the interviews to the expected norms.
   a. What similarities exist between the norm and those interviewed?
   b. What differences exist between the norm and those interviewed?
   c. Discuss whether the differences can be attributed to

their state of singleness.
3. Design a teaching plan for a middle-age adult that reflects a maximum level of health promotion.
4. Analyze mortality and morbidity data in your county and rank the order of the 10 most prevalent health problems.
5. Using a community service directory for your county, match available services to the needs identified in the survey of mortality and morbidity data. If gaps are noted, what services would you recommend to overcome this deficit?
6. Consult the most recent annual report of the State Department of Public Health and compare state and national incidence figures for the five leading causes of death in your state vs. the nation.

BIBLIOGRAPHY

Aaronson LS and MacNee CL: The relationship weight gain and nutrition in pregnancy, Nurs Res 38(4):223, 1989.

Adelmann PK, Antonucci TC, Crohan S, Coleman LM: A causal analysis of employment and health in midlife women, Women Health 16(1):5, 1990.

Adler RC: From DX (diagnosis) and RX (prescription) to RFX (risk factor reduction) = a new prescription for health patients, Fam Community Health 11(4):1, 1989.

Aiken LH: AIDS: the health policy context, Fam Community Health 12(2):1, 1989.

Allan JD: Identification of health risks in a young adult population, J Community Health Nurs 4(4):223, 1987.

Americans with Disabilities Act of 1990, Pub No 101-336, 104 Stat 327 Washington, DC, 1990, U.S. Government Printing Office.

Anderson R: Is the problem of noncompliance all in our heads? Diabetes Educ 11(1):31, 1985.

Anthony, JC and Petronis KR: Cocaine and heroin dependence compared: evidence from an epidemiologic field survey, Am J Public Health 79(10):1409, 1989.

Archer VE: Psychological defenses and control of AIDS, Am J Public Health 79(7):876, 1989.

Bachrach LL: Homeless women: a context for health planning, Milbank 65(3):371, 1987.

Bassuk EL and Rosenberg L: Why does family homelessness occur?: a case-control study, Am J Public Health 78(7):783, 1988.

Becker MH and Joseph JG: AIDS and behavioral change to reduce risk: a review, Am J Public Health 78(4):394, 1988.

Berkseth JK: Public health nursing for America's children, Public Health Nurs 2(4):222, 1985.

Bowels CL and Carwein VL: Survey of baccalaureate nursing schools' guidelines/policies on AIDS, J Nurs Educ 27(8):349, 1988.

Brody EM, Johnsen PT, and Fulcomer MC: What should adult children do for elderly parents?: opinions and preferences of three generations of women, J Gerontol 39(6):735, 1984.

Carter ER: Quality maternity care for the medically indigent, MCN 11:85, 1986.

Castro FG, Newcomb MD, and Cadish K: Lifestyle differences between young adult cocaine users and their nonuser peers, J Drug Educ 17(2):89, 1987.

Centers for Disease Control: *Chlamydia trachomatis* infections: policy guidelines for prevention and control, MMWR 34(suppl):535, 1985.

Centers for Disease Control: Update: acquired immunodeficiency syndrome—United States, 1981–1988, MMWR 38(14):229, 1989.

Chattopadhyay B, Fricker E, and Gelia CB: Incidence of parasitic infestations in minority travellers to and new immigrants arriving from the third world countries, Public Health 102:245, 1988.

Chavez LR, Cornelius WA, and Jones OW: Mexican immigrants and the utilization of U.S. health services: the case of San Diego, Soc Sci Med 25(1):93, 1985.

Chi PS: Medical utilization patterns of migrant farm workers in Wayne County, New York, Public Health Rep 100(5):480, 1985.

Chirikos TN: Accounting for the historical rise in work-disability prevalence, Milbank Q 64(2):271, 1986.

Cleary PD: Education and the prevention of AIDS, Law Med Healthcare, 16(3-4):267, 1988.

Clemen-Stone S, Eigsti DG, and McGuire SL: Comprehensive family and community health nursing, ed 3, St Louis, 1991, Mosby-Year Book, Inc.

Colosi ML: AIDS: a question of human rights versus the duty to provide a safe workplace, J Ambulatory Care Manage 11(4):63, 1988.

Combs-Orme T, Reis J, and Ward LD: Effectiveness of home visits by public health nurses in maternal and child health: an empirical view. Public Health Rep 100(5):490, 1985.

Cordes SM: Biopsychosocial imperatives from the rural perspective, Soc Sci Med 21:1373, 1985.

Cornell JT, Frame PS, and Franks P: Effectiveness of tuberculin skin test screening in a rural family practice, J Fam Pract 21(6):455, 1985.

Cross CK and Hirschfield RMA: Epidemiology of disorders in adulthood: suicide. In Klerman GL, Weissman MM, Appelbaum PS, and Roth LH, editors: Psychiatry: social, epidemiologic and legal psychiatry, vol 5, New York, 1986, Basic Books.

Curry M: Nonfinancial barriers to prenatal care, Women Health 15(3):85, 1989.

DeFrank RS and Stroup CA: Teacher stress and health: examination of a model, J Psychosom Res 33(1):99, 1989.

Deutsch FM, Brooks-Gunn J, Fleming A, Ruble D and Strangor C: Information-seeking and maternal self-definition during the transition to motherhood, J Pers Psychol 55(3):420, 1988.

Eisenberg M: The logotherapeutic intergenerational communications group. Int Forum Logotherapy 2(2):23, 1979.

Erikson E: Childhood and society, New York, 1950, WW Norton.

Erikson EH: Reflections in adolescent psychiatry: developmental and clinical studies, vol 11, Chicago, 1983, University of Chicago Press.

Falck VT: A re-evaluation of urban vs rural as ways of life: implications for health educators, Hygiene 4(4):40, 1985.

Fine MA, Schwebel AI, and Meyers LJ: The effect of world views on adaptation to single parenthood among middle-class adult women, J Fam Issues 6(1):107, 1985.

Fineberg HA: The social dimensions of AIDS, Sci Am 259(4):128, 1988.

Frankl V: Man's search for meaning, New York, 1959, Simon & Schuster.

Frankl V: The doctor and the soul, New York, 1973, Random House.

Frankl V: The unconscious God, New York, 1975, Simon & Schuster.

Forbes KR and Wagner EL: Compliance by Samoans in Hawaii with service norms in pediatric primary care, Public Health Rep 102(5):508, 1987.

Friedman GD et al.: CARDIA: study, design, recruitment and some characteristics of the examined subjects, J Clin Epidemiol 41(11):1105, 1988.

Friedman SM, DeSilva LP, Fox HE, and Bernard G: Hepatitis B screening in a New York City obstetrics service, Am J Public Health 78(3):308, 1988.

Goff W and McDonough P: A community health approach to AIDS: caring for the patient and educating the public, J Community Health Nurs 3(4):191, 1986.

Gomberg ESL: Suicide risk among women with alcohol problems, Am J Public Health 79(10):1363, 1989.

Grieco AJ and Kowalski W: The care partner. In Burnstein L, Grieco A, and Dete M, editors: Primary care in the home, Philadelphia, 1987, JB Lippincott.

Guide to clinical preventive services: report of the U.S. Preventive Services Task Force, Baltimore, 1989, Wilkins & Wilkins.

Helgeson DM and Berg CL: Contracting: a method of health promotion, J Community Health Nurs 2(4):199, 1985.

Hibbard JH: Social ties and health status: an examination of moderating factors, Health Educ Q 12(1):23, 1985.

Hirschfield RMA and Davidson L: Risk factors for suicide. In Frances AJ and Hales RE, editors: Review of psychiatry, vol 7, Washington, DC, 1988, American Psychiatric Press.

Holcomb NE and Ahr PR: Arrest rates among young adult psychiatric patients treated in inpatient and outpatient settings, Hosp Community Psychiatry 39(1):52, 1988.

Johns J: Self-care today: in search of an identity, Nurs Health Care 6(3):153, 1985.

Knaub PK: Growing up in a dual-carrier family: the children's perceptions, Fam Relations 35(3):431, 1986.

Kolata G: Is the war on cancer being won? Science 233:543, 1985.

Laitman L: An overview of a university student assistance program, J Am Coll Health 36(2):103, 1987.

Lambert CE and Lambert VA: Psychosocial impacts created by chronic illness, Nurs Clin North Am 22(3):527, 1987.

Lawson BZ: Work-related post-traumatic stress reactions: the hidden dimension, Health Soc Work 12(4):250, 1987.

Lee BA: Stability and change in an urban homeless population, Demography 26(2):323, 1989.

Levinson DJ et al.: The seasons of a man's life, New York, 1978, Ballantine Books.

Levinson DJ: The concept of adult development, Am Psychol 41(1):3, 1986.

Lipkin M and Williams S: Psychosocial issues, In Bernstein L, Grieco A, Dete M, editors: Primary care in the home, Philadelphia, 1987 Lippincott.

Lisansky ES: Suicide risk among women with alcohol problems, Am J Public Health 79(10):1363, 1989.

Looney KM: The respite care alternative, J Gerontol Nurs 13(5):18, 1987.

Lurie N, Manning WG, Peterson C, Goldberg GA, Phelps CA, and Lillard L: Preventive care: do we practice what we preach? Am J Public Health 77(7):801, 1987.

Lynam M: Support networks developed by immigrant women, Soc Sci Med 21(3):327, 1985.

Marvin C and Slevin A: *Chlamydia:* cause, prevention and cure, MCN 12:318, 1987.

Maslow AH: Motivation and personality, New York, 1970, Harper & Row.

Milio N: The profitization of health promotion, Int J Health Serv 18(4):573, 1988.

Montana DE: Predicting and understanding influenza vaccination behavior: alternatives to the health belief model, Med Care 24(5):438, 1986.

Moskop JC: AIDS and public health, Death Studies 12:417, 1988.

Neugarten BL and Neugarten DA: The changing meanings of age, Psychol Today 21(5):29-33, 1987.

Newcomb MD and Bentler PM: Drug use, education aspirations, and work force involvement: the transition from adolescence to young adulthood, Am J Community Psychol 14(3):303, 1986.

Nichols JN, Wright LK, and Murphy JF: Proposal for tracking health care for the homeless, J Community Health 11(3):204, 1986.

Niskala H: The role of community health nurses in cardiac rehabilitation, Home Healthc Nurse 5(3):10, 1987.

Nolan JW: Developmental concerns and the health of midlife women, Nurs Clin North Am 21(1):151, 1987.

Norbeck JS and Anderson NJ: Psychosocial predicators of pregnancy outcomes in low-income Black, Hispanic and White women, Nurs Res 38(4):204, 1989.

Orem D: Nursing concepts of practice, New York, 1985, McGraw-Hill.

Orr J, Neuberger J, Rowden R, Cumberlege J, and Flint C: Retracing our cultural roots, Nurs Time 83(11):22, 1987.

Oswald SK and Williams HY: Community health nursing in workplace health programs: rationale and ethics, J Community Health Nurs 4(3):121, 1987.

Owen AY and Frankle RT: Nutrition in the community, ed 2, St Louis, 1986, Mosby-Year Book.

Pang KY: The practice of traditional Korean medicine in Washington, DC, Soc Sci Med 28(8):875, 1989.

Papalia DE, Olds SW, and Feldman RD: Human development, New York, 1989, McGraw Hill.

Patton L: Setting the rural health services research agenda: the congressional perspective. Health Serv Res 23(6):1005, 1989.

Perez-Stable EJ, Slutkin G, Paz A, and Hopewell PC: Tuberculin reactivity in United States and foreign-born Latinos: results of a community-based screening program, Am J Public Health 76(6):643, 1986.

Peters DA: Development of a community health intensity rating scale, Nurs Res 37(4):202, 1988.

Phillips BU: The forgotten family: an untapped resource in cancer prevention, Fam Community Health 11(4):17, 1989.

Popendorf W, Donham KJ, Easton DN, and Silk J: A synopsis of agricultural respiratory hazards, Am Ind Hyg Assoc J 46(3):154, 1985.

Rakowski W: Personal health practices, health status, and expected control over future health, J Community Health, 11(3):189, 1986.

Redman BK: New areas of theory development and practices in patient education, J Adv Nurs 10:425, 1985.

Robertson MJ and Cousineau MR: Health status and access to health services among the urban homeless, Am J Public Health 76(5):561, 1986.

Robinson CH, Lawler MR, Chenoweth WL, and Garwick AE: Normal and therapeutic nutrition, ed 17, New York, 1986, Macmillan.

Rogers JC and Dodson SC: Burnout in occupational therapists, Am J Occup Ther 42(12):787, 1988.

Rowland D and Lyons B: Triple jeopardy: rural, poor and uninsured, Health Serv Rep 23(6):975, 1989.

Safer DJ: Substance abuse by young adult chronic patients, Hosp Community Psychiatry 38(5):511, 1987.

Sakala C: Community based, community oriented maternity care, Am J Public Health 79(7):897, 1984.

Schlossberg VK: Taking the mystery out of change, Psychol Today 21(5):74, 1987.

Selder FE: Life transition theory: a resolution of uncertainty, Nurs Health Care 10(8):436, 1989.

Selye H: Stress and holistic medicine, Fam Community Health 3:85, 1980.

Sheehy G: Pathfinders, New York, 1981, William Morrow & Co.

Shimizu H, Mack TM, Ross RK, and Henderson BE: Cancer of the gastrointestinal tract among Japanese and White immigrants in Los Angeles County, J Nat Cancer Instit 78(2):223, 1987.

Smith KG: The hazards of migrant farm work: an overview for rural public health nurses, Public Health Nurs 3(1):48, 1986.

Susser E, Struening EL, and Gonover S: Psychiatric problems in homeless men, Arch Gen Psychiatry 46(9):845, 1989.

Swift JS, Colvin C, and Mills D: Displaced homemakers: adults returning to college with different characteristics and needs, J Coll Student Personnel 28(4):343, 1987.

Topf M: Personality hardiness, occupational stress, and burnout in critical care nurses, Res Nurs Health 12:179, 1989.

Travelbee J: Interpersonal aspects of nursing, Philadelphia, 1966, FA Davis.

Turner SL, Bauer G, McNair E, McNutt B, and Walker N: The homeless experience: clinic build-ing in a community health discovery-learning project, Public Health Nurs 6(2):97, 1988.

U.S. Department of Commerce, Bureau of the Census: Statistical abstract of the United States, ed 109, Washington, DC, 1989, U.S. Government Printing Office.

Vega WA, Kolody B, Valle R, and Hough R: Depressive symptoms and their correlates among immigrant Mexican women in the United States, Soc Sci Med 22(6):645, 1986.

Von Windeguth BJ and Urbano MT: Cocaine abusing mothers and their infants: a new morbidity brings challenges for nursing care, J Community Health Nurs 6(3):147, 1989.

Waldron I and Jacobs JA: Effects of multiple roles on women's health: evidence from a national longitudinal study, Women Health 15(1):3, 1989.

Wayne R: Rural trauma management, Am J Surg 157:463, 1989.

Weaver DA: Case review: cocaine-induced chest pain and myocardial ischemia, J Emerg Nurs 14(4):203, 1988.

Weiten W: Psychology: themes and variations, Pacific Grove, CA, 1989, Brooks/Cole Publishing.

Winter L, Goldy S, and Baer C: Prevalence and epidemiologic correlates of *chlamydia trachomatis* in rural and urban populations, Sex Transm Dis 17(1):30, 1989.

Wolfgang AP: The health professions stress inventory, Psychol Rep 62:220, 1988.

The Older Adult

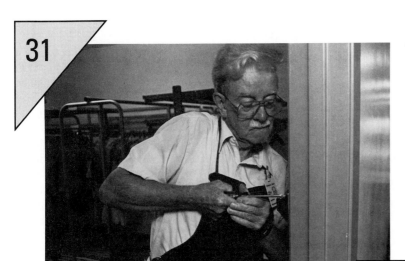

Delois H. Skipwith

OBJECTIVES

After reading this chapter, the student should be able to:

List two demographic facts about older adults.

Describe at least two common myths or stereotypes about the older adult.

Identify two personal biases about aging.

Discuss the role of the community health nurse in providing care for older adults who have at least one major health problem.

Describe at least three possible effects of health promotion activities for older adults.

Name at least three community resources and services available for the care of the elderly.

Identify at least three losses that older adults may incur.

List three nursing interventions that could assist the older client to cope with each of the three losses names.

KEY TERMS

abuse of the elderly
activity theory
acute brain syndrome
aging network
Alzheimer's disease
autoimmunity theory
chronic brain syndrome
confusional states
dementia

depression
developmental or continuity theory of aging
drug resistance
disengagement theory
eight stages of life
life expectancy
psychotropic
retirement

respite care
self-esteem
senility
stress management
substance abuse
time management
wear and tear theory
widowhood

T he elderly are the fastest growing population in the United States. Increased longevity is often accompanied by a higher incidence of chronic disease, which results in a substantial challenge to the health care system. Technology can keep people alive much longer, yet care is costly and often uncomfortable. This chapter discusses the following questions: Who are the older adults? What major health problems accompany their increasing longevity? What are appropriate community health nursing interventions in these situations? What community programs, resources, and legislative support are available to make one's older years more worthwhile?

DEMOGRAPHY

Historically, the elderly have been described as people who are age 65 years or older. In the early 1900s, 1 in every 25 people was 65 years of age and over, compared with the 1984 rate of 1 in every 8 people. The 65-years-and-older age group numbered 28 million in 1984 and had increased to 29.8 million by 1987. By the year 2010, the number of Americans 65 years of age and over will drastically increase to a rate of 1 in 7. By 2050, 1 in every 5 persons is expected to be 65 years of age and over (U.S. Senate, 1986). (The increasing growth rate of the older population is shown in Table 31-1.)

In 1986, the life expectancy at birth was 78.3 years for women and 71.3 years for men. In 1987 the median age of the U.S. population was 32 years; the projected increase for the year 2000 is 36 years, and 42 years for the year 2050 (U.S. Senate, 1986; U.S. Bureau, 1987). Analysis of gender distribution indicates that the 65-years-and-older segment of the population is about two thirds female (approximately 15.2 million women and 10.2 million men). A breakdown of the older population into smaller age segments illustrates that women outnumber men throughout later life (Table 31-2).

Blacks constitute the largest minority in the United States, with a total of 28.1 million in 1983. Of this number

2.3 million or 8% are age 65 years and older (U.S. Bureau, 1984). Asians and Pacific islanders account for 6% of the 65-years-and-older population, and native Americans and Hispanics account for 4% each (Need for Long-term Care, 1981). Statistics show racial and ethnic differences in life expectancy, gender distribution, and median age.

Life expectancy at birth for blacks is less than for whites; however, this gap is narrowing. The 1940 life-expectancy margin of 11 years held by whites over blacks decreased to 5.6 years in 1983. After the age of 80 years, life expectancy is higher for blacks than whites. In 1987, the median age for blacks was 27.2 years and 33 years for whites. Black females have gained the largest increase in life expectancy, with an increase of 5.5 years from 1970 to 1983. The 1987 ratio of 65-years-and-older black males to black females is 67.1:100 (U.S. Bureau, 1984: U.S. Bureau, 1987).

The educational level of the elderly population has also improved. The median level of education was 11 years in 1983 and increased to 12 years for persons 65 years of age and older in 1987. Differences in education levels exist between elderly blacks and whites. About 33% of older whites and 66% of older blacks did not attend school beyond the eighth grade (U.S. Senate, 1986; U.S. Bureau, 1987).

Social Security payments and Medicare have benefited the elderly economically. Only 7.2% of older adults lived below the poverty level in 1987, (U.S. Bureau, 1987). Racial and gender differences are found in the economic status of elderly people. In 1987, approximately 5% of elderly whites and 24% of elderly blacks lived below the poverty level. In 1986, white men 65 to 69 years of age had a median income of $14,041, whereas the median income for black and Hispanic men was $7,078 and $8.083, respectively. Elderly women constitute 72% of the elderly poor. In 1986, elderly women had a median income of $6,425 as compared with $11,544 for elderly men (U.S. Senate, 1987).

The older adult in the United States lives in a culture oriented toward youth, productivity, and rapid paces. This orientation influences the goods and services produced and marketed, as well as the work and recreation options available.

A youth-oriented attitude may convey to older adults that they are not respected or valued and that declining health,

TABLE 31-1
Older population growth and projections

Year	Number (in thousands)	Percentage of total population
1900	3084	4.0
1920	4933	4.7
1940	9019	6.8
1960	16,560	9.2
1980	25,544	11.3
1990	31,697	12.7
2000	34,921	13.0
2010	39,195	13.8
2020	51,422	17.3
2030	64,581	21.2
2040	66,988	21.7

Adapted from U.S. Bureau of the Census, Current population reports, Series P-23, No. 138, Demographic and socioeconomic aspects of aging in the United States, US Government Printing Office, Washington, DC, 1984.

TABLE 31-2
Number of men per 100 women in 1984

Age group	Number of men
65-69	81
70-74	72
75-79	63
80-84	53
85-89	43
90-94	36

From the U.S. Bureau of Census: Current population reports, Series P-25, No 952, estimates, Washington, DC, 1984, U.S. Government Printing Office.

health problems, and health issues are "natural" or just "old age." Some health problems go undetected, are mislabeled or misdiagnosed, or are ineffectively treated. There are fewer adequately prepared health care providers for the older segment of the population than for other age groups. Additionally, the allocation of resources—type, amount, and location—may indicate to older adults that their needs go unmet. Although many demographic and social changes are beginning to alter this youth-oriented attitude, much work is needed to create an attitude recognizing the social worth of all age groups.

Knowledge of the role of the elderly in different cultural and ethnic groups is essential for providing quality care. Across cultures and ethnic groups, the roles of the elderly in family relationships as storers and transmitters of knowledge and information are evident. The black U.S. family honors its older members for their "adaptation" to many crises and struggles, for their strong religious affiliations, and for the life expectancy crossover phenomenon (that is, blacks aged 80 years and older live longer than whites).

In Asian-American families, the older adult man may give up status and responsibility to his wife and oldest son. Many older Chinese men live alone by choice and because of cultural beliefs, whereas in Japanese culture the young are expected to respect and care for their elders.*

Mexican-Americans often view health and illness as a balance-imbalance between the will of God and their own behavior. Additionally, children are expected to care for the aged, and there is little use of nursing homes (Ebersole and Hess, 1990). Chapter 6 gives additional information on the influence of culture in determining the community health nursing role.

Changes in social expectations and life-styles of aged persons partly determine the dominant needs and issues for the group. Members of the generation who were young during the 1960s and who were characterized as rebellious and concerned with rights and freedom will differ greatly in character, expectations, and social participation at 65 years of age than members of the Depression era generation who are now a part of the older population. Young people of the 1990s will age with an entirely different set of issues and concerns—influenced by education, consumerism, the financial problems of inflation and unemployment, and health consciousness.

MYTHS AND STEREOTYPES

In recent years, aging as a life process has received greater focus and study. The earlier lack of emphasis on this population group perpetuated many myths and stereotypes. The public often views old people as persons who wear glasses, are hard of hearing, are bald or have grey hair, have wrinkled skin, and are crippled. How many times have these illusions been depicted as typical of old people in dramas, drawings, and other works? The characteristics of older people portrayed on television and the public's conversation and jokes about older people dehumanize and unfairly label this group.

A popular myth is that most older people are institutionalized, yet only about 5% of elderly persons actually reside in institutions (U.S. Senate, 1986). Another common myth is that the elderly are poor. The majority of older adults (93%) live above the poverty level (U.S. Bureau, 1987). However, this figure does not negate the severity of the problems stemming from poverty, such as living in older houses in deteriorating neighborhoods, having limited access to transportation, and receiving poor health care.

The myth of the inability of the elderly to learn has serious consequences for the health of elderly persons. Health education opportunities for the elderly are often neglected because providers believe that "they can't learn." Yet investigations have shown that older adults are capable of learning, and when learning problems occur, they are generally associated with other conditions that interrupt health such as hearing or vision loss. Adjustments are needed in the attitudes of both the educators and the learners.

Older people have also been unfairly characterized as "bad drivers." However, the biggest automobile accident problem for people over 65 years of age is being injured as a pedestrian. In reality the 15- to 24-year-old group has the highest motor vehicle death rate (Healthy People, 1979).

The perception of older people as "chair rockers" is contradicted by Harris' survey (1975). Harris' study revealed that people 65 years of age and older are thought to spend 42% of their time "sitting and thinking" and 27% of their time "doing nothing," whereas they actually spend only 31% of their time "sitting and thinking" and 15% "just doing nothing." Older people's actual activities include at least 20% of their time gardening, caring for others, walking, and participating in organizations and hobbies.

Additional myths center on sexuality. Sexual drive and sexual activity are present in old age, with changes in the level of sexual activity resulting from physiological causes, sociocultural perspectives, or both. Health problems and medications can alter sexual activity, as can availability of a mate, stereotypes, privacy, and living arrangements.

DEVELOPMENTAL TASKS AND THEORIES OF AGING

The developmental tasks of old age and the potential problems associated with them are shown in Table 31-3 on p. 548.

Psychological theories of aging try to describe the aging process and explain behaviors observed during this life phase. Cummings and Henry (1961) proposed the *disengagement theory of aging*. Withdrawal is a key concept in this theory. The disengagement theory postulates that aging people withdraw from customary roles fulfilled during middle years and invest themselves in more self-focused activities. Withdrawal and self-examination are protective mechanisms that allow the individual to establish a new balance and adapt to the many changes of aging. Additionally, withdrawal of society from the aged creates a state of mutual withdrawal.

The *activity theory*, states that continuing activities during middle age is a requirement for successful aging. The active old person who maintains social relationships, is involved in community activities, travels, and has many hobbies and interests is considered the model old person (Havighurst, 1963).

---

*In Japanese culture, children tend to assume responsibility for aging relatives rather than expecting them to live alone and care for themselves.

TABLE 31-3
Developmental tasks and potential problems of the elderly

Tasks	Potential problems
Adjusting to decreasing health and physical strength	Hypochondria, anger, anxiety, chronicity, grief, depression, low self-esteem, loss of health
Adjusting to retirement and reduced income	Loss of status, poverty, rejection, low self-esteem
Adjusting to death of a spouse	Loss of spouse, grief, guilt, loneliness, depression
Acceptance of self as an aging person	Rejection, low self-esteem
Maintaining satisfactory living arrangements	Dependency, isolation
Realigning relationships with adult children	Conflict, hostility, rejection, loneliness, isolation
Finding meaning in life	Guilt, despair, suicide

The *developmental* or *continuity theory of aging* emphasizes continuing an individual's unique traits, characteristics, and habits into the later years without much change from earlier age. Interiority, which emphasizes the importance of a personal system of values, self-examination, and individuality is a key concept in this theory (Neugarten, 1964). This theory is a balance between the disengagement and activity theories.

The *eight stages of life* (Erikson, 1963) provides another perspective for viewing aging. In this theory, timing, sequential order of movement, and accomplishment of certain critical tasks are essential for moving from one life stage to the next. Aging is viewed as the successful resolution of the conflict between the critical tasks of integrity and despair. Positive resolution results in people who are content with life and whose relationships involve a mixture of leading and following. The individual who suffers from despair regrets that life cannot begin again, be better, and that the remaining years are too few.

Physiological theories explain aging as stemming from a breakdown in the performance of bodily organs and systems (Steffe, 1984). The *wear and tear theory* of aging emphasizes that aging is a programmed process in which cells are constantly wearing out, affected by harmful stress factors and the accumulation of harmful by-products. The autoimmune reaction is the basis of the *autoimmunity theory* of aging (Ebersole and Hess, 1990). With increased age, normal cells within the body are not recognized by the body as its own, and the body sets off a protective mechanism, forming antibodies against the "unknown cells."

Somatic mutation theory is based on the premise that mutation or genetic damage from radiation exposure will produce functional failure and death. There is limited evidence to support this theory.

The *error theory* explains aging as resulting from errors in the protein molecules in the genetic makeup. The erroneous molecules are multiplied until death results. This theory has limited evidence to support it.

Functional changes and declines resulting from changes in neurons and hormones form the bases for the *neuroendocrine theory*. The signal and response timing mechanisms of the body are impaired. Decline also is central to the immunological theory of aging in which the functional capacity of the immune system declines with age. In the *free radical theory*, aging is related to the production rate of free radicals or the escape and accumulation of chemically reactive molecules (Cristofalo, 1988).

Although these theories provide some explanations for the aging process, no one theory completely explains the aging process for all people. However, theories of aging are still important to nursing because they can provide a framework within which practice decisions can be made.

HEALTH PROMOTION

Physical, as well as psychosocial or developmental, changes accompany aging. The observed changes represent the cumulative and lifelong effects of heredity, environment, nutrition, rest, activity, and altered health status. Both men and women experience some changes in hair color and distribution. The thinning epidermis, dehydrated dermis, lessened blood supply, loss of skin elasticity, and reduction and loss of subcutaneous fat culminate in wrinkles. The skin surrounding the eyes is affected by aging. Lines about the lateral canthus of the eyes form shapes resembling crow's feet. The gastrointestinal tract changes during aging are the result of a reduction in the senses of smell and taste and decreased gastric and intestinal secretion and motility. These changes, in addition to those listed in the box at right, represent some of the changes that affect the body. Increased efforts to educate the elderly about normal changes during aging must become a priority nursing intervention.

A life-style of healthy habits during the elderly years contributes to the well-being of older adults because the continuation of healthy habits and the addition of age-specific habits improve the quality and quantity of life. Aging can be healthy, and old age is not synonymous with ill health or a pronouncement "to take it easy and retire to the rocking chair." Moderation in exercise, diet, and alcoholic beverage consumption and meaningful activities provide for days of meaningful living. Regular physical checkups, adherence to prescribed treatment regimens, and healthy life-styles must replace expressions such as "medicine won't do any good," "I haven't seen a doctor in so many years, why see a doctor now?," and "I've just got a few years left, so I can eat and do what I please." Discussions of health education topics concerning nutrition, sleep patterns, exercise, older adult development and changes, health care costs, and self-care strategies need to be directed to both elderly individuals and groups.

NORMAL CHANGES IN AGING

INTEGUMENTARY SYSTEM

Hair and nails: hair thin and gray, receding hairline, thicker nails

Skin: wrinkles, thinning, drier, easily bruised, decreased perspiration, spotty pigmentation

SENSORY SYSTEM

Sight: increased opacity of lens, grayish white corneal ring, less tearing, droopy eyelids, inability to focus on near objects

Hearing: slight decline in hearing (especially for high frequency tones)

Touch: decreased differentiation of cold, heat, and touch sensations

Smell: diminished sense of smell, prominent or protruding nose

Taste: diminished taste bud sensations, less saliva, dry mouth

MUSCULOSKELETAL SYSTEM

Flabby muscles, less energy and more frequent fatigue, slower and shorter gait, less swinging of arms, stooped posture, loss of height, some rubbing of articular cartilage in joints, stiffening of joints, porous and lighter bones

CARDIOVASCULAR-RESPIRATORY TRACT SYSTEM

Lessened vital capacity, decreased chest movement, slower pulse, increased systolic and decreased diastolic pressures, poor reaction to increased and sustained demand on heart activity

GASTROINTESTINAL-GENITOURINARY TRACT SYSTEM

Decrease motility of gastrointestinal system (organ) function, less secretion of digestive enzymes and acid secretions, slower emptying of stomach, decreased filtering ability of urinary system, polyuria, drier vaginal mucosa, enlarged prostate glands

NERVOUS SYSTEM

Atrophy of brain cells, slower reflexes

Immunization

Immunization against influenza is a special safeguard for older adults with chronic illnesses and respiratory problems such as emphysema. Pneumonia vaccines also are available. Older adults should discuss the advisability of influenza and pneumonia immunization with their private physicians in view of the existing controversy about the use of such preventive measures.

Nutrition

As discussed in Chapter 34, a balanced diet including the four food groups is essential to good nutrition. Nutrients such as protein, minerals, calcium, and vitamins must be included in sufficient amounts, which are generally considered the same as for younger people. A diet pattern of three meals per day is just as important during the later years as during the earlier years. Modification of caloric intake is necessary to keep off excess weight because the physical activity of many older adults declines. Adequate hydration with sufficient amounts of water is a good nutritional practice.

Sociological, economic, and biological factors contribute to the eating habits of older persons. Some of these factors are living arrangements, availability of transportation, limited income, dental health, sense of smell and taste, digestion, and myths about nutrition. Some typical statements of older adults are "I don't feel like cooking just for myself. I just eat something light like cereal, soup, and sometimes some vegetables," "I don't like to eat alone," "I don't have an appetite; nothing tastes good." Health status, physical activity, cultural practices, individuality, and physiological changes of aging must also be considered in determining nutritional requirements. Attractive meals, companionship, and good dental health and digestion make mealtimes healthy and enjoyable.

MAJOR HEALTH PROBLEMS

Although many older adults enjoy good health, approximately 80% of the group over age 65 years has at least one chronic health problem. One half of the elderly population is limited in an activity of daily living, and 18% of this same group cannot carry on a major activity (Healthy People, 1979). Cardiovascular, arthritic, and visual problems are the three most frequently reported activity-limiting conditions experienced by this age group (Need for Long-term Care, 1981).

The major causes of death in people over age 65 years are heart disease, malignant neoplasms, and cerebrovascular diseases (U.S. Senate, 1987: U.S. Bureau, 1984). Other leading causes of death for the elderly are shown in Table 31-4. Table 31-5 on p. 551 discusses selected health problems and nursing management of these conditions.

PSYCHOSOCIAL ASPECTS OF AGING
Coping with Retirement

The ability to successfully adjust to *retirement* is affected by health status, income, number of situational changes and quality of personal relationships. The ability to manage time effectively, flexibility, ability to relinquish the work routine, and anticipation and realistic expectation for retirement are other factors. The community health nurse has an important role in elderly people's adjustment. The best preparation for retirement occurs years before the event. Good health practices, for example, begin in utero and continue throughout life. However, circumstances, life-style choice, and other factors sometimes create health problems. In these instances the individual has to learn to adapt to illness. Chronic health problems must be dealt with through life-style adjustments and management of prescribed regimens.

The community health nurse can often provide direction and guidance to the retiree and the family. Professional support for the family is an important nursing role that benefits both the retiree and the family. For example, the community health nurse who speaks to a group of preretirees at a local industry may provide them with information about

TABLE 31-4
Sex ratio of mortality from leading causes of death—United States, 1985

Cause of death	Ratio of male to female mortality (%)				
	All ages*	55-64	65-74	75-84	85 and over
All causes	175	184	181	163	128
Diseases of heart	195	260	202	156	117
Malignant neoplasms	148	140	168	194	191
Cerebrovascular diseases	117	134	131	115	90
Accidents and adverse effects	278	262	185	180	169
Chronic obstructive pulmonary diseases and allied conditions	223	166	225	307	363
Pneumonia and influenza	180	210	211	184	149
Diabetes mellitus	105	102	101	101	94
Suicide	384	348	483	781	1204
Chronic liver diseases and cirrhosis	223	234	203	182	176
Atherosclerosis	131	228	178	124	97
Nephritis, nephrotic syndrome, and nephrosis	153	131	148	162	181
Homicide and legal intervention	328	337	246	171	129

*Adjusted on basis of age distribution of the United States total population, 1940.
Adapted from unpublished data from Division of Vital Statistics, National Center for Health Statistics; and Statistical Bulletin, Metropolitan Life, 69(1):21, 1988.

normal expectations and behaviors, *time management,* and other issues often excluded in the customary financial planning programs for preretirees. Educating people about the normal changes of aging, health, retirement, and problems of aging promotes understanding, caring, and positive actions. Two critical aspects of adjustment to retirement are how effectively the retiree learns to restructure time and the quality of personal relationships.

Managing Time

Retirement, formally institutionalized in the United States by the passage of the Social Security Act in 1935, generally occurs at the age of 65 years. Considering the present life expectancy, a person can anticipate living for at least several years in retirement. At the moment of retirement, the worker is confronted with the loss of a job, a reduction in income, and the loss of and altered relations with co-workers. Time becomes available, and the individual asks, "What will I do with all of this time?"

Time management is therefore crucial for older adults. They must be motivated to arise and meet the day's challenges and opportunities. Many do not possess leisure-time skills; consequently, they feel alienated, lonely, and unhappy with the increased time available in later years. Loneliness is one consequence of inadequate, pleasureless, or absent interpersonal relationships. Many older adults mask loneliness with various complaints such as insomnia, indigestion, muscular aches, and general malaise. Realistic plans for meaningful activities during retirement must be made. Senior centers offer a social outlet, as well as other services.

Mrs. A, who has to take a taxi to the center, makes the trip on Monday, Wednesday, and Friday to avoid being home alone and thinking and grieving about her deceased husband. Participation in crafts, water exercise, and health education programs have proved to be an effective use of her time. Other people, like Mr. J, Miss T, and Mrs. O, gain purpose and meaningfully use time by volunteering to serve juice, set the table, help in the kitchen, or do the "Thoughts for Living" at the nutrition center. Additionally, they have earned hours as Retired Senior Volunteer Program (RSVP) workers and are publicly recognized for their contribution.

The retired person should plan for ways to satisfy basic needs, further develop as a total person, and derive happiness from living, in addition to planning for fun, entertainment, and leisure. A meaningful activity is one that is consistent with the life-style, interests, resources, and health of the older adult. Health-promoting leisure behaviors for older adults generally include physical fitness activities; visiting (in person or via the telephone) with relatives and friends; arts and crafts such as painting, sewing and ceramics; viewing television; reading; and travel. The development of new interests should be encouraged. The community health nurse can provide referrals and information about available community activities. Many organizations, such as nutrition centers, community schools, and multipurpose senior centers, provide places for older adults to meet.

Realignment of Relationships

Retirees must often reconsider the relationships between themselves and significant others, including spouse, family, and neighbors. Family relationships represent one of the challenges of this age period. Retired people must learn to live with or without their spouse. A man who has spent many years working away from home must now spend many

TABLE 31-5
Major health problems in the older adult

Problem	Percentage	Community health nursing roles
Hypertension	39.4 (1986)	Monitor blood pressure and weight; educate about nutrition and antihypertensive drugs; teach stress management techniques; promote an optimal balance between rest and activity; establish blood pressure screening programs; assess the client's current life-style and promote life-style changes; promote dietary modifications by using techniques such as a diet diary
Cancer	Varies according to type of cancer	Obtain health history; promote monthly breast self-examinations and yearly pap smears and mammograms for older women; promote regular physical examinations; encourage smokers to stop smoking; correct misconceptions about the processes of aging; provide emotional support and quality care during diagnostic and treatment procedures
Arthritis	48 (1987)	Help adult avoid the false hope and expense of arthritis quackery; educate adult about management of activities, correct body mechanics, availability of mechanical appliances and adequate rest; promote stress management; counsel and assist the family to improve communication, role negotiation, and use of community resources
Visual impairment (e.g., loss of visual acuity, eyelid disorders, opacity of the lens)	9.5 (1987)	Provide support in a well-lighted, glare-free environment; use printed aids with large, well-spaced letters; assist adult with cleaning eyeglasses; help make arrangements for vision examinations and obtain necessary prostheses; teach the adult to be cautious of fraudulent advertisments
Hearing impairment (e.g., presbycusis)	29.6 (1987)	Speak with clarity at a moderate volume and pace and face the audience when performing health teaching; help make arrangements for hearing examination and obtain necessary prostheses; teach the adult to be cautious of fraudulent advertisements
Confusional states	Unknown	Provide complete assessment; correct underlying causes of disease (if possible); provide for a protective environment; promote activities that reinforce reality; assist with adequate personal hygiene, nutrition, and hydration; provide emotional support to the family; recommend applicable community resources such as adult day care, home health aides, and homemaker services
Alzheimer's disease	Unknown†	Maintain optimal functioning, protection, and safety; foster human dignity; demonstrate to the primary family caregiver techniques to dress, feed, and toilet the adult; provide frequent encouragement and emotional support to the caregiver; act as an advocate for the client when dealing with respite care and support groups; ensure that the client's rights are protected; provide support to maintain family members' physical and mental health; maintain family stability; recommend financial services if needed
Dental problems	Varies according to problem	Perform oral assessment and refer as necessary; emphasize regular brushing and flossing, proper nutrition and dental examinations; encourage clients with dentures to wear and take care of them; allay fears about dentists; help provide access to financial services (if necessary) and access to dental care facilities
Drug use and abuse	31 (1986)	Obtain drug history; educate adult about safe storage, use of drug, drug-drug and drug-food interactions, and general information about the drug (such as drug name, purpose, side effects, and dosage); instruct adult about the presorting technique (using small containers with one dose of drug that are labeled with specific administration times)
Substance abuse	Unknown‡	Arrange and monitor detoxification if appropriate; counsel adults about substance abuse; promote stress management to avoid the need for drugs or alcohol; encourage adult to use self-help groups such as Alcoholics Anonymous and Al-Anon; educate the public about the dangers of substance abuse

*National Center, 1987; Includes year data collected.
†Unknown because of problems of early recognition and accurate diagnosis.
‡Statistics are difficult to determine because the elderly abuser often lives alone.

hours at home; this requires adjustment. The woman who has been home alone must now become accustomed to having her husband underfoot all day. Families in which both adults work must also adjust to increased leisure time.

Another aspect of family relationships after retirement is the relationship realignment between aging parents and their adult children. Issues of role reversal, dependency, conflict, guilt, and loss require recognition and resolution.

The community health nurse must consider the parent who has always met the needs of each household member and who now needs assistance with feeding, bathing, dressing, and mobility and must rely on the adult children to accomplish such daily tasks. The reversal of "helper-helpee" roles can create an environment of kind caring and love or one of hostile dependency. Many community health nurses hear that "when parents grow old they are just like children experiencing second childhood." These phrases contribute to the decline in self-esteem, self-worth, and equalitarian relationships.

A second issue, guilt, is dominant in adult children who think such thoughts as "If only I had 'come sooner,' made the aging adult move in with us, or realized that the behaviors were symptoms of a problem rather than meanness, stubbornness, or cantankerousness." The community health nurse can assist adult children with their middle-life crises, as well as be a resource for helping with the problems of their parents' tasks and crises. The effects on younger children and adolescents also must be managed. Nursing strategies for providing knowledge about normal developmental needs throughout the life span, communication, conflict resolution, and valuing other people are essential in working with multigenerational families.

Living on a fixed income is another important issue for retirees. Many retirees receive Social Security benefits and employment-related pensions. An additional segment may have savings or rental or other supplemental income. Thus budget planning and wise shopping can help those on a fixed income. Some older people supplement their income with part-time work or the exchange of services such as cooking, shopping, childcare, or home cleaning. Other income extenders include food stamps and Supplemental Security Income (SSI) for eligible individuals.

Maintaining Self-Esteem

Self-esteem is critical in the later years of life. Elderly people must often modify the criteria they use to evaluate themselves to reflect their changed position. Community health nurses should encourage planned activities and programs, satisfying interpersonal relationships, good health, quality housing, adequate income, and suitable transportation to promote increased self-esteem (Schwartz, 1978). Other activities include recognition of achievements; providing positive feedback; granting respect and courtesies; promoting choice, decision making, and control; and encouraging and facilitating interpersonal relationships. An observant community health nurse can comment on certificates, rewards, and pictures that may be visible in the living environment. Encouragement for work or volunteer services that use existing knowledge and skills can be valuable; for example, a retired teacher might tutor a group of school children,

another might teach a special hobby to older adults at the multipurpose senior center, a carpenter might assist in building shelves for the display of the center's produced items, and an annual bazaar and sale of crafts might be run by an older business enterpreneur. Each one can be recognized for at least one desirable trait and thereby feel needed and valued. Additionally, the community health nurse must remember the small yet significant value of addressing older adults with appropriate titles such as Mr., Mrs., Miss, Dr., Rev., and Father. Policymakers should be aware of the effect of policies on elderly adults. Policies can implicitly state that "we care about you," "old people are of value to this country," and "minority producers and consumers also have clout."

Coping with Loss and Grief

Loss and grief are often experienced by elderly adults and threaten the maintenance of self-esteem. Loss of roles through retirement, health from chronic illnesses, and death of a spouse are just a few of the losses. Women are at higher risk for loss of a spouse because women outnumber men and live longer. Married women can expect to live some of their later years in widowhood. Additionally, remarriage following widowhood is less frequent in women because there are fewer older men, and older men generally select younger women as spouses.

The beginning phase of grief is characterized by a person experiencing shock, disbelief, and denial. Sadness and crying follow as people become fully aware of the reality of death. The survivors carry out the ritual of a funeral and other culturally meaningful practices as part of the grieving process. The steps of living alone, relinquishing the lost spouse, and reinvesting in something and someone else awaits the widow or widower. Nursing activities of providing correct information, a sense of reality, supportive listening, and caring during periods of crying and other emotional releases are essential to healthy grieving. The community health nurse can be a caring individual and provider when the family and friends have returned to their routine activities and the mourner is left alone to deal with problems of loneliness, social isolation, altered finances, changed living arrangements, and a new identity.

After sustaining a major loss, life problems may mount so that some older adults see ending their own lives as a viable alternative. There is an alarming suicide rate in the elderly. The suicide rate of white males over 65 years of age (41.6 of 100,000) is approximately four times the national rate (11.6 of 100,000), with blacks and women committing fewer suicides (National Center, 1987). Early recognition of danger signs and timely interventions can decrease the problem. Clues to the potential for suicide include a refusal to eat, medication misuse, and noncompliance with health-sustaining treatment regimens. During contacts with older adults, community health nurses should watch for suicide risks, recognize and compliment clients on areas of individual worth and esteem, and encourage meaningful activities and associations.

Time is important in healing the wound of loss and in allowing for successful grieving. Self-help groups and counseling may be beneficial during this phase for assisting the remaining spouse to cope with loss without feeling guilty or losing self-esteem. Factors such as fewer marriages, co-habitation, more divorces, childlessness, geographic mobility, financial instability, and improved educational and health status present special challenges in planning care for future widows or widowers. People must be educated to plan for their later years in life-style choices that are made throughout life. Preparation for widowhood must include financial and psychosocial planning.

Dealing with Depression

Depression is a common health problem of the aged but is often masked by other complaints and problems. Signs include complaints of sadness, insomnia, anorexia, weight loss, and constipation. Frequently these complaints are undervalued and labeled as normal complaints of old age or as hypochondria.

Treatment of the problem must include a thorough history, counseling, and careful use of medication. Assessment can be made using questions such as the following: Do you awaken during the early morning hours and find yourself unable to return to sleep? Is it hard to "get going" in the morning? Do you feel better as the day progresses? Have your appetite and food intake changed from their usual patterns? Do you have crying spells?

Community health nurses can help older adults adjust to the changes of aging, cope with declining years and health, and view life as meaningful and valuable by aiding in arranging an activity schedule including rest periods, teaching normal expectations of aging and signs of impending health problems, and devising ways of managing financial demands with a fixed income. Nurses, as sensitive listeners, can be partners for older adults in the life-review process. The life-review process, including reminiscing about past joys, accomplishments, and disappointments, is helpful to the older adult in reconciling unresolved conflicts, bringing order to life, relinquishing life, and preparing for death.

The community health nurse may determine that the client is unresponsive to nursing interventions and that additional care is warranted. Referral to a community mental health center, physician, or hospital may be needed. The community health nurse should maintain contact with the referral agency so that continuity of care is provided. Additionally, a record of the care rendered by the community health nurse should be sent, with the written permission of the client, to the referral agency to avoid unnecessary delays and duplications.

Abuse of the Elderly

As described in Chapter 24, family violence continues to be a serious community problem, whether it is violence of a child, a spouse, or an elderly member. Abuse of the elderly can be physical, psychological, or material abuse, as well as violations of the rights for safety, security, and adequate health care. The classic profile of the elderly victim of abuse is generally an older woman with mental or physical impairments who lives with an adult child or other relative. Abusers are often middle-age women, who are related or unrelated caretakers and who often are experiencing considerable stress. Other contributory factors include financial status, interpersonal conflicts, life responsibilities, health,

and dependency (Elder Abuse, 1980). Often out of fear, the abused person denies that abusive acts are occurring. The victim's helplessness and resignation to abuse increase as the victim tries to protect both self and the caretaker.

Using a family-oriented approach, interventions include counseling for both the abused and the abusers and teaching stress management techniques. In selected instances, placement of the abused adult in a protected setting outside of the home, family vacations from the older adult, and sharing of responsibilities among children may be necessary.

Criminal Victimization

Many elderly individuals are the victims of confidence games, manhandling, fraudulent consumerism, and crimes against persons and property. The fear of crime prevents many elderly persons from leaving their homes, thus making them prisoners. The frail, sensory-impaired, poor, older woman who lives alone is a prime candidate for criminal victimization. Physical injury often results from the criminal activity. The popularity of confidence games or swindle tactics such as "bank examiner–crooked bank employee" and "pigeon drop–good faith money" continue to be major threats to the security of older adults. The bank examiner–crooked bank employee game consists of a stranger posing as a bank examiner, federal agent, or special police officer who tells the older adult the story of trying to catch a crooked bank employee and needing the older person to withdraw a large amount of cash money from the bank to trap the employee. The pigeon drop–good faith money swindle involves a stranger approaching an elderly person with the pretense of having found a large sum of money that will be shared with the elderly person; however, the elderly person first must withdraw some money from the bank to show good faith. The elderly person may even be given an envelope, allegedly containing the money, and be instructed not to open the envelope, which actually contains cutup paper.

The community health nurse can caution elderly clients about home repair rip-offs, admitting strangers into one's residence, withdrawing large sums of money from the bank on the request of a stranger, flashing or displaying large sums of money, leaving car or house doors unlocked, and walking alone in dimly lighted, deserted areas. Older adults may need assistance in reading and understanding legal papers and transactions. They also should be taught how to evaluate and use products.

HEALTH CARE USE AND COSTS

As a group, older persons are major users of health services. Persons 65 years of age and older averaged 9.1 physician visits in 1986. Although the elderly make up approximately 12% of the population, they are responsible for about 19.6% of physician visits. Hospitalization statistics indicate that the 65- to 74-year-old age group had an average hospital stay of 8.2 days in 1985, whereas persons 75 to 84 years old averaged 9.1 hospital days. The length of the hospital stay increased to 9.6 days for adults 85 years of age and older. Although hospital stays are relatively short, multiple admissions per year are common (National Center, 1987).

Soaring health care costs continue to be a problem for all age groups but are of particular concern for the elderly, who usually have at least one chronic health problem. Health care costs and expenditures for the elderly are approximately one third of the nation's total health care expenditure, yet they only account for 12% of the population. Although the elderly pay for part of their health care costs (25%), public funds such as Medicare and Medicaid are the major sources.

In April 1983, Public Law 98-21 of the Social Security Amendments was signed into law. Title VI of this law stipulates that Medicare reimbursement for hospital inpatient services be on a prospective payment system (Smith, 1985). This payment system, or Diagnostic Related Groups (DRGs), has created a national health care revolution. The DRGs reimbursement approach is based on payment of a predetermined amount for the care of persons who have a medically related diagnosis and treatment and a similar length of hospital stay. Gender and age factors are also considered in the classification of a person into any of the 467 diagnostic groups. In addition to reimbursement for health care, the system also reviews quality assurance and use (Chapter 4 provides further discussion of DRGs.)

Many changes in the health care system have been attributed to DRGs. The most notable is the earlier discharge of clients. More formal and informal caregivers are required to provide services to recovering individuals. When available, the family has become an even greater partner in health care delivery. However, the increased number of women who are employed outside the home creates a major barrier to providing continuing care at home to elderly persons who have experienced a brief hospitalization or early discharge or who need a longer recuperation. Furthermore, bureaucratic barriers are encountered if the need for home health care exceeds the provisions as designated by Medicare guidelines and time frames. The needs of the elderly as listed by Auerbach (1986) are for chronic illness monitoring, supportive services, and acute, posthospitalization care. Medicare categorizes this type of care as requiring unskilled nursing except during the immediate postacute phase, which creates many difficulties for elderly people, their families, and home health care agencies. It is not uncommon for a home health care nurse to be assigned an elderly person who undergoes intravenous therapy and parenteral nutrition and has a respirator. The need for professional nursing services has grown more intense with these health care changes.

Futurists have predicted that during the next decade that changes in eldercare will occur in the structuring, use, and financing of health care and in the type and number of health care providers. The health care structure will change from a separate system of acute care, long-term care, and social and support services to a central entry system of coordinated care and services. Federal funding for eldercare will be reorganized and there will be an increased sharing of costs among the elderly, public sources, and private corporations. Use of health maintenance and preferred provider organizations will grow. Regulations, incentives, consumerism, and quality control will be hallmarks of the health care system for the elderly. The providers of care increasingly will be professional nurses, physician assistants, allied health professionals, paraprofessionals, and volunteers (Dychtwald and Zitter, 1988; Selker and Braoski, 1988). Ed-

ucation and training of these providers will be essential to improving the health care and quality of life for older persons.

HOME HEALTH SERVICES

Many elderly persons require daily care from a home health care professional and supportive assistance from home health aides. Home health care services combined with homemaker services prevent or delay institutionalization for older adults who need some assistance with self-care and other activities of daily living and some care for chronic health problems. Agencies providing home health care, homemaker services, or both may be governmental, proprietary, or hospital based and funded. The combined staff may include a nurse, social worker, physician, occupational therapist, and aide. Some states and agencies require some type of training program and certification for home health care aides. Home health care is covered by Medicare for the person meeting a requirement for skilled care. The care is provided by a professional nurse, home health aide working under the direction of the professional nurse, or both. The aide performs personal hygiene tasks, measures vital signs, and gives technical care. In contrast to the home health care aide, the homemaker aide, whose services are not covered under Medicare, does light housework and cooking. The visiting nurses' association, community health nurses from local public health departments, and nurses from private agencies provide professional nursing services to homebound persons needing skilled care.

Chapter 4 contains more information on the economics of health care. Attention to policy issues, problem resolutions, instructions at the time of discharge, and advocacy activities is essential to an effective community health care practice. Community health nurses are a vital link in the health care system; they provide care, institute preventive measures, and reduce functional impairment.

ALTERNATIVES TO INSTITUTIONALIZATION

Day care centers, day hospitals, respite care, and congregate housing are aimed at delaying or preventing institutionalization. Adult day care centers associated with health care institutions or ambulatory care settings and multipurpose adult day care centers are two models of adult day care (Emick-Herring, 1983; Koenen, 1980). Health-oriented day care centers provide health and physical rehabilitation, whereas multipurpose day care centers provide social activities and interaction. Day care centers serve the person who has some physical or mental limitation that interferes with totally independent living and who needs social, nutritional, or recreational services. Day care centers also allow the permanent caretaker to use day hours for work or other activities. The day hospital is directed toward providing day health services to a person who can live at home during the evening. The respite care program provides care for the dependent older person while the permanent caretaker has time off for rest, recuperation, recreation, or an emergency. The services may be used for several days to a week; however, the services provide only time-limited care, and their goal is the return of the dependent older person to a refreshed caretaker.

Congregate housing is an alternative living arrangement that provides shelter and supportive services to assist the elderly in effectively managing community living. This type of housing arrangement is best suited for the older adult who is independent or semi-independent and has some functional impairment or social deprivation but is otherwise healthy. Congregate housing may include single or multiple units arranged into a community with some commonly shared areas, such as recreational facilities.

The alternatives to institutionalization have disadvantages. Problems of eligibility, cost, access, service limitations, and the impact of long-term disability and care on the client and the family exist and are challenges to the health care system. Should chronic care receive only marginal support and importance? Should eligibility guidelines eliminate more people from services? Should a family that chooses to keep the older person at home be penalized? Is the older adult forced into a more dependent role just to obtain minimal help? The political, professional, ethical, and legal ramifications of each answer must be examined.

LONG-TERM CARE IN INSTITUTIONAL SETTINGS

When situations of declining health, depleted physical, financial, and human resources, and increased dependency occur, institutionalization in a long-term care facility may become a necessity. A long-term care facility may become a necessity. A long-term care facility provides long-term or extended residential, intermediate, or skilled nursing care, medical care, and personal and psychosocial services. The level and type of services offered determine the criteria that clients must meet to satisfy local, state, and federal requirements. Additionally, federal Medicare and Medicaid guidelines and regulations must be met by participating agencies. Guidelines at each level—local, state, and federal—generally address the type of client; staff qualifications and ratio; environmental regulations; health care; client rights; and food, recreational, and social services. Individual needs and resources determine which type of facility is most appropriate for the client.

The decision to institutionalize a client is usually a difficult one for the client and the family. The client may experience a sense of helplessness, a loss of control, independence, and love, and an overwhelming feeling of abandonment. Going to a "nursing home" or an "old folk's home" is viewed as a "last resort." The giving away of possessions and selling of the "home house" indicate that the client is going away, never to return to familiar or loved surroundings. The family has to cope with feelings of conflict, ambivalence, blame, guilt, and helplessness. The community health nurse must support the family members, understanding that they have made the best decision for their situation. The community health nurse can facilitate the expression of feelings by such phrases as the following: "It is usually hard to place a loved one in a nursing home. I wonder what it is like for you?" "Sometimes families have second thoughts about putting a loved one in a nursing home." "I imagine this is a difficult time for you." The family and the older adult must be encouraged to talk *with* each other and not just *to* each other. Listening and hearing become important as the family seeks the best answer.

The community health nurse also must be an advocate for the family, a negotiator between the older adult and other family members, and a resource person. Family contacts should be followed up with visits, telephone calls, or both to determine what actions have been taken by the family and if additional assistance is needed. During each encounter with the family, the community health nurse must remember to apply the concepts of choice, rights, responsibility, and decision making to assist the family in formulating a practical solution. The admission of the client to the long-term care facility is not the termination of care to the family. The family needs the nurse during this period of crisis and adjustment.

Long-term care facilities cannot be discussed without considering the image of such facilities. Many years ago these facilities were referred to as "nursing homes", yet neither the staffing pattern nor activities demonstrated much "nursing" or "home." Perhaps the first effort at changing the image of these facilities would be to change the name. A second factor would be to look at staffing and mechanisms for recruiting and retaining capable professional nurses for these facilities. Third, the public needs to be educated about the different types of facilities and how to select the most appropriate facility according to the needs and preference of the individual. The public must also change its values about long-term care facilities so that adequate resources are provided to correct some of the problems of the long-term care industry. The combined forces of the population growth pattern, the prevalence of chronic illnesses, and social forces such as working women, an increasing divorce rate, and a declining birth rate require that the long-term care industry be modified and that alternative resources be created.

HOSPICE

A hospice is a community resource available for the care of the terminally ill. A hospice program has a family orientation and is concerned with the special needs and care of the terminally ill person. The quality of life and decision making for the family and individual are focal points in the delivery of medical, nursing, spiritual, and social care by an interdisciplinary team. Hospice programs may be hospital based or exist separately. Many elderly persons experiencing the later stages of a terminal illness may view this community resource as an answer to the wish to live and die with comfort and dignity and to having their family at their side. Additional information about hospice care is available in Chapter 42.

LEGISLATION AND COMMUNITY RESOURCES AND PROGRAMS

The legislative and political aspects of aging pervade every other aspect of aging. Programs such as Social Security, Older American's Act, and Medicare have altered some of the issues of later life and will continue to do so. Nurses should be informed about the legislative process and legislation and policies that influence health care in general and the elderly population in particular.

The Social Security Act became law in August 1935 during the administration of Franklin D. Roosevelt. Eligibility for Social Security, a general public retirement pension, is based on previous work history and age. There are also survivor, disability, and health benefits. The Social Security Act has been amended in several significant ways. Two key amendments, Medicare in 1966 and Supplemental Security Income (SSI) in 1974, have special importance for the elderly. The Supplemental Security Income (SSI) includes a federal supplement to adults with inadequate incomes.

In 1966 Medicare was instituted as a health insurance program for older Americans. Covered services include hospitalization, skilled nursing home care, physician's services, and home health care. The services not covered by Medicare are so great that they are frequently referred to as "Medi-gap." Many private insurance companies have programs specifically designed to cover these services.

Medicaid as a health care program for the poor, exclusive of age eligibility, is administered by individual states. These programs, in addition to Social Security benefits, have meant an improved life-style for the poor, including improved health care, food, shelter, and clothing.

The Older American's Act of 1965 and its amendments established the United States Administration of Aging, which deals with program funding, training, and research. The responsibility for coordinating and planning services for the elderly—such as multipurpose senior centers, nutrition centers, employment, and transportation services at a local level—is vested in the Area Agency on Aging (AAA). Multipurpose senior centers created by Title V of the Older American's Act provide health, social, legal, educational, and recreational services. Title VII of the Older American's Act provides nutrition programs for the elderly. Nutrition services are offered in group settings or are delivered to people at home via Meals on Wheels. In addition to partially meeting individual nutritional requirements, socialization and education needs are met. The Older American's Act Amendments of 1981 provide a state ombudsman program for long-term care facilities and boarding homes.

Major legislations enacted during the 1980s included the Health Insurance Continuation Act of 1986; the Nursing Home Reform Act of 1987; and the Pension Reform and Spousal Impoverishment Protection of 1988. The aims of these legislations are the provision of expanded health insurance coverage, the improvement of health care, and the protection of personal assets.

AGING NETWORK

The aging network includes organizations concerned with advocacy, special populations, and volunteer services by older people. As of 1969, two components of the National Older American Volunteer Program are Retired Senior Volunteer Program and Foster Grandparents Program. Volunteer activities in hospitals, schools, nursing homes, and other settings are provided by members of the Retired Senior Volunteer Program (RSVP). Persons who are 60 years of age and older may volunteer their services. These volunteers are provided transportation and meals in connection with their volunteer activities. The Foster Grandparents Program offers an opportunity for older people and children to mutually share, meet needs, and experience gratification across

generations. The Gray Panthers, organized by Margaret (Maggie) Kuhn, began as an advocacy group for change and social justice. Currently, the combined assets and forces of young and old are directed toward investigative research, legislative action, monitoring of services to the aged, and organization of training for the Gray Panthers network (Kuhn, 1976). The National Council of Senior Citizens (NCSC) was founded in 1961 out of the need to defeat the American Medical Association's campaign against Medicare, thereby becoming one of the first senior powers (Kleyman, 1974). The Older Women's League (OWL) was founded in 1980 by Tish Sommers and Laurie Shields to address the special needs of midlife and older women.

Awareness of and sensitivity to the needs of black Americans and concern about national goals and the necessity for activities to address these needs stimulated Hobart Jackson to organize the National Caucus on the Black Aged (NCBA). The NCBA is an advocacy group for the improvement of the quality of life for older persons of minority groups (Jackson, 1976). Other organizations concerned about issues involving the aged include the American Association of Retired Persons (AARP) and the National Retired Teachers Association.

Four White House conferences on aging have been held, one each decade beginning in 1950, to hear concerns and issues of importance to older Americans and to propose plans for national policies on aging for the next decade. The 1981 conference centered on the theme "The Aging Society: Challenge and Opportunity." The conference focused on more than 600 recommendations; however, the following recommendations were highlighted: strengthen the Social Security system, prohibit mandatory retirement, increase the availability of home and community-based health care, and emphasize preventive health care. A national policy on aging that emerged from this fourth conference has the following goals (Final Report, 1981):

1. To provide the elderly with the maximum opportunity to live an independent and healthy life and to encourage them to remain in the economic and social mainstream.
2. To provide economic, medical, and social support to the elderly who need help.
3. To encourage serious discussion of the choices we must make as a result of the very large baby boom generation that will become elderly in the twenty-first century.

The health objectives for the nation's elderly population for the year 2000 include the five areas of health status, risk reduction, public awareness, professional awareness, and services and protection (Public Health, 1989). The objectives focus on increasing the active life expectancy, reducing the incidence and limitations of major health problems and improving health counseling, geriatric training, and policymaking.

Nurses can be advocates for the elderly through cooperative efforts with advocacy groups that influence health and social policies. Nurses can also serve as sources of health information for organizations concerned with the well-being of aged persons.

CLINICAL APPLICATION

A referral was made to the City Home Health Care Agency for Mrs. Rose Lee, a 70-year-old woman who has had essential hypertension since age 35 years. Mrs. Lee has also suffered from arthritis since age 60 years. She was admitted to the hospital twice in the past 6 months for treatment of uncontrolled hypertension. On the last admission, her blood pressure was 190/100, pulse 100, and respiration rate 28 and her temperature was normal. She was prescribed methyldopa (Aldomet) (250 mg. b.i.d. by mouth) and hydrochlorothiazide (Hydro Diuril) (50 mg qd by mouth). She was told to consume a low-sodium diet.

When Mrs. Lee was visited in her home by the home health care nurse 1 week after discharge from the hospital, the nurse found more pills in the medicine bottles than should have been present had Mrs. Lee been taking the medication as prescribed. Her blood pressure was still elevated and she had minimal knowledge of what constituted a low-sodium diet. When the nurse talked with her about her illness, how she felt, and how she was managing it, Mrs. Lee responded, "I feel fine some of the time; this medicine doesn't help me any" and "Sometimes I don't take my medicine, but I feel fine usually."

The nursing diagnosis was: noncompliance to prescribed medicine related to nonacceptance of a chronic illness. The nurse established with Mrs. Lee the following goals:

1. She will take the antihypertensive medicine as prescribed for at least 3 months. (This will be evaluated by the number of pills in the bottles at each nursing visit, by patient self-report, and by a decrease in blood pressure to the range of 150/90 to 160/90.)
2. Mrs. Lee will talk about her ideas, feelings, and fears related to her diagnosis.

Specific nursing actions to be taken included: (1) assist Mrs. Lee to develop a medication record system using specific medication times and a medication calendar check-off list; (2) determine the number of antihypertensive pills taken and when; (3) discuss with the pharmacist the use of easy to open medication containers; (4) take and record lying, sitting, and standing blood pressure and pulse at least once per week; (5) help Mrs. Lee discuss her ideas, feelings and actions related to her chronic illness; (6) teach Mrs. Lee and one family member or significant other about medications, food, and their relationship to essential hypertension.

One month later when the nurse made a follow-up home visit, she found that Mrs. Lee's blood pressure was 150/90 and had been close to that reading for the past 3 weeks as evidenced on a chart that the patient was keeping. According to Mrs. Lee's medication chart and the number of pills remaining in the bottles, she had been taking the medication correctly. In the follow-up discussion, Mrs. Lee talked about how hard it is to follow a low-salt diet, but described specific recipes that she had followed and acknowledged that she was making progress here also.

The nurse planned to continue monthly home visits to determine if Mrs. Lee was able to comply with her treatment regimen and also to support and encourage her in the actions that would help to maintain a lowered blood pressure.

SUMMARY

Older Americans are influencing the cultural orientation of this country, as seen in efforts to prevent polarization between generations and to educate the public about and change attitudes toward the elderly, which encourage a perception of the elderly as diverse people who are a national resource and asset. Many minority groups, such as blacks, Hispanics, Native Americans, and Pacific Asians, honor and respect the elderly for their unique needs and assets. The myths of older adults as institutionalized, poor, unable to learn, accident prone, passive, and sexless are being replaced with new knowledge, perceptions, and attitudes. The valuing of "oldness" will possibly increase as the elderly population continues to grow, with members of the baby boom generation reaching age 65 years during the twenty-first century. The theories of aging—including the disengagement, activity, continuity, and developmental and biological theories—will be tested as explanations are sought for the aging phenomenon. The developmental task of adjusting to declining health, death, retirement, and changing interpersonal relationships will be addressed for its contribution to health aging.

The major health problems of this population are heart disease, malignancies, and cerebrovascular diseases.

Health problems such as arthritis, sensory impairments, and confusion limit activity and affect comfort and independence. Decreasing functional dependency is one goal in the improvement of the health of older adults, enabling them to function at their optimal physical, social, and psychological level.

Criminal victimization, drug misuse, abuse from relatives and institutional caregivers, and social isolation are psychosocial issues affecting the health and quality of life of aged persons. An interdisciplinary approach to solving these problems is necessary to prevent occurrences at epidemic levels. Health, social, and political organizations must join forces to fight abuse and victimization.

Health promotion involves adequate nutrition; a balance of exercise, rest, and activity; immunizations against influenza and pneumonia; assistance with time management; and optimum self-esteem. These are central to healthy older adults, for whom the dream of retirement and "lots of time on hand" has become a reality.

Community health nurses as caregivers must assist older adults to capitalize on their assets and guide them in coping with the process of living with chronic illnesses and disabilities. A life theme of moderation, variety, and balance contributes to healthy older years. The art of decision making, the privilege of choice, and the responsibility of self-discipline are essential in solving problems of living and aging.

KEY CONCEPTS

The elderly are the fastest growing population in the United States. Their increased longevity and the accompanying high incidence of chronic disease pose a substantial challenge to the health care system. Technology can keep people alive much longer, yet such care is costly and often uncomfortable.

In recent years, aging as a life process has received greater focus and study. The earlier lack of emphasis on this population group perpetuated many myths and stereotypes.

According to Erikson's theory, aging is viewed as the successful resolution of the conflict between the critical tasks of integrity and despair.

Physical, as well as psychosocial or developmental, changes accompany aging. The observed changes represent the cumulative and lifelong effects of heredity, environment, nutrition, rest, activity, and altered health status.

Although many older adults enjoy good health and freedom of activity, approximately 80% has at least one chronic health problem.

The ability to successfully adjust to retirement is affected by factors such as health status, sufficient income, number of situational changes, quality of personal relationships, ability to manage time effectively, flexibility, ability to relinquish the work routine, and anticipation and realistic expectation for retirement.

Older persons are major users of health services. Persons aged 65 to 74 years average 9.1 physician visits annually. Although the elderly constitute approximately 12% of the population, they are responsible for about 19.6% of physician visits.

The legislative and political aspects of aging pervade every other aspect of aging.

The myths of older adults as institutionalized, poor, unable to learn, accident prone, passive, and sexless are being replaced with new knowledge, perceptions, and attitudes. The valuing of "oldness" will possibly increase as this nation's elderly population continues to grow.

LEARNING ACTIVITIES

1. Develop a hypothetical chart that identifies the developmental tasks of the older adult; Identify potential problems that might interfere with accomplishing the task.

2. Make a developmental task chart for a client with whom you have been working and enumerate the problems you have observed resulting from inability to satisfactorily master the developmental task(s).

3. Based on the problems with completing developmental tasks

identified in the preceding activity, develop a nursing plan of action for at least two of these problems.

4. Interview two elderly people and determine what myths and stereotypes they perceive younger people hold about them.

5. Read your local newspaper to find at least three stories that discuss older adults. Do the stories portray them in a positive or negative way?

BIBLIOGRAPHY

Auerbach M: Changes in home health care delivery, Nurs Outlook 33:290, 1986.

Cristofalo VJ: An overview of the theories of biological aging. In Birren JE and Bengtson V, editors: Emerg Theories Aging, New York, 1988, Springer.

Cummings E and Henry WE: Growing old: the process of disengagement, New York, 1961, Basic Books.

Dychtwald K and Zitter M: Changes during the next decade will alter the way eldercare is provided, financed, Mod Health C 18(16):38, 1988.

Ebersole P and Hess P: Toward health: aging human needs and nursing response, St Louis, 1990, Mosby-Year Book.

Elder abuse, Washington DC, 1980, Office of Human Development Services, Department of Health and Human Services.

Emick-Herring BC: Adult day care: support system for disabled elderly and their caregivers, Rahabil Nurs 8:29, 1983.

Erickson EH: Childhood and society, New York, 1963, WW Norton.

Final report: the 1981 White House Conference on Aging, Washington DC, 1981, Department

of Health and Human Services.

Havighurst RJ: Successful aging. In Williams RH, Tibbilts C, and Donahue W, editors: Process of aging, vol 1, New York, 1963, Atherton Press.

Healthy people: background papers. Washington, DC, 1979, Public Health Service, Office of the Assistant Secretary for Health and Surgeon General, Department of Health, Education, and Welfare.

Jackson HC: Black advocacy: techniques and trials. In Kerschner PA, editor: Advocacy and age, Los Angeles, 1976, The University of Southern California Press.

Kleyman P: Senior power, San Francisco, 1974, Glide Publications.

Koenen RE: Adult day care: a northwest perspective, J Gerontol Nurs 6:218, 1980.

Kuhn ME: What old people want for themselves and others in society. In Kerschner PA, editor: Advocacy and age, Los Angeles, 1976, The University of Southern California Press.

National Center for Health Statistics: Advance report of final mortality statistics, vol 33, Hyattsville, MD, 1984, U.S. Public Health Services.

National Council on Aging: The myth and reality

of aging in America, Washington, DC, 1975, The Council.

Office of Human Development Services: Need for long-term care information and issues, Washington, DC, 1981, Office of Human Development Services.

Neugarten BL: Personality in middle and late life, New York, 1964, Atherton Press.

Public Health Service, U.S. Department of Health and Human Services: Promoting health/preventing disease: year 2000 objectives for the nation (draft), Washington, DC, 1989, U.S. Department of Health and Human Services.

Schwartz AN: Counselling the older adults. In O'Brien B, editor: Aging, today's research and you, Los Angeles, 1978, The University of Southern California Press.

Selker LG and Broski DV: An aging society, Gerontol Geriatr Educ 8(3/4):107, 1988.

Smith CE: DRGs: making them work for you, Nurs 85 15:34, 1985.

Steffl B: Theories of aging: biological, psychological, and sociological. In Steffl B, editor: Handbook of gerontological nursing, New York, 1984, Van Nostrand Reinhold.

U.S. Senate Special Committee on Aging: Trends and projections, Washington, DC, 1986, The Committee.

U.S. Bureau of the Census: Statistical abstract of the United States, ed 105, Washington, DC, 1984, The Bureau.

U.S. Bureau of the Census: Statistical abstract of the United States, ed 105, Washington, DC, 1987, The Bureau.

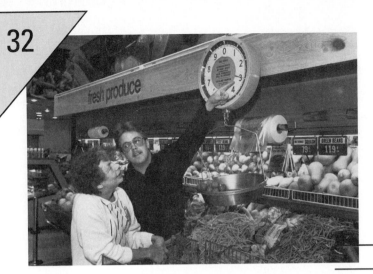

32

The Developmentally Disabled Population

Marcia Cowan

OBJECTIVES

After reading this chapter, the student should be able to:

Define the term *developmental disability*.

Discuss the recent changes in the definition and their effect on the number of children categorized as developmentally disabled.

List at least five categories of conditions that might cause a child to be developmentally disabled.

Discuss three preventive measures that might reduce the number of children identified in these categories.

Discuss the concept of family-centered, community-based care for the developmentally disabled child.

Identify the role of community health nurses in caring for people with developmental disabilities.

Plan a hypothetical program for providing support to families with a member who is developmentally disabled.

KEY TERMS

cerebral palsy
Child Abuse Amendments of 1984
Denver Developmental Screening Test (DDST)
developmental disability
Developmental Profile II

Education for All Handicapped Children Act (PL 94-142)
family-centered care
independent living
learning disabilities
mental retardation

retinopathy of prematurity
social isolation
spina bifida
trisomy 21 (Down's syndrome)
very low–birth-weight

T hroughout history, people with handicaps have been denied rights and privileges afforded to others. Government efforts to ensure that developmentally disabled individuals are treated with dignity and offered the same opportunities of other citizens have not been undertaken until recently. In 1962, President Kennedy's Panel on Mental Retardation made 95 recommendations to ensure humane and appropriate care for the developmentally disabled. These recommendations formed the basis for much of the federal policy currently in effect (Braddock, 1986).

Many children and adults with developmental disabilities are mainstreamed into the community as a result of federal policies and a changing consciousness among the general public. They are likely to live at home, attend public schools, and participate in community health programs. Nurses are in a key role to provide the leadership needed to improve the quality of life for this population. Nurses work with the family, other health care providers, and representatives of community agencies to provide education and health assessment, to assist in family adaptation, and to identify available resources to integrate those with special needs into the community.

The term *developmental disability* refers to a variety of conditions, both mental and physical, that interfere with the ability of an individual to function successfully in society. Public Law (PL)95-602 (Comprehensive Rehabilitation Service Amendments of 1978) gives the following definition:

A developmental disability is a severe, chronic disability of a person which:

A. Is attributable to a mental or physical impairment or a combination of mental and physical impairment
B. Is manifested before the person attains 22 years of age
C. Is likely to continue indefinitely
D. Results in substantial limitations in three or more of the following areas of major life activity:
   1. Self-care
   2. Receptive and expressive language
   3. Learning
   4. Mobility
   5. Self-direction
   6. Capacity for independent living
   7. Economic sufficiency
E. Reflects the person's need for a combination and sequence of special, interdisciplinary or generic care, treatment, or the services which are of lifelong or extended duration and are individually planned and coordinated.

The definition previously used by governmental agencies specified conditions such as cerebral palsy, mental retardation, autism, and epilepsy. The current definition eliminates the need for a specific diagnosis. Expanding the age of onset from 18 to 22 years of age increased the number of people who qualify for resources.

The current definition emphasizes the inability to function in three or more areas of major life activities. The conditions that may interfere with adequate function include environmental deprivation and biological impairment.

Environmental deprivation may involve intellectual impairment resulting from limited opportunities or stimulation to learn. A number of studies, such as Project Headstart, show the short-and long-term benefits of preschool enrichment for environmentally disadvantaged children. The results seem to depend on continued support during school years (Denhoff, 1981).

Biological impairments include genetic, metabolic, neurological, or anatomical defects. A number of coexistent conditions may serve to impair function.

In contrast to the term, *developmental disability, developmental delay* is a broader term referring to a failure to meet developmental landmarks or milestones. Delays do not always indicate a developmental disability. Neither term specifies a diagnosis for the underlying cause of the delay or disability.

Many people who fall within the category of developmental disability are classified as being mentally retarded. *Mental retardation* refers to intellectual function that is below average and coexists with adaptive deficits. Mental retardation is categorized based on intelligence quotients (IQ) derived from standardized testing. The definition approved by the American Association on Mental Deficiency (1983) recognizes an IQ of less than 70 as significantly subaverage.

SCOPE OF THE PROBLEM

The problems associated with developmental disabilities are complex, far-reaching, and profound. There are millions of developmentally disabled people in the United States, and the provision of services for them carries exceptional costs. The actual number of disabled people varies according to the definition used and measurement techniques. As many as 20% to 25% of the population may have a physical or mental handicap (Perry, 1989). The types of disabilities are diverse. Mental retardation, considered the most common disability, actually only comprises 1% to 1.6% of the population (Scheerenberger, 1987; Castellani, 1987). The number of disabled people is increasing as a result of improved medical technology, enabling survival at birth and throughout the life span. Meeting demands for services has led to growing expenditures at the federal, state, and local levels. Government spending for developmental disability programs increased approximately 150% between 1962 and 1984 (Castellani, 1987).

Before 1970, the focus for this population was services and income support. Civil rights and protection from discrimination dominated in 1970 through 1990. The problems for the 1990s will be the balancing of civil rights and service provision in an atmosphere of financial constraints.

CAUSES OF DEVELOPMENTAL DISABILITIES

Definitive causes for developmental disabilities are known in only about 25% of the cases. Of this small percentage, the causes are usually categorized as chromosomal aberrations, neural tube defects, and central nervous system damage occurring in the perinatal period, including the sequelae of premature birth.

Trisomy 21 (Down's syndrome) is the most commonly found chromosomal abnormality. It is estimated to occur at a rate of 1 to 1.2 per 1000 livebirths. Maternal age has been demonstrated to be closely related to the incidence of this condition, which increases markedly when the mother is past age 35 years. However, only 20% of the children with trisomy 21 are born to mothers who are older than 35 years, which is probably the result of the increased availability of genetic screening (Hook, 1982).

Neural tube defects occur at a rate of 1 to 2 per 1000 livebirths and encompass anomalies ranging from anencephaly to spina bifida occulta. *Spina bifida,* currently the second most common birth defect, usually involves serious physical handicaps and may include mental retardation. In addition, 70% of children with myelomeningocele, the most severe form of spina bifida, also have hydrocephaly. Medical complications include serious infections and renal failure and are major causes of morbidity and mortality during infancy and early childhood (Nelson and Crocker, 1983). Early surgical intervention and infant stimulation programs have improved the outlook for these children. However, treatment is expensive, difficult for some families to obtain, and emotionally stressful for the entire family. The constant care, prolonged grief, and financial burden create a tremendous problem for the child and the family.

Most children who have spina bifida are of normal intelligence, but because of severe physical problems, it is difficult to find suitable educational programs for them. Consequently, they may have lower IQ test scores simply because physical limitations prevent them from participating in educational activities.

Very low–birth-weight infants (less than 1500 g) are generally considered to be at risk for developmental disabilities. Although advances in neonatal care have improved the survival rate of these infants, recent studies show a 10% to 19% incidence of severe neurological handicaps, intellectual handicaps, or both, and the incidence of severe handicaps reaches 22% to 35% for infants weighing less than 750 g (Hack and Fanaroff, 1988). Problems encountered include hydrocephaly, cerebral palsy, mental retardation, and sensory impairment, especially involving hearing and vision. It is estimated that 500 to 600 infants are blinded each year by *retinopathy of prematurity* (Phelps, 1981). Alterations in parent-infant interaction that occur as a result of prematurity may also place infants at risk for developmental delay.

Maternal infections during pregnancy that can result in developmental problems include rubella, cytomegalovirus, and toxoplasmosis. Infectious agents, chemicals, drugs, and physical agents can all be considered teratogens. Teratogens are any agents or factors that cause permanent alterations of the fetus in form or function during prenatal development. The extent of damage is determined by the systems developing in the embryo or fetus at the time of exposure. Severe infections and metabolic disorders, including phenylketonuria and hypothyroidism, can lead to central nervous system damage during infancy.

Central nervous system damage may result in *cerebral palsy*, a disorder of movement and posture. Damage resulting in cerebral palsy may occur prenatally, perinatally or in childhood. Birth asphyxia and prematurity are the two major risk factors in the cause of cerebral palsy (Paneth, 1986). Mental retardation occurs in 50% of affected individuals (Taft & Matthews, 1983).

Some children who have *learning disabilities* may also be classified as developmentally disabled. Because *learning disability* is a poorly defined term, prevalence figures vary widely. The child's performance may be affected in specific areas of neurological function such as memory, language, selective attention, perception, and motor abilities. Areas of emotional function may also be involved, including social perception and the ability to interact with peers. Learning disabilities include a broad range of problems that may interfere with a child's ability to function normally in society (Levine, 1980).

PREVENTION
Primary Prevention

To be effective, preventive measures must begin with education of the parents before conception. Social behavior, environmental factors, family mores, and moral issues are parts of this complex problem. Technological advances, research, and improved standards of living have contributed to increased infant survival rates and to a longer life span for most people, yet a large number of children continue to have developmental disabilities.

Family planning services, genetic counseling, comprehensive prenatal care, immunizations, decreasing use of drugs and alcohol, and continuing research are all preventive means that need to be used to the fullest extent. It has been predicted that the number of developmentally disabled children could be reduced by one half if all the available knowledge was now applied.

Nurses play a vital role in preventive measures before conception through family planning and counseling with high-risk parents such as teenagers, women over 35 years of age, and families with histories of developmental disabilities.

Prenatal care that begins early and continues throughout pregnancy has been a vital factor in the prevention of problematic pregnancies and births. Included in this care is identification of mothers at risk for having a child with a developmental disability. This list includes women age 35 years and older; women who have had a child with a congenital abnormality; and those with a history of drug abuse, alcoholism, infectious diseases, environmental exposure to toxic substances, or premature births.

Families at risk need support from the nurse. They may need information, referral, encouragement, or a combination of these to seek and follow through with services that are available. Amniocentesis is frequently suggested to these families. Parents need to understand the procedure, its purpose, and its value.

If the fetus is at risk for or has an actual developmental disorder, the possibility of abortion presents a difficult decision for most parents. The nurse must be skilled in supporting the parents in the decision they make.

Secondary and Tertiary Prevention: Early Intervention and Prevention of Further Disability

Early intervention programs seek to stimulate the development of children who are not progressing at an appropriate rate of motor, cognitive, language, or socioemotional development. Interventions are ideally aimed at promoting

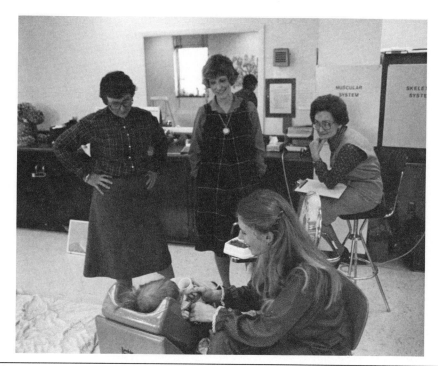

FIGURE 32-1

Interdisciplinary team evaluation.

optimal development, prevention of secondary disabilities, and improvement of family function. Programs are based on theories that stimulation strengthens functional connections or enhances the development of new pathways in the central nervous system. Studies of the effectiveness of such programs are plagued with problems related to numbers and outcome criteria; however, these studies generally find improvements in personal and social skills and in family interaction.

Prevention of further disabling conditions is a sound reason for recommending early intervention programs. Although much controversy still exists about the value of early stimulation for the child with a developmental disability, its importance has been recognized by many nurses working with these children and their families.

Early intervention services may include nursing, occupational therapy, physical therapy, speech pathology, child development, social work, nutrition, psychology, audiology, and medicine. The interdisciplinary team works together to promote all areas of development. Nursing services may include case management, health assessment, dealing with actual or potential health problems, administration of medications or treatments, and collaboration with other team members to develop family service plans. Figure 32-1 depicts an interdisciplinary team evaluation; in Figure 32-2, the occupational therapist is adapting a stroller to provide appropriate positioning for the child.

Early intervention programs can be beneficial for both the child's development and the parent's feeling of competence as illustrated by the following case study.

A 10-month-old child was brought to a university-affiliated program by the mother through a referral from a community health nurse. When examined by the nurse, this child, Amy, could not lift her head, did not attend well to voice commands, and had a weak sucking reflex. The mother was distraught, discouraged, and physically exhausted. She had accepted the physician's diagnosis that Amy had severe brain damage and had been giving the medications as ordered for her child. She had continued to care for her like a newborn infant but expressed the need to know what she could do to help her child.

A team of experts evaluated the child, and a program was designed with the participation of the mother. The program involved some visits to the center for demonstration and reinforcement, but most of the activities prescribed were carried out in the home by the parents. The nurse at the center coordinated the program with the community health nurse, family, and the center.

Progress was slow for Amy, but it did occur. Within 3 months she was lifting and turning her head in response to sound. Moreover, socialization was seen as she began to respond positively to her parents with some eye contact and facial expressions.

Experiences such as this demonstrate that many of these children can be helped through early stimulation programs. The value to the family is inestimable. This young mother appeared to have a new lease on life as a result of the progress made by her child.

Early and continuous assessment of these children aids in identifying other problems, such as hearing or visual deficits. Recognition and treatment should enhance the learning ability of the child. Figures 32-3 and 32-4 illustrate the assessment of motor and speech function. Encouraging the parents to keep the child under medical supervision can prevent the development of further physical problems. Physical stimulation helps to prevent contractures and to strengthen the muscular development of the child. Nutri-

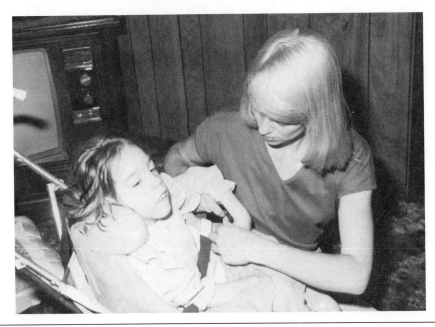

FIGURE 32-2

Occupational therapist performing an intervention.

tional counseling, intellectual stimulation, and up-to-date immunizations are also valuable components of a preventive program for these children.

ROLE OF THE COMMUNITY HEALTH NURSE

The community health nurse caring for a child with a developmental disability must have a sincere concern for the child and family. The child with a problem must first be viewed as an individual worthy of dignity and capable of living for a purpose.

Ideally, physicians and hospital personnel work closely with the community nurse so that referral of the child from hospital to home is made early in the child's life. The community health nurse should visit the child and the parents while they are in the hospital. This provides an opportunity for the community health nurse to meet the medical team and the nursing staff. The community health nurse should have access to all the medical information and the medical plan for the child so that steps for the child's care within the community can be coordinated.

Information acquired from observations, interviews, and test results is used to develop care plans for the child. Often the community health nurse is the health care coordinator for the child and the family. Assessment skills, knowledge of community resources, familiarity with the medical plan, and effective communication abilities are essential assets for such a coordinator.

Developmental Assessment

Nurses are responsible for pediatric screening and assessments beginning in the immediate neonatal period and continuing throughout childhood. Several conditions that categorize a child as developmentally disabled can be identified at birth, but many do not become apparent until the child is older. Developmental and behavioral assessments are performed by nurses to provide early detection of developmental disabilities and as a part of the ongoing care for disabled children and adolescents.

Developmental assessments and adaptive behavior judgments are made by observing the child in the home, physician's office, school, or clinic. One or several tools may be used by the nurse to validate observations. The *Denver Developmental Screening Test (DDST)* is one of the simplest and most economical measures to identify developmental delays for the child from birth to 6 years of age. The test can be administered in less than 30 minutes and identifies many of the strengths and weaknesses of the child. Four areas of evaluation included in the DDST are personal/social, fine motor/adaptive, language, and gross motor development. The test may be used repeatedly to plot the individual child's development over a period of time. Instructions for using the test are written on the back of each form.

The DDST must be administered by the examiner to one child at a time. Some items required direct observation of performance, and others may be reported by the parent. The test yields reliable information that can be most helpful as a screening tool. The DDST may be administered by nonprofessionals with minimal training and is relatively inexpensive. It is used effectively to identify developmental delays or for follow-up assessments. The test does not measure intelligence quotient, and those who use the DDST should explain its purpose clearly to the parents to lessen the tension associated with any examination.

The *Denver Prescreening Developmental Questionnaire (PDQ)* is a short version of the DDST designed to identify children who need further testing with the DDST. It is designed for children 3 months to 6 years of age and is a series of questions designed to be answered with a "yes" or "no" by the parent or caretaker. The test requires less than 10 minutes to complete. Referral is recommended for any child

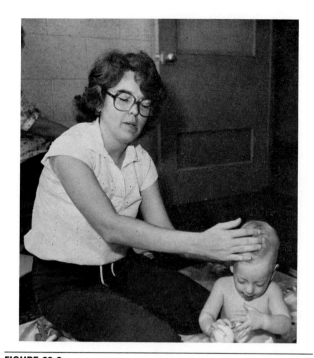

FIGURE 32-3

Assessment of motor function.

with six or fewer "yes" answers. (See Appendix K, and use source for DDST.)

The *Developmental Profile II* is an assessment tool based on the responses of the mother or caretaker to questions posed by the nurse. It is a single test that has been used effectively for a number of years for screening purposes and has been a reliable and valid tool. This standardized test can be used to evaluate children from birth to preadolescence. The test provides developmental age scores in the following five categories: physical/motor, self-help, social, academic, and communication skills. The test can be administered after a short training period and is relatively inexpensive. The evaluation is made in an interview and can be completed in approximately 30 minutes. Parent responses to the questions can yield valuable information that can be used in developing a program for the child. Referrals for further evaluation or placement into programs for children can be made using this instrument. (See Appendix K for source.)

The American Association on Mental Deficiency has designed two instruments to assess the development of children or adults. Both instruments are called the AAMD Adaptive Behavior Scale. The first version of the test was designed to be used by staff members who work with clients in institutions. The later version, the *Public Schools Version*, was designed to be used by schoolteachers or school nurses. Either test yields valuable information that can be used to develop appropriate care plans for children or adults. (See Appendix K for source.)

Several guides, such as the Portage Guide, the Washington Guide to Child Development, and the Hawaii Early Learning Profile Activity Guide (HELP) are useful for nurses planning developmental activities for children.

Sources for these guides are in Appendix K. Each of these guides gives specific steps that parents or teachers can follow to help a child learn a particular skill or advance his or her development. Most are easy to understand and simple to use. No one guide meets every need, so the nurse must use a repertoire of tools.

Health Maintenance and Promotion

Nurses providing care for persons with developmental disabilities assess growth, maturation, and general well-being to help prevent further alterations in health status. Regularly scheduled health assessments can provide early recognition and treatment of problems and serve as the basis for wellness counseling and preventative care. The families of developmentally disabled children, adolescents, and adults have many of the same health promotion and counseling needs as other families; however, these needs are often overlooked because of the emphasis placed on the disability. Additionally, health promotion may be more complex in light of the disability. Alterations in activity and rest patterns, health maintenance, and elimination, potentials for injury, and knowledge deficits should be considered as potential nursing diagnoses.

Sleep patterns should be assessed and problems discussed with parents. Issues such as resistance to going to bed, sleeping in the parent's bed, and night wakening should be managed by establishing a consistent bedtime routine and positively reinforcing appropriate sleep behaviors.

Independence in health maintenance is an important goal for the family and the developmentally disabled individual. Topics for teaching should include the management of minor illness, including temperature assessment, and guidelines for seeking medical attention. Families should be encouraged to participate in cardiopulmonary resuscitation (CPR) training. As the child becomes more independent in activities of daily living, behaviors that promote wellness should be encouraged. Health education related to appropriate food choices, oral hygiene, exercise, grooming, stress management, and the avoidance of substance abuse and smoking should be addressed.

Elimination patterns may vary according to the individual's disability and life-style. Inactivity, ineffective gastrointestinal muscle tone, and inadequate fluid or nutrient intake may predispose the individual to constipation. Medical problems or medications may cause diarrhea. Interventions such as dietary modifications, increasing activity, use of medications, and skin care may be indicated. Toilet training will often need to be addressed with caregivers. It may be necessary to adapt the bathroom to facilitate appropriate positioning. Assisting the family to determine readiness for training includes assessment of the following areas: cognitive awareness of elimination, an established pattern of voiding and elimination, and ability to communicate the need. Programs of behavior management, including rewarding appropriate behaviors, may be sufficient to accomplish toilet training. However, with severe disabilities, bowel and bladder management programs may be indicated.

Safety issues should be based on the individual's developmental status. As developmental gains are attained, families need to become aware of the changing safety issues.

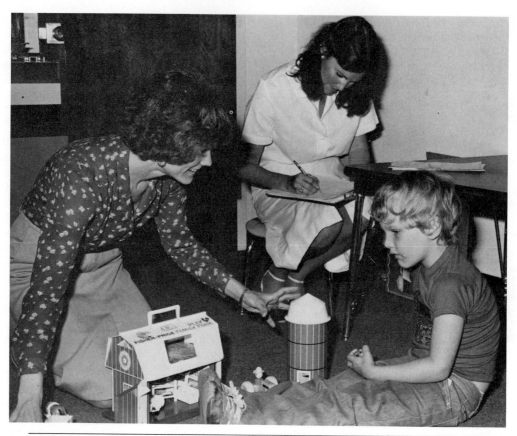

FIGURE 32-4

Speech evaluation

As the child becomes mobile, poison prevention, electrical safety, and falls should be addressed. Car restraints are a critically important issue. It may be necessary to work with other disciplines, such as physical therapy or occupational therapy, to provide adaptive automobile seating. Older children and adults should be taught the importance of using seat belts.

Health education related to the diagnosis of the disability is important. Explanations of the diagnosis should be provided for the family and for the child as he or she develops to a level of understanding. Encouraging questions and providing appropriate educational materials will increase awareness of the cause and nature of the disability. Parenting issues, such as behavior, temperament, and discipline, may constitute another area of knowledge deficit. Families may need guidance and support in determining realistic and appropriate expectations for their child.

Nutritional Assessments

Nutritional problems are common in developmentally disabled people, particularly when physical handicaps are involved. Adequate nutrition is critical to the well-being and health maintenance of the individual. Protein intake directly affects the function of the immune system and influences the prevention of illness. Adequate protein intake is also important for ensuring brain growth during infancy and early childhood. Appropriate fluid and caloric intake is essential for growth in childhood and adolescence. Caloric intake is also essential in maintaining the energy level that is important to a sense of well-being.

The nutritional needs of the developmentally disabled and the effect of various conditions have not been well researched. The problems that arise are quite diverse. Overnutrition may be a problem if physical activity is restricted because of the disability, as in spina bifida. In other situations, caloric expenditure may be increased by excessive movement, as in cerebral palsy (Dietz and Bandini, 1989).

Assessment of nutritional status includes measuring weight and height regularly and comparing with standardized measures. Children and adolescents who fall below the tenth percentile, fail to maintain a steady growth curve, or are above the ninetieth percentile may be exhibiting abnormal patterns of growth and need further evaluation.

The adequacy of the diet should be evaluated. A 3-day intake diary maintained by a consistent caregiver is most accurate; however, a 24-hour recall may be sufficient. It is important to differentiate between the food that is offered and what is actually consumed. The amount of time the caregiver must spend feeding is another area of focus. Feeding times may be so prolonged that they interfere with family maintenance or opportunities for other interaction with the child. Behavioral problems related to feeding may also arise as the child realizes that refusal to eat, regurgitation, and rumination are attention getting behaviors.

Feeding interventions may be multidisciplinary in scope, and referral to physical therapy, occupational therapy, and speech therapy are frequently beneficial. Diverse feeding strategies are available; selection should be based on the nature of the problem. Thickening liquids with cereal or wheat germ may improve swallowing abilities. Providing jaw support by placing the caregiver's fingers under the chin or along the mandible may improve jaw closure, swallowing, and chewing. Adaptive seating may be required to ensure appropriate positioning to facilitate swallowing, head control, and body support. Specialized utensils may increase the client's independence in self-feeding skills. Thick-handled spoons, utensils with straps that attach to the arm or hand, dishes with guards that assist scooping foods, and many other forms of adaptive equipment are available. Oral exercises may be used to improve oral-motor function and to decrease tactile defensiveness around and in the mouth.

Caloric intake may need to be adjusted. Caloric restriction may be appropriate for clients with limited mobility who are no longer actively growing. Strategies to increase caloric intake may be necessary for children, adolescents, and the elderly with disabilities. Consultation with a dietitian is recommended. Strategies may include increasing the frequency of feedings, selecting higher caloric density food choices, and using additives (commercially prepared or products such as Karo syrup, Instant Breakfast, or corn oil) and special formulas.

Tube feedings may be instituted when oral motor problems or structural defects interfere with the maintenance of nutritional status. Nasogastric or orogastric tubes may be placed intermittently for each feeding. Other clients may require gastrostomy feedings. Families need ongoing education and support regarding the techniques and care of these feeding interventions.

Breast-feeding a developmentally disabled infant may provide fullfillment of prenatal hopes and dreams at a time when disappointment prevails. Breast milk provides the infant with antibodies and nutrients most suited to growth and health. Mothers may need to pump milk to be bottle-fed or tube fed to the infant temporarily while oral-motor mechanisms are developing or during hospitalizations. This may still be a very satisfying experience for the mother. The community health nurse may find resources to assist breast-feeding mother's through lactation consultants at area hospitals, at regional perinatal centers, or through local La Leche League groups.

Family Assessment and Support

Many professionals enter the lives of people with developmental disabilities, but the ultimate responsibility for the health, development, social, and emotional needs belongs to the family. The community health nurse must practice family-centered care to enable families to assume the role of advocates, decision makers, and caregivers. Families will be faced with balancing plans of care from many professionals and the needs of the rest of the family. Recognizing and supporting the family's role means sharing information and including them in all aspects of planning. Working effectively with families begins with an understanding of the reactions to the diagnosis of a developmental disability.

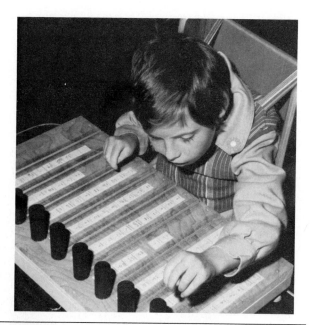

FIGURE 32-5

Coordination training.

Parents' Reactions

Parents react to the knowledge of having a developmentally disabled child in a fairly predictive manner, according to Rosen (1955). These stages are:

1. Awareness of a problem
2. Recognition of the basic problem
3. Search for a cause
4. Search for a cure
5. Acceptance of the problem

The time involved in moving from one stage to another varies with each family. *Awareness* may come early in the life of the child, particularly with the child with a physical handicap. If the problem is mental, awareness may come as late as the beginning of school. Denial and anger are the dominate emotions during the awareness stage.

Recognition of the basic problem, the second stage, helps the parents gain insight and motivates most to *seek a cause,* the third and perhaps most difficult stage in the parents' reactions. Mothers tend to blame themselves, and the inability to cope with an unknown cause leads to poor adjustment. This often manifests in misplaced hostility, anger, or self-pity. Many parents exhaust all their financial, physical, and emotional resources trying to find a reason for the child's problem.

Searching for a cure, the fourth stage, can also lead to family destruction. Hoping that each new drug, therapy, or published bit of research will help the child, many families travel from one physician to another, from city to city, and from school to school only to find little real help. The despair and grief are overwhelming for many. These families need support from the social worker, nurse, or other professionals.

The final stage, *acceptance* of the problem, takes much time. Often it is years before the parents can accept the

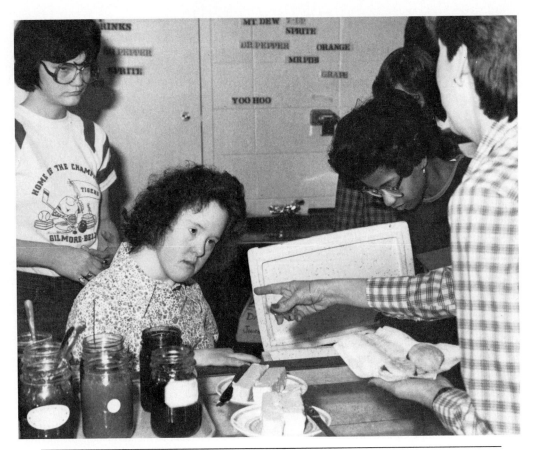

FIGURE 32-6

Activities of daily living laboratory.

reality of the child's problem. It is only when they have accepted the problem that they can begin to actively participate in the therapeutic plan of care. Until that time, their grief interferes with their ability to completely understand the information being shared with them. Their participation in the care of the child is essential, and professionals must be aware of the personal struggle the parents face every day as they live and work with the child.

Olshansky (1962) proposed that chronic sorrow is the natural response to a child's disability. He disputed the idea that families move through stages toward a plateau of acceptance of the problem. Instead, he suggested that families continue to move back and forth between the stages of grief and adjustment. Periodic crises will reevoke feelings of intense grief, anger, guilt, hostility, and denial. These periods may coincide with various developmental milestones such as birthdays, the beginning of school, or graduation. Sharing their feelings with other parents and professionals can provide a great deal of support during these periods. When families feel they have adjusted to the situation, they function most smoothly.

It is important for the nurse to respect the various routes taken by families to adapt to their needs and overcome their challenges. How families cope is strongly influenced by their cultural and socioeconomic background. Listening may be the nurse's most effective strategy.

Assessment

Complete family assessments are critical for the nurse providing services for developmentally disabled clients and their families. Particular emphasis should be placed on areas that are unique to these families. Areas that may be more problematic for these families include interactions between family members and division of responsibilities. It is also important to determine how realistic the family's perceptions of and expectations for the developmentally disabled individual are and to assess how each member copes with having a disabled family member. The nurse should assess family functions and the ability of family members to carry on roles within and outside of the family. Support systems should be defined and evaluated for effectiveness. Management of conflicts, stresses, and crises should be described. Each family member's perceptions of the strengths and weaknesses of other family members and of themselves should be discussed.

Intervention

Responding to the needs of families who have children with developmental disabilities begins with recognizing, appreciating, and validating the pain they experience (Tudor, 1981). From the moment the family members learn that they have a "less than perfect" child they need a nurse who is sensitive to their grief.

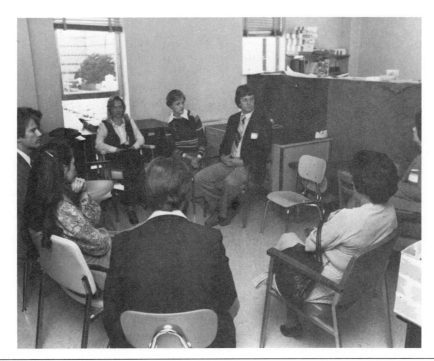

FIGURE 32-7
Parent group.

Planning strategies that support the child and the family should be based more on the development and abilities the child has than on disability. Focusing on the positive qualities of the child first is one concept that can be shared with the family.

Nurses must identify interventions that assist the child to develop to his or her highest level of health, independence, and growth. It is sometimes difficult for parents to encourage independence in children who have problems. Nurses may plan activities that help the child build necessary skills, such an improving coordination (Figure 32-5). Independence is fostered as the child develops self-help skills by learning to manage activities of daily living (Figure 32-6). Parents can foster independence at home by giving responsibilities to the child, such as household chores and simple meal preparation.

Parents need to be supported by their extended families, friends, and others who have experienced similar problems. Small groups of parents of developmentally disabled children can share their problems and their joys. Voluntary groups such as those sponsored by the Association for Retarded Citizens groups, the Spina Bifida Association, and the Cerebral Palsy Organizations provide a mechanism for communication. As seen in Figure 32-7, parent support groups are vital in working with families of developmentally disabled children. The nurse should encourage the parents to join these groups and share their experiences with others.

Parents are also helped by continued participation in the normal day-to-day activities of the community. They should be encouraged to find responsible babysitters and respite care services so that they have time to spend with other children, their spouse, and friends.

Families should be encouraged to seek out community resources that provide recreational activities for the disabled. Participation in community activities can strengthen the individual's self-esteem and enhance the family's sense of belonging. Many areas offer horseback riding, day camps, and sports programs at minimal or no cost. The nurse may identify programs by contacting local Special Olympics, Association for Retarded Citizens, Easter Seal Society, or other special interest groups.

An exemplary program is the Recreation Ranch in Signal Mountain, Tennessee, which offers therapeutic recreational activities for children and adults with special needs. Sports and games, horseback riding, hiking (including special wheelchair trails), arts and crafts, dancing, drama, independent-living classes, and special self-awareness classes are offered (Figures 32-8 and 32-9). The program is financially supported by the community and offers individuals the opportunity to enjoy the same recreational benefits as those who are able bodied.

Siblings face special challenges as a part of a special-needs family. They need to be educated to understand the nature and cause of the disability. Even the youngest of children may share feelings of denial and guilt. Normal issues within families, such as sharing parental time and sibling rivalry, take on extra dimensions when a family member is disabled. The Sibling Information Network (Appendix H) offers a quarterly newsletter for families and professionals.

Adolescence and Adulthood

To provide anticipatory support and guidance, the community health nurse must have an understanding of the needs

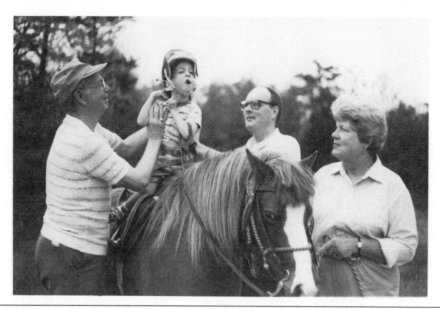

FIGURE 32-8

Horseback riding program for developmentally disabled children. *(Courtesy Recreation Ranch, Signal Mountain, TN.)*

of developmentally disabled adolescents and adults and their families. Families of older children with disabilities may experience periods of stress during the adolescent years and at the onset of adulthood. These may be times when families receive less support and may have difficulty obtaining needed services. Parents are often concerned about the adolescent's social, sexual, marital, and vocational possibilities. At this time, the nurse may need to help the family discuss concerns openly and realistically, to offer information they may lack, and to help them find available resources.

Frequently the physical growth of the developmentally disabled adolescent is normal. The adolescent must adapt to body changes, often without the ability to fully understand the implications of those changes. Information about reproduction and sexuality is needed by both the family and the adolescent. It is important to help the family and the adolescent understand the normality of sexuality and to find appropriate behaviors that are acceptable within the family structure. Family planning referrals may be appropriate. The family and the adolescent should be made aware of the possibility of sexual abuse.

Social isolation often occurs as the adolescent's social and emotional development lags behind peers. Parents are often concerned that the adolescent or young adult is lonely, and these concerns should be addressed. Families should be encouraged to participate in school and community programs that offer opportunities for peer interaction.

As adulthood approaches, families are often concerned about vocational programs and living arrangements. The current tendency is to place disabled adults into institutions because of limited services available as transition occurs from school systems to adult service programs (Black et al., 1985). Vocational skills are often encouraged in the school

setting (Figure 32-10); in reality, it may be difficult to find a job or work setting. Care of adults with developmental disabilities reflects three major trends: the increasing number of developmentally disabled adults residing in communities, the increasing advocacy for the rights of developmentally disabled citizens, and the increasing numbers of elderly developmentally disabled adults.

Adult service programs are insufficient in many states to meet educational, vocational, and housing needs. Further job training is often needed but unavailable after the age of 22 years. Waiting lists for group homes prevent more developmentally disabled adults from living away from home. Sheltered workshops or supported employment situations need expansion in many communities.

Many of the increased number of developmentally disabled persons remaining in or returning to the community from institutions reside with family members or in group facilities. Currently, the majority of those residing in institutions are severely retarded. They have limited self-care and adaptive skills, complex medical problems, or family stressors that interfere with home placement. However, strengthening community services for the individual and the family may promote the trend of home care. Needed services include medical care, sheltered housing, and counseling (Black et al., 1985).

Because developmentally disabled adults have the right to marry and have children, more information is needed about the childrearing abilities of disabled parents. There is insufficient research to predict the possibilities of developmental delay or disability in the offspring of these parents or to suggest the range of supportive services that may be necessary.

Seltzer (1985) estimated that there are as many as 460,000 developmentally disabled adults over the age of 55 in the United States. Unlike most elderly persons, these persons generally do not have children or a spouse to provide assistance or support. Addressing the needs of this population can help plan for the anticipated increase in their numbers, resulting from increased survival rates. Providing services will require the coordinated efforts of federal, state, and local agencies.

The goal of care for all the developmentally disabled people in our society is to assist the individual to live a productive life. All are not able to achieve the goal of *independent living,* but many are capable of living a productive life with help from the community.

THE ROLE OF FEDERAL PROGRAMS

Federal assistance programs for mental retardation and developmental disabilities operate in three major areas: income support, provision of service programs and facilities, and protection of rights. Federal programs were initiated in 1935, by the legislative mandate of Title V of the Social Security Act, which required states to identify and provide services to crippled children. Amendments to the original act have provided increased authorization of services for developmentally disabled children and families.

Income maintenance programs include expansions of the Social Security Act in 1950 to include disabled persons. The Supplemental Security Income Program (SSI) was enacted in 1972, and for the first time disabled children became eligible for benefits. By 1984 this program was providing financial assistance to an estimated 588,000 mentally retarded citizens. Expansion of the Food Stamp program in 1979 authorized changes that increased the eligibility of disabled persons, providing benefits to group-home residents (Braddock, 1986).

A landmark act was passed by Congress with enactment of the Education for All Handicapped Children Act (PL94-142) in 1975. This act provides "education for every child, regardless of handicaps, in the least restrictive environment possible." Implementation has increased state education expenses and the responsibilities of teachers and nurses in school settings. Each state may implement programs to respond to individual needs and restrictions. For example, in Virginia, several counties employ pediatric nurse practitioners to manage the students with special needs. In other states, school nurses and community health nurses are meeting the needs of this population. Often the nurse is responsible for teaching school staff specialized care techniques and coordinating the specialty services a child may need.

The Education of the Handicapped Act (PL99-457) of 1986 offers incentives to states to provide services to disabled children younger than 6 years of age. It requires a system to identify children, evaluate family needs, and provide a statewide central directory of early intervention services and resources that are available within each state. In South Carolina, families and professionals have access to the directory through a toll-free telephone number. Other states have adopted this model of implementation (Mayfield-Smith et al., 1990). Information about access to central directories is available through public health departments and other community health agencies.

The Developmental Disabilities Assistance and Bill of

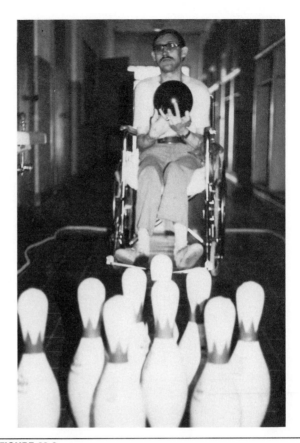

FIGURE 32-9

Adults in wheelchairs enjoy bowling in a specially constructed alley. *(Courtesy Recreation Ranch, Signal Mountain, TN.)*

Rights Act and the Older Americans Act require states to develop plans to meet the needs of the aging developmentally disabled population. This population is likely to increase as improved health care services and better living conditions increase the average life span of the disabled population (Janicki et al., 1985).

Two major legislative efforts involve the rights of the disabled. The Child Abuse Amendments of 1984 (known as the Baby Doe Rule) contains provisions prohibiting the withholding of medical treatment from infants born with mental and physical disabilities. The Rehabilitation Act of 1973 prohibits discrimination against handicapped individuals who are otherwise qualified to participate in programs, employment, or activities receiving federal funds (Braddock, 1986). Current legislation seeks to expand the prevention of discrimination to include businesses and agencies not receiving federal monies.

Although federal spending for service programs and income supplementation has increased, money for research and training of professionals in this field has declined. Continued advances in the prevention of disabilities and the provision of quality services depends on financial support, ongoing research, and the education of professionals (Braddock, 1986).

The largest portion of federal dollars spent in this area in 1985 was for reimbursement for institutional care. Federal

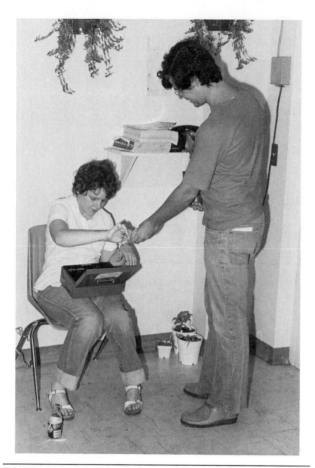

FIGURE 32-10

Teenagers practicing sales skills.

efforts were then redirected to focus on assistance to community and local programs. For example, in 1989 legislation was enacted to focus on the costs and benefits of respite care programs (Overview of Respite Care Programs, 1990).

There is a wide variation in individual state's implementation of programs, leaving gaps in services provided. Respite care services, home health nursing, multidisciplinary support in school services, and vocational training programs are only a few of the many services that must be available in communities. Nurses need to be aware of the availability of services and income support programs and should serve as advocates for the population with special needs as state and local policies are developing.

THE FUTURE

Plans for the health field must include both children and adults who have developmental disabilities. These individuals are increasingly living in the community and are cared for by their families and local agencies. Support of families through adequate funding for community services, provision of respite care to relieve families from the ongoing burden of constant care, continuation of research into causes and preventive measures, and increased recognition of the rights of this population are concerns that must be addressed by any group that is involved in planning care for people with developmental disabilities. The community as a whole must

not lose sight of the needs of these individuals as they grow from childhood to adulthood and into old age. Far too often in the past, recognition has been given to disabled children, but as they age, they receive less and less attention. Community health nurses can help add meaning to the lives of these individuals and their families.

CLINICAL APPLICATION

A referral was made to a public health department from a nearby regional level III neonatal intensive care unit regarding discharge plans for a developmentally delayed infant. The infant, Joel, was born at 27 weeks of gestation and had remained in intensive care for 7 months. His hospital course was complicated by hyaline membrane disease, bronchopulmonary dysplasia, and intraventricular hemorrhage. At the time of discharge, Joel was receiving neither supplemental oxygen nor medications and was taking all of his feedings orally. There were strong indications of spastic diplegia, and he was diagnosed as having severe retinopathy of prematurity with the expectation of eventual blindness. Family financial resources were extremely limited. Although Medicaid coverage was available for subsequent needs, the family owed over $100,000 to the hospital. Joel's 17-year-old mother, Mary, was unmarried. Joel's grandmother would babysit while Mary finished high school. Joel's father, who was also 17 years old and unemployed, had not been active with Mary and her mother in the hospital discharge planning program. His involvement with Mary and Joel was expected to be minimal. The hospital was seeking a home evaluation before discharge.

The community health nurse planned to evaluate the safety of the home environment and to begin her assessment of the family's understanding of the situation and their concerns. She found that Joel's mother and grandmother were optimistic about the future and delighted to bring him home after such a long hospitalization. They recognized that he would probably suffer motor and visual impairments, yet they wanted to participate in a program to help him develop to his best potential.

The nurse also assessed knowledge of infant care and availability of infant care items. The nurse recommended the purchase of a cool mist humidifier. Because the family had been so involved in providing Joel's daily care in the nursery, they had become skilled in this area and no knowledge deficits were identified.

In planning for early intervention services, several factors were considered. Joel's family expressed a desire for developmental services. Joel's chronic lung disease made him susceptible to complications of respiratory tract infections, making it unwise to expose him to groups of young children. Lack of financial resources limited access to services. Available community resources were center-based, offered no provision for home programs, and primarily served children ages 3 to 6 years. The neonatal intensive care unit (NICU) follow-up clinic was a multidisciplinary program that could offer periodic evaluations and recommendations for developmental intervention. The health department staff—the nutritionist, physical therapist, and nurse—would receive recommendations from the hospital and follow-up program staff to develop a home program for Joel. Later the com-

SAMPLE DEVELOPMENTAL PROGRAM FOR JOEL

GOAL	INTERVENTION	TARGET DATE	EVALUATION
Joel will respond to auditory, visual, and tactile stimuli that indicates he is going to be picked up. Caregivers will recognize Joel's cues indicating that he wants to be picked up (holding arms out). Joel will demonstrate decreased extensor tone when lifted from supine. Family will use appropriate handling techniques to facilitate Joel's motor and cognitive development: lifting Joel up.	Before lifting Joel, talk to him about "up," smile at him, and touch him gently. Do not lift him until he indicates a response by cooing, smiling back, or lifting his arms. If he does not give a response, prompt him by guiding his arms forward at the shoulders. When lifting Joel, do not encourage extension; place your hands behind his shoulders and roll him forward, keeping his head and shoulders flexed.	2 weeks	Family consistently demonstrates appropriate lifting technique for Joel. Joel brings his hands forward when signaled that he will be picked up. Caregivers recognize Joel's cues indicating that he wants to be picked up.

munity developmental center would serve as the main program.

During the week following Joel's discharge from the hospital, he was seen at the health department by the pediatrician and nurse to establish a baseline health appraisal. The DDST was administered using Joel's corrected age (birth age in weeks minus number of weeks premature). Results showed delays in all areas. Nutritional assessment showed that weight gain was only minimally acceptable but consistent with the growth demonstrated in the hospital. Feeding practices were assessed; Joel continued to take a high calorie formula and rice cereal with a spoon. He tired easily with feedings and was fed small amounts on a frequent schedule. Joel's immunization status was also reviewed. He had received a DPT vaccine in the nursery at 5 months of age but had not been given oral polio vaccine (OPV). An immunization schedule was established. Mary and her mother had concerns about his irregular sleeping habits and irritability. The nurse counseled them regarding behavioral and environmental interventions to promote a more organized sleeping pattern. Before the family left the clinic, the nurse checked Joel's position in his carseat and made recommendations about support for correct posture.

The physical therapist and nurse made a home visit in the following week to assess the family's success with interventions begun in the nursery and their readiness to continue the program. Mary and her mother demonstrated the exercises the hospital physical therapist had taught them. They expressed a desire to set goals, including: fostering appropriate parenting skills, developing Joel's awareness of sensory stimuli, and facilitating optimal motor functioning. Examples of interventions for promoting development included recognizing Joel's behavior cues (for hunger, sleepiness, overstimulation, boredom), offering auditory and tactile stimulation in addition to visual stimulation, and demonstrating handling techniques that promote appropriate muscle tone (see box above). Joel's mother, father, and grandmother were taught how to incorporate the interventions into Joel's playtimes and daily care. Assessment of

the family's coping abilities continued to indicate that the family was adjusting to the complexity of Joel's care and his physical and sensory limitations.

The nurse planned to continue biweekly home visits with the physical therapist to develop further intervention techniques and establish goals in self-help, social, emotional, cognitive, and language skills. Periodic evaluations were performed by the multidisciplinary staff at the follow-up clinic. In collaboration with the physician and nutritionist, the nurse also planned a schedule of health appraisal, nutritional assessments, and family assessments to identify health problems and to guide well-child care.

At Joel's 1-year health assessment (9 ¾ months corrected age), Mary was upset about Joel's delays. The nurse encouraged her to discuss her frustrations and pointed out the progress Joel had made. Mary expressed anger and guilt and was unable to handle the constant demands placed on her. She was having difficulty understanding her own feelings, because she usually seemed able to adjust to everything. The nurse supported her in her grief responses and helped her recognize that she was experiencing natural emotions that other parents had also described. The nurse helped her to realize that, although she accepted Joel's limitations, she might experience times of intense pain and grief. The nurse recommended that Mary and other family members attend parent–support-group meetings through the community's developmental program.

◊   ◊   ◊

The preceding case study illustrates the role of the community health nurse in providing care for developmentally disabled children and their families. The nurse is often responsible for the coordination of services, the provision of well-child care, the assessment of health status, and the implementation of interventions. The key to the management of care is the involvement of the family in mutual goal setting and the recognition and support of appropriate coping mechanisms of family members. Use of multidisciplinary resources is essential.

SUMMARY

Recognition of the need for community health nurses to become more skilled in meeting the requirements of developmentally disabled individuals and their families has led to greater interest and desire to learn more about this population. Concern and commitment to care can be augmented through the use of specific techniques and the study of problems that have currently become increasingly apparent in communities. With emphasis on care of the developmentally disabled child or adult at home and in the community, nurses must familiarize themselves with the resources available and must plan experiences to enhance their ability to provide professional service for this group. These goals can be accomplished through the cooperative efforts of the service and educational groups found in all the states. Nurses working in harmony with professionals in other fields can help provide a brighter future for our developmentally disabled population and their families.

KEY CONCEPTS

Providing care for those who are developmentally disabled is a goal that has been emphasized by the federal government for many years. It is a broad goal and encompasses the work of many people in a variety of professions.

Nurses are in a key role to provide services that have a positive impact on communities.

Definitive causes for developmental disabilities are known in only about 25% of the cases. Of this small percentage, the causes are usually categorized as chromosomal aberrations; neural tube defects; central nervous system damage occurring in the perinatal period, including the sequelae of premature birth; neonatal infection; and metabolic disorders.

To be effective, preventive measures must begin with education of the parents before conception.

The role of the community health nurse in the care of the child with a developmental disability must be built on a sincere concern for the child and family. The child with a problem must first be viewed as an individual worthy of dignity and capable of living for a purpose.

Nurses providing care for persons with developmental disabilities are involved in assessments of growth, maturation, and general well-being to prevent further alterations in health status.

Adequate nutritional status is critical to the well-being and health maintenance of the client; diverse problems may exist in the developmentally disabled population.

The nurse must practice family-centered care, which empowers families to assume the responsibilities of advocacy, decision making, and caregiving.

Complete family assessments are critical for the nurse providing services for developmentally disabled clients and their families.

Intervention strategies for assisting families to cope include listening, focusing on the abilities of the client, encouraging independence, referral to support groups, and using community resources.

To provide anticipatory support and guidance, the community health nurse must understand the needs of developmentally disabled adolescents and adults and their families.

Federal programs for the care of developmentally disabled children were initiated by the legislative mandate of Title V of the Social Security Act. This act required states to identify and provide services to crippled children. Through the years federal programs have been expanded to provide services to many more children.

LEARNING ACTIVITIES

1. Divide the class into two groups and debate the following issue: Children with developmental disabilities should or should not be mainstreamed into the schools.

2. Make a home visit with a nurse who has a developmentally disabled client and assess how this person's presence (1) affects the family and (2) affects (or alters) the home and (3) what physical, emotional, and financial costs are involved for the family.

3. Using a telephone book or community resources directory, list and evaluate the services available for developmentally disabled people and their families. Include fees, location, and range of services. What gaps, overlaps, or both exist in your community? What resources are available for (1) prevention, (2) assessment, (3) intervention, and (4) follow-up care?

4. Practice using at least two of the developmental assessment tests described in this chapter.

BIBLIOGRAPHY

American Association on Mental Deficiency: Classification in mental retardation. Washington, DC, 1983, The Association.

Black MM et al: Individual and family factors associated with risk of institutionalization of mentally retarded adults, AM J Ment Defic 90:271, 1985.

Braddock D: Federal assistance for mental retardation and developmental disabilities. II. The modern era, Ment Retard 24:209, 1986.

Castellani P: The political economy of developmental disabilities, Baltimore, 1987, Brookes Publishing.

Denhoff E: Current status of infant stimulation or enrichment programs for children with developmental disabilities, Pediatrics 67:32, 1981.

Dietz WH and Bandini L: Nutritional assessment of the handicapped child, Pediatr Rev 11:109, 1989.

Hack M and Fanaroff A: How small is too small?: considerations in evaluating the outcome of the tiny infant, Clin Perinatol 15:773, 1988.

Hook EB: Epidemiology of down syndrome. In Pueschel S and Rynders JE, editors: Down syndrome—advances in biomedicine and the behavioral sciences, Cambridge, 1982, The Ware Press.

Janicki MP, Ackerman L, and Jacobson JW: State developmental disabilities, aging plans and planning for an older developmentally disabled population, Ment Retard 23:297, 1985.

Levine MD: The child with learning disabilities. In Scheiner AP and Abroms IF, editors: The practical management of the developmentally disabled child, St Louis, 1980, Mosby–Year Book.

Mayfield-Smith KL, Yajnik GG, and Whiles DL: Information and referral for people with special needs: implications for the central directory of Public Law 99-457, Infants Young Children. 2:69, 1990.

Nelson R and Crocker AC: The child with multiple handicaps. In Levine MD et al., editors: Developmental and behavioral pediatrics, Philadelphia, 1983, WB Saunders.

Olshansky S: Chronic sorrow: a response to having a mentally defective child, Soc Casework, 43(4):190, 1962.

Overview of respite care programs, GAO/R-HRD-90-125, 1990. Washington, DC, US Government Printing Office.

Paneth N: Etiologic factors in cerebral palsy, Pediatric Annals 15:191, 1986,

Percy SL: Disability, civil rights, and public policy, Tuscaloosa, AL, 1989, University of Alabama Press.

Phelps DL: Vision loss due to retinopathy of prematurity, Lancet i:606, 1981.

Porter P: The role of the independent community nurse practitioner in providing services to the developmentally disabled children and their families, Nurs Clin North Am 15:419, 1980.

Rose TI: The education of all handicapped children act (PL 94-142): new responsibilities and opportunities for the school nurse, J Sch Health 50:30, 1980.

Rosen L: Selected aspects in the development of the mother's understanding of her mentally retarded child, Am J Ment Defic 59:522, 1955.

Scheerenberger RC: A history of mental retardation, Baltimore, 1987, Brookes Publishing.

Seltzer MM: Informal support for aging mentally retarded persons, Am J Ment Defic 90:259, 1985.

Shelton TL, Jeppson ES, and Johnson B: Family centered care for children with special health care needs, Washington DC, 1987, Association for the Care of Children's Health.

Taft LT and Matthews WS: Cerebral palsy. In Levine MD et al., editors: Developmental and behavioral pediatrics, Philadelphia, 1983, WB Saunders.

Tudor M: Child development, New York, 1981, McGraw-Hill Book Co.

Wallace HM, Gold EM, and Lis E: Maternal and child practices: problems, resources and methods, Springfield, IL, 1973, Charles C Thomas Publisher.

Whaley LF and Wong DL: Nursing care of infants and children, ed 3, St Louis, 1987, Mosby–Year Book.

Zelle RS and Coyner AB: Developmentally disabled infants and toddlers, assessment and intervention, Philadelphia, 1983, FA Davis.

PART SIX

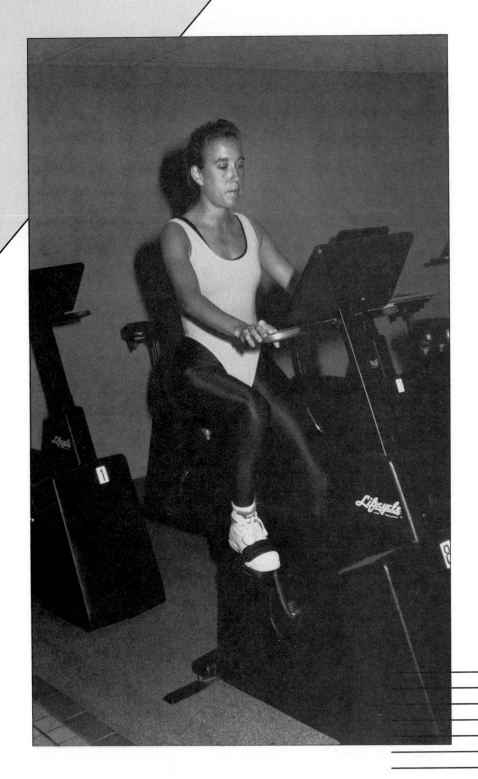

Tools and Techniques for Health Promotion

I
t has been estimated that the affect of the medical care system on usual indexes for measuring health is about 10%. The remaining 90% is determined by factors over which health care providers have little or no direct control, such as lifestyle and social and physical environmental conditions. This text focuses on the processes and practices for promoting health, principally by the community health nurse, who is considered an ideal person to personally demonstrate and teach others how to promote health. To be effective, health promotion requires that people cease focusing on how to "fix" themselves and others only when they detect physical and emotional disequilibriums and that they, instead, assume personal responsibility for health promotion. Such a change in emphasis requires that health care providers incorporate health promotion techniques into their practice.

The chapters in this section document the effectiveness of health promotion and describe specific strategies that community health nurses can practice and teach to clients. The benefits of self-care are described in Chapter 33, followed by chapters that emphasize the way in which nutrition, exercise, stress management, and crisis intervention can be incorporated into a plan for personal and client-centered health.

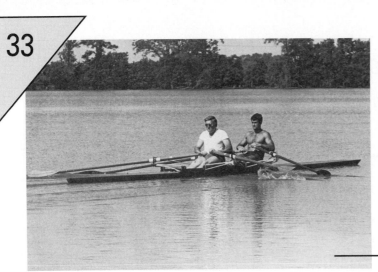

33

Self-Health Care Through Risk Appraisal and Reduction

Jean Goeppinger

Karen T. Labuhn

OBJECTIVES

After reading this chapter, the student should be able to:

Identify factors influential in the development and practice of self-health care.
Define self-health care.
Relate self-health care to risk appraisal and reduction.
Compare and contrast methods of appraising individual health risks.
Describe methods of assessing aggregate and community health risks.
Compare and contrast methods of reducing health risks.
Develop an argument for community health nursing roles in risk appraisal and
    reduction.

KEY TERMS

health-risk appraisal	microlevel interventions	risk appraisal and reduction
macrolevel interventions		self-health care

A marked resurgence of interest in *self-health care* is apparent. Many Americans exercise regularly, maintain their weight at recommended levels, and deliberately attempt to manage their stress. Some drive at reduced speeds, drink fewer alcoholic beverages than in the past, and no longer smoke. Others jog on country lanes and in city parks, participate in structured physical fitness programs, patronize natural foods stores, practice organic gardening, and engage in a variety of relaxation techniques at home and at work.

Newspaper articles and radio and television programs provide evidence of this growing popular interest in *self-health care,* as does the rapid proliferation of commercial weight-reduction programs, smoking cessation plans, health spas, and worksite health-promotion programs (Glasgow and Terborg, 1988). A similar increase in the interest of nurses—nurses in practice, education, and research—is evident. The recent work of Orem (1985), Pender (1987), McBride (1987), and Woods (1989) is illustrative.

This chapter focuses on *self-health care* through *risk appraisal and reduction.* The context within which health-*risk appraisal and reduction* has developed is described, and the scientific basis is discussed. A variety of methods for appraising and reducing health risks at individual and community levels is explained. Finally, suggestions for applications of these methods are given, with specific references to community health nursing practice.

SELF-HEALTH CARE

The concept of people helping themselves in health matters is not new. Very likely the practice of self-health care began before recorded history. Early references appear in ancient Greek, Chinese, and Hebrew writings. Americans have been involved since colonial times.

History

References to self-health care in classical literature include mythical and religious elements, as well as pragmatic components. For instance, in Greek literature the goddess Hygeia represented the belief that humans could remain healthy if they lived rationally. Certain activities of daily living, such as exercise, were considered essential to the maintenance of health; tributes to Hygeia were also important. Similarly, in biblical times, various food laws were instituted that promoted health.

With the later development of a scientific and biological orientation toward disease, self-health care was gradually deemphasized. A focus on treatment and cure displaced the original goals of health protection and illness prevention. This focus encouraged a growing dependence on health professionals.

During the last three decades, self-health care has reemerged as an important factor in health care. In some cases it is competing with, if not supplanting, professional care. For example, some versions of self-health care emphasize lay diagnosis and self-treatment, as opposed to professional diagnosis and collaborative management. Other more conservative versions focus on teaching people how to work with their health care providers. In either case the professional health care system is dramatically affected. Professional roles are being renegotiated, and the structure of the existing health care system is changing. The rapid growth of health maintenance organizations (HMOs) and other prepaid medical plans reflects the development of one such self-health care model, emphasizing collaboration between consumers and providers.

The revitalization of self-health care in the United States may represent a cyclical recurrence of the more general self-help theme. Americans on the frontier did not have the benefit of expert advice nor were they often close to professional medical help. In the true spirit of Jacksonian democracy, they not only depended on themselves but often scorned advice from outsiders. In health matters, as in other areas, the older, wiser, and more experienced family members were the experts. They may have consulted the medical encyclopedia on the parlor bookshelf or used folk remedies. In either case self-health care retained its original religious links. Early popular self-health care books, such as the *Primitive Physic* by John Wesley (1747), were recommended regularly at prairie revivals.

The reemergence of the self-health care movement also was accelerated by the political climate of the 1960s and 1970s. Authority, in general, was challenged. Racial minorities began to demand their rights in the 1960s; women, patients, and the elderly began to make their demands public in the 1970s. A challenge to the professional health care system, which many believe exemplifies elite rather than democratic control, is illustrated clearly in the ideology of self-health care. Illich, for example, wrote, "The medical establishment has become a major threat to health. The disabling impact of professional control over medicine has reached the proportions of an epidemic" (Illich, 1976, p. 3). Illich chastised U.S. health professionals and society for robbing individuals of their self-health care skills. He warned that politicians and legislators may promote self-health care because of their interest in cost containment rather than a genuine belief in individuals' abilities to preserve health.

Other self-health care advocates believe that modern medicine has been given too much credit for improvements in health. McKinlay and McKinlay (1977) have argued that the main contributors to the decline in mortality at the turn of the century seem to have been better standards of living, including improvements in sanitation, personal hygiene, and diet, which have led to a more favorable balance in the host-agent-environment relationship. Conclusions such as these have been drawn for chronic illnesses, as well as for communicable diseases. Wildavsky (1977) asserted that the medical system affects only 10% of the variability in health indicators such as infant mortality, disability days, and adult mortality. He attributed the remainder to factors over which physicians lack control—"from individual life-style (smoking, exercise, worry), to social conditions (income, eating habits, physiological inheritance), to the physical environment (air and water quality)" (p. 105).

In the political arena, these conclusions were supported first by LaLonde in *A New Perspective on the Health of Canadians* (1974). As the Canadian Minister of National Health and Welfare, LaLonde urged a more comprehensive approach to health care. He identified four major determi-

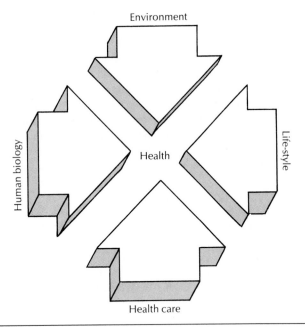

Environment

Human biology

Health

Life-style

Health care

FIGURE 33-1

Determinants of health. *(Adapted from LaLonde M: A new perspective on the health of Canadians, Ottawa, 1974, Government of Canada).*

nants of health: human biology, environment, life-style, and health care (Figure 33-1). LaLonde's ideas also influenced policymakers in the United States. The three major categories of health risks delineated in the Surgeon General's Report, *Healthy People* (Department of Health, Education and Welfare, 1979), were inherited biological factors, the environment, and behavioral factors. These are identical to LaLonde's first three major determinants of health. More recently, the objectives listed in *Healthy People:2000* address factors in all four categories that compromise the health status of Americans (Department of Health, Education, and Welfare, in press).

Definition

Despite its renewed popularity, the concept of self-health care lacks a consistent definition. Labels for the concept also vary, from life-style management to self-care, self-health care, and self-health management.

Lorig (1980) developed a conceptual paradigm that is very useful for comparing and evaluating the various perspectives on self-health care. The paradigm includes four dimensions: the instigator of care, the target of care, the goal of care, and the type of knowledge on which care is based. Most commonly the instigators of self-health care are lay persons who carry out health care for themselves. When compliance behaviors are included as a component of self-health care, however, the instigators may be health professionals.

Self-health care may be targeted toward the individual, the community, or the society. Approaches by primary care providers are generally directed toward the individual; they focus on changing health beliefs and behaviors. From a public health and political perspective self-health care emphasizes community responsibility and social change rather than individual reform.

Goals of self-health care can be directed toward health promotion or disease prevention, early detection, and treatment. The goal of *risk appraisal and reduction* usually involves primary prevention or early detection and treatment of health problems.

Interpretations of the final dimension of Lorig's paradigm, the knowledge base of self-health care, have changed over the decades. Whereas early self-health care practices often were based on religious or philosophical tenets, current self-health care primarily has a scientific base with strong cultural and folk-medicine overtones.

Contemporary literature about self-health care emphasizes varying dimensions of Lorig's paradigm. Orem, a commonly cited nurse theorist, uses the term *self-care* to describe activities that individuals initiate and perform on their own behalf to maintain life, health, and well-being (Orem, 1991). According to Orem, the nursing profession is essential because individuals are not always self-sufficient. Consequently, although self-health care is a lay responsibility, professional contributions may be required. Orem's focus is on the individual, and the basis of self-health care is scientific.

This conceptualization of self-health care is quite restrictive. A more complete definition includes the full range of possibilities. *Self-health care* then encompasses all those activities that people can do for themselves, individually or collectively, in a variety of health and illness matters. These activities complement professional health care services. They may be directed toward the individual, community, and society and are based on various combinations of scientific, religious, philosophical, and cultural influences (Goeppinger, 1982, p. 380). In the following discussion, we consider risk appraisal and reduction in light of this broad perspective on self-health care.

Risk Appraisal and Reduction

Risk appraisal and reduction is a quantitative approach that health professionals can use to help individuals and groups maximize their self-health care activities. It compares information supplied by individuals about their health-related practices, health habits, demographic characteristics, and personal and family medical history with data from epidemiological studies and vital statistics. It uses the comparison to predict individuals' risks of dying, provide recommendations for reducing risks, and promote healthful behavior changes. The goal of risk appraisal and reduction is the prevention or early detection of disease. The knowledge base for this approach is the scientific evidence regarding the relation between risk factors and mortality and the effectiveness of planned interventions in reducing both risks and mortality.

Since the early 1970s risk appraisal and reduction have gained popularity among health professionals. This trend has been influenced by three factors: (1) the renewed emphasis on health promotion and disease prevention; (2) epidemiological studies that have provided an empirical data base for making predictions from risk appraisal methods; and (3) a proliferation of risk appraisal tools for use in clinical practice. The health insurance industry also has recognized the potential of risk reduction for cost containment and has promoted the approach in occupational and health care settings.

Two of the most influential epidemiological studies of health risks are the Framingham Heart Study, initiated in 1949, and the Human Population Laboratory's longitudinal survey of Alameda County, California residents, initiated in the early 1970s. Both of these studies have supported the hypothesis that selected risk factors are directly related to morbidity and mortality.

In the Framingham Heart Study, 5209 adult residents of a small town in Massachusetts agreed to be followed over their life spans to help researchers identify factors contributing to the development of coronary heart disease and high-blood pressure. The subjects received periodic health and life-style assessments, and morbidity and mortality statistics were collected. The longitudinal study was successful in meeting its objectives. Heart disease was found to be more prevalent among persons who had high-blood pressure, high-cholesterol levels, low levels of exercise, and who smoked. Obesity also was identified as a contributor to high-blood pressure and elevated cholesterol levels and thus to heart disease (Haynes, Feinleib, and Kannel, 1980).

The Alameda County Study was also designed as a prospective study; it included a probability sample of 6928 subjects (Breslow, 1972). In this study a number of social and behavioral factors were studied in relation to mortality. The health behaviors studied included eating three meals daily at regular intervals, eating breakfast, sleeping 7 to 8 hours a night, using alcohol moderately, exercising regularly, not smoking, and maintaining a desirable height to weight ratio (Belloc, 1973). Results from follow-ups of the sample have consistently shown that cigarette smoking, alcohol consumption, physical exercise, hours of sleep, and weight in relation to height are related to mortality (Cohn, Kaplan, and Cohen, 1988; Kaplan and Camacho, 1983; Wiley and Camacho, 1980; Wingard, Berkman, and Brand, 1982).

Also in the Alameda County Study, social factors were identified as being important influences on health. Renne (1974) found that the strength of social networks (such as marriage, contact with close friends and relatives, church membership, and ties with formal and informal groups) was inversely related to mortality. These findings were initially received with a great deal of controversy. However, they encouraged the inclusion of social and environmental variables, as well as personal behaviors, in health-risk appraisals. Subsequent studies have verified the early findings (Kotler and Wingard, 1989).

Findings from large scale surveys such as the Framingham and Alameda County studies prompted a number of intervention trials that focused on reducing health risks. Some studies that attempted to evaluate community-based interventions were the Stanford Heart Disease Prevention Program (Farquhar et al., 1990), the North Karelia Study (Puska et al., 1983), and the Pawtucket Study (Lasater et al., 1984)

The findings of the initial three-community study conducted by Stanford University researchers (Maccoby et al., 1977) were encouraging. This study tested the impact of a mass media campaign alone and in conjunction with face-to-face instruction. The intervention including both mass media and face-to-face instruction was found to be a more effective method of inducing change in three cardiovascular risk factors—cigarette smoking, systolic blood pressure, and serum cholesterol—in the two intervention communities than in the community receiving the media campaign alone.

Subsequently, the Stanford Five-City Project was initiated (Farquhar et al., 1985). The two treatment cities received a low-cost, comprehensive intervention program based on principles from social learning theory (Perry, Baranowski, and Parcel, 1990), a communication-behavior change model, community organization, and social marketing. Once again, risk factor changes in plasma cholesterol, blood pressure, smoking rate, and resting pulse rate were observed (Farquhar et al., 1990). These resulted in substantial decreases in composite mortality risk scores and coronary heart disease mortality risk scores (of 15% and 16%, respectively) (Farquhar et al., 1990, p. 362).

Positive results likewise were found in the North Karelia Study (Puska et al., 1983). Citizens of North Karelia, a rural area in Finland, experienced extraordinarily high mortality from cardiovascular disease in the early 1970s. At this time more than half of North Karelian men smoked. They ate large amounts of animal fats and had grossly elevated serum cholesterol levels. In addition, many suffered from untreated hypertension. The government initiated an intervention program at both individual and community levels to assist individuals in modifying their high-risk behaviors.

The North Karelia Project involved extensive retraining of health professionals; reorganization of public health services; production of low-fat dairy products and low-fat, low-salt sausages; and the development of community health education programs. Follow-up studies demonstrated that the prevalence of the three major risk factors for cardiovascular disease decreased much more in North Karelia than in a comparison county (Puska et al., 1983).

The Pawtucket Study is an ongoing intervention project in a Rhode Island community that traditionally has had very high rates of cardiovascular disease. As in the North Karelia Study, the interventions in Pawtucket are directed toward both individuals and the community. The news media, churches, social groups, and business community have been actively involved in risk–reduction-education activities. For instance, the food industry offers "Heart Healthy" food items and menus, and there are extensive campaigns to inform citizens about their cholesterol levels and other cardiovascular risk factors (Lefebvre et al., 1986). The final results of this study have not been reported, but the study has been publicized widely and has served as a model for many other risk-reduction projects.

These studies, among others, have provided a beginning scientific knowledge base for the implementation of risk-appraisal and risk-reduction programs. However, information on the relative effectiveness of specific interventions in reducing risks remains limited (Schoenbach, Wagner, and Beery, 1987). Still, most health professionals agree that we cannot afford to postpone intervention efforts. Nurses must carefully examine research findings and act prudently. They can promote action against risk factors based on careful

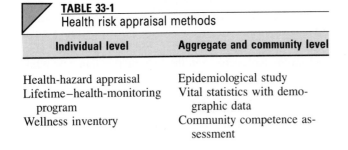

TABLE 33-1
Health risk appraisal methods

Individual level	Aggregate and community level
Health-hazard appraisal	Epidemiological study
Lifetime–health-monitoring program	Vital statistics with demographic data
Wellness inventory	Community competence assessment

interpretation of the available data, while energetically seeking better evidence. In the following sections, methods of risk appraisal and reduction are discussed, and both their strengths and limitations are highlighted.

METHODS OF HEALTH RISK APPRAISAL

In *health-risk appraisal,* data about health risks experienced by an individual or group are collected and analyzed, and a health-risk profile is generated. Health-risk appraisal may be carried out on both individual and community levels (Table 33-1). A clinical approach is commonly used to identify the presence or absence of risks at the individual level, and epidemiological approaches are frequently used to identify risks at the community level. Both of these approaches are important to community health nurses.

Appraising Individual Health Risks

At least three types of individual health-risk appraisal approaches are common: the health-hazard appraisal and its many versions; the lifetime–health-monitoring program; and wellness appraisals or inventories. Each type of risk appraisal is rather complex, and only the basic concepts and procedures are described in this chapter. Fuller explanations can be found in the references cited at the end of the chapter. Some examples of risk appraisal tools are shown in Appendix C.

Health-Hazard Appraisal (HHA)

Among the earliest proponents of individual health-risk appraisal were two family physicians who called their approach *prospective medicine* (Robbins and Hall, 1970). Unlike physicians in conventional curative practice, they wanted to deal with an individual's health from the perspective of what was likely to occur, rather than what had already happened. They recognized that most chronic diseases have a predictable sequence and that the characteristic precursors of many diseases can be monitored and controlled. The natural history of one such illness, arteriosclerotic heart disease, is diagrammed in Figure 33-2.

Robbins and Hall (1970) put the concept of prospective medicine into practice by developing a method of profiling risk, called the health-hazard appraisal. The objectives of the health-hazard appraisal are to: (1) assess the total risks to a client's health based on knowledge of the client, the natural history of certain diseases, and the major causes of mortality for aggregates of the client's age, sex, and race; (2) initiate life-style changes in the client to avoid disease precursors or to minimize their pathogenic influence; and (3) institute medical treatment and life-style changes as early in the course of disease as possible.

To accomplish these objectives, data are collected by a self-administered questionnaire, basic laboratory tests, and clinical examination. The questionnaire elicits information about personal characteristics and behaviors known to predict health status. The laboratory testing is limited to obtaining the serum cholesterol level; and the physical examination consists of height, weight, and blood pressure measurements.

These personal data then are compared with data compiled from the 10 major causes of death of an aggregate of the same age, sex, and race as the client. Based on the comparison of data, the client's appraisal and achievable ages are calculated. The appraisal age is the health age of the average person in the client's racial, sex, and age aggregate or group with a similar risk profile. For example, a 20-year-old white woman might have an appraisal age of 15 if she has good health habits and no family history of chronic disease. Another 20-year-old white woman might have an appraisal age of 26 if she smokes, fails to wear a seat belt while driving, does not perform regular self–breast examinations, and has a family history of hypertension. Achievable age refers to the health age the client could achieve by modifying health hazards. The second woman's achievable age would be considerably lower than her appraised age.

After Robbins' and Halls' initial work, health-risk appraisal (HRA) tools proliferated rapidly. The National

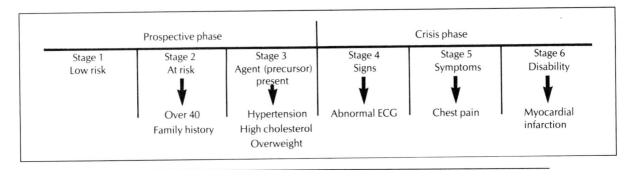

FIGURE 33-2

Natural history of arteriosclerotic heart disease.

Health Information Clearinghouse identified 50 different HRA instruments in 1986, and Smith, McKinlay, and Thorington (1987) included 41 computer-scored HRAs in their instrument validation studies. HRA instruments vary in their intent and methods. Some are medically focused; others include risks related to mental, social, and environmental health; and still others include risk assessments and wellness appraisals. The Life-style Assessment Questionnaire (National Wellness Institute, Inc., 1988), for example, includes a wellness inventory, a health-risk appraisal, and a "topics for personal growth" section. Only data from the health-risk appraisal portion, however, are compared with mortality data. The current version (1988) provides users with a sample action plan to increase their levels of wellness, as well as summaries of the results from the wellness-inventory, health–risk appraisal, and personal-growth sections.

Special versions of health-hazard appraisals have been developed for children and adolescents. The Know Your Body program, developed by the American Health Foundation in New York City (Williams, Carter, and Eng, 1980), was designed to identify chronic disease risk factors in school children who are 11 to 14 years of age. The children receive feedback and health prescriptions in a "health passport." The University of Florida 4-H for Life Appraisal (Moody et al., 1979) provides teenagers with health-risk profiles and educational messages regarding their health behaviors.

One of the most comprehensive health-risk appraisals is the Healthier People Questionnaire developed by the Carter Center of Emory University and the Centers for Disease Control (CDC). The Healthier People Project was initiated in 1986 to 1987 after a decade of developmental work by the CDC and a network of state health departments and collaborating universities and after completion of the Risk-factor Update Project (Breslow et al., 1985). Healthier People is a comprehensive program for health-risk appraisal and reduction that is available to the public. The program includes the computer-scored Healthier People Questionnaire and five sets of materials to facilitate easy use. The user materials include: (1) instructions on how to administer the questionnaire and use the software, (2) guidance in planning and implementing a comprehensive health promotion program, (3) procedures for modifying the software for special population groups, (4) epidemiological data and mortality tables used to support Healthier People, and (5) software design information for programmers.

The intent of the Healthier People project is to provide a methodologically sound health-risk appraisal instrument for public use and to facilitate development of effective risk-appraisal and risk-reduction programs. The Healthier People project disseminates its materials through a network of local health departments and universities and sponsors frequent user workshops. Information can be obtained from state health departments or from the Health-Risk Appraisal Program, The Carter Center of Emory University.*

---

*Address: Health Risk Appraisal Program, The Carter Center of Emory University, 1989 N. Williamsburg Drive, Suite E, Decatur, GA 30033; telephone, (404) 872-2100.

Lifetime Health Monitoring Program (LHMP)

Because a substantial portion of a health professional's time is spent in evaluating the health of apparently well people (often considered the "worried well"), Breslow and Somers (1977) proposed a lifetime–health-monitoring program. Like the health-hazard appraisal, it uses clinical and epidemiological data to identify specific needs for health care. However, it does more than assess individual health risks; the lifetime–health-monitoring program provides a detailed list of recommendations for preventive measures appropriate to each of 10 different age groups. Many of these preventive measures are routine nursing interventions. For example, recommendations for women who are 40 to 49 years of age include tests for hypertension and malignancies of the breast, cervix, and gastrointestinal tract and counseling on changing nutritional needs, physical activity, and the use of cigarettes, alcohol, and drugs (Breslow and Somers, 1977).

In the 1980s, lifetime–health-monitoring programs for use in specific settings were developed. In such cases the known risk profile of the group being monitored is used to modify screening recommendations for the general population. Guidotti (1983) describes a lifetime–health-monitoring program that was developed for managers in an occupational setting. Because the managers were shown (in health surveys) to be heavier smokers and coffee drinkers than other white-collar employees in the company, these behaviors and psychological stress factors were taken into consideration when developing the monitoring program.

Wellness Inventories

The various wellness inventories are slightly different from most health-risk appraisal instruments and the lifetime–health-monitoring program. They tend to define health risks more broadly and emphasize lay control. The health-hazard appraisal is designed to avert disease and premature death. Wellness appraisals may encourage disease prevention, but they do so by advocating health enhancement or promotion.

Typical wellness inventories include a wide range of personal self-health care behaviors. For example, Clark's Wellness Assessment (1981) has six categories: eating well; being fit; feeling good; caring for self, others, or both; fitting in; and being responsible. Ardell (1977) includes inventories related to self-responsibility, nutritional awareness, physical fitness, stress management, and environmental sensitivity. Travis' Wellness Self-Evaluation (1977) includes a Life Change Index, an Eating Habits Survey, a Wellness Inventory Symptom Checklist, a Medical History, a Purpose in Life Test, Stress Assessments, and a Creativity Index. The Wellness Inventory of the Lifestyle Assessment Questionnaire (National Wellness Institute, Inc., 1988) covers six dimensions: physical, social, emotional, intellectual, occupational, and spiritual. Unlike these instruments, the health-hazard appraisal assesses only those health behaviors that have clearly documented relationships to disease.

Advantages

Risk-appraisal instruments are convenient tools that can be used to determine individual health risks. Because these instruments also recommend preventive actions, they may support the individual's self-health care efforts. Nurses also receive support and direction in their educational activities. Studies of health-risk appraisals in clinical settings indicate that clients who complete the instruments generally are more aware of their health risks (Avis, Smith, and McKinlay, 1989; Bartlett, Pegues, Shaffer, and Crump, 1983; Schultz, 1984), are more willing to discuss their health behaviors (Skinner, Allen, McIntosh, and Palmer, 1985), and in some cases initiate suggested changes (Bartlett et al., 1983; Schultz, 1984). Risk appraisals also may be useful for measuring the effectiveness of planned interventions for risk reduction. Completed by individuals and groups at different time periods, they provide feedback about how behavioral changes have influenced health risks and life expectancy.

Limitations

Despite these advantages, practitioners should be aware of the limitations of risk-appraisal instruments. Some of these limitations are inherent in the tools themselves, whereas others relate more to problems in usage (Kirscht, 1989). Actual tool limitations include: (1) the questionable validity and reliability of some of the instruments, (2) the inconsistency with which different appraisal instruments measure and analyze health characteristics, and (3) a general overemphasis on life-style factors and lack of attention to other important risks such as environmental hazards and inadequate health care (Smith, McKinlay, and McKinlay, 1989; Smith, McKinlay, and Thorington, 1987; Meeker, 1988). Instruments may be particularly weak in measuring risks such as smoking, alcohol consumption, or violent behavior (Killeen, 1989).

Because of the methodological limitations of some risk appraisal tools, practitioners are advised to obtain information about the reliability and validity of a specific tool before attempting to use it. Information should be available to assess the overall strengths and limitations of the tool, as well as its advantages and disadvantages for specific populations.

The best results can often be obtained by using health-risk appraisals in conjunction with clinical observation and assessment. Although educational messages may have a great impact on some individuals, other persons may deny or avoid the implications (Becker and Janz, 1987). Even when individuals are motivated by health-appraisal feedback, they may not have the behavioral skills necessary to initiate and sustain changes in life-style. This is especially true regarding those behaviors that are difficult to change, such as smoking habits.

Another limitation of health-risk appraisals is that they are probably more suitable for use with middle-age people than for those younger than 35 years of age or older than 65 years of age (Doerr and Hutchins, 1981). They provide little statistical incentive to the very young to change poor health habits because the effects of life-style illness are usually detected in middle to late adulthood, and with persons over 65 years of age the risk factors themselves are not as good predictors. In addition, existing appraisals are probably not particularly useful for minority ethnic or blue-collar populations. In one study blue-collar employees could not understand many of the words in the CDC Health-Risk Appraisal (Shy et al., 1985). Among African-Americans, their use is compromised by the inadequacy of epidemiological data on certain risk factors such as homicide and the lack of available and accessible health services, especially for the poor. In addition, individual life-style change is limited by the realities of living as a minority group member in systems that limit participation in decision making and restrict economic and educational opportunities and in environments where external threats to health, such as violence, are common (Rowley et al., 1985).

Studies show that risk appraisals are most effective when they are followed by a well-planned risk-reduction program (Schoenbach, Wagner, and Beery, 1987; Doerr and Hutchins, 1981). Some examples of risk-reduction methods are discussed later in this chapter.

Appraising Community Health Risks

Health-risk appraisals can be used at the community and aggregate levels to estimate risks for a number of chronic diseases, accidents, and acts of violence. Three basic approaches to establishing such risks include: (1) epidemiological studies, health surveys using risk appraisal instruments, and morbidity and mortality statistics; (2) vital statistics showing demographic correlates of health and illness; and (3) community competence levels reflecting a community's ability to identify and resolve problems of community life, including those related to health (Table 33-1).

The use of mortality data and, to a lesser extent, morbidity figures to establish aggregate measures of health risk is a useful approach. Similarly, the results of health-risk appraisals for a given population may be compiled to form a composite picture of risk. The use of health-risk appraisals to assess group risks in occupational settings has become especially popular (Sherman, 1990; Chenoweth, 1989). The risk profiles for the total employee group in a company or a particular occupation are used to assess needs for system-wide intervention programs. Individuals completing the risk appraisal instruments generally are given clear and comprehensive feedback and guidance on how to modify their behavioral health risks (Conrad, 1987; Smeltzly, 1985).

The assessment and feedback concerning occupational health risks is often less optimal. An exception to this is a combined employee health risk–occupational hazard appraisal initiated by the New York City Health Department Laboratory. Individual employees completed the CDC's health-appraisal tool. They then were interviewed by health educators, and detailed workplace appraisal questionnaires were completed. Over 600 workplace problems were identified. The most frequently reported problems were lack of adequate ventilation, poor safety procedures and education, job stress, unclean rest rooms, and noise. Following the interviews, walk-throughs of problem areas were completed, and remedial actions were taken by management (Koplin, Davidow, Backman, and Escobar, 1988).

An example of health-risk appraisal by a governmental agency is Ohio's Health Risk Prevalence Survey, conducted in the early 1980s under funding from the Centers for Disease Control. In this study a random sample of 607 Ohio residents age 18 years and older were polled by telephone, using random digit dialing techniques. A standardized health-risk appraisal instrument was used to collect descriptive statistics on selected risk factors.

Among other findings, the study revealed very high rates of smoking, low use of protective devices such as smoke detectors, and a generally low level of awareness about preventive measures. Goals set as a result of the study included: (1) removing economic barriers impeding the installation of smoke detectors in homes, (2) initiating health education at an early age to counter smoking trends, and (3) encouraging more adult self-determination in reducing health risks (Chen and Bill, 1983).

The concept of lifetime-health monitoring can be applied at the community level. National health objectives and model standards established by state health departments (American Public Health Association, 1985; Wisconsin Department of Health and Social Services, 1990) encourage public health practitioners to monitor their populations for health problems that are high priorities. An example is a project conducted by the CDC and the Oregon Health Division of the Indian Health Service. In this project, all infant birth weights and prenatal visits from 1973 to 1986 were monitored to assess the effectiveness of the Yellowhawk Indian Health Center's maternal–child-health program in relation to 1990 national objectives. Findings from the project showed that the number of low birth-weight infants had declined over the 13-year period. There was a significant increase in the number of Indian women who received prenatal care in the first trimester, although the 1990 objective (that 90% of mothers would receive prenatal care) was not met. New initiatives to meet this objective were identified. The Indian Health Service also began work on a surveillance system to monitor the rates of smoking and alcohol use during pregnancy (Campbell, Kimball, Helgerson, Alexander, and Goldberg, 1989).

The use of demographic data that have a documented relationship to health status and illness can also be helpful in estimating health risks at the community level. Dependency ratios, socioeconomic status indexes, race, gender, and education levels supply valuable information in identifying community health risks. A community with a high unemployment rate, for example, will have a higher level of health risk than one with little unemployment.

The third approach, the use of community competence levels, has been proposed and tested (Goeppinger and Baglioni, 1985) but not widely used. The potential use of this approach is described in Chapter 16. Community competence is considered a correlate, if not an actual indicator, of the population's health; thus, low levels of community competence should be associated with increased morbidity and mortality risks. Like demographic measures, community competence may be an important contextual variable, occurring at the community process level. The possible use of demographic data and community competence levels to assess community health risks needs further study. Just as critical is the need to develop methods for combining health-risk appraisals with high-quality risk-reduction programs.

METHODS OF HEALTH-RISK REDUCTION

As might be expected, successfully reducing health risks is even more difficult than is their adequate appraisal. Broad risk-reduction efforts focus on minimizing risks for specific health problems and maximizing positive aspects of any of the four determinants of health: human biology, life-style, environment, and health care (Figure 33-3). *Microlevel interventions,* those performed at the individual or small group level, are most feasible in the areas of human biology and life-style. *Macrolevel interventions,* those carried out at the community or societal level, are essential in the areas of environment and health care delivery. Both microlevel and macrolevel interventions may be required to sustain health-risk reduction. Individuals can initiate positive changes in life-style and may even be successful in improving their health care resources, but without corresponding changes at the community or societal levels, these improvements may be very difficult to maintain. Similarly, legislation to control environmental hazards can be implemented, but without cooperation from individuals, these efforts will be ineffective.

Microlevel Interventions

Microlevel interventions are the most popular approaches for achieving health-risk reduction. Most of these interventions essentially require persons to modify risk behaviors in their individual life-styles. The philosophical premise is that people can and do use their own self-interest, knowledge, creativity, and resources to achieve risk reduction. Other persons, including health professionals, may take supportive roles in the efforts to reduce health risks, but the locus of control for change rests with the individual. Microlevel intervention programs directed toward exercise and fitness, nutrition and weight control, smoking cessation, stress management, automobile safety, and other preventive measures are common in health care settings and in many educational and occupational settings. Some of the intervention strategies used to modify life-style behaviors include individual and group counseling, educational programs and materials, behavior modification, contracting, referral to community resources, self-management, and mass media programs (Schultz, 1984).

Pender has categorized intervention strategies that are useful for initiating behavior change at the individual level as: (1) self-confrontation, (2) cognitive restructuring, (3) modeling, (4) operant conditioning, (5) counterconditioning, and (6) stimulus control (1987, pp. 259). Self-confrontation is based on the premise that individuals make changes when they recognize inconsistencies within their own beliefs, values, and behaviors or between their own behaviors and those of persons whom they emulate. Providing written feedback from health-risk appraisals is an example of an attempt to induce behavior change through self-confrontation. The use of nationally known athletes to communicate health messages about the dangers of drugs through the mass media is another example.

Strategies using cognitive restructuring attempt to teach clients to think more rationally and thus increase control over their lives and health. Rational thinking about obesity and weight loss is reflected in the following statement, "I

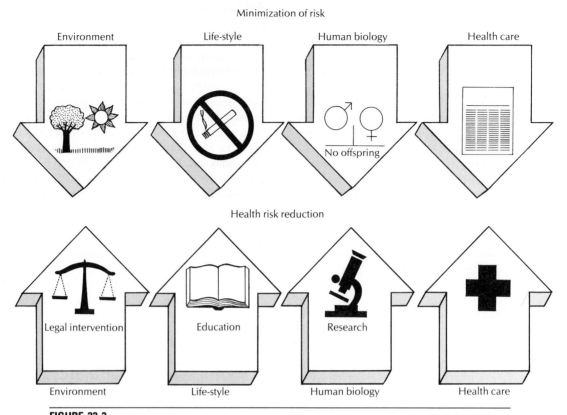

FIGURE 33-3

Aims of health-risk reduction.

have difficulty controlling my between-meal snacking." In the same situation, the statement "I'll never be slender; I've always been chubby," exemplifies irrational thinking. Focusing initially on modifying a single behavior, snacking, is more reasonable than changing one's body image.

Modeling is a common strategy used to help individuals or groups modify their behaviors. The person desiring to modify a particular behavior and reach a specific goal is given opportunities to observe the behavior of other persons who have achieved the goal. The person then practices the desired behavior, identifying with the role models. Modeling is especially helpful when persons are unsure of the behaviors required to reach a specific goal. The learning of social skills, beginning in early childhood and continuing in adult life, entails much modeling. Alcoholics Anonymous and other self-help groups successfully use modeling (among other strategies) to support their group members, as do arthritis self-care programs (Goeppinger, Arthur, Baglioni, Brunk, and Brunner, 1989). In these programs, the lay leaders who have arthritis serve as models, or behavioral examples, of healthy arthritis self-care. The modeling of both health-protecting and health-promoting behaviors is also common to the professional nurse's role. For example, nurses are expected to not smoke, to eat a more balanced diet, and to exercise more regularly than the public.

Some of the most effective self-modification strategies

use operant conditioning, which is based on the principle that behavior is determined by its consequences. As a result, health-generating behaviors must be identified and rewards provided. Practitioners who use operant conditioning need to be well informed about methods to increase individuals' awareness of health-generating and health-damaging behaviors, the appropriate use of rewards, and the gradual shaping of health behaviors. Pender (1987, p. 268) suggests that the client should control the selection of behaviors to be changed and the rewards to be received. Positive reinforcements are better motivators of behavior change than negative reinforcements. Clients should decide, for instance, how they will reward themselves for achieving their exercise goals. Some may select a financial reward; others may request verbal praise from their nurses.

Counterconditioning, or systematic desensitization, focuses on breaking an undesirable bond between a stimulus and a response. The response represents an irrational or maladaptive response to a specific situation, such as immediately lighting up a cigarette when becoming anxious or angry. The goal of counterconditioning in this example might be to replace the maladaptive response with a relaxation response. Imagery, biofeedback, or progressive relaxation techniques might be used to help promote tension release. These techniques frequently are used in stress management programs.

Stimulus control, the final self-modification strategy identified by Pender (1987), focuses on the antecedents rather than the consequences of behavior. By changing the events that precede behavior, it is theoretically possible to decrease or eliminate undesired behavior and to increase desired outcomes. To use stimulus control successfully, the client must have accurate information about the desirable and undesirable behaviors and must arrange for environmental cues to be encountered in such a way as to promote only the desired behavior. Internal cues to action include perceptions and affective states. External cues include interactions with others, media communications, and visual or other stimuli. Nurses can assist clients in achieving stimulus control by providing correct information, giving appropriate cues, and helping clients eliminate any barriers to change.

Changes in health behavior may be transitory. If they are to result in risk reduction, changes in health behaviors must be maintained and incorporated into generalized life-style modifications. Pender notes that other microlevel intervention strategies may be helpful in maintaining healthful behavior change: making the behavior change public, habit formation, recording progress, and intermittent rather than continuous reinforcement (Pender, 1987, pp. 278).

Microlevel interventions also may be targeted to the area of human biology. The application of knowledge from human genetics is one example of individual change. Individuals with sickle cell anemia, for instance, could be counseled about the risks of their children inheriting the disease or sickle-cell trait.

The effectiveness of any of these strategies varies depending on the targeted behaviors, the client characteristics, and the intervention setting. Health-risk appraisals combined with various educational programs, individual and group counseling, or both have been shown to be effective in both clinical and occupational settings (Becker and Janz, 1987; Pilon and Renfroe, 1990; Schoenbach, Wagner, and Beery, 1987). In general, life-style changes that entail the introduction of new behaviors (such as preventive dental visits, self-breast examination, and seatbelt use) are more amenable to educational approaches than are changes that require giving up negative habits. The modification of long-term addictive behaviors such as cigarette smoking and drug or alcohol abuse usually requires a combination of education efforts, behavioral modification strategies, and ongoing interpersonal support.

Despite the difficulties in effecting behavior change, many nurses are implementing risk-appraisal and risk-reduction programs. One example of a successful program is a home-based personal screening and counseling program designed for union employees and their families (Acquista, Wachtel, Gomes, Salzillo, and Stockman, 1988). In this program, nurse practitioners interview the program participants in their homes, using a health-appraisal tool, and complete physical examinations, collect blood for cholesterol testing, and provide instructions on collection of stool samples. Following this, any detected health problems are discussed, and if there is sufficient interest referrals are made to health education courses. Follow-up calls and counseling are initiated at 3 weeks, 6 weeks, and 1 year after the visit.

Nurses also play a key role in another innovative program, the Family High-Risk Program at the Utah Department of Health (Beck et al., 1988). In this program, a health family-tree questionnaire is used to identify families at risk for cancer and other chronic diseases. The questionnaire is given to senior high school students in their science classes. Families who have a strong positive history for specific chronic disease are referred to the local health department for follow-up by a professional nurse. The nurses have developed standards of care for each disease, and they counsel individuals and families on their risks, needed screening, and behavioral risk-reduction measures. The standards of care are similar in concept to Breslow's and Somer's lifetime–health-monitoring guidelines, discussed earlier in this chapter.

Macrolevel Interventions

Macrolevel interventions, those aimed at the societal level, are less popular than those directed toward individual change. It is certainly easier to assume that individuals are responsible for their own health risks. However, individuals have only limited control. For example, how can an individual be held solely responsible for reckless driving when overly powerful automobiles continue to be manufactured? Or, how can persons who live in impoverished and volatile neighborhoods take sufficient preventive action to protect themselves from physical attack?

Obviously, to be effective in reducing health risks, many changes in life-style require concurrent societal level changes. In her book, *Promoting Health Through Public Policy* (1981), Milio points out the realistic limitations of microlevel interventions. She argues for a more ecological focus, in which there is greater emphasis on creating healthy environments for individuals and groups. Jeffrey (1989) also argues that appreciating both individual and population views is important to the development of action strategies that will reduce risk behaviors as public health problems. The effectiveness of community organization and development in initiating societal level changes and improving the health of population groups at-risk has been documented (Minkler, 1990).

In areas such as the environment, societal change is essential. Only legislation to control environmental hazards from chemical and physical agents will reduce mortality caused by occupationally induced cancer. The need to earn enough to purchase basic necessities prevents many persons from quitting jobs with well-established health risks. As a result, the risks themselves, rather than the individual's exposure to them, must be altered.

Clean air and water and safe jobs require group action. State legislation mandating the inspection of wells and the laboratory examination of well water is a traditional example of risk-reducing surveillance. Negotiations between the United States and Canada on the pollution of the Great Lakes are a creative example of group action for environmental health at the international level. Recent studies of inner-city violence (Tardiff, Gross, and Messner, 1986) also represent attempts to deal with health problems on the macrolevel.

The current initiatives of antismoking groups to effect smoking bans in businesses and other public places is another example of collective group action directed toward change at both the community and societal levels. Although various individuals and groups have differing opinions concerning the best strategies for meeting their goals, significant progress in implementing antismoking policies has occurred. Successes in lobbying against the tobacco industry have been much slower, however, and the goal of a smokefree society remains elusive.

Similarly, macrolevel interventions are necessary in the health care delivery system. Young mothers, living in rural areas and heavily dependant on working family members and friends for transportation to well-baby clinics, cannot be expected to keep appointments made between 9 AM and 5 PM on weekdays. Clinic staff and administrators must, instead, change the days and hours of service so that they are more accessible to clients.

Multilevel Change

It is clear that effective risk reduction involves health-generating changes at both the individual and societal levels. Change requires the community health nurse to use multiple intervention strategies, such as individual behavioral contracts, the establishment of coalitions, the use of small interacting groups, and cooperation with lay advisors, the mass media, public policy, and legislation.

The community health nurse's unique synthesis of clinical and population-focused skills provides a strong knowledge base for applying risk-appraisal and risk-reduction methods. At the microlevel, community health nurses might use health-hazard appraisals, wellness inventories, or a lifetime health-monitoring program to strengthen their assessment of clients' health risks. Clients then could be counseled regarding their self-care needs, and interventions could be planned collaboratively to reduce health risks. The community health nurse might also seek opportunities for intervening in educational and occupational settings. Here, health-risk appraisals might be used to identify group risks, as well as individual risks, and interventions could be planned to reduce or eliminate the risks.

At the macrolevel, nurses can use data from surveys, compiled statistics, and community assessments to identify the most significant health hazards for a given population. They can work with other health professionals and community leaders in planning system-wide interventions to reduce these hazards. These interventions may involve political and legislative activities and education programs. Successful attempts to intervene at the macrolevel will be especially rewarding because large numbers of persons can benefit from these efforts. Societal-level interventions are more fully discussed in Chapter 7 and 16. The following example illustrates the nurse's role in risk appraisal and reduction.

CLINICAL APPLICATION

Sally Jones is a community health nurse employed by a rural county health department in the eastern United States. She has worked in the community for a number of years and is knowledgeable about the demographic and health characteristics of the local population, as well as community resources and leadership patterns. Ms. Jones' typical work week entails involvement in wellness clinics in the small towns in her district, a number of home visits, visits to two local schools, consultation with lay community leaders, planning with other health professionals, and occasional meetings with elected officials to lobby for specific health legislation.

Ms. Jones recognizes the potential usefulness of risk-appraisal tools to strengthen her health assessments and intervention efforts. In health clinics and home visits, she has begun educating her clients about the concept of health risks and uses a lifetime health-monitoring schedule to advise them about preventive self-health care. She also encourages her clients to complete health-risk appraisals, wellness inventories, or both, providing guidance on the selection of instruments that are most meaningful for the individual's age and overall living situation.

One appraisal completed by Stanley Hess, a 30-year-old truck driver, revealed an appraisal age of 43 years and an achievable age of 25. He had a sedentary job that kept him apart from his family for long periods, drank 25 to 40 bottles of beer a week, never wore a seatbelt, was hypertensive (blood pressure 200/160), smoked two packs of cigarettes a day when he was "on the road," and drove 198,000 miles annually. Mr. Hess was at greater risk than his contemporaries for motor vehicle accidents, arteriosclerotic heart disease, suicide, cirrhosis of the liver, stroke, and cancer of the lungs.

Despite these ominous findings, Mr. Hess was somewhat motivated to improve his health situation. He very much wanted to be a good parent and role model for his two sons and to please his wife and family. His wife had previously established a trusting relationship with the community health nurse. Both Mr. and Mrs. Hess thus were quite receptive to the nurse's comments when the health appraisal was reviewed.

In planning interventions to reduce this client's health risks, Ms. Jones first assisted him to identify those risks he actually wanted to change and those he considered modifiable. She then worked with him, his wife and family, and his employer in developing a plan that would begin to bring his appraisal age down to the desired achievable age. A behavioral contract between Ms. Jones and Mr. Hess was developed to assist in goal attainment (Pender, 1987; Schultz, 1984). Because several of the client's health risks involved long-term habits, such as smoking and alcohol abuse, referrals to community agencies and programs were made to assist with risk reduction. Ms. Jones kept in close contact with Mr. Hess to encourage and support his active involvement in these programs.

Working in the school setting provided Ms. Jones with another opportunity for using health-risk appraisals. In one of the parent-teacher organization's meetings, she introduced the idea of risk appraisal. This resulted in a lively discussion concerning health-promotion topics. Subsequently, Ms. Jones worked in collaboration with several teachers to plan a program for family risk appraisal and reduction based in the school.

Because there was interest in testing the effectiveness of risk appraisals and various educational and counseling methods in reducing the identified health risks of the students' families, the nurse helped to design an intervention program to meet these goals. She sought advice from a nurse researcher at a nearby university in designing the experimental program. After the program was initiated, Ms. Jones was contacted by one child's father who expressed interest in developing a similar risk-reduction program for employees in his small industrial plant. He believed that risk reduction would be quite difficult but he was willing to give it a try. This contact resulted in collaborative planning between Ms. Jones, an occupational health nurse in the area, an experienced health educator, and the interested employer.

Ms. Jones eventually was successful in convincing county health department officials to conduct a prevalence survey in her community to identify community-wide aggregate health risks. This, she reasoned, would provide useful data for planning health promotion and disease prevention programs and for documenting the need for increased funding and legislation to support the necessary changes. Plans to seek state funding for the survey were begun. Ms. Jones requested to be actively involved in planning the survey because she wanted to ensure that environmental risks, as well as life-style factors, were adequately assessed. Excited about this new venture, she began considering how she would convince others of the potential impact of macrolevel interventions.

SUMMARY

This chapter presented risk appraisal and reduction as important ways for community health nurses to assist individuals, families, aggregates, and community groups to improve their self-health care. Past and present self-health-care activities were discussed, and risk appraisal and reduction was described. Four areas in which self-health care can be targeted were reviewed: human biology, environment, life-style, and health care. The environment and life-style were emphasized as expecially important to risk appraisal and reduction because of our growing abilities to successfully modify risks in these areas. A number of methods of appraising individual, aggregate, and community-level health risks are available for nurses in practice, as are examples of innovative intervention strategies. Microlevel and macrolevel interventions were described and compared. The necessity of intervention at multiple levels was stressed. The chapter concluded with an illustration of how one community health nurse went about appraising and reducing risks at the individual and group levels.

KEY CONCEPTS

The debate between the critics and proponents of self-health care is important. It suggests that, despite the rhetoric of support and recent progress, important questions still remain.

The revitalization of self-health care in the United States may represent a cyclical recurrence of the more general self-help theme.

Risk appraisal and reduction is an approach that health professionals can use to help individuals and groups maximize their self-health care.

In health-risk appraisal, data about health risks experienced by an individual or group are collected and analyzed, and a health-risk profile is generated. Health-risk appraisal may be carried out on an individual and community level.

At least three types of individual health-risk appraisal tools are common today. These include the Health-Hazard Appraisal and its many versions, the Lifetime–Health-Monitoring Program, and wellness appraisals or inventories.

The overall objective of lifetime–health monitoring is to focus routine health evaluations on the specific problems most likely to occur at a given age and thus to better prevent these problems.

Health-risk appraisals can be used at the community or aggregate level to estimate risks for a number of chronic diseases, accidents, and acts of violence.

As might be expected, the successful reduction of health risks is even more difficult to achieve than is the adequate appraisal of risks. Broad risk-reduction efforts focus on minimizing risks for specific health problems and maximizing positive aspects of any of the four determinants of health: human biology, life-style, environment, and health care.

The community health nurse's unique synthesis of clinical and aggregate skills provides a strong knowledge base for applying risk appraisal and reduction methods.

LEARNING ACTIVITIES

1. Read any of the recent legislative proposals for federal health insurance. Note the position on self-health care taken and implied in the legislation and outline the supporting argument. Identify the key factors (such as religious beliefs, professional attitudes, scientific knowledge) in the argument.

2. Interview a nurse, client, physician, and businessperson about their views of self-health care. Ascertain their beliefs about each of Lorig's four dimensions of a comprehensive self-health care definition: instigator, target, goal, and knowledge base.

3. Attend a meeting of Weight Watchers, TOPS, Reach for Recovery, or a similar self-help health group. Identify several key themes of the meeting and discuss how they exemplify both self-health care and risk appraisal and reduction.

4. Complete any two of the Health-Risk Appraisal forms included in Appendix C. Compare and contrast them on the breadth of health risks covered, the extent to which they require professional involvement, and the ease with which they can be completed.

5. Interview a school health nurse, a home health care or visiting nurse, or an occupational health nurse about nursing roles in risk appraisal and reduction. If these roles are not now a part of the job description of the nurse you are interviewing, sketch a revised job description that includes such roles.

BIBLIOGRAPHY

Ardell DB: High level wellness: an alternative to doctors, drugs, and disease, Emmaus, PA; 1977, Rodale Press.

Acquista VW, Wachtel TJ, Gomes CI, Salzillo M, and Stockman M: Home-based health risk appraisal and screening program, J Community Health 13(1):43, 1988.

American Public Health Association: Model standards: a guide for community prevention health services, ed 2, Washington, DC, 1985, The Association.

Amler RW, Moriarty DC, and Hutchins EB, editors: Healthier people, Decatur, GA, 1988, The Carter Center of Emory University HRA Program.

Avis NE, Smith KW, and McKinlay JB: Accuracy of perceptions of heart attack risk: what influences perceptions and can they be changed? Am J Public Health 79(12):1608, 1989.

Bartlett EE, Pegues HU, Shaffer CR, and Crump W: Health hazard appraisal in a family practice center: an exploratory study, J Community Health 9(2):135, 1983.

Beck S, Breckenridge-Potterf S, Wallace S, Ware J, Asay E, and Giles RT: The family high-risk program: targeted cancer prevention, Oncol Nurs Forum, 15(3):301, 1988.

Becker MH, and Janz NK: Behavioral science perspectives on health hazard/health risk appraisal, Health Serv Res 22(4):537, 1987.

Belloc NB: Relationship of health practices and mortality, Prev Med 2(1):67, 1973.

Breslow L: A quantitative approach to the World Health Organization's definition of health: physical, mental, and social well-being, Int J Epidemiol 1(4):347, 1972.

Breslow L, Fielding J, Afifi AA et al.: Risk factor update project: final report. Atlanta, GA, 1985, U.S. Department of Health and Human Services, Centers for Disease Control, Center for Health Promotion and Education.

Breslow L and Somers AR: The lifetime health-monitoring program: a practical approach to preventive medicine, N. Engl J Med 296(11):601, 1977.

Campbell BC, Kimball EH, Helgerson SD, Alexander IL, and Goldberg HI: Using 1990 national MCH objectives to assess health status and risk in an American Indian community, Public Health Rep 104(6):627, 1989.

Chen MS and Bill D: Statewide survey of risk factor prevalence: the Ohio experience, Public Health Rep 98(5):443, 1983.

Chenoweth D. Nurses' intervention in specific risk factors in high risk employees: an economic appraisal, AAOHN J 37(9), 367-373.

Clark CC: Enhancing wellness: a guide for self-care, New York, 1981, Springer Publishing.

Cohn BA, Kaplan GA, and Cohen RD: Did early detection and treatment contribute to the decline in ischemic heart disease mortality?: prospective evidence from the Alameda County Study, Am J Epidemiol 127(6):1143, 1988.

Conrad P: Wellness in the work place: potentials and pitfalls of work-site health promotion, Milbank Q 65(2):255, 1987.

Department of Health, Education and Welfare: Healthy people: the Surgeon General's report on health promotion and disease prevention, DHEW Pub No (PHS) 79-55071, Washington, DC, 1979, U.S. Government Printing Office.

Department of Health, Education and Welfare: Healthy people 2000, Washington, DC, U.S. Government Printing Office (in press).

Doerr BT and Hutchins EB: Health risk appraisal: process, problems, and prospects for nursing practice and research, Nurs Res 30(5):299, 1981.

Farquhar JW et al.: Effects of community-wide education on cardiovascular disease risk factors: the Stanford Five-City Project, JAMA 264(3):359, 1990.

Farquhar JW et al.: Stanford Five-City Project: design and methods, Am J Epidemiol 122(2):323, 1985.

Goeppinger J: Changing health behaviors and outcomes through self-care. In Lancaster J and Lancaster W, editors: Concepts for advanced nursing practice: the nurse as a change agent, St Louis, 1982, Mosby–Year Book.

Goeppinger J, Arthur MW, Baglioni AJ Jr, Brunk SE, and Brunner CM: A reexamination of the effectiveness of self-care education for persons with arthritis, Arthritis Rheum 32(6):706, 1989.

Goeppinger J and Baglioni AJ Jr: Community competence: a positive approach to needs assessment, Am J Community Psychol 13:507, 1985.

Glasgow RE and Terborg JR: Occupational health promotion programs to reduce cardiovascular risk, J Consult Clin Psychol 56(3):365, 1988.

Guidotti TL: Adaptation of the lifetime health monitoring concept to defined employee groups not at exceptional risk, J Occup Med 25(10):731, 1983.

Haynes SG, Feinleib M, and Kannel WB: The relationship of psychosocial factors to coronary heart disease in the Framingham Study III: eight-year incidence of coronary heart disease, Am J Epidemiol 111:37, 1980.

Illich I: Medical nemesis: the expropriation of health, New York, 1976, Random House.

Jeffrey RW: Risk behaviors and health: contrasting individual and population perspectives, Am Psychol 44:1194, 1989.

Kaplan GA and Camacho T: Perceived health and mortality: a nine year follow-up of the Human Population Laboratory cohort, Am J Epidemiol 117(3):292, 1983.

Killeen ML: What is the health risk appraisal telling us? West J Nurs Res 11(5):614, 1989.

Kirscht JP: Process and measurement issues in health risk appraisal (editorial), Am J Public Health 79(12): 1598, 1989.

Koplin AN, Davidow B, Backman P, and Escobar V: The combined employee health risk: occupational hazard appraisal— the New York City experience, J Public Health Policy 9(1):42, 1988.

Kotler P and Wingard DL: The effect of occupational, marital and parental role on mortality: the Alameda County Study, Am J Public Health 79(5):607, 1989.

LaLonde M: A new perspective on the health of Canadians, Ottawa, 1974, Government of Canada.

Lasater T et al.: Lay volunteer delivery of a community-based cardiovascular risk factor change program: the Pawtucket Experiment. In Matarazzo JD, Weiss SM, Herd JA, Miller NE, and Weiss SM, editors: Behavioral health: a handbook of health enhancement and disease prevention, Silver Spring, MD, 1984, John Wiley & Sons.

Lefebvre RC et al.: Community intervention to lower blood cholesterol: the "Know Your Cholesterol" campaign in Pawtucket, Rhode Island, Health Educ Q 13(2):117, 1986.

Lorig K: Arthritis self-management: a joint venture— a multiple outcome patient education evaluation, doctoral dissertation, Berkeley, CA, 1980, University of California—Berkeley.

Maccoby N, Farquhar JW, Wood PD, and Alexander J: Reducing the risk of cardiovascular disease: effects of a community-based campaign on knowledge and behavior, J Community Health 3(2):100, 1977.

McBride S: Validation of an instrument to measure exercise of self-care agency, Res Nurs Health 10(3):311, 1987.

McKinlay JB and McKinlay SM: The questionable contribution of medical measures to the decline of mortality in the United States in the twentieth century, Milbank Q 55(3):405, 1977.

Meeker WC: A review of the validity and efficacy of the health risk appraisal instrument, J Manipulative Physiol Ther 11(2):108, 1988.

Milio N: Promoting health through public policy, Philadelphia, 1981, FA Davis.

Minkler M: Improving health through community organization. In Glanz K, Lewis FM, and Rimer BK, editors: Health behavior and health education: theory, research, and practice, San Francisco, 1990, Jossey-Bass Publishers.

Moody L et al.: A computerized health profile model for adolescents. In Proceedings of the 15th meeting of the Society of Prospective Medicine, Bethesda, MD, 1979, Society of Prospective Medicine.

National Wellness Institute: Lifestyle assessment questionnaire, Stevens Point, WI, 1988, The Institute.

Oregon Health Division: Health objectives for the year 2000: report of the Oregon Health 2000 Project, Portland, OR, 1988, The Division.

Orem D: Nursing: concepts of practice, New York, 1985, McGraw-Hill Book Co.

Pender NJ: Health promotion in nursing practice, Norwalk, CT, 1987, Appleton & Lange.

Perry CL, Baranowski T, and Parcel GS: How individuals, environments, and health behavior interact: social learning theory. In Glanz K, Lewis FM, and Rimer BK, editors: Health behavior and health education: theory, research, and practice, San Francisco, 1990, Jossey-Bass Publishers.

Pilon BA and Renfroe D: Evaluation of an employee health risk appraisal program, AAOHN J 38(5):230, 1990.

Puska P et al.: Change in risk factors for coronary heart disease during 10 years of a community intervention programme (North Karelia Project), Br Med J (Clin Res) 287(6408):1840, 1983.

Renne KS: Measurement of social health in a general population survey, Soc Sci Res 3:25, 1974.

Robbins LC and Hall JN: How to practice prospective medicine, Indianapolis, 1970, Methodist Hospital of Indiana.

Rowley DL et al.: Are current health risk appraisals suitable for black women? In Proceedings of the 21st annual meeting of the Society of Prospective Medicine, Bethesda, MD, 1985, Society of Prospective Medicine.

Schoenbach VJ, Wagner EH, Beery WL: Health risk appraisal: review of evidence for effectiveness, Health Serv Res 22(4):553, 1987.

Schultz CM: Lifestyle assessment: a tool for practice, Nurs Clin North Am 19(2):271, 1984.

Sherman Z: Health risk appraisal at the worksite, AAOHN J 38(1):18, 1990.

Shy CM et al.: Project to modify the CDC Health risk appraisal for blue collar workers. In Proceedings of the 21st annual meeting of the Society of Prospective Medicine, Bethesda, MD, 1985, Society of Prospective Medicine.

Skinner HA, Allen BA, McIntosh MC, and Palmer WH: Lifestyle assessment: just asking makes a difference, BR Med J 290:214, 1985.

Smeltzy J: Employee health promotion: the Hennepin Wellway program, Am J Public Health 75(7):785, 1985.

Smith KW, McKinlay SM, and McKinlay JB: The reliability of health risk appraisals: a field trial of four instruments, Am J Public Health 79(12):1603, 1989.

Smith KW, McKinlay SM, and Thorington BD: The validity of health risk appraisal instruments for assessing coronary heart disease risk, Am J Public Health 77(4):419, 1987.

Tardiff K, Gross E, and Messner SF: A study of homicides in Manhattan: 1981, Am J Public Health 76(2):139, 1986.

Travis JW: Wellness workbook for health professionals, Mill Valley, CA, 1977, Wellness Resource Center.

Wesley J: Primitive physic: or, an easy and natural method for curing most diseases, London, 1747, Thomas Trye.

Wildavsky A: Doing better and feeling worse: the political pathology of health policy, Daedalus 106:105, 1977.

Wiley JA and Camacho TC: Life-style and future health: evidence from the Alameda County Study, Prev Med 9(1):1, 1980.

Williams CL, Carter BJ, and Eng A: The "Know Your Body" program: a developmental approach to health education and disease prevention, Prev Med 9(3):371, 1980.

Wingard DL, Berkman LF, and Brand RJ: A multivariate analysis of health-related practices: a nine-year mortality follow-up of the Alameda County Study, Am J Epidemiol 116(5):765, 1982.

Wisconsin Department of Health and Social Services: Healthier people in Wisconsin: a public health agenda for the year 2000—report of the Division of Health, Madison, WI, 1990, The Department.

Woods N: Conceptualization of self-care: toward health oriented models, ANS 12(1):1, 1989.

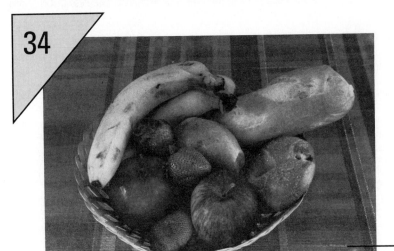

34

Health Promotion Through Nutrition, Exercise, and Sleep

Kathleen Beckman Blomquist

OBJECTIVES

After reading this chapter, the student should be able to:

Discuss reasons nurses should be knowledgeable about nutrition, exercise, and sleep.

Discuss changes in the dietary habits of Americans that could significantly reduce the incidence of leading diseases.

Analyze factors influencing food consumption.

Discuss the origin and usefulness of the RDAs.

Use dietary guidelines and the nursing process to plan and evaluate diets.

Evaluate physiological and psychological benefits of exercise.

Design exercise programs for individuals and groups of people.

Assist clients to improve sleep and rest patterns.

Use the nursing process to help clients engage in healthy behaviors.

KEY TERMS

aerobic exercise
anorexia
Basic Food Groups
bulimia
cooldown
Dietary Guidelines for Americans
exercise
food exchange system

Meals on Wheels
NREM sleep
nutrients
nutritional assessment
obesity
physical activity
physical fitness
Recommended Dietary Allowances (RDAs)

REM sleep
sleep deprivation
Special Supplemental Food Program for Women, Infants, and Children (WIC)
target heart rate
warmup
vegetarians

H ilda and Carl Willow are 60 years old, moderately obese, and mildly hypertensive. Mrs. Willow has trouble sleeping. Their physician tells them that if they will lose some weight and get some exercise, they might not have to take medication to control their blood pressures. The Willows provide an example of the challenge nurses in the community face in promoting the health of people with chronic diseases caused by sedentary lifestyles and inadequate dietary practices. Nurses play a major role in primary prevention of chronic disease by encouraging people to be more active and eat properly. Community health nurses are often the only contact community residents have with the health care system. Through health promotion programming, nurses can have great impact on the health of community groups.

This chapter discusses current trends in nutrition, exercise, and sleep, and the role of nurses in educating community residents about these lifestyle issues. The chapter concludes with the health promotion program planned with Mr. and Mrs. Willow.

PROMOTING HEALTH THROUGH NUTRITION

Nurses are concerned about the nutritional status of all their clients. All people eat to stay alive, and what is eaten affects health from conception through old age. Throughout the world, chronic malnutrition affects physical and mental development. In industrialized societies, diet-related conditions are among the leading causes of disease and death (Scrimshaw, 1990).

Many diet-related diseases result from nutritional excesses rather than undernourishment. Coronary heart disease, the number-one killer in the United States, is linked with excessive intake of saturated fats and cholesterol. Cancer is linked to high-fat, low-fiber diets, and alcohol consumption. High blood pressure, a risk factor for strokes, is associated with intake of excessive calories and salt. Liver disease is associated with heavy alcohol consumption. Diabetes mellitus is associated with excessive calorie intake and subsequent obesity.

Because of frequent and extended contact with clients in the community, nurses have excellent opportunities to provide information and counseling about the role of nutrition in health promotion and prevention of illness. Knowledge and skills related to nutrition enable community health nurses to:

1. *Answer questions clients ask about nutrition.* The media bombard people with nutrition information. People are interested in and sometimes confused about the relationship of nutrition to health. They expect nurses to be able to answer questions and resolve confusion.

2. *Provide appropriate dietary advice.* Community health nurses should be familiar with basic dietary principles so they can counsel healthy people as well as those with disease conditions.

3. *Recommend age-appropriate diets and eating strategies.* Nutritional requirements change throughout life. Nurses knowledgeable about the special needs of infants, children, adolescents, pregnant and lactating women, and adults of all ages can improve the nutritional health of these groups.

4. *Prevent and treat diseases.* Diet is an important factor in the etiology and treatment of many disease conditions. Nurses care for healthy and ill clients through nutritional counseling and referral to community resources. Appropriate diet prevents or delays symptoms of disease and supports the body in recovery. Anticipatory guidance is an important aspect of care. For example, women planning pregnancy, people having elective surgery, and middle-aged and aging persons benefit from nutritional guidance. Some nutrition resources, such as emergency food pantries, offer food. Other resources provide mechanisms for extending food dollars, such as the federal government's Food Stamp program. Information is offered by nutritionists at health departments, county extension offices, and private agencies such as the American Dairy Council, the American Health Association, and food manufacturing companies.

5. *Identify and appropriately refer malnourished clients.* Dietitians and nutritionists are trained to assess clients' diets and help clients meet their nutritional needs. Appropriate referral to these specialists improves health care services.

6. *Evaluate current research studies.* Controlled studies in clinical nutrition are difficult to design, conduct, and interpret because of the complexity of diets and the variations in nutritional needs of individuals due to age, sex, activity, and physical condition. Three questions can be asked when evaluating research studies related to nutrition:

   What kind of evidence has been presented relating a specific nutrient to a certain disease process?

   What is the quality (strength) of this evidence?

   What are the possible risks and benefits of increasing, reducing, or eliminating the specific nutrient from the diet?

The answers to these questions assist nurses in determining the validity of claims made about dietary practices. By combining knowledge of nutrition principles with this analysis of information, community health nurses can help clients to understand the difference between proven and unsubstantiated nutrition information (Burtis, Davis, and Martin, 1988; Nestle, 1985).

Factors Influencing Diet

What people eat is determined by a variety of factors including biological needs, psychological characteristics, sociocultural influences, and environmental aspects. Research in the area of nutrition is rapidly producing new information, some of which contradicts old ideas. Politics, economics, and social norms influence the growing, marketing, distribution, and consumption of food products. Figure 34-1 summarizes some factors that influence food selection and ultimately the health of a population. Dietary counseling should be based on an understanding of the biological, psychological, sociocultural, and environmental factors influencing food selection and eating behaviors.

Biological Factors

The human body requires certain nutrients to maintain health. Appendix J15 summarizes the nutrients needed for

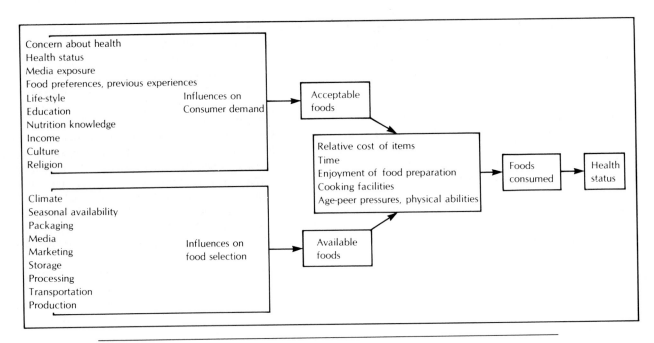

FIGURE 34-1

Factors influencing food selection.

growth, development, and repair of body structures and maintenance of body processes. Level of activity and stress, age and rate of growth, genetics, and a variety of factors such as temperature, taste, and smell affect intake of food. In addition, medications, tobacco, alcohol, and caffeine affect absorption of vitamins and minerals (Williams, 1988).

Psychological Factors

Eating behavior is affected both by positive emotions, such as enjoyment and tranquility, and negative feelings like anger and insecurity. Food may represent rewards, comfort, and security. Habits, such as skipping breakfast or taking regular mid-morning coffee and donut breaks, are important factors in determining eating behavior. They require little or no conscious thought and often result in poor dietary practices. Two other important factors are self-esteem and knowledge about nutrition. Both affect the foods a person selects.

Sociocultural Factors

The cultural and ethnic backgrounds of clients play a major role in food selection and eating behaviors. Many cultural practices have evolved because they are healthful (Wilson, 1985). Recognition of and respect for these food preferences are important for nurses counseling clients in the community. Nurses should gather information about the nutritional value of ethnic foods, tailor recommended changes as much as possible to cultural practices, and encourage major changes only when foods are clearly hazardous to the health of clients. Working with a client of a particular ethnic group for whom a specific diet has been recommended can be quite a challenge for the community health nurse and requires the nurse, client, and the client's family to work as a team. For example, the diet recom-

mended for an Hispanic client with hypertension will be quite different from that of a hypertensive Japanese client.

The number of vegetarians has increased rapidly over the past few years partly in response to information about the relationship of animal fat to cardiovascular disease. Vegetarians, especially those who eat no dairy products or eggs, must plan meals that contain essential amino acids, vitamins, and minerals. Meals will supply essential amino acids if they include legumes (such as soy beans, other beans, or peas) and whole grains, nuts, or seeds. Calcium, iron, vitamin D, and vitamin B_{12} intake may be deficient in some vegetarian diets, especially for growth and development of children and adolescents and for the health of pregnant women (Dwyer, 1988).

Environmental Factors

Cost, accessibility, convenience, and safety are major factors influencing food selection and eating behavior. With rising food prices, consumers attempt to get the most for their money. Unfortunately, foods high in nutritional value, such as fruits and grains, may be more expensive than highly refined sugar products and may require more preparation. Consumers often buy foods that are easy to prepare but are high in calories and fats and low in nutritional value. By being familiar with cultural preferences and available resources, nurses can assist clients to select menus that are nutritionally sound. For example, nurses may recommend seasonal fruits and vegetables to minimize cost and maximize nutritional value; they may recommend that less expensive cuts of meat be purchased by low-income families or that beans be used as a source of protein in the diet of vegetarians. Nurses should be ready to assist with food preparation when they introduce new foods.

Accessibility is a major factor in food selection. Many

low-income families have limited mobility and must rely on local merchants. Small local stores tend to be more expensive than supermarkets. Planning meals over several days and shopping less often, but in larger stores, may help clients learn to plan more nutritious, less expensive meals.

Convenience also plays a large part in food selection. Many women work outside the home, so families today eat more meals that are quickly and easily prepared. They are also eating "out" more often. Counseling regarding the nutritional value, deficiencies, and excesses of convenient and "fast-food" menus is an important function of community health nurses.

Safety of food and water is not usually a problem for families in the United States because of the network of inspection services. However, the number of chemicals in use is increasing rapidly. The ability to detect potentially harmful substances is improving, and all community residents, especially health professionals, should be alert to the potential for contamination of air, water, and foods. In homes, nurses can teach families about food preparation and storage to ensure that food is not spoiled. For example, nurses can discuss with families how to prepare and store lunches taken to school or work.

Recommended Dietary Allowances

Recommended dietary allowances (RDAs) are the amounts of essential nutrients considered adequate to meet the known nutritional needs of most healthy persons. The RDAs are developed by a committee of scientists designated by the National Academy of Sciences' Food and Nutrition Board. The Committee bases its recommendations on a review of the world's literature on nutrient requirements, paying particular attention to new findings.

The RDAs were first published in 1943 and have been revised about every five years to include new scientific information. The 10th edition was released in 1989. This revision was scheduled to be published at the end of 1985, but the proposed changes were rejected by the Food and Nutrition Board because the committee's suggestions altered the concept of RDA from that of meeting nutritional needs for nearly all healthy people to "protecting practically all healthy persons against nutritional deficiencies."

Changes made in the 10th edition of the RDAs include increases in recommendations for calcium and vitamin C. Decreases in recommendations were made for iron for women of childbearing age as well as for sodium, vitamins B_6 and B_{12}, folate, magnesium, and zinc. RDAs were set for the first time for vitamin K and selenium.

The RDAs will continue to evolve as new information becomes available. Topics of current interest include developing guidelines for fats, carbohydrates, and additional minerals, and specific RDAs for all nutrients for the elderly. The current RDAs do not reflect the new thrust of reducing risk for chronic disease through diet.

The RDAs are recommendations for the average daily amounts of nutrients that population groups should consume over a period of time. Consistent consumption of less than 70% of the RDA for a vitamin, mineral, or protein is cause for concern. Although it is almost impossible to exceed the RDA limits with foods alone, people who take vitamin and mineral supplements should be aware of possible toxic effects of fat-soluble vitamins (A, D, E, and K) at levels above five times the RDA and of some minerals at three times the RDA (Monsen, 1989).

Since nutrient needs vary by sex and stage of life, the RDAs give recommendations for nutrients by sex and age groups. Appendix J15 lists the RDAs for nutrients for adult men and women. Nutrition texts list the RDAs for the various age and sex groups. The RDAs that appear on food labels use the highest RDA of a nutrient for any group.

The RDAs are used by federal, state, and local health and welfare agencies for licensing and certification standards for day care centers, schools, nursing homes, and other group feeding programs. They are used to interpret food consumption records, evaluate adequacy of food supplies in meeting nutritional needs, establish guides for public food assistance programs, evaluate newly developed food products, establish guidelines for nutritional labeling of foods, and develop nutrition education programs.

Dietary Guidelines

Practical food guides have been developed to assist health care workers with nutrition education. Such tools include the basic food groups, the food exchange system, and the Dietary Guidelines for Americans.

The United States Department of Agriculture identified the Basic Food Groups as a guide for planning a well-balanced diet. Although this guide has its limitations, it provides a practical, general basis for planning meals and evaluating a person's overall food intake. Table 34-1 outlines the basic food groups and summarizes appropriate food groups.

Another food guide in general use, especially for modified diets such as for diabetics or the obese is the food exchange system. There are six food groups in this system: milk, vegetables, fruits, breads and other starches, meats and other protein foods, and fats. These foods are grouped according to their similarity in calories and food values, so a set portion (amount) of food from each group can be traded off ("exchanged") in meals. This provides an easy way for anyone to learn to balance a meal. Most nutrition texts provide exchange lists.

The Dietary Guidelines for Americans were developed by the United States Departments of Agriculture and Health and Human Services in 1980 and revised in 1985 and 1990. They recommend changes in food intake to improve the health of the population. No guidelines guarantee health or well-being, and individuals vary widely in their food needs, but these general statements about variety and moderation can help people improve nutritional intake.

Statements that comprise the Dietary Guidelines for Americans and some suggestions for nurses to assist clients to follow the guidelines are described in the following paragraphs (Pennington, 1989; USDA and USDHHS, 1985, 1990; Williams, 1988).

Eat a variety of foods. About 40 different nutrients are needed to maintain health and no single food can supply all the essential nutrients in the amounts needed. To ensure variety, teach clients to select foods from all of the major food groups on a daily basis.

Maintain ideal weight. Obesity is associated with chronic disorders, such as hypertension, diabetes, and heart disease. Each person's "ideal" weight must be determined individually, since many factors are involved, such as body composition, body metabolism, genetics, and physical activity. The following formulas can be used to roughly calculate

ideal weight with a 10-pound leeway (Anderson, 1989):

Males: 106 pounds for the first 5 feet and add 6 pounds for each additional inch of height.

Females: 100 pounds for the first 5 feet and add 5 pounds for each additional inch of height.

For example, ideal weight for a woman who is 5 feet 8

TABLE 34-1
The basic food groups

Food group	Main nutrients	Daily amounts
Vegetables	Vitamin A Vitamin C (ascorbic acid) Folate Magnesium Fiber	3-5 servings 1 serving equals: ⅓ cup raw or cooked vegetables 1 cup raw leafy vegetables Include: 1 dark green or deep yellow vegetable or fruit rich in vitamin A, at least every other day
Fruits	Vitamin C Fiber	2-4 servings 1 serving equals: ¼ cup dried fruit ½ cup cooked fruit ¾ cup juice 1 whole piece of fruit 1 melon wedge
Breads, cereals, and other grains	Thiamin Niacin Riboflavin Iron Protein	6-11 servings of whole-grain, enriched, or restored 1 serving equals: 1 slice bread 1 oz (1 cup) ready-to-eat cereal, flake or puff varieties ½-¾ cup cooked cereal ½-¾ cup cooked pasta (macaroni, spaghetti, noodles) Crackers: 5 saltines, 2 squares graham crackers, etc.

Meats
  Beef, veal, lamb, pork, poultry, fish, eggs
 	
  Alternatives: dry beans and peas, nuts, peanut butter
	Protein
	Iron
	Thiamin
	Niacin
	Riboflavin
		2 or more servings
		1 serving equals:
		2-3 oz lean, boneless, cooked meat, poultry, or fish
		2 eggs
		1-1½ cup cooked dry beans or peas
		4 tbsp peanut butter
		½-1 cup nuts

Milk	Calcium Protein Riboflavin Potassium Zinc	Children under 9: 2-3 cups Children 9 to 12: 3 or more cups Teenagers: 4 or more cups Adults: 2 or more cups Pregnant women: 3 or more cups Nursing mothers: 4 or more cups (1 cup = 8 oz fluid milk or designated milk equivalent) 1 serving equals: 1 cup milk, skim milk, buttermilk ¼ cup dry skimmed milk powder ½ cup evaporated milk 1½ oz cheese 2 oz processed cheese 1 cup yogurt 2 cups cottage cheese 1 cup custard/pudding 1½ cups ice cream 1 cup ice milk
Fats, sweets, and alcoholic beverages		Avoid

From U. S. Department of Agriculture, Home and Garden Bulletin #23 2-1, April, 1986.

inches tall is $100 + (8 \times 5) = 140$; plus or minus 10 pounds gives a range of 130 to 150 pounds.

Suggestions on ways to improve eating habits, such as eating slowly, preparing smaller portions, avoiding second helpings, and concentrating on eating rather than reading or watching TV may be useful to overweight clients. Eating frequent meals may help underweight clients gain weight.

Avoid too much saturated fat and cholesterol. Americans maintain a high-fat diet. Some people do not tolerate much fat, and increased fat intake leads to high levels of blood lipids and cholesterol, which are associated with higher risk of heart disease. People should get less than 30 percent of their calories from fat, with only 10 percent coming from animal fat and tropical oils. To assist families in lowering fat intake, nurses can suggest the following:

Choose lean meat, fish, poultry.

Trim excess fat off meats and remove skin from chicken.

Cook meats on racks that allow fat to drain off.

Stretch meat portions by mixing meats with grains and vegetables in mixed dishes.

For protein, eat legumes such as soybean substances, other beans, and peas.

Use no more than three eggs per week.

Eat organ meats (e.g., liver) very infrequently.

Limit intake of hydrogenated margarines, shortenings, coconut oil, and foods made from such products.

Use low-fat milk and dairy products.

Prefer baking, broiling, or boiling over frying.

Read labels carefully to determine both amounts and types of fats contained in foods.

Eat foods with adequate starch and fiber. Complex carbohydrates, such as whole grain cereals and breads, beans, peas, fruits, and vegetables, are better sources for energy than are fats and sugars and contain many essential nutrients and fiber. The average American diet is low in fiber because many processed and refined foods are eaten. Fiber improves bowel functioning and contributes to cholesterol and blood sugar control (Anderson, 1989). Nurses can encourage clients to:

Choose whole grain breads and pastas instead of white breads and refined pastas.

Eat two or more servings of fresh fruits daily.

Frequently eat dark green leafy vegetables and deep yellow vegetables, dry beans, and peas.

Eat starchy vegetables such as potatoes and corn.

Eat brown rice instead of white refined rice.

Choose baked potatoes with skins instead of mashed potatoes.

Eat whole grain cereals such as corn, wheat, and oats for breakfast.

Avoid too much sugar. The major health hazard resulting from eating too much sugar is tooth decay. If sugar creates excess calories, obesity results. Each American eats over 100 pounds of sugar per year. To avoid excess sugar, nurses can recommend that people:

Use less of all sugars including white, brown, and raw sugars, honey, and syrups.

Eat fewer foods containing sugar, such as candy, soft drinks, ice cream, and cake.

Read food labels for clues to sugar content. If sucrose, glucose, maltose, dextrose, lactose, fructose, or syrup appear first, or if several of these sugars are listed, the product contains a large amount of sugar.

Select fresh fruits or fruits canned without sugar.

Avoid too much sodium. Many processed foods contain added sodium, and most Americans eat more sodium than they need. Lower sodium intake by cooking without salt, adding little salt to foods at the table, limiting intake of salty foods, reading labels to determine the amount of sodium in processed foods, and being aware of sodium content in water and medications.

If you drink alcohol, do so in moderation. Alcoholic beverages are high in calories and low in nutrients. Limited food intake may accompany heavy drinking. Alcohol contributes to chronic liver disease, neurological disorders, and throat and neck cancer. Encourage clients to drink fewer than two alcohol-containing drinks per day. Nurses working with clients who drink excessively can consider help from community resources such as Alcoholics Anonymous or local mental health centers.

In addition to these suggestions, the USDA revised its Hassle-Free Daily Food Guide in 1991 to make it a total, easy-to-follow plan. The latest version, *USDA's Food Guide—A Pattern for Daily Food Choices,* is shown in Table 34-1. This guide increases fruit and vegetable servings from 4 servings to 5 to 9 servings per day and increases bread and cereal from 4 servings to 6 to 11 servings per day. The aim of these changes is to limit fat while increasing carbohydrates.

There are several important points to keep in mind:

1. The guide is not meant for infants.
2. No one food group provides all essential nutrients.
3. No one food is absolutely essential to good nutrition.
4. Variety is essential.

The keys to making the plan work are variety, balance, and moderation.

Using the Nursing Process to Promote Sound Nutrition

Since most meal planning and preparation occurs in the home, community health nurses can provide nutrition education during home visits. Physicians, dietitians, nutritionists, and home economists often assist in resolving nutritional problems and related diseases. However, the responsibility for identification of problems frequently rests with community health nurses who use the nursing process to detect and intervene in nutritional difficulties encountered by individuals, families, and groups in the community.

Assessment and Diagnosis

Nutritional assessment of an individual or group of people should include biological, psychological, cultural, and environmental factors. Review of the person's medical history may identify conditions that place the client at risk for malnutrition. Some of these conditions include hypermetabolic states, compromised digestive or resorptive capacity, chronic or acute diseases associated with abnormal nutrient intake or loss, recent major surgery, or a treatment plan with nutritional implications, such as chemotherapy, radiation, or multiple drug therapies. Side effects of some medications cause nutritional problems or symptoms of nutri-

TABLE 34-2
Clinical signs of nutritional status

Features	Good	Poor
General appearance	Alert, responsive	Listless, apathetic; cachexia
General vitality	Endurance; energetic; sleeps well at night; vigorous	Fatigues easily, no energy, falls asleep, looks tired, apathetic
Weight	Normal for height, age, body build	Overweight or underweight
Skin	Smooth, slightly moist; good color	Rough, dry, scaly, pale, pigmented, irritated; petechiae, bruises
Posture	Erect, arms and legs straight, abdomen in, chest out	Sagging shoulders, sunken chest, humped back
Muscles	Well developed, firm	Flaccid, poor tone; undeveloped, tender
Skeleton	No malformations	Bowlegs, knock-knees, chest deformity at diaphragm, beaded ribs, prominent scapulae
Legs and feet	No tenderness, weakness, or swelling; good color	Edema, tender calves; tingling, weakness
Nervous control	Good attention span for age; does not cry easily; not irritable or restless	Inattentive, irritable
Hair	Shiny, lustrous; healthy scalp	Stringy, dull, brittle, dry, depigmented
Neck glands	No enlargement	Thyroid enlarged
Skin on face and neck	Smooth, slightly moist; good color; reddish pink mucous membranes	Greasy, discolored, scaly
Eyes	Bright, clear; no fatigue circles	Dryness, signs of infection, increased vascularity, glassiness, thickened conjunctivae
Lips	Good color, moist	Dry, scaly, swollen, angular lesions (stomatitis)
Tongue	Good pink color; surface papillae present; no lesions	Papillary atrophy, smooth appearance; swollen, red beefy (glossitis)
Gums	Good pink color; no swelling or bleeding; firm	Marginal redness or swelling; receding, spongy
Teeth	Straight, no crowding; well-shaped jaw; clean, no discoloration	Unfilled cavities, absent teeth, worn surfaces; mottled, malpositioned
Abdomen	Flat	Swollen
Gastrointestinal function	Good appetite and digestion; normal, regular elimination	Anorexia, indigestion, constipation or diarrhea

Modified from Williams SR: Basic nutrition and diet therapy, ed 7. St. Louis, 1984, The CV Mosby Co.

tional problems and should be considered when doing physiological assessment. For example, antibiotics may cause stomatitis, nausea, vomiting, gastritis, or diarrhea; and steroids may cause digestive tract disturbances or interfere with protein, lipid, and electrolyte utilization (Burtis, Davis, and Martin, 1988; Williams, 1988).

Community health nurses should be alert to the possibility of eating disorders such as anorexia (fear of gaining weight and disturbances in perception of body) or bulimia (binge eating often followed by self-induced vomiting, fasting, use of laxatives or diuretics, or vigorous exercise), especially in young women or athletes in sports with weight categories (such as wrestling or boxing). Bulimia is much more common than anorexia and is often associated with alcohol abuse or depression. Assessment includes evaluating the client's concept of weight and self image, relationships with family members, and use of alcohol and drugs, as well as checking on nutritional deficiencies through physical exams (Edelstein, Haskew, & Kramer, 1989). A physical examination can enable the nurse to document signs and symptoms of inadequate nutrition. Table 34-2 summarizes clinical signs of nutritional status.

During interviews with clients about food intake, nurses can obtain information on patterns of eating, food aversions, intolerances, and difficulties in eating or digesting certain foods. Some key questions to ask during nutritional assessment are listed in the box at right.

During the assessment and diagnosis phase, the nurse may ask the client to keep a food diary of all foods and beverages consumed, the time of day foods are eaten, and environmental and emotional aspects of the eating situation. The nurse and client can review the diary together to identify eating and food selection patterns and to plan interventions.

Assessment and diagnosis that focus only on the foods eaten but ignore the cultural, environmental, and economic influences on dietary habits fail to provide an adequate basis for planning nursing interventions. Information must be obtained regarding food preferences, preparation time, cost, availability, daily meal patterns, physical limitations, and environmental constraints (e.g., lack of running water). In addition, the client's relation to the family and community as a whole must be considered to gain an understanding of all influences on food selection and eating behaviors. For example, before helping a client with hypertension in selecting a low sodium diet, the nurse should gather information and state diagnoses regarding such variables as the

---

KEY QUESTIONS TO ASK DURING NUTRITIONAL ASSESSMENT

How much do you weigh and how tall are you?

What is the most you have ever weighed? When and under what circumstances?

Has your weight changed recently? How much? Any idea why?

Do you follow a special diet at home? Type?

Are there any foods you avoid? What and why? (aversions, intolerances, allergies, culture)

Have you recently experienced nausea, vomiting, diarrhea, constipation, chewing or swallowing problems?

Have you experienced any changes in your appetite? in food intake?

Are you taking any vitamins or nutritional supplements? Type?

What is your occupation? Usual activity?

Are you being treated for any disease? taking any medications?

Have you had surgery? When and type?

Recall all the food you have eaten in the past 24 hours.

---

major foods eaten, the client's eating patterns (food prepared at home vs. meals eaten out), family support of the dietary changes for one member (how willing other family members are to alter their diets), and cultural influences (e.g., an ethnic diet high in sodium).

Planning

The information gathered and organized during assessment and diagnosis guides plans for nutrition education. Whether working with individuals, families, or groups, community health nurses must consider the concerns, interests, and priorities of the potential audience when planning interventions. Clients may have limited food choices because of the cost and availability of foods, or they may be confused over advertising claims.

During the planning phase of the nursing process, include all individuals who will be affected by the proposed nutritional changes. For example, when assisting an adolescent to plan a weight reduction diet, include family members responsible for selecting, preparing, and financing the food. Inclusion in the planning process generally encourages participation in implementation of the diet.

In the planning phase, additional resource persons such as nutritionists, physicians, and social workers are consulted to assist in meeting the identified needs of the clients. Special needs of clients may be met by community nutrition resources or government aid programs. For example, poor pregnant women and families with low-birth-weight infants may be eligible for the Special Supplemental Food Program for Women, Infants, and Children (WIC), commonly administered through local health departments. Elderly clients confined to their homes may benefit from Meals on Wheels, a local program in which one hot meal and sometimes a cold breakfast and sack lunch are brought to their homes daily. Poor families may be able to obtain food stamps to extend their food dollars. Local food banks offer food in times of crisis, and soup kitchens at community centers or churches offer free meals.

Implementation

The nursing process culminates in the implementation and evaluation of the plan jointly developed by nurses, clients, and their families. Involving clients and their families in the planning phase, setting reasonable and achievable goals, and suggesting incorporation of self-rewards into the plans keep clients interested and motivated during implementation of the nursing care plan.

Evaluation

How clients and their families perceive the benefits of the proposed changes is essential to success. Discussion and feedback about progress are important. Progress can be monitored and modifications made to ensure maximum benefit from the nursing interventions. Evaluation at the conclusion of nursing interventions provides nurses and clients with valuable information about the degree to which objectives and client needs have been met, what strategies were effective, and any further data collection and planning that is needed.

To evaluate progress, community health nurses may ask clients to keep food diaries for one or more days each week. Nurses can use data in the diaries to educate and reinforce clients and their families about a balanced diet.

Weight Control

Obesity is generally defined as being 20% or more overweight. Heredity, interpersonal factors (e.g., family problems, anxiety, unrealistic expectations of self and others), sociocultural factors (such as food selection or preparation practices), and environmental factors have been identified as probable causes of obesity. Numerous studies have suggested that it is more important to deal with personal, social, and environmental influences rather than with biochemical causes of obesity.

Because of their holistic approach to care, nurses can be quite effective in assisting obese people to lose weight. Assessment of the individual desiring weight loss is essential to developing an individualized, effective program. In addition to gathering data regarding current dietary practices and sociocultural influences, nurses should also consider the client's past weight loss efforts. Persons who derive the greatest benefits from a weight reduction program exhibit adult-onset rather than adolescent-onset obesity; they report fewer previous attempts to lose weight; and they are more adept at self-reinforcement (Pender, 1987). The box on p. 600 offers suggestions for controlling weight.

Although controversy exists regarding the value of many nutrients, little doubt remains that nutrition plays a vital role in maintaining health. Attempts are being made to link diseases with dietary practices, and the government has made recommendations regarding the nutritional intake and elimination of excesses from the American diet.

The concept of physical fitness and its relation to health promotion and maintenance is also receiving much attention. The next section of this chapter focuses on exercise.

TIPS TO CONTROL EATING AND WEIGHT

Decrease fat and sugar in recipes.

Set realistic goals. Two pounds per week is reasonable weight loss. Use charts to visualize progress. Plan rewards for certain loss levels.

Eat regularly—3 or more small meals per day. Skipping meals promotes binging.

Eat small portions of all nutritious foods and favorite foods.

Slow down when eating: count bites, chews, or swallows; put utensils down between bites; pay attention to your food so your brain knows you have eaten; leave the table when full.

When you want a snack, wait 10 minutes and distract yourself. The urge to eat may pass.

Have a small snack of fruit or salad to control hunger before cooking or going out to eat.

Keep the serving plates out of reach at the table. At social events, stand a distance away from the food table.

Shop only once per week at a supermarket rather than the corner store to control expenses and limit "impulse buying."

Buy groceries from a list; shop *after* a meal.

Put food out of sight; serve in covered dishes; store in non-see-through containers.

Minimize tasting when cooking; don't lick serving utensils before washing them.

When cleaning up, scrape leftovers into storage containers, the dog's dish, or garbage—don't eat leftovers after your meal.

Exercise daily. Increase exercise when weight loss plateaus.

Gather support. Join Weight Watchers. Start a weight loss program or contest at your workplace or church. Ask family members to help through regular praise and rewards.

PROMOTING HEALTH THROUGH EXERCISE

Exercise promotes physiological and psychological health. Community health nurses are in prime positions to observe activity patterns and problems of individuals and groups. By recognizing the potential benefits of exercise, innovative and vitally important nursing interventions can be planned.

The majority of American adults are concerned about their physical fitness and think that regular exercise is essential to good health. However, only about one-third of all adults participate in exercise on a weekly basis, and only 10% exercise at levels recommended for cardiovascular fitness. Well educated, affluent, young adults have increased their exercise participation. Americans over 50 have limited knowledge of the kinds and amounts of activity needed to maintain physical fitness, and many believe that exercise may be dangerous (Dishman, Sallis, and Orenstein, 1985; Public Health Service, 1990).

Physical activity is movement produced by skeletal muscles that results in energy expenditure. Exercise is physical activity that is planned, structured, and repetitive and is designed to improve or maintain physical fitness (Powell and Paffenbarger, 1985). Physical fitness is a set of physiological attributes, some of which are health related. Fitness is defined as the ability to perform moderate to vigorous levels of physical activity without undue fatigue and the capability of maintaining such ability through life (American College of Sports Medicine (ACSM), 1990). The skill-related measures of physical fitness required for performance of particular sports or activities are agility, balance, coordination, speed, power, and reaction time. The measures of physical fitness important for health are cardiorespiratory endurance, flexibility, body composition, muscular endurance, and muscular strength. Table 34-3 defines each of these measures and lists ways to evaluate them. Levels of physical fitness range from high to low, and the measures may differ greatly; for example, a person may be strong but not flexible.

TABLE 34-3
Health-related physical fitness measures

Measure	Definition	Evaluation
1. Cardiorespiratory endurance	Ability of the circulatory and respiratory systems to supply fuel during sustained physical activity and to eliminate waste products that produce fatigue	Maximum or submaximum oxygen uptake tests on treadmill or cycle ergometer; 12-minute run
2. Muscular endurance	Ability of muscle groups to exert external force for many repetitious or successive exertions	Isokinetic tests; number of repetitions of pull-ups, sit-ups, or lifts of light to moderate weights
3. Muscular strength	The amount of external force that a muscle can exert	Weight lifts by particular muscles or groups of muscles
4. Flexibility	The range of motion available at a joint	Flexometer tests; sit and reach tests
5. Body composition	Relative amounts of muscle, fat, bone, and other vital parts of the body	Underwater weighing; skinfold pinch test

Modified from Caspersen CJ, Powell KE, and Christenson GM: Physical activity, exercise, and physical fitness: definitions and distinctions for health-related research. Public Health Rep 100:126-131, 1985.

Effects of Exercise

Exercise has both physiological and psychological effects. Both should be considered during nursing assessment, diagnosis, planning, intervention, and evaluation.

Physiological

Nurses recognize the detrimental effects of prolonged bed rest and the resultant lack of exercise. Venous thrombosis, orthostatic hypotension, a progressive increase in heart rate, and a reduction in the strength of skeletal muscles are a few of the problems associated with inactivity. In recent years much research has been conducted to demonstrate a cause-and-effect relationship between physical inactivity in ambulatory populations and specific disease processes. Although no unequivocal relationships have been demonstrated, physiological responses and benefits from exercise have been determined as shown in Table 34-4. Mounting epidemiological evidence suggests that physical inactivity is related to the occurrence of several diseases that are major causes of death and disability in the United States. The relationship between activity and coronary heart disease has been studied the most extensively. Other studies suggest that physical activity also contributes to prevention and control of diabetes mellitus, hypertension, and osteoporosis (Bouchard, Shephard, Stephens, et al., 1990; Pollock and Wilmore, 1990).

Psychological

Claims have been made that exercise produces a variety of psychological benefits. Some of the claims come from anecdotes and self-reports, whereas others have been demonstrated in research studies. The effects may be caused by biochemical changes resulting from the exercise, or by the perceptions of the individual, or a combination of both. Many people claim that they "feel better" when they exercise regularly. Exercise increases arousal, which improves alertness and mood. It enhances self-esteem and body image by increasing the ability to undertake physical and mental work. Regular exercise also tends to control stress, relieve depression and anxiety, and lessen the frequency of minor medical complaints and subsequent absence from work. Cognitive functioning and psychomotor abilities in children, retarded persons, and geriatric clients are enhanced by exercise (Ryan and Allman, 1989; Shephard, 1983).

Potential negative psychological effects of exercise include mental fatigue and compulsiveness, self-centeredness, and competitiveness, all of which affect work and family life. It is not clear whether exercise causes the negative behavior or if certain personalities are predisposed to abuse exercise as a way of coping with other problems (Bouchard et al, 1990; Morgan and Goldston, 1987).

Although the psychological benefits of exercise and physical fitness have been studied in a variety of settings, no exact mechanisms of action have been discovered. Individual differences in expectations, beliefs, coping patterns, and initial fitness potentially affect benefits derived from exercise.

Potential Hazards of Exercise

Exercise can provide many benefits, but it also carries

TABLE 34-4

Responses of body systems to exercise

System	Changes due to conditioning
Muscles and locomotive organs	Increased strength of muscles, bones and ligaments
	Increased volume and tensile strength of tendons and ligaments
	Increased thickness, compressibility, and contact area of articular cartilage
	Increased capillary density (number of capillaries per square millimeter of muscle tissue)
Neurological	Hypertrophy of synapse of nerve fiber with muscle fiber
	Increased ability for motorneurons to be stimulated frequently
	Increase in number of fibers contracting at one time
	Faster reaction time
Blood	Increase in total hemoglobin
	Increase in plasma volume
	Increased speed of formation of red blood cells
Heart	Increase in size and weight of heart muscle and chambers, especially the left ventricle, due to increased muscle volume
	Increased maximum stroke volume and resting stroke volume (about 150%)
	Decrease in heart rate at rest (due to larger stroke volume)
Circulatory	Decrease in blood pressure, if hypertensive
	Increased ability of capillaries to supply blood to working muscles
Respiratory	Increase in maximum oxygen uptake
	Increase in efficiency and endurance of ventilation muscles
Miscellaneous	Increase in ability of cells to utilize sugar in the diabetic, lowering the amount of insulin needed
	Lower risk of colon cancer due to faster GI transit time
	Lower risk of breast cancer, possibly due to control of obesity
	Increase in lean body mass and decrease in fat, if caloric intake is unchanged
	Increase in fatigue threshold—may be psychological, owing to willingness to exert and practice doing so

risks. Client education regarding risks of exercise and how to minimize them should be part of a fitness program. Common problems associated with exercise and related nursing interventions are summarized in Table 34-5 on p. 602.

Fitness Evaluation

The stimuli for many of the health benefits of exercise are not well defined. Many of the health effects may be related more to physical or mechanical stress placed on the muscles, connective tissue, or skeleton than to increased energy ex-

TABLE 34-5
Common exercise-related problems and suggested nursing interventions

Problem	Probable causes	Nursing interventions
Nausea and/or vomiting	Delayed gastric emptying secondary to exercise	Encourage client to exercise on an empty stomach
Dehydration	Inadequate fluid intake	Encourage client to drink fluids (preferably water) before, during, and after exercise
Fatigue, lightheadedness	Overexertion	Teach client to exercise at an intensity at which he can easily talk and is not breathless; teach client to do body and mind checks every few minutes to become aware of symptoms of overexertion and slow down if necessary
Orthopedic injuries	Overuse or misuse	Teach client to warm up before vigorous exercise, gradually increase intensity and duration of exercise over several months, and rest if muscle or joint discomfort develops. Teach appropriate first aid and follow-up measures
		Teach client to run whenever possible on smooth asphalt or cinders rather than concrete or uneven grass, and to wear proper shoes
Injuries related to heat	Inadequate training Inadequate precautions	Encourage clients to exercise during cool parts of day; lower intensity during hot, humid weather. Teach signs, symptoms and first aid for heat stroke and heat exhaustion
		Encourage water intake
Injuries related to cold	Inadequate precautions	Teach client to wear extra clothing during cold weather, perform frequent body checks for sensation, and exercise during warmer parts of day

penditure (Haskell, 1985). Nurses should inform clients that increasing activity even slightly improves both physiology and mental status and is likely to promote further activity. Aiming for major changes in exercise may not be as effective as planning small changes. Nurses should also ask about activity at work when assessing overall physical fitness. Waitresses, carpenters, city mailmen, and nurses are physically active at their jobs.

Exercise is a safe activity for most people. A healthy individual under age 35 can usually begin an exercise program without a physical examination if the exercise proceeds gradually and the individual is alert to unusual signs or symptoms. Requiring someone to consult a physician before beginning any type of program may deter the person from exercising at all, which is more detrimental to health than beginning without medical approval. The Physical Activity Readiness Questionnaire (British Columbia Department of Health, 1975, cited in Shephard, 1988) may be used to screen people for an exercise program. If a person answers "yes" to any of these questions, he or she should postpone plans for vigorous exercise until given clearance by a physician:

1. Has your doctor ever said you have heart trouble?
2. Do you ever suffer from pains in your chest?
3. Do you often feel faint or have spells of dizziness?
4. Has a doctor ever told you that you have a bone or joint problem, such as arthritis, which has been or could be aggravated by exercise?
5. Is there a good physical reason not mentioned here why you should not follow an activity program even if you wanted to?
6. Are you over age 65 and not accustomed to vigorous exercise?

Individuals should be examined by a physician before beginning a program involving vigorous exercise if they smoke or if any coronary risk factors are present, such as high blood pressure, elevated cholesterol, abnormal resting EKG, or a family history of cardiovascular disease prior to age 50; or if they have pulmonary diseases or metabolic diseases such as diabetes mellitus, thyroid disorders, renal disease, or liver disease.

Exercise Recommendations

The American College of Sports Medicine (1990) has made the following recommendations for quantity and quality of exercise for developing and maintaining cardiorespiratory fitness and body composition.

Type of Activity

Activities that improve cardiovascular endurance and functional capacity are recommended. These are activities that use large muscle groups, can be maintained for prolonged periods, and are rhythmical and aerobic in nature, such as walking, hiking, jogging, running, swimming, skating, bicycling, rowing, cross-country skiing, and skipping rope. Various endurance game activities such as dancing, figure skating, soccer, and tennis are also beneficial if done on a continuous basis over a period of time (Fig. 34-2). Competitive aspects of exercise should be minimized to reduce risk to participants.

Intensity

Physical activity should elevate heart rate to between 60% and 85% of age-predicted maximum heart rate. A formula for determining the target heart-rate range is shown in the box at right. An important aspect of planning intensity of

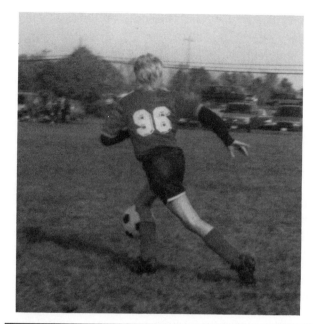

FIGURE 34-2

Competitive sports provides opportunities for regular exercise.

exercise is to teach clients how to take their pulses so they can monitor themselves. The most difficult problem in designing exercise programs is the prescription of appropriate intensity. Target heart rate range is one way of estimating intensity. However, Gaesser and Rich (1984) found that after 18 weeks, middle-aged men who exercised five times per week at 40% of maximum oxygen uptake had just as great aerobic fitness improvement as men who exercised at 80% of maximum oxygen uptake. Their fitness did not increase as rapidly, but they attained the same level at the end of the program. People who start an exercise program at low fitness levels can achieve a significant training effect with heart rates as low as 40% to 50% of maximum. However, people who begin a fitness program at higher levels of fitness require higher training heart rates to improve fitness.

Perceived exertion (light, moderate, heavy, very heavy) can be used by clients to gauge intensity. Clients exercising at perceived heavy or very heavy levels may not be exer-

cising safely, are at risk for musculoskeletal injury, and probably will not continue the exercise program (ACSM, 1990).

Frequency

Exercise is recommended three times per week for conditioning. Initially a day of rest should follow each day of exercise. The benefits of training peak at a frequency of five workouts per week; those who exercise more often than that do not improve fitness at a faster rate. (ACSM, 1990).

Duration

Fifteen to sixty minutes of continuous aerobic activity is recommended. Aerobic activity for twenty to thirty minutes results in a conditioning effect. Lower intensity activities over longer durations are recommended because of the potential hazards of high intensity activity. In addition, when persons perceive the activity as too intense, they are less likely to participate.

Rate of Progression

Progression in an exercise program is dependent on an individual's initial fitness level, health status, age, and goals. The initial phase should result in minimal muscle soreness and should include low-level aerobic activities, light calisthenics, and stretching. Discomfort is associated with starting an exercise program without time for physiological adaptation. During the improvement phase, intensity is increased to the targeted heart rate, and duration of exercise is increased every two to three weeks until a satisfactory level of fitness is achieved. To maintain the fitness level, workouts are continued. Different aerobic activities may be substituted for variety, but duration and intensity of workouts should not be increased.

Components of an Exercise Program

An exercise program should include (1) a warm-up period, (2) aerobic exercise, and (3) a cool-down period. The exercise session should gradually progress from a low to a vigorous level of activity and then slowly return to a low activity level (ACSM, 1990; Nieman, 1990; Pollock and Wilmore, 1990).

Warmup

The warm-up period lasts five to twenty minutes and begins with slow motion, low intensity activities like those planned for the aerobic workout. If desired, calisthenics, stretching, and flexibility exercises can be done when the muscles are warm. The duration and intensity of each of these activities depends on environmental conditions, the individual's functional capacity and symptomatology, and exercise preferences. For participants who require or prefer greater amounts of muscle strength or endurance, additional calisthenics and exercises using weights may be included when muscles are warm. Weight lifting with light weights and many repetitions firms muscles with less danger of injury to muscles or joints than lifting heavy weights. However, weight lifting is not recommended for persons with hypertension, arrhythmias, or poor cardiac reserve. Warm-up exercises increase respiration, circulation, and body tem-

---

FORMULA FOR DETERMINING TARGET HEART RATE

220 minus age = age-predicted maximum heart rate
Maximum heart rate × 0.60 = minimum aerobic effect heart rate
Maximum heart rate × 0.75 = target heart rate
Maximum heart rate × 0.85 = maximum safe heart rate

For example, the maximum heart rate for a 45-year-old man is 175; the heart rate for minimal aerobic effect is 105; and the maximum safe heart rate is 149. Target heart rate to be attained during aerobic activity after the initial weeks of conditioning is 131.

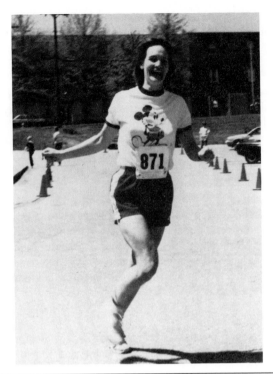

FIGURE 34-3

Regular running or jogging is a popular form of exercise for people of all ages.

perature and gently stretch ligaments and connective tissue to prepare them for more vigorous activity. Proper warm-up activities decrease the probability of injury.

Aerobic Exercise

The endurance or aerobic phase of conditioning includes activities involving large muscle groups to produce heart rates of targeted intensity for desired duration. One or a combination of activities such as brisk walking, running, swimming, climbing stairs, jumping rope, dancing, tennis, soccer, or hockey can be performed (Fig. 34-3).

Cool-down

The cool-down period includes exercises of diminishing intensities, such as slower jogging or walking, stretching, and in some cases, relaxation activities. A cool-down period of five to ten minutes allows body temperature and heart rate to decrease slowly. This prevents blood pooling in the lower extremities, reducing the potential for dizziness. Metabolites of muscle activity are oxidized so pain and muscle stiffness are less likely.

Motivation for Exercise

Even the best exercise program will fail if people are not motivated to initiate or follow it. Because community health nurses work closely with individuals and groups over extended periods of time, they can tailor exercise programs to specific needs and motivators. When planning exercise programs, three aspects should be considered: (1) the person's characteristics and social support system; (2) the exercise

setting; and (3) the characteristics of the physical activity (Gavin, 1988).

Characteristics of People

People who begin and will adhere to exercise programs are those who perceive that they lack activity and express a desire for improvement in health, fitness, and/or mental working capacity. They feel they can control their health and that exercise will affect their health. They feel they have or can learn the skills needed to exercise successfully and can recover from relapses of inactivity. They have support of significant others and see exercise as a way to socialize and vary their routines. Many who exercise have done so sometime in their past. Enjoyment of the activity and feelings of well-being tend to be stronger motivators for participation in exercise than concerns about improvements in health. Persons most likely to drop out are obese and feel less well; they are precisely the people who need the activity the most. The challenge for community health nurses is to increase awareness and perceptions of control, teach skills, and gather support for clients to increase their activity levels. Role modeling exercise is also important. Nurses can show clients the benefits of regular exercise.

Characteristics of Settings and Programs

Important aspects of the exercise setting are: (1) convenient hours and accessible facilities; (2) leaders who individualize the programs and offer choices to participants, provide reinforcement, and serve as models; (3) activity partners who expect to have each other's company while exercising; and (4) plans for time constraints and various weather conditions. Programs that help people anticipate problems and learn how to deal with them — such as walking in a mall in bad weather, taking turns watching children, or climbing steps for 20 minutes in a hotel when traveling — are more likely to result in adherence.

Exercise Characteristics

Activities that are perceived as uncomfortable will not be performed. A program begun with too much intensity will produce dropouts quickly or may produce injuries that prohibit continuation. People may be unwilling or unable to incorporate structured exercise into weekly routines but might be willing to increase daily activity. Some examples include walking to a nearby store rather than driving or taking a bus; parking in a corner of the parking lot rather than next to the building entrance; climbing stairs rather than riding elevators or escalators; taking a walk during work breaks or meals; or doing yard work rather than delegating it to someone else. Community health nurses can use their creativity to help clients increase activity in ways that are acceptable.

No motivators are effective in all situations, but the following suggestions can help community health nurses promote exercise (Blomquist, 1986; Estok and Rudy, 1986; Fixx, 1980; Franklin, Gordon, and Timmis, 1989; Travis and Ryan, 1988):

1. *Involve clients in the planning process.* Clients provide nurses with clues to the types of activities they may enjoy as well as barriers that may inhibit their

participation.

2. *Select activities that have already been mastered.* Clients may become discouraged and quit if they are unable to master a new skill (such as swimming). The nurse should also be alert to clients' desires to learn new skills. Above all, exercise should be fun.

3. *Fit the exercise program into the individual's present lifestyle.* Programs that require minimal alterations in a person's life-style will meet with less resistance than those demanding greater changes.

4. *Plan the exercise activities at the same time every day or each week to help in establishing a routine.* When exercise becomes a habit, a person will be more likely to continue.

5. *Develop realistic, achievable goals.* Clients are likely to participate when a particular goal is in sight. Some clients enjoy plotting their progress on a graph so that achievement is easy to see. Plotting the number of minutes of exercise or the miles walked is one way of determining progress toward goals and offering recognition.

6. *Establish rewards.* At the beginning of the week, clients may set goals and rewards for meeting the goals. Companies can offer monetary rewards for miles employees walk, run, or swim and "well-pay" for employees who are neither absent nor tardy for a specified period of time. Facilities can offer T-shirts proclaiming achievements of goals (such as 100-mile clubs). People can make contracts with themselves, with friends, or with their community health nurse.

7. *Encourage and reinforce.* Nurses should let clients know that the positive aspects of exercising are readily apparent in their appearance, in modification of smoking or eating habits or in other outward measures.

8. *Teach self-management techniques.* Teaching participants to encourage and reinforce themselves may help them maintain enthusiasm. Nurses can encourage clients to praise themselves at intervals, use relaxation and persuasion techniques, and plan personal rewards for milestones. Another technique is to have clients plan game-like activities or look for things while walking or running, such as flowers, cloud formations, or wildlife.

9. *Acknowledge the disadvantages of exercise.* Preparing clients for the daily aggravations of exercise while at the same time expounding on the positive aspects not only protects the nurse's credibility but also helps prevent discouragement with the program. Clients should be advised to respect pain and other warning signs. Exercise helps people tune in to messages from their bodies.

10. *Use exercise as social time.* Individuals may find it more difficult to abandon the program if others are depending on them. Groups, clubs, and teams promote social interaction, cooperation, fun, and variety. Group discussions provide opportunities for comparing notes with peers; setting goals; sharing thoughts, feelings and strategies about exercise; and modeling desirable behaviors. The aspect of competition should be minimized.

11. *Integrate music into the exercise program.* Music facilitates movement, relieves boredom, and may distract the individual from the repetitive nature of some exercises. People are often amazed at the number of rope-jumps or sit-ups they are able to complete while listening to energetic music.

12. *Enlist the support of companies and community organizations to provide additional motivations.* Discounts on insurance rates, free group exercise programs, and free clinics in which exercise-related problems can be discussed may be incentives to exercise.

13. *Serve as a role model to clients.* The nurse's enthusiasm for exercise and example of fitness will act as a motivator.

14. *Offer role models to clients.* Enlisting the help of people of all ages who exercise regularly will show clients the benefits of exercise.

PROMOTING NUTRITION AND EXERCISE IN THE COMMUNITY

Community health nurses can play an important role in promoting community health through diet and exercise. The public is increasingly interested in nutrition and physical fitness because of strong epidemiological and clinical evidence that supports diet and exercise as ways to prevent chronic disease. Community programs may involve collaboration with other health professionals and leaders in industry, schools, and the community.

Health Professionals

Advice from physicians and nurses can influence clients to make life-style changes. As age increases, professional advice becomes more important. Clients want and expect advice about how to stay well in addition to advice on managing symptoms of chronic and acute diseases more common in older people. Health professionals sometimes do not teach clients about the benefits of changes in diet or exercise because they lack knowledge or confidence that they can help the clients change (Powell, Spain, Christenson, and Mollenkemp, 1986). Most health care providers can make an impact on the lifestyle behaviors of clients. Community health nurses can develop nutrition and fitness programs aimed at increasing knowledge and changing behaviors of community residents and health professionals. Health professionals are important role models in the community.

Worksite

The worksite is an ideal place to promote good nutrition and increase physical activity because a large percentage of the population is employed, spending approximately one-third of the day at work. Offering opportunities for nutritious food choices and physical activity provides economic and performance benefits both for employees and employers.

Nutrition can be addressed at the worksite because most employees eat at least one meal there. Nurses can help businesses offer nutritious meals in company cafeterias.

"Heart-healthy" stickers can be used on labels of low-fat foods and nutrition information can be listed on menus. Nurses can encourage companies to provide refrigerators and microwave ovens for storage and preparation of food. They can assist employers in planning nutrition education programs and can provide appropriate materials to distribute to employees in eating places or in paycheck envelopes. Companies can be encouraged to sponsor corporate weight reduction programs, such as Weight Watchers, or group weight reduction contests.

Companies can create fitness rooms with mats and equipment or can develop outdoor trails for walking and jogging, possibly including exercise stations. The Cabinet for Human Resources in the Kentucky state capital provides an example of what employers can do to encourage exercise. Each morning a question is posted in the basement of the huge building and employees are encouraged to walk down during work breaks to see it. In the afternoon the answer is posted and curious employees again walk the halls and stairs. Health promotion personnel have been delighted with the number of people who make the long walk twice daily through the halls and up and down the stairs to find the daily question and its answer (personal communication, Phyllis Skonacki, Director, Health Promotion Branch, Cabinet for Human Resources, Frankfort, KY).

Successful health promotion programs have strong leadership, convenient facilities, ongoing recruitment, long-term commitment, varieties of program options, systems for employee recognition, and plans for involvement of family members (Wood, Olmstead, and Craig, 1989). Community health nurses can work with businesses to promote health in the workplace. Assessment of employee nutrition and fitness levels, needs, and desires, as well as the planning, implementation, and evaluation of employee health programs are activities that fall within the scope of community health nursing practice.

Schools

The nation's schools underpin the effort to achieve national health goals. Programs in schools can provide children with knowledge and skills for a lifetime of nutritious food choices and physical activity.

School nurses can work with planners of school lunches (and in some places, breakfasts) to offer nutrition education along with healthful food choices. For example, as in work-site cafeterias, stickers can indicate low-fat, heart-healthy foods, and menus can offer information on nutrition. Special weeks can be declared in which the amount of vitamin A for all foods is listed one week, vitamin C another week, and iron another week. In this way children are not overwhelmed with information and can learn to discriminate which foods are more nutritious. Questions can be posted around the cafeteria which ask children to apply the information offered in the serving line. Nurses can also work with parent groups through PTA nutrition education sessions and by offering special programs on nutrition and general health promotion to community residents at schools.

Studies indicate that active adults developed activity patterns and attitudes in childhood. Physical education requirements vary greatly among school districts. Physical education programs are not conducted daily and tend to emphasize team sports, which build skill, rather than individual sports, which build aerobic fitness (Simons-Morton et al, 1988). Pressure on schools to emphasize basic academic skills and reduce costs has placed physical education programs in jeopardy. Community health nurses working in schools can be instrumental in promoting exercise both in formal physical education classes and during recess times. Nurses also can work with parent groups to increase exercise of families and work with school officials to open school exercise facilities to community residents.

Community

The largest number and variety of health promotion programs are offered by community agencies. Grocery stores and supermarkets have rich potential as sites for nutrition education because customers represent all segments of society and may shop several times per week. Nurses working with grocery store managers and local media can develop programs to increase knowledge of nutrition and modify food choices (Light et al., 1989). Examples include regular columns on nutrition and modifying eating habits in local newspapers, mini-classes in grocery stores, information on nutrition offered with samples of food, and bulletin boards with nutrition tips at checkout stands. Many voluntary groups in the community offer nutrition literature and resources. Examples are the American Dairy Council, the American Heart Association, the American Cancer Society, weight loss programs, 4-H, and Homemaker programs. Federal, state, and local government agencies such as county extension offices and county and state health departments have nutrition experts who can offer programs and printed materials for distribution to community residents.

Exercise programs are offered by city parks and recreation departments, nonprofit private agencies such as YMCAs and YWCAs, educational institutions such as local colleges, local clubs (skiing, bicycling, running, swimming, tennis, dancing), and for-profit health and fitness clubs. Many communities provide a variety of facilities for exercise including bike paths, fitness courses, swimming pools, courts for basketball, volleyball, and tennis, soccer and football fields, and open fields for other games. Many shopping malls open early for walking. Nurses can assess the community to determine gaps in facilities and programs and coordinate efforts to expand exercise options for all age groups. By enlisting support of community groups and government agencies, community health nurses can spearhead campaigns to educate community residents about the benefits of exercise and how to begin exercise programs. Media campaigns can increase awareness about available facilities, the need for additional facilities, and the benefits of exercise and proper nutrition. Health fairs in shopping areas, churches, and community centers can offer fitness assessments (e.g., cardiovascular, body-weight, flexibility, and strength) and educational programs. Emphasis can be placed on neutralizing perceived barriers and portraying exercise as sociable, enjoyable, and part of a balanced lifestyle. Walk-a-thons, bike-a-thons, and runs to support worthy causes increase awareness, interest, and participation exercise.

TABLE 34-6
Types of sleep

Type	Characteristics	Time
Sleep latency	Awake before sleep begins	10 minutes
NREM Sleep	A quiet brain in a moveable body	60-90 minutes for all 4 stages
Stage I	Sensation of floating	4 minutes
Stage II	Eyes roll back and forth	64 minutes
Stage III	Deep relaxation; only loud noise or physical jolt will awaken; emergence of EEG delta waves	7 minutes
Stage IV	Deep sleep; slow EEG delta waves	15 minutes
REM Sleep	An active brain in an immobile body; EEG arousal and heightened physiological activity; increased cerebral blood flow; episodic fluctuations in heart rate, blood pressure, breathing, and sexual arousal; vivid dreaming; lack of muscle movement	20 minutes

PROMOTING HEALTH THROUGH REST AND SLEEP

Rest and sleep are required for health, and most people spend from one-quarter to one-third of their lives sleeping. Sleep habits can be disrupted by work schedules, travel, illnesses, stress, food, drugs, lack of exercise, and pain, as well as by environmental factors such as noise, uncomfortable sleeping quarters, temperature, and crowding. If headaches and the common cold are excluded, problems associated with sleeping are among the most frequent of health complaints. Insomnia (inability to sleep), narcolepsy (inability to control falling asleep), myoclonis (kicking), bruxism (grinding teeth), sleep apnea (stopping breathing), sleepwalking, and nightmares are a few of the recognized sleep disorders (Biddle and Oaster, 1990).

Disturbed sleep results in daytime drowsiness and inability to function well. The true test of sleep deprivation is how well one functions during waking hours. Sleep deprivation of 72 hours results in fatigue, irritability, feelings of persecution, and misinterpretation of stimuli. Sleep deprivation of 150 hours may result in brief psychotic episodes (Mendelson, 1987).

Sleep is an active process of the nervous system, the body, and the mind. Sleep has many functions. It is restorative. The rates of cell division and protein synthesis increase during sleep, and sleep promotes recovery of physiological, neurological, and psychological states. It is protective; humans and animals sleep to avoid exhaustion of the body and brain. It also promotes energy conservation. Animals with high metabolic rates have longer total sleep times. Sleep seems to be an instinct like thirst and hunger. Sleep can be viewed as a shift in the delicate balance between two opposing forces: an arousal or vigilance enhancing force (waking system) and a low-vigilance or desensitization force (sleeping system). A variety of substances, primarily neurotransmitters, play pivotal but incompletely understood roles in sleep and wakefulness (Biddle and Oaster, 1990).

Human sleep is of two kinds: nonrapid eye movement (NREM) sleep and rapid eye movement sleep (REM). In NREM sleep the quiet brain is in a moveable body. The four stages of NREM sleep are described in Table 34-6, including the light sleep of stages I and II and the deep sleep of stages III and IV. In REM sleep, the brain is active, but the body is immobile. Dreaming occurs during REM sleep.

Normal adults have several cycles of sleep each night (or each usual long sleep-period) beginning with NREM stages 1 through 4, followed by a return to stage II, and then REM sleep. The total cycle time is 1 to 2 hours with 25 percent of total sleep in REM sleep. Time in stage III and IV sleep decreases and REM sleep time increases through the night (Biddle and Oaster, 1990; Dinner, Erman, and Roth, 1989; Shaver and Giblin, 1989).

Sleep requirements and patterns vary with individuals and change with age. In general, total sleep requirments are greatest in infancy and decrease in childhood (Figure 34-4). Sleep needs remain relatively stable through the young

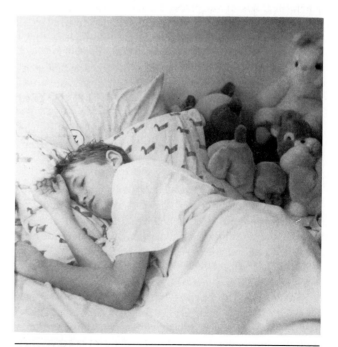

FIGURE 34-4

Total sleep requirements decrease in childhood from what was needed in infancy.

SUGGESTIONS FOR IMPROVING SLEEP

Keep regular hours of sleep and predictable times for going to bed and arising. If you spend time trying to fall asleep, retire later but arise at the regular time.

Regular naps may be included, but napping may cause delay of nighttime sleep.

Perform regular bedtime rituals, such as brushing teeth, bathing, donning pajamas, reading, or listening to soft music.

Reserve the bedroom for sleeping and sex. To associate the bedroom with sleeping, do not regularly eat, watch TV, or read in bed.

Sleep in a safe and comfortable bed in a quiet room with comfortable lighting, temperature, and humidity.

Plan time to relax before bedtime. Relaxation exercises, such as deep breathing or contracting and relaxing muscle groups from feet to head, may be helpful.

Exercise during the day, but not just before bedtime.

Drink beverages containing caffeine only in the morning.

Limit use of alcohol, cigarettes, and drugs. Be aware of the effects of medications such as steroids, beta blockers, and hormone replacements on sleep.

Get help for troubling medical conditions such as heart irregularities, breathing difficulties, urinary problems, or pain.

Use sedatives and hypnotics sparingly. They lose effectiveness quickly, induce tolerance, and can lead to significant problems.

Do not drink fluids for several hours before bedtime; empty bladder before going to bed.

Do not consume a heavy meal before bedtime. Warm milk or other noncaffeinated beverage may aid sleep.

Do not lie in bed if you are unable to sleep; get up and do something monotonous.

Do not be concerned about sleep unless it is disrupted for several days. Worry may create further sleep disruption.

One long night seems to compensate for several short nights. Plan for an occasional long night of sleep.

---

adult years until old age when sleep needs may change. Normal total sleep time for young adults is six to nine hours, but there is much variation among individuals.

Older adults have longer sleep latency and more stage I and II (lighter) sleep. REM sleep time declines and occurs earlier in the night. Because older people experience less deep sleep, they wake up more often at night and may need more bed time to satisfy their sleep needs (Muncy, 1986).

A comprehensive sleep and activity assessment may provide clues about sleep problems. Keeping logs of daily activities, sleep conditions, sensations upon awakening, and general feelings of sleepiness during the day will give direction to nurses and clients about ways to improve sleep. Information included in a sleep diary could include times of sleeping and waking up at night and during the day; food, drink, and drugs ingested during the day; physical and mental activity; and stress and concerns. Often an assessment reveals causes of sleep disruptions which can be modified to improve sleep and rest. The box offers suggestions for improving sleep and rest. Community health nurses can promote health by helping clients of all ages improve sleep.

CLINICAL APPLICATION

Hilda Willow is a 60-year-old married grandmother with mild hypertension (150/95). She is 5 feet 3 inches tall and weighs 160 pounds. She is depressed and having trouble sleeping. The primary care physician at the health department has referred Mrs. Willow to the community health nurse for assessment of her depression and guidance in a weight reduction and activity program.

The nurse learns that Mrs. Willow is a homemaker who lives with her husband, Carl, a butcher in a local supermarket. Carl is also obese and hypertensive. They have three adult children—one in another state and two nearby. They frequently care for their two grandchildren, aged 2 and 4. The Willow home is a small, immaculate bungalow with flower boxes. Mrs. Willow welcomes the nurse and laments

that she has been on a diet most of her life but continues to get "a little fatter every year." She is worried about her own and her husband's high blood pressure because her father has had several strokes and has been an invalid in a nursing home for two years. She is tired all the time.

The nurse and Mrs. Willow discuss Mrs. Willow's daily routine, her activity, and her concerns, as well as the kinds of foods she eats, how she prepares them, and the milieu of the eating situation. The nurse asks Mrs. Willow to keep a food intake-, sleep-, and activity-log for 1 week to discuss at the next visit.

The next week Mrs. Willow and the nurse review the log and discover that Mrs. Willow engages in very little physical activity, naps for two hours each afternoon, eats small amounts of food almost continuously during the day, enjoys foods that are high in fat and salt, and drinks about six cups of coffee during the day. Mrs. Willow is quite surprised at these findings and indicates interest in making changes in her diet, sleep, and exercise patterns. She says her husband wants to help and has suggested they take walks each evening because it would be good for both of them. With the baseline data of the diet/activity/sleep log, the nurse and Mr. and Mrs. Willow are able to plan and implement a program that helps them both lose weight and control their blood pressure without medication. The new focus and activities help Mrs. Willow sleep more soundly and her symptoms of depression lessen.

Assessment and Diagnosis

Information was obtained from Mrs. Willow regarding when, where, why, and what cues or stimuli led to eating; what or who were reinforcers for the Willows; and how these reinforcers could be mobilized. The wife and husband were willing to help each other, and they found support in the daughter whose children they frequently cared for. Environmental and financial supports and barriers were identified. The Willows have adequate food preparation and storage facilities and live in a clean, safe neighborhood. They have a restricted income but are accustomed to watching how money is spent. Both read and write at a high school level and have social and vocational skills. Both have a history of dieting with little success but have many health, function, and body image reasons for wanting to lose weight now.

Planning and Contracting

Three major tasks to be accomplished during this phase were (1) making a problem list and setting priorities ranking goals in terms of degrees of difficulty; (2) establishing contracts that were written and specific and were mutually agreed upon; and (3) discussing the expectations of the Willows and the nurse. The nurse asked the Willows to keep records for self-monitoring. She initially visited them weekly to monitor progress and assist with future planning. A typical one-week contract relating to diet called for Mrs. Willow to keep a record of foods eaten and the milieu for the week, focusing on eliminating half of the between-meal snacks. According to the terms of the contract the nurse brought information on low-calorie, low-fat cooking methods and food seasonings to replace salt. A contract related to activity called for Mrs. Willow to walk for 15 minutes at a comfortable pace three times in the next week, to record when and where she walked and any thoughts, feelings, or questions she had to discuss with the nurse. During the planning phase, the nurse explored use of community resources such as the nutritionist at the health department, Weight Watchers programs, and local senior citizen programs related to nutrition and exercise.

Involvement of the clients in developing plans and contracts is essential. Building client self-esteem and self-confidence is an important objective in planning and intervention activities. During the process the nurse teaches clients how to change and monitor their own lifestyle behaviors.

Intervention

During the intervention phase, the nurse gave the Willows information about nutrition and exercise programs and taught them how to learn new behaviors, how to problem-solve, how to cope with relapses, and how to reinforce their healthful behavior. Specific topics related to nutrition included low-calorie cooking (especially decreasing fat content to less than 30% of total calories); choosing healthful, varied foods; tips on stimulus control such as chewing gum or singing while cooking; eating only in the kitchen or dining room; recognizing eating, exercise, and sleep patterns; and finding patterns that produced a loss of no more than two to three pounds (1 kg) per week. Exercise-related subjects were numerous and included taking the pulse; determination of activity to induce conditioning without discomfort; discussion of equipment relevant to desired activity (e.g., shoes and bicycles); safety (including weather, night activity, pollution, animals, and carrying identification); scheduling (preferably before meals or at least 1 to 2 hours after meals); control of soreness by limiting intensity and performing adequate warm-up and cool-down; companions and competitiveness; fluid intake in hot weather; and ideas for motivation and variety. Sleep-related information regarded cutting down on caffeine, especially in the evening, increasing exercise, and shortening naps; information about changes in sleep needs with age was also conveyed.

Evaluation

A variety of methods of evaluation was used, including nutrition and activity knowledge, activity level changes, weight loss and body dimension changes, blood pressure levels, modification of eating and activity patterns based on diet/activity/sleep logs, expressed feelings of well-being, and abilities to problem-solve and manage relapses.

Nurses helping clients with weight management and exercise programs influence them by modeling health behaviors. Modeling helps nurses bring behaviors to the attention of clients, shows them how to perform healthy behaviors, and demonstrates examples of the rewards of healthy lifestyles. Besides being a good model, a nurse should develop knowledge of nutrition and exercise as well as skills in rapport, patience, flexibility, and awareness of the ways clients can be helped to succeed. Nurses must not consider noncompliance as a reflection on their ability, but rather as an impetus for more creativity and teamwork with clients (White, 1986).

SUMMARY

This chapter has described current trends in promotion of health through nutrition, exercise, and sleep. Health promotion involves collaboration by clients, nurses and other health care professionals. It is often community health nurses who first come into contact with individuals and groups in need of nutritional, exercise, and sleep guidance. Nurses can play important roles by increasing awareness of benefits of and resources for nutrition and exercise, identifying risk factors, educating and motivating individuals and groups, and interpreting research findings. No diet plan or exercise prescription works for all people at all times, but through the use of the nursing process, nurses can assist people to develop personalized plans for health promotion.

KEY CONCEPTS

Frequent and extended contact with clients in the community affords nurses excellent opportunities to provide information and counseling regarding the role of nutrition, exercise, and sleep in the promotion of health and prevention of illness.

In industrialized societies, diet-related conditions are among the leading causes of disease and death. Many of these result from nutritional excesses rather than undernourishment.

Knowledge and skills related to nutrition enable nurses to assess clients of all ages, provide them with anticipatory guidance and recommended diets, answer questions, refer malnourished clients, and evaluate research studies.

What people eat is determined by a variety of factors, including biological needs, psychological variables, sociocultural influences, and environmental aspects such as price, availability, and storage facilities.

The cultural and ethnic backgrounds of clients play a major role in food selection and eating behaviors. Recognition and respect for these food preferences are important for nurses counseling clients.

The Recommended Dietary Allowances (RDAs) are the levels of intake considered adequate to meet the known nutritional needs of practically all healthy persons.

The Dietary Guidelines for Americans are general recommendations from the Federal government for food intake to promote health and prevent disease.

Through the nursing process, community health nurses are able to detect and intervene in nutritional difficulties encountered by individuals, families, and groups in the community. Nutritional assessment of an individual or group should include biological, psychological, cultural, and environmental factors. Most meal planning and preparation occur in the home, so community health nurses have many opportunities to provide nutrition education when making home visits.

Counseling regarding the nutritional value, deficiencies, and excesses of convenient and "fast food" menus is an important function of community health nurses.

Obesity, defined as being 20% or more overweight, is the result of hereditary, sociocultural, psychological, and environmental influences as well as physiological functioning. Nurses can assist people with weight loss through individualized and group programs.

Well-educated, affluent young adults have increased their level of exercise. Americans over 50, however, have a limited awareness of the kinds and amounts of activity needed to maintain physical fitness, and there is a widespread belief within that age group that exercise may be dangerous.

The skill-related measures of physical fitness are agility, balance, coordination, speed, power, and reaction time. The health-related measures of physical fitness are cardiorespiratory endurance, flexibility, body composition, muscular endurance, and muscular strength.

Exercise has both physiological and psychological benefits. Both should be considered during nursing assessment, diagnosis, planning, implementation, and evaluation.

Exercise recommendations can be made regarding type of activity, intensity, frequency, and duration, as well as rate of progress.

Components of a fitness program are warmup, aerobic workout, and cool-down.

Fitness program planners should consider characteristics of the participants and their social support systems, the exercise setting, and the physical activity itself.

Community health nurses can collaborate with other health professionals and leaders in industry, schools, and the community to promote nutrition and physical fitness.

Sleep is an active process of mind and body, and sleep disorders are common health complaints.

Sleep is designated as nonrapid eye movement (NREM sleep with four stages) and rapid eye movement (REM) sleep.

Normal total sleep time for adults is 6 to 9 hours, and the test of sleep deprivation is how well one functions during waking hours. Community health nurses can offer suggestions for assessment and improvement of sleep and rest for clients.

LEARNING ACTIVITIES

1. Keep a food diary for 1 week. Record the types and amounts of foods, times and situations of eating, and personal thoughts and feelings while eating. Analyze the diary for nutritional adequacy. How does your diet compare with the RDAs for your age and sex, the four food groups, and the Dietary Guidelines for Americans? Where could improvements be made? How will you motivate yourself to have a better diet?

2. Select two cultures and compare their diets. What similarities can be seen? Identify factors influencing food selections in both cultures. What changes might be recommended to improve nutritional adequacy?

3. Keep an activity and sleep log for 1 week. Analyze your activity and determine how you might get the recommended amount of exercise and sleep. Plan an exercise program for yourself and get started.

4. Select an article regarding nutrition or exercise in a current lay publication and analyze the information provided and how it might be understood by people with little background in nutrition or exercise.

5. Plan a lifestyle change program aimed at weight reduction and improvement in physical fitness for a 45-year-old man who is 30 pounds overweight and has not exercised vigorously in 15 years.

6. Analyze the lifestyle of a friend who complains of being tired all the time. Offer suggestions to improve sleep.

7. Survey local businesses and industries to discover what health promotion programs are available and how they are used.

8. Assess the facilities and resources for exercise in your community.

9. Work with a local grocery store to offer nutrition information to customers.

10. Talk with a school nurse to learn what nutrition, exercise, and health promotion programs are available in the schools.

BIBLIOGRAPHY

American College of Sports Medicine 1990: The recommended quantity and quality of exercise for developing and maintaining cardiorespiratory and muscular fitness in healthy adults, Med Sci Sports Exerc 22:265-274, 1990.

Anderson JW: Be heart smart . . . the HCF way to a healthy heart, Lexington, Ky, 1989, The HCF Nutrition Research Foundation, Inc.

Biddle C and Oaster TRF: The nature of sleep, J Am Assoc Nurse Anesth 58:36-44, 1990.

Blomquist KB: Modeling and health behavior: Strategies for prevention in the schools, Health Educ 17(3):8-10, 1986.

Bomar PJ, editor: Nurses and family health promotion: Concepts, assessment, and interventions, Baltimore, 1989, Williams & Wilkins.

Bouchard C, Shephard RJ, Stephens T, et al: Exercise, fitness, and health, Champaign, IL, 1990, Human Kinetics Publishers.

Burtis G, Davis J and Martin S: Applied nutrition and diet therapy, Philadelphia, 1988, WB, Saunders.

Caspersen CJ, Powell KE and Christenson GM: Physical activity, exercise, and physical fitness: Definitions and distinctions for health-related research, Public Health Rep 100:126-131, 1985.

Dinner DS, Erman MK and Roth T: Help for geriatric sleep problems, Patient Care 23(8):74-85, 1989.

Dishman RK, Sallis JF and Orenstein DR: The determinants of physical activity and exercise, Public Health Rep 100:158-171, 1985.

Dwyer JT: Health aspects of vegetarian diets, Am J Cl Nut 48:712-738, 1988.

Edelstein CK, Haskew P and Kramer JP: Early clues to anorexia and bulimia, Patient Care 23(13):155-175, 1989.

Estok PJ and Rudy EB: Jogging: Cardiovascular benefits and risks, Nurse Pract 11(5):21-27, 1986.

Fixx J: Jim Fixx's second book of running, New York, 1980, Random House.

Franklin BA, Gordon S and Timmis GC: Exercise in modern medicine, Baltimore, 1989, Williams & Wilkins.

Gaesser GA and Rich RG: Effects of high- and low-intensity exercise training on aerobic capacity and blood lipids, Med Sci Sports Exerc 16:269-274, 1984.

Gavin J: Psychological issues in exercise prescription, Sports Med 6:1-10, 1988.

Haskell WL: Physical activity and health: Need to define the required stimulus, Am J Cardiology 55:4D-9D, 1985.

Light L, Portnoy B, Blair JE, Smith JM, Rodgers AB, Tuckermanty E, Tenney J and Mathews O: Nutrition education in supermarkets, Fam Comm Health 12:43-52, 1989.

Mendelson WB: Human sleep: Research and clinical care, New York, 1987, Plenum.

Monsen E: The 10th edition of the recommended dietary allowances: What's new in the 1989 RDAs?, J Am Dietetic Assoc 89:1748-1752, 1989.

Morgan WP and Goldston SE: Exercise and mental health, New York, 1987, Hemisphere Publishing.

Muncy JH: Measures to rid sleeplessness, J Geron Nurs 12(8):6-11, 1986.

Nestle M: Nutrition in clinical practice, Greenbrae, Calif., 1985, Jones Medical Publications.

Nieman DC: Fitness and sports medicine: An introduction, Palo Alto, CA, 1990, Bull Publishing Company.

Pender N: Health promotion in nursing practice, New York, 1987, Appleton & Lange.

Pennington JAT: The Food and Drug Administration and dietary guidelines, Fam Com Health 12:33-41, 1989.

Pollock ML and Wilmore JH: Exercise and health in disease: Evaluation and prescription for prevention and rehabilitation, Philadelphia, 1990, WB, Saunders.

Powell KE and Paffenbarger RS: Workshop on epidemiologic and public health aspects of physical activity and exercise: A summary, Public Health Rep 100:118-126, 1985.

Powell KE, Spain KG, Christenson GM and Mollenkamp MP: The status of the 1990 objectives for physical fitness and exercise, Public Health Rep 101:15-21, 1986.

Public Health Service: Promoting health/preventing disease: Year 2000 objectives for the nation, Washington, DC, 1990, USDHHS.

Ryan AJ and Allman FL: Sports medicine, San Diego, 1989, Academic Press.

Scrimshaw NS: Nutrition: Prospects for the 1990's, Annual Rev Public Health 11:53-68, 1990.

Shaver JLF, and Giblin EC: Sleep, Ann Rev Nursing 7:71-93, 1989.

Shephard RJ: Physical activity and the healthy mind, Can Med Assoc J 128:552-530, 1983.

Shephard RJ: PAR-Q, Canadian home fitness test and exercise screening alternatives, Sports Med 5:185-195, 1988.

Simons-Morton BG, Parcel GS, O'Hara NM, Blair SN and Pate R: Health-related physical fitness in childhood: Status and recommendations, Ann Rev Public Health 9:403-425, 1988.

Travis JW and Ryan RS: Wellness workbook, Berkeley, Calif, 1988, Ten Speed Press.

U.S. Department of Agriculture and U.S. Department of Health and Human Services: Nutrition and your health: Dietary guidelines for Americans, Home and Garden Bulletin No. 232, ed 2, 1985; ed 3, 1990.

White JH: Behavioral intervention for the obese client, Nurse Pract 11(1):27-34, 1986.

Williams SR: Mowry's basic nutrition and diet therapy, St. Louis, 1988, The CV Mosby Co.

Wilson CS: Nutritionally beneficial cultural practices, World Rev Nutrition Dietetics 45:68-96, 1985.

Wood EA, Olmstead GW and Craig JL: An evaluation of lifestyle risk factors and absenteeism after two years in a worksite health promotion program, Am J Health Prom 4:128-133, 1989.

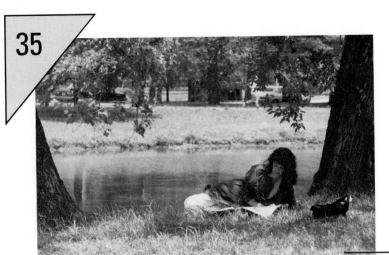

35

Stress Management and Crisis Intervention

Phyllis Graves

Jeanette Lancaster

OBJECTIVES

After reading this chapter, the student should be able to:

Define stress
Describe the physical and psychological response to stress
Discuss burnout and how it relates to stress
Identify five alternatives for managing stress
Recognize the characteristics of crisis
Contrast maturational crisis and situational crisis
Describe two anticipatory guidance activities to prevent the occurrence of a crisis
Discuss the focus of crisis intervention and the roles of the nurse and the client

KEY TERMS

active listening
adaptation
assertiveness
biofeedback
broken record
burnout
creative imagery
crisis
crisis intervention

crisis phases
fogging
hardiness
homeostasis
maturational crisis
meditation
negotiating
perfectionism
primary crisis
  prevention

progressive relaxation
secondary crisis
  prevention
situational crisis
stress
stress management
stressor
tertiary crisis
  prevention
thought-stopping

L aura went to her neighbor Alice's home in tears. As they sat down over coffee, Laura said, "I burned the beans I was cooking for supper. Yesterday, the vacuum broke and this week John came home with a note from his teacher about the fights he has been in. Nothing is going right." After talking awhile, Laura noticed Alice's flat appearance. "What is your problem, Alice?" Alice said that her husband had lost his job and without an income they would lose their house and car.

Both Laura and Alice have problems. Laura is suffering from stress; Alice is in crisis. A community health nurse aware of these situations can assist both women to cope. The first part of this chapter discusses ways to help clients and nurses manage stress effectively through assertiveness, changes in thoughts and attitudes, support networks, relaxation, effective communication, meditation, imagery, and biofeedback. The second part deals with crisis theory and identifies ways to help clients cope with life circumstances that may seem unbearable.

STRESS MANAGEMENT
Nature of Stress

Stress occurs when physical or emotional demands are placed on people, usually requiring the person to change (Selye, 1974). The level of stress depends largely on the person's appraisal or perception of the situation. Perception of stress depends largely on predictability (the degree to which people can anticipate the occurrence of an event), social context (the psychosocial setting or factors present in the environment), and control (the degree to which one can alter a situation or event). The effects of stress are less disruptive when the onset is expected or preceded by some warning. The social context of a stressor influences the reaction. A person's own loud music is more tolerable than music coming from someone else's apartment. Small children running and yelling are generally better tolerated by their parents in their own homes than by others in a crowded restaurant. In addition, the degree of perceived control influences how a situation is interpreted. For example, listening to loud music in one's own car may be less stressful than if the music were playing in a public building. The volume could be turned down in the car but not in the building.

The rate of change and meaning of the event also influence whether people feel stressed. The greater the number of life changes during a period of time, the more likely the person is to develop a stress-related illness (Rahe, 1978). The ability to cope with stress largely depends on the person's perception of the event. Some people seek stress because they are challenged by new or unusual experiences. Bruhn (1987) discusses novel stress as being a situation that a person does not routinely experience. He says that some novel stress situations are created through normal developmental events, while others are created by people (e.g., mountain climbers, race car drivers, and others who seek to stretch their past performance limits). What is stressful for one person may be energizing for another. For example, meeting deadlines, writing papers, and speaking in public affect people in different ways. Each person responds differently to stress because of the interplay of such factors as genetics, organ vulnerability, general state of health, fitness,

sociocultural background, and previous experience with stress.

Not all stress is bad. Stress is especially useful in times of danger, when people need to mobilize physical and emotional forces for their own defense. In tolerable levels, stress is a motivator; it keeps people moving toward goal accomplishment and prevents boredom and feelings of uselessness. Selye (1974) described a positive form of stress as being "*eustress.*" The "eu" means good or positive, as in euphoria. This form of stress results from an optimistic orientation toward life events combined with the ability to regulate one's life and alter attitudes to view stress positively rather than negatively (Petosa, 1985). Stress-related problems occur when the degree of stress remains high for a prolonged period of time.

Stress Response

Stress theory is based on the concepts of *adaptation* and *homeostasis*. People attempt to adapt to their stressors to maintain balance. Stressors elicit both psychological and physiological responses. Selye (1978) identified the general adaptation syndrome (GAS), in which physiological responses in the nervous and endocrine systems alert people to either *distress* or eustress. These sensations produce a wide range of feelings, varying from joy to fear. They serve as a mechanism to alert individuals to summon their resources to fight stress. The physiological changes caused by stress are nonspecific and affect the entire body.

The stress occurs as the body attempts to normalize after its previous state of homeostasis has been disrupted. When people are in distress too long or intensively, the GAS becomes less effective and makes a person vulnerable to mental or physical illness. The body responds to stress in three phases:

1. *Alarm reaction:* physiological indications of alertness during which defense mechanisms are mobilized.
2. *State of resistance:* a state in which the individual resists the alarm and fights back to normal.
3. *Stage of exhaustion:* a point when stress is sustained, and adaptation energy is depleted.

To minimize the effect of stress, interventions should prevent a person from reaching exhaustion. People need to be aware of internal and external stress-producing events and recognize their personal signs of stress accumulation. Essentially, stress is a response to a stressor, and can be caused by either internal or external sources.

The bodily reaction to stress typically includes increases in the following:

1. Metabolism (oxygen consumption)
2. Blood pressure
3. Heart rate
4. Rate of breathing
5. Amount of blood pumped by the heart
6. Amount of blood pumped to the skeletal muscles

During a stress response the hypothalamus is stimulated, which in turn stimulates the *autonomic nervous system* (ANS) and the anterior pituitary gland. Stimulation of the ANS causes the heart to speed up, the digestive systems to slow down, and epinephrine and norepinephrine to be released. When the anterior pituitary gland is stimulated, it releases *adrenocorticotropic hormone* (ACTH), which subsequently stimulates the cortex of the adrenal glands and causes the release of steroids or anti-inflammatory hormones. A second hormone, *somatotropin* (STH), is also released from the anterior pituitary gland and stimulates the growth of the body as a whole and increases the activity of proinflammatory corticoids (Selye, 1978).

When the sympathetic portion of the ANS is activated, a "fight-or-flight" reaction is manifest in the accelerated heart rate, increased respiration, and redistribution of blood from peripheral areas of the body into the head and trunk.

This reaction to stress originally evolved to help humans escape from predators. Once safe, escapees were able to proceed with their normal routines when the physical effect wore off. Today we have the same physiological response to stress, but the kinds of stressors we encounter are different.

The autonomic response occurs quickly and lasts only a short time; the endocrine response initiates more slowly and lasts longer. Setting off this response many times over a long period has a wear-and-tear effect on the body; eventually it lowers resistance to diseases. The hormones flowing through the system, along with the accompanying tensions, also have a psychological effect. Over a period of time, the chain reaction of the stress response can cause depression, irritability, nervousness, apathy, sleep difficulties, and changes in smoking, eating, and drinking habits.

Stress Identification

Stress cannot and should not be avoided; it can and should be successfully managed. All machines wear out with excessive use, and the human body is no exception. Selye (1978, p. 405) states that the critical first step in managing stress is "to know thyself." Everyone is familiar with the sensation of being keyed up from nervous tension. This feeling has a physiochemical basis. It is often difficult to learn to "tune down" or decelerate the pace of life. Simple rest is no panacea for managing stress. Successful stress management balances activity and rest to meet the individual's requirements.

Although each person reacts in a unique way to stress, several commonly observed physical, behavioral, and emotional indicators of increased stress are depicted in the box on this page.

A key part of stress diagnosis is determining if perceptions are accurate. Occasionally a person's anxiety during a stressful event diminishes the ability to assess reality accurately. For example, passing remarks of co-workers or supervisors may be viewed negatively if the person overhearing the remarks is tired or feeling worthless. It is important to remain as objective as possible when stress is present.

Once it is determined that one's perceptions are accurate, the next phase of stress identification includes locating the source of the stress. The following questions may be useful:

1. Is the stress work-related?
2. Is something going on in one's personal life that is worrisome or unfavorable?
3. Is the stress a combination of personal and professional demands?

INDICATORS OF STRESS

PHYSICAL

1. Elevated blood pressure
2. Increased muscle tension (neck, shoulders, back)
3. Elevated pulse and/or increased respiration
4. "Sweaty" palms
5. Cold hands and feet
6. Slumped posture
7. Tension headache
8. Upset stomach
9. Higher pitched voice
10. Change in appetite
11. More frequent need to urinate
12. Restlessness
13. Difficulty in falling asleep or waking up; frequent awakening
14. Dry mouth and throat

BEHAVIORAL

1. Decreased productivity and quality of job performance
2. Tendency to make mistakes; poor judgment
3. Forgetfulness and blocking
4. Diminished attention to detail
5. Preoccupation, daydreaming, or "spacing out"
6. Inability to concentrate on tasks
7. Reduced creativity
8. Increased use of alcohol and/or drugs
9. Increased smoking
10. Increased absenteeism and illness
11. Lethargy
12. Loss of interest
13. Accident proneness

EMOTIONAL

1. Emotional outbursts and crying
2. Irritability
3. Depression
4. Withdrawal
5. Hostile and assaultive behavior
6. Tendency to blame others
7. Anxiousness
8. Feeling of worthlessness
9. Suspiciousness

---

4. Does the person who is feeling the stress set unrealistic goals and standards?
5. Does the person resist change because it is threatening?
6. Does the person feel anxious a lot of the time?

Stressors

Stressors are internal or external factors that cause physical or emotional coping reactions. Some stressors are positive (a job promotion) while others are negative (an injury). People may respond differently to the same stressor. Hardiness is considered a motivating factor in resolving stressful situations and in adapting to health problems (Pollock, 1989). The hardy person recognizes that "he is expected to use judgment and make good decisions (control), to become

TABLE 35-1
Categories of stressors

Category	Example
BIOPHYSIOLOGICAL-CHEMICAL	
Toxic substances	Medication
	Chemical additives
	Drugs
	Excesses of alcohol
	Nicotine
	Caffeine
	Insecticides
	Air pollution
Insufficient exercise, rest or relaxation	Working overtime
Poor nutrition	Overeating
Trauma	Injury
	Bacteria
Weather changes	Temperature extremes
Noise	Living in house on busy street
Crowded living conditions	Large family in small apartment
Radiation	Exposure at work
PSYCHOSOCIAL-CULTURAL (SOCIETAL, SITUATIONAL OR PERSONAL)	
Negative emotions	Anger, frustration, hopelessness
Economic changes	Loss of job
Dissatisfaction with self	Obesity
Changing social values and attitudes	Teenage pregnancy
Violence	Rape victim
Role conflict, ambiguity, overload	New mother returning to work
Change	New job
Labeling and prejudice	Job discrimination
Low self-esteem, perfectionism	Need to control or be controlled

actively involved with others in various activities of life (commitment), and to perceive change as ultimately beneficial to personal development (challenge)" (Pollock, 1989, p 54). Hardiness is considered the key personality resource enabling some people to adjust or to benefit from stressors while others seem to respond negatively.

Stressors can be grouped into two major categories: biophysiological-chemical, and psychosocial-cultural. Table 35:1 lists examples of each type of stressor.

Stress Management Techniques

According to Donnelly (1980a), there are two ways of dealing with stress: reactive and active. Reactive techniques are based on the belief that stress is inevitable and that a person must simply sit back and wait for "it" to happen. This view is similar to the flight response to stress. People who behave in a reactive way simply take what comes along. For example, they work late when the poor planning of others causes extra work. They blame themselves for all that goes wrong at home, school, or work. When self-blame and overconscientiousness fail, the reactive person may lash out

at others in an irrational or aggressive manner or may escape by using drugs or alcohol, overeating, smoking, or oversleeping. The reactive pattern can lead to chronic fatigue, irritability, depression, feelings of inadequacy, and finally stress-related diseases such as colitis or hypertension.

The alternative is to gain control and assume an active role in fighting stressors. The ability to fight stressors, however, does not depend only on one's willingness to assume responsibility. Complex, interrelated factors also play a part. These include past experiences in assuming responsibility; cultural variables, which may or may not sanction certain behaviors; and the availability of support systems. For example, people are more likely to continue stress-reducing behaviors such as managing diet and regularly exercising if friends or family members actively encourage them or join in the effort.

Some of the generally accepted methods for managing stress appeal more to some cultural and socioeconomic groups than others. People with limited education and restricted incomes may not know about or have access to techniques such as biofeedback, progressive relaxation, or yoga.

The following are four general ways to deal with stress:
1. Alter exposure to stress by establishing priorities and setting limits (Sutterly, 1986).
2. Alter the environment so that it is less stressful.
3. Change one's own beliefs and/or behavior so that situations are perceived differently, resulting in different responses.
4. Learn to reduce physiological response to stress by countering the long-range effects.

There are many ways to manage stress. People have preferences and find some methods more successful than others. Also, certain techniques require more skill and resources than others. A variety of techniques will be discussed to equip the community health nurse with choices for developing personal stress management programs with clients. Some general principles of stress management are presented on the next page.

The nursing process may be used to determine the most appropriate method for stress reduction. The assessment phase includes questions such as the following:
1. What specific demands is the person experiencing?
2. What are perceived as stressors?
3. How has the person previously coped with stressful situations?
5. What support systems have assisted in the past?
6. Is the discomfort proportional to the event?
7. What are the person's current resources, limitations and level of motivation?

The stress reduction plan is unique for each client, depending on the level and nature of stress, the person's interest and motivation to reduce stress, and the skill in practicing stress-reducing activities on a regular basis.

Various strategies can be used to reduce stress including diet, exercise, recreation, assertiveness, changing one's thoughts and attitudes, relaxation, meditation, imagery, and biofeedback. Techniques that require special training include hypnosis, acupressure and therapeutic touch. These are beyond the scope of this text.

STRESS MANAGEMENT TIPS

1. Get to know your body so that you can recognize the first signs of stress. (Have clients recall their last stressful situation and describe their physiological reaction.)
2. Learn to relax. Deep breathing is a natural relaxant.
3. Practice simple relaxing exercises.
4. Exercise. Take a brisk walk, run, play tennis, or dance to stimulate blood flow.
5. Learn to smile and laugh and to balance work and recreation. (Ask clients to recall the last time they had fun, what they were doing, and how they felt.)
6. Learn to worry effectively by doing something about it. (Instruct clients to talk out their worries with people they trust and respect.)
7. Learn to accept things and people. Some situations are beyond your control. (Instruct people to change their attitudes about a situation or to develop a stress-reduction plan.)
8. Take one thing at a time. A sure way to become overwhelmed is to find yourself in the middle of a dozen projects.
9. Give in once in a while and try to avoid getting angry. Once you are angry you are conquered, because the ability to think clearly and rationally is diminished in the face of anger.

Assertiveness

Assertiveness means standing up for one's own rights without violating the rights of others. Assertive behavior is learned, and it involves taking responsibility for one's decisions and actions (Bond, 1988a). In contrast, aggressiveness is described as behavior that does not respect the rights of others and conveys an attitude of "what you have to say is less important than what I have to say." Nonassertive or submissive behavior involves giving in and reflects lack of self-respect.

Assertive behavior is a direct way to handle stress. Just as people say "ouch" when they are hurt, an assertive response clearly indicates feelings and desires (Palmer and Deck, 1987). Assertiveness requires two key skills: thought substitution and assertive responses. Thought substitution replaces negative, often erroneous, beliefs with valid, objective perceptions of self. This allows the person to feel equal to others. Assertive responses reflect behaving as an equal. Skills for being assertive include non-verbal aspects of behavior, speaking clearly, active listening, and assertive responses.

NON-VERBAL ASPECTS OF BEHAVIOR. As the old saying goes, "a picture is worth a thousand words"; likewise, body language communicates more clearly than do words. The way a person stands, his posture, whether he looks directly at the other person, his facial expression and his voice tone and loudness all tell how he feels about himself. The most persuasive stance is to stand erect, look the other person straight in the eye and speak in a clear tone, avoiding distracting, nervous gestures like wringing hands or biting nails.

SPEAKING CLEARLY. Assertiveness requires honest, straightforward, and prompt communication of beliefs, ideas, plans, or feelings. Sitting and stewing simply increases stress. Assertive people say what they want clearly and precisely, in as few words as possible (Baugh, 1989). If the response they get is an icy stare, they stand firm and repeat what they said. They remain calm, stick to the facts, and use "I" statements (Cornell, 1985). Sentences that start with "you" immediately put the other person on the defensive. A person owns his own thoughts and feelings by saying "I think," "I need," or "I'm angry." The goal is to convey one's thoughts and feelings, explain why one is upset, and state the desired outcome.

ACTIVE LISTENING. Assertiveness means not only speaking but also listening carefully. Many people, while appearing to listen, are instead thinking intently about what they want to say next. *Active listening*, essential to discovering the other person's needs and values, includes letting the speaker know he was heard. Feedback to the speaker includes paraphrasing what was heard, asking for clarification or more information, or indicating either agreement or disagreement with the message.

ASSERTIVE RESPONSES. The most useful assertive responses for nurses to use and to teach clients are:

◇ Learning to say no
◇ Fogging
◇ Broken record
◇ Negotiating

Nurses and clients have the right to make choices and establish priorities. The word "no" is one of the most difficult words for some people to use. When deciding how to respond to a request, a person should be sure he understands exactly what is being asked. He should listen carefully and ask questions for clarification. If he decides to say no, he should do so in a clear, concise way using an "I" statement (Bond, 1988b), such as "I cannot do that for you, but I will ask . . . " In saying no, it may be useful to briefly explain the reason. If saying "I'm sorry" helps in saying "no," then do so. It is often helpful to suggest alternatives when the answer to a request is "no." For example, the request may be reasonable, but the deadline is the problem; perhaps the deadline can be changed. If the deadline cannot be changed, offering the names of other people may be helpful.

Fogging is the technique of agreeing in principle in response to criticism. It is called "fogging" because the criticized person generates a barrier that is similar to a bank of fog to disguise his reaction. Fogging is not direct nor does it really deal with the underlying issue; however, it diffuses the emotion associated with criticism. For example, an employee who arrives ten minutes late for the first time in five weeks is asked by his supervisor, "You never get here on time; how can we rely on you?" A fogging response would be "I was late today."

A *broken record* response involves repeating a word or phrase used by the other person over and over without getting angry until the person finally acknowledges having heard. The broken-record technique is especially useful for people who have trouble saying "no." A good exercise is to devise a short sentence and repeat it in broken-record fashion. For example, if asked to make an additional home visit on a day that clearly is already filled with assignments, one can try repeating a phrase such as "I would like to help you by making the home visit, but I simply cannot add another patient today"; and then, "I am sorry that I cannot add another patient visit today."

NEGOTIATING. is a strategy that uses principles of communication, conflict resolution, and assertiveness. Timing is important in negotiation. Also important is identifying and dealing with people's problems separately from the situation being negotiated. One should find out the interests of all people involved. What is at stake? What are the shared interests of all participants? It is best to identify all possible options that might be acceptable to the parties involved rather than immediately assuming there is only one right solution. Brainstorming is effective in identifying options, and it should be followed by turning the options into proposals and beginning the process of finding the proposal most acceptable to all participants (Dainow, 1986).

Negotiation is a process, not an event. Before beginning to negotiate, participants should gather all relevant information in order not to appear confused and poorly prepared. Throughout the process it is essential to practice active listening to hear exactly what the opponent is really saying.

Changing Thoughts and Attitudes

Changing thoughts and attitudes is an essential part of stress management. It is important to handle stressors as they occur and to deal directly with feelings in order to avoid bottling up thoughts or emotions. It is also important to find something to substitute for troubling thoughts. Nothing erases unpleasant thoughts more effectively than conscious efforts to focus on positive things. Adams (1980) describes a process for shifting attitudes to deal more effectively with feelings:

1. Notice the feeling or sensation by being consciously aware that something is occurring.
2. Give the feeling a label such as anger or happiness.
3. Decide whether or not the feeling or cluster of feelings is appropriate to the perceived situation.
4. Give expression to feelings in a way that is safe, that will get what is wanted or needed, and that will do no harm to others. It is much more appropriate to talk with people about anger than to become physically aggressive.

"The most effective way to change the way you feel is to change the way you think" (Montgomery, 1987, p. 859). *Thought-stopping* is a behavior therapy technique used to help people control obsessive and phobic thoughts (Wolpe, 1969). Thought stopping uses the command "stop" or some other distraction to interrupt an unpleasant thought. The unpleasant thought is then replaced with an accurate and positive assertion.

PERFECTIONISM. often leads to a negative view of oneself. Typically, perfectionists are conscientious, hard-working people who compulsively attempt to meet unrealistic goals. They always aim for perfection and are never content to settle for merely the "good." The perfectionist's striving is often created by "all-or-none thinking": the person either wins or loses, fails or succeeds. One critical remark will make the person feel like a failure.

Other types of thinking and negative internal messages that increase stress include:
◊ Absolutizing—thinking there is only one right way
◊ Awfulizing—turning problems into catastrophes
◊ Shoulds—beliefs that one ought to do things that are really beyond one's abilities

In thought substitution, people listen to what they say to themselves, identify negative statements, and substitute positive ones. For example, "shoulds" can be changed into "wants." When people eliminate perfectionism, shoulds, absolutizing, and awfulizing, they free up considerable energy and are often more productive than ever before.

Creating and Using Support Networks

One of the best ways to cope with stress is to seek support from members of a reliable and caring work, family, or social group. Everyone needs someone to trust and talk to about stress-producing situations without fear of rejection or retaliation. Talking with one or more members of a trusted support network provides opportunities for testing reality, obtaining valued feedback, working through feelings, and constructively planning future actions.

A support network is a resource pool on which one can selectively draw to provide support and strength. People need several options in their resource pool so they do not consistently draw on the same person. This variety also ensures that the person assumes responsibility for choosing how to deal with situations and does not delegate them to the support system. Clients should be guided in identifying the support networks currently available. Who are the members of their support network? How many people can they call on in a crisis or a stressful situation?

The purpose of support groups is to assist members in growing and developing through people who understand and who care about one another. Usually, a common bond holds the members of a support group together. In many groups there are no meeting agendas, but rather the goal is to support, encourage, and at times challenge one another. Seashore listed the following four functions of a support group (1980, p. 157):

1. *Reestablish competence:* In times of high stress, people often devalue their ability and fail to recognize their own strengths.
2. *Maintain high performance:* In good times when excessive stress is not present, support groups help members "keep their batteries charged."
3. *Gain new competencies:* Some members of the group may be better able to challenge, teach, or motivate others.
4. *Achieve selected objectives:* Group membership can help in the clarification, formulation, and refinement of short-term and long-term objectives.

Group members can help identify the selection of an ineffective coping mechanism and assist members in learning and practicing new responses.

Often people think that they have behaved so badly that no one else could possibly understand, much less accept them. Community health nurses for many years have recognized the value of group sessions in helping clients deal

---

PROGRESSIVE RELAXATION: MODIFIED APPROACH FOR COMMUNITY HEALTH NURSING PRACTICE

This activity simply involves relaxing one step at a time, as follows:

1. Sit or lie in a comfortable position.
2. Close your eyes.
3. Concentrate on breathing easily.
4. Once your body feels calm, instruct all bones and muscles of the lower body to relax in the following order:
   - a. Feet
   - b. Ankles
   - c. Lower legs
   - d. Knees
   - e. Upper legs
   - f. Hips
5. Shift attention to the upper parts of your body, instructing all bones and muscles to relax in the following order:
   - a. Hands
   - b. Wrists
   - c. Lower arms
   - d. Elbows
   - e. Upper arms
   - f. Neck
   - g. Shoulders

By this time, your arms and legs should feel heavy and unmovable. However, if you become uncomfortable, shift your position. Then continue with step 6.

6. Spend some time concentrating on relaxing the main part of your body, instructing each organ and all muscles to be relaxed.
7. Relax your head muscles in the following order:
   - a. Jaws
   - b. Face
   - c. Scalp
8. With the relaxation process complete, spend a few minutes focusing on (but not altering) your breathing, which probably has become quite shallow.
9. Gradually increase your breathing to "get the blood flowing again." To prevent dizziness, take one or two relatively deep breaths before standing up.

---

with problems. Group experiences have included successes with people dependent on alcohol and/or drugs, those with problems of obesity or major chronic illnesses, those suffering the loss of a child or spouse, and victims and/or perpetrators of abuse.

Stress management groups offer a rich potential for clients and nurses. These groups can be oriented toward discussions, activities, or a combination of both. Group membership is a natural and desirable social phenomenon. Groups can promote a healing by providing opportunities for self-understanding and acceptance.

Support systems help people reestablish their competence during times of high stress as well as serving as sources of strength and encouragement during ordinary situations. Clients need to rely on support systems sparingly so that they are not "worn out" by giving such assistance. A support system should be maintained in times of homeostasis as well as when under stress.

Relaxation

Relaxing tends to be cast aside in the busy hustle and bustle of life. Many people view relaxing as a waste of time rather than an opportunity for unwinding and passively dealing with the stresses of life.

Community health nurses are in an ideal position to teach relaxation techniques. Before teaching them, however, they should learn and practice the techniques themselves.

Relaxation exercises are simply "journeys into self," which provide a mechanism for unwinding. The primary purpose of relaxation is to relieve muscle tension and induce a quieting response so that the body can rebuild needed energy resources. Nurses can assist clients through teaching and role modeling to assume a mental state of relaxation. One form of relaxation, progressive relaxation, is discussed in some detail.

PROGRESSIVE RELAXATION. Progressive relaxation reduces stress by altering the relation between muscle and psychological tension in order to monitor and control stress levels. Jacobson (1974) did extensive research on mind/muscle interaction and suggested that anxiety and relaxation are

mutually exclusive. Progressive relaxation is a method of combating tension and anxiety by systematically tensing and relaxing muscle groups.

Progressive relaxation, a rudimentary form of biofeedback, is based on the person's ability to feel the contrast as each of fourteen major muscle groups is tensed and then immediately relaxed. The procedure follows a systematic format moving from the feet to the head (see Brallier's (1982) adaptation of Jacobson's technique in the box above.) This form of relaxation is within the scope of nursing practice and has been successful in treating clients with borderline hypertension, headaches, insomnia, and anxiety.

Before progressive relaxation is implemented, assessment should include a history and a determination that this technique is appropriate. The nurse should also verify that there are no contraindications to the relaxation of certain muscle groups. For some types of low back pain, strengthening rather than relaxing certain muscle groups is preferred (Richter and Sloan, 1979). Planning and implementation are consistent with all other forms of relaxation. In the evaluation phase, the nurse should carefully observe any factors that may have compromised the effectiveness of this technique.

During the tension phase of progressive relaxation, cramps may occur in the neck, calves, feet, or any other muscle group. These cramps can often be avoided by reducing the intensity and duration of tension. If cramps do occur, the client should move or rub the affected muscle, relax for a few minutes, and then continue.

Some people have difficulty tensing certain muscle groups and may need assistance in developing an alternative tensing pattern. Others have difficulty following instructions. Some people prefer to keep their eyes open during early sessions so that they can model after the nurse. This also may decrease their fear of the unknown (Richter and Sloan, 1979). Other clients have strange or unfamiliar feelings such as a floating sensation during progressive relaxation. If this occurs, they may need to become reoriented to their surroundings. The following approach, meditation, is often used in combination with progressive relaxation.

Meditation

Meditation is a form of self-discipline that helps people achieve inner peace by focusing uncritically on one thing at a time (Kneisl, 1988). The state of meditation is one of deep rest where the heart rate slows, the body uses less oxygen, and blood lactate decreases remarkably. Meditation is used to treat insomnia, asthma, addictions to food, alcohol, tobacco, and other drugs, and to help prevent hypertension and heart disease.

Meditation exercises are easy to learn, take only a few minutes each day, require no special equipment, and can be done in almost any quiet and private place. The four major requirements for meditation are:

◊ A quiet place
◊ A comfortable position
◊ A focused thought
◊ A passive attitude

The focused thought refers to a mental device or mantra, a word or sound that is repeated with each exhalation. Frequently used mantras are: "one," "I am relaxed," or "I am." Four steps to meditation are:

1. Sit quietly in a comfortable position with eyes closed.
2. Using progressive relaxation, deeply relax all muscles beginning with the feet and moving to the face.
3. Breathe through the nose being consciously aware of the breathing pattern. While exhaling, mentally say the word "one."
4. Continue the breathing process of step 3 for 10 to 20 minutes, but do not set an alarm; open your eyes to check the time. When finished, remain seated several minutes with your eyes closed, and then a few minutes more with the eyes open.

Meditate in a quiet place, free from distractions. Avoid meditating within two hours after a heavy meal, since digestion interferes with the ability to relax.

Creative Imagery or Visualization

Creative imagery is a way to help people in creating a milieu for their own healing processes to occur. The concept behind creative imagery is that "the body is equipped to heal itself from every manner of disorder, and that under most circumstances the body requires no special instructions to accomplish this feat" (Achterberg and Lawlis, 1980, pp. 55-56). Mental images of events or places use the senses mentally and consciously to alter bodily functioning (Achterberg and Lawlis, 1980). The concept of creative imagery involves any or all five of the senses. Although this concept is often used in attaining and maintaining health, it is also useful for psychotherapy and spiritual care.

Visualization exercises help to demonstrate the relation between the mind and the body. When the mind focuses on a peaceful and tranquil scene, the body tends to respond by relaxing. Nurses can assist clients to relax by suggesting that they visualize a place they would like to be. The mental image should be specific and detailed to encourage active participation in the process. For example, a client might find the seashore relaxing. First the nurse asks the client to imagine sitting beside the sea listening to the many sounds. Next, the nurse instructs the client to ask questions such as the following: What kinds of sounds are most prominent at the sea? How do I feel as I sit, listen, and look at the calm, gently moving blue sea?

The research by Simonton, Simonton, and Creighton (1978) demonstrated the use of visualization in treating cancer. They combined visualization with other methods of cancer treatment, including radiation and chemotherapy. The patients were taught to visualize their concern in an attempt to combat the disease. "For many cancer patients, the body has become the enemy. It has betrayed them by getting sick and threatening their lives. They feel alienated from it and mistrust its ability to combat their disease" (Simonton et al. 1978, p. 125). These researchers devised a cancer treatment program based on the assumption that relaxation helps to reduce fear, which can itself become overwhelming. They combined progressive relaxation with mental imagery and recommended that patients practice this program 3 times a day for 10 to 15 minutes. Several principles form the foundation for this relaxation and mental imagery program. By forming an image of a desired event, people can make a personal statement of what they want to occur. By repeating the statement, clients come to expect that the desired event will occur and begin acting in ways consistent with the achievement of the desired outcome.

These same approaches can be used in dealing with arthritis. Clients can be instructed to picture their joints as being irritated and having many small granules on the surface. Next they are urged to see their white blood cells coming in, cleaning up the debris, and smoothing over the joint surfaces. Finally they visualize themselves as being active and free of joint pain.

Relaxation and mental imagery can decrease fear by enabling people to take responsibility for and control of themselves. These processes can also bring about an attitude change, moving from despair or despondency to anticipation and the will to live. They can also promote physical changes that enhance the immune system and can be a basic method for stress reduction.

Biofeedback

The basic principles of biofeedback are (1) monitoring a physiological index that is sensitive to stress, (2) feeding the information back to the person involved, and (3) using the information as a guide to alter the physiological state. Biofeedback provides immediate confirmation of personal control. Various stress reactions have been effectively controlled with biofeedback, including excessive anxiety, phobias, tension, headaches, insomnia, essential hypertension, bruxism (teeth grinding), colitis, ulcer, and menstrual distress.

Through *biofeedback* electronic sensors can make people aware of normally unconscious processes. Alpha brain waves, muscle tension, and skin temperature are often used to provide people with an immediate interpretation of their bodily reaction. One popular way to use biofeedback is by using an electromyograph, a machine designed to gauge the state of muscle tension by detecting electrical signals through the skin. Biofeedback helps people learn to reduce mounting tension.

Several simple procedures, which require no machinery, may be used to detect responses to stress. It is common practice for nurses to monitor clients' reactions by noting changes in breathing, heart rate, and blood pressure. Clients can easily be taught to monitor pulse as a gauge of their emotions. Clients can also be taught to use a sensitive thermometer for measuring skin temperature of the fingers. It is important to tape the thermometer firmly to the finger to obtain an accurate reading.

Another variation of temperature monitoring includes the warming of hands via biofeedback. Before warming the hands, the person's palmar skin temperature of the index finger should be measured using a standard thermometer. Readings below 85°F indicate distress. Once the temperature is recorded, the person can be taught to raise it by a variety of relaxation techniques, including sitting or lying in a comfortable position with shoulders relaxed and attention focused on slow, even breathing. The next step in warming the hands includes concentrating on and repeating the phrase, "My arms and hands are heavy and warm."As relaxation occurs, the hands begin to warm and may tingle as the temperature rises. Temperature should be recorded before and after each session to motivate and encourage the participant.

If the person's blood pressure is elevated considerably, medication is initially used to bring it under control before entry into the biofeedback program. Clients are aided in identifying their personal sources of stress, what physiological changes they typically experience in response to stress, and what changes can be made either in their lifestyles or in their responses to the stressor. With this reasonably simple, painless method, clients can be taught to control hypertension while simultaneously reducing their reliance on drugs.

Burnout: Ineffective Coping with Stress

The term *burnout* was coined by psychologist Herbert Freudenberger in 1975 to describe a reaction to excessive job-related stress (Bunch, 1983). It may also be observed in individuals who suffer major losses, such as a job or a close family member, within a short time span, or in persons experiencing chronic illness. Whatever the cause, the person experiencing burnout is unable to respond successfully to stress.

Both internal and external stressors contribute to burnout. Inadequate leadership, poor working conditions, long hours, heavy workloads, lack of control over work, and bureaucratic procedures are examples of external stressors. Internal stressors include the need for autonomy, respect, recognition, feelings of competence, and involvement in meaningful activities (Bunch, 1983).

The physiological components of burnout include cardiac irregularities and electrolyte imbalance (hypokalemia), which may result in decreased cardiac output. Additional physical symptoms include fatigue, gastrointestinal problems, persistent colds, back pain, weight loss or gain, loss of appetite, susceptibility to infections, headaches, insomnia, dyspnea, or angina.

Physical signs are generally accompanied by several behavioral symptoms including irritability, rigid thinking and general resistance to new ideas or proposed changes, finding fault easily with other people, or displaying a generally negative and cynical attitude. Other behavioral indicators of burnout are absenteeism, tardiness, decreasing accuracy, and a tendency to "take problems home." The person approaching burnout becomes increasingly exhausted physically and emotionally and, in general, begins to show lack of respect, empathy, or warmth for others. For nurses these signs of burnout are often followed by decisions to leave the profession, seek administrative positions, or use drugs or alcohol to cope with the stress.

Burnout is common among human service workers who spend considerable time and energy helping others. An unfortunate aspect of burnout is that the people who suffer from it tend to be those the organization values most highly. Victims of burnout typically are high achievers who thrive on accomplishments.

Three categories of events have been found to be instrumental in precipitating burnout among health care workers.

1. Environmental deficits, such as insufficient supplies or equipment, poor physical layout of the institution, and a shortage of staff.
2. Professional relationships characterized by ineffective communication or personality conflicts.
3. Relationships with clients and families in which the nurse identifies with the client and feels guilty that the best possible care is not being given.

Ironically, increased knowledge can precipitate burnout. As health care technology has improved, greater knowledge is available on preventing and treating diseases. Nurses know what they could or should do; yet lack of time, energy, commitment, or resources prevent them from taking the necessary actions. A failure to act leads to stress, especially if lack of action brings about untoward results. For example, Ms. Smith, a home health care nurse, was visiting an elderly client to change her indwelling catheter. Ms. Smith brought only one sterile catheter kit. She had considered stopping by the office to get an extra catheter, but she was running late. Unfortunately, Ms. Smith dropped the sterile catheter onto the floor just as she was about to insert it. Because of her tight schedule, Ms. Smith picked up the contaminated catheter and used it. The following week Ms. Smith visited the client and saw signs indicating a urinary tract infection. She felt depressed, guilty, and overwhelmed by her inability to effectively manage her time and use good judgment. If Ms. Smith continued to have many days like the one described, she would be a likely candidate for burnout.

Coping with burnout includes the same basic stress management techniques as those previously discussed. These efforts begin with self-awareness to recognize accumulating stress, followed by a carefully developed intervention plan with exercise, recreation, open communication, group or individual support, outside interests and resources, and the recognition that burnout does not result from "bad" people but from "bad" situations. The box at right summarizes steps for self-management of burnout, focusing on both prevention and intervention.

Coping with a Community Stressor

This chapter has dealt with stress assessment and management on an individual level. However, the importance and complexity of community stressors should not be underestimated. Factors such as crowding, excessive noise, and

---

SELF-MANAGEMENT FOR BURNOUT

1. Know yourself; pay attention to your feelings to see what sets off negative feelings.
2. Delegate whenever possible; do not try to do everything for yourself and others.
3. Recognize that burnout is a function of poor situations, and work to change them.
4. Plan a variety of self-care activities to increase resistance to stress.
5. Vary the amount and type of client contact so you are not consistently caring for the same kind of people. Staff members working in tense clinical situations may plan regular, brief "time-outs" to mobilize their personal resources.
6. Keep work and home separate. Leave feelings and problems in the proper place.
7. Form a peer support group to discuss reactions and feelings about work.
8. Negotiate roles and responsibilities to do what you feel competent to do.
9. Regularly show appreciation to others; positive expressions can become contagious.

---

climate influence the community's level of stress. Other community stressors can include high crime rates, chemical and other pollution, natural and man-made disasters, poverty and homelessness, economic down-turns resulting in company closings and lay-offs, or school closings.

Far more research has been conducted on how individuals cope with the stressors of daily life than on how people cope with community stressors. Bachrach and Zautra (1985, p. 127) define community stressors as "problems that affect a large number of people in a given area . . . [which] cannot be readily resolved by the individual alone and thus require collective action." These stressors may be acute or chronic and may originate either within or outside the community.

Whether a stressor causes either a physical or mental reaction depends upon what other things residents are dealing with, the availability of social supports, previous successful coping experiences, and the residents' confidence-level in their ability to cope. For example, consider two similar events in nearly identical mid-western towns. In 1988 a tornado heavily damaged over 100 homes in an Illinois town (Town A) of 7500 people. At that time the town's churches opened their facilities to residents who needed food, clothing, and places to sleep. Town leaders realized they had handled this situation effectively; however, they had done so by instinct rather than through a disaster plan. Over the next year, town officials developed a disaster plan that included volunteers and a range of available facilities.

In 1990, due to weeks of heavy rains on previously drought-plagued land, the rivers in this same town and those in Town B, 50 miles away, overflowed and caused substantial flood damage. As might be expected, Town A fared much better than Town B. A disaster plan was ready and, equally important, residents believed they could cope because of their successful experience two years earlier.

Areas in which community health nurses could participate in planning with community groups to decrease stress and physical vulnerabilities include:

1. Opposing stress-producing projects: When community residents feel threatened by the construction of facilities such as airports, shopping areas, highways, or chemical disposal facilities, community health nurses can assist with developing group cohesion so residents can work in concert to oppose the projects.
2. Programs for special populations: Community awareness and organized neighborhood protection programs can reduce crime toward vulnerable groups such as children, the elderly, and shopkeepers running small businesses that have few employees present at any given time.
3. Legislation affecting social practices such as the legal drinking age, use of seatbelts, and possession of firearms can decrease community stress and vulnerability.
4. Regulations: Regulatory bodies can be urged by community pressure to enforce building and fire safety codes, investigate accidents in a timely fashion, and increase support for educational and social programs.

The role of the community health nurse in stress reduction extends to individuals, groups, and communities. Although the challenge is complex, the rewards for successful stress management are great.

CRISIS INTERVENTION

Stress, while debilitating and difficult, does not have the same impact on people or communities as does a crisis. Crisis is a term commonly used in our society for an instance in which circumstances are suddenly altered. There can be events that are not in themselves crises but which may predispose individuals, families, and communities to crises. The nature and characteristics of a crisis are distinct from other changes in circumstances. A crisis progresses through a series of identified phases, each with its own possibilities for intervention.

Crisis intervention techniques can be used by health professionals, non-health professionals, and volunteers trained to assist individuals or groups in crisis. Crisis intervention helps clients resolve situations so that they are stronger after the crisis than they were before. Responsible community health nurses are aware of facilities available for crisis prevention and intervention and can help clients gain entry to those resources.

The remainder of this chapter considers the nature, characteristics, and phases of crisis and the types of crises that individuals, families, and communities experience. An overview of crisis intervention is presented, and the concepts of primary, secondary, and tertiary prevention are discussed. A case illustrates how community health nurses can use the nursing process in crisis intervention.

Nature of Crisis

An essential property of crisis is the potential for promoting growth. Crises present challenges and call for new responses (Rapoport, 1965). Assisting people in crisis to achieve growth is an important role for community health nurses.

Caplan (1964), a leader in the development of crisis theory, described crisis as an "upset," or disequilibrium in a steady state, occurring when usual problem-solving strategies are ineffective. Typically, a problem situation causes a change in equilibrium. The affected person responds with a previously successful problem-solving or coping strategy to reinstitute a state of balance. Because of the magnitude of the crisis, the person's usual strategies are ineffective, leading to an intense level of disequilibrium. New strategies for problem-solving must then be initiated. The effectiveness of the identified and new strategies leads to one of three potential outcomes. (1) Effective strategies often lead to psychological growth and an improved state of functioning. Crises provide opportunities for people to learn new coping mechanisms that can be applied to other situations. (2) The person returns to the level of functioning before the crisis, with no appreciable gain or loss. (3) The person functions at a lower level after the crisis. When the new strategies are ineffective or the problem continues or intensifies over time, the risk of major psychological disorganization increases.

As with individuals, when families and communities experience problems that are not solved by usual coping strategies, a crisis occurs, offering the possibility for growth and improved function and the danger of major disorganization.

Characteristics of Crisis

The duration of the state of disequilibrium, the individual's perception of the event and problems, and the functioning pattern of the individual are characteristics of a crisis. A crisis may also affect the ability of many people to think clearly, as well as evoke the presence of strong subjective feelings and the occurrence of stressful physiological symptoms.

The degree of disequilibrium is related to the duration of the crisis. Most crises tend to be temporary and self-limiting and last between four and six weeks; thus a successful or unsuccessful resolution is reached within a relatively short period of time. For the community health nurse this means that intervention must be prompt and concentrated in a brief time span.

Whether or not an event and its problems lead to crisis depends on the perception and coping abilities of the individual. For example, if a man loses his job after 20 years with a company and has no experience with unemployment, he may experience a crisis. However, for a high school student who works only for additional spending money, job loss is much less likely to be followed by crisis.

The pattern of functioning is also affected in a state of crisis (Caplan, 1964). The level of function decreases and associated disorganization occurs. Even routine tasks may not be effectively completed. Recognition of this impairment of functioning level is exemplified by the custom in many communities of taking food to the homes of families who have experienced events such as death, accident, or serious illness. Families in crisis are not expected to function at the same level as before.

People in crisis feel helpless and often seek assistance in relieving their misery. They feel pain and a need to resolve the situation (Lawler and Yount, 1987). The increased need for assistance and the increased receptivity to interventions are both important factors for nurses working with those in crisis. Christensen and Harding (1985) illustrated these facets of crisis. A family receiving hospice care refused to allow the nurse to demonstrate a bed bath until the client's first episode of incontinence. For this family the incontinence was the event that precipitated a crisis. At this point the family quickly learned the skills that allowed them to cope with similar events.

Lindemann's (1979) work with the victims of the Coconut Grove fire is a classic study of individuals in a crisis and provides an understanding of psychological and physiological responses. Fire engulfed a Boston nightclub on November 28, 1942, during the celebration of the Harvard-Yale football game. The magnitude of the fire was tremendous, and the death toll reached 491; only 39 people survived. Responding to a request for psychiatric assistance, Lindemann worked with the burn victims, their relatives, and the relatives of those who died. Physical and psychological reactions were noted. Frequent physical responses included sighing respiration, exhaustion, lack of strength, and altered gastrointestinal patterns. Common activities such as walking resulted in exhaustion. However, even with the exhaustion, there were feelings of restlessness and the need for activity. Routine tasks were sought but were carried out with much effort. Psychological responses in the crisis of acute grief included guilt, hostility, and preoccupation with the image of the deceased.

Although Lindemann found that reactions to the crisis usually followed closely after the precipitating event, there were instances of delayed responses. An individual's need to deal with a pressing problem was a factor in the delay. One example involved an adolescent girl who was burned and whose parents were killed in the Coconut Grove fire. Two younger siblings were her chief concern during her hospitalization and resettlement time. Only after more than two months did she show depression, frequent crying, and other symptoms of grief.

Another example of a crisis situation occurred in a New Jersey suburb in which three girls were raped within the same day (Underwood and Fiedler, 1983). The entire community was in a state of fear, and The Community Mental Health Center initiated a multi-focus program to cope with the crisis of rape. Meetings were begun for parents, which focused on communicating with children of various ages, correcting misinformation, and reinforcing the *amount of control children possess,* for example, telling an adult or running away. Police, the county prosecutor, counselors from the local women's crisis center, and mental health professionals participated in presentations to the community, which consisted of a filmstrip, videotapes, and written materials; an educational coloring book was prepared for children. Initiating the effort shortly after the assaults and involving a variety of agencies contributed to the success of the intervention.

The problems resulting in crisis stem from events of loss, threat of loss, or overwhelming challenge. Losses such as the death or incapacitating illness of a significant other are not the only events that can precipitate crisis. A desirable event, such as an important new job, may produce a crisis for a person who lacks effective coping strategies. Problems

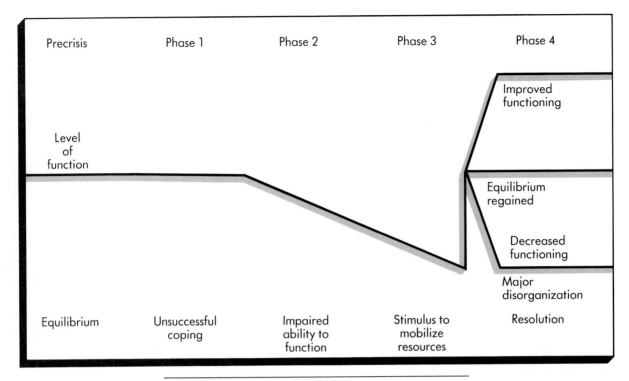

FIGURE 35-1

Phases of crises.

that could arise following a much desired promotion include establishing relations with new peers and former co-workers, changes in family life-style, and changes in social obligations. Associated problems are inevitable once a significant event has occurred, and crisis can result if adequate coping strategies are absent.

Another feature of crisis is "cognitive uncertainty" (Spradley, 1990 p. 328), in which the individual in crisis cannot predict the outcome of the situation. This uncertainty increases the tension of the person in crisis, who may experience feelings of helplessness and ineffectuality (Caplan, 1964). In addition, feelings of anxiety, guilt, fear, or shame can occur. For instance, if a child is severely injured while playing, the parents may feel guilty and think that the accident could have been prevented if they had been more attentive.

Individuals in crisis often exhibit physiological symptoms, and these vary from person to person according to individual responses to stressors. Sleep disturbances, gastrointestinal symptoms, muscle tension, shortness of breath, irritability, need for routine activity, and exhaustion are among the possible manifestations. For example, a widow said that the night after her husband died she had been able to sleep only intermittently, and at 4 am she had begun cleaning the kitchen.

Phases of Crisis

Caplan (1964) describes progression of an individual through a crisis in four phases (Figure 35-1). In phase 1 a problem is encountered, and tension increases. This causes the person to recall coping strategies that have been successful in the past. When past strategies do not solve the

problem, phase 2 follows, with a further rise in tension. In phase 2 disequilibrium is evidenced by characteristic psychological and physiological crisis responses and impaired ability to function. Phase 3, with another rise in tension, stimulates the individual to mobilize resources. Activities in phase 3 can include awareness of previously overlooked aspects of the problem, redefining the problem, setting aside irrelevant aspects, or developing new problem-solving mechanisms. If the strategies used in phase 3 are successful, the problem will be resolved and the individual will either return to the previous state of equilibrium or move to an improved level of functioning. If the strategies of phase 3 are not successful, phase 4 follows. With continuation of the problem, lack of success in resolution, and increased tension, a breaking point is reached, and the result is major disorganization with accompanying decreased functioning.

Types of Crisis

Crises may be categorized as maturational or situational. Additional classification labels a crisis as internal or external, depending on the origin of the event precipitating it. Examples of external precipitating events include termination of employment, death of a spouse, or severe injury to one's child. Internal events occur when individuals question their relationship to life and their place in it. Internal events concern decisions, such as deciding to end one's marriage or deciding to terminate a pregnancy.

Maturational Crises

Throughout life, people are faced with transitions when moving from one stage of development to the next. Devel-

---

NORMAL STATES OF TRANSITION

Infancy to toddler
Toddler to preschool
Preschool to school age
School age to adolescence
Adolescence to adult
Adult to middle age
Middle age to old age

From Erikson E.: Childhood and society, New York, 1950, W.W. Norton & Co., Inc.

STAGES OF FAMILY LIFE

Stage 1—Married couples
Stage 2—Childbearing families
Stage 3—Families with preschool children
Stage 4—Families with schoolchildren
Stage 5—Families with teenagers
Stage 6—Families launching young adults
Stage 7—Families with middle-aged parents
Stage 8—Families with aging family members

From Duvall EM and Miller BC: Marriage and family development, ed 6, New York, 1985, Harper & Row, Publishers, Inc.

opmental psychologists such as Erikson (1950) have identified normal major states of transition (see box). Maturational, or developmental, crises occur during natural transitions in the developmental process. Entering school, marrying, and retiring are examples of events that can lead to maturational crises.

Because these transitions can be anticipated, measures can be taken to lessen their impact. For example, discussion groups for young teenagers can ease the transition into adolescence. Pre-retirement programs can help individuals cope with the problems of old age.

As with all crises, maturational crises hold the possibility for growth and the danger of stagnation or regression. Adolescents confront issues such as dating, sexual activity, and career choice; young adults face establishing their own households, securing jobs, and possibly having children. Marsha is an example of someone in maturational crisis. Marsha had only completed one year of college when she was suspended because of her grades. She was faced with finding a job and supporting herself while losing her best friend, who had married and moved to another state the previous month. Marsha is moving from the life state of adolescence to adult. How she copes with this crisis will determine the remainder of her life and her ability to cope. (Problems across the life span are considered in Part Five).

Situational Crises

Situational, or accidental, crises follow unanticipated, uncontrollable events. Divorce, death, illness, and natural disasters are examples of events that can lead to situational crises.

Unlike maturational crises, situational crises are frequently sudden and unexpected; thus anticipatory guidance is not always possible. Prompt contact and early intervention can assist in coping with a situational crisis. Centers for battered women, laryngectomy self-help groups, and rape crisis centers are examples of organizations developed to assist individuals to cope with specific events that can lead to situational crises.

Some events that lead to situational crises occur precipitously, whereas others have some lead-time, which can be used to avert or lessen their impact. For example, relocation of an elderly person may cause disequilibrium and subsequent situational crisis (Rosswurm, 1983). Community health nurses have several opportunities to assist with elderly people who are being relocated. Encouraging older people to discuss what the move means to them and their thoughts

and feelings can assist in promoting a realistic perspective of the situation. In addition, several visits to the new residence before the move will not only orient the person to the new surroundings but will also allow him to actively participate in planning the move. Bringing familiar furniture and treasured belongings to the new residence can also ease the transition. The community health nurse, the elderly person, the family, and the staff of the institutions can work together, discussing strategies for coping with the move and the new situation.

Maturational-Situational Crises

If an unexpected, hazardous event occurs during transition from one maturational state to another, an individual who normally could complete the necessary developmental task may experience crisis (Moynihan and Hayes, 1982). If coping mechanisms are depleted in dealing with the situational event, the developmental task will not be achieved. On the other hand, if all coping mechanisms are devoted to the maturational task, it is not possible to adequately cope with the situational event. For example, a young man who is engaged and just beginning to establish his career became partially paralyzed in an accident. He has experienced events that could lead to a combined maturational-situational crisis. Not only is he in the developmental process of establishing a career and achieving intimacy, but he must also cope with the changes caused by his paralysis. Strategies for coping with both the maturational and situational events are necessary.

Families and Crisis
Maturational Crisis

Family life is a dynamic cycle requiring readjustments as one phase is completed and another begins. Typically, periods of relative calm are followed by more intense activity at family-life transition times. As with individuals, families may face maturational or situational crises. And like individuals, families progress through developmental stages, each presenting a unique set of circumstances and requiring new coping strategies. For successful progression through the developmental stages, all family members must cope with the new situations. Each developmental stage requires members to relinquish some previously held roles and to assume new roles.

Duvall and Miller (1985) developed an eight-stage family life cycle. The family life stages are listed in the box.

These stages are predictable, and anticipatory guidance can help families cope with the inherent problems of each stage. Programs designed to promote growth through the family developmental process include premarital conferences, classes on preparation for parenthood, parenting groups, and classes that focus on preparing for retirement. If a family successfully progresses through the developmental stages, the individual family members and the whole family grow.

A family crisis can also result from an event within the family (intrafamilial) or outside the family (extrafamilial) (Smitherman, 1981). Examples of intrafamilial events include the birth of a baby or the youngest child getting married. Extrafamilial crisis may be precipitated by loss of a job or rape and can result in increased cohesiveness among the family members.

The following are examples of families in crisis. John, aged 20, and Sarah, aged 19, brought home their newborn infant one week ago. Jonathan is a normal, active newborn. Sarah's mother will meet her new grandchild for the first time today. John is late for work and Sarah is in tears. Jonathan is in one of his usual moods, crying. Sarah tells John, "He is not normal, he needs to be fed at least every 3 or 4 hours, and he has to be changed all the time. I thought you fed a baby breakfast, lunch, and dinner and changed them three times a day. I can never get a night's sleep." John said, "He is tough. Maybe we will get used to him after awhile."

Mable and Lee have been married 30 years. Their youngest child, a daughter, has just married. Their house no longer has children living in it. Mable is sad and cries most days. Lee says he wishes Mable would snap out of it and be a companion to him. Mable seldom cooks, no longer keeps the house looking neat and clean, and dresses in old clothes. This, too, is a family in crisis.

Situational Crises

Situational crises affecting families can occur in any developmental stage. Stressful unanticipated events that can precipitate a family crisis include the birth of a premature infant, the death of a family member, a diagnosis of serious illness, or relocation. Even events that are planned may result in a family crisis if family resources are insufficient for effective coping. Although anticipatory guidance is not always possible for family situational crises, resources are available to assist families confronted with stressful situations. People who have experienced a particular event often band together to form an organization of support for others facing the same situation. Organizations for families of retarded children, hyperactive children, cancer victims, and children lost as a result of sudden infant death syndrome have been useful in crisis intervention.

Not all families that encounter stressful events experience crises, and some families are more prone to crisis than others. Whether a crisis occurs depends on the nature of the event, the family's perception of the event, and the family's coping resources (Hill, 1965). If a family defines an event as threatening and impossible to overcome, crisis is more likely than if an event is seen as a challenge to be met. Effective communication, coalition formation, and the abil-

ity to work together toward a goal are internal resources that aid families in averting crises (Hall and Weaver, 1974). Nurses can assist families to cope by using interventions such as objective clarification of events, promoting development of internal family resources, and referring to community resources.

Events such as unemployment and natural disaster hold the potential for crisis. In recent years sudden unemployment has been experienced by many, and often by thousands in the same community. This affects not only the worker, but also all family members and family-unit functioning (Voydanoff, 1983). The unemployed person loses the role associated with a job as well as relationships with his employer and coworkers. In addition, roles at home change in regard to responsibility for household chores. A previously unemployed spouse may need to seek employment. Adolescent children may be required to alter educational plans and obtain part-time work.

A family affected by a disaster, such as a fire destroying their home, faces many adjustments. Relocation places the family in an unfamiliar residence. This is especially difficult if the family includes an infant or an elderly or disabled member. Belongings accumulated over a lifetime may be lost when a home is destroyed, and insurance may be insufficient to replace the home and lost furnishings.

An organized effort to aid families at risk of situational crises occurred in Israel during the Yom Kippur War in 1973 (Caplan, 1976). Caplan, an expert in crisis intervention, worked in Israel at the time and implemented actions of intervention for families of soldiers killed in the war. These interventions could be used in similar situations, such as the 1991 war in the Persian Gulf.

The first action Caplan took was to ensure that families were linked to significant others who could provide emotional support and assistance. This began by assembling family members in one location to inform them of the soldier's death. External support was simultaneously provided by friends, neighbors, and members of religious congregations. Nurses in the community and other health care providers monitored the status of bereaved families to identify those who needed additional attention. For most families, no additional crisis intervention was required.

Five other actions guided families that needed further assistance. The first of these was to limit aid to only those who truly needed help. This meant that careful assessment was required to identify families at greatest risk of disequilibrium from the effects of the war.

Another measure was to avoid using psychiatric labels for families struggling to cope with their loss. Families were treated and referred to as normal people under stress rather than as dysfunctional families or as people who were ill.

The third subsequent intervention was to enlist professional and nonprofessional community volunteers to act as interveners. As community members they could understand the nature of the crisis and convey sincere empathy; they were easily accessible and usually knowledgeable about available resources and services. Community health nurses were among the health professionals who provided crisis intervention.

As a fourth action, Caplan established mutual self-help

groups and support networks. By joining others that had experienced the same loss, families could mobilize energy for coping and gain group support.

The final action was to provide assistance to the supporters. People helping others to cope with crises often feel drained of their energy. Unless the supporters receive nurturing, they are prime candidates for burnout or high stress reactions. Expert consultation was made available to community health nurses and others working with bereaved families in the crisis.

As with individuals, situational and maturational crises can occur simultaneously in a family. For example, job loss at the time a family's first child is born would require adaptation to developmental and situational events. Both types of crises require involvement of all family members and additional strategies to cope successfully.

Communities and Crisis
Maturational Crises

Communities are also at risk for both maturational and situational crises through processes such as growth, expansion, and retrenchment. Growth early in the life of a community often takes place when people in the region move to a concentrated area. As a community grows, formal governmental structure is needed, as well as health care, education, safe water supply, sewage disposal, utilities, public safety, fire protection, and transportation. Unless problems resulting from growth are successfully solved, stagnation or loss of population will result. The American West is dotted with ghost towns that did not cope with developmental events.

Diversification and growth continue during expansion. A community originally established on one or two economic bases, such as manufacturing or agriculture, could expand and become a center for a variety of activities including education, medical care, trade, and industry. The diversification would bring people of different cultural backgrounds, talents, and experiences into the community. Basic services must then expand and be blended into the life of the community. During successful expansion, basic needs are met and the community is richer for the contributions of the newcomers. Crisis can arise when any basic need is not met or when there is conflict among the various segments of the population.

With retrenchment, population and economic support for basic needs are lost. Loss of population can result from movement to suburbs and/or loss of economic bases, such as industries closing. Individuals who are elderly, poor, or have few job skills are less likely to leave a community. If the needs of those remaining in a community are not met, crisis can result.

Young people predominate in growing communities; thus maternal and child services are especially needed. These services include facilities for prenatal care, well-child care, and day-care, as well as for school health and disabled children. As communities and their populations mature, there is greater need for chronic illness services and programs for the elderly.

Anticipatory preparation to avoid crisis in the growth and expansion stages of a community can include forecasting the population growth and planning and providing facilities to accommodate that growth. In retrenchment, financial support must be found to provide basic services. One example of a revenue source for such communities is a local tax on all income earned within the community. In this way people who are employed in the community but choose to live outside the area contribute to meeting the needs of the community. Communities in retrenchment as a result of the loss of an economic base often begin aggressive programs to attract new businesses and industry to the area.

By becoming active members of boards and committees charged with the responsibility for planning and providing basic services, community health nurses can make health needs known and can play a part in developing coping strategies to prevent a maturational crisis in the community. Political activity by nurses through election to public office or support of candidates for public office can also influence the development of a community.

Situational Crises

A situational crisis in a community can result from an event such as a natural disaster or the sudden influx of a large number of refugees. When these unexpected events lead to crisis, resources beyond the community are needed to successfully resolve the situation.

An example of a community disaster was the San Francisco earthquake of 1989. Langley Porter Psychiatric Hospital provided help to those in crisis (Garrison, 1990). Personnel, including nurses, staffed the hospital's crisis hot line. By telephone, they would give educational information and suggestions for self-care. For those who needed further assistance, outpatient appointments were arranged for individual or group crisis intervention. In response to the calls of approximately a dozen businesses, professional staff held group sessions for employees whose earthquake experience prevented them from returning to work. As could be expected in a crisis situation, the number of telephone calls diminished after 4 weeks.

Intervention in situational crises in communities includes mobilization of local disaster plans and assistance from governmental and voluntary agencies. Community health nurses are involved in maintaining or restoring the health of citizens affected by disaster. In shelters, they work to assist parents to care for their children, to meet the needs of the chronically ill so that complications do not occur, and to provide support or identify support systems to prevent individual and family crises. As part of the health department, the Red Cross, or voluntary organizations, community health nurses work at all levels, from making policy to rendering direct service in a community crisis.

Techniques of Crisis Intervention

Because crisis is temporary, intervention is aimed at promptly assisting the individual, family, or community to resolve the situation so that growth is achieved once equilibrium has been regained. In crisis intervention, clients need to acquire support and coping mechanisms to resolve specific situations. The following summary of crisis intervention is based on the work of several authors (Aguilera and Messick, 1990; Caplan, 1964; Schwenk and Bittle, 1979).

Crisis intervention is a short-term method focused on solving immediate problems. The usual length of a crisis with or without intervention is four to six weeks. To be effective in preventing disorganization, intervention must take place while disequilibrium is present. Unlike psychotherapeutic techniques, which are long-term and focus on the past, crisis intervention is short term, includes one to six contacts, and focuses on the present.

Crisis intervention can be used by health professionals, non-health professionals, and specially trained volunteers. Nurses, physicians, psychologists, and social workers are among the health professionals who use crisis intervention. Many non-health professionals, such as police, clergy, and teachers, are confronted with crisis situations in the course of their work. Trained volunteers in rape crisis centers and drug abuse facilities use crisis intervention skills, as do self-help groups for people who have experienced a traumatic event, such as a mastectomy or the birth of a disabled child.

Because of their educational backgrounds, acceptance by clients, and frequent encounters with individuals and families in crisis, community health nurses can be an integral part of a community's crisis intervention efforts. They may provide crisis intervention to individuals, families, and groups; participate on crisis intervention teams; and serve on committees that manage crisis programs.

To provide specific crisis intervention services, crisis teams may be formed. The composition of the team depends on the purpose of the service and the available resources. A crisis team at a drug abuse facility could consist of a psychiatrist, nurse, social worker, and rehabilitated drug abuser. Members of a team draw upon their own unique experiences as well as their crisis intervention expertise. Leadership of the team is assumed by the member who can best assist the particular client in resolving the crisis.

Community health nurses and other trained health professionals function as crisis intervention therapists. In crisis intervention, assessment of the client and the problem is the first step in the initial contact. Information is gathered regarding (1) the precipitating event, (2) resulting problem(s), (3) onset of the crisis, (4) impact of the crisis on the life of the client, (5) impact of the crisis on the life of significant others, (6) previous coping strategies, (7) strengths of the client, (8) individuals in the client's life who can provide support, and (9) risk of homicide or suicide.

Assessment of the client in crisis reveals an identifiable history. (Brownell, 1984). The individual has experienced a distressing event followed by ineffective attempts to cope. The client perceives the event as significant and his attempts to cope with the event ineffectual, and he feels helpless and anxious. The nurse explores the stressor event and its meaning to the client and the family. They review the resultant problems, as well as past attempts to deal with them and the coping mechanisms that were used. Strengths of the client and external supports are also identified.

To assess potential for suicide or homicide, direct and specific questions are asked (Aguilera and Messick, 1990). Are you considering suicide? Are you planning to kill someone else? If so, how and when? The more specific the plan and the more lethal the method, the greater the risk of suicide

(Dixon, 1979). Clients at risk of harming themselves or others are candidates not for crisis intervention but for referral for psychiatric evaluation and possible hospitalization.

With candidates for crisis intervention, information obtained during assessment is organized and presented to the client so that the relationships among the event, the problems, and the crisis are evident. This organized summary allows the client to validate the information and serves as a therapeutic technique for a person who does not recognize the relationships among the components of the crisis. To plan the intervention the problem must be broken into manageable parts.

The intervention techniques used in crisis are varied and include listening actively with concern, helping the client express feelings, exploring new ways of coping, helping the person find and use supports, and assisting him to gradually accept reality. The nurse and client set immediate goals, explore workable plans of action, and select specific actions. The client leaves the session with certain tasks to perform. In crisis intervention the therapist is an active and direct participant. For example, the therapist may contact community agencies that require referral from a health professional. However, the resolution of the crisis ultimately rests with the client. In crisis intervention the assessment remains focused on the crisis situation. As in other community health nursing interactions, the client is an active participant in planning, intervention, and evaluation.

In the first contact it is important to focus on the crisis. The therapist and client should be aware that crisis intervention lasts at most only a few weeks. For some clients, one contact provides the assistance necessary to resolve the problem. In future contacts, progress in using new coping methods and meeting goals is reviewed, and the therapist reinforces the client's success. Other aspects of the crisis problem are explored in manageable parts, and ways of coping are considered. Throughout crisis intervention, individuals and/or groups who can provide support are identified and mobilized. The length and frequency of client contacts with the therapist depend on the nature of the crisis but usually range from one to six contacts.

In the final interview, the client's achievements are reinforced by summarizing the new strategies that were attempted—successful and unsuccessful—and the progress that was made. To help the individual maintain the achieved level of function, realistic plans for the future are discussed. The client who achieves resolution of a crisis at an improved level of function has experienced growth and gained coping mechanisms that can prevent a crisis in the future.

The process of crisis intervention parallels the nursing process of assessment, diagnosis, planning, intervention, and evaluation. Steps in crisis intervention are shown in the box on p. 628.

Crisis intervention may be provided in individual, family, or group settings, depending on the need of the client and the availability of services. One example of group intervention following a community disaster with crisis potential is seen in the efforts of a Washington, D.C. area Health Maintenance Organization (HMO) after a Hanafi Muslim sect seized and held hostages for more than a day and a half (Sank, 1979). Mental health professionals from the HMO

THE FIVE STEPS OF CRISIS INTERVENTION

ASSESS

Clarify precipitating event
Explore meaning of event to the client
Identify problems
Identify present and past coping strategies
Identify resources

DIAGNOSE

Clearly define the problems
Label the problems

PLAN

Separate problems into manageable parts
Explore alternative coping methods
Set goals
Define specific tasks to meet goals

INTERVENE

Formulate an objective statement of the situation
Carry out tasks to meet goals
Mobilize resources

EVALUATE

Appraise progress toward goals
Evaluate the success of coping methods used
Reinforce the progress made

---

offered the released hostages eight group sessions that began four days after the ordeal. During the group sessions the former hostages discussed their perceptions of the event, their feelings while being held hostage, resultant problems since their release, and methods of coping with those problems. The aims of the intervention were to provide support for the ex-hostages and to assist them in developing the coping skills necessary to deal with problems resulting from the traumatic event.

Three aspects of crisis increase the possibility of favorable resolution through crisis intervention (Caplan, 1964). First, the outcome of the crisis is most often determined by factors occurring during the crisis, not by the client's past experiences or the nature of the events leading to the crisis. Developing new ways of coping and mobilizing support can provide internal and external factors that favor a successful outcome. Second, the client in crisis has an increased desire for help and is more likely to seek and accept crisis intervention. Third, clients in crisis are more open to influence by others than they are in periods of equilibrium. Therapists skilled in crisis intervention have a unique opportunity to influence crisis outcome.

Primary, Secondary, and Tertiary Prevention in Crisis Intervention

Just as community health nurses work to prevent disease and injury, they also work to prevent crisis. Primary prevention is the attempt to avert crisis in stressful maturational and situational circumstances. Secondary prevention entails identifying people in crisis early and initiating intervention promptly in order to effect successful resolution. Tertiary prevention consists of rehabilitation by mental health specialists when resolution of a crisis has resulted in a level of function that is lower than the pre-crisis level and that is accompanied by major disorganization.

Community Resources

The nature and scope of crisis resources in a community depend on the size of the community, the crisis needs, and the available interest and expertise. The community health nurse in a rural community may be the only available health care professional but need not be the only resource. Other professionals such as ministers, cooperative extension agents, or locally based home economists employed by the state university may provide primary and secondary prevention. For example, the cooperative extension agent works on a daily basis with homemakers and has an educational background that includes knowledge of individual and family development. Parenting classes and groups to discuss transitions in family life are examples of activities that may be conducted by cooperative extension agencies. When organizing crisis resources in a rural community, the community health nurse should consider both professionals and volunteers.

In larger communities, resources for crisis include both official and voluntary agencies. The health department and mental health center are two agencies that may offer programs of primary and secondary prevention for individuals and families. In health departments, community health nurses participate in assessing needs for crisis services and diagnosing specific areas for intervention as well as planning, conducting the interventions and evaluating the actions. Mental health centers and private psychiatric facilities offer assistance to clients who experience decreased levels of function accompanied by disorganization following crisis resolution.

Voluntary agencies in a community are concerned with a wide variety of conditions including drug abuse, birth defects, mental retardation, child abuse, and rape. Services provided by these agencies range from distributing information to sponsoring support groups to offering crisis intervention. In some communities, traditional agencies are expanding the scope of services to include crisis assistance. For example, some Young Women's Christian Associations (YWCAs) offer help to battered women. Religious institutions may also offer programs of primary prevention. Community health nurses have opportunities to support voluntary crisis efforts by joining the organization, serving as consultants, accepting board positions, and providing direct services.

Those with serious mental illnesses can also experience crisis (Stroul, 1988). One community facility for assisting these people is residential crisis housing. In a small network or single-home setting, the seriously mentally ill are given support and protection.

At the very least, community health nurses provide primary prevention services and are familiar with the resources for secondary and tertiary crisis prevention. For effective referral to a community resource, the community health nurse must know the specific services of the agency, eligibility requirements for clients, and the procedures for obtaining services. If the community health nurse does not provide crisis intervention, prompt and appropriate referral of clients in crisis is needed.

CLINICAL APPLICATION

The following example illustrates secondary crisis intervention by a community health nurse. A summary of the nursing process used in this situation follows the example.

Susan Jones, a community health nurse employed by a county health department, had been assigned several new clients. Among them was 23-year-old Betty Steward, an unmarried mother of a 4-year-old girl and pregnant for the second time. A review of Betty's record revealed that she was in her thirty-ninth week of pregnancy and had missed her clinic visit the previous week. A home visit was planned. On arriving at the home, Susan was greeted by a young woman with uncombed hair and a rumpled housecoat; she was obviously not pregnant. Betty said she had delivered twin boys 3 days earlier, and she and her sons had arrived home that day. Betty's daughter, Karen, was at home and eager to show her brothers to the nurse. Susan's examinations of Betty and the infants revealed no physical problems. As Susan talked with Betty, she noted Betty's slow movements and sad expression. Susan told Betty she looked sad and asked if there was a problem. Betty began to cry and said that throughout the pregnancy she had planned to give the new infant up for adoption; but when the twins were born she thought they were "special" and changed her mind. Now she was uncertain of her decision and felt overwhelmed.

Although Betty's only income had been child support from Karen's father, she felt that Karen needed her at home during the preschool years and was unemployed at the time of pregnancy. However, she had looked forward to the time when Karen would enter school. Betty would then get a job, and their situation could improve. Keeping the infants meant loss of a goal. In addition, she expressed concern about her ability to provide for the infants. Since she had not expected to keep the infants, she had no care items. The only formula was the take-home package from the hospital, and there was little food in the house. Betty repeatedly said she needed to decide whether or not to keep the twins. Susan inquired about individuals in Betty's life who had helped her to make decisions in the past. She responded that she had neither family nor friends with whom she could discuss the situation. Her minister, however, was a person she trusted and who had helped previously.

The plan developed by Susan and Betty was for Betty to contact her minister and meet with him. Susan was to contact a community agency to arrange for emergency formula, supplies for the infants, and food for Betty and Karen. If Betty decided to keep the infants, further plans would be made on the next visit. They agreed that Susan would return in 2 days; if Betty needed her before then, she would call.

On Susan's next visit Betty was smiling and said that after talking with her minister she had made a final decision and would keep the twins. Her biggest problem was how she would provide for them because she did not want to get a job and leave them. Susan informed Betty about Aid to

Families with Dependent Children and told her how to go about contacting a social worker. Susan was to call the social worker so that he would expect Betty's call, and Betty would arrange for an appointment. The next visit was scheduled for a week later.

By the next visit, Betty had seen the social worker and arrangements had been made for interim assistance and ongoing assistance. Betty's present concern was providing a suitable environment for the children. When asked what kind of place she would like, her response was a clean place that did not have roaches and mice, which were her main objections to the present house. They discussed options for the problem, and the decision was that Betty would contact the landlord and request that he have the pests exterminated. Because Betty had little experience taking assertive action with someone she considered an authority figure, they role-played the contact with the landlord. The next visit was scheduled for 3 weeks later.

At the next visit Betty, neatly dressed, met Susan at the door and began to tell her about the telephone call to the landlord. She related that she had been firm in her request for extermination services and, as a result, the landlord agreed. She proudly showed Susan the twins and her cleaner house. Susan commended Betty for the progress she had made and spoke of her recent achievements. Although life with her daughter and the infants was not without problems, Betty was successfully coping with the situation. As a result of her contact with her minister, members of the congregation had come to visit, and Betty talked of her plans to participate in church activities. With the present situation resolved, they agreed upon routine health care plans for the family, and Betty was to contact Susan if assistance was needed in the future.

The steps in the nursing process—assessment, nursing diagnosis, planning, intervention, and evaluation—are reviewed here in relation to the previous example. The first step in the nursing process is assessment, and Susan began assessment of the Steward family by checking the biophysical status of the mother and infants. Assessment of the emotional status revealed problems subsequent to the birth of twins. Further assessment revealed lack of coping strategies and loss of a life goal, leading to a diagnosis of crisis. There was no evidence that Betty was suicidal or would have harmed others. Using crisis intervention, the remainder of the first visit focused on the problems associated with the crisis. Assessment included identification of individuals who could be of support, and this revealed Betty's relationship with the minister.

Plans were jointly developed by Susan and Betty, with priorities established so that problems of greatest importance were dealt with first. Consistent with crisis intervention, problems were considered in manageable parts. Implementation of the plans involved active participation by the nurse and client and allowed Betty to develop new coping skills; the role-playing to prepare Betty for the contact with her landlord was an example. In the last contact, Betty's successful efforts and achievements were reviewed and reinforced, and plans for the future were discussed.

Throughout the crisis period, reassessment, client participation in planning, intervention, and evaluation occurred. The last visit reviewed progress and future plans.

In this case study the client successfully resolved the problems resulting from the birth of the twins and developed new coping strategies.

SUMMARY

Stress can cause considerable mental and physical wear and tear. People respond to stress differently based on their own needs and resources for adapting to changing life events. Stress is manifested in a variety of ways: physically, behaviorally, and emotionally. Each person tends to develop a unique way of handling stress. The magnitude of the stress response to changes in life events and expectations can be minimized by a variety of stress management techniques including relaxation, creative imagery, use of support networks, exercise, diet, and assertive behavior. Community health nurses can play a vital role in teaching stress-reduction techniques.

In contrast to stress, crisis is an upset in a steady state of functioning: a disequilibrium resulting from problems that follow an event of significance to the person and for which coping skills are inadequate. With crisis there is the opportunity for growth and the achievement of a higher level of psychological functioning if successful resolution occurs; and, on the other hand, the possibility of a decreased level of psychological functioning and disorganization if resolution is unsuccessful. Community health nurses can participate in assessment, diagnosis, planning, intervention, and evaluation of crisis events and services for individuals, families and communities. Community health nurses may provide direct interventions or refer people in crisis to agencies that can more effectively meet their needs.

KEY CONCEPTS

Stress and its effects on health and well-being are key areas of concern for community health nurses.

Stress is often present and influences the ability to cope, adapt, and lead a productive life; thus the nature of stress, stressors, the stress response, levels of stress, and sources of stress have implications for community health nurses.

Stress is directly or indirectly related to many illnesses.

People respond differently to stress depending on their past experiences, the predicability and rapidity of the onset of stress, the context in which it occurs, and the degree of control they have.

In tolerable levels, stress is a motivator.

Assertiveness is a skill that nurses can use and teach their clients for assistance in stress management.

Aggressive behavior, unlike assertiveness, occurs when people infringe on the rights of others while standing up for their own rights.

Changing one's thoughts and attitudes is an essential part of stress management.

One of the most effective ways of coping with stress is by seeking support from members of a caring family, social, or work group.

Progressive relaxation provides a way of reducing stress by altering the relation between muscle and psychological tension.

Burnout is one negative consequence of excessive job-related stress.

The role of the community health nurse in stress reduction deals with individuals, families, groups, and entire communities.

An essential property of crisis is the potential for promoting growth. Assisting people in crises is a part of the community health nursing role.

People in crisis feel helpless and often desire assistance in relieving their misery.

Crises may be maturational or situational. Maturational, or developmental, crises occur during natural transitions in the developmental process.

Unlike maturational crises, situational crises are often sudden and unexpected and require more emotional reserves for effective coping.

Because a crisis is a temporary state of being upset and in disequilibrium, the aim of intervention is to promptly assist the person, family, or community to resolve the situation so that growth can occur when equilibrium is reestablished.

Crisis resources in a community depend on the size of the community, crisis needs, and the expertise of the people involved.

LEARNING ACTIVITIES

1. Ask three people other than fellow nursing students or faculty how they would define stress. Ask each to describe the last time a stressful event occurred and what was done to resolve the situation.

2. For two weeks, keep a log of the stressors that affect you. List what worked to resolve the stress and also what you tried that was less successful.

3. Drive through your community and identify at least five sources of biophysiological-chemical stress.

4. For a week, observe the behavior of at least two people with whom you have frequent contact, such as a classmate or family member. Note whether the person's responses to others were assertive, aggressive, or passive. Identify if the results were positive or negative. If negative, what other alternatives existed?

5. Recall a crisis situation. If no real crisis can be recalled, think about situations from books, television, or other media. Put yourself in the place of the person most directly involved and describe how that person perceived the event; identify the person's coping strengths; and describe what worked or did not work to resolve the crisis.

6. In your community, identify two programs that offer anticipatory guidance for maturational crises or programs that are currently unavailable but could be instituted.

7. Using a newspaper account of a crisis, identify what the role of the community health nurse would be with the individual, group, or community.

BIBLIOGRAPHY

Achterberg J and Lawlis F: Bridges of the body-mind; behavioral approaches to health care, Champaign, Ill, 1980, Institute for Personality and Ability Testing.

Adams JD: Understanding and managing stress: a workbook in changing life styles, San Diego, Calif, 1980, University Associates.

Aguilera D and Messick J: Crisis intervention theory and methodology, ed 5, St. Louis, 1990, Mosby-Year Book, Inc.

Bachrach KM and Zautra AJ: Coping with a community stressor: the threat of a hazardous waste facility, J Health Soc Behav 26(2):127-141, 1985.

Baugh C: Practical ways to assert yourself, Nursing 89 19(3):57, 1989.

Bond M: Understanding assertiveness, Nurs Times 84(9):61, 1988a.

Bond M: Saying no assertively, Nurs Times 84(14):63, 1988(b).

Brallier LW: Successfully managing stress, Los Altos, Calif, 1982, National Nursing Review.

Brownell MJ: The concept of crisis; its utility for nursing, ANS 6:10, 1984.

Bruhn JG: The novelty of stress, Southern Med J 80:1398-1406, 1987(11).

Bunch D: Are you ready to explode? Burnout may make you feel that way, AAR Times 7:21-24, 1983.

Caplan G: Principles of preventive psychiatry, New York, 1964, Basic Books, Inc, Publishers.

Caplan G: Organization of support systems for civilian populations. In Caplan G and Killilea M editors: Support systems and mutual help: multidisciplinary explorations, New York, 1976, Grune & Stratton, Inc.

Cornell D: How to talk back without raising your voice, RN 48(3):13, 1985.

Christensen S and Harding M: Integrating theories of crisis intervention into hospice home care teaching, Nurs Clin North Am 20:499, 1985.

Cobb S and Lindemann E: Neuropsychiatric observations after the Coconut Grove fire. In Lindemann E, editor: Beyond grief, New York, 1979, Jason Aronson.

Dainow S: Assertiveness: believe in yourself, Int Nurs Rev 33:171-177, 1986 (6).

Dixon S: Working with people in crisis, St. Louis, 1979, The CV Mosby Co.

Donnelly GF: Why you just can't take it anymore! . . . coping, RN 43:34-37, 1980a.

Duvall EM and Miller BC: Marriage and family development, ed 6, New York, 1985, Harper & Row, Publishers, Inc.

Erikson E: Childhood and society, New York, 1950, WW Norton & Co.

Garrison S: Telephone interview, San Francisco, CA, 1990.

Hall J and Weaver B, editors: Nursing of families in crisis, Philadelphia, 1974, JB Lippincott Co.

Hill R: Generic features of families under stress. In Parad H, editor: Crisis intervention: selected readings, New York, 1965, Family Service Association of America.

Jacobson E: Progressive relaxation: a physiological and clinical investigation of muscular states and their significance in psychology and medical practice, ed 3, Chicago, 1974, University of Chicago Press.

Kneisl CR: Stress management. In Wilson HS and Kneisl CR, editors: Psychiatric Nursing, ed 3, Menlo Park, CA, 1988, Addison-Wesley Publishing Co. p. 763.

Lawler TG and Yount EH: Managing crisis effectively: An intervention model, JONA 17(11), 39-43, 1987.

Lindemann E: Symptomatology and management of acute grief. In Lindemann E, editor: Beyond grief, New York, 1979, Jason Aronson.

Montgomery CL: Battling the awfulist, absolutist "shoulds", Am J Nurs 87(6):859, 1987.

Moynihan MM and Hayes ER: Combined developmental-situational events: a theoretical model for nursing practice and research. In Infante MS, editor: Crisis theory: a framework for nursing practice, Reston, Va, 1982, Reston Publishing Co., Inc.

Palmer ME and Deck ES: Teaching your patients to assert themselves, Am J Nurs 87(5):650, 1987.

Petosa R: Eustress and mental health promotion, Health Values 93:7, 1985.

Pollock SE: the hardiness characteristic: A motivating factor in adaptation, Adv Nurs Sci 11(2):53, 1989.

Rahe RH: Life change and illness studies: past history and future directions, J Human Stress 4:3-16, 1978.

Rapoport L: The state of crisis: some theoretical considerations. In Parad H, editor: Crisis intervention: selected readings, New York, 1965, Family Service Association of America.

Richter JM and Sloan R: Stress: a relaxation response, Am J Nurs 79:1960-1964, 1979.

Rosswurm MA: Relocation and the elderly, J Gerontol Nurs 9(12):632, 1983.

Sank LI: Psychology in action: Community disasters, Am Psychol 34:334, 1979.

Schwenk TL and Bittle SP: Applicability of crisis intervention in family practice, J Fam Pract 8:1151, 1979.

Selye H: Stress without distress, Philadelphia, 1974, JB Lippincott Co.

Selye H: The stress of life, ed revised, New York, 1978, McGraw-Hill Book Co.

Simonton CO, Simonton S and Creighton J: Getting well again: a step by step self help guide to overcoming cancer for patients and their families, Los Angeles, 1978, JP Tarcher, Inc. (Distributed by St. Martin's Press, Inc, New York.)

Smitherman C: Nursing actions for health promotion, Philadelphia, 1981, FA Davis Co.

Spradley BW: Community health nursing: concepts and practice, ed 3, Glenview, Illinois, 1990, Scott Foresman/Little Brown, & Co.

Stroul BS: Residential crisis services: a review, Hospital Community Psychiatry 39(10):1095-99, 1988.

Sutterly DC: Stress management: grazing the clinical turf, Holistic Nursing Practice 1:36-53, 1986.

Underwood MM and Fiedler N: The crisis of rape: a community response, Community Ment Health J 19:227-230, 1983.

Voydanoff P: Unemployment: family strategies for adaption. In Figley CR and Cubbin HI, editors: Stress and the family, vol 2, New York, 1983, Brunner/Mazel, Inc.

Wolpe J: The practice of behavior therapy, 1969, Pergamon Press.

PART SEVEN

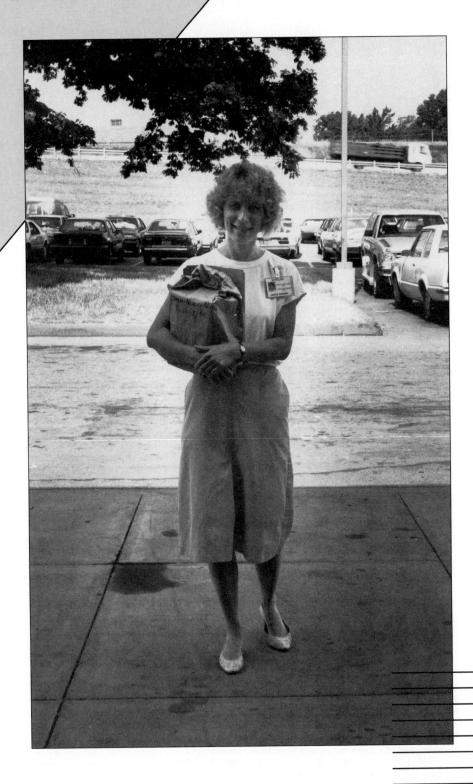

Diversity in the Community Health Nursing Role

At one time the role of the community health nurse primarily included visiting clients at home and identifying cases of communicable disease; over the decades the role has become multi-faceted. As the health care delivery system has changed and the field of public health has expanded, nursing education has evolved to embrace many levels of preparation. Through these levels of education, nursing practic᠎ has expanded to include preparing nurses to function in a variety of clinical speciaɩty areas. In addition, nurses are prepared to function as personnel managers, educators, consultants, and case managers. As a result of their level of education, community health nurses find that a variety of clients comprise their case load including individuals, families, groups, and communities.

With increasing emphasis being placed on the community client, community health nurses recognize that in order to address community health issues the nurse must be able to meet the needs of the individuals, families, and groups who are the nucleus of the community. Unlike the past, when the primary practice setting for the nurse was the hospital or public health agency, nurses find their clients in multiple practice settings. Regardless of type of client, practice setting, specialty area of practice, or the functional role the nurse may be filling, the community health nurse acts as advocate for clients in meeting their needs through the health care system.

This section offers discussions of the functional roles of personnel manager, consultant, and case manager, with specific emphasis on the development of the advocacy role in community health practice. Throughout the text, content is applicable to a variety of practice settings, including the more traditional public health practice arena such as the health department. Aside from the official agencies, a few multiple practice settings with the closest association to community health nursing have been chosen for presentation (e.g., school health, occupational health, home health, and primary health care settings).

Finally, as community health has become a recognized clinical specialty in nursing, the roles of community health clinical nurse specialist and family nurse practitioner have evolved in recognition of the diversity and expansion of knowledge in this field of practice. In addition to being direct care givers, these nurses provide leadership and direction and serve as facilitators to clients as they provide primary preventive and other health care services.

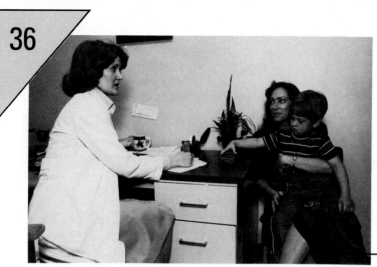

36

The Community Health Nurse Clinician and Family Nurse Practitioner in Primary and Ambulatory Care

Cynthia S. Selleck

Ann T. Sirles

Rebecca H. Sloan

OBJECTIVES

After reading this chapter, the student should be able to:

Briefly discuss the historical development of the roles of the clinical nurse specialist and nurse practitioner.

Describe the educational requirements for the community health clinical nurse specialist and family nurse practitioner.

Discuss the four credentialing mechanisms in nursing as they relate to the role of the clinical nurse specialist and family nurse practitioner.

Compare and contrast the various role functions of the community health clinical nurse specialist and family nurse practitioner.

Identify potential arenas of practice for the clinical nurse specialist and family nurse practitioner.

Explore current issues and concerns relative to the practice of the community health clinical nurse specialist and family nurse practitioner.

Identify five stressors that may affect community health nurses in expanded roles.

KEY TERMS

administrator
block nursing
certification
clinical nurse specialist
  (CNS)
clinician
collaborative practice
consultant
educator

family nurse
  practitioner (FNP)
health maintenance
  organization
independent practice
Indian Health Service
institutional privileges
joint practice
liability
National Health
  Service Corps

nurse practitioner (NP)
parrish nursing
prescriptive authority
professional isolation
protocols
researcher
satellite clinics
third-party
  reimbursement

Social changes and changes in health problems over the past century have redefined the pattern of health care in this country. One result of these changes was the introduction of primary care. Although there have been many definitions of primary care, the American Nurses Association (ANA, 1985) defines it as "continuous and comprehensive care, including all the services necessary for health promotion, prevention of disease and disability, health maintenance, and in some cases rehabilitation." Primary care is comprehensive, coordinated, and continuous, and it requires collaboration among many health professions (ANA, 1985).

The philosophy of primary care is similar to that of primary nursing, which has become a popular method for delivering nursing care to clients in a variety of settings, particularly the hospital. The primary care system includes all types of ambulatory care that begins when the client requests health care from a provider in a clinic or office setting within a community. The client contributes to and receives care, and the provider is not only available, but has authority, autonomy, and accountability.

In 1980, Andrus and Mitchell reported that 25% of physicians in the United States practiced in primary care. By 1982 the percentage of physicians in primary care had risen to 40% (American Medical Association, 1984). A growing population, increasing health care costs, and consumer demand for more health-related services prompted the belief that one profession alone could not provide primary care for the health and illness needs of the population (Davidson and Lauver, 1984). It was predicted that by 1990 the United States would experience an oversupply of physicians and that there would no longer be a need for nurses to provide primary care services. Although the total number of physicians has increased, the need for nurses specializing in primary or ambulatory care has also increased. By expanding their existing skills, nurses are uniquely qualified to plan and provide primary care, using other care providers as consultants.

This chapter provides historical perspectives on the educational preparation of the community health clinical nurse specialist (CNS) and family nurse practitioner (FNP) in primary and ambulatory care. Functions in advanced practice and arenas for practice are discussed. Issues and concerns, role negotiation, and areas of role stress relative to the community health CNS and FNP are also discussed.

HISTORICAL PERSPECTIVE

Changes in the health care system and nursing have occurred in the past few decades because of a shift in societal demands and needs. Trends that have influenced the new roles of the CNS and NP include improvements in technology, self-care, cost-containment measures, accountability to the client, third-party reimbursement, and demands for humanizing technical care.

The CNS role began in the early 1960s and grew out of a need to improve patient care. CNSs educate patients and their families, provide social and psychological support to patients, serve as role models to nursing staff, consult with nurses and staff in other disciplines, and conduct clinical nursing research (Elder and Bullough, 1990). Although

CNSs were making strides in advanced nursing practice before the introduction of NPs, the NP movement hastened the development of the CNS role and provided credibility for advanced practice (Kitzman, 1989).

In the United States during the 1960s, a shortage of physicians occurred, and there was an increasing tendency among physicians to specialize. The number of physicians who might have provided medical care to communities and families across the nation was thus reduced. As this trend continued, a serious gap in primary care services developed (Bullough, 1980).

Demographic factors also influenced the evolution of nonphysician providers. Although the number of medical personnel in primary care was decreasing, the population was increasing. The lower socioeconomic groups in the inner cities and rural areas were most affected by these changes. Additionally, the median age of the population was steadily rising, resulting in a higher proportion of aged persons; the aged often suffer from chronic disease or the infirmities of old age, and this is complicated by dwindling financial resources and other social problems. Access to primary care for these two groups is a nationally recognized problem.

The NP movement was begun in 1965 at the University of Colorado by Dr. Henry Silver and Dr. Loretta Ford. They determined that the morbidity among medically deprived children could be decreased by educating community health nurses to provide well-child care to children of all ages. Nursing practice for these pediatric nurse practitioners included the identification, assessment, and management of common acute and chronic conditions, with appropriate referral of more complex problems (Silver, Ford, and Stearly, 1967). As a profession, nursing's priorities have traditionally been to care for and support the well, the worried well, and the ill, in both physiological and psychological terms. Nurse practitioners could offer health-focused care, psychological support, and physical care services previously provided only by physicians. Preparing nurses as primary care providers was not only consistent with traditional nursing but also responsive to society's critical need for primary health care services, including health promotion and illness prevention (Davidson and Lauver, 1984; Kozlowski, 1990).

The physician assistant (PA) role was initiated at Duke University in 1965. This program was intended to attract ex-military corpsmen for training as medical extenders (Fisher and Horowitz, 1977). Nurse practitioners are often combined into a single category with other nonphysician providers and are erroneously portrayed as physician extenders. This misinterpretation of the intended role is addressed by one of the movement's founders, Dr. Loretta Ford (1986).

As conceptualized, the nurse practitioner was always a nursing model focused on the promotion of health in daily living, growth and development for children in families as well as the prevention of disease and disability. It evolved from such societal needs and opportunities as nursing's development as a discipline and a profession, not because there was a shortage of physicians. Nor did our early plans include preparing nurses to assume medical functions. Our interests were in health and prevention for aggregate populations in community settings including underserved groups. These were the hallmarks of community health nursing.

These innovative programs, directed at resolving the problems of physician shortage and access to primary care for rural and other medically underserved populations, attracted the interest of the federal govenment. A report issued by the Department of Health, Education, and Welfare, *Extending the Scope of Nursing Practice* (1971), helped convince Congress of the value of NPs as primary care providers. The Nurse Training Act of 1971 (PL 92-150) and the comprehensive Health Manpower Act of 1971 (PL 92-157) provided educational funding for many NP and PA programs through the 1970s and into the 1980s. When the market for medical specialties was saturated and the costs of hospital-based health care reached critical levels, primary care began attracting greater numbers of physicians. Competition among physicians in primary care is increasingly evident today.

The NP movement has created several types of NPs. Currently in the United States there are programs preparing family nurse practitioners (FNP), adult nurse practitioners (ANP), pediatric nurse practitioners (PNP), school nurse practitioners (SNP), geriatric nurse practitioners (GNP), obstetric and gynecologic nurse practitioners (OGNP), family planning nurse practitioners (FPNP), emergency nurse practitioners (ENP), and nurse midwives (NM). While the FNP is a specialist in providing primary care to individuals and families throughout the life span, NPs from other programs are specialists in providing primary care to select groups of individuals.

EDUCATION

Educational preparation for the community health CNS includes a master's degree with study of scientific content as well as advanced clinical practice in the nursing specialty of community health nursing. In addition to performing the functions of the generalist in community health nursing, specialists possess "substantial clinical experience with families and groups; expertise in the formulation of health and social policy and the assessment of the health of a community or population; and proficiency in planning, implementation, and evaluation of population-focused programs" (ANA, 1986). The community health CNS's skills are based on knowledge of epidemiology, demography, biometry, community structure and organization, community development, management, program evaluation, and policy development. In addition, CNSs in community health nursing are involved in research, theory testing, theory development relative to their specialty areas, and health policy development (ANA, 1986).

In contrast to the CNS, educational preparation of the NP has not always been at the graduate level. Early NP programs were continuing education certificate programs, and the baccalaureate degree was not always a requirement. The recent trend, however, has been toward graduate education for NPs. More than 80% of NP programs are now at the master's level, with only a few certificate programs still operating (Geolot, 1987).

The objectives of NP programs are to teach nurses to (1) assess normalcy, health deviations, and health risks; (2) provide anticipatory guidance, counseling about health maintenance, and disease prevention; (3) develop and implement therapeutic plans for selected health problems and clients; and (4) consult with and refer to other disciplines and collaborate with nurses in community agencies for client care that represents special needs or is beyond the NP's expertise (Davidson and Lauver, 1984). In addition, graduate programs also prepare NPs to assume the indirect nursing care roles of educator, administrator, researcher, and consultant (ANA, 1987).

CREDENTIALS

The academic degree and accreditation are important to the community health CNS and FNP; however, licensure and certification affect their practice most directly. Certification examinations for these nurses are offered by the ANA through the Division of Community Health Nursing. The purpose of professional certification is to confirm knowledge and expertise and provide recognition of professional achievement in a defined area of nursing. Certification is a means of assuring the public that nurses who claim competence at a certain level have had their credentials professionally verified (ANA, 1985). Although certification itself is not mandatory, several state boards of nursing require that nurses in advanced practice, particularly those in an NP role, be nationally certified as a prerequisite to practice.

The ANA began its certification program in 1973 and has offered NP certification examinations since 1974. The FNP examination was first offered in 1976. Since 1985 the basic qualifications for certification as an FNP have been a baccalaureate degree in nursing and successful completion of a formal FNP program. Beginning in 1992, a master's or higher degree in nursing is required for all NP exams.

Family nurse practitioners make up the largest group of NPs certified through the ANA, and since 1982 the percentage of NPs seeking FNP certification has been consistently higher than that for other NP certification exams (Knutson, 1989; Wilbur et al., 1990). As of August 1989, 5595 FNPs had been certified through the ANA.

Although the ANA has offered specialist certification since 1976, the first certification exam for clinical nurse specialists in community health nursing was not offered until October 1990. Qualifications for this examination include a master's or higher degree in nursing with a specialization in community/public health nursing practice or a baccalaureate degree in nursing and a master's or higher degree in public health. The second option is available only through the 1993 test administration. The applicant must also meet a practice requirement of an average of 12 hours per week and a minimum of 1400 hours in the specialty since receiving the master's degree.

Certification for the community health CNS and FNP is for 5 years. To maintain certification, the nurse must submit documentation of current RN licensure and meet a practice and continuing education requirement within the specialty area.

THE ADVANCED PRACTICE ROLE

Master's degree programs in community health nursing may prepare CNSs or FNPs. Debate on the similarities and differences in these two roles has taken place over the past decade. The roles are merging and many common features exist, but there are still important differences in role functions in community health nursing.

Clinician

Most differences between the roles of the community health CNS and FNP are seen in clinical practice. Although the CNS's practice includes nursing directed at individuals, families, and groups, the primary responsibility is promoting and maintaining the health of a population as a whole (ANA, 1986). The CNS's primary "client" is the community or an aggregate of the community, and the goal is to reduce the amounts of disease, premature death, discomfort, and disability within that community or population (ANA, 1986). Practicing within the role of clinician, the community health CNS is involved in conducting community assessments; identifying needs of populations at risk; and planning, implementing, and evaluating population-based programs to achieve health goals.

The FNP uses physical, psychosocial, and environmental assessment skills to manage common health and illness problems of clients of all ages and both sexes. The FNP's primary "client" is the individual and family. In the direct role of clinician, the FNP assesses health risks and health and illness status, as well as the response to illness of individuals and families. The FNP also diagnoses actual or potential health problems; decides on treatment plans jointly with clients; intervenes to promote health, protect against disease, treat illness, manage chronic disease, and limit disability; and evaluates with the client and other primary health care team members the effectiveness, comprehensiveness, and continuity of the intervention (ANA, 1985).

The ability of FNPs to diagnose and treat has increased the provision of primary care, teaching, and compliance. Although physician input may be necessary at times, the nurse can usually carry out the treatment regimen and establish the relationship of primary care giver. Frequently, the FNP will use protocols or algorithms that have been previously agreed upon by the physician and FNP. These documents serve as standing orders for the management of certain illnesses. Protocols allow the FNP to diagnose and treat client problems and are required by some states to regulate NP practice.

The primary health care team may consist of a variety of members who usually have specialized and complementary skills that strengthen the team. Adding nurses to the health care team increases the diversity and quality of primary care services. The use is cost effective when the needs of the client and community are matched with the provider who can best meet those needs. Community health CNSs and FNPs practice as colleagues with physicians and other health care providers, and they must develop strategies for effectively combining their expertise.

Within the past several decades there has been a growing belief that the most effective way of dealing with major health problems is through prevention. This requires refocusing the health care system, teaching people that they control their own health, and encouraging health promotion and health maintenance behaviors. It has been predicted that there will be an even greater emphasis on community-based care and that nursing will be increasingly viewed as the key to addressing many of the health care problems that plague society in the 1990s (Maraldo, 1990). Clients will become actively involved in self-care and will be more conscious of the cost and quality of the health care services they receive.

Educator

Nurses in advanced practice function in several indirect nursing care roles. The educator role of the community health CNS and FNP includes client education and professional nursing education.

As the population grows more conscious of health and fitness, educating clients and the community about good health habits becomes increasingly important. The CNS identifies areas of educational need within the community and assists with teaching new knowledge. The CNS and FNP enhance wellness and contribute to health maintenance and promotion by teaching the importance of good nutrition, physical exercise, stress management, and a healthy lifestyle. They provide education about disease processes and the importance of following treatment regimens. In addition, they provide anticipatory guidance and educate clients on the use of medications, diet, birth control methods, and other therapeutic procedures. They also counsel clients, families, and the community on the importance of assuming responsibility for their health. Frequently nurses in advanced practice are resources for educating community groups and organizations on different aspects of health and self-care.

As professional nurse educators, the CNS and FNP provide formal and informal teaching of staff nurses and undergraduate and graduate students in nursing and other disciplines. They also serve as role models by instructing students in advanced practice in the clinical setting.

Administrator

The community health CNS and FNP may function in administrative roles. As health administrators, they may assume the responsibility for all administrative matters within the setting. They may be responsible for and have direct or indirect authority and supervision over the organization's staff and client care. In this capacity, nurses in advanced practice in community health nursing serve as decision makers and problem solvers. They may also be involved in other business and management aspects such as supporting and managing personnel; budgeting; establishing quality control mechanisms; and influencing policies, public relations, and marketing (ANA, 1985; Felton et al., 1985).

Consultant

Consultation is an integral part of practice for the community health CNS and FNP. Consultation involves problem solving with an individual, family, or community to improve health care delivery. Steps of the consultation process include assessing the problem, determining the availability and feasibility of resources, proposing solutions, and assisting with implementation, if appropriate (ANA, 1985).

The CNS and FNP may serve as formal or informal consultants to other nurses, providing them with information on improving client care. They may also consult with physicians and other health care providers or with organizations or schools. The exchange of professional expertise among colleagues should be encouraged. It is especially important for nurses in advanced practice to make their contributions known to other members of the primary health care team.

Researcher

Improvement in nursing practice depends on the commitment of nurses to developing and refining knowledge through research (ANA, 1986). Practicing CNSs and FNPs are in ideal positions to identify researchable nursing problems. They can use research findings and apply them to the community health practice setting.

In *Characteristics of Master's Education in Nursing* (1987), the National League for Nursing stated that graduate programs in nursing should prepare students to identify researchable nursing problems and participate in research studies in advanced nursing practice. All CNSs and most FNPs are trained in the research process and can conduct their own investigations, answering questions relevant to nursing practice and primary care. Identifying, defining, and investigating clinical nursing problems and reporting findings foster collegial relationships with other professions and contribute to health care policy and decision making.

Publishing clinical research findings is beginning to be a priority of practicing nurses. Molde and Diers (1985) suggested that future research be theory-based, involving prudent clinical insight and meticulous design. They also suggested that clinical research holds the greatest promise for advancing the work of NPs.

ARENAS FOR PRACTICE

The market for FNPs has continued to expand. Organized health care settings such as Health Maintenance Organizations (HMOs), outpatient clinics, and private practice settings have evidenced an increased need for nurse practitioners (Shanks-Meile et al., 1989). Positions for FNPs may vary greatly in terms of scope of practice, degree of responsibility, power and authority, working conditions, creativity, and reward structure (Edmunds, 1983). These factors and their effect on practice are influenced by Nurse Practice Acts and other legislation (e.g., reimbursement and prescriptive privileges) that govern the legal practice of nursing in each state.

As the health care structure continues changing to decrease costs and increase accessibility to health care, the FNP and the CNS in community health nursing will find increasing opportunities for practice. The following areas include traditional and more recent practice settings for community health nursing.

Private Practice

Research indicates that the opportunities for FNPs increased in private practice settings throughout the 1980s. This trend is expected to continue (Shanks-Meile et al., 1989). In medical private practice settings, the FNP or CNS may be the only professional nurse. When the FNP role is not clearly understood or accepted by the physician and office staff, conflict and dissatisfaction are inevitable. Role negotiation is essential before entering into an employment contract in this situation.

Joint Practice

Joint practice between nurses and physicians is considered to be the most appropriate model for the delivery of primary health care services (National Joint Practice Commission, 1977). However, there must be a true collaboration between medical and nursing practitioners. Unfortunately a collaborative practice model is not always found where nurses and physicians practice together. A study by McLain (1988) suggests that despite the positive attributes nurse specialists bring to the practice of primary health care, "there remain deeply embedded beliefs and behaviors associated with the traditional hierarchical relationship between medicine and nursing." Physicians have usually been taught to promote and maintain a hierarchical relationship with other disciplines. There must be clear communication among FNPs, CNSs, and physicians so that there is mutual understanding and respect for each practitioner's role and contribution to the care of clients.

Currently, the CNS role in joint practice is not as clearly defined in private practice as that of the FNP. This will change as health care continues to shift from primarily acute care settings such as hospitals to innovative models of community-based preventive care.

Independent Practice

Nurses form independent practices for several reasons, including personal or professional desire to break new ground for nursing and to meet health care needs within a community. It is important to investigate the state's nurse practice act to determine the limitations and legal ramifications of this arrangement. For example, FNPs may provide a more comprehensive array of health services in states where they have legislative authority to prescribe drugs. Currently, no states provide this privilege for CNSs without NP certification. However, nurses in many states have successfully lobbied for third party reimbursement for all RNs who provide currently reimbursable services (Pearson, 1991). The independent practice option is more likely to be chosen by FNPs and CNSs in states that have established legislation to facilitate this nursing practice.

Implementing the independent practice model requires planning and financial resources. Along with the legal and philosophical issues of functioning independently to provide nursing services, nurses must also consider financial aspects. In an area of the Southeast where costs are generally lower than in the rest of the country, it was estimated that the cost to open a private nursing practice in an office setting is more than $30,000 for the first year (Sirles and Smith, 1990). This cost did not include salaries, marketing of services, or retainer fees for attorneys or accountants.

Even in areas where third-party payers do not reimburse for services by nurses, CNSs and NPs have successfully established private practices. Nurses who correctly assess and identify their markets and implement realistic business plans make incomes comparable to what they would earn as employees. However, it may take 3 to 4 years to determine the profitability of independent practice (Pearson, 1986).

Another option for FNPs and CNSs interested in independent practice is to contract with physicians or organizations to provide certain services for their clients or staffs. Nurses need to define a service package and market it attractively. An example is providing a home visit to new parents after 2 weeks to assess the newborn, respond to parental concerns, and provide counseling and anticipatory guidance about nutritional, developmental, and immunization needs. This service may be marketed to pediatricians and family practice physicians who would offer or recommend the service to their clients as an option. An FNP may negotiate with a local school board to provide preschool children with health examinations or physical assessments before beginning participation in sports. CNSs may develop health and safety programs on accident prevention and health promotion activities for small companies that provide time and resources (Grove and Pruitt, 1984). Home health nursing agencies may also use consultants to provide skills and educational workshops for their staffs. Although contracting services requires a market survey and considerable planning, it does not involve the costs of maintaining a practice setting.

Despite legal and financial deterrents, nurses find independent practice gratifying because they can practice autonomously within a nursing model. It is not known whether an independent nursing practice can be profitable in the long term. The cost-effectiveness and health care outcomes of clients receiving health care from nurses practicing independently are also unknown.

Institutional Settings
Ambulatory/Outpatient Clinics

FNPs and CNSs may be employed in the primary care unit of an institution (e.g., the ambulatory center or outpatient clinic). A decline in the number of inpatients and increased competition among hospitals for the available market are incentives to develop alternative services. Expanding health care delivery by providing outpatient services also provides referrals for inpatient services (Lamper-Linden, Goetz-Kulas, and Lake, 1983). Ambulatory/outpatient facilities are cost-effective and can improve the hospital's image in community service.

Hospital clinics generally provide hospital referral, hospital follow-up care, and health maintenance and management for nonemergent problems. The population served is usually more culturally and economically diverse and represents a larger geographic area than that served by private practices. In these outpatient settings, FNPs typically practice jointly with physicians to provide acute and chronic primary health care. Hospital acute care outpatient services may include clinics for general-medicine or family practice, or specialty-oriented clinics, such as pediatric, obstetric-gynecological, and ENT clinics. Outpatient clinics organized for chronic care may be problem-oriented (e.g., hypertension, diabetes, or AIDS clinics).

FNPs and CNSs have the greatest impact in chronic care. For chronic diseases such as hypertension, diabetes, and AIDS for which no cures presently exist, the nursing emphasis on self-care, education, and health promotion may be more beneficial than medical care alone in preventing complications and containing costs. Client care is further enhanced by the CNS's knowledge of community resources and collaboration with nurses in community agencies.

When developing a model for providing direct care in an outpatient ambulatory setting, FNPs should adopt the principles of primary nursing as much as possible. They need to ensure that health promotion and disease prevention services are incorporated into each client's plan of care. For example, if a woman's only contact with a health care pro-

vider is in the hypertensive outpatient clinic, there should be a procedure to offer a yearly Pap smear and routine adult immunizations (Gonzalez, Ranney, and West, 1989). Similarly, when a client's condition requires home visits, FNPs can consult with the CNSs who can arrange the necessary community referral or provide the home care while acting as the liaison between the outpatient department and the home.

Job satisfaction in these institutional ambulatory/outpatient settings often depends on how effectively FNPs and CNSs can define their functions and responsibilities. Communicating their roles to the clinic staff and providers is critical to their effectiveness (McLain, 1988; Paradise and Kendall, 1985).

Satellite outpatient clinics are often an extension of the hospital's outpatient services to an outlying suburban or rural population. In rural satellite clinics, FNPs may practice alone or with a physician present for a part of each week. The use of FNPs or CNSs depends on the extent that third-party payers, especially Medicare and Medicaid, will reimburse the institution for services provided by nonphysician providers.

Emergency Departments

Persons without accessible health care, such as the medically uninsured and the homeless, frequently do not seek health care services until they become ill. Hospital emergency departments are increasingly used for non-emergent primary care. Although this is an inappropriate use of expensive health resources, it is a result of the current system, which limits access to routine and preventive health care.

Emergency services often require long waits for persons presenting with nonemergent problems. Medical treatment is usually provided with little or no counseling or guidance. FNPs in these settings see clients with nonemergent problems and provide the necessary treatment and appropriate counseling. CNSs may also help to educate clients on the importance of health care and how to gain access to the health care system. CNSs' knowledge of community resources helps ensure that, if possible, psychosocial needs are assessed and met. CNSs can act as liaisons for community programs that serve the needs of special populations. Through hot lines and direct communication with service organizations, CNSs can often provide immediate access to assistance.

For FNPs and CNSs practicing in emergency departments, continuing education in trauma nursing is appropriate. Cross training, whether learned on the job or through continuing education, is increasingly encouraged by institutions as an effective cost-containing measure.

Long-Term Care Facilities

The Bureau of the Census estimates that between 4% and 5% of Americans over age 75 reside in nursing homes. It is estimated that by the year 2025, persons 65 and older will make up approximately 22% of the total population of the United States (Torrey, Kinsella, and Taeuber, 1987).

Gerontology is an increasingly important field of study, and many courses are available on health needs of the elderly. FNPs and CNSs with an interest in geriatrics will need to continue their education in this area to increase their effectiveness. Many FNPs and CNSs view long-term care facilities as exciting areas for practice. Federal legislation provides reimbursement for NPs and CNSs associated with physicians to provide care to clients in Medicare-certified nursing homes and to recertify eligible clients for continued Medicare coverage. In long-term care facilities where clients are not ambulatory, FNPs and CNSs associated with a medical practice may make regular nursing home rounds, assess the health status of clients, and provide care and counseling as appropriate. In long-term care facilities in which the residents are more ambulatory, FNPs and CNSs contract with the primary care physicians to provide health maintenance and other primary care services to their nursing home clients.

CNSs in a long-term care facility typically assume maximum responsibility and function with a great deal of independence (Edmunds, 1983). FNPs and CNSs benefit clients by reducing the number of acute infections and complications, thus having a positive impact on both the quality and the cost of care (Grzeczkowski and Knapp, 1988). CNSs are more likely to assume major administrative responsibilities; FNPs are more likely to have major clinical responsibilities. Both FNPs and CNSs can serve as role models and consultants to the nursing staff.

The health needs of special populations such as the institutionalized elderly receive a great deal of public and policy-making attention. Providing services to the elderly presents an opportunity for FNPs and CNSs to demonstrate their effectiveness in increasing quality of care while containing the costs of long-term care (Molde and Diers, 1985).

Industry

The National Health Council estimates that 11,100 deaths and 1.8 million disabling injuries can be attributed annually to on-the-job accidents (U.S. Bureau of the Census, 1989). Thousands of new cases of disease and death occur each year from occupational exposures. With rising insurance premiums and health care costs, more companies are becoming self-insured and providing comprehensive on-site primary health care services. Worksite health programs offer new areas for nursing practice and considerable cost savings for corporations (Touger and Butts, 1989).

CNSs and FNPs are increasingly useful in occupational health programs as business and industry seek ways to control their health care costs. The CNS in an industrial setting would assess the health needs of the organization based on claims data, cost/benefit health research, results of employee health screening, and the perceived needs of employee groups. With their advanced administrative and clinical skills, CNSs plan company-wide health programs. The CNS would be responsible for the overall implementation and continuing evaluation of health programs.

FNPs in occupational settings generally practice independently, with physician consultation as needed. The health and welfare of the worker is a major concern; therefore concentration is on health maintenance. Responsibilities for maintaining employee health include direct nursing care for on-the-job injuries. Often clinical responsibility extends to monitoring nonoccupationally related illnesses

such as diabetes and hypertension. Employees may elect to see the FNP for common problems and see a physician for more complicated problems (Dellinger, Zentner, McDowell, and Annas, 1986). FNPs, like CNSs, may also have program planning responsibilities. In terms of administration, however, FNPs are more likely to function in the day-to-day operations of the health service to oversee the ordering and monitoring of supplies, keep daily logs, and collect data required by federal and state regulations for occupational health and safety. The role of the occupational health nurse is discussed in chapter 41.

Government

U.S. Public Health Service

The U.S. Public Health Service operates two services: the National Health Service Corps, which places health practitioners in federally designated areas with shortages of health manpower, and the Indian Health Service, which provides health services to Native Americans.

During the 1970s, both the Corps and the Indian Health Service offered to pay to educate RNs to be nurse practitioners if they would promise to work for a designated period of time with the Public Health Service. These programs were discontinued during the 1980s when the emphasis was on physician recruitment. In 1988, Congress reauthorized two loan repayment programs—one with the Corps and one with the Indian Health Service.

The only nurses who are currently eligible for the loan repayment program are experienced BSN graduates and MSN graduates prepared as NPs, midwives, or anesthetists. Nurse anesthetists and BSN graduates are primarily sought by the Indian Health Service. Congress is currently considering the addition of a scholarship program for FNPs, nurse midwives, and physician assistants who promise to work for the Public Health Service.

Depending on the needs of the area, an FNP employed by the Public Health Service may be the only health care provider in the setting or may practice with a group of providers to serve a rural or Native American population.

Armed Services

The increased availability of physicians reduced the active recruitment of nurses in advanced degree programs that the armed forces had conducted during the 1980s. Currently the Army, Navy, and Air Force have programs providing educational leave and tuition to pursue advanced degrees for nurses on active duty. NPs are used in ambulatory clinics serving enlisted personnel and their dependents.

CNSs are used by the armed forces in the broad scope of community health nursing. The role of the community health CNS is so valued that they receive promotions without having to change their basic role as client and family advocates in the community.

Public Health Departments

Public health departments are increasingly employing community health nurses with master's degrees. These CNSs and FNPs need administrative and clinical skills to work collaboratively with physicians and to manage and implement clinical services provided by the health departments.

Home care and hospice services are nursing sections in many public health departments and require the services of community health nursing specialists.

Health departments also provide primary care services in well-child clinics, family planning clinics, and general adult primary care clinics. A public health department may use FNPs and CNSs, depending on the size of the department, the department's health priorities in the community, and financial constraints.

Schools

School health nursing involves comprehensive assessment and management of care, with particular emphasis on health education to promote healthy behaviors in children and their families (Igoe, 1975). CNSs and FNPs may be employed as school health nurses by school boards or county health departments to provide specific services to schools. These services usually include confirming that immunization status is current and performing hearing and vision screening. More progressive school systems employ an on-site nurse at each school within their jurisdiction. School-based health services are generally staffed by CNSs and/or nurses prepared as school, pediatric, or family nurse practitioners. Services provided by these advanced practitioners include not only basic health screening but also monitoring of children with chronic health problems and securing health care for children with limited access to medical care. These nurses work collaboratively with parents, community leaders, educators, and physicians to ensure that each child within the school community receives needed services. Community health CNSs and NPs are well suited to manage school health services.

Other Arenas
Health Maintenance Organizations

HMO practices emphasize health promotion and disease prevention services to reduce health risks and avoid expensive medical care. FNPs are often employed in HMOs to provide cost-effective basic health care services.

A concept similar to the HMO is the Preferred Provider Organization (PPO). Formation of nursing PPOs has begun (Pearson, 1986), but their future is unknown. Nursing PPOs provide unique opportunities for FNPs and CNSs. They need to offer unique services that produce measurable client outcomes and are cost efficient. For example, a nursing PPO for corporate clients maintained itself with reimbursement fees 20% below physician costs for the same services (Mahoney, 1988).

Home Health Agencies

Major legislative changes in Medicare and third-party reimbursement for hospital services have resulted in unprecedented growth in the home health care industry (Kent and Hanley, 1990). The opportunities for FNPs and CNSs in the home health care market continue to expand. Home health care is less expensive than extended hospitalization and thus is an attractive option for third-party payers (Kent and Hanley, 1990). Additionally, equipment and drug companies are developing products for home use, physicians and hospitals are exploring the development of home services, and consumers are demanding greater availability of services.

Because of their knowledge and skills in the following areas, FNPs and CNSs are well-qualified to provide home health care that yields positive outcomes for clients and their families: (1) public/community health principles, (2) family and individual counseling skills, (3) health education and strategies for adult learning, and (4) increased decision-making.

Correctional Institutions

The organizational structure of prisons and jails has long been a barrier to providing or improving health care. Inmates are a population with health needs that can be met by CNSs and FNPs.

Research in this area is limited but has demonstrated that NPs have had a positive effect in correctional health programs. One correctional system reported that its capacity for primary care doubled and the cost of each client visit decreased by one-third (Hastings, Vick, Lee, et al., 1980). The technical quality of primary care also continued to improve over a 3-year period, while client outcomes, satisfaction levels, and overall mortality rates remained unchanged. In the same study the suicide rate also dropped. The real challenge for future research is to evaluate the reasons for these findings.

Community health CNSs would be an asset within prison systems, planning and implementing coordinated health programs that would include health education as well as health services. Where personnel resources are limited, CNSs can provide counseling for inmates and their families to prepare prison clients for transition to the community upon their release.

Parrish Nursing

Parrish nursing, more recently referred to as *block nursing,* is an innovative nursing model designed to allow the elderly to stay in their homes when they are not totally independent.

The beginning of block nursing was seen in the earliest days of professional nursing, when people sought service on a fee basis from nurses who lived in their community. The present model arose from a study by the U.S. General Accounting Office (GAO) conducted in 1979. The study showed that 20% to 40% of the elderly in nursing homes could have remained in their own homes had they received some support services (Martinson et al., 1985). More recent block nursing models involve FNPs and CNSs collaborating in the case management of individuals and families in a specific geographic area. These individuals and families receive professional nursing assessment and care from the FNP, while the CNS mobilizes and coordinates community agencies and volunteers to provide needed supportive services.

An evaluation of a block nursing program in Minnesota revealed that 85% of those served would have been institutionalized without the block nursing services and that the total cost of living for families with block nursing was 24% less than it would have been for custodial care in nursing homes (Jamieson, 1990). Federal agencies and private foundations have granted funds to communities to form block nursing programs (Jamieson, 1990). Block nursing may be a future trend that will offer unique opportunities for CNSs and FNPs.

ISSUES AND CONCERNS
Legal Status

The legal authority of nurses in advanced practice is determined by each state's nurse practice act and, in some states, by additional rules and regulations for practice. Community health CNSs have less need than FNPs for expanded practice within the traditional nursing domain. The community health CNS role involves acting as a consultant-facilitator, and guidelines for practice are more frequently defined by the nurse practice act (Hanson and Martin, 1990). In the 1970s, regulations for the direct care role performed by FNPs and NPs, including diagnosis and treatment, were less defined in state nursing laws than they are today, and the legal statuses of NPs and FNPs were being questioned. Since 1971, when Idaho revised its nurse practice act to include the practice of NPs, states have amended their nurse practice acts or revised their definitions of nursing to reflect the new nursing roles. In a 1991 survey by *Nurse Practitioner: The American Journal of Primary Health Care,* it was reported that NPs in 35 states were regulated by the Board of Nursing through specific regulations; in 7 states, NPs functioned under a broad nurse practice act; and in 8 other states, they were regulated by both the Board of Nursing and the Board of Medicine (Pearson, 1991).

Legislative authority to prescribe has changed dramatically in the last several years. By 1990, 35 states had prescriptive authority for NPs, and 7 other states were seriously considering the issue (Pearson, 1991). Although legal problems and unresolved disputes still exist in a few states, tremendous gains have been made because of nurses' active involvement in the political and policy-making arenas.

Reimbursement

The third-party reimbursement system in the United States, both public and private, is complicated. As health care costs rise at an average of 10% per year, many people need a third-party payer to receive health care services (Grace, 1990). Third-party reimbursement is a concern primarily to NPs because of their role in providing direct care. When FNPs provide services that are categorized as reimbursable but cannot collect from insurers unless the claim is filed by a physician, it is viewed by nurses as exploitation of themselves and the public. Exploitation of nurses occurs when fees are collected by one professional (the physician) for services performed by another (the FNP). Exploitation of the public occurs because clients must seek care from providers whose fees will be honored by insurers. Since over half of all personal health care services are financed by third-party payers, providers must be eligible for third-party reimbursement to be economically solvent. This limits alternatives in health care by discouraging independent practice by nurses (Griffith, 1982).

The Rural Health Clinic Services Act of 1977 (PL 95-210) was the first breakthrough in third-party reimbursement for nurses in primary care roles. The law authorized Med-

icare and Medicaid reimbursement to qualified rural clinics for services provided by NPs and PAs, regardless of the presence of a physician (Wasem, 1990). The intent of the act was to improve access to health care in some of the nation's underserved rural areas; however, its use from state to state has varied dramatically. Recent legislative changes, including the coverage of services by certified nurse midwives (CMN), clinical psychologists, and social workers, have improved the effectiveness of the Rural Health Clinic Services Act for reimbursement options.

Nurses can change reimbursement policies using legislative and nonlegislative strategies. Because they create a more permanent solution, legislative strategies are preferred (Streff and Netzer, 1990). As of 1990, 23 states had legislation concerning third-party reimbursement to NPs. Twenty-five states had rules and regulations allowing NPs to receive direct Medicaid reimbursement; and insurance companies in 8 states were providing direct reimbursement to NPs without legislative mandates to do so (Pearson, 1991).

Institutional Privileges

Because of their direct care role, FNPs in community health are more concerned than CNSs about institutional privileges. It is often difficult for FNPs to obtain hospital privileges through the nursing departments within institutions where their clients are admitted. The traditional hospital nurse is automatically responsible to and governed by the department of nursing as a condition of employment. However, if an FNP is employed in a private joint practice with a physician, there is rarely a mechanism for clinical privileges to be granted by the department of nursing because the nurse is not employed by the hospital. There are two reasons for providing a mechanism for community-based FNPs to gain access to their hospitalized clients. First, if people are allowed to choose or purchase direct nursing care, access by FNPs to hospitalized clients is a necessity. Second, nursing must be accountable for and regulate the practice of its practitioners. No other group can knowledgeably review or set forth the standards for nursing practice (Manley, 1981). Because NPs in primary care usually work to keep clients out of hospitals, staff privileges are not a priority for many FNPs (Richards, 1984).

Many institutions grant clinical privileges to nonphysicians, including nurses, through the department of medicine. The *Accreditation Manual for Hospitals,* published in 1976 by the Joint Commission on Accreditation of Hospitals (JCAH), states that hospitals, within their bylaws and rules and regulations, will have their medical staffs define privileges for nonphysician practitioners and identify the roles and responsibilities of the medical staff in relation to the nonphysician practitioners. A medical staff definition adopted by JCAH in 1984 directed hospitals to be more permissive in granting nonphysicians medical staff privileges (Richards, 1984). However, these policies limit nursing's autonomy and professional responsibility within the hospital setting. They also decrease an institution's ability to monitor the nursing care that is provided by nurses who have been granted clinical privileges under medical authority.

Since the nursing department is responsible for establishing and upholding nursing care standards within an institution, nurses should have the authority to grant or deny nursing privileges for all nurses within the setting, regardless whether they are employed by the institution (Manley, 1981).

The importance of state legislation and the role of the professional organization in encouraging institutional privileges cannot be minimized. Legislative action, changes in nurse practice acts, Federal Trade Commission intervention, consumer demands, and pressures by nonphysicians will increase FNPs' direct client access (Durham and Hardin, 1985).

The changing economy and health care trends are altering the role of the traditional hospital. With competition for clients and nonhospital care increasing, hospitals are more willing to consider alternatives to the medical model. Efforts to obtain third-party reimbursement for care provided by FNPs must continue, because few hospitals will encourage admission and treatment of clients who cannot pay.

Employment and Role Negotiation

For NPs and CNSs to collaboratively provide comprehensive primary care, they must understand and develop negotiation skills. Positive working relationships with health professionals, organizations, and clients require role negotiation, particularly when few guidelines exist or a role is new and undeveloped. NPs and CNSs need to assess the internal politics of the organization as part of their role negotiation. Networking is another necessary skill. Forums, joint conferences, collaborative practice, and research provide opportunities to expand their functions (Forbes et al., 1990).

Because FNPs and CNSs often seek employment, as opposed to being sought by employers, assertiveness is needed. Increased economic constraints and new health care legislation have reduced the visibility of job opportunities. FNPs and CNSs should feel comfortable about marketing their skills. Marketing strategies should be designed to project an image that reflects achievement. In assessing and analyzing the needs of target markets they must balance professional, institutional, and target group goals (Andreoli, Carollo, Pottage, 1988).

Providing copies of credential documents and samples of professional accomplishments such as audiovisual materials, client education packets, and history and physical tools, helps in obtaining a job and negotiating future roles. FNPs and CNSs should keep folders containing examples of all professional activities that may be used for prospective employment, while not overselling their position. Names, addresses, and telephone numbers of professional and personal references should be furnished only after permission has been obtained. A business card left at the conclusion of the interview is another way of increasing visibility.

ROLE STRESS

Stressors directly affect nurses in advanced practice. In addition to legal issues, factors causing stress include professional isolation, liability, collaborative practice, conflicting expectations, and professional responsibilities. Strategies to reduce stress have been so extensively discussed that "burnout" is a section in the Cumulative Index to Nursing and Allied Health (Hutchinson, 1987). FNPs and CNSs should identify self-care strategies to cope with predictable stressors.

Self-care strategies promote a sense of control and well-being. They require vigilance, self-evaluation, and a belief in the importance of self-care. Job satisfaction is affected by positive self-care outcomes. Personal control or power leads to professional power, which expands the FNP and CNS roles and further fosters professionalism.

Professional Isolation

Professional isolation is a source of conflict for FNPs and CNSs. Because they practice across all age groups, FNPs and CNSs are likely to be sought for remote practice employment sites. Rural communities that cannot support a physician, for instance, may find the FNP an affordable and logical alternative for primary care services. The autonomy of practice in these sites attracts many FNPs and CNSs, who may fail to consider the disadvantages of isolated practice. Long drives, long hours, lack of social life and cultural activities, and lack of opportunity for professional development are often experienced by these rural practitioners.

Additionally, nurses may experience isolation even though they are team members in collaborative practices because they fill unique positions. Specialization and advanced practice in nursing require a pioneering spirit. FNPs and CNSs can lead the profession by being involved in the following issues (Styles, 1990):

1. Professional unity
2. Professional education
3. Clinical research
4. Legal scope of nursing practice
5. Cost-effective, high-quality health care
6. Professional autonomy
7. Ethical issues in clinical practice
8. Reimbursement
9. Compensation
10. A comprehensive system of credentialing to promote quality assurance in advanced practice.

FNPs and CNSs must also consider family members and their needs. The long hours, social isolation, lack of cultural activities, child care, and quality of school systems are important issues for every family. These sources of stress that lead to job dissatisfaction can be reduced or eliminated by negotiating the employment contract to include educational and personal leaves. Back-up providers during times of leave ensure that health services are not compromised (Sirles, 1981). FNPs and CNSs who choose isolated employment settings should consider their own needs as well as those of the community and should negotiate accordingly.

Liability

All nurses are liable for their actions. Because more legal action is appearing in the judicial system, specifically concerning NPs and CNSs, the importance of liability and/or malpractice insurance cannot be overemphasized. Although malpractice insurance is not a prerequisite to functioning as an FNP or CNS, most nurses carry their own liability insurance. It is in the best interest of FNPs and CNSs to thoroughly investigate the coverage offered by different companies rather than to assume that the coverage is adequate. Practitioners who function without a physician on site are particularly vulnerable.

NPs who have been successful in defending themselves against charges of illegal practice emphasize the importance of clear, objective documentation of clinical findings, therapy, counseling, and when appropriate, physician consultation. Charting should be a habitual practice for nurses in expanded roles.

The scope of the FNP's and CNS's authority determines the liability standards applied. The limits of each practitioner's authority are legislated by individual states (King and Sagan, 1989).

Collaborative Practice

The future of FNPs and CNSs depends upon whether they make a recognizable difference in the health of families and communities and on their ability to practice collaboratively with physicians. Collaborative practice denotes a collegial relationship with mutual trust and respect. Working out a collaborative practice takes a considerable amount of time and energy. Until such practice relationships evolve within joint practice situations, the quality health care that nursing and medicine can collaboratively provide will not be achieved. The arrangement demands the professional maturity to work together without territorial disputes, and the structure and philosophy of the organization must support joint practice as a mechanism for health care delivery. The growing pains of establishing such a practice produce stress for all involved; however, the results and benefits to clients and professionals are worth the effort (Steel, 1986).

Conflicting Expectations

Services provided by FNPs and CNSs in health promotion and maintenance are often more time-consuming and complex than just the management of clients' health problems. FNPs and CNSs frequently experience conflict between their practice goals in health promotion and the need to see the number of clients required to maintain the clinic's economic goals. The problem is compounded when the clinic administrator or physician views FNPs or CNSs only as medical extenders and reimbursement to them is limited. A practice model that can assist nurses in integrating health promotion and maintenance activities as well as medical case management into each client visit uses (1) flexible scheduling; (2) health maintenance flow sheets; and (3) problem-oriented recording with nursing goals and plans prominently displayed in the health record.

Professional Responsibilities

Professional responsibilities contribute to role stress. Most states require FNPs and CNSs in expanded roles to be nationally certified and to maintain certification. Recertification requires documentation of continuing education hours in primary care topics. Because the practitioner is in a minority role in nursing, continuing education may not be locally available and may require travel and lodging expenses in addition to time away from practice. Anticipating professional responsibilities and attendant expenses in financial planning decreases these concerns. Negotiating with the employer for educational leave and expenses should be part of any contract.

Quality of client care, however, cannot be measured or ensured by continuing education or credentials. Professional responsibility includes monitoring one's own practice according to standards established by the profession.

A quality assurance process with peer review is another professional responsibility for FNPs and CNSs. This process should evaluate need, cost, and effectiveness of care in relation to client outcomes (Cassidy and Freeman, 1990). The difficulties of the peer-review quality assurance process include the time and distance involved in traveling to widely separated clinics as well as the need to plan the reviews to minimize interference with individual schedules.

Self-review can also serve as a quality assurance process. A group of nurse practitioners at the Johns Hopkins Hospital developed a performance appraisal tool that is used to reflect the practitioner's role and practice setting. This tool is divided into four categories: clinical, leadership, education, and professional activities (Levitt et al., 1985).

A mechanism for self-review is the chart-audit, using protocols to measure quality of care. Many states require protocols for practicing in an expanded role. Although there are many published protocols to guide practice, the physician and the FNP or CNS who work together must adapt protocols according to the diagnostic scope and treatment regimes of their practice. Client history, diagnostic findings, indications for consultation and referral, client education relative to treatment, prevention, and follow-up should all be clearly defined within each protocol.

TRENDS

Andreoli and Musser (1985) discuss trends that may affect the future of nursing, emphasizing that the future will belong to nurses who develop skills and behaviors to meet health care needs. Computer use will continue to increase. This challenge requires continuing education as well as computer literacy and proficiency skills to assist FNPs and CNSs in developing, implementing, and maintaining computer software programs oriented to nursing care. CNSs and FNPs can also help health agencies to evaluate software to manage cost-effective, quality health care.

Additionally, Mahoney (1988) challenges practitioners to be cost-sensitive providers, stimulating competition in an effort to lower overall health care costs. As knowledgeable professionals, practitioners can provide information that will assist clients in making informed health care choices.

CLINICAL APPLICATIONS
Case One: Family Nurse Practitioner

Julia Andrews is a master's level FNP who practices with two board-certified family practice physicians in an urban office. Julia has her own appointment schedule and sees 12 to 15 clients on an average day. Although she sees some acutely ill clients, most of her appointments are for routine health maintenance visits for both adults and children. The two physicians also refer clients to Julia for management of stable chronic health problems like hypertension and diabetes. Referral of these problems by the physicians did not begin until Julia had been with the practice for about a year.

During the first months in practice, Julia assessed the numbers and types of patient problems seen in a typical week. She found that hypertension was the most frequent chronic problem. Julia reviewed a sample of records of hypertensive clients and found that many had recorded blood pressures indicating uncontrolled hypertension. After her assessment, Julia negotiated with the physicians to randomly assign 30 hypertensive clients to her for follow-up care. Nine months later, Julia was able to show that blood pressure measurements were lower in her group of clients than in a randomly selected group of 30 clients managed by the physicians. Also, her group of clients indicated a high degree of satisfaction with her care and were more informed about their medications than the physicians' clients. It was also noted that clients seen by Julia were more likely to be up-to-date on Pap smears and immunizations. By doing the study, Julia confirmed her belief that clients with chronic problems have as much or more need for nursing care as medical care. The physicians now also refer clients to Julia for weight loss, smoking cessation, and diabetes education. Because of limited time, Julia chose to assess these clients for their readiness to make lifestyle changes and then assist them in choosing an appropriate program from those offered by community agencies or private groups.

One of Julia's goals as an FNP in private practice was to use her knowledge of community resources to serve the needs of clients. She has contracted with the agencies and programs to which she refers for written assessments of clients' progress. Julia stays current with the strategies used in the various community programs so that she can reinforce teaching during the clients' office visits. The practice also contracts with two local small industries to provide preemployment physicals and office visits for employees with nonemergency job-related injuries. Julia has talked with the physicians and the manager of one of the industries about conducting an on-site health screening program. The first phase, assessing the needs of the employees, is in the planning stage. Through the state nurses' association, Julia has had opportunity to network with other nurse practitioners, including those in occupational health nursing. One of the occupational health nurses has offered Julia consultation services as a professional courtesy.

Julia has demonstrated her value to the practice in several ways. She has formed working relationships with community health resources, made significant contributions to the quality and diversity of health care offered by the practice, and has involved the practice in an outreach program to small industry; additionally, she has contributed to the physicians' practice in terms of leveraging their time, increasing income, and enhancing professional satisfaction.

Case Two: Clinical Nurse Specialist

Martha Corley is a community health CNS who coordinates the after-care services for a community hospital's early discharge patients. Martha has worked with the nursing staff to develop a nursing history form to identify family and social supports available to patients who are likely to need nursing or supportive care for a limited time after discharge. With this and additional information from head nurses, Martha visits selected patients to begin discharge planning.

She consults with each patient and family to validate assessed needs. The physician is also consulted about medical therapies to be continued at home. Martha has access to nurses and other resources throughout the community who accept cases on contract. She outlines the initial care plan with the nurse case-manager assigned to the patient and receives regular progress reports. Martha continually evaluates the aftercare service, assessing patient and family satisfaction by questionnaire and by telephone. Patient outcome data on medical complications and/or rehospitalization is also used to evaluate the service.

Evaluation indicates that the after-care program is meeting a need for families in the community. Martha believes her expertise in community health nursing has been of critical importance to the after-care program.

As shown by these descriptions, the diverse roles of the CNS and FNP are evident in the community and within a structured health care system.

SUMMARY

The shortage of physicians during the 1960s created problems of access to primary care services. NPs and PAs were viewed as an answer to the medical shortage. As nurses became knowledgeable and comfortable with the assessment and management skills of their role in primary care, it became apparent that their major contribution was not in the acute care management functions they performed but in the nursing skills they brought to primary care.

The expanded nursing role is one of the most comprehensive roles in primary care. FNPs specialize in the ambulatory health management of the family unit. Family dynamics, family assessment, growth and development, and management of common acute and stabilized chronic health problems provide the framework for the primary care nursing practice of FNPs. Within this framework are the components of health maintenance and management, which focus on health problems in children, women, adults, and the aged. CNSs have skills in community assessment and proficiency in planning, implementing, and evaluating population-focused programs and can contribute greatly to the primary care team. In addition, they possess substantial clinical knowledge and use an epidemiological approach in the formulation of health and social policy.

The expanded role of community health nurses, particularly FNPs, remains controversial. Are they practicing medicine or nursing? Should they practice independently or jointly? How should they be educated? What is their legal relationship to the physician? Do they make a contribution to the health of people to whom they provide services? Since the introduction of the NP role, these questions have not yet been fully answered. There is a limited amount of nursing research with implications relative to the roles and functions of nurses in expanded practice. Studies directed toward outcome as well as process of care are greatly needed. A long-range, follow-up evaluation of the impact of nurses in advanced practice in community health is also necessary. To remain viable in the health care system, especially in this time of cost containment, community health FNPs and CNSs must be valued by clients for meeting health care needs not addressed by others.

KEY CONCEPTS

Social changes and changes in health problems over the past century have redefined the pattern of health care in this country.

Primary care is comprehensive, coordinated, and continuous, and it requires collaboration among many health professionals.

Trends such as an increase in technology, self-care, cost-containment measures, accountability, third-party reimbursement, and demands for humanizing technical care have influenced the new roles of the CNS and NP.

Educational preparation of the CNS has always been at the graduate level, whereas this has not been true of NP preparation; 80% of NP programs are now at the master's degree level.

Specialty certification through ANA began in 1976 for FNPs and in 1990 for community health CNSs.

The roles of NP and CNS are merging and many common features exist, but there are still important differences in role functions in community health nursing.

The major role functions of the FNP and CNS in community health nursing are clinician, consultant, administrator, researcher, and educator; typically, the FNP spends a greater proportion of time in direct care clinical activities and less time in indirect activities, whereas the proportion of time is distributed more evenly across direct and indirect practice activities for the CNS.

Major arenas for practice for FNPs and CNSs in community health include private practice, institutional settings, industry, government, public health departments, and schools; increasingly both are found in HMOs, home health, correctional health, and parrish nursing.

Legal status, reimbursement, institutional privileges, and role negotiation are important issues and concerns to nurses who practice in an advanced role in community health nursing.

Major stressors for FNPs and CNSs include professional isolation, liability, collaborative practice, conflicting expectations, and professional responsibilities.

The expanded nursing role in community health nursing is one of the most comprehensive roles in primary care, yet it remains controversial.

To remain viable in the health care system, community health CNSs and FNPs must be seen and valued by clients for meeting health care needs not addressed by others.

LEARNING ACTIVITIES

1. Explore the development of the community health FNP and CNS roles locally.

2. Compare and contrast the local, state, and national movement related to advanced practice in community health nursing.

3. Investigate graduate programs in community health nursing within the state or region to determine the requirements for admission, the type of degree awarded, and whether or not FNP and/or CNS preparation is available.

4. Review your state's nurse practice act and any rules and regulations governing advanced practice roles.

5. Negotiate a clinical observation experience with an FNP and a CNS in community health nursing and compare and contrast their roles.

BIBLIOGRAPHY

American Medical Association: Physician characteristics and distribution in the U.S. 1983 edition. Survey and Data Resources, 1984.

American Nurses' Association: The scope of practice of the primary health care nurse practitioner, Kansas City, Mo, 1985, The Association.

American Nurses' Association: Standards of community health nursing practice, Kansas City, Mo, 1986, The Association.

American Nurses' Association: Standards of practice of the primary health care nurse practitioner, Kansas City, Mo, 1987, The Association.

Andreoli KG and Musser LA: Trends that may affect nursings' future, Nursing & Health Care, 6(1):47–51, 1985.

Andreoli KG, Carollo JR, and Pottage MW: Marketing strategies: Projecting an image of nursing that reflects achievement, Nursing Administration Quarterly 12(4):5–14, 1988.

Andrus LH and Mitchell FH: Change processes in primary care. In Renihardt AM and Quinn MD, editors: Family-centered community nursing: a sociocultural framework, St. Louis, 1980, The CV Mosby Co.

Bullough B, editor: The law and the expanding nursing role, ed 2, New York, 1980, Appleton-Century-Crofts.

Cassidy DA and Friesen MA: QA: applying JCAHO's generic model, Nursing Management 21(6):22–27, 1990.

Davidson RA and Lauver D: Nurse practitioner and physician roles: delineation and complementarity of practice, Res Nurs Health, 7:3–9, 1984.

Dellinger CJ, Zentner JP, McDowell PH and Annas AW: The family nurse practitioner in industry, AAOHN J 34(7):323–325, 1986.

Durham JD and Hardin SB: Nurse psychotherapists' experiences in obtaining individual practice privileges, Nurs Pract 10(11):62–67, 1985.

Edmunds M: Models of clinical practice, Nurse Pract 8(9):59, 1983.

Elder RG and Bollough B: Nurse practitioners and clinical nurse specialists: are the roles merging?, Clin Nurse Specialist 4(2):78–84, 1990.

Extending the scope of nursing practice: Department of Health, Education, and Welfare, Washington, D.C., 1971, US Government Printing Office.

Felton G, Kelly HD, Renehan K and Alley J: Nursing entrepreneurs: a success story, Nurs Outlook 33(6):276, 1985.

Fisher DW and Horowitz SM: The physician's assistant: profile of a new health profession. In Bliss AA and Cohen ED, editors: The new health professionals, Germantown, MD, 1977, Aspen Systems Corp.

Forbes KE, et al: Clinical nurse specialist and nurse practitioner core curriculum survey results, Nurse Pract 15(4):43, 46–48, 1990.

Ford LC: Nurses, nurse practitioners: the evolution of primary care, (Book review). Image 18(4):177–178, 1986.

Geolot D: Nurse practitioner education: observations from a national perspective, Nurs Outlook 35:132–135, 1987.

Gonzalez JJ, Ranney J and West J: Nurse-initiated health promotion prompting system in an internal medicine residents' clinic, Southern Med J 82(3):342–344, 1989.

Grace H: Can health care costs be contained?, Nursing & Health Care 11(3):123–130, 1990.

Griffith HM: Strategies for direct third-party reimbursement for nurses, Am J Nurs 82:408, 1982.

Grove SK and Pruitt SS: The health care needs of small company employees, Home Healthcare Nurse 2(5):32, 1984.

Grzeczkowski A and Knapp M: The gerontological nurse practitioner as director of nursing in the long-term care facility, Nurs Management 19(4):64B–64F, 1988.

Hanson C and Martin LL: The nurse practitioner and clinical nurse specialist: should the roles be merged?, J Am Acad Nurse Pract 2(1):2–9, 1990.

Hastings GE, Vick L, Lee G et al.: Nurse practitioners in a jailhouse clinic, Med Care 18(7):731–744, 1980.

Hutchinson S: Self-care and job stress, Image 19(4): 192–196, 1987.

Igoe JB: The school nurse practitioner, Nurs Outlook 23:381, 1975.

Jamieson MK: Block nursing: Practicing autonomous professional nursing in the community, Nursing & Health Care 11(5):250–253, 1990.

Joint Commission on Accreditation of Hospitals: Accreditation manual for hospitals, Chicago, 1976, The Commission.

Kent V and Hanley B: Home health care, Nursing & Health Care 11(5):234–240, 1990.

King EW and Sagan PR: Nurse practitioner liability and authority, Nurs Ad Q 13(4):57–60, 1989.

Kitzman HJ: The CNS and nurse practitioner, In AB Hamric and JA Spross, editors: The clinical nurse specialist in theory and practice ed 2, Philadelphia, 1989, WB Saunders.

Knutson K: What's in a name?, American Nurses' Association Council of Primary Health Care Nurse Practitioners Newsletter 12(3):3–4, 1989.

Kozlowski D: Nurse practitioners: 25 years of quality health care, American Nurses' Association Council of Primary Health Care Nurse Practitioners Newsletter 13(7):4, 1990.

Lamper-Linden C, Goetz-Kulas J, and Lake R: Developing ambulatory care clinics: nurse practitioners as primary providers, J Nurs Adm 13(12):11–18, 1983.

Levitt MK, Stern NB, Becker KL, et al.: A performance appraisal tool for nurse practitioners, Nurs Pract 10(8):28–33, 1985.

Mahoney DF: An economic analysis of the nurse practitioner role, Nurse Pract 13(3):44–45, 1988.

Manley MV: Clinical privileges for nonhospital-based nurses, Am J Nurs 81:1822–1825, 1981.

Maraldo P: The nineties: a decade in search of meaning, Nursing & Health Care 11(1):11–14, 1990.

Martinson I, Jamieson M, O'Grady B and Sime M: The block nurse program, J Community Health Nurs 2(1):21–29, 1985.

McLain B: Collaborative practice: the nurse practitioner's role in its success or failure, Nurse Pract 13(5):31–32, 34–35, 38, 1988.

Molde S and Diers D: Nurse practitioner research: selected literature review and research agenda, Nurs Res 34(6):362, 1985.

National Joint Practice Commission: Statement on joint practice in primary care: definition and guidelines, Chicago, 1977, The Commission.

National League for Nursing: Characteristics of master's education in nursing, New York, 1987, The League.

Paradise RL and Kendall VM: Ambulatory care: primary nursing brings continuity, Nurs Management 16(12):27–30, 1985.

Pearson LJ: Nancy Dirubbo: Fighting for the rights of NPs in private practice, Nurse Pract 11(9):56–61, 1990-91.

Pearson LJ: 190–91 update: how each state stands on legislative issues affecting advanced nursing practice, Nurse Pract 16(1):11–18, 1991.

Richards G: Nonphysician practitioners make slow headway on staff privileges, Hospitals 58(24):82–86, 1984.

Shanks-Meile SL, Shipley AC, Collins PA and Tacker A: Changes in the advertised demand for nurse practitioners in the United States, 1975–1986, Nurse Pract. 14(9):41–2, 44, 49, 1989.

Silver HK, Ford LC and Stearly SA: A program to increase health care for children: the pediatric nurse practitioner program, Pediatrics 39:756–760, 1967.

Sirles A: The potential for the family nurse practitioner in the community, Ala J Med Sci 11(3):229, 1981.

Sirles AT and Smith AE: The administrative and clinical requisites to the implementation of a family nursing center. Paper presented at the Second Annual Family Health Nursing Conference, University of South Florida College of Nursing, Tampa, Fla, April 20, 1990.

Steel J, editor: Issues in collaborative practice, Orlando, Fla, 1986, Grune & Stratton.

Streff MB and Netzer R: Third-party reimbursement. In J.C. McCloskey & H.K. Grace, editors: Current issues in nursing, St. Louis, 1990, Mosby–Year Book, Inc.

Styles MM: Nurse practitioners creating new horizons for the 1990s, Nurse Pract 15(2):48–57, 1990.

Torrey B, Kinsella K and Taeuber C: An aging world, Washington, D.C., 1987, U.S. Department of Commerce, Bureau of the Census.

Touger GN and Butts JK: The workplace: an innovative and cost effective practice site, Nurse Pract 14(1):35–42, 1989.

U.S. Bureau of the Census: Statistical abstracts of the United States: 1989 ed 109, Washington, D.C., 1989.

Wasem C: The Rural Health Clinic Services Act: a sleeping giant of reimbursement, Journal of the American Academy of Nurse Practitioners 2(2):85–87, 1990.

Wilbur J, Zoeller LH, Talashek M and Sullivan JA: Career trends of master's prepared family nurse practitioners, Journal of the American Academy of Nurse Practitioners 2(2):69–78, 1990.

37

The Community Health Nurse Manager

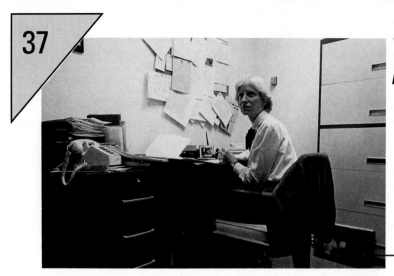

Roberta K. Lee

OBJECTIVES

After reading this chapter, the student should be able to:

Distinguish between the concepts of leader and manager in community health nursing;

Describe the history of management and organization theory;

Apply general systems theory to community health nursing management;

Apply concepts of the management process to community health nursing;

Apply concepts of intervention in public health to community health nursing;

Describe applications of nursing care delivery models in community health nursing;

KEY TERMS

accountability	functional nursing	personal health services
administrator	general systems theory	
ambulatory clinic	health education	primary nursing
authority	home visiting	program budget
block nursing	human resources planning	responsibility
budget		screening clinic
district nursing	leader	sensitive screening test
effective	management process	specific screening test
efficient	manager	strategic plan
financial resources planning	mobile clinics	tactical plan
follower	nursing care delivery model	team nursing
formal structure	organization theory	public health services

T he managerial role of the community health nurse varies tremendously. Some factors that influence the management role include the size and complexity of the organization, the organization's mission and goals, the organizational setting (Fenton, et al., 1988), and the nurse's job description. Understanding the relationships among leaders, followers, managers, and administrators in community health nursing is important. This chapter describes these roles and their interrelationships, briefly reviews organizational theory, and describes the application of the management process within the context of community health nursing.

Leadership is the ability to influence the behavior of others (e.g., colleagues or clients) toward the achievement of a mutually established goal. The leader and follower roles are determined by people's interactions within groups. In contrast, the roles of manager or administrator are jobs within an organization. The role of the manager is to coordinate the efforts of lower level employees (subordinates) to achieve the goals of the organization.

The roles of leader and manager and the roles of follower and subordinate have common characteristics. For example, both leaders and managers are concerned with coordinating individual efforts to achieve goals. The sources of their power, however, are very different. A leader's power is informal and is given to the leader by followers. The manager's power base is formal and is given by the employing organization. Ideally, people with informal leadership skills will be selected for formal management positions in an organization. Unfortunately, this does not always occur.

People selected for management positions in organizations are expected to be skilled in areas such as program development, personnel, and financial management. Depending on the size of the organization and its function, managers may rely more on clinical than management information for problem solving.

Figure 37-1 illustrates the relationship between clinical and management knowledge for the roles of staff nurse, supervisor, and administrator. When an organization is relatively large, these roles and the types of clinical and management responsibilities are very different.

A staff nurse's major responsibilities are providing nursing care to many clients effectively and efficiently. In the management sense, effectiveness means that the nurse assists the client and family to accomplish mutually agreed-upon goals that are consistent with the goals of the organization. Efficiency means that responsibilities are managed in a way that maximizes productivity. Productivity is usually measured by the number of clients served per unit of time (such as average number of clients served per day).

Supervisory roles, especially for middle-level supervisors, require excellent clinical skills as well as management education and expertise (Knollmueller, 1986, 1988). Supervisors guide clinical nursing decisions, manage staff nurses, participate in the management of the organization, and interpret management policies and decisions to staff nurses.

The executive role primarily requires management knowledge and skills. Executives prepare information to document the organization's effectiveness (Porter, 1987) and efficiency for its constituents, usually represented by an elected or appointed board of directors.

Pickett (1980) notes that although most texts on public health administration describe large "ideal" health departments, the most prevalent form of health departments in the United States is the county health department. County health departments are most commonly staffed by one nurse and one sanitarian. The position of public health officer frequently rotates among physicians living in that county. In this situation, community health nurses provide services to clients and manage the organization. They act as clinician, manager, and administrator.

HISTORY OF ORGANIZATION AND MANAGEMENT THEORY

The history of organization theory has three phases: (1) the scientific or classical period, (2) the human relations period, and (3) the contemporary period.

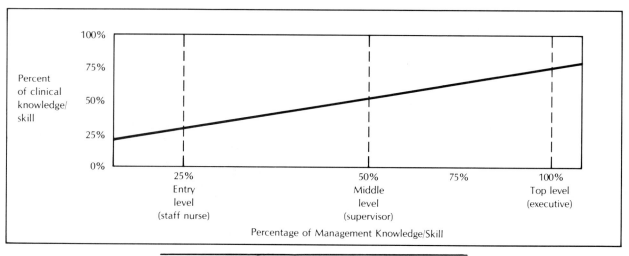

FIGURE 37-1

Clinical and management knowledge.

Scientific Period

The scientific period (approximately 1900 to 1935) is characterized by efforts to understand the relationships between administrative functions (described by Fayol as planning, organizing, directing, and controlling) and production. F.W. Taylor, an engineer, made major contributions to organization theory (Filley and House, 1969). During this period, workers were seen as motivated only by economic rewards, and the organization was characterized by (1) a clearly defined division of labor with highly specialized personnel, and (2) a distinct hierarchy of authority (Etzioni, 1964). Administrative duties, according to classical or scientific thinking, include study of the work, deduction of the "best" or most efficient procedure, selection of the right person(s) for the job, and training personnel in the proper method.

During the scientific period several significant contributions were made to the conceptualization of organizations and administration, including the delineation of management functions; the development of concepts of authority, responsibility, and accountability; and viewing the organization as one unit or entity. Limitations, however, included an incomplete understanding of worker motivations, especially those of non-salaried workers, and the concept of a one-way (administrator to employee) direction for administrative functions.

Human Relations Period

The second major phase in the development of organization theory, the human relations period, began with the writing of Barnard in 1938, who described the interrelationships among the individual, the organization, and the informal organization. Barnard's work, and its extension by Simon in 1947 (Filley and House, 1969), emphasized the human dimension of organizations. This shift in theory was strengthened by the social movement toward formal organization of labor, the emergence of labor unions (e.g., the Wagner Act of 1935), and the Hawthorne studies. These experiments suggested that productivity was affected by attitudes of individuals and the social situation within work groups as well as mechanical efficiency in the plant (Filley and House, 1969).

Contemporary Period

The studies in organization theory that were completed following the Hawthorne findings ultimately concluded that there were limits to the belief that the happy worker or work group is necessarily productive. In the contemporary period, theoretical perspectives regarding administration reflect a blend of the research about types of organizations and research done in organizations. Behavioral science research has contributed to contemporary thinking about administering an organization. One theory that arose from the contemporary period is general systems theory, which can be used to describe community health nursing management.

General Systems Theory

General systems theory states that organizations consist of elements in mutual interaction (Henry et al., 1989). Systems theory uses a general (macro) rather than a specific (micro) perspective by demonstrating overall relationships among the components of the whole organization. According to Stevens (1985), a systems model has at least eight categories of information. One of these is the input-transformation-output process. This can apply to community health nursing.

In community health nursing, the input component includes financial, environmental, staffing, and other resources needed to produce services. In the transformation phase the organizations, personnel, information, and knowledge combine to create an output of community health nursing services (Figure 37.2). An example of the transformation of inputs to the outputs of a community nursing service is illustrated by the following:

There was a request for community health nursing to respond to the need for scoliosis screening in a community's public schools. The Board of Education had eliminated many school nurse positions and lacked sufficient school nurse personnel to screen the large student population. An ad hoc committee of community health staff nurses was selected and was asked to make a recommendation to the nurse administrator. The committee recommended that the community health agency provide school health services (including scoliosis screening) to all public schools.

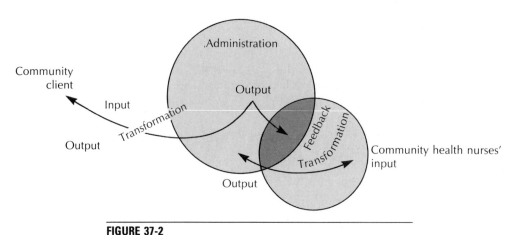

FIGURE 37-2

Transformation phase.

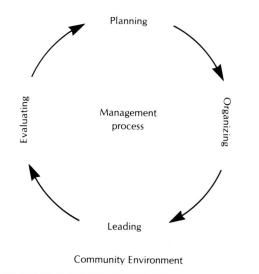

FIGURE 37-3

Management cycle.

In this example, inputs include the request for service from the community (the environment) and the knowledge of the nursing personnel. These were transformed into a recommendation to restructure the delivery of nursing services to the school-age population in the community.

This story also illustrates the interaction between the system's components—the community health organization and the community. The community health organization considered the community's specific request (input) for scoliosis screening. The screening request provided input to the organization, which then requested additional information from the nursing service. Nursing's information and expertise (inputs) were transformed and expressed in a recommendation. The recommendation, viewed by the nurses as a final output, was an additional input to the organization. The program for the community was the organization's output.

THE MANAGEMENT PROCESS

Like the nursing process, the management process is a systematic, cyclical method for solving problems (Figure 37-3). The management process includes four major functions: planning, organizing, leading, and evaluating. The major concern of management is to provide community health nursing services effectively and efficiently. In management theory, effectiveness is measured by comparing the organization's performance with its philosophy, goals, and objectives. In community health nursing, effectiveness relates to the nurse's role in reduction of risk factors, morbidity, and mortality in the population. According to management theory, efficiency relates to attaining goals in ways that minimize costs and maximize benefits. Costs include salaries, fringe benefits, equipment, supplies, secretarial services, and office space and maintenance.

Planning

Often planning results in change by creating, revising, or eliminating resources available to members of a community. The community health nurse must be knowledgeable about change theory and develop skill in its application to practice.

Planning was not emphasized as much in the past as it is today. Planning involves deciding what will be done (goals and objectives) and how it will be done. It is a managerial function that occurs at all levels within an organization. Planning is probably the most time consuming and most complex of the management process functions. As a concept, it is similar to primary prevention. Planning can be classified as either strategic or tactical (Newman, Warren, McGill, 1987).

Strategic planning is the process that determines basic organizational goals and directions. It is long-term and includes ends (outcomes) as well as means (processes). Community health nurse managers use epidemiological data and community assessment data to develop strategic plans. For example, if the firearm mortality data in Figure 37-4 represented the community, the community nurse executive may include as an objective in the strategic plan reduction of firearm mortality among males aged 15 to 24.

In contrast, tactical planning uses shorter time frames, a narrower scope, more attention to detail and is more flexible (Newman, Warren, and McGill, 1987). An example of the tactical phase of planning is the work involved in establishing programs to reduce risk factors for firearm mortality in the target population.

At all levels of management, the planning process requires decision-making skills. Like the nursing process, planning begins with assessment of the relevant information. All information needed may not be available; and it is common to prepare a plan based on partial information, implement the plan, and not achieve the desired objectives. Critically reviewing all aspects of the plan, including the objectives and the plan itself, is necessary to identify and solve planning problems.

An example of the importance of planning can be shown in the following situation:

Prompted by a nursing student's assessment that hypertension was prevalent in their apartment complex, some senior citizens requested the local health department to set up a weekly blood pressure screening clinic in their building. Assuming the student had validated the findings, a district nursing supervisor assigned a staff nurse to set up such a clinic each Thursday and to notify the residents about the service. The clinic was set up and notices were sent out. After three weeks, only four residents had attended. There were numerous phone calls from local physicians questioning the need for this clinic. The drug store and a neighborhood center less than three blocks away notified the administrator that they did free blood pressure screening.

A plan to set up a blood pressure screening clinic had been made. Management of the clinic was assigned to the staff nurse, who was responsible for conducting the clinic. However, evaluation of the clinic six weeks later indicated that it was a "failure." In this case, incomplete assessment of the situation had led to the mistaken conclusion that an unmet need existed. Although the tactical plan for actual implementation of the clinic was appropriate, its establishment was an inappropriate strategic plan in this situation.

The following example shows a situation where the strategic plan was appropriate:

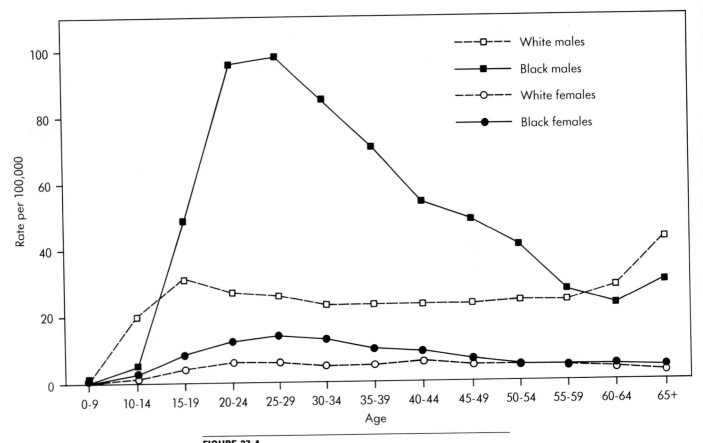

FIGURE 37-4

Firearm mortality rates by race and sex, United States, 1986.

A community health nurse was making home visits to several elderly persons who had initially been referred to the agency for medical and nursing care problems. Over time, their medical and nursing care problems were resolved. However, the nurse was reluctant to stop services because these people were socially isolated and valued the interpersonal contact the nurse provided. The nurse discussed this problem with representatives of a local church. The church planned and implemented a "Friendly Visitor" program to socially isolated elderly people who were referred and introduced by the nurse. The nurse then discontinued nursing care to these families.

This demonstrates success in planning. In both examples, the tactic to implement the clinic and program were adequate. However, in the first example, the strategy was inappropriate because it duplicated a service that was already available. In the second example, the nurse helped plan a new and appropriate community service, and the result was successful from the viewpoint of strategic planning.

Planning for Nursing Care

Staff nurses in community health agencies contribute to the organization through planning. An example of day-to-day planning is managing work activities. The community health nurse is frequently assigned to clinics, which operate on a regularly scheduled basis, or to home visits and other activities. Effective and efficient use of time is essential.

For example, arriving at a family's home without essential equipment may require a return trip to the office. In this situation, lack of planning results in waste of the nurse's time (salary) and excess travel costs (the nurse's salary associated with travel time and actual travel expenses). The client's time is also wasted with nonproductive visits, and nursing care for other clients may have to be postponed.

Community health nurses also plan for comprehensive client care. The nurse may call a meeting of all agencies that are providing services to an individual or family to establish a plan of care. Planning objectives may include coordinating services and ensuring the client's needs are met. Interagency conferences are especially common for multiproblem families.

Another aspect of planning includes personal planning. If the nurse is expected to provide transportation during the work day, vehicles must be adequately maintained, maps are needed, and local weather conditions must be checked. For example, community health nurses in Minneapolis must winterize their vehicles in October to prepare for the winter ice and snow.

Community health nurses are frequently involved in planning for established clinics, such as child health and antepartum clinics, and for sporadic clinics, such as health fairs. Planning for these services involves marketing and advertising, arranging for space and equipment, planning for staff and volunteers, record keeping, and follow-up of clients.

Financial Resources Planning

Planning is incomplete without a budget. Simply stated, a budget is a plan stated in financial terms, and it identifies the costs associated with implementing the plan. Implementing any type of program requires money. In community health, funding comes from several resources. Adequate funding for programs is essential for successful community health organizations.

A budget is required by law, and regardless of the organization, the nurse needs to know how much money is available and required for nursing services. Budgets can be classified as program budgets or departmental budgets.

In a program budget, expenses and income are related to a specific service, such as a rubella immunization program. A program budget directly relates financial planning to the evaluation of program outcomes. For example, the costs of a hypertension screening program are directly related to the "savings" associated with reducing the incidence of cardiovascular disease mortality and morbidity (Hypertension Detection and Follow-Up Program, 1979). The major disadvantage of program-based budgeting is that a separate budget is required for each program. A multiservice agency may have 40 or 50 separate programs and budgets, which increases the cost of managing the total organization.

The departmental budget shows the services to be provided in return for the funds available or income generated by each department in the organization (such as community nursing, laboratory, and sanitation). The advantage of departmental budgeting is that it provides more exact information on the cost per unit of services. Disadvantages include the difficulty of developing this type of budget and the danger of placing equivalent values on different services (e.g., comparing the cost per rubella immunization with the cost per home visit by the nursing department). A more appropriate focus would be to compare outcomes, such as increased levels of immunization of children after new mothers have been taught the need for immunizations by nurses.

The way financial resources are obtained frequently determines which budgeting method will be used. For example, Medicare requires specific budgeting procedures that are very different from budgets generated for grant applications.

Human Resources Planning

The heart of any service organization is the human resources that have been attracted to the organization: the human knowledge and skills available that will plan and implement programs. In human resources planning the type, classification, availability, and combination of needed personnel must be identified. Depending on the needs of the programs, the staff usually includes professional and nonprofessional personnel.

Establishing policies, procedures, and job descriptions is also part of human resources planning. Job descriptions define employee work, the work-role relationship, and areas for performance evaluation. Policies and procedures provide guidelines for employees when implementing programs. They also help set standards of behavior in the relationship between a community and the organization.

Personnel need to be used appropriately. For example, in a large child health clinic with technicians, volunteers, and other nonprofessional staff members, community health nurses are poorly used if they set up the clinic, make appointments, clean the room and order supplies. Another example is using a community health nurse to do mass vision-screening when volunteers, school health aides, or other technical personnel can be taught the procedure under the nurse's direction.

Organizing

Once the plan, money, and personnel are available, the next step is organization. Organizing involves arranging and defining the relationships among personnnel and other resources.

Formal and Informal Structure

The organization of any agency involves a formal and informal structure, and the nurse must be aware of both. Communication must occur not only within a program or department but also with other units of the organization and among individuals and agencies outside the organization. The system must effectively use selected and trained personnel and available resources.

Nursing Care Delivery Models in Community Health

The work of community health nurses, especially in large agencies, is often organized using a nursing care delivery model. These models facilitate supervision of employees and assignment of specific work tasks to individuals.

The type of nursing care delivery model used by an agency is related to the size and complexity of the organization. Small organizations often employ only one staff nurse; large agencies may employ more than a hundred nurses. Nursing staff members frequently have multiple assignments, including both clinics and home visits. The amount of the nurse's time spent in a clinic versus the home varies greatly (Cayner, 1985), depending on the service offered.

PRIMARY NURSING. Small agencies usually use a variation of the primary nursing model. In this method the individual nurse is responsible for individual clients and families who are referred to the agency for service and who meet the agency's admissions standards, which often include a geographic factor. In community health, this method is called district nursing. The nurse may be responsible for all cases within the agency's jurisdiction. District nursing is similar to primary nursing in that the client usually has only one nurse, who assumes total responsibility for the client's care. Block nursing (Bremer, 1987, 1989; Corcoran et al., 1988; Jamieson, 1989) is a contemporary term for district nursing.

If several nurses are employed and the geographic area is large, it is common to divide the area and assign a nurse to each division. This nursing care delivery model reduces travel time and travel expense. It requires each nurse to be skilled in nursing care of all client-family problems that may occur.

FUNCTIONAL NURSING. The functional nursing method assigns staff nurses and other personnel to functions such as client medications, treatments, hygiene, and teaching. Functional nursing has its roots in the scientific period of management theory, which focused on identifying the most efficient "assembly line." It is used by some agencies, especially those whose focus is home care of sick individuals. The client and family may receive care from a staff nurse responsible for nursing care planning and teaching, a practical nurse who alternates with the staff nurse and provides medications and treatments, and a home health aide who assists with hygiene and homemaker services. This nursing care delivery model can be justified when the use of lower-salaried personnel offsets the additional staff members' travel costs.

A variation of the functional approach is to assign staff according to client diagnostic categories. In this approach, one nurse may be assigned to all clients with tuberculosis, and a different nurse's assignment may be limited to antepartum clients. This model tries to improve nursing care quality by employing nurses with special expertise in major clinical problems rather than expecting each nurse to maintain competence in all categories. This approach is often combined with the primary or district method.

Team Nursing

In the team nursing model, a team of staff provides nursing care to a group of clients. The staff's work is coordinated by a designated team leader. Some community health agencies, especially larger agencies, have adapted team nursing to the community setting.

One type of team approach is a combination of team nursing and district nursing. Staff members are assigned to a geographic area to provide care to all clients in that area. A team leader, usually an experienced community health nurse, is appointed. This position is a permanent assignment similar to the position of head nurse in a hospital. Depending on the agency's policies, nurses may be assigned to their own case load. The team leader may assign clients with certain nursing care problems to less experienced staff to develop the staff nurse's skills. In this situation, the team leader should plan for time to adequately supervise the inexperienced staff nurse so that the nurse learns and quality assurance objectives are ensured.

In another variation of the team approach, the team leader has the responsibility of nursing care planning and scheduling home visits. A master schedule is developed, and team members are assigned to clients or families on a daily or weekly basis. Team members do not have permanent case loads. This application is more commonly found in hospital-based home care organizations where staff move from the hospital to the home environment when providing nursing care. In this situation, the team leader assumes greater responsibility for coordinating care for each client and family and determining which personnel should be assigned. This approach is similar to the case method of delivering care that was popular in hospitals in the 1920s.

These nursing care delivery models have been applied to home visits in the past and are still in use in community health nursing. Because of the high cost of delivering services in the home, administrators have urged the expansion of clinics and other approaches that increase the number of clients seen per day.

Leading

With an appropriate plan and a clearly defined organization, the community health nurse directs implementation of the plan. The concept of leadership is broader than the concept of management. Managers establish and require adherence to policies and procedures to meet organizational goals. Managers have the formal authority of the organization to direct and evaluate the work of subordinate employees.

Leaders try to develop fresh approaches to long-standing problems and to create new options to resolve problems. These new options are not always consistent with organizational goals. An effective leader shapes ideas into images that excite people and only then develops choices to implement the conceived ideas. Followers support a leader's ideas and their implementation. In the small public health organization, a nurse's leadership affects other persons, groups, and organizations in the community.

Nurse managers will see that all referrals are handled and that a systematic approach is used to carry out each request. If managers are leaders and use leadership skills, they can create an environment that allows creativity and risk-taking to meet the requirements of the organization. Leaders and managers differ in their views of their work. Leaders often view work as an enabling process, involving an interaction of people and ideas to establish strategies and make decisions. Managers often view work as the accomplishment of organization goals.

Community health nurses display leadership activities constantly as they implement nursing care. Community health nurses should learn about their leadership style and the likely consequences associated with that style by using available self-tests (Kirkpatrick, 1987). Staff members also need to understand the leadership style of the nurse manager and their own behavior as followers to promote effective functioning.

Evaluating and Controlling

Community health nurse managers are responsible for ensuring that there is an ongoing evaluation of the implemented plan. The community health agency is accountable to the community for the quality of its care, and accountability is ensured by an effective evaluation process. Evaluation includes examining the original plan and its rationale, the organization of a program, its financial and human resources, and to what extent goals were achieved. Evaluation may determine that there is a need for reorganization. Standards for evaluation of the community nursing service have been developed by the American Nurses Association and the National League for Nursing in collaboration with the American Public Health Association (see Appendix).

MANAGEMENT PROCESS IN COMMUNITY HEALTH
Community Health Values

The management process involves consideration of community health values (e.g., primary health care), providing services that will benefit the entire community at the least expense, and prevention (Beauchamp, 1980; Lanik and Webb, 1989; Jenkins, 1989). Medical care organizations value providing services to individuals and treatment of illness. It is important to understand the effects these values have on community health nursing management.

Community Health Goals

In community health organizations, it is desireable to specify organizational goals and objectives in terms that describe a community's health. Miller and Moos (1981) note renewed interest in using measures of community health such as rates of morbidity and mortality to define an organization's objectives and program outcomes. For example, if a community has a high fertility rate among adolescents, a reduction of the rate could be an objective of the public health agency. Developing and implementing a health services program for adolescents, including family planning services, could then be a program strategy for achieving the objective.

Community Health Interventions
Regulations

Community health nurses may be involved in implementing regulations for a communicable disease case and contact follow-up, especially for infectious hepatitis and tuberculosis. In these situations, the public health concern is protection of the noninfected members of the community by adequately treating diagnosed cases and identifying, diagnosing, and potentially treating people who have been exposed. All states have communicable disease regulations as part of their public health laws. When functioning as a regulator, the community health nurse must implement the regulations legally and uniformly.

It is possible for a regulation to become outdated not only because the regulation is old, but also because improved prevention and treatment have eliminated a disease from the population. For example, because of the virtual elimination of smallpox worldwide, immunizations are no longer required for school children or for travelers to foreign countries. In such cases, nurses may be involved in the political process of changing the laws and regulations.

Community health nurses are also involved in implementing legally required screening programs and following potential or identified cases. An example is metabolic screening of newborn infants for phenylketonuria (PKU) and other inherited diseases. Because of shorter hospitalization for child birth, community health nurses are frequently involved in obtaining blood tests and following up on infants with suspicious or positive test results. Although it may appear expensive to implement this legislation, screening is less expensive than chronic, long-term medical care for persons with untreated PKU.

Community health nurses may also be employed in positions in which regulation is the major job responsibility. Nurses are involved with other interdisciplinary team members in regulating the hospital and nursing home industries. The role is to verify that organizations meet or exceed established standards.

Nurses sometimes collaborate with other community health professionals to improve services in a community. For example, environmental health professionals may be involved in implementing regulations affecting day care facilities. A community health nurse working with that team may have opportunities to improve health practices in day care facilities by providing education to the day care staff on managing ill children, identifying children who are neglected or abused, preventing injuries, and promoting normal growth and development.

When nurses implement regulations, self-management, including interpersonal communication, is important. Although there are laws to protect the health of citizens, everyone may not agree that the laws and regulations are appropriate. Some people may believe that their individual rights are improperly constrained when they are faced with regulations. Others may resist because they are misinformed. The community health nurse should be sensitive to these issues and provide information to gain cooperation from the concerned individuals. Adopting a collaborative, assisting approach results in cooperation more frequently than a controlling approach. However, if the individual and family continue to refuse required service, the community health nurse needs to use the resources available in the community, such as referring a family that is noncompliant with PKU screening to child protective services.

Depending on the specific goals and objectives of the organization, community health nurses may be highly involved in regulatory strategies to promote community health. Assessing clients and their families for signs of neglect and abuse or assessing a work environment for minimal hygiene standards is part of every community health nurse's practice. However, community health nurses tend to perceive themselves as service providers rather than service regulators.

Health Services

Providing personal health services, especially to the medically indigent or disadvantaged, has not been highly valued among public health professionals. However, most community health programs are heavily involved in this intervention strategy (Pickett, 1980). Community health nurses are especially involved in managing the delivery of personal health services. Among the several methods of service delivery are ambulatory clinics, mobile clinics, screening clinics, and home-based services.

AMBULATORY CLINICS. In this approach, clients are scheduled for ambulatory clinic services at a central location. Personnel may include physicians, nurses, aides, nutritionists, social workers, and volunteers. Especially for child and adult health screening or immunizations, these clinics are managed by nurses, either alone or with clerical staff. Clinics may be located in small communities or in suburban areas. The organization arranges for space, and the nurse brings the appropriate supplies. Appointments may be scheduled or may be on a drop-in basis.

Using clinics to increase nurse efficiency has advantages and disadvantages. Nurse travel time is reduced, but client travel time is increased. Travel to a clinic site may be difficult or impossible for some clients. It is difficult to assess the home environment during a clinic interview. If drop-in appointments are allowed, maintaining consistent client charts and assessing the client-family history are problems. Some clients attend nurse-managed clinic appointments and find that they need physician evaluation, which may require an additional trip to another location. In some areas, it is difficult to find adequate facilities to provide clinic services. Finally, immediate access to a physician (e.g., in the case of an allergic reaction to an immunization) may be difficult to accommodate.

With any clinic setting, time management may be a problem. In large clinics that use a variety of health professionals a triage system is usually necessary. The nurse may be responsible for determining whether a visit with the nutritionist is necessary for the client. In complex clinics, priorities are frequently established to assist the nurse in triage. For example, a pregnant woman might be referred for nutrition services only if her hematocrit is below 34% or if she gains more than 5 pounds in 1 month. Volunteers are also used in clinic situations and can be very helpful by performing nonnursing tasks such as registering clients, measuring height and weight, and putting clients in the examination rooms. However, it can take a tremendous amount of work to organize, schedule, and supervise volunteers.

Recording data can be another problem in the clinic setting. Nurses must complete a client's record before beginning to interview the next client. If a nurse interviews 20 antepartum clients or the mothers of 50 children before immunizations, it is not possible to complete client records accurately at the end of the clinic session.

MOBILE CLINICS. Specially equipped mobile vans have been used to provide mobile clinic services. They decrease the problems of inadequate physical facilities and transportation of supplies and increase the opportunity to provide services in a greater variety of geographic areas. With this approach, it is essential to communicate the scheduled locations well in advance. The costs of adequately outfitting and maintaining mobile clinics can be high.

SCREENING CLINICS. Management of screening clinic operations is not very different from any other type of clinic. However, there are differences in planning the procedures and follow-up. The purpose of screening clinics is the early detection of specific health problems. Screening clinics may be single-purpose or multipurpose (multiphasic). The multiphasic screening clinic screens individuals for more than one health problem or risk factor during one clinic encounter. Computerized multiphasic screening programs are a recent approach (U.S. D.H.H.S., 1985), and these can be used in many settings.

Important issues must be considered in planning screening clinics. Screening is intended to identify unrecognized or undiagnosed disease or risk factors in aggregates of the population. Since most diseases are rare (occurring in less than one person per thousand) the proportion of a population to be diagnosed is small compared with the population risk. Therefore, the target population for screening is usually quite large. It is essential to use a screening test that can be administered quickly and inexpensively. Sensitive screening tests (which correctly classify infected persons as diseased) and specific screening tests (which correctly classify healthy persons) are necessary. Most screening tests have some disadvantages. Planning for screening clinics should include procedures to minimize the problems associated with misclassification. An example would be a screening test that is highly sensitive but not highly specific for AIDS infection; in this case a positive HIV-III test reliably predicts an AIDS infection, but a negative HIV-III test does not ensure noninfection. If the test is negative, the

client should be advised that the test could be wrong and additional testing or counseling should be arranged.

Other aspects of planning include establishing a method for recording, reporting, and following-up people with positive screening tests. Marketing the screening program involves informing the target population about the availability of screening and working with others such as physicians and neighborhood leaders, for support for the screening clinic. Notifying the target population may mean advertising in the media (including radio, television, and newspapers). It may also mean personal contact with each person in the eligible population by letter or telephone.

Planning for follow-up care or the definitive diagnosis of people with positive tests is as important as any other aspect of screening. However, it is often minimally addressed in the planning process. In many screening clinics, follow-up care is limited to interpreting the test results to the person and advising people with positive tests to seek further evaluation. However, it may be necessary to contact persons with positive tests once again: this contact would determine whether the advice to seek further evaluation had been followed and to learn the results of the evaluation. It is also necessary to rate existing community resources for the client's evaluation and necessary treatment. For example, the Hypertension Detection and Follow-Up Program (1979) illustrated the benefits that could be obtained through population-based screening, referral, treatment, and follow-up. This program found that overall mortality as well as cardiovascular mortality could be reduced if hypertension was detected and effectively treated.

HOME VISITS. Managing a home visit schedule, especially one that involves clients needing health promotion and others with communicable diseases, can be complex. The problems encountered in a hospital environment (the need to return to the nurse's station to obtain additional equipment or the delay in changing a dressing because the client has gone to physical therapy) are heightened in the community setting. Many organizations have policies to prioritize clients. The guidelines involve the client's physical and psychosocial condition and the organization's past experiences with the client. If the client is new to the organization, the priority for service is usually high, and contact should occur within 24 hours of the referral. Once a thorough assessment has been completed and a plan of care established, predicting the type and frequency of additional home visits is easier. The information available to the nurse on the referral form is often limited to the person's name, address, and reason for the visit. A thorough assessment is thus essential. A prompt assessment also promotes rapid feedback to the person or organization that initiated the referral. Informal data suggest that a prompt response to people who refer clients including information about the client situation tends to result in future referrals. For an organization whose main income is from home care, maintaining referral networks is important. Rapid response to referrals and rapid feedback are important management aspects of the community nurse's role.

Harris (1987) states that when planning for the home visit, nurses should realize that new clients frequently require about twice the average visit time. The usual 30 to

45 minutes is doubled in completing the admission and data base assessments and establishing a relationship with the client and family. More time is also required when two people (e.g., mother and infant) require assessment.

Community health nurse's must also be knowledgeable about other community resources. Some communities publish books about the services available in the community. Other communities have an "information and referral" service that functions as a clearing house for information about available services. It is more efficient to telephone the information and referral service than to telephone ten agencies to find out if a particular client's needs can be met.

The need for efficiency in home visiting also applies to time spent recording, completing billing records, consulting with other professionals, supervising home health aides, and telephoning. Hemphill et al. (1988) advocate the use of flow sheets to increase recording efficiency. Using patient classification systems and focused recording for service evaluation is becoming common (Weidmann and North, 1987; Harris, 1985; Kosidlak and Kerpelmann, 1987). Community health nurses should be skilled in using dictating machines and computers for recording their reports.

Monitoring and improving the effectiveness and efficiency of community health nursing is accomplished through supervision (Knollmueller, 1988). Home visiting as an intervention strategy is generally an independent nursing activity, and many community health nurses enjoy the autonomy it affords. However, when nurses are confronted with new client situations, it is difficult to know whether the assessment data are accurate and complete and whether the nursing diagnosis and intervention plans are appropriate. It is likely that no one else knows the family and thus the only set of client data is that collected by the nurse. In these situations, community health nurses should seek supervision, which may include telephone conferences, office conferences, and joint home visits. A positive supervisor-nurse relationship makes it easier for nurses to obtain assistance in non-routine client situations.

In organizations that employ many community health nurses, it is possible to share complex clients with another staff nurse. Examples of appropriate situations include (1) families with a history of child abuse, especially if home visits have been ordered by juvenile courts or if legal proceedings are anticipated, (2) families that are caring for terminally ill family members at home, and (3) clients or families who require complex interventions from multiple agencies. Sharing cases like these can help reduce the nurse's frustration and potential for burnout.

Although it is necessary to be informed about changes in nursing and to maintain licensure in some states, continuing education can be complex in community health nursing, especially if the nurse visits clients with a wide variety of nursing diagnoses. Organization-sponsored staff development activities are one way to maintain competence. Attending staff development programs offered by hospitals is another method. Regular reading of professional journals and active involvement in professional associations are also beneficial. Many community health nurses also identify expert nurses in the local area and develop informal consulting relationships with them. Thus, when the nurse needs help

with a specific nursing care problem, expert advice may be obtained by telephone.

From the perspective of administration, home care tends to be viewed as an expensive approach to delivering nursing care. In some cases it is the only available approach. In others, home visiting continues because it is a tradition. Since the development of diagnosis-related groups, delivery of home care services has dramatically changed (Humphrey, 1988). Most agencies are now proprietary or are managed by hospitals.

Health Education

Health education implies education of the entire community about health. It is different than teaching an individual on a one-to-one basis. Presenting information verbally is one teaching strategy. Instructional strategies for health education also include video productions for television and preparing posters and pamphlets for different settings.

Community health nurses are frequently involved as content experts in preparing media productions. In this situation, nurses may work with photographers, graphic artists, and others to develop instructional materials that are relevant, accurate, and marketable. Community health nurses may also use these materials in instructing individuals and groups about health matters. It is appropriate for the nurse to maintain a file of pamphlets and other materials to use in implementing teaching plans with clients, families, and other groups. Clients may find they have questions later, when the nurse is not available. If instructional materials are given to clients, the information is available at any time.

Research

Community health nurses are often involved in research. This may include participation in data collection activities (e.g., completion of communicable disease reports), development of epidemiological studies of specific diseases, or studies of nursing care problems. In most communities it is relatively simple to monitor age, race, and sex-specific causes of mortality. Information about morbidity is much more difficult to obtain.

The community health nurse often uses epidemiological data to identify groups in the population that are at higher risk of developing specific health problems (Figure 37-4). These data identify target populations for intervention. Understanding incidence, prevalence, risk factors, and rates of a disease is essential in developing appropriate intervention strategies and methods of evaluating the interventions. For example, if a nurse determines that the adolescent firearm homicide mortality rate in the community is high, it may be appropriate to intervene. In this situation, the immediate target population is all adolescents. A secondary target population may be elementary school children; teaching them ways to resolve conflicts could be a prevention strategy. The nurse should identify the risk factors associated with adolescent firearm mortality and generate a list of possible intervention strategies, classifying them as primary, secondary, or tertiary preventions. Next the nurse would establish goals, objectives, and evaluation criteria and prepare budget estimates. It is essential to establish a method for collecting surveillance data. Community health nurses are frequently

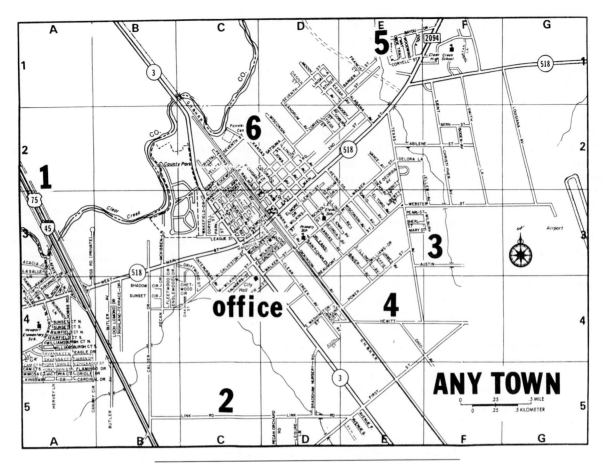

FIGURE 37-5

Anytown, USA.

are frequently involved in collecting surveillance data, especially when existing data collection systems are inappropriate or inadequate.

Participating in epidemiological investigations may lead to the development of new community health services or other interventions. Nurses must consider the ethical dilemmas associated with participation in these studies. A current example is the epidemiological research regarding AIDS. In studying the epidemiology of this public health problem, investigators are monitoring entire populations, usually on a voluntary basis, for HIV-III antibodies. Identifying this subpopulation and its characteristics and monitoring the group prospectively is important to fully understanding the AIDS epidemiology. However, what measures should be taken to ensure confidentiality for persons who volunteer to be screened? If screening is included as part of a pre-employment examination, should the employer have access to the test results? What services should be available to persons with positive tests? What services should be available to sexual partners of persons with positive tests? Responding to these and other ethical questions before initiating research, surveillance, and possibly intervention projects is a professional responsibility.

CLINICAL APPLICATION

A community health nurse plans to visit the following six clients today. After reading the case summaries, the reader

should plan the sequence of visits. The nurse must include 30 minutes for lunch and return to the office by 3:30 PM for a staff meeting. Figure 37-5 is a map showing the location of the nurse's office and the clients' homes (corresponding by the client numbers that follow).

1. Miss James is a 16-year-old who delivered a 6-lb, 3-oz son at County Hospital last night. She had no prenatal care. She lives with her parents. She signed out of the hospital 8 hours after delivery. This is the nurse's first visit.

2. Mr. Andrews has severe chronic obstructive lung disease. He is on 2 to 4 litres of oxygen per nasal cannula at home. He sees no reason to quit smoking at this late date. You have been instructing his wife in the use of a home intermittent positive pressure breathing device and in chest physical therapy. She has called to report that he has had a temperature of 102 degrees since yesterday.

3. Bill McKay is a 6-year-old who was born with myelomeningocele. He is paraplegic. You are instructing his new foster mother on catheterization. She is doing well.

4. Mrs. Fristan is a 53-year-old insulin-dependent diabetic. She has a draining, gangrenous right foot. The culture report is antibiotic-resistant staphylococcus aureus. You are to soak the foot and apply a dressing. She is scheduled to leave the house for hyperbaric oxygen therapy at 1:00 PM.

5. Mr. Landers is a 70-year-old man with serious chronic

congestive heart failure who lives alone. He is an alcoholic who alternates between sobriety and beer-and-pretzel binges. When you call to arrange the appointment, you note he is short of breath and you hear gurgling as he breathes. He is complaining of chest pain.

6. Mrs. Stoddard is at 28 weeks gestation with twins. She is on bed rest and home-monitoring for premature labor. She has called, frantic because the two older children are both running high fevers and are very irritable. She mentions that her baby-sitter's children just got over chicken pox.

Planning

After reviewing these case summaries, it may be very tempting to advise driving immediately to Mr. Landers's or Miss James's home, depending on one's personal view about the priority needs of these clients. However, it would be wise to take a few minutes to plan the schedule for the day.

Care for patients who are experiencing life-threatening health problems should not wait until the community health nurse can arrive to assess their condition. In this situation, the nurse's most appropriate response is to telephone the physician or hospital to arrange for an ambulance. Or the nurse can call the community's emergency medical services (EMS) team.

Organizing

Three clients have high priority for visits early in the day. They are Miss James, Mr. Andrews, and Mr. Landers. The next step in setting up appointments is to consider geography and establish a visit sequence that will minimize travel time. The remaining clients, except for Mrs. Fristan, could be seen at any time, depending on the efficiency of travel time. Mrs. Fristan should probably be seen last to minimize the possibility that the nurse could inadvertently infect another client. Isolation procedures in the home environment are often difficult.

Mr. Andrews and Mr. Landers may also require longer-than-average visits. The available information suggests that the nurse may need to refer these clients to the physician, pharmacy, and possibly the hospital for additional services. Many community nurses carry notebooks with information about each client (if client records are not available in the home) so that the referral process can be expedited from

the client's home rather than waiting until the nurse returns to the office.

Implementing

Although the nurse plans to visit each of these clients today, the plan must be flexible. The nurse may anticipate that a home visit will last 30 minutes but, after arriving at the client's home, could find that the visit will require more time. For example, assume that the nurse telephones Mr. Landers's physician before the visit, anticipating arrangements for hospitalization. The physician, however, orders serial doses of Lasix to be given in the home until diuresis occurs. The visit may not require additional time, depending on how many doses will be needed and on whether this therapy is effective. The nurse may receive a telephone call at a patient's home and find that an additional client requires a home visit that day. It may be necessary to reschedule or work overtime, depending on the situation.

Evaluating

In managing a caseload of clients, evaluation includes the services provided to several individuals and their families.

SUMMARY

Until recently, sophisticated management concepts have not been applied to community health nursing. Articles about computerization of records, development of client classification systems (including DRGs) and outcomes are relatively new in the community health nursing literature. The sophistication of community health nursing research, regarding both practice and management, will likely increase in the coming years.

Values about community and health have shaped a philosophy of public health and a set of basic intervention strategies. These intervention strategies (regulation, service, education, and research) are broader than those typically associated with nursing. Additionally, service is most commonly given to the individual client and family. Nurses employed in community health most frequently intervene with clients; however, these clients receive nursing service because they are members of target populations. Application of the nursing management process by community health nurses within public health is essential to the client, the agency, and the community.

KEY CONCEPTS

Leadership implies the ability to influence the behavior of others (colleagues or clients) to achieve a mutually established goal or objective.

The role of the manager is to coordinate the efforts of subordinates to attain goals and objectives as determined by the organization.

Strategic planning is long-range and includes ends (outcomes) and means (processes). In contrast, tactical planning uses shorter time frames, narrower scope, more attention to detail, and more flexibility.

In the program budget, expenses and income are related to a specific service. The performance budget clearly and concisely shows services to be provided in return for available funds or generated income.

The heart of any service organization is the people that have been attracted to the organization.

Organizing involves arranging and defining the relationships among personnel and other resources by establishing a structure.

The type of nursing care delivery model used by an agency is related to the size and complexity of the agency.

In small agencies, the nursing care delivery model most frequently used is a variation of primary nursing.

The functional nursing care delivery model assigns staff nurses and other personnel to client functions such as medications, treatments, hygiene, and teaching clients.

In the team nursing-care delivery model, a team of staff nurses provides nursing care to a group of clients.

The concept of leadership is broader than the concept of management. Leaders strive to develop fresh approaches to long-standing problems and to create new options to resolve problems.

Evaluation includes reexamining the original plan, its rationale, the organization, its financial and human resources, and the degree to which goals were achieved.

Public health work may be defined as an interdisciplinary activity that seeks to provide the greatest good for the greatest number of people at the least cost, with the purpose of maintaining or improving the level of health in a population.

LEARNING ACTIVITIES

1. Interview some community health nurses and have them describe their work relationships within their organization(s) and with other community agencies. Diagram these relationships to identify the community health nurse's work environment or system.

2. Read the job description for a community health nurse manager or administrator. Identify the types of planning that are required in the position.

3. Discuss the plan for assigning work to staff nurses in the agency where you have clinical experience. Identify the nursing care delivery model used by the agency.

4. Assess community need and identify a program that should be developed. Prepare a brief plan for the program (goals, objectives, financial and human resources, and evaluation criteria). Describe how you visualize the management role of the community health nurse in this program.

5. Write a four-paragraph paper (one paragraph each on planning, organizing, leading, and evaluation) describing how you have managed nursing care in the clinical component of your community health nursing course.

Bibliography

Beauchamp DE: Public health and individual liberty, Annu Rev Public Health 1:121-136, 1980.

Bremer A: A description of community health nursing practice with the community-based elderly, J Community Health Nurs 6(3):173-184, 1989.

Bremer A: Revitalizing the district model for the delivery of prevention-focused community health nursing services, Family and Community Health 10(2):1-10, 1987.

Cayner A: Home visiting by public health nurses: a vanishing resource for families and children, zero to three, National Center for Clinical Infant Programs 6(1), 1-7, 1985.

Corcoran J, Hill N, Credle J, et al: Improving the delivery of services in a local health department: Integration versus block, Public Health Nursing 5(2):76-80, 1988.

Dawson J: The use of computers in public health

nursing: today or tomorrow, Canadian Nurse, 81:40-43, 1985.

Etzioni A: Modern organizations, Englewood Cliffs, NJ, 1964, Prentice-Hall, Inc.

Fenton MV, Rounds L, and Iha S: The nursing center in a rural community: The promotion of family and community health, Family and Community Health 11(2):14-24, 1988.

Filley A and House RJ: Managerial process and organizational behavior, Glenview, Ill, 1969, Scott, Foresman & Co.

Freeman RB: Community health nursing practice, Philadelphia, 1970, WB Saunders.

Harris MD, Peters DA, Yuan J: Relating quality and cost in a home health care agency, Quality Review Bulletin 13(5):175-81, 1987.

Henry B, Arndt C, DiVincenti M, Marriner-Torney A: Dimensions of Nursing Administration: Theory, Research, Education, Practice, Cam-

bridge, Mass, 1989, Blackwell Scientific Publications.

Humphrey CJ: The home as a setting for care: clarifying the boundaries of practice, Nursing Clinics of North America 23(2):305-314, 1988.

Hypertension Detection and Follow-up Program Cooperative Groups: Five-year findings of the hypertension detection and follow-up program, I and II, JAMA 23:2562-77, 1979.

Jamieson M, Campbell J, and Clarke S: The block nurse program, Gerontologist 29(1):124-127, 1989.

Kirkpatrick TO: Supervision: A Situational Approach, Boston, 1987, Kent Publishing Co.

Knollmueller RN: Community health nursing supervisor: a handbook for community/home care managers, New York, 1986, National League for Nursing.

Knollmueller RN: Reshaping supervisory practice in home care, Nurs Clin North Am 23(2):353-362, 1988.

Kosidlak JG and Kerpelmann KB: Managing community health nursing: A personal computer tool for assessing, monitoring, and planning the distribution of public health nursing resources at the community level, Computers in Nursing 5(5):175-180, 1987.

Lancaster JM: Systems theory and the process of change. In Lancaster J and Lancaster W, editors: Concepts for advanced nursing practice: the nurse as a change agent, St. Louis, 1982, The CV Mosby Co.

Lanik G and Webb AA: Ethical decision making for community health nurses, J Community Health Nurs 6(2):95-102, 1989.

Miller CA and Moos MD: Local Health Departments, Washington, DC, 1981, American Public Health Association.

Newman WH, Warren EK, and McGill AR: Process of management: strategy, action, results, Englewood Cliffs, NJ, 1987, Prentice-Hall, Inc.

Pickett G: The future of health departments: a governmental presence, Annual Review of Public Health 1:297, 1980.

Porter EJ: Administrative diagnosis—implications for the public's health, Public Health Nursing 4(4):247-256, 1987.

Ramsey County Public Health Nursing Service: Health-specific family coping index, Unpublished manuscript, St. Paul, Minn, 1983.

Stevens BJ: Nurse as executive, Rockville Md, 1985, Aspen.

Weidmann J and North H: Implementing the Omaha classification system in a public health agency, Nurs Clin North Am 22:971-979, 1987.

38

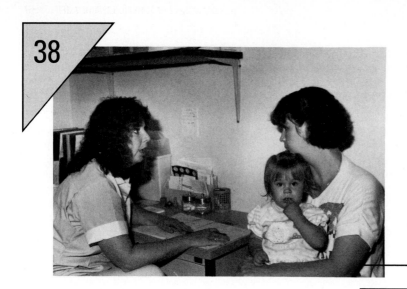

The Community Health Nurse Consultant

Marcia Stanhope

Rena Alford

OBJECTIVES

After reading this chapter, the student should be able to:

Describe the meaning of consultation in community health nursing practice.
State the major goals of consultation.
Discuss theories of consultation and their applicability to community health nursing practice.
Apply the principles of process consultation in community health nursing practice.
Compare and contrast the internal and external nurse consultant functions.
Discuss the educational requirements and practice arenas for the nurse consultant.
Identify consultant and client responsibilities in the process.

KEY TERMS

acceptant intervention mode	consultation	political process model
catalytic intervention mode	consultative contract	power/authority
client population	doctor-patient model	prescriptive intervention mode
client responsibilities	generalist	process model
conflict sources	goals/objectives	purchase model
confrontation intervention mode	morale/cohesion	specialist
	norms/standards	theory-principles intervention mode
	nurse consultant	

N urses have skills that make them valuable contributing members in their work setting and in the community. The specific skills helpful in the community include nurses' preparation for comprehensively assessing all factors that influence individual, family, group, and community health status; nurses' ability to plan, implement, and evaluate goals and programs for individuals, groups, families, and communities as units of service; and nurses' extensive knowledge of community resources and the referral process. These skills can give nurses the expertise and information to function as consultants to individuals, families, groups, or community clients, as well as to other health and social service providers.

This chapter focuses on the definition and goals of consultation models relevant to community health nursing, principles relating to process consultation, and the scope of the nurse consultant role. Baccalaureate-prepared community health nurses often find themselves in a consultant role, either temporarily or permanently. The purpose of the discussion is to define consultation as a community health nursing role. Whether the nurse is the consultant or is receiving consultation services, this chapter will prepare the nurse to be an effective consultant or to use the services of a consultant appropriately.

DEFINITIONS AND GOALS

Like many other concepts, consultation has a variety of definitions. Schein (1969) described it as a process involving a set of activities on the part of the helper that assists the client to perceive, understand, and act on events occurring in the client's environment. Caplan (1970) defined it as a process in which a specialist identifies ways to handle work problems involving the management of clients or the planning and implementation of programs. Others refer to consultation as an interpersonal interaction between the person with expert knowledge and a client, helping the client make constructive behavioral changes (Clark, 1983; Oda, 1982; Rogers, 1987).

The *goal* of consultation is to stimulate clients to take more responsibility, feel more secure, deal constructively with their feelings and with others in interactions, and internalize flexible and creative skills. The functions of a consultant differ from the role functions of administrator, supervisor, coordinator, planner, educator, researcher, or client advocate because consultation typically is a temporary and voluntary relationship between a professional helper and a client. This relationship is a cooperative effort between the consultant and client, who share equally in resolving a problem.

ASSUMPTIONS OF CONSULTATION MODELS

PURCHASE

1. The client correctly diagnoses the problem.
2. The client correctly communicates the needs to the consultant.
3. The client correctly assesses the consultant's expertise to provide the information or perform the service.
4. The client knows the consequences of having the consultant provide the information or the consequences of implementing the services suggested by the consultant.

POLITICAL PROCESS

1. A persistent pattern of human relationships exists in consultation, which is influenced by power and authority.
2. The consultant is an agent acting on behalf of or for another.
3. Manipulation, influence, and negotiation are acceptable ways to control differences, reach settlement, and exchange expertise.
4. Participants in the bargaining system benefit from the system.
5. Open and closed issues exist in the bargaining situation.

PROCESS

1. Clients often do not know what the problem is and need assistance in problem diagnosis.
2. Clients are not aware of the services a consultant may offer and need assistance in finding proper help.
3. Clients want to improve situations and need guidance in identifying appropriate methods to reach goals.
4. Clients can be more effective if they learn to diagnose their own strengths and limitations.

5. Consultants usually cannot spend enough time learning all variables that may help or hinder suggested courses of action, so they need to work with the client, who has intimate knowledge of the effects of proposed courses of action.
6. The client who learns to diagnose situation problems and who engages in decision making about alternative courses of action will be actively involved in implementing actions for problem resolution.
7. The consultant is an expert in problem diagnosis and in establishing an effective helping relationship and passes these skills to the client.

MENTAL HEALTH

1. The consultant does not accept direct responsibility for implementing remedial action for the client.
2. Professional responsibility for the client remains with the consultee.
3. The consultant may clarify, diagnose, and advise about care.
4. The consultee is free to accept or reject all or part of the consultant's advice.
5. The consultant does not exercise administrative or coercive authority.
6. The consultant is not liable for client outcomes unless advice is followed by the consultee.

DOCTOR-PATIENT

1. The client is willing to reveal information needed by the consultant to make an appropriate diagnosis.
2. The consultant, through observations, gets an accurate picture of the problem.
3. The client accepts the diagnosis and the prescription offered by the consultant.

Although consultants are commonly thought to be "outside resource persons" (i.e., not part of the power system in the work setting), this may not apply to the community health nurse consultant. The community health nurse's job responsibilities include internal and external consultation. For example, a nurse may be employed to consult with other nurses in the agency about client care problems or may, as an employee of the health department, serve as a consultant to a local retirement center about the public health care needs of its residents.

If the community health nurse is an internal consultant, the nurse is employed on a full-time salaried basis by a community agency in which the consultation takes place. If the community health nurse is an external consultant, the nurse is employed temporarily on a contractual basis by the client. The client of the external nurse consultant may be a colleague, another health provider, or a community group or organization. The nature of the consultative relationship should not change the goal of consultation.

CONSULTATION MODELS

Although nursing's involvement in consultation has expanded, few data are found in the literature about the effect of the nurse consultant on health care delivery. Selected models of consultation are discussed to provide a basic understanding of approaches for establishing the consultation relationship. (See box on p. 663.)

The Purchase Model

Purchase model consultation (Figure 38-1) is defined as the purchase (hiring) of a professional helper by a client to provide expert information or expert service (Schein, 1969). Others refer to this particular model as "expert consultation"

(Lareau, 1980; Oda, 1982). Buyers may be individuals, groups, or organizations. In this model the client defines the need for the consultant. The need is defined as information the client seeks or an activity the client wants implemented. The advantage of the popular purchase model is that the client does not have to spend time or energy in solving the identified problem, because that is the responsibility of the "expert consultant." The disadvantage of the model is that the client may question the consultation's quality if the client has identified the wrong problem or does not like the consultant's solution.

An example of use of the purchase model to *provide information* to the buyer follows. The public health department supervisors may employ a consultant to instruct them in designing a method for improving nurse productivity. The client has defined the problem before employing the consultant and has determined that the consultant's knowledge is needed to provide a solution.

An illustration of a consultant purchased to provide *services* is seen in a case in which the community health nursing staff members request a consultant to analyze their caseloads to establish client-mix guidelines for future case assignments. The nurse consultant may need to review records for age, sex, diagnosis, physical activity, and client service demands to arrive at a client classification system to be used for distributing equitable caseloads. The staff has determined the need for an expert consultant's active participation in finding and implementing a solution to the problem.

Although the purchase model is often used by consultants and clients, the consultant enters the picture at the point of implementing a solution to the problem. This model may be unsatisfactory in effectively and efficiently identifying and resolving client problems. Once the consultant has im-

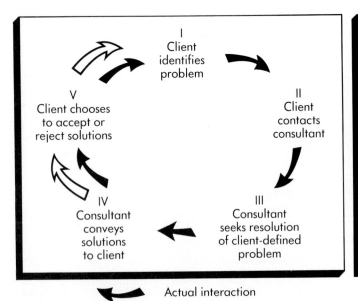

FIGURE 38-1

The purchase model.

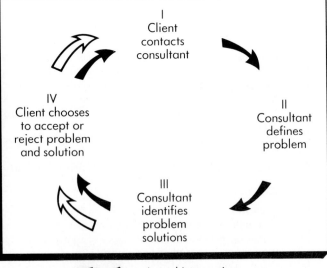

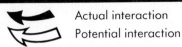

FIGURE 38-2

The doctor-patient model.

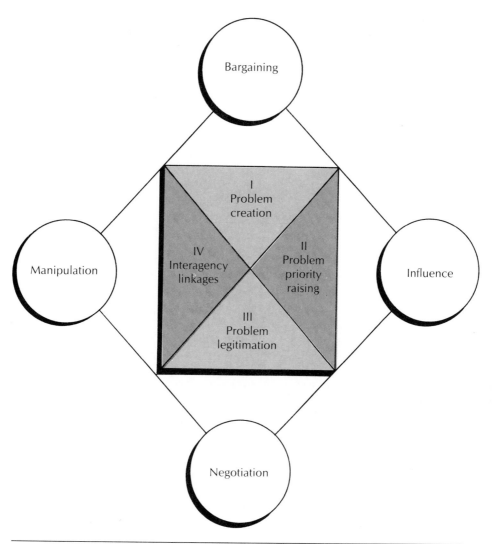

FIGURE 38-3

The political process model.

plemented steps to solve the problem, the client must live with the consequences of the changes. While this is often used in community health, it is not viewed as the best model.

The Doctor-Patient Model

Another popular consultative model is the *doctor-patient model* (Figure 38-2), in which the consultant is employed by the client to find the problem and offer solutions without assistance from the client (Schein, 1969). Again, the major advantage of this model from the client's viewpoint is the limited time and energy required of the client.

This model is often applied in nursing situations requiring consultative services. The director of nursing at the public health department calls in a nurse consultant from the local university. Nurse performance is poor, according to the director, and the nurse consultant is asked to diagnose what is wrong with the department. In this example the nursing director is the client and the staff nurses are the "patient." The staff nurses must provide the data that will identify the problem for the consultant (doctor). If the problem is found

to be poor administrative organization and direction rather than lack of quality performance by the staff, the administrator may be reluctant to accept the diagnosis. Since the client and the "patient" are reluctant to be part of the assessment of the problem, the goals of consultation cannot be met.

The Political Process Model

Consultation has been described as a political process (Baizerman and Hall, 1977; Hendrix and LaGodna, 1982). The *political process model* (Figure 38-3) is a bargaining process in which expertise, organizational position, and personal and organizational reputation are the currency of the bargaining between consultant and consultee. Each actor attempts to maximize his currency at a minimum cost (Baizerman and Hall, 1977, p. 143).

The political process model assumes that the consultant has four major functions:

1. *Problem creation:* defining and legitimizing the problem.

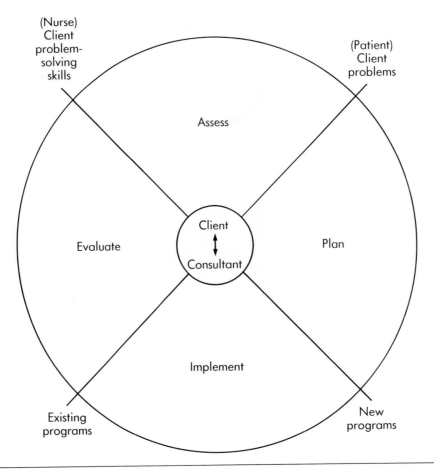

FIGURE 38-4

The mental health model.

2. *Priority raising:* raising the problem as a priority to get action within the consultee agency.
3. *Legitimation:* validating or redefining the problem to arrive at a solution or continued bargaining.
4. *Interagency linkages:* creating and sustaining interagency linkage.

For example, a staff nurse in the local public health department may have noticed an increasing number of homeless persons among the caseload. The nurse requests and is given permission to call in a member of the local government to assist in finding data that will show homelessness to be a major local problem *(problem creation)*. The consultant is asked by the staff nurse (consultee) to present the facts and alternative actions to the agency administration *(priority raising)*. The administration has ignored the need for a program for years because the administration's policy is that homelessness is a social problem and not a health issue. The consultant presents data to indicate the nature of homelessness and the health-related problems *(legitimation)* and suggests a joint program to be sponsored by the health department and the local government *(interagency linkage)*. The political process model is viewed as a process more applicable to the community client than to the individual or family client where interagency linkage may be a major issue.

Mental Health Model

According to Caplan (1970, p. 17), consultation may be limited to an interaction between two professionals: the consultant who is the specialist and the client who requests the consultant's help to solve a current work problem. The problem may be related to the management or care of clients or the planning and implementing of a program. The primary goal of the *mental health model* (Figure 38-4) is increased effectiveness in the work setting through communication between a mental health specialist and other professionals. Problems that may be resolved by applying this model are mental health problems of clients, promotion of mental health in clients, or interpersonal aspects of the work setting (Caplan, p. 28).

While Caplan intended this model to be applicable in dealing with mental health issues, the model has been adapted for use in many settings (Hoffman, 1988). The model can be effective and appropriate in community health nursing.

The following examples show the four types of consultation described by Caplan. They are appropriate for use in community health settings by community health nurses. In *client-centered case consultation* a community health nurse may be having difficulty working with a client recently discharged from the local psychiatric hospital. The client is

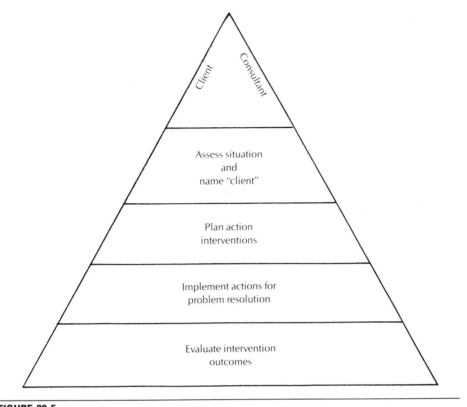

FIGURE 38-5

The process model.

noncompliant in following the prescribed care regimen. The mental health nurse makes a home visit with the community health nurse, assesses the client's mental health status, makes a diagnosis, and prescribes written recommendations for the community health nurse to follow in managing the client's care.

As an example of *consultee-centered case consultation*, an AIDS program nurse works with a group of community health nurses throughout the state who express a lack of "professional objectivity" in working in the home with AIDS clients. The program nurse reviews the latest information on AIDS, universal precautions, disease transmission, and techniques for working with AIDS clients in the home. The purpose of the discussions is to relieve the nurses' anxiety about working with these clients by providing objective data regarding the care of clients with AIDS.

With *program-centered administrative consultation*, the consultant is invited by an administrator to advise regarding resource needs to set up a nurse-managed clinic for the homeless in a community where the homeless population is growing. In *consultee-centered administrative consultation* the director of nursing asks the consultant to work with him to develop problem solving strategies which can be used with a group of supervisors to enhance their interpersonal interactions.

The Process Model

Schein's definition (1969) describes a process consultation model. The major goals of the *process model*, as seen in Figure 38-5, are to assist the client to assess both the problem and the kind of help needed to resolve the problem. Problem solving is a key tool used in process consultation. Both the consultant and the client participate in the problem-solving steps that lead to changes or to actions for problem solution.

In this model, the consultant is a resource person whose primary goal is to provide the client with choices for decision making. As shown in Figure 38-4, the process consultation model includes the same steps as the nursing process, establishing a nurse-client interaction to assess the problem, plan and implement actions, and evaluate the outcomes of nursing interventions. Nursing interventions may be described as direct client care or as consultation activities, depending on the goal of the intervention. Because process consultation closely parallels the nursing process, this model is viewed as the most appropriate model to apply in nursing. The analysis and synthesis of the process consultation model by Blake and Mouton (1983) serves as the basis for the following discussion and application of this model.

PROCESS CONSULTATION—FOCUS AND PRINCIPLES

Process consultation involves a temporary relationship between client and consultant for the purpose of bringing about *change*. Consultation may be *proactive* or *reactive*. *Proactive consultation* is directed toward anticipating a future problem and taking steps to prevent it. *Reactive consultation* is directed toward curing an existing problem through therapeutic intervention. For example, a board developing a new retirement center contacts the community health nurse to assist with options for future nursing and health care for the residents. The board wishes to be *proactive* and plan for the needs of the residents before opening the center. Conversely, the administrator of a minimum security prison has found that inmates are missing work for minor health problems and that health screening program-costs are skyrocketing, because the prison must contract with individual providers to offer these services. The community health nurse is asked to help administration explore solutions to the problem. The prison administration is *reacting* to an existing problem requiring immediate intervention.

Client Population

One of the most important decisions a nurse makes before accepting or writing a consultative contract is to identify the client in the situation. A client of the community health nurse may be an individual, a family, a group within the agency, a community group, or a community organization. The client is identified by determining who in the situation has the problem and needs to change. For example, the staff nurse at the district health department is resistant to working in the clinic caring for clients with sexually transmitted diseases because of a fear of working with AIDS victims. The state-level community health nurse consultant may negotiate a contract with the staff nurse to deal with these feelings and to arrive at alternative methods for problem solution. It would not be worthwhile for the consultant to contract with the director of nursing or the nursing supervisor to solve the staff nurse's personal problem. Contracts with management may make the staff nurse more resistant to assigned duties.

As a second example, a school health nurse receives an inquiry from the school board about ways to get parents to support the hearing and vision screening programs of the schools. The nurse decides that the consultative contract needs to include representatives of the school board and representatives of the parents group to find effective answers to the question. The nurse realizes that time would be wasted and resistance to change would still be present if the focus were only on one group at a time. If the nurse were to meet separately with the parent group, they may decide the school board should employ someone to do the screening; at the school board meeting the nurse could find that the board does not have the money to employ persons to do all of the screening but is willing to employ one person to coordinate the parents' efforts. After expending much energy meeting with both groups separately, the nurse would find that by being a messenger between the two groups rather than a facilitator for problem solving, the consultant role has been diluted. On the other hand, by meeting with both groups together the nurse can serve as a resource in helping the parents and school board to explore all available alternatives for solving the problem.

Intervention Modes

Once the client has been identified, the nurse must decide the best method(s) for intervening in the problem situation. Blake and Mouton (1983) describe five basic intervention modes or techniques that can be applied to the process consultation model: acceptant, catalytic, confrontation, prescriptive, and theory-principles. These are summarized in Table 38-1.

The *acceptant intervention mode* is a process of clearing emotional reactions so that more objective problem solving can begin. The use of this intervention mode to solve problems benefits the client by improving self-acceptance, spontaneity, emotional health, appropriate situational emotional responses, and the ability to objectively define and deal with problem situations.

The disadvantages of the intervention mode are twofold. The cathartic process of expressing emotions may assist the client in accepting the circumstances leading to the problem rather than in taking actions to correct the problem, and the emotional catharsis may be viewed by others as a hostile and aggressive act (Blake and Mouton, 1983). For example, Jane is a staff nurse who, in interaction with a consultant, realizes that she is not motivated to increase her productivity because she never gets positive reinforcement from her supervisor. However, she may not wish to change the situation because of reluctance to discuss the problem with her supervisor. Conversely, Jane may learn to be assertive and show the supervisor evidence of quality client care during the supervisor-nurse evaluation conference. The supervisor may interpret Jane's behavior as aggressive and out of character and my penalize the nurse further with a poor evaluation.

The *catalytic intervention mode* is a situation in which the consultant assists clients to broaden their views of existing situations by gaining additional information or by integrating existing data (Blake and Mouton, 1983). The consultant assists the client to (1) strengthen perceptions about problems by improving available information, (2) break down barriers to communication by identifying inadequate communication processes and procedures, and (3) raise the awareness level of all involved regarding the problem issue.

In the catalytic intervention mode the consultant is seen as a facilitator providing the client with the information needed to solve a problem. The lack of information, however, may be the symptom, not the problem. The disadvantage of having the consultant improve information-flow is that the client may rely on the factilitator for the data rather than becoming efficient in finding solutions to future problems (Caplan, 1970; Blake and Mouton, 1983).

In a local public health department the director of nursing received resignations from all nursing staff members on the home health care team. The director called the state health department and requested the home health nurse consultant be sent to provide assistance in problem-identification and solution. The nurse consultant planned interviews with the staff nurses to determine the cause of resignations. After sharing the information with the director, a staff meeting was called so that the director could discuss problems with the staff and suggest solutions. The consultant served as a facilitator in the meeting to promote discussion between the staff and the director. After the meeting, the consultant assisted the director in analyzing the content of the meeting. Three months later a related communication problem occurred with the same group. Rather than seek the causes of the problem, the director phoned for the consultant to return to find the causes and solutions.

The *confrontation intervention mode* presents the client

TABLE 38-1
Consultive intervention modes

Intervention mode	Definition	Problem example	Consultant actions
Acceptance	Consultant urges client to share feelings to move to more objective problem solving.	1. Determining who's the boss. 2. Feeling of powerlessness to change the situation.	1. Attempt to understand the client's feelings about the situation. 2. Listen actively. 3. Encourage the client to talk. 4. Try to clarify the client's feelings and help the client to accept the feelings. 5. Refrain from agreeing or disagreeing with the client's situation. 6. Encourage the client to explore ways of dealing with the problems. 7. Listen for more data to reveal the total scope of the problem.
Catalytic	Consultant broadens client's knowledge of problem by offering new data or clarifying existing data	1. Standards are violated/changed. 2. Inability to meet goals or objectives.	1. Set a nonauthoritarian tone for the interaction by beginning the intervention with social conversation. 2. Ask the client to describe the situation and use the description as a basis for the interaction. 3. Suggest data-gathering techniques that may provide new information of interest to the client. 4. Provide support to the client as the client attempts to accurately perceive the problem. 5. Avoid specific suggestions for problem solving or resolution. 6. Encourage the client to make decisions about problem resolution.
Confrontation	Consultant presents clients with indisputable facts.	1. Additional insight needed. 2. Unwillingness to solve problem.	1. Continually question clients about their description of the situation. 2. Present data and logic to test clients' chosen courses of action. 3. Challenge clients' chosen courses of action. 4. Probe for motives and causes of present situation. 5. Provide own thoughts about situation without personally attacking clients' values.

Continued

TABLE 38-1
Consultive intervention modes—cont'd

Intervention mode	Definition	Problem example	Consultant actions
Prescriptive	Consultant tells client how to solve problem.	1. Inability to cope. 2. Needs immediate answer.	1. Probe for data about the client's situation. 2. Act authoritatively. 3. Control by telling the client how the problem is to be perceived. 4. Tell the client the best solutions. 5. Remind the client if he is procrastinating in implementing actions. 6. Offer praise if the client does exactly what the consultant wants done.
Theory-principles	Consultant teaches how to solve problem using theories or principles.	1. Additional insight needed. 2. Lack of knowledge to solve problem.	1. Introduce theories for problem solving to the client. 2. Use techniques to assist the client to internalize theories. 3. Provide strategies for practical application of the theories, such as problem situations or critiques of applications. 4. Offer support when the theory is applied in the actual problem situation.

Adapted from Blake R and Mouton J: Consultation, ed 2, Reading, Mass, 1983, Addison-Wesley Publishing Co, Inc.

with facts that reveal the client's values and assumptions in ways that are undeniable and indisputable (Blake and Mouton, 1983). This intervention mode provides clients with an objective look at how their values and beliefs control their behavior. By looking at present behavior, the consultant can examine alternative values with the client to redirect behavior toward improved methods of problem solving. The disadvantage to this mode is that the client may not wish to participate in interactions that may be interpreted as criticism (Blake and Mouton, 1983).

In the previous example, the consultant may have found that the staff nurses were going to resign their positions because they viewed the director's decisions as autocratic and uncompromising. On the second visit to the agency, the consultant could confront the director with these observations. The director may deny the behavior and point out evidence of having acted democratically. As a result of the confrontation, the director may regard the consultant's observations as a personal affront or be willing to examine and analyze the discrepancies between the perceived and the actual behavior.

The *prescriptive intervention mode* requires less collaboration between consultant and client because the consultant explicitly tells the client how to solve the problem (Blake and Mouton, 1983). The prescriptive mode is best used along with other intervention modes, such as acceptant or catalytic. If clients do not participate in problem solution, they will not be able to solve future problems and may not

follow the prescriptions offered. The advantage of the prescriptive intervention mode is its usefulness in situations where clients have lost confidence in their ability to solve problems or have given up in despair (Blake and Mouton, 1983).

In the example, the nurse consultant has decided the best method of dealing with the problems between the home health staff and the director is to present a prescription for behavioral conduct to be implemented by the director and the staff. The consultant tells the group when and how follow-up evaluation will be conducted to look at the progress of both parties in resolving their differences.

Use of the *theory-principles intervention mode* requires that the client learn theories, such as behavioral theory, and their application to problem solving. This intervention mode introduces the theories after clients have shared their usual methods of problem solving. It also allows the client to apply the theories to problem situations while developing skills in problem diagnosis and solution. The major problem with this intervention mode is determining how to help the client internalize use of the theory for practical application, thus removing the abstract aspects that theories usually involve (Blake and Mouton, 1983).

Before using this mode with the home health staff and director, the consultant may present a conference on leadership theories and principles as well as a discussion of the inherent responsibilities in administrative decision making. The consultant may be able to show both parties that leadership styles should vary with the types of decisions to be made and with the people who are to be affected by the decision.

Use of Intervention Modes

The use of a particular intervention mode is decided by two factors: the client and the problem. Blake and Mouton (1983) have identified four categories of problem issues: power/authority, morale/cohesion, norms/standards, and goals/objectives.

The *power/authority* issue becomes a question of who has the right to be the boss and who has the right to make decisions. The *morale/cohesion* problem occurs when the client has lost confidence in the ability to solve problems and feels powerless to take action. The *norms/standards* problems occur when group norms or professional or organization standards are violated or changed. Problems related to *goals/objectives* usually involve establishing new goals, changing goals, or being unable to meet them.

Several intervention modes may be used with each of the problem issues. When the consultant is trying to decide which intervention mode to use, the client and the nature of the problem must be considered. Although there are exceptions, when the problem with a client is identified as a morale/cohesion problem or a power/authority issue, the most common intervention may be the acceptant mode because the issue generally causes feelings that block action in decision making. When a norms/standards or goals/objectives problem is the issue, the catalytic mode may be the choice to strengthen the client's perceptions of the most effective decision-making methods. The theory-principles intervention mode may be helpful regardless of the problem, especially when additional insights are needed. However, the prescriptive mode may *not* be helpful unless the client is unable to cope with the situation and needs immediate direction or answers to solve the problem. (Blake and Mouton, 1983).

THE COMMUNITY HEALTH NURSE AND USE OF PROCESS CONSULTATION
The Consultative Contract

The consultative relationship is based on expectations. The consultant has expectations concerning time, reimbursement, resources, and the participation of the client in the process. Clients have expectations about what they will gain from the consultative relationship. Although nurses are beginning to contract for their services, it is more commonplace for consultants to have written contracts. Discussing the terms of the *consultative contract* makes expectations more explicit, reduces the likelihood of violations of contract terms, and reduces the risk of additional demands being made on either party. Areas that should be included in the written consultative contract are: (1) the goals of the client and consultant; (2) the identified problem; (3) the consultant's resources; (4) the time commitment; (5) limitations of the contract; (6) cost; (7) conditions under which the contract may be broken or renegotiated; (8) intervention modes to be used; (9) expected benefits for the client; (10) methods of data collection to be used; (11) client resources; (12) potential interventions; (13) methods of evaluation of the interaction; and (14) confidentiality. An example of a

consultation contract that may be used to establish a consultant-consultee relationship appears in the clinical application at the end of this chapter.

Writing a contract for consultative relationships has a number of advantages. The contract terms assist the consultant in determining the number of hours that must be devoted to the interaction and in identifying needed resources and out-of-pocket expenses required to complete the interaction. Negotiation of the contract assists the client in identifying realistic expectations of the consultant and firmly establishes what the consultant will and will not do. The client has the opportunity during the negotiation to place limits on what the consultant can do, and the contract allows for future renegotiation of terms.

Consultation Phases

Consultation involves seven basic phases:
1. Initial contact with the client
2. Definition of the relationship
3. Selection of a setting and approach
4. Collection of data and problem diagnosis
5. Intervention
6. Reduction of involvement and evaluation
7. Termination

The initial contact is made when the client or someone in a family, group, or community communicates with the nurse about a potential problem that requires intervention. The communication may be person-to-person during a home visit, may be written, or may occur by telephone. On initial contact, the client and the nurse have an exploratory meeting to define the problem, assess the nurse's ability to help, assess the nurse's interest, and formulate future actions.

At the initial meeting, the consultee will want to inquire about the nurse's expertise, personality characteristics, and interpersonal style. If the nurse has little experience with the type of problem presented, the client may wish to seek assistance elsewhere. Also, if the nurse is quick to make decisions and has a directive approach, the client who has a more laissez-faire philosophy may have difficulty accepting the nurse's approach. Conversely, the nurse may conclude that the situation holds little interest or is not within the nurse's expertise and will want to recommend someone else to work with the client.

If the nurse decides at the initial meeting that the real client has been identified, the terms of the relationship will be discussed. The nurse consultant will find out what the client expects to gain from the relationship and will establish terms for the interaction.

Finally, in the initial exploratory meeting the setting for the consultation will be decided upon, the time schedule will be set, the goals of the interaction will be established, and the mode of intervention will be chosen.

When the terms of the contract are agreed upon, the data gathering methods will be part of the agreement. The nurse may find it essential to gather more data before diagnosing the problem. Data gathering methods used by consultants include direct observation, individual and group interviews, use of questionnaires or surveys, and tape recordings. While data are being gathered, as well as after the diagnosis has been finalized, the nurse will be actively engaged in the intervention mode chosen for the interaction.

After fulfilling the terms of the contract, the nurse must be concerned with disengagement or reducing the amount of involvement with the client. The disengagement process requires mutual agreement between the nurse and client consultee that involvement should be reduced. The amount of continuing involvement that is wanted should be checked at varying intervals during the consultative relationship. At these points, contract renegotiation may take place. Determinants of continued involvement include, but are not limited to, the client's willingness to continue, the value of the interaction for client and nurse, and situational changes that may have occurred.

Before termination, the number of contacts between nurse and consultee should be decreased. The continued but decreased contacts will allow each side to evaluate the effectiveness of the intervention. During the disengagement period the nurse reassures the client that future interactions are possible at the client's discretion. When the agreed-upon period of disengagement has passed, the relationship is terminated (Beare, 1988; Blake and Mouton, 1983; Reinert, 1989; Schein, 1969). The nurse typically provides the consultee with a written summary of the findings and recommendations resulting from the interactions during the disengagement and termination phases.

Consultation includes the formal interaction phases of: *trust-building*, which includes the initial contact, definition of the relationship, and selection of the setting and intervention approach; *problem solving*, which includes gathering data, formalizing the problem, and intervening; and *closure*, which involves disengagement and termination.

Client Responsibilities

The consultative relationship depends on the interaction between the nurse and the client. Although the consultative contract defines the terms of the relationship, the client can assist in making the consultative process a successful interaction.

Initially the client must determine who can best assist in solving the client problem: an internal or external consultant. An internal nurse consultant knows the organization and the values of the organization and the staff, is a team member, has expertise, and is probably committed to helping solve internal problems. The external nurse consultant brings new ideas and a broader regional or national prospective, has new or proven strategies to offer, can bring objectivity to the problem, and has a short-term, less expensive commitment to the organization (Collins, 1989; Noble, 1988).

The client can have an efficient, effective consultation by recognizing that the problem belongs to the client and the nurse's role in solving the problem is limited. Once the problem has been accepted, the client can offer an agenda to maximize the nurse's time, identify key people to work with the nurse, and offer a written summary of issues to be addressed and questions to be answered. The client should also remain open to all proposed suggestions or solutions, summarize the content of the nurse's visits and need for follow-up, clarify disputed findings and recommendations with the nurse, and try out the proposed solutions after examining the benefits and consequences of implementing them (Collins, 1989; Novle, 1988; Schaffner, 1989).

Consultant Responsibilities

In addition to the nurse's responsibilities negotiated in a contract with a client, the nurse must be aware of the "goodness of fit" between the nurse and client. The nurse should work with clients and problem issues that are congruous with the nurse's philosophy, personality characteristics, and interpersonal style. The nurse should develop visibility within the nursing profession, the organization, or the community as a person with expert knowledge and skills who can serve as a facilitator or resource within a specialty area. However, a nurse consultant should not be so specialized that she is useful only to a limited range of clients; rather, she should develop a reputation of taking opportunities that are consistent with her skills.

To develop a credible reputation, a nurse must clarify all role expectations with the client and present accurate credentials and skills, maintain a professional image, and complete assignments in an agreed-upon time frame. The nurse should also thoroughly assess the consultative situation and collect all essential data, be available for follow-up, and use a written evaluation tool to assess the fulfillment of mutual expectations (Beare, 1988; Beecroft, 1988; Reinert, 1989).

Examples of Consultation

Five examples of consultative interventions are described in the following discussion.

Intervention: prescriptive
Client: Director of Nursing
Consultant: internal
Problem: norms/standards

The client telephoned the state nursing consultant and requested a meeting at the local health unit. The purpose of the meeting was to review serious problems the local nursing staff was having in meeting program standards and requirements, as identified in a recent audit. The nurse consultant, Elizabeth, met with the client, Maggie, and reviewed her findings, sharing her analysis of the problems and contributing factors. The central problem was defined as inconsistent supervision of staff with a need for role clarification of supervisory responsibilities. Maggie was immobilized by the situation. Elizabeth directed Maggie to restructure the supervisory job descriptions to clearly reflect supervisory roles and expectations; she also recommended giving supervisors written performance evaluations and guidelines for improving staff performance. Elizabeth maintained contact with Maggie until termination of the consultation occurred and corrective action was completed.

Intervention: acceptant
Client: staff nurse
Consultant: internal
Problem: morale/cohesion

Elizabeth received a phone call from staff nurse Susan requesting a meeting to discuss problems that Susan was experiencing in her job situation. Susan was obviously under stress as evidenced by the immediacy of the requested need for the meeting. Susan talked about her perceived inability to communicate with administration, the effect of these feelings on her ability to function, and her perception of being out of control in the job situation. Susan had decided that resignation was her only alternative. Elizabeth listened and provided a non-threatening opportunity for Susan to verbalize freely. Elizabeth did not agree or disagree with Susan's perceptions of the job situation or respond to her direct question about resignation. Elizabeth focused on Susan's perceived problems with the job and her feelings about her performance. She then attempted to clarify events described by Susan and to keep events in perspective. Finally, Elizabeth explored with Susan ways in which she might improve communication with administration. Ultimately, Susan decided to choose resignation as the solution.

Intervention: catalytic/theory-principles

Client: community group

Consultant: external

Problem: goals/objectives

Josie was consulted by a representative of a local community hospital. The hospital staff and the pediatrician had expressed concern about child-neglect problems the hospital was seeing and about the lack of information on the part of many mothers about basic child care. Acting as a facilitator, Josie recognized that the problem involved not only the single community hospital but two other community hospitals as well as the county department of social services, the health department, and the county home extension office. These groups were identified by Josie as having the potential to influence the identified health issue.

Josie contacted the agencies and requested that a representative from each be present at a planning meeting. At the initial meeting Josie, acting as a resource, presented the magnitude of the infant morbidity and mortality problem within the county, presented data for three years regarding the causes of infant mortality, and raised the issue of preventive intervention through a hospital discharge system. Hospitalization and discharge of the newborn were identified as prime times to provide parents with information on basic child care and local resources.

The client group believed that educational materials were not designed for the level of understanding of many parents in a rural multi-income-level area. The decision was made by the group to develop a county-specific, newborn hospital-discharge packet that was easily understandable and provided county-specific resource information. Through a series of five or six meetings the group reviewed and selected the most significant principles from an extensive literature review and applied them to their identified local health issue. They subsequently developed a discharge planning model with community-wide applicability. During disengagement the group renegotiated with Josie to evaluate the application of the model at the end of a three-month period.

Intervention: confrontation

Client: departmental group

Consultant: internal

Problem: power/authority

The Director of Nursing asked for consultation to help the health department program supervisors assume management-supervisory responsibility for their staff. The lack of management responsibility was having a domino effect on program standards, fiscal accountability, and nursing practice standards. In an initial meeting with the director, the consultant determined that the client was the supervisory group, not the Director of Nursing.

The consultant then met individually with supervisors to determine their perceptions of the administration's expectations in the area of program management. Using client care findings on a record audit and an audit of staff evaluations, the consultant revealed the managerial problems of each supervisor and shared these findings in the individual conferences. Reasons offered by the supervisors for lack of involvement in management functions included excessive caseload, lack of clear understanding of their management functions and of the expectations of administration, and insecurity in management techniques.

The consultant met with the supervisors as a group. At this point the consultant specifically reviewed the management tasks for which the supervisors would be held responsible by administration and reviewed the organizational structure and the line authority held by each supervisor. The consultant also reviewed the supervisors' caseloads and the amount of projected time they needed to perform managerial functions. The consultant-client relationship was to be continued monthly for a maximum period of six months, at which time the contract would be renegotiated or terminated.

Intervention: catalytic

Client: community agency

Consultant: external

Problem: goals/objectives

The consultant was contacted by the Family Practice Center to discuss the issue of adolescent pregnancy problems in the county and the Family Practice Center's involvement in providing an adolescent maternity service clinic within a residency training program. A meeting was scheduled during which the nurse consultant presented adolescent pregnancy data for the county, outlined the local health department's role in adolescent prenatal services and the current adolescent prenatal caseload, and provided data that projected the caseload and service demands the adolescent clinic would be expected to meet. The center staff, health department staff, and consultant made a site visit to observe an adolescent prenatal clinic at another medical center.

As a result of several additional meetings, the consultant negotiated a collaborative arrangement between the health department and the Family Practice Center. The services to be provided included short-term nursing education, social work, and nutrition support services. The consultant assumed the facilitator role and continually clarified the ongoing developmental and agency commitments (goals) in this collaborative effort. The adolescent prenatal clinic was initiated with the aid of the short-term commitments that grew out of the interagency relationships. After the clinic was established, health department services were withdrawn and replaced by the Family Practice Center staff as scheduled. The consultant's relationship continued for approximately six months and was terminated after meeting a request from the center staff for evaluation.

THE NURSE CONSULTANT

As previously stated, *nurse consultants* in the community health setting may function as internal consultants employed on a full-time basis by an organization for the purpose of helping the staff in problem solving; or nurses may be employed as external consultants with a contractual arrangement to assist an individual, group, or community organization to find solutions to existing problems. Nurses may provide consultation for a wide range of issues related to community health nursing, or they may narrow their scope of expertise and provide consultation only in an identified specialty area.

The Internal Nurse Consultant: Generalist vs. Specialist

How a health agency provides services determines the specific framework in which a consultant functions. An agency that delivers care similar to an official generalized community health service will most likely employ a generalist nurse who provides traditional or comprehensive community health nursing consultation for a broad range of community health activities.

A community health agency that provides a programmatic approach or specialized approach to the delivery of community health services, such as family planning, maternity, child health, crippled children services, school health, or home health, will tend to employ *specialist* consultants; these may have skills and specialized training in primary clinical areas (e.g., the clinical nurse specialist in pediatrics) in addition to broad community health expertise.

The degree to which the agency is involved in specific primary care areas influences the use of the specialized consultant. Agencies providing primary health care require a consultant with both a knowledge of community health practice and specialized knowledge in a clinical area. This is also a requirement in agencies involved in long-term and home health care.

Role Functions

The community health nurse consultant employed within an official health agency functions as an internal consultant to the employing agency. As a representative of the agency, the nurse provides nursing and community health consultation to colleagues, other disciplines, agency administration, and other health and human service agencies and/or community groups. Two primary roles of the internal consultant are **resource person** and **facilitator** (Pati, 1980). Both roles emerge because of the availability of the nurse to the agency and community.

The *resource role* has traditionally been associated with the community health nurse consultant within and outside of the official health agency. Because of new and varied health delivery models within communities, the resource role has assumed increased significance. With knowledge of available resources, the nurse can identify deficiencies and gaps in service, identify the critical services provided by the health delivery systems, and promote the integration of these services in meeting health or social needs of the population.

The nurse consultant as a *facilitator* assists staff nurses, administration, groups, and organizations to solve problems relating to the needs of clients, staff, or the organization. Performing the facilitator function, the consultant guides the staff nurse in solving problems about individual client and family needs, health needs of a group of clients, or professional concerns and attitudes. The consultant may assist supervisors, managers, directors, and administrators to solve problems about personnel, program needs, orga-

nizational goals, community relationships, and client population needs. The consultant may also assist communications between the employing agency and other facilities or health providers in the community.

Role Relationships

The consultant's role with nursing administration and staff is determined by the organizational structure. The internal consultant is generally responsible to and strongly influenced by nursing administration and agency administration. The nursing administration's framework for nursing practice, goals for nursing service, and the role the consultant is to assume should be clearly defined before employment. Personnel responsible for nursing practice should be clearly defined for the consultant, the supervising staff, and the staff nurses. The internal consultant may not have formal authority but informally will have responsibility for making changes in nursing practice (Kohnke, 1978). The perception on the part of the staff nurse regarding the consultant's alignment with administration, as "eyes and ears" of administration, is a definite factor in the staff's relationship with the consultant; this factor will depend on the consultant-consultee relationship developed and established by the consultant.

A generalist nurse in an official community agency is often required to function in a dual supervisor-consultant role. Supervision means decision making and implementation of activities in an ongoing relationship, which is the opposite of consultation. Functions of the supervising role could replace the consultative role, and the staff could perceive the supervisor/consultant as being directly aligned with administration. Quality communication is vital.

A number of allied health professionals are functioning within community health practice: clinical social workers, nutritionists, occupational therapists, physical therapists, health educators, home economists, and home health aides. The community health nurse and the allied health providers share mutual skills and commitment to community health practice and provide specific professional skills to mutual clients, families, and each other. The nurse consultant provides consultation to the allied health provider and serves as a resource and content-person to these professionals in the areas of community health nursing practice. In a facilitator role, the nurse can enhance the efficient use of other health providers and often prevent "turf" issues. The consultant's broad knowledge base and multi-disciplinary approach to health care helps to ensure the effective use of allied health providers and also promotes more efficient use of nursing personnel.

Conflict Sources

The internal consultant as a representative of the employing agency has implied authority that may result in conflict between the consultant and the consultee. The amount of conflict depends on the centralization or decentralization of the health agency and the degree of autonomy of the individual units in the organization. One way to decrease potential conflict is to clearly define the role the consultant is to assume. For example, in one state the state health department has jurisdiction over all the county health departments (centralized). The state has decided to make all the county health departments autonomous in their delivery of health services; this aspect is decentralized. The state health department will continue to advise the county units about delivery of services but will not supervise the delivery of care. Nursing in the county units will have its own directors, and the nursing consultants at the state level will be used as resource persons and facilitators.

While the state health department was centralized and provided direct supervision to the counties for delivery of health care, the state family planning consultant was also responsible for supervising the county health department staff members who were responsible for delivery of family planning services. In the decentralized system, the supervisory functions are removed from the consultant's responsibilities and the consultant helps the work of other nurses by offering advice and information that will assist them in understanding how to do their work. The administrative or managerial strength of the individual unit can also determine the role the consultant may assume and the involvement of the consultant in an implementation role.

The External Nurse Consultant

When the community health nurse consultant is contacted by an agency or organization other than the employing agency, the nurse consultant is considered an outsider to the organization and an external consultant.

Role Functions and Relationships

Again, the external nurse consultant acts as a **facilitator** or a **resource** person. The external nurse consultant may represent the employing agency and provide information to the consultee for the planning of interagency programs to meet population needs. The external nurse consultant may serve as a resource to health educators, health planners, school personnel, psychologists, audiologists, counselors, dentists, social workers, physicians, legislators, and probation officers, providing data about individual client, group, or community needs.

The external consultant may be asked to serve as facilitator to an official agency board to solve problems about community health priorities. Similarly, the consultant may be asked to serve as a facilitator or resource person to a voluntary agency, such as the American Red Cross or the American Heart Association.

Consultants from federal agencies are often used in community health as external nurse consultants. The nurse consultant from the federal agency may come to the local or state agency to serve on request as facilitator or resource person helping with program planning, development, and implementation. The primary role function of this consultant is to serve as a resource person, although the consultant may facilitate movement toward identifying actual program objectives.

The role relationships of the external consultant with groups or individuals are determined by the client, whether individual or group. The principles and process of consultation are the same for either the internal or external consultative functional framework. One of the principle differences between the internal and external consultant is that the external consultant has less time to collect the data needed to identify the problem.

Conflict Sources

The external consultant only has assumed authority, which may result in conflict for the consultant and the client (Polk, 1980). Since the consultant is external, the client may not feel obligated to implement the agreed-upon actions. In many instances the consultant may hold a complementary role to the client, such as a community health nurse as consultant to the school health nurse.

Although equal sharing and input should guide the consultant-consultee relationship, conflict may arise if the school nurse interprets the community health nurse consultant's involvement as an invasion of territory. One way to prevent potential conflict is to clearly establish the terms of the contract for the consultant-client interaction. For example, the community health nurse consultant is called by the school health nurse. The school nurse needs input from the consultant about developing and implementing a health education program for sexually transmitted diseases. The terms of the contract stipulate that the consultant will provide input on how to develop and implement the program and the school health nurse will do the work of the program. Thus, the consultant is not involved in the program and the school nurse's turf is protected.

The consultative relationship is also time-limited. The consultant may not have enough time to identify all variables in the situation to arrive at a diagnosis of the real problem. The client may be frustrated in attempts to make changes suggested by the consultant and may offer resistance because the real problem did not surface during the consultant-client interaction.

Power Issues

Role relationships are often affected by the power that clients perceive the nurse consultant possesses. Consultants' advice is frequently followed because of perceived *expert power*. The client feels that the consultant possesses superior knowledge or skills and is trustworthy and credible. Expert power is often assigned to the external consultant.

The nurse consultant may be defined as having *legitimate power* as a direct result of the internal consultant's role in the organization. In this instance the client may believe the consultant has the right to influence decisions.

The *label of referent* or *mentor power* may be assigned to an external consultant because of an affiliation with other well-known consultants or a national organization. The ability of the consultant to persuade clients to follow prescriptions by offering reasons, new techniques, or methods of problem solving may establish the consultant's *informational power*.

Funding Implications

In the last decade, funding mechanisms have promoted the position of specialist consultant in some community health departments. Title X of the Social Security Act included provisions for funding of family planning services. This funding mechanism is one way a federally funded community health service promoted the use of specialist consultants within a specific area of community health care. The funding mechanism gave rise to use of the family planning nurse practitioner. To meet the agency needs, consultants with special skills and expertise in reproductive health were employed by official health agencies. Similarly, Title V of the Social Security Act provided funding that traditionally focused on more generalized services to mothers and children and resulted in the use of the nurse consultant for crippled children and the school health nurse consultant. The Medicare funding in 1965 for home health care gave rise to the home health services consultant with community skills in medical and surgical nursing practice. Current Medicare funding provides nurse consultants for personal care aide services in the home and nurse consultants for AIDS-related programs.

The impact of state's block grant funding for primary care and the move of some health agencies from specific programs to more integrated service delivery will affect the role and use of nurse consultants in official community health agencies. The competition for limited health dollars, the increasing focus on the at-risk population, the anticipated surplus of physician manpower, and the shortage of nurses are going to affect the specialist-versus-generalist consultant role in official health agencies.

As federal, state, local, and private funding becomes more competitive, fewer external nurse consultants may be used. If an external nurse consultant is employed, costs for the consulting services must be built into the client's budget. These future limited funds may be reserved for program implementation rather than for contracting with consultants. Although all external nurse consultants do not receive direct reimbursement for their services, the needs of the employing agency for internal consultation may become greater and the agency may not be willing to pay, either in time or travel, for the consultant to be away from the organization.

Educational Requirements

The educational requirements for the community health nurse consultant are primarily determined by two factors: the practice setting and the client population. The community health nurse with undergraduate preparation may serve as a generalist nurse consultant to individuals, families, and groups of clients with an identified health problem such as hypertension or diabetes. The consultant serves either as a facilitator to seek a problem-solution or as a resource to provide for community referral. This nurse may also consult with other health provider agencies involved with client groups, such as the hospital, ambulatory clinics, the private physician, and the physical therapist.

The community health nurse consultant who has graduate preparation with a generalist or specialist clinical and functional focus has expert knowledge in the application of the theories of change, group, systems, interaction, motivation, communications, behavior, management, and epidemiology. This kind of nurse also has in-depth knowledge of family and individual development, advocacy, and health and nursing issues (Kohnke, 1978). This nurse may be an internal or external consultant serving as an expert resource person or as a facilitator to client groups.

Practice Arenas

The nurse who wishes to become a consultant will find employment opportunities with philanthropic organizations, government agencies, private enterprise, and voluntary and professional organizations.

The federal government employs nurse consultants in many branches of the Public Health Service. The Division of Nursing of the Health Resources and Services Administration employs a group of nurse consultants to serve as resource persons for education. The Health Care Financing Administration employs nurse consultants to serve as resource persons for programs such as home health. Many state health departments employ clinical specialist consultants who serve as facilitators and resource persons to local health departments regarding program needs (e.g., child health). State health departments also employ clinical nurse consultants to serve as resource persons to such agencies as schools and rehabilitation centers. Local city, county, and district health departments employ nurse consultants—usually generalists—who help staff members in meeting client and program needs.

Private organizations use the expertise of nurses in consultation with clients of the organization. Publishing and audiovisual equipment companies employ nurses who serve as resources and facilitators for persons interested in writing or developing audiovisuals or for persons who require assistance in the use of the companies' products. Pharmaceutical companies and health care supply and equipment companies employ nurse consultants for similar purposes.

Private philanthropic organizations, such as the Robert Wood Johnson Foundation, may use nurse consultants to serve as resource persons for health care or education programs funded by the organizations; professional organizations, such as ANA and NLN, offer nurse consulting services to clinical agencies (e.g., home health) and to education institutions that require assistance in setting program standards or in readying themselves for accreditation review.

An employment arena that is becoming more popular to nurse consultants is the private consulting firm. Private health care consulting firms, numbering over 200 in the nation's capital alone, offer assistance to individuals, groups, institutions, and government organizations in setting health care priorities; writing goals, standards, policies, and procedures; developing better managerial solutions for program efficiency; and planning health care programs. Nurses may incorporate their own private consulting firms to provide services directed toward nursing issues (Braddock and Sawyer, 1985; Hoffman, 1988; Reinert and Buck, 1989; Wright, 1981).

Approximately five percent of nurses perceive their role to be that of nurse consultant. Although third-party reimbursement may not be readily available, direct reimbursement by clients acknowledges the increasing expertise of nurses to solve problems related to the complex health care delivery system. This example of the growing entrepreneurship in nursing promotes professional recognition, association among nurses and other professions, and autonomy and authority to act for clients; it also enhances nursing's economic equality in the health care delivery system (Hoffman, 1988).

Similarly, voluntary organizations (e.g., the American Red Cross) may employ nurses to serve as resource persons in the development of local programs such as blood banks. The World Health Organization may employ nurses to serve as resources and facilitators to third world countries in the development of health care programs. Community health nurses, undergraduate and graduate, are prepared to meet the challenges of these employment arenas because of their expertise in comprehensive client assessment and in program development and evaluation, and because of their extensive knowledge of the use of available resources.

CLINICAL APPLICATION

The manager of a small housing project approached the local university's College of Nursing for assistance with health promotion and health monitoring activities for the project residents. Many of the residents were elderly with chronic illnesses; most were living on fixed incomes and were ten to fifteen miles from medical facilities. The community health faculty member assigned Patricia, a community nursing student, to *assess* this community's request for consultation.

Patricia arranged for a meeting with the housing manager to discuss the problem, *assess* her ability to help with the problem, and explore the client's expectations for herself or for the College of Nursing. As a result of these discussions the contract shown in the box on p. 678 was developed by Patricia.

After careful consideration, Patricia and the manager determined that a survey of residents' needs and facility resources would assist them in *planning* the alternatives they could explore for providing health monitoring to the residents.

With the approval of the community health faculty member, Patricia and her fellow students agreed to *implement* a health screening survey project and to collect data about the housing project, such as the physical facilities, the available equipment and supplies, and staff available to volunteer assistance with health screening and promotion activities. They also collected data on existing relationships with community referral sources, money available to support the program, and the attitude of staff and residents toward such a

program. Anticipated outcomes to be *evaluated* for the consultation included recommending to the project management a permanent health monitoring clinic within the facility, using one of several options: the development of a nursing clinic with the College of Nursing; contracting with the health department to provide the service; employing staff at the housing project to implement the clinic; or establishing a clinic staffed with volunteer nurses from the community.

At the *evaluation conference,* Patricia and her colleagues shared the results of their data-gathering activities. After careful consideration of the data, the housing project manager decided a permanent health clinic was essential for the residents. A review of the budget revealed that money was available to employ a full-time nurse to staff the clinic at the housing project.

SUMMARY

This chapter has outlined and discussed the definitions of consultation, consultation models, principles of process consultation, intervention modes, determinants of intervention modes, client populations, various frameworks for nurse consultation, academic preparation, and practice arenas for nurse consultants. The practical application of the consultative process in community health is reflected in the varied practice situations discussed in this chapter.

As qualified nurse consultants become more readily available, the acceptance by administrators and staff of this concept as a critical component of nursing practice is essential. With continually diminishing health dollars and the focus on fiscal accountability, the cost effectiveness of the nurse consultant is another factor affecting acceptance. The client's involvement in problem identification, selection and use of the consultant, and commitment to implementing workable solutions is necessary to ensure the most effective use of the consultant's and the client's time and resources.

CONSULTATION CONTRACT

Client name C. Jones, Manager

Address Housing Project

Phone 333-0000

Consultant name P. Smith, Nursing

Address College of Nursing

Phone 333-1000

Estimated costs (external consultant only) $500
   (including *phone, secretarial assistance, preparation, supplies, travel expenses* and *consultant sessions*)

Client problem definition 85 unit housing project. 75% elderly residents with chronic illnesses and limited income. 10-15 miles from health facilities. Exacerbations undetected and/or chronic illnesses go unresolved until acute state of illness.

Suggested intervention mode Catalytic/Prescriptive

Client goals

A healthier population through accessible and on-going health monitoring

Scope of consultation (time and no. of sessions)

3 planning and data gathering sessions in 6 weeks; 3 evaluation sessions at 2 to 3 week intervals during data collection; final evaluation session

Consultant resources (e.g., computer, secretary, library)

Computer to analyze data; library; assistance from faculty; staff to collect data (3 students)

Contract renegotiation and termination terms

Renegotiation at 2 to 3 week evaluation conferences. Termination at final evaluation conference.

Client resources (e.g., records, secretary, copy)

Project records available to collect data; secretary to type survey questionnaires; conference room for interviews; final report types; supplies.

Anticipated client benefits

Housing project will have identified plan for meeting health needs of residents. Residents will have a permanent health monitoring program.

Contract limitations (e.g., who, what, when, how will data be shared)

Survey of resident's health, housing project staff, administration, and resources by the CHN students. Report to manager and college faculty.

Potential interventions (e.g., report shared with administration; meeting held with staff)

Meetings with staff and residents to get input about best method to solve problem. Review of resources to find housing project's potential for solving own problem.

Consultant goals

Collect data as outlined.

Assess and define problem.

Identify resources for solving problem.

Prescribe best method for meeting residents' health care needs.

Data collection methods

Interviews staff, manager, local health care representatives

Surveys residents

Questionnaires

Meetings staff, residents, manager, faculty

Phone n/a

Contract evaluation

At end of 12 weeks will look at potential alternatives; choose one that is satisfactory to residents, staff, and management.

KEY CONCEPTS

The goal of consultation is to stimulate clients to take responsibility, feel more secure, deal constructively with their feelings and with others in interaction, and internalize skills of a flexible and creative nature.

The major goals of the process model are to assist the client to assess both the problem and the kind of help needed to solve the problem.

Purchase model consultation involves the hiring of a professional helper to provide expert information or service.

In the doctor-patient model, the client hires the consultant to find the problem and offer solutions without background data or assistance from the client.

The mental health model limits consultation to an interaction between professionals.

Consultation has also been described as a political process.

Five basic intervention modes or techniques applied to process consultation are acceptant, catalytic, confrontation, prescriptive, and theory-principles.

The use of a particular intervention mode is based on two factors: the client and the problem.

Four categories of problem issues are power/authority, morale/cohesion, norms/standards, and goals/objectives.

The process of consultation involves seven basic phases: initial contact, definition of the relationship with the client, selection of a setting and approach, collection of data and problem diagnosis, intervention, reduction of involvement and evaluation, and termination.

Nurse consultants may function as internal consultants within an organization or as external consultants from outside the client organization.

Educational requirements for the nurse consultant are primarily determined by two factors: the practice setting and the client population.

LEARNING ACTIVITIES

1. Interview one or more practicing community health staff nurses. Ask them to describe the activities of their jobs that could be categorized as consultation. During the interview attempt to determine the following:

   a. How they define consultation.

   b. The goals they are attempting to attain in the related consultative activities.

   c. The model they seem most likely to apply in their consultation.

   d. The intervention modes they practice.

   e. Whether their activities are of a generalist or specialist nature

and of an internal or external consultative nature.

   f. The strengths and limitations they perceive in themselves regarding their consultative functions (e.g., educational, experiential, organizational, relational, economic).

2. Interview one or more community health nurse consultants. During the interview, attempt to determine the answers to the aspects examined in the preceding activity.

3. After gathering data from your interviews and reading the material in this chapter, choose a definition of consultation that you think is most applicable to community health nursing practice.

BIBLIOGRAPHY

Baizerman M and Hall W: Consultation as a political process, Community Ment Health J 13(2):142-149, 1977.

Baradell J: Client-centered case consultation and single-case research design: application to case management, Arch Psychiatr Nurs 4(1):12-17, 1990.

Beare P: The ABCs of external consultation, Clinical Nurse Specialist 2(1):35-38, 1988.

Beecroft P: The consultant's image, J Nurs Adm 18(2):7-10, 1988.

Beyerman K: Consultation roles of the clinical nurse specialist: a case study, Clinical Nurse Specialist 2(2):91-95, 1988.

Blake R and Mouton J: Consultation, ed 2, Reading, Mass, 1983, Addison-Wesley Publishing Co, Inc.

Braddock B and Sawyer D: Becoming an independent consultant: essentials to consider, Nurs Econ 3(6):332-335, 1985.

Caplan G: The theory and practice of mental health consultation, New York, 1970, Basic Books, Inc, Publishers.

Clark M: The nurse educator in an expanded consultant role, The Journal of Continuing Education in Nursing 14(4):5-7, 1983.

Collins B: Do you need an external consultant? A model for decision making, Clinical Nurse Specialist 3(2):91-96, 1989.

Crowley A: Day care center directors' perceptions of the nurse consultant's role, Journal of School Health 60(1):15-18, 1990.

Hendrix M and LaGodna G: Consultation: a political process aimed at change. In Lancaster J and Lancaster W, editors: Concepts for advanced nursing practice: the nurse as a change agent, St. Louis, 1982, The CV Mosby Co.

Hoffman S and Fonteyn M: Third party reimbursement for CNS consultation, Nurs Econ 6(5):245-247, 274, 1988.

Hough A: The nursing consultant role, Nursing Management 18(6):69-72, 1987.

Kohnke M: The case for consultation in nursing: design for professional practice, New York, 1978, John Wiley & Sons.

Lamb H and Peterson C: The new community consultation, Hosp Community Psychiatry 34(1):59-63, 1983.

Lareau S: The nurse as clinical consultant, Topic Clin Nurs 2:79-84, Rockville, Md, 1980, Aspen Systems Corp.

Lippitt R and Lippitt G: Consulting process in action. In Jones I and Pfeiffer J editors: The 1977 annual handbook for group facilitators, San Diego, Calif, 1977, University Associates, Inc.

Miller L: Resistance to the consultation process, Nursing Leadership 6(1):10-15, 1983.

Novle J and Harvey K: Selecting and using a nursing consultant, Nurs. Econ. 6(2):83-85, 1988.

Oda D: Consultation: an expectation of leadership, Nursing Leadership 5(1):7-9, 1982.

Parsons W, Myrick R, and Gunnoe J: The case of Mr. W. mental health consultation, Journal of Gerontological Nursing 14(8):14-17, 1988.

Pati B: Nursing consultation: a collaborative process, J Nurs Adm 10(11):33-36, Nov. 1980.

Reinert B and Buck E: Issues in liability insurance and the nursing consultant, Clinical Nurse Specialist 3(1):42-45, 1989.

Rogers M and Trimmell J: Maximizing the use of the clinical nurse specialist as consultant, Nurs Adm Q 12(1):53-58, 1987.

Schaffner J: The consultation you don't want: taking charge, J Nurs Adm 17(8):6-7, 1987.

Schein E: Process consultation: its role in organization development, Reading Mass, 1969, Addison-Wesley Publishing Co, Inc.

Schilling K: The consultant role in multidisciplinary team development, Intern Nurs Rev 29(3):73-75, 96, 1982.

Stanley M: Critical care nurse as home health care consultant, Critical Care Nurse 8(8):74-75, 78-80, 1986.

Stone L: Consultation builds success for nurses, Nursing Success Today 1:23-29, 1984.

Wright BL: The nurse consultant, Canadian Nurse 77(2):34-36, Feb 1981.

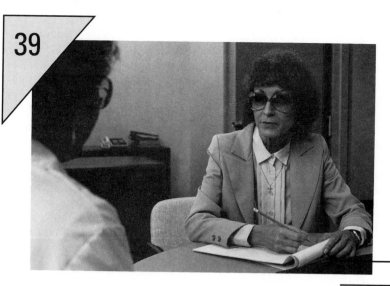

39

Promoting Continuity of Care: Advocacy, Discharge Planning, and Case Management

Ann H. Cary

OBJECTIVES

After reading this chapter, the student should be able to:

Define continuity of care, advocacy, discharge planning, and case management.

Identify the models of delivery and scope of nursing practice for each.

Identify the common factors and differences in process and activities for advocacy, discharge planning, and case management.

Analyze the legal and ethical implications of assuming the roles of advocate, discharge planner, and case manager.

KEY TERMS

abandonment	direct care	mediator
accountability	discharge planning	minimum data set
advocacy	episodic care	negligence
affirming	distributive	obstructors
aftermath	dissenters	ombudsman
aggressive behavior	empathy	passive behavior
amplification	empowerment	politics
assertiveness	gatekeeper	problem solving
attentive	helping relationship	rapport
brainstorming	indirect care	referral
case management	informal caregivers	rescuers
enduring care	information-exchange	self-determination
clarification	integrative	self reflection
collaboration	intercessor	supporting
congruence	interdisciplinary	territorialism
constituents	liability	validation
continuity of care	managed care	
coordination		

Contents of this chapter may reflect contributions of Ellen Kent Bailey and Sharon Sheahan from editions 1 and 2 of this text.

ADVOCACY

F or community health nurses, advocacy involves diverse activities, ranging from self-exploration to lobbying for health policy. Advocacy is essential for practice with clients and their families, communities, organizations, and colleagues on an interdisciplinary team. The functions of advocacy require scientific knowledge, expert communication, facilitation skills, and problem-solving and affirmation techniques. As the *Code of Nurses* (1985) states,

" . . . the goal of nursing actions is to support and enhance the client's responsibility and self-determination." (p.i)

However, this goal is a contemporary one. As Nelson (1988) indicates, the perspective regarding the advocacy function has shifted through time. The nurse advocate has been described in earlier writings as one who acted on behalf of or interceded for the client. As example of the *intercessor* role is the community health nurse who calls for a well-child appointment for a mother visiting the family planning clinic when the mother is capable of making an appointment on her own.

The evolution of the advocate role to that of *mediator* by the nurse advocate is described as a response to the complex configuration of social change, reimbursers, and providers in the health care system (Winslow, 1984). Mediation is an activity in which a third party attempts to provide assistance to those who may be experiencing a conflict in obtaining what they desire. The goal of the nurse advocate as *mediator* is to assist parties to understand each other on many levels so that agreement upon an action is possible. In the instance of a nurse as case manager for a health care organization, mediation activities between an elderly client and the payor (HMO), could accomplish the following results: the client may understand the options for community-based skilled nursing care; and the payor may understand the client's desires for a less restrictive environment for care. While the case manager as mediator does not *decide* the plan of action (in contrast to the role of arbitrator), he facilitates the decision-making processes between the parties so that the desired care can be reimbursed within the continuum of options.

In contemporary practice the nurse advocate places the client's rights as the focus of priority. The goal of *promoter* for the client's autonomy and self-determination may result in an optimal degree of independence in decision making. In the case in which a group of young pregnant women is the collective "client," the nurse advocate's role may be to inform the group of the benefits and consequences of breastfeeding their infants. However, if the new mothers decide upon formula feeding, the nurse advocate should support the group and continue to provide parenting, infant, and well-child services.

This proposition shows a different perspective of the nurse as advocate. It holds that the nurse's role as advocate may demand a variety of functions which are influenced by the client's physical, psychological, social, and environmental abilities. The nurse adapts the advocacy function to the client's dynamic capabilities as he follows a trajectory of health states. Even clients who desire access to more substantial health promotion activities can benefit from a partnership with the nurse advocate. Promoting a client group's access to onsite physical fitness programs in the occupational setting or supporting parents' and students' concerns about the high fat content of vending machine cuisine in the school system can stimulate the advocacy role in community health nurses. With the cost of health care expected to exceed a trillion dollars annually before the year 2000 and consumers assuming a larger financial portion of the care they choose, the *"promoter"* role of advocacy for those clients capable of autonomy is expected to intensify.

Conflict Potential
Roles

Nurses must be aware of available sources of support for fulfilling the advocacy role. Sources include each of the following: the *Code for nurses with interpretive statements* (1985); state practice acts; guidelines from the National Society of Patient Representatives; the American Nurses Association; *Standards of practice for community health nurses* (1986); the employing organization's *"bill of rights"* and philosophy, position descriptions, and employee evaluation criteria; external accreditation, certification, and licensure criteria for the employing organization; state health codes; the nurse's own philosophical basis of practice; and nursing theories.

Conflict can arise from two situations: advocates as adversaries and advocates as rescuers. When fulfilling the role of client advocate (as people who inform and support clients and affirm their decisions), nurses may be seen as adversaries to a client's family, other providers, or other organizations such as insurance companies. When advocates' actions are viewed as conflicting with another's interests, problems can arise.

Legal precedent for the nurse's role in client advocacy has been indirectly interpreted in the highly publicized case of *Jolene Tuma vs. the Idaho Board of Nursing*. This is an example of the plight of one nurse who encountered legal difficulties in her actions as client advocate. An elderly female patient was acutely ill with a type of cancer of the blood cells. The patient's physician informed her of the need for chemotherapy and outlined its side effects. Although the patient agreed to take the drugs, she eventually told Tuma of her negative feelings about taking them. Tuma informed her of alternative forms of treatment, including nutritional therapy and the use of Laetrile. The patient asked the nurse to explain these treatments to her son, who then told the physician. The physician brought charges against Tuma to the Idaho State Board of Nursing, who found her guilty of "unprofessional conduct." Her nursing license was suspended for three months. Upon appeal, the Idaho Supreme Court ruled that the Board of Nursing had been wrong in its action since the definition of what constituted "unprofessional conduct" was not clear in the Board's guidelines. No rules or regulations in the state's practice act had been found that prohibited Tuma's actions. (Creighton, 1984; Gargaro, 1978; Tuma, 1977).

Another conflict that can develop in the advocacy role is when nurses act as *rescuers* (Kohnke, 1982). A nurse who makes decisions for clients rather than supporting their decision making rescues them from self-determination and the consequences of their decisions. This places the nurse in the position of being blamed for any negative consequences experienced in a situation. Nurses can be viewed as scapegoats by clients, payors, families, and communities. Nurses who believe that their knowledge allows them to know and make decisions on the client's behalf may be more concerned with their own authority than with clients' needs and desires.

Position

A nurse employed in a position of *client advocate, patient representative, case/care manager, discharge planner, ombudsman, patient hostess,* or *organizational liaison* may experience conflicts related to functions, authority, and accountability.

Functions of nurses may vary from aiding their clients by promoting and protecting their interests to smoothing over conflicts between the clients and other parties so that the other parties benefit (Robinson, 1985). The *authority* to promote a client's self-determination may be covertly or overtly challenged by others. Informing a client about options and consequences which influence his decision may conflict with another party's needs. If the advocate's authority promotes desires or demands that are incongruous with the organization's goals, authority may be diminished. Nurses must be aware that having authority to perform the role can place them in conflict with higher authorities. This may cause problems with those having greater authority (physicians, administrators, and payors) and those with equal or less authority (interdisciplinary peers, clients, and families).

Accountability is needed in every profession. Advocates are answerable to their employees, peers, and clients. Problems will arise when nurses cannot show accountability to everyone's satisfaction. If advocates have more clients than they can handle, accountability for quality can create personal conflict.

Politics is defined as the "total complex of relations between people and society . . . the art and science of guiding and influencing policy" (Webster, 1984). Nurses must be aware that politics can greatly influence their actions. For example, when the advocacy role involves a subgroup in the community, the nurse's actions may come into conflict with the prevailing community policies.

There is a real potential for conflict in the community health nurse's role and position of advocate. By anticipating, assessing, diagnosing, and evaluating the situations likely to promote conflict, the nurse advocate can judge the impact of conflict management strategies. Scientific knowledge of community, interpersonal, and organizational systems and skillful performance in advocacy activities are critical in promoting self-determination in clients. Where dilemmas are uncovered and laws exist which are ambiguous or nonsupportive of the nurse advocate role, changes must be made (Brooke, 1988).

The Process of Advocacy

The goal of advocacy is to promote self-determination in a *constituency*. The constituency may be a client, family, peer, group, or community. The process of advocacy was defined by Kohnke (1982) to include *informing* and *supporting*; affirming is the third essential part of advocacy. All three activities are more complex than they may initially seem, and they require self-reflection on the part of the nurse as well as skill development as the process unfolds.

Self-reflection or self-exploration is a process of examining one's knowledge, attitudes, and behaviors in light of one's self and other values and expectations. Nurses may be unclear about their knowledge and knowledge deficit areas. While some attitudes and beliefs are readily known to self, others are more covert and inapparent. Behaviors usually reflect attitudes, but in some cases the attitudes are not very clear to the actor until exploration and reflection have been done. The value of self-exploration and reflection for the nurse in an advocacy role comes with being in touch with one's responses to others' choices in self-determination activities. It is often easier for the nurse to *inform, support,* and *affirm* another person's decision when it is congruent with the nurse's values. But when clients make decisions that are within their value systems which run counter to the values of the nurse, the advocate may feel conflict in contributing to the process of informing, supporting, and affirming those decisions. Promoting self-determination in others demands a philosophy of free choice once the information necessary for decision making has been discussed.

Informing

Knowledge is essential, but not sufficient, to the outcome of decision making. The interpretation of knowledge will be tempered by the client's values and meanings assigned to it. The interpretation of facts is the result of both objective and subjective processing of information. The subjective dimension greatly influences client decisions.

Informing clients about the nature of their choices, the content of those choices, and the consequences to the client is not a one-way activity. The information exchange process is composed of interactions which reflect three processes: *amplification, clarification,* and *verification. Amplification* is a process that occurs between the nurse and client to assess the needs and demands that will eventually frame the client's decision. Information is exchanged from both viewpoints. While the exchange may be initiated at the objective, factual level, it will likely proceed to incorporate the subjective perspectives of both parties.

The information exchanged between the parties is important to consider. Guidelines include the nurse's need to:

1. Assess the client's present understanding of the situation;
2. Provide correct information;
3. Communicate with the client's literacy level in mind, making the information as understandable as possible;
4. Utilize a variety of media and sources to increase the client's comprehension;
5. Discuss other factors that affect the decision, such as financial, legal, and ethical issues; and

6. Discuss the possible consequences of a decision.

The tone of the *amplification* process can direct the remainder of the informational exchange. It is important to relate with clients in a manner that reflects the advocate's endorsement of their self-determination. Setting aside the time necessary to listen to clients is critical. The client will feel that he is part of a mutual process if the nurse can engage him during the information exchange with a message that says "I respect your needs and desires as I share my knowledge with you." Non-verbal behaviors including direct eye contact, sitting at the client's level, arriving and concluding at a prescribed time, as well as verbal patterns that will foster exchange (open-ended statements, questions, probes, reflections of feelings, and paraphrasing) convey the interactive promotion of self-determination.

A client may not desire the exchange of information because of lack of self-esteem, fear of the information, or inability to comprehend the content of the communication. In such a case, the focus will be to understand the client's desire for no information and to express to the client the consequences of such inaction. The nurse may invite the client to ask for the information exchange at a later time, when he is ready, and can intermittently check with the client whether information exchange and amplification is desired. In these cases, the nurse should document the implemented nursing actions to reflect the procedures discussed above. This can reduce the basis for litigation and misunderstanding by other parties.

Clarification is a process in which the nurse and client strive to understand meanings in a common way. Clarification builds on the breadth and depth of the exchange developed in amplification to determine if the parties understand each other. During this process, misunderstandings and confusions will be examined. The goal of clarification is to avoid confusion between the parties. To foster clarification, nurses can use certain verbal prompts:

"What do you understand about . . . "
"Please tell me more about how you . . . "
"I don't think I am clear. Let me explain the situation in another way . . . As an example . . . "
"What other information would be helpful so that we both understand?"

Verification is the process used by the nurse advocate to establish accuracy and reality in the informing process. If the nurse discovers that a client is misinformed, he may return to the clarification or amplification stage and begin the process again. Verification produces the chance for the advocate and client to examine "truth" from their perspectives, which may include knowledge, intuition, previous experiences, and anticipated consequences. The advocate does not sanction the outcome. In true self-determination, the client sanctions the outcomes.

In reality, promoting a client's self-determination may take the advocate and client through the information exchange process a number of times as new dimensions or obstacles to an issue develop. Information exchange is a critical process for advocacy and is applicable to all advocacy constituents: individuals, families, groups, and communities.

TABLE 39-1
Nursing process and advocacy process

Nursing process	Advocacy process

Assessment/diagnosis	Information exchange
	  Gather data
	  Illuminate values

Planning	Generate alternatives & consequences Prioritize actions

Implementation	Decision making
	Support of client
	  Assure
	  Reassure

Evaluation	Affirmation
	  Evaluation
	  Reformulation

Communication that seeks to amplify, clarify, and verify knowledge, beliefs, and behaviors is used throughout both processes.

Supporting

The second major process, supporting, involves upholding a client's right to make a choice and to act on the choice. People who become aware of clients' decisions fall into three general groups: *supporters*, *dissenters*, and *obstructors*. Supporters approve and support clients' actions. Dissenters do not approve and do not support clients. Obstructors cause difficulties while clients try to implement their decisions.

Kohnke (1982) points to the need for the nurse advocate to implement several actions that fulfill the supporting role. Assuring clients that they have the right and responsibility to make decisions and reassuring them that they do not have to change their decisions because of others' objections are important interventions.

Affirming

The third process in the advocacy role is affirming. It is based on an advocate's own belief that a client's decision is consistent with the client's values and goals. The advocate validates that the client's behavior is purposeful and consistent with the choice that was made. The advocate expresses a dedication to the client's mission, and there may be a purposeful exchange of new information in order that the client's choice remains viable. Recognizing that a client's needs may fluctuate with changing resources, the affirmation activity must encourage a process of reevaluation and rededication to promote self-determination.

The importance of affirmation activities cannot be emphasized strongly enough. Many advocacy activities stop with assuring and reassuring, but affirmation is often critical in promoting a client's self-determination. Table 39-1 compares the nursing process with the advocacy process.

The following case study demonstrates how the community health nurse can use the process of advocacy to assist a client in reaching a decision.

The community health nurse operating an immunization clinic for residents of a city's homeless shelter has encountered an unemployed mother and her three children who have come to receive polio vaccines so the children can enter school near the shelter. During the interview the nurse discovers that the mother is concerned about the heating system and environment at the shelter. All three of her children are asthmatics and from the time they were forced to seek residence in the shelter, the children—particularly the youngest—have had multiple, acute episodes of asthma. When she shared her observations with a few of the other shelter inhabitants, they dissuaded her from complaining to the manager, since he had not shown any action on prior complaints of dust, mold, and inadequate heating; in fact, he had previously told the residents they would be evicted if they made any "noise" to the city about the conditions. Adding to their intimidation was the fact that there was a waiting list for the shelter, the only one in the city.

The nurse set up an appointment with the mother the next day to provide time to adequately explore and exchange information about the situation. The goal of the appointment was to provide an opportunity for information sharing. The nurse did not know whether the mother would be capable of making a decision at the conclusion of the appointment.

During the interview the nurse explored the client's perception of the problem. The nurse provided information about precipitating factors for asthma attacks and care-measures. The nurse provided "user friendly" written materials and pictures that had been supplied by a pharmaceutical company and answered the mother's questions. During the amplification process the nurse explored with the client her financial status as it related to housing, her legal status as a resident, and the relationship she had with other residents and the manager; she also obtained a description of the environment, the timing and intensity of the asthma episodes, and their impact on the children and herself. The nurse explored the mother's reactions to her children's increasing attacks, her dependency on the shelter at this point in her life, and her abilities for decision making and autonomy. At the conclusion of the visit the nurse asked the client to think about the positive and negative consequences of living at the shelter and to be prepared to discuss them the following day.

At the next visit, the nurse and client generated a list of positive and negative experiences and their consequences on the children. The client clarified the legal, environmental, and physical information she received from the nurse. The nurse clarified the mother's financial status and corrected a perception she had previously misinterpreted about guilt on the mother's part. The client and nurse restated to each other their understanding of the concerns and consequences, and they verified the reality and accuracy of the dimensions and consequences of the situation. The Community Health Nurse began to promote the client's decision-making powers in light of the information and their discussion and also helped her explore the options and consequences of these powers.

Because the nurse engaged the information-exchange process, this facilitated the client's understanding of the information and her feelings related to the dilemma. The mother made the decision to discuss her concerns with the manager. During the support phase of the nurse advocate's plan, she found the client experiencing reactions from supporters, dissenters, and obstructors. She assured the client of the normalcy of these anticipated behaviors and discussed alternate plans to meet her goals. The nurse reminded the client of her legal rights and reinforced the client's decision to consult with a legal aid organization. During the process of affirmation, the advocate provided verbal and behavioral evidence of her support for the client's decision. When a new housing code went into effect, she provided information to the client and discussed the impact this would have on the client's goals. They investigated alternate housing resources where the client could have more control over environmental factors affecting the health of her children. Upon their realization that no changes were possible for at least six months, the mother adjusted her goals and elected to participate in a new group-home option.

The advocate's role in the decision-making process is not to tell the client which option is "correct" or "right." The advocate's role is to provide the opportunity for information exchange, arming the client with tools that can empower him in making the best decision from his perspective. Enabling the client to make an "informed decision" is a powerful tool for building self-confidence. It gives the client the responsibility for selecting the options and experiencing the success and consequences based on current data.

Clients are empowered in their decision-making when they can recognize events that are beyond their control and can link chance occurrences with predictable events to make decisions they want. Sophistication decision-analysis techniques are beyond the scope of this book. Most involve mathematical calculations based on assigned values and are grounded in Operation Research literature.

Nurses can promote client decision-making through the following: the information-exchange process; promoting the use of the nursing process; incorporating written techniques (contracts, lists); reflection and prioritization; and using role playing and sculpturing to "try on" and determine the "fit" of different options and consequences for the client. By engaging clients in the information-sharing process and assisting them to recognize the progression of activities they experience as they build their "informed decision making base," the nurse advocate is empowering clients with skills that can strengthen their autonomy and confidence in the future.

Advocacy is a complex process. The balance between "doing for" and "promoting autonomy" can be precarious and is influenced by the client's physical, emotional, and social capabilities. The goal of advocacy is to promote the ultimate degree of self-determination possible for the client given the client's current and potential status; for most clients this goal can be realized.

For cases in which clients are comatose, unborn, or legally incompetent, nurse advocates have unique functions. The advocate's role is usually determined by the legal system; however, there are cases in which nurses must decide what roles they will play. These are areas requiring intensive self-exploration, research, and collaboration with professionals, family members, and significant others.

Skill Development

Skills needed by the nurse advocate are not unique to their profession. Nursing demands technical, relational, and problem-solving skills. Advocacy requires applying nursing skills to promote self-determination. However, there are several other skills that are necessary and well-defined.

Advocates must be open-minded and aware of people, society, and social order (Kohnke, 1982). Knowledge of nursing and knowledge from other disciplines is essential for the advocacy role in establishing authority and developing skills. Highly developed communication skills and a strong sense of self-esteem and professional confidence are also needed (Webb, 1987). The capacity for assertiveness for personal rights and the rights of others is essential.

The Helping Relationship

The helping relationship is defined as a relationship in which one participant helps the other to develop appreciation, expression, and more functional use of his inner resources (Rogers, 1961). A nurse's role in the helping relationship is to promote the client to make informed decisions. The client's role is to understand his needs and desires, obtain needed information, and use the information to make and implement decisions. The helping relationship is generally a process rather than a one-time event; it involves sequential actions and practices progressing toward a goal.

The helping relationship begins when a client or another person seeks out the nurse advocate. It can also be initiated through a case-finding process. Certain clients may be at higher risk when advocate functions are not available. For example, uninsured clients may encounter significantly greater barriers in their access to health care services than insured clients.

Four advocate skills can facilitate the goals of the helping relationship:

1. Establishing rapport: Rapport can be characterized by showing interest, responsiveness, and sensitivity, and it promotes trust, acceptance, and understanding. Rapport is conveyed in facial expressions and gestures, and it is fostered by asking pertinent questions, restating points, summarizing, and reflecting feelings.
2. Showing empathy: Empathy involves putting oneself in another's place. Advocates achieve empathy by trying to see the world from the client's viewpoint. They are "with" the client's experience. Clients experiencing difficult challenges to health maintenance, health protection and terminal disease may believe they have unique confusing feelings and perspectives when attempting to make informed choices. The skillful use of empathetic verbal and non-verbal reactions lets the client know he is being understood, and this can promote the effectiveness of the helping relationship.
3. Being congruent and genuine: Congruence implies honesty, sincerity, and spontaneity. Advocates do not create an illusion of advocacy. Rather, they are authentic, precise, and consistent in promoting clients' autonomy. Actions must be consistent with words, and verbal and nonverbal behaviors should match.

TABLE 39-2
Assertive communication components (Angel and Petronko, 1983)

Empathetic message*	I understand that. . . .
	I know you feel. . . .
Description of the situation/feeling	I purchased this. . . .
	I feel that. . . .
Expectations	I would like a new one.
	I would like this client to be seen next.
	I would like you to bring your records from your last visit.
Consequences	
Positive	I will do business with you again.
	I think his pain can be relieved much more quickly.
Negative	I cannot admit you without your record.

*Nonessential component

Advocates must be genuine in thinking, believing, and taking actions to promote clients.

4. Being attentive: Advocates who are involved in a client's communication are attentive. They are listening for what is said, how it is said, and what is omitted. It is through the skills of attentiveness that the advocate understands the client and his capacity. Attentiveness includes attention to the verbal and nonverbal, including such things as words, tone of voice, pace, volume, facial expressions, eye contact, posture, and gestures.

Assertiveness

"Assertiveness is open, honest and direct communication that takes into consideration your own personal rights as well as the rights of others" (Angel and Petronko, 1983, p. 7). Assertiveness is crucial in the role of advocate and should not be used to gain control but rather to relate to others respectively and effectively. Advocates can model assertive behaviors for clients and teach them assertive skills to promote self-responsibility. Clients may be encouraged to do the following:

- Use "I" statements in which they take responsibility for their messages.
- Avoid "you" statements, which place blame on the other person;
- Describe the situation and state what they want;
- Use an empathetic component if they feel it and want to convey it;
- When learning assertive communication, plan what they will say and practice through role playing, rehearsal, writing the responses, or speaking in front of a mirror.

Assertive behaviors have both verbal and nonverbal components. Table 39-2 illustrates verbal components of assertive behavior. Table 39-3 compares various nonverbal components of passive, assertive, and aggressive behavior.

When promoting self-determination, nurses may also

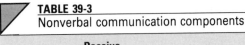

TABLE 39-3
Nonverbal communication components

Passive	Aggressive	Assertive
Nervous laughter	Abruptness	Using a well-modulated voice
Shifting weight from one foot to another	Slamming objects	Firm manner
	Using profanity	
Leaning against an object	Pointing	Maintaining an upright position
Wringing hands	Loudness	Maintaining an appropriate social distance
Slouching	Staring	

teach assertive communication skills. When nurses model the behavior, clients quickly learn what the process looks like and how the results appear. Rehearsing, role playing, and written practice will promote a smoother delivery of clients' messages with others.

Systematic Problem Solving

The nursing process—assessment, diagnosis, planning, implementation, and evaluation—is an example of a problem-solving model that can be used in the advocacy role. Advocates can be particularly helpful with *illuminating values,* and *generating alternatives.*

Illuminating Values

The values people hold affect their behavior, feelings, and goals. In the process of amplification, clarification, and validation, the advocate understands a client's values. Through the process of self-revelation, an emerging value (environment, people, cost, quality) may become more apparent to a client. This can impact in two ways. The client may be able to focus on actions consistent with the value, or the value may lend confusion and assist him in prioritizing action. Values can also change as new or relevant data is processed. The advocate's role is to assist clients in discovering their values, and this can be particularly demanding in the information exchange and affirmation process.

Generating Alternatives

Clients and advocates may feel limited in their options if they generate solutions before completely analyzing the problems, needs, desires, and consequences. Several techniques can be used to generate alternatives, including brainstorming and a technique known as the problem-purpose-expansion method. Brainstorming is an activity in which the nurse, client, professionals, or significant others generate as many alternatives as possible, without critical evaluation. Brainstorming creates a list which can subsequently be examined for the critical elements the client seeks to preserve (such as environmental preferences or degree of control). The list can be analyzed according to the consequences, the probability of chance events occurring, and the effect of the alternatives on self and others.

The problem-purpose-expansion method is a way to broaden limited thinking (Volkema, 1983). It involves restating the problem and expanding the problem statement so that different solutions can be generated. For example,

if the problem statement is to convince the insurance company to approve a longer hospital stay, the nurse and client have narrowed their options. However, if the problem statement is to make the client's convalescence as optimal and safe as possible, there are a number of solutions and options such as:

Obtaining extended care institutional placement;
Obtaining home health skilled services;
Obtaining M.D. home visits;
Paying for custodial care;
Paying for private duty skilled care;
Obtaining informal caregiving.

Conflict Management

Advocacy involves helping clients to manage conflicting needs and scarce resources. Techniques for managing conflict encompass the range of active communication skills. These skills are directed toward learning all parties' needs and desires, detecting their areas of agreement and disagreement, determining their abilities to collaborate, and assisting in discovering alternatives and valuable activities for reaching a goal. Mutual benefit with limited loss is a goal of conflict management.

Conflict and its management will vary in intensity and energy in a number of ways. Figure 39-1 illustrates one view of the activities of the continuum of conflict and conflict management.

The effort needed to manage a conflict depends on different factors: the existence of evidence to support facts, and objective/subjective perceptions of the parties involved.

Negotiating is a strategic process used to move conflicting parties toward an outcome. The outcome can vary from one in which one party enlarges its share at the other's expense *(distributive outcomes)* to one in which mutual advantages override individual gains *(integrative outcomes).* Integrative outcomes are usually based on problem-solving and solution-generation techniques (Bisno, 1988).

The process of negotiation can be characterized in three stages: prenegotiation, negotiation, and aftermath. Prenegotiations are activities designed to get parties to agree to collaborate. Parties must see the possibility of achieving an agreement and the costs of not achieving an agreement. Preparations must be made as to time, place, and ground rules concerning participants, procedures, and confidentiality.

The negotiation stage consists of phases in which parties

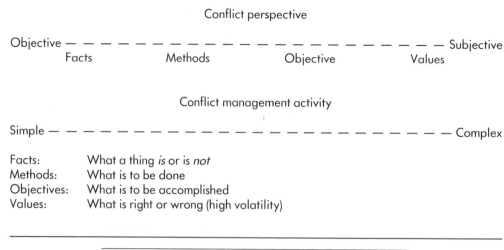

FIGURE 39-1

Conflict and conflict management continuum.

must develop trust, credibility, distance from the issue (to limit the feeling of "one best way"), and the ability to retain personal dignity. Bisno (1988) characterizes the phases as the following:

Phase 1: Establishing the issues and agenda. This is accomplished by identifying, clarifying, presenting, and prioritizing the issues.

Phase 2: Advancing demands and uncovering interests. Negotiations center around presenting parties' interests and differentiating parties' demands and positions.

Phase 3: Bargaining and discovering new options. *Debates* include gathering facts based on reasoning that will generate understanding and promote relearning. *Bargaining* reduces differences on issues by giving or removing rewards or desired objects. Creating new solutions or options through brainstorming, reflective thinking, and problem-purpose-expansion techniques is important in achieving options that provide mutual benefits.

Phase 4: Working out an agreement. This may involve settling on some but not all points. Parties can agree to reexamine the issues later, and steps for implementation and follow-up must be clarified.

The aftermath is the period following an agreement, in which parties are experiencing the consequences of their decisions. The reality of their decisions may lead to a re-evaluation of their values.

Thomas and Kilmann (1974) postulate that in a conflict situation parties engage in behaviors which reflect the dimensions of assertiveness and cooperation. Assertiveness is the ability to present one's own needs. Cooperation is the ability to understand and meet the needs of others. Each person uses a predominant orientation and secondary orientation to engage in conflict (see box). The importance of the Thomas-Kilmann categories is that there is a whole repertoire of orientations one can use and that each orientation can be valuable in a given situation.

CATEGORIES OF BEHAVIORS USED IN CONFLICT RESOLUTION

Competing	An individual pursues his concerns at another's expense.
Accommodating	An individual neglects his own concerns to satisfy the concerns of another.
Avoiding	An individual pursues *neither* his concerns nor another's concerns.
Collaborating	An individual attempts to work with others toward solutions which satisfy the work of both parties.
Compromising	An individual attempts to find a mutually acceptable solution that partially satisfies both parties.

Modified from: Thomas KW and Killman RH: Thomas-Killman Conflict Mode Instrument, New York, 1974, Xicom, Inc.

Clearly, flexibility in the advocate's conflict management behavior can facilitate an outcome that meets the client's goals. Helping parties to navigate the process of goal attainment requires effective personal relations, knowledge of the situation and alternatives, and a commitment to the process of advocacy.

The Impact of Advocacy

Advocacy empowers clients to participate in problem-solving processes and decisions about health care. Clients try to understand changing opportunities in the health care system for access, utilization, and continuity of care, while nurse advocates promote client control of morale, life satisfaction, self-esteem, and adherence to therapeutic regimes (Kohler, 1988). Clients are part of larger systems: the family, the work environment, and the community. Each system interacts with the client to shape the available options through resources, needs, and desires. Each system will also exhibit both confirming and conflicting goals and processes that need to be understood for client self-determination to be successful. For example, the practice of advocacy among minority groups may entail the ability to focus attention on the magnitude of problems caused by diseases affecting minority clients. It also mandates the planning, development, and implementation of programs that assure access and utilization to reduce collective morbidity and preventable deaths (Lythcott, 1985). Whether the client is an individual, family, group, or community, the advocacy function can promote the interest of self-determination that characterizes progressive societies.

Advocacy is not without opposition. Clients and advocates may find barriers to services, vendors, providers, and resources. A community may experience a shortage in nursing home beds, a child care facility may experience staffing shortages, a family may not have the financial resources to keep a child at home, and a client may find that the school system cannot fund a full-time nurse for its clinic. The reality of scarce resources constitutes a difficult barrier for advocates. However, it is often events such as these that stimulate a community's self-determination and innovative actions to correct gaps in service.

Advocates' accountability to employer goals and client goals can result in ethical concerns. A nurse advocate employed by an institution may experience conflict between the institution's financial need to limit services to nonpaying clients and the nurse's personal responsibility to provide information to clients about legal procedures to use when access to care has been denied.

Informed consent can cause another ethical concern. Clients may seek information from advocates about practice patterns and outcomes for medical options they are considering. How and to what extent clients are informed must be reconciled by the advocates.

Accepting referral fees from organizations that admit clients, presents a particularly difficult dilemma for advocates. Advocates can benefit from strong professional and ethical decision-making capabilities and access to consultation for support when faced with such conflicts.

Advocacy is a philosophy and standard of practice for community health nurses. It is a complex process weighted with legal and ethical implications. Nurses are encouraged to reexamine their care regularly in light of promoting clients' self-determination. The assimilation of skills in advocacy, communication, and conflict management is a career-long process that can result in higher levels of satisfaction and quality of life for clients, families, organizations, and communities.

CONTINUITY OF CARE

Continuity of care has been defined as a goal (Hartigan and Brown, 1985, Buckwalter, 1985) and as a process (Tebbitt, 1981; ANA, 1975; Urbanic et al., 1985). As a goal, it should meet three requirements:

1. Linkages should exist among health care providers (individuals and organizations in the community) and should be clearly identified.
2. Services offered by each provider must contribute to

the health status of the client.
3. There must be identifiable processes (planning, coordinating, communicating, referral, and follow-up) to achieve improved health status in a community.

As a process, continuity of care has been described as the coordination of activities involving clients, providers, and payors to promote the delivery of health care. Building a care system that is client-centered necessitates flexibility, interaction, and supportiveness, and it requires four elements (Vladeck, 1987):

1. Combining and integrating payment sources for services (Medicare, medi-gap policies, and out-of-pocket).
2. Integrating documentation and record-keeping data systems; i.e., creating communication systems and a common language among those involved in care.
3. Identifying someone to manage the activities.
4. Providing interdisciplinary and informal caregiving teamwork.

It is not coincidental that the interest in continuity of care has blossomed with the expansion of options in the current health care system. As different provider systems crystallize within health care choices, the inevitable byproducts are fragmentation, duplication, and gaps in service delivery. Donabedian (1987) notes that the elements of continuity, teamwork, and coordination are indicators of quality in health care. In the changing health care system, services must be carefully coordinated in tandem and without fail if clients are to receive quality care.

With the health care industry in transition and not expected to restabilize soon, certain trends will portend the value of continuity of care:

◊ Health continues to be a high-priority expenditure by consumers—12% of the GNP in 1985; 20% of the GNP by the year 2000.
◊ Innovations of new health-care product lines and recycling of matured health care services are expected.
◊ A shift to capitation and prepayment of services is occurring.
◊ There is a push to increase the efficient use of all resources providing care in the continuum.
◊ Escalation of the entrepreneurial spirit in designing and managing community health services is evident.

A free-market attitude is consumer-driven. The value of health care services for consumers is the result of price and quality:

$$Value = Price + Quality$$

Community health nurses who can deliver well-coordinated care options at a competitive price will be valued professionals in the emerging health care system.

Continuity of care can be viewed from many perspectives. Payors may view it as a method to control costs. Consumers may see it as promoting their rights to make choices or control access. Providers may understand it as the opportunity to help clients tethered to their systems of delivery. Regardless of perspective, nurses are the ideal professionals to direct the leadership and delivery efforts toward the goal of continuity of care, which is to provide efficient and effective use of limited health care resources.

To achieve continuity of care, nurses may be involved in three activities: advocacy, discharge planning, and case management. In this section, the latter two activities will be discussed. *Standard VIII—Continuity of Care* serves as a guideline for those activities (ANA, 1986):

> The nurse is responsible for the client's appropriate and uninterrupted care along the health care continuum and therefore uses discharge planning, case management, and coordination of community resources.

In addition, the American Association for Continuity of Care is endorsing a certification process for continuity of care providers (discharge planners) to be implemented in the future (Poe, 1990).

Discharge Planning

Discharge planning is an essential component of nursing practice and should be a part of every health care delivery structure. It can be a process and an organized unit of service in a facility. Discharge planning is a segment of the continuity of care process, and it prepares the client for the next phase of care through organized planning and coordination of resources. It is client-oriented, promotes clients' self-determination, and facilitates access and options during service delivery and after discharge. The development of the plan of care is a confidential, organized, interdisciplinary process that recognizes client preferences, needs, and potential (Russ, 1989). Donabedian's (1987) notions of team-hood, coordination, and continuity are explicit in this perspective of discharge planning.

The historical roots of discharge planning go back more than 150 years (Shamansky, Boase, and Horan, 1984). Discharge planning was anchored in social services in the early twentieth century. The first social service department in a hospital was established in 1905 by a nurse at Massachusetts General Hospital (Cagan & Meier, 1979). A review of the literature of the first half of the twentieth century suggests that this period was characterized by premature discharge, gaps in service, and social causes of diseases (Shamansky, et al., 1984). The 1940s and 1950s brought federal support to the expansion of health care institutions through the Hill-Burton Act and Kerr-Mills Legislation. More health care facilities and services became available. The hospital became the focus of health care delivery. The 1960s and 1970s brought Social Security legislation to cover hospital, physician, and other health care services for those eligible for Medicare, Medicaid, and other federal benefits programs. Reimbursement for the utilization of these expanded services became available. Today, reimbursement has shaped utilization and discharge patterns for consumers. Some examples of regulations from the legislation that have shaped the structures and delivery of discharge planning for clients in the 1990s include the mandated existence of discharge planning in all Medicare-certified hospitals, specifications of minimum data sets on all discharged clients, and the requirement of issuing a written statement on discharge rights. This legislation resulted from concerns on the part of consumers and organizations regarding the system of reimbursement for Medicare patients. Implemented in 1983 and increasingly adapted as a reimbursement method by other insurers, the payment system resulted in patients being prematurely discharged or dumped from institutions without adequate planning for their acute aftercare needs (AHA, 1987; HCFA, 1986; Chakrabarty, Beallor, and Pelle, 1988; GAO, 1987). If historical precedent is any indication, the federal and accreditation mandates for the existence and process of documented discharge planning will eventually be required for any organization or provider in the community delivering health care services. As a condition for reimbursement, this method is a powerful driver of care standards.

National organizations have endorsed concepts and standards for discharge planning. The National League for Nursing (NLN) instituted a recommendation as early as 1966 for discrete discharge planning programs staffed by full-time nurses. The American Nurses Association (1975) endorsed the existence of continuity of care and discharge planning programs in institutions and community agencies. Professional Practice standards appeared in 1986 (ANA, 1986). The American Association for Continuity of Care published *Standards for Hospital Continuity of Care* in 1986. In 1987, the Medicare Conditions of Participation and the Joint Commission on the Accreditation of Healthcare Organizations (JCAHO) included discharge planning activities in their minimum standards. The 1990 edition of the Community Health Accreditation Program (a subsidiary of the NLN) includes discharge planning in its standards.

The mandate for discharge planning services is clear and has created the need for program development and personnel who are conceptually and practically prepared to perform discharge planning activities that can foster continuity of care. McNulty (1988) indicates that 56% of all discharge planning services have been initiated since 1984. In 1982, nurses constituted 25% of the discharge planning workforce. This number rose to 45% by 1988. Social work professionals constituted 47% of these positions in 1988 (Feather, 1985; 1988). The trend for nursing leadership in discharge planning positions is projected to rise through the 1990s as lengths of stay decline, health care options expand, acute care cases are managed in community-based services, and undergraduate and specialty graduate programs for nurses in this area become more available.

Goals and Process

The goal of discharge planning is to promote continuity of care. Discharge planning facilitates the appropriate transition of clients to other settings for care.

Certain characteristics are important for nurses to include in their discharge-planning philosophy:

1. The client is the focus of the process. Values, desires, and needs of the client are essential in planning. The client, significant others, and legal representatives should be active participants in the process.
2. Basic client needs at the time of discharge can be identified before or at admission. While a client is receiving services, needs must be monitored.
3. The use of screening criteria to automatically begin a discharge process should be implemented carefully and evaluated periodically.
4. Discharge planning is a multidisciplinary process that depends on collaboration and clear verbal, nonverbal, and written communication among all participants.

TABLE 39-4
Nursing process and discharge planning

Nursing process	Discharge planning process	Activities
Assessment	Preadmission process	Perform high-risk or referral-source screening
	Admission	Perform self-referral screenings and professional and family referrals during early portion of contact; perform discharge-planning rounds; gather comprehensive assessment data
	Duration of service	Monitor client's desires and needs; perform interdisciplinary family, and client assessment conferences; document
Diagnosis	Identify and substantiate potential and actual problems	Observe and gather interdisciplinary, family, and client data; cluster signs and symptoms; document
Planning	Design discharge plan and set goals	Perform interdisciplinary, family, and client conferences; consult standards of care; analyze resources for appropriateness and availability; prioritize choices; set immediate and long-range goals; design realistic time-frames; determine gaps in service; explore reimbursement sources; designate responsibilities; define communication and feedback processes; document
Implementation	Test action plan; revise as contingencies demand	Monitor ability of client and family to engage in actions; conduct interdisciplinary, family, and client conferences; monitor changes in needs, desires, and goals; perform education, coordination, and referrals; monitor changes in resource capabilities; document
Evaluation	Measure results; incorporate adjustments	Conduct interdisciplinary, family, and client conferences; gather data from referral sources, physicians, clients, and families; examine degree of goal attainment; examine readmissions and morbidity data; examine the client's regained functional status; examine use of unplanned resources; measure outcomes against standard care; document

5. The presentation of care options upon discharge requires current knowledge of providers, programs, resources, reimbursement, procedures, quality, accessibility, and appropriateness of the options.

6. Clients should make informed decisions about their discharge options. They should demonstrate an understanding of costs, professionals involved, length and duration of services, risks, benefits, and legal implications.

7. Discharge planning occurs in any service a client enters, including clinics, managed care organizations, and schools.

The process of discharge planning begins before admission if possible. The nursing process is inherent. Table 39-4 shows appropriate activities that support the discharge planning process and how they relate to the nursing process.

Teamwork and Collaboration

The activities of many disciplines are needed for successful discharge planning. The client, family, significant others, and community organizations contribute to achieving the goal. Physicians, nurses, and social workers are usually the disciplinary members in the process. Each has an expertise or scope over which he exerts control. The physician may serve as a gatekeeper, writing the orders to discharge from and admit to; or the physician may play a more intensive role in the process of education, diagnosis of discharge needs, and referral sources. The discharge planning nurse engages in the process illustrated in Table 39-4 above.

The social worker may also engage in the discharge process, offering unique social service and discipline-based knowledge that augments the expertise of nurses and other practitioners. A complementary approach by the team, in which the expertise and abilities of each member combine to produce a comprehensive, validated discharge process, is effective. Otherwise, territorial conflicts can serve as barriers to collaboration.

Figure 39-2 portrays the sequential yet reciprocal process of collaboration and is illustrated in six stages and activities (Androwich and Cary, 1989). The goal of communication in the collaborative developmental process is to promote amplification, clarification, and verification of all team members' perspectives. While communication is an essential component in collaboration, it is not sufficient to result in or maintain collaboration. The box lists the six stages and activities within each stage which are proposed to result in collaboration (Cary and Androwich, 1989). Although the collaboration model recognizes the contributions inherent in joint decision making, one member of the team should be accountable to the system and the client and should be responsible for monitoring the entire process.

Providers of continuity of care are uniquely positioned to encounter conflict on a daily basis. Competing needs, resources, organizational demands, and professional role boundaries among team members present opportunities and pitfalls for conflict management and collaboration. Figure 39-3 examines the stimuli for conflict and the domains for competing demands experienced by discharge planners.

Collaboration is enhanced during discharge planning if team members respect one another's roles and functions, if they are prepared for and open to problem-solving, and if

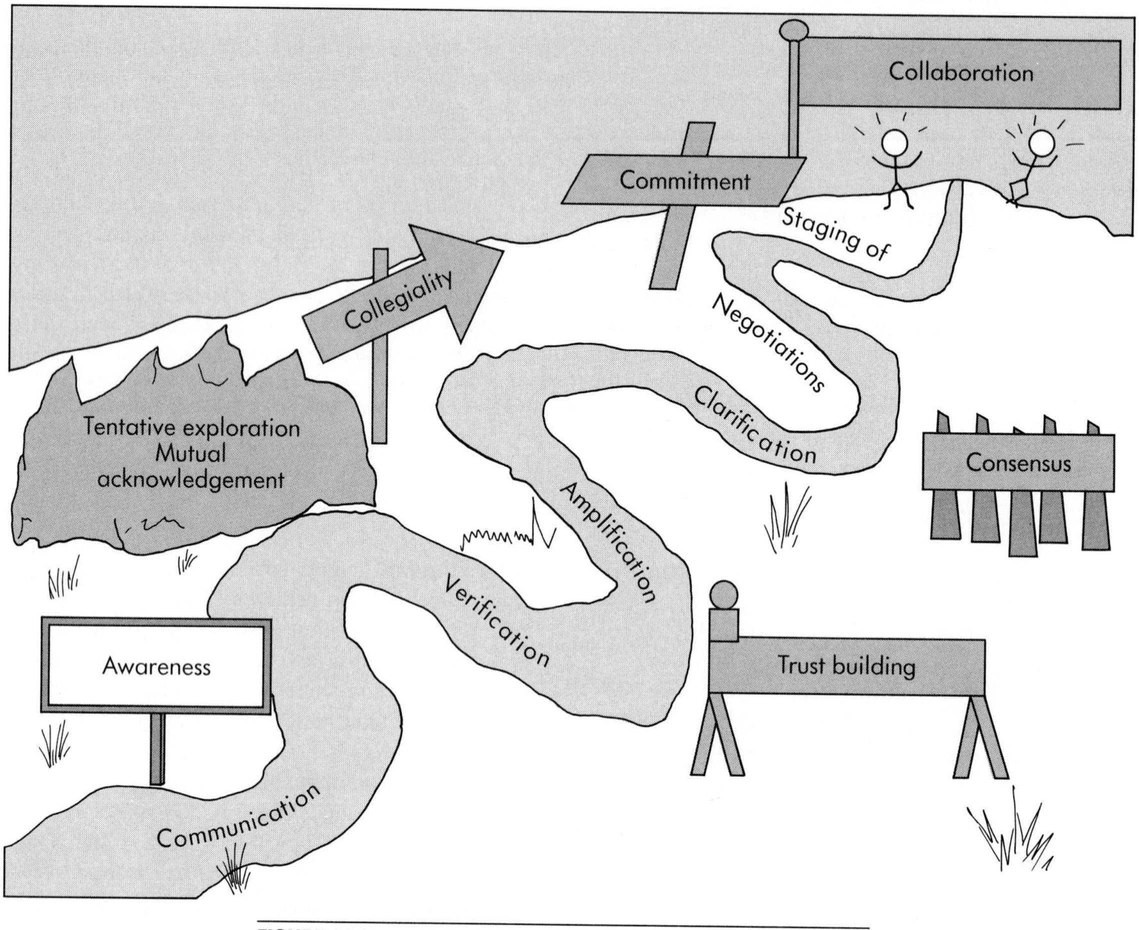

FIGURE 39-2

Collaboration is a sequential yet reciprocal process. *(From Cary A and Androvich I, 1989. A collaboration model: a synthesis of literature and research survey. Paper presented at the Association of Community Health Nursing Educators Spring Institute, Seattle, June 1989.)*

STAGES OF COLLABORATION

AWARENESS

Make a conscious entry into a group process; focus on goals of convening together; generate definition of collaborative process and what it means to team members.

TENTATIVE EXPLORATION AND MUTUAL ACKNOWLEDGEMENT

Exploration

Disclose professional skills for the desired process; disclose areas where contributions cannot be made; disclose values reflecting priorities; identify roles and disclose personal values including time, energy, interest, resources.

Mutual acknowledgement

Clarify each member's potential contributions; verify the group's strengths and areas needing consultation; clarify member's work style, organizational supports, and barriers to collaborative efforts.

TRUST BUILDING

Determine the degree to which reliance on others can be achieved; examine congruence between words and behaviors; set interdependent goals; develop tolerance for ambiguity.

COLLEGIALITY

Define the relationships of members with each other; define the responsibilities and tasks of each; define entrance and exit conditions.

CONSENSUS

Determine the issues for which consensus is required; determine the process used for clarifying and decision making to reach consensus; determine the process for reevaluating consensus outcomes.

COMMITMENT

Realize the physical, emotional, and material actions directed toward the goal; clarify procedures for reevaluating commitments in light of goal demands and group standards for deviance.

Collaboration

A process of joint decision-making reflecting the synergy that results from combining knowledge and skills.

From Cary A and Androwich I: A collaboration model: a synthesis of literature and research survey, Paper presented at the Association of Community Health Nursing Educators Spring Institute, Seattle, June. 1989.
Mueller WJ and Kell B: Coping with conflict, Englewood Cliffs NJ, 1972, Prentice Hall, Inc.

---

they are committed to the goals of the discharge plan. Client information presented in team conference may include the following:

1. Sociodemographics: Includes name, residence, birthdate, gender, marital status, religious preference, race, education, employment status and site, health care coverage, languages spoken, income, and financial status.
2. Health status: Includes diagnoses, procedures, known health problems and risk factors affecting postdischarge needs, level of consciousness, and cognitive/behavioral factors affecting discharge needs.
3. Functional status: Includes eating, bathing, dressing, toilet use, bowel and bladder management, transferability, locomotion, and instrumental activities of daily living (such as meal preparation, medication administration, telephone use, housekeeping, shopping, handling finances, and transportation use). Medical restrictions that alter functional status are also discussed.
4. Environmental barriers: Includes living arrangements, location, barriers, and presence of others in home setting.
5. Nursing and other care requirements: Includes skin, nutrition, hydration, respiratory, and elimination requirements, as well as medications. Educational needs, durable medical equipment needs, and therapy or service needs (such as P.T., O.T., S.T., S.W., R.T., M.H., aide, or household services) are also discussed.

6. Family and community support: Includes sources and the ability and willingness of primary supports. Community services used before admission are also listed.
7. Goals and preferences of the patient, family, and significant other.
8. Goals, options, and resources (informal and formal).

Institutions have their own tools that address many of these areas. In some institutions these areas are rated to optimize discharge-planning services and to classify discharge plan activities. The Omaha Classification Scheme lists 44 nursing diagnoses, 15 community health parameters, and 4 domains that organize information on clients in a community health setting (see Chapter 14). Peters (1988) cited this *Scheme* as advantageous in standardizing language and required data elements for discharge-planning clients.

It is clear that teamwork and collaboration demand knowledge and skills about clients, health status, resources, treatments, and community providers. The ability to assess clients' and families' complex needs encompasses knowledge of intrapersonal, interpersonal, medical, nursing, and social dimensions. The demonstration of team member and leadership skills in facilitating a goal-directed group process is essential. It is unlikely that any single professional possesses the expertise required in all dimensions. It is likely, however, that the synergy produced by all can result in successful strategies for discharge planning.

Referral and Coordination

Referral and coordination are major parts of discharge planning action. A *referral* sends or directs clients for in-

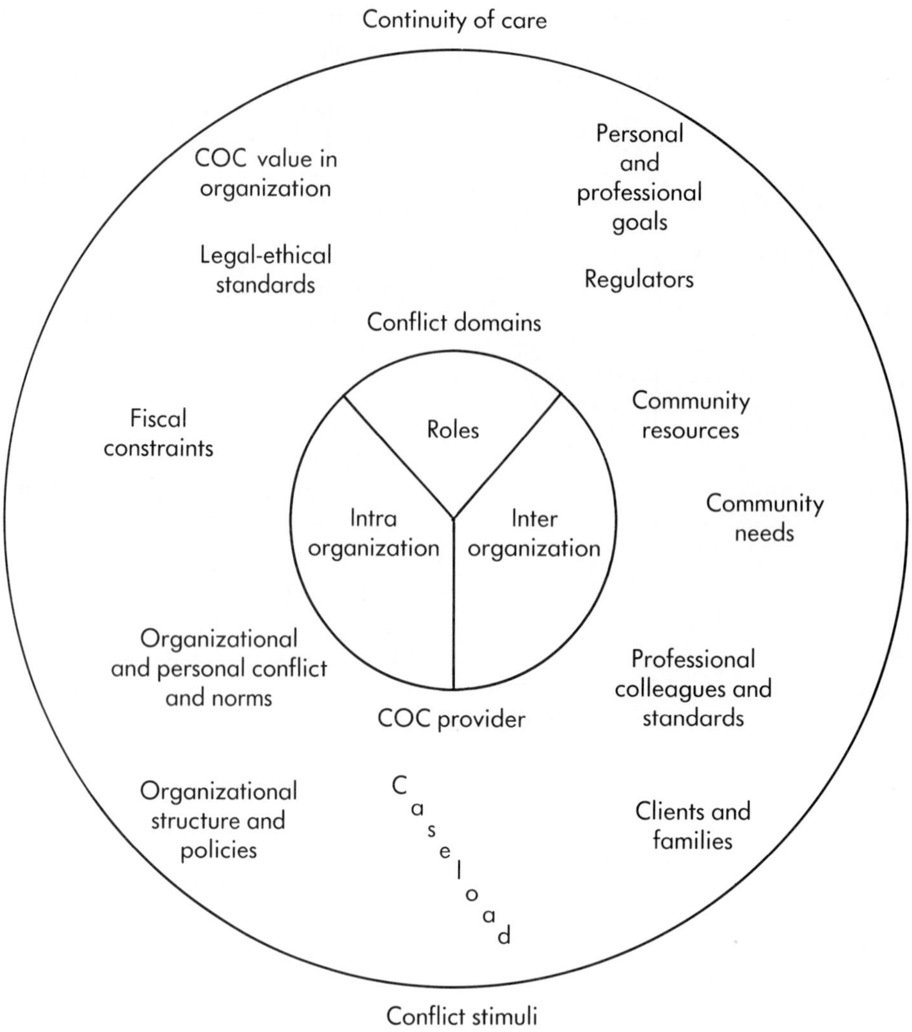

Continuity of care

COC value in
organization

Legal-ethical
standards

Personal
and
professional
goals

Regulators

Conflict domains

Fiscal
constraints

Roles

Community
resources

Community
needs

Intra
organization

Inter
organization

Organizational
and personal conflict
and norms

COC provider

Professional
colleagues and
standards

Organizational
structure and
policies

Case load

Clients and
families

Conflict stimuli

FIGURE 39-3

Conflict stimuli model for continuity of care providers.

formation, treatment, assistance, support, or help with decisions. A referral should be written and supplemented with a documented conversation. Verbal interaction clarifies the written referral.

Discharge planners may receive or initiate referrals. Referral processes are characterized as *open* or *closed*. In an open referral system, anyone can initiate a referral for discharge planning. In a closed referral system, only designated individuals can write an order that begins the discharge planning process. Use of the latter process is declining in institutions. Characteristics of quality referrals include the following:

◇ The client's documented agreement to the referral
◇ A signed *release of information* to accompany the referral
◇ Accurate and comprehensive information about the client
◇ Direct knowledge of the client
◇ Knowledge of availability, cost, and quality of the referred resources

◇ Use of tracking and monitoring methods to determine the status of activity on the referral
◇ Follow-up and feedback components from the referent, referral source, and client.

The referral process should be discussed with physicians, staff, and clients before beginning. Wherever possible, options for referral sources should be objectively presented to the client, and the client should be able to choose among the options that meet the goals. A copy of the referral, communication about the referral, and the outcome evaluation of the referral should be documented in the client's record. Referral sources can benefit from a periodic assessment of their capabilities in meeting the needs of clients. The box shows examples of community resources that can be referral sources.

The definition of *coordination* is less precise. Some authors include the supervision of paraprofessionals in their definitions (Cloonan and Shuster, 1989) while others include the actual delivery of direct care (Campbell and Patton, 1985; Capitman, Haskins, and Bernstein, 1986).

EXAMPLES OF COMMUNITY RESOURCES

ADVOCATES

American Civil Liberties
Long-term Care Ombudsman
Local Government Citizen's Advocacy
Department of Social Services
State Public Service Commission

ALCOHOL & DRUG ABUSE

Alcoholics Anonymous
Comprehensive Care
Detoxification Programs
National Council on Alcoholism
Narcotics Anonymous
Rehabilitation Counseling Centers

CHILD CARE

Department of Social Service
Salvation Army
Neighborhood Organizations

CHILDREN'S SERVICES

Adoption Teams
Local Government Children's Services
Foster Care
Crisis Drop-in Centers

COMMUNITY EDUCATION

American Red Cross
Dairy & Food Nutrition Council
March of Dimes
Parents-in Training Programs
Parents-Plus for Handicapped

HEALTH

Local Medical Center
American Cancer Society
American Lung Association
Cancer Information Services
Hospice Agencies
Diabetes Foundation
Physicians for Medical Assistance
Health Department
Muscular Dystrophy Association
Veterans Hospitals
Home Health Agencies
Nursing Homes
Hearing & Speech Services
Child Development Center
Council for Blind
Mental Health Facilities
Shriner's Hospitals

COUNSELING

Alternatives for Women
Comprehensive Care
Catholic Social Services
Department of Social Services

Family Counseling Services
Life Educators
Government Psychological Service Center
Veterans Centers

EDUCATION

Vocational Technical Schools
Preschool for Handicapped
Hearing & Speech Center

ELDERLY

Senior Citizens Center
Alzheimer's Association
Community Service Nutritional Programs
Senior Citizen Employment Services
Creative Living Center
Public Housing
Reassurance Phone Service (Red Cross)
Home Care
Nursing Homes
Health Department Social Security Administration
Council on Aging

EMPLOYMENT

Community Service Employment Programs
Local Government Employment & Training Centers
Workshops for Mentally Handicapped
Private Employment Agencies
Vocational/Rehabilitation Services

FINANCIAL AID

Department Social Insurance
Salvation Army
Unemployment Insurance

HUMAN ABUSE

Local Government Children's Services
Crimes Against Children
Department of Social Service
Protective Services
Local Child Abuse Council
Rape Crisis Center
YWCA Spouse Abuse Center

LEGAL

Juvenile Service Center
Legal Aid Services

PREGNANCY/CHILDBIRTH

Pregnancy Help Center
Birthright Organizations
Planned Parenthood Association
Right to Life

Continued.

EXAMPLES OF COMMUNITY RESOURCES—cont'd

HOTLINES

Adoption
Adult Abuse
American Cancer Society
Child Abuse
Crisis Intervention
Help Line (General)
Parental Help Line
Poison Control
Toxic Chemical National Response Center
Rape Crisis Center
Spouse Abuse Crisis Center

HOUSING

Association for Retarded Citizens
Community Action
Local Government Division of Housing Grants
Hospital Hospitality Houses
Housing Authorities
Human Rights Commission
Ronald McDonald Houses
Salvation Army

SELF-HELP

Al-Anon
Alternatives for Women
Alliances for Mentally Ill
Alzheimer's Societies
Compassionate Friends for Bereaved Parents
Smoking Cessation Programs
I Can Cope Education Programs for Cancer
Lost Chord Club
Parents Anonymous
Parents Without Partners
Parkinson's Disease Support
Prison Family Support
Reach to Recovery
United Ostomy Association
Widows Helping Widows

TRANSPORTATION

Local Bus Service
Salvation Army
Wheels (Red Cross)

Coordination

Coordination has a history in public health nurse's actions in the Hull House and Henry Street Settlements. Nurses coordinated the care and community resources for immigrant and low socioeconomic families in these areas.

Coordination is a nursing activity that includes planning, linking clients with services, and communicating information among clients and providers. Research has found that five activities comprise nursing-coordination activities: completing required paperwork, supervising staff, exchanging information, arranging services, and collaboratively planning care (Cloonan, 1990). The coordination activities performed within these categories include telephone calls, meetings, correspondence, trips or visits outside the employment site, and paperwork.

Coordination has also been termed *indirect care,* in contrast to direct care (providing technical skills, teaching, and counseling). Although direct care activities are more tangible and are seen as reimbursable, indirect care activities are essential to the outcomes of nursing care. Coordination may involve 12%-44% of nursing time and is labor-intensive (Mor et al., 1985; Banfield, 1987).

Care coordination is costly. Weiss (1987) suggests that attention to the coordination function is not appropriate for every client, especially not for the independently functioning person. People with functional limitations, chronic conditions, long-term needs, and lack of family support can benefit from directed coordinated efforts. Discharged patients can have several needs. Kromminga and Ostwald (1987) found that clients of an agency's discharge-planning service involving a local hospital had a mean of 5.8 needs per client. Clients who encounter barriers to access, utilization, reimbursement, or appropriate providers are more likely to ben-

efit from coordination. Each agency will have its own philosophy on the importance and manpower dedicated to this function. For community health nurses, professional standards support the role and functions of coordination. In tandem with other activities, a nurse's responsibility is to participate in the coordination of care with other providers in order to achieve the goal of continuity of care.

Screening Criteria

Nurses should evaluate the appropriateness of using screening criteria to guide the initiation of a discharge planning process. Examples of screening criteria are shown in the box. Nurses should also examine these criteria to identify potential post-discharge problems. In a research study done with an elderly population, Johnson and Fethke (1985) found four categories of variables related to post-discharge problems:

1. CLIENT'S SELF-ASSESSMENT OF GENERAL HEALTH: Clients' and professionals' assessments of general health even in the presence of disability were positively related to long-term health outcomes.
2. COMPLEXITY OF MEDICAL SITUATION: Risk factors include five or more diagnoses, medications scheduled at times other than mealtime, and frequent changes in medication doses.
3. HISTORY OF INABILITY TO MAINTAIN HEALTH: Characteristics include the presence of mental status deficits, repeated hospitalization within the last year, and use of community agencies before admission.
4. EXCESSIVE CLIENT NEEDS: The abilities of family members and informal caregivers were exceeded (Johnson and Fethke, 1985).

SCREENING CRITERIA

Admitted from another health care setting	Progressive diseases
Age (very young to very old)	Chronically ill or debilitated
No known relatives or address	Permanently disabled
Developmental delays	Multiple medical diagnoses
Lives alone or with incapable caregiver	Multiple therapy needs
Terminal illness	Special equipment or supplies
Recently discharged from acute care facility	Radical/mutilating surgery
Trauma/rape or substance-abuse victims	Psychiatric disorders
Pregnant minors	Very low birth weight, failure to thrive, congenital anomalies
Persons with Acquired Immunodeficiency Syndrome	Inadequate financial resources
Open/infected wounds, ostomies	Inadequate health care reimbursement
Drainage tubes	Cognitive deficits
Intravenous or entero feedings	Functionally impaired
History of noncompliance	Transplants
Repeated readmissions for same problem or its sequelae	High technology needs
Behavioral problems	Potent, experimental, or multiple medications
	Knowledge deficits

Provider Models and Functions

Community health nurses provide discharge planning services in several settings. Planning for the post-discharge needs of clients is a standard professional practice of all nurses.

The *consultative model* is used by nurses who advise and support the discharge planning activities of the professional, organization, or team. They may advise and assist others in solving particular challenges and barriers to their discharge planning goals, and they may develop resource information and educate personnel who perform the discharge-planning tasks.

In many community health agencies, discharge planning is the responsibility of the primary nurse, team leader, or case manager. In this *direct service model* it is viewed as an essential component of the nursing process and is a part of direct client care activities. Some community health agencies are removing discharge planning from the functions of nurses' daily responsibilities by forming separate teams of liaison, coordinator, and/or discharge planning nurses within the organization; these are seen as better able to handle complex discharge-planning activities.

Community health organizations may also use these teams to contract with other agencies to perform discharge planning within those agencies. *Partnership* models provide continuity of care through multi-organizational discharge planning contracts.

Challenges to Effective Discharge Planning

Conflicting goals can often reduce the effectiveness of discharge planning if not managed appropriately. Examples include the following:

1. Client/family/legal representative: Participants who are unaware of the potential benefits of improving their health may refuse services. Not having everyone's consent can interfere with planning, and the discharge goal will not be met. Intrafamily and in-tergenerational conflict can increase barriers to the discharge plan. Individual and family coping responses to health care delivery may limit responsible decision-making and planning. Participants' lack of knowledge and financial resources may increase difficulties.

2. Systems support: Discharge planning typically operates in an organization, and value of the planning depends on its ability to support the goals, mission, and plans of the organization. When discharge planning is undervalued, the activities can suffer from a lack of human resources, funding, and support of decision making. Discharge-planning activities are rarely income-generating, but they are often cost-effective. Documentation that supports the value of discharge-planning activities is critical to promote the program.

3. Interdisciplinary support: Role clarification, mutual support, and open feedback can reveal the value of team members in achieving the discharge goal. When problems among team members affect the group's functioning, discharge planning goals are often sabotaged.

4. Health care system: Health care policy today can be summed up as inconsistent, unclear, and contradictory. It is often cost-driven while denigrating quality. High technology has prolonged life and decreased mortality rates while in some cases it has prolonged iatrogenic morbidity. Today's clients are both victims and benefactors of health care policy. Rules for reimbursement, qualifications for access and utilization, and poorly distributed services variously lead to overutilization, underutilization, and gaps in care. The lack of community support services is a formidable barrier to the discharge goal. Problem solving skills to negotiate these barriers to care are essential.

Legal Issues

Hogue (1989) cites two major legal issues associated with discharge-planning activities: (1) liability for premature discharge, negligence, or abandonment, and (2) freedom of choice, fraud, and abuse.

Liability exists when three conditions are met: (1) the provider had a duty to give reasonable care; (2) a breach occurred in the duty, either through an act or an omission to act; and (3) the act or omission caused injury or damage to the client.

Negligence can occur if providers discharge clients from service when there is a need for additional clinical care. Responding to pressure from payors to discharge clients when payors stop payment for care poses legal risks. In *Wickline vs. The State of California,* the California Supreme Court ruled that providers of care have an obligation to warn payors when they make payment decisions that are adverse to treatment needs.

Abandonment occurs when the following three conditions are met: (1) the provider unilaterally ends the provider-patient relationship; (2) care is terminated without reasonable notice; and (3) further care was required.

To avoid charges of abandonment, discharge planners should offer clients the option of paying privately for care when third-party payment ends; provide reasonable written notice of the option to pay privately when this occurs; and establish a process to ensure that this duty is fulfilled.

Freedom of choice is guaranteed in Medicare and Medicaid statutes. Clients have the right to choose their own providers, and discharge planners must honor the stated choices of clients. The Medicare and Medicaid Patient and Protection Act of 1987 requires that providers disclose to clients their investment interests in the referral sources. Kickbacks or rebates to providers in exchange for referrals are prohibited because these activities constitute fraud and abuse.

Case Management

Case management is another activity that promotes continuity of care. Simmons and White (1988) argue that case management differs from discharge planning in its breadth of activity. Discharge planning is applied to an episode of illness or health deficit that plans for the care of clients after discharge. Case management imposes longer-range support as the client uses the health care system. The authors illustrate the differences as "episodic care" (discharge planning) vs. "enduring care" (case management). However, the terms discharge planning, case management, and managed care are often used interchangeably in the literature.

Case management is defined by the AHA (1986) as the process of planning, organizing, coordinating, and monitoring services and resources needed to respond to an individual's health care needs. It supports the effective use of health care and social services. A comparison of case management and the nursing process is shown in Table 39-5. The ANA (1988) describes the continuity, quality, and cost-containment aspects of case management as follows: "A health care delivery process whose goals are to provide quality health care, decrease fragmentation, enhance the client's quality of life, and contain costs." Secord (1987) defines case management as a systematic process of assessment, planning, service coordination, referrals, and monitoring that meets the multiple service needs of clients. The National Council on Aging (1988) states that case management involves assessment, planning care, arranging and monitoring service, and reassessing needs.

Case management as described above is not synonymous with *managed care*. Managed care is an organized program to control access and use of health services. It is designed to ensure the medical necessity of proposed services and the delivery of the most cost-effective level of care (AHA, 1986). Another term for managed care is *utilization management* (Secord, 1987). Examples of managed care organizations are

---

TABLE 39-5
The nursing process and case management

Nursing process	Case management process	Activities
Assessment	Casefinding; identification of and incentives for the target population; screening and intake; determination of eligibility; assessment	Develop networks with target population; disseminate written materials; seek referrals; apply screening tools according to program goals and objectives; use written and on-site screens; apply comprehensive assessment methods (physical, social, emotional, cognitive, economic, and self-care capacity); perform interdisciplinary, family, and client conferences
Diagnosis	Identification of the problem	Determine conclusion based on assessment; use interdisciplinary team
Planning	Problem prioritizing; planning to address care needs	Validate and prioritize problems with all participants; develop activities, timeframes and options; gain client's consent to implement; have client choose options
Implementation	Advocation of clients' interests; arrangement of delivery of service; monitoring of clients during service	Contact providers; negotiate services and price; coordinate service delivery; monitor for changes in client or service status
Evaluation	Reassessment	Examine outcomes against goals; examine needs against service; examine costs; examine satisfaction of client, providers, and case manager

health and social health maintenance organizations (HMOs and SHMOs). Activities used to achieve the goals of managed care include preauthorization for care, second surgical opinions, continued stay reviews, medical case management, bill auditing, and retrospective review. Many insurance companies, employers, and health care activists are demanding the implementation of a managed care approach in health care policies. As major purchasers of health care insurance, employers view managed care programs as critical for the survival of the health care benefit option.

The historical development of case management is strongly rooted in social services, nursing services, and client advocacy groups. Elements of case management have been provided throughout the 19th and 20th centuries by social workers, public health nurses, community health and social agencies, discharge planners, clergy, volunteers, charitable groups, and individual private practitioners. Case management projects were funded by the federal government in 1971 to test mechanisms for integrating delivery of health and social services to clients. The 1980s brought the federal and foundation funding of "channelling" projects, some of which had discrete case management activities as the hallmark of their programs. These demonstration projects attempted to substitute community care options for nursing home care for older persons. The demonstrations were intended to show reduced costs and improved quality of life for the frail elderly. However, an evaluation of the National Long Term Care Demonstration by Kemper (1988) revealed that in these projects the benefits were not necessarily in the cost-saving areas:

1. The costs of *additional* community services and case management were not offset by the costs of nursing home use; i.e., *total costs increased;*
2. Informal caregiving (family, friends, others) was not substantially reduced by expanded formal caregiving;
3. Channelling had benefits for the clients, family, and friends. These benefits were increased services, reduced un-met needs, increased confidence in care, and increased satisfaction with life.

Though these studies did not support case management and expanded community services as being cost neutral (since one cost did not offset the cost of another), they demonstrated that clients and caregivers experienced greater access and satisfaction with care and quality of life. Hurley, Paul, and Freund (1989) examined primary care case management (PCCM) with Medicaid patients for which the case manager functioned in a narrow "gatekeeper" role of authorizing access to referral sources. Their findings of case management/gatekeeper activities suggested that PCCM affected utilization patterns. However, when the gatekeeping function was not accompanied by financial risk-sharing, these programs did not save money.

Nurses need to evaluate the outcomes of their case management activities. Case management is a standard of practice for nurses. It embodies the philosophy of what nurses believe clients should be entitled to. Smith (1989) has questioned whether the benefits of case management will stimulate the public to finance it. As nurses become part of the evolution of case management programs, they are responsible for evaluating its cost and quality components.

Case Management Process

Components of the case management process have been identified by Polich, Parker, Iversen, and Korn (1989) and White (1986). These are illustrated in Table 39-5 and compared to the nursing process components. The core components of case management as illustrated by Secord (1987) appear in Figure 39-4.

Case management can be initiated at a number of entry points in the continuum of care. The box illustrates an example of service negotiation options for a person with AIDS.

Roles and Characteristics

Case management is part of the practice of community health nurses, along with the delivery of skilled nursing care. It is labor intensive, time consuming, and costly. Because of the increasing number of clients with complex problems in nurses' caseloads, the intensity and duration of activities required to support the case management function may soon exceed the demands of direct care. Management and clinicians in community health are exploring different models to make case management more efficient.

Case manager duties and responsibilities include the following (AHA, 1987):

Client evaluation	Treatment plan coordination
Family evaluation	Monitoring client progress
Provider evaluation	Ancillary service coordination
Communication facilitation	Cost-benefit analysis assistance

Characteristics of the role include the following (Weil, 1985):

1. The technical qualifications to understand and evaluate specific diagnoses (generally requires clinical credentials and experience);
2. Conversance in language and terminology (able to understand and explain to others in simple terms);
3. Assertiveness and diplomacy with people at all levels;
4. The ability to objectively assess situations to determine the appropriateness of case management;
5. Knowledge of available resources and the strengths and weaknesses of each;
6. Familiarity with employee benefits, eligibility, and insurance concerns;
7. The ability to act as advocate for the client and payor in models relying on third-party payment; and,
8. The ability to act as a counselor to clients, providing support, understanding, information, and intervention.

Models and Provider Practices

There are three predominant models of case management: the *brokerage model*, the *prior authorization model*, and the *consolidated direct service model* (Quinn and Burton, 1988). Examples of these three models are shown in the box. In the brokerage model a client's access to services is strengthened by linking the client, funding, and service providers into a network of medical, nursing, social, and supportive services. No direct care is given to the client by the organization, which only accesses and coordinates services. In some cases the organization pays directly for the services.

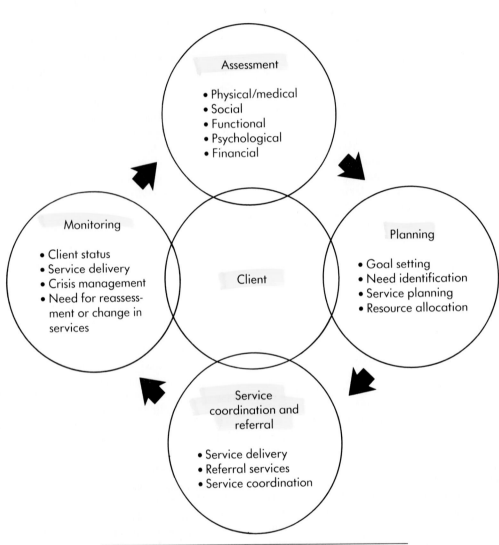

FIGURE 39-4

Core components of case management. *(From Secord, L.J.: Private case management for older persons and their families, Excelsior, Minn., 1987, Interstudy.)*

THE AIDS SERVICE CONTINUUM

PRIMARY MD

Diagnosis
Treatment
Referral

INPATIENT ACUTE CARE

Attending MD
Consultants
Primary care team (RN, SW, CNA)
Ancillary therapists (physical/occupational/speech/nutrition/respiratory therapy)
Lab/pharmacy/infection control
Housekeeping/central
Supply/laundry/dietary

CLINICS

AIDS, STD
General Medicine
Hematology/Oncology
Neurology
Pulmonary
Gastroenterology
Dermatology
Mental Health
Subspecialties, and so forth

VOLUNTEER ORGANIZATIONS

AIDS Education and PHIV support groups
Emergency shelter, clothing, and food projects
"Buddy" system
AIDS housing for end-stage disease ("Hospice")
AIDS chaplaincy

HOME CARE

Registered nurse
Social worker, by referral
Homemaker/home health aide
Ancillary therapists (as above, though may be different individuals)
Durable medical equipment/Pharmacy/lab

HOSPICE

Registered nurse
Social worker
Homemaker/home
Health aide
Chaplain
Bereavement staff
Volunteers
Medical director
Ancillary therapists (as above, though may be different individuals)
Durable medical equipment/pharmacy/lab

INDEPENDENT COUNSELING

Diagnostic
Financial
Legal
Drug abuse
Family planning
Psychologic

From Ryndes T: Coalition model of case management for care of HIV-infected persons, QRB (615(1):4, 1989.

MODEL EXAMPLES

BROKERAGE

Private case management firm, private case manager; *Project Open* of Mt. Zion Hospital in San Francisco; *Triage* in Connecticut

PRIOR AUTHORIZATION

New York Project Access; State-Administered Preadmission Screening Program (PAS); insurance companies

DIRECT SERVICE

Community health agency offering case management services; HMOs; ONLOK Community Care Organization in California

---

The prior authorization model requires that a client's access to service be screened and approved to determine the appropriate level of care. For example, if a client was designated for nursing home placement, the case manager would determine whether community support services or nursing home placement would be warranted. This model attempts to delay institutionalization and substitute alternative services. The use of this model may be required by certain payors (Medicaid, insurance companies, and managed care systems).

The consolidated direct service model pools funds and provides comprehensive services to clients within their organizations. This model provides both direct service and case management services.

Practice models of case management also vary. The traditional casework model places the client at the center of priority. One nurse provides all case management activities for the client. A variation on the traditional approach involves other professionals consulting in the case. A contrasting practice model features highly specialized functions of case managers. Individual staff members are responsible for specific tasks, but no single case manager is responsible for the entire process. For example, one nurse may be handling assessments, diagnoses, and care planning because of the advanced professional judgements required. Others may handle intakes or perform paperwork referral functions for the system.

In examining the infrastructure of case management, Pol-

CASE MANAGEMENT PROGRAMS

PUBLIC NONPROVIDERS

- State nursing home preadmission screening programs (not available in all states)

Area agencies on aging (Title III of Older Americans Act [1965]; controlled and designated by all states)

PRIVATE NONPROVIDERS

- Private case management (Polich et al, 1989) (Most firms in business around 5 years; 65% are for-profit; provide complete range of services but most contract-out medical assessments; sources of referral are from physicians and other clients; employ case managers with postgraduate degrees; small caseloads [1 to 20 cases/month]; common fee $75 to $100 per hour; payment paid out of pocket by client or family caregiver)
- Family members

ACUTE PROVIDER-BASED SYSTEMS

- HMOs/SHMOs
- Hospitals (small number)
- Geriatric assessment units
- Veterans Administration

LONG-TERM CARE PROVIDER-BASED SYSTEMS

- Home health care
- Adult day care
- Hospice

ich, Parker, Iversen, and Korn (1989) found growth in the number of case management programs over the years, even without formal funding. These have been organized into four categories and reflect a variety of approaches (see Box). So many variations exist in these programs that it has been said, "If you have seen one case management program, you have seen one case management program." National case management standards such as those developed by the National Institute of Community-Based Long-Term Care (NICLC), an affiliate of the National Council on Aging, and those issued by the American Nurses Association (1988) should serve as valuable guides to consumers, referral sources, and insurers to identify, understand, and evaluate the case management process.

Conflicts: Legal and Ethical Considerations

Advocacy and professional practice in case management promote the potential for conflict in several areas. When case managers are also service providers it may be difficult to be impartial and objective designators of service. Manipulating a client into accepting services violates the client's autonomy. The distinction between advising, persuading, and manipulating vulnerable clients is narrow (Kane, 1989). Case managers who function in a gatekeeping role must be fair in recommendations about who gets resources and must provide equitable ways to resolve disputes while controlling costs and ensuring quality. Case managers with considerable purchasing power can purchase services from providers with higher standards.

Saue (1989) notes that court cases influence the legal considerations of case managers. When courts find that cost considerations affect medical care decisions, all parties to the decision will be liable for resulting damages. Guidelines to reduce risk exposure include the following:

1. Clear documentation of the extent of participation in decision making and reasons for decisions;
2. Records demonstrating accurate and complete information on interactions and outcomes;
3. Use of reasonable care in selecting referral sources, which may include verification of licensure of providers;
4. Written agreements when arrangements are made to modify benefits other than those in the contract;
5. Good communication with clients; and,
6. Informing clients of their rights of appeal.

CLINICAL APPLICATION

The community health nurse from the public health department was conducting her regularly scheduled blood pressure clinic in a local apartment cluster. Mrs. B., a 45-year-old woman had attended for the last 2 months. During one visit, Mrs. B. complained of feeling dizzy and forgetful. She could not remember which of her six medications she had taken during the last few days. Her blood pressure readings on reclining, sitting, and standing revealed gross elevation. The nurse and Mrs. B. discussed the danger of her present status and the need to seek medical attention. Mrs. B. called her physician from her apartment, and the nurse discussed the data findings with him. Reluctantly, Mrs. B. agreed to meet the physician in the emergency room and the nurse, with Mrs. B.'s consent, arranged for her transportation.

While in the emergency room, Mrs. B. manifested the progressive signs and symptoms of a CVA. After hospitalization, she lost her capacity for expressive language and demonstrated hemiparesis and loss of bladder control. Her cognitive function became intermittently confused, and she was slow to recognize her physician and neighbors who came to visit. The clinic nurse contacted the discharge planner, a nurse from the health department's discharge-planning team contracted to the community hospital. She suggested that Mrs. B. be screened and assessed for post-hospital care options as early as possible because she lived alone and family members resided out of town.

The discharge planner confirmed the referral and requested a written report from the clinic nurse. Mrs. B. met many of the screening criteria indicating she could benefit from the service. The discharge planner worked with the unit nurses, physician, social workers, speech therapist, physical therapist, client, family members (long distance by phone), the utilization review nurse, the insurance company, and the clinic nurse to determine Mrs. B's post-discharge prognosis, the desires that she and her family had for aftercare, and the appropriate, reimbursable levels of care options. With the recommendations produced from the interdisciplinary and family conferences and with the client's and family's consent, the discharge planner initiated the referrals for home health care (skilled and supportive services) and meals-on-wheels. Family members agreed to come from out of town for 3 weeks to assist in Mrs. B.'s care and assess the adjustment to home supportive care. All supports were in place at the time of the client's discharge, and home health care (R.N. and aide service) and meals-on-wheels were initiated within 6 hours of discharge. Therapies began within 48 hours.

Mrs. B. could be maintained at home with informal and formal caregiving systems in place. However, the situation and level of care were not static. It became apparent that family caregiving could not continue because members lived too far away. Mrs. B. had residual functional and cognitive deficits that would demand longer-term care. The home health agency nurse managing Mrs. B.'s care delivery communicated regularly with the insurance company to convey her status and prognosis. She held interdisciplinary team conferences with service providers and formulated community and institutional options for appropriate levels of care. Mrs. B. and family members were educated, advised, and supported to examine their goals and options and to formulate alternative options for remaining at home. The client and family selected a case management firm to guide them in the selection and access to care that would promote Mrs. B.'s optimal function.

The nurse case manager screened the client for eligibility for the service. A self-pay option was arranged, based on a sliding scale. The case manager worked with the physician, home health nurse, therapists, social worker, client, and family to conduct a comprehensive assessment of current status and predicted prognosis. She presented her findings to the client and family, the home care nurse, and the insurance company. With the clients' and family's permission, she negotiated with the insurance company to reimburse for selected community-based services for six months as an alternative to institutionalization. She arranged for transportation, adult day care, cognitive stimulation sessions, environmental improvements to accommodate functional status, and an emergency response system device. With the assistance of church volunteers, support and monitoring of instrumental activities of daily living were provided. The original clinic nurse monitored the client's response during her weekly blood pressure clinics. The case manager coordinated, referred, monitored, and evaluated service delivery as related to the client's and family's goal to maintain the client in her residence. At the conclusion of the 6-month contract with the nurse case manager, the client was able to reduce the degree of formal support and assume more direction in her own management so that she could remain in the community. The case manager terminated her services with the client until a further need might be identified.

SUMMARY

As the U.S. health care system undergoes significant changes, the goal of achieving continuity of care for clients will provide a greater challenge for nursing practice. Clients are receiving larger amounts of health care within the community and are often challenged to gain access to a myriad of providers and new services. For those clients without health care reimbursement and who have inadequate payment options, access and utilization of essential services is frustrating. Many clients will continue to experience inadequate health care in the absence of community health advocacy and appropriate attention to activities assuring continuity of care.

Continuity of care for clients encountering the fragmented delivery of health care can be achieved by a particular emphasis in the community health nurse's scope of practice. Advocacy, discharge planning, and case management are three essential components of nursing practice. For the individual and family client, continuity of care reflects uninterrupted and coordinated access to services that will promote optimal level of functioning within the system. For the community, continuity of care encompasses systems of health care and social service delivery that enable the health status of the community to improve over time and in accordance with standards for a healthy community. Whether viewed as a direct or indirect service by nurses, the provision of services promoting continuity of care is critical to the standard of practice and to the outcomes of nursing services in the community.

KEY CONCEPTS

An important role of the community health nurse is that of client advocate.

The goal of advocacy is to promote the client's self-determination.

Advocacy involves the skills of informing, supporting, and affirming.

When performing in the advocacy role, conflicts may emerge regarding the full disclosure of information, territoriality, accountability to multiple parties, legal challenges to clients' decisions, and competition for scarce resources.

Amplification, clarification, and verification are three communication skills necessary in the advocacy process.

Additional skills important in fulfilling the role of client advocate include the helping relationship, assertiveness, and problem solving.

Being assertive requires verbal and nonverbal communication that conveys the expression of self.

Problem solving is a systematic approach which includes understanding the values of each party and generating alternative solutions.

Brainstorming and problem-purpose-expansion are two techniques to enhance the effectiveness of problem-solving skills.

During conflict, negotiations can move conflicting parties toward an outcome.

Prenegotiation, negotiation, and aftermath are three phases of managing a conflict.

Each individual has a predominant orientation when engaging in conflict: competing, accommodating, avoiding, collaborating, or compromising.

Collaboration may result by moving through seven stages: awareness, tentative exploration and mutual acknowledgement, trust-building, collegiality, consensus, commitment, and collaboration.

Continuity of care is a goal of community health nursing practice. It requires making linkages with services to improve the health status of the client.

As the structure of the health care system moves toward delivering more services in the community, the achievement of continuity of care will present a greater challenge.

Continuity of care can be achieved through three nursing activities: advocacy, discharge planning, and case (care) management.

Discharge planning is inherent in the nursing process and prepares the client for the next phase of care.

Discharge planning is typically an interdisciplinary process in which the client is the focus of the discharge plan.

Documentation of discharge planning activities and outcomes is essential to community health nursing practice.

Major skills used in discharge planning include teamwork and collaboration, referral, screening, assessment, coordination, and evaluation.

Case management and care management are synonymous terms for the systematic process of assessment, planning, service coordination, referral, and monitoring that meets the multiple service needs of clients.

While care management is enduring or continual, discharge planning is episodic.

Community health nurses have within their scope of practice both discharge planning and case management.

Nurses functioning as advocates, discharge planners, and case managers need to be aware of the ethical and legal issues confronting these component of their practice.

LEARNING ACTIVITIES

1. Observe a typical workday of a community health nurse, noting the types of activities that are done in coordinating and care managing, as well as the amount of time that is spent in these areas. Interview several staff members to determine whether they perceive that their time spent in care coordination is changing.

2. Initiating, monitoring, and evaluating referrals are essential components of community health nursing practice. Describe a client situation and the *referral process* that might occur in the following practices:
   a) A school nurse in an elementary school; a high school.
   b) An occupational health nurse in a hospital; a manufacturing plant.
   c) A nurse working in a well-child clinic.

   d) A case manager employed by a health maintenance organization.

3. The values and beliefs held by a community health nurse influence the nurse's ability to be an advocate for clients. Discuss your values and beliefs about health care issues and how they may impact on your ability to be a client advocate.

4. Read the following article. Discuss your reactions:
   a) If I were in that situation, I believe I would . . .
   b) Comment on the ethical issues and responses of the staff in the nursing home relative to the performance of the advocacy role.
   Kayser-Jones J, Davis A, Weiner CL, and Higgins SS: An ethical analysis of an elder's treatment. Nurs Outlook, 37(6):267, 1989.

BIBLIOGRAPHY

American Hospital Association: Case management: an aid to quality and continuity of care, Chicago, 1987, AHA Council Report.

American Hospital Association: Discharge hospital patients: legal implications for institutional providers and health care professional, Report of the Task Force in Legal Issues and Discharge Planning, Legal memorandum number nine, Chicago, 1987, The Association.

American Hospital Association: Glossary of terms and phrases for health care coalitions, Chicago, 1986, AHA Office of Health Coalitions and Private Sector Initiatives.

American Nurses Association: Continuity of care and discharge planning programs in institutions and community agencies, Kansas City, Mo, 1975, ANA.

American Nurses Association: Code for nurses with interpretive statements, Kansas City, Mo, 1985, The Association (Publ No G-56).

American Nurses Association: Nursing case management, Kansas City, Mo, 1988, The Association.

American Nurses Association: Standards of community health nursing practice, Kansas City, Mo, 1986, The Association.

American Nurses Association: Standards of home health nursing practice, Kansas City, Mo, 1986, The Association.

Angel G and Petranko DK: Developing the new assertive nurse—essentials for advancement, NY, 1983, Springer Publishing Co, Inc.

Banfield S: A management system analysis, Caring 6:45-50, 1987.

Bisno H: Managing conflict, Beverly Hills, Ca, 1988, Sage Publications.

Bremer A: A description of community health nursing practice with the community-based elderly, J Community Health Nurs 6(3):173-184, 1989.

Brooke PS: Informed consent: an ethical dilemma having life/death and legal implications, Clinical Nurse Specialist 2(3):157-161, 1988.

Brooten D, Brown LP, Munro BH, et al: Early discharge and specialist transitional care, Image 20(2):64-68, 1988.

Brooten D, Kumar S, Brown L, et al: A randomized clinical trial of early hospital discharge and home followup of very low birthweight infants, New Engl J Med 315 934-939, 1986.

Buckwalter KC: Exploring the process of discharge planning: application to the construct of health. In McClelland E, Kelly K, and Buckwalter KC, editors: Continuity of care: advancing the concept of discharge planning, Orlando, Fla, 1985, Grune & Stratton, Inc.

Cagan J and Meier PA: A discharge planning tool for use with families of high risk infants, J Obstet Gynecol Nurs 8:146-8, 1979.

Campbell J and Patton M: External evaluation of the St. Anthony Park Block Program Report, 1985.

Capitman JA, Haskins B, and Bernstein J: Case management approaches in coordinated community-oriented long-term care demonstrations, Gerontologist 26(4):398-404, 1986.

Cary A and Androwich I: A collaboration model: a synthesis of literature and a research survey, Paper/Presentation at the Association of Community Health Nursing Educators Spring Institute, Seattle, Wash, June 1989.

Chakrabarthy C, Beallor GN, and Pelle D: A multidisciplinary approach to continuing care planning. In Volland PJ, editors: Discharge planning: an interdisciplinary approach to continuity of care, Owings Mills, Md, 1988, National Health Publishing.

Cloonan P: A study of care coordination provided by home health nurses, Unpublished dissertation, 1990, University of Virginia.

Cloonan P and Schuster J: Care coordination: a resource-intensive component of home health nursing practice, Public Health Nursing 7(4): 204-208, 1990.

Conference Report to Accompany H.R. 5300, OBRA, 1986.

Corcoran S: Decision analysis: a step-by-step guide for making clinical decisions, Nurs and Health Care 7:149-154, 1986.

Creighton H: RN advocate and the law, Nurs Management 15(12):14-17, 1984.

Desimone BS: Between a rock and a hard place . . . life as a facility-based care manager, The case manager 1(1):12-15, 1990.

Donabedian A: Some basic issues in evaluating quality of health care. In Rinke L, editor: Outcome Measures, New York, 1987, National League for Nursing.

Feather J: Discharge planning education: results of a national survey, New York, 1988, Western New York Geriatric Education Center.

Feather J and Nichols LO: Hospital discharge planning for continuity of care: the national perspective. In Hartigan EG and Brown DJ, editors: Discharge planning for continuity of care, New York, 1985, NLN, 71-77.

Forchuk C, Beaton S, Crawford L, et al: Incorporating Peplau's theory and case management, J Psychoso Nurs 27(2):35-38, 1989.

Gargaro WJ: Update on Tuma case, Cancer Nursing 1(6):466-468, 1978.

Gibson JI: Continuity of care and ethics, Continuing Care 9(4):11-14, 1990.

Government Accounting Office: Access to post-hospital care, Maryland, 1987, US General Accounting Office.

Gray B: Collaborating: finding common ground for multiparity problems, San Francisco, 1989, Jossey-Bass Publishers.

Green JH: Long-term home care research, Nurs Health Care 10(3):139-144, 1989.

Handy J: Private case management, Home Health Management Advisor 3(7):1,4, 1990.

Hanson PC: Quality assurance: a strategic guide for discharge planning professionals, Eagan, Minn, 1988, Healthcare Management Services.

Hartigan EG: Discharge planning: identification of high risk groups, Nursing Management 18(12):30-32, 1987.

Hartigan EG and Brown DJ: Definitions, goals, benefits and principles. In Discharge Planning for Continuity of Care, 1985, NLN Publishing.

Health Care Financing Administration: Uniform needs assessment tool, Unpublished manuscript, 1989.

HCFA Lists Questionable Discharges and Transfers as Top PRO Priority, Discharge Planning Advisor in Hospital Peer Review, Winter, p 4-6, 1986.

Hogue EE: The legal risks of discharge planning, The Next Step 6(1):1-4, 1989.

Humphrey CJ and Milone-Nuzzo P: Home care nursing—an orientation to practice, Norwalk, Conn, 1991, Appleton-Lange.

Hurley RE, Paul JE and Freund DA: Going into gatekeeping: an empirical assessment, Q R B 15(10):306-314, 1989.

Jandt FE: Win-win negotiating: turning conflict into agreement, New York, 1985, John Wiley & Sons.

Johnson N and Fethke CC: Postdischarge outcomes and care planning for the hospitalized elderly. In McClelland E, Kelly K and Buckwalter KC editors: Continuity of Care, Orlando, Fla, 1985, Grune & Stratton, Inc.

Kane R: Case management: ethical pitfalls in the road to high quality managed care. In Fisher K and Weisman E, editors: Case management: guiding patients through the health care maze, Chicago, 1989, JCAHO, 27-32.

Karp HB: The art of creative fighting, The 1983 Annual for facilitators, trainers and consultants, LaJolla, California, 1983, University Associates.

Kayser-Jones J, Davis A, Weiner CL, Higgins SS: An ethical analysis of an elders treatment, Nursing Outlook 37(6):267-270, 1989.

Kemper P: The evaluation of the national long-term care demonstration-overview of the findings, Health Serv Res 23(1):161-173, 1988.

Knollmueller RN: Case management: what's in a name? Nurs Management 20(10):38-42, 1989.

Kohler P: Model of shared control, J Gerontol Nurs 14(7):21-25, 1988.

Kohnke MF: Advocacy risk and reality, St. Louis, 1982, The CV Mosby Co.

Kongstvedt PR: The managed health care handbook, Rockville, Md, 1989, Aspen Corp.

Kromminga SK and Ostwald SK: The public health nurse as a discharge planner: patients perceptions of the discharge process, Public Health Nursing 4(4):224-229, 1987.

Lythcott GI: Health advocacy among minority groups. In Marks JH, editor: Advocacy in health care, Clifton, NJ. 1985, Humana Press.

McNulty EG: Discharge planning models. In Volland PJ, editor: Discharge planning, Owings Mills, Md, 1988, National Health Publishing.

MacAdams M and Capitman J: Case management for elders expands hospital boundaries, Continuing Care 8(7):25-26, 1989.

Melynk KAM: Barriers: a critical review of recent literature, Nursing Research 37(4):196-200, 1988.

Mor V, Schwartz R, Laliberte L, and Hiris J: An examination of the effect of reimbursement and organizational structure on the allocation of hospice staff time, Home Health Care Services Quarterly 6(1):1985.

Mueller WJ and Kell B: Coping with Conflict, Englewood Cliffs, NJ, 1972, Prentice Hall, Inc.

The National Institute of Community-Based Long-Term Care: Care management standards: guidelines for practice, Washington, DC, 1988, National Council on the Aging, Inc.

National League for Nursing: Steering Committee of the NLN Division of Nursing: Statement of Continuity of Care, New York, 1966, NLN.

National Society of Patient Representatives: The patient representative in the hospital, Chicago, AHA.

Nelson ML: Advocacy in nursing, Nursing Outlook, 36(3):136-141, 1988.

O'Hare PA: Developing discharge planning programs: current and future models and strategies. In O'Hare PA and Terry MA, editors: Discharge planning, Rockville, Md, 1988, Aspen Corp.

O'Mara L: Taking the guesswork out of OBRA'87, Continuing Care 10(2):12-14, 1991.

Palmer ME and Deck ES: Teaching your patients to assert their rights, Am J Nurs 87(5):650-654, 1987.

Poe C: Back to school? Putting certification for discharge planners to the test, Continuing Care. 9(3):20-24, 35, 1990.

Peters D: Minutes of the Second Meeting of the Advisory Panel on the Development of Uniform Needs Assessment Instrument(s), August 3-4, 1988, p. 31, Washington, DC, US Government Printing Office.

Polich CL, Parker M, Iversen LH, and Korn K: Case management for long-term care, Excelsior, Minn, 1989, Interstudy.

Quinn J and Burton JS: Case management: a way to improve quality in long-term care. In Fisher and Weisman, editors: Case management: guiding patients through the health care maze, Chicago, 1988, Joint Commission on the Accreditation of Health Care Organizations.

Robinson MB: Patient advocacy and the nurse: is there a conflict of interest? Nursing Forum 22(2):58-63, 1985.

Rogers C: On becoming a person, Boston, 1961, Houghton Mifflin Co.

Rorden JW and Taft E: Discharge planning guide for nurses, Philadelphia, 1990, WB Saunders Co.

Russ GH: Principles and definitions related to discharge planning and continuity of care, Paper presented at The Institute for Discharge Planning, Buffalo, N.Y., June, 1989.

Russ GH: Discharge planning policy and procedure manual.

Ryndes T: Coalition model of case management for care of HIV-infected persons, QRB 15(1):4-8, 1989.

Sager D: The business of case management, The Case Manager, 1(1):36-40, 1990.

Saue JM: Legal issues related to case management. In Fisher K and Weisman E, editors: Case management: guiding patients through the health care maze, Chicago, Ill, 1989, JCAHO. 87-92.

Secord LJ: Private case management for older persons and their families, Excelsior, 1987, Interstudy.

Shamansky S, Boase JC, Horn B: Discharge planning: yesterday, today and tomorrow, Home Healthcare Nurse 3(3):14-21, 1984.

Simmons J: Admissions and screenings, Continuing Care, 9(4):15, 16, 18, 1990.

Simmons JH: Risks, rights, realities, Continuing Care 9(2):18-21, 34, 1990.

Simmons WJ and White M: Case management and discharge planning—two different worlds. In Volland P, editor: Discharge Planning: Owings Mills, Md, 1988, National Health Publishing.

Slevin AP and Roberts AD: Discharge planning: a tool for decision making, Nursing Management 18(12):47-50, 1987.

Smith G: Using the public agenda to shape PHN practice, Nurs Outlook 37(2):72, 1989.

Sonsel GE: Case management in a community-based AIDS Agency, Q R B 15(1):31-36, 1989.

Tebbitt BV: What's happening in continuity of care? Supervisor Nurse 12:226, 1981.

Terry MA: Essential considerations in setting up a discharge planning program. In O'Hare PA and

Terry MA, editors: Discharge planning, Rockville, Md, 1988, Aspen Corp 33-65.

Thomas KW and Kilmann RH: Thomas-Kilmann Conflict Mode Instrument, New York, 1974, Xicom, Inc.

Tuma JL: Letter to the editor, Nurs Outlook 25(9):546, 1977.

Urbanic B and McKeehan K: Forward. In McClelland E, Kelly K and Buckwalter K, editors: Advancing the concept of discharge planning, San Diego, Ca, 1985, Grune & Stratton.

USD HHS, PHS Healthy people 2000, 1990, Rockville, Md, US Government Printing Office.

Vladeck BC: The continuum of care: principles and metaphors. In Evaswick CJ and Weiss LJ, editors: Managing the continuum of care, Rockville, Md, 1987, Aspen.

Volkema RJ: Problem-purpose expansion: a technique for reformulating problems, Unpublished Manuscript, 1983, University of Wisconsin, Eau Claire.

Webb C: Professionalism revisited, Nursing Times 83(35):39-41, 1987.

Webster's Ninth New Collegiate Dictionary, Springfield, Mass, 1984, Merriam-Webster, Inc.

Weil M, Karls JM, et al: Case management in human service practice, San Francisco, 1985, Jossey-Bass Publishers.

Weiss LJ: Care coordination: an integration mechanism. In Evashwick CJ and Weiss JL, editors: Managing the continuum of care, Rockville, Md, 1987, Aspen Corp.

Wickline vs California, 118 Cal Rptr 661 (Ct App 1986).

Wickline vs California, 183 Cal App 30 1175, 228 Cal Rptr 661, cert dismissed, 239 Cal Rptr 805, 741, p 2d, 613 (1986).

Winslow GR: From loyalty to advocacy: a new metaphor for nursing, Hastings Center Report 14:32-40, 1984.

Zappe C and Epstein D: Assertive training, J Psychosoc Nurs 25(8):23-26, 1987.

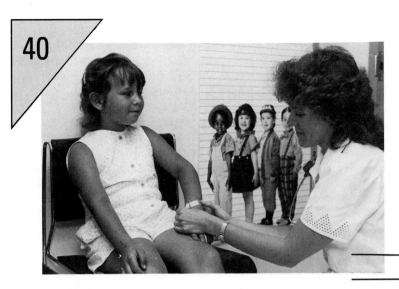

40

The Community Health Nurse in the Schools

Judith B. Igoe

Sudie Speer

OBJECTIVES

After reading this chapter, the student should be able to:

Describe the functions of school nurses as clinicians and managers.
Examine the three core components of school health.
Identify health-related behaviors and risk factors that contribute to school failure.
Identify and discuss two of the health services provided in schools.
Explain the basic requirements for administration of medications in schools.
Discuss the school health implications of the Individuals with Disabilities Education Act (PL 94:142).
Cite three general goals of health education
Describe a health education program that empowers the consumer to use the health system effectively.
Explain the four essential steps involved in managing a school health program.
Describe one innovative approach to the planning, organization, and delivery of school health programs.

KEY TERMS

Absenteeism
Area education agencies (AEA)
Boards of cooperative education services (BOCES)
Case finding
Case management
Certificates of Immunization Status
Community health nurse specialist for school-aged youth
Controlling
Counseling
Directing

Early Periodic Screening Diagnosis and Treatment Program (EPSDT)
Employee health
Health education
Healthy school environment
Individuals with Disabilities Education Act (P.L. 94:142)
Individual Education Plans (IEP)
Individual Family Service Plans (IFSP)
Means-tested entitlement program
Neurodevelopmental evaluations

New morbidities
Nontraditional health facilities
Organizing
Planning
Primary health care services
School-based health centers/clinics
School nurse practitioner
School nurse-teacher
Screening
Self-help
Vague nonspecific health complaints

"Children as children are constantly growing and developing. This basic dynamic characteristic accounts for both their increased vitality and vulnerability and requires specific health approaches in relation to the child's changing needs" (Child Health USA, 1989, p. 6).

In the United States 46,222,124 children and adolescents attend approximately 110,000 public and private schools (Digest of Educational Statistics, 1989). Although these girls and boys can be described as relatively healthy individuals, the stresses of rapid growth and development and societal pressures create health problems.

HEALTH PROBLEMS OF SCHOOL-AGE CHILDREN

School nurses are in a unique position to help children manage these health problems and to provide health education so that children can enjoy good health throughout their school age and adult years. The box lists the leading health problems of children, by age groups. It is interesting to note that for school-age children these problems vary substantially between the younger years (5 to 12) and the adolescent years (13 to 19). For children, accidents, cancers (including leukemia), influenza and pneumonia, homicides, upper respiratory infections, malnutrition, and dental disease are the major problems that interfere with their health and school attendance. For adolescents, pregnancy, alcohol and drug abuse, accidents, suicide, homicide, and venereal disease are the most common conditions that lead to school failure.

Since 1977, acute respiratory diseases have consistently been the main reason for absence from school because of illness. In 1987, 182 school days per 100 children were lost because of respiratory diseases. Asthma and chronic bronchitis were the leading chronic conditions limiting children's activity (Health: United States, 1989).

The nutritional problems seen in schools may have changed, but they still exist. Today fewer children are undernourished; modern problems are related to overconsumption and imbalances in the types and amounts of food. Many children consume foods high in sugar, fat, and salt and thus increase their risk of becoming obese and acquiring diabetes, heart disease, hypertension, and other chronic degenerative diseases later in life (Guide to Clinical Preventive Services, 1989). Childhood obesity is a serious problem for children aged 2 to 9 years, particularly for females and Hispanic children (Child Health USA, 1989).

Many children and adolescents have vision and hearing problems. In 1981, state maternal and child health agencies reported that over 250,000 school-age children who received vision screening required treatment. The prevalence rate for myopia ranges from 6% to 20% with the higher rates occurring in children and youth aged 10 to 14 years (Committee on Vision, 1989). The National Society for the Prevention of Blindness (NSPB) estimates that 1 in 500 school children in the United States is partially sighted (Harley, 1983). Hearing loss occurs in 6% of children of all ages, and 0.87% of children are diagnosed as legally deaf (Northern, 1989).

Alcohol is still the most widely abused substance among teenagers and drug abuse continues. However, recent studies show that alcohol and drug use has declined for this age group. Among high school seniors, 6.9% reported drinking alcohol daily and 41.2% reported that they had five or more drinks at one time during the previous 2 weeks in 1979. By 1988, 4.2% of these students reported daily drinking (a decline of 39%), and 34.7% indicated they had five or more drinks in the previous 2 weeks (a decline of 16%) (Health: United States, 1989, pp. 70-71).

Use of marijuana and cocaine also decreased from 1977 to 1988. The National Center for Health Statistics reported that marijuana use dropped from 9% in 1977 to 2% in 1988. Cocaine use by adolescents was also reported to be less, declining from 6.7% in 1985 to 3.4% in 1988 (Health: United States, 1989, pp. 70-71). Not only is the use of alcohol and drugs among those aged 12 to 17 years reported to be down, the awareness of the risks involved in these behaviors also has generally increased (Health: United States, 1989, pp. 70-71).

Unfortunately, this profile of declining drug and alcohol use does not hold true for younger students. In 1987 reports of 8th and 10th graders' daily drinking habits indicated an increase of 35%, and 6% of 8th grade students and 15% of 10th grade students interviewed indicated they had used

---

LEADING AGE-SPECIFIC HEALTH PROBLEMS OF CHILDREN 1-19 YEARS OF AGE

EARLY CHILDHOOD (1-4 years)	CHILDHOOD (5-12 years)	ADOLESCENCE (13-19 years)
Accidents	Accidents	Pregnancy
Infectious diseases	Cancers, including leukemia	Alcohol
Child abuse	Influenza and pneumonia	Drug abuse
Lead poisoning	Homicide	Accidents
Development lag	Infections including ear, nose, and throat	Suicide
	Malnutrition	Homicide
	Dental disease	Venereal disease
		Dental disease
		Mental/emotional problems
		Sports injuries

Modified from Dever A: Epidemiology of health service management, Rockville, Md, 1984, Aspen Systems Corp.

marijuana during the previous month. Reports of cocaine use ranged from 5% among 8th graders to 9% among 10th graders (Health: United States, 1989, pp. 70-71).

In 1985, 1,031,000 teenagers became pregnant; of these, 31,000 were younger than age 15. The outcomes included 477,710 live births; 416,170 induced abortions; and 137,120 spontaneous abortions. For children aged 15 to 19 years, one American teen in 10 becomes pregnant each year as compared with fewer than one in 20 in Canada, England, and France (Child Health USA, 1989).

Each year, 2.5 million teenagers in the United States are infected with a sexually transmitted disease. Seventy-five percent of all sexually transmitted diseases occur among those aged 15 to 24 years (Prevention 84/85:21-27). As of April 1989, 1561 cases of Acquired Immune Deficiency Syndrome (AIDS) were reported in children younger than 13 years of age and there were 372 cases of AIDS reported in adolescents aged 13 through 19 years. Most of the cases in children under 13 years of age involve babies and toddlers. Whereas the majority of cases of AIDs occurring in whites are related to blood product exposure, the majority of cases in blacks and Hispanics are a result of sexual activity and drug use (DHHS, 1989, pp. 20, 33).

Although adolescents are at risk for HIV infection, they are not well informed about its prevention (Stoto, Behrens, and Rosemont, 1990, p. 155). Consequently, the American School Health Association suggests a broad-based health education approach, addressing the subject of sexually transmitted diseases (STD) in all grades. Financial resources to provide education about AIDS prevention have been substantial, and these funds provide the opportunity for increasing this type of health instruction.

Children do not benefit as much from school when they are not feeling well and are absent. According to Klerman (1988), "Educators believe that students who miss more than 10 days in a 90-day semester (11% of school days) have difficulty in staying at grade level." In 1986, the National Health Survey (NHIS) estimated that students ranging in age from 5 to 17 years lost 226.4 million days of school or 5 days per child. (A missed class day in this instance is classified as an absence only when it occurs as the result of an acute or chronic health condition.) The absentee rate for girls is slightly higher than for boys, and the rate for whites is somewhat higher than for blacks. Children who miss school have a higher rate of visits to the school nurse than other students (Klerman, 1988). Excessive school absence in intermediate and high school often is the result of factors outside the health care sphere. Chaotic family environments, lack of achievement motivation, understaffed and uninviting schools, and other societal problems are the major reasons for repeated absences, school failure, and early school leaving (Klerman, 1988).

Poor children and adolescents are at highest risk for absenteeism and therefore need and deserve special attention from the school nurses. These children often have serious ear infections that will eventually lead to hearing loss if left untreated (Flinn, 1989). Others have repeated upper respiratory infections, bouts with allergies, dental decay, skin disorders, and other clinical disorders that will result in extended periods of absenteeism if diagnostic and treatment

services are not readily available. These students are four times as likely to miss school because of their ailments. They are also two to three times more likely to have a health condition that limits their school activity and are twice as likely to have mental health problems (Starfield, 1982). They frequently go without health care because they are uninsured, and they may fail academically, perhaps because adult supervision is lacking. Some are homeless and do not attend school regularly. Others live in homes in which English is a second language and the child does not speak enough English to understand class discussions. Therefore, they soon lose interest in attending school.

Today, 20% to 25% of school children in the United States are poor; minority youth are most often members of this group (Current Population Reports, 1988). In 1987, the poverty rate for Hispanics was 2.7 times that for whites but less than the poverty rate for blacks (Christian Science Monitor, 1989). Because poor children often are enrolled in the federally sponsored free breakfast and lunch programs offered at schools, school nurses can discreetly use enrollment rosters for these programs to identify those students who are in special need of school health care and access to community health services. Measures should be taken to reduce physical and emotional health problems and poor health habits among these children and youth. Offering diagnostic and treatment services at school may be necessary for these students if no other sources of health care are available in the community. For these girls and boys, these health-related risk factors often set in motion a cycle of absenteeism and school failure.

In addition, children and adolescents want and need to address their own problems. Several surveys of school-age youth reveal that they are interested in learning about health and that health topics are most often at the top of their priority lists. When more than 3000 high school students were surveyed to determine the health needs with which they wanted help, the top five identified were acne, sex education, depression, obesity, and parental disagreements (Family Health, 1979).

The modern health problems of school-age children involve social, emotional, behavioral, and technological issues that require a complex range of services delivered by individuals and systems in a flexible, coordinated, and collaborative manner. Many practitioners, educators, and policymakers have concluded that the school nurse is a key figure in meeting many of the health care needs of students, especially those who are at high risk (Califano, 1986).

The number of students who have disabilities and chronic health conditions and are enrolled in regular school has increased since the enactment of the Education for All Handicapped Children legislation (PL 94-142) in 1975. Over a million more children now have access to a free and appropriate education than previously had access. From 1977 to 1978, about 8.6% of students received special education because of their disabilities; 11.1% received these services in 1987 to 1988. Most of this increase is attributed to the preparation of children identified as learning disabled, which rose from 2% of all children in 1977 to 1978 to 5% of all children in 1987 to 1988 (Digest of Educational Statistics, 1989).

Scientific advances and improved technology make it possible for low birthweight babies to survive, for students with chronic and terminal illnesses to enter remission and live with their diseases, and for severely physically disabled youth to communicate with others. The largest category of students eligible for services under PL 94-142 have specific learning disabilities and are usually in good health. However, the health problems experienced by those who do need nursing care at school (related services) has become increasingly complex. The proportion of school-aged children limited in activity by special health needs and reporting to school increased from 4% in 1975 to 6% in 1985 (Kovar, 1988). Among the treatments and procedures some students require at school are medications; bladder catheterization; endotracheal suctioning; colostomy, ileostomy, and ureterostomy care; and nasogastric tube feedings (American Nurses' Association, 1983).

At the time of the reauthorization of PL 94-142 in 1991, this legislation was retitled the Individuals with Disabilities Education Act (IDEA). This federal law guarantees a free public education and related services for every disabled child from 5 to 21 years of age. The IDEA bill PL 101-476 identifies a number of related services including health care, physical therapy, occupational therapy, speech therapy, and psychological services. In addition each state has its own plan for implementing this legislation, which can be more specific. In some states, like Colorado, school nursing services are designated as a type of health services that must be available for these students.

HISTORY OF SCHOOL NURSING

Lillian Wald, the nursing director of Henry Street Settlement House in New York City discovered a 12-year-old boy excluded from school because of eczema:

> In the early 1900s, I had been downtown only a short time when I met Louis. An open door in a rear tenement revealed a woman standing over a washtub, a fretting baby on her left arm, while with her right hand she rubbed at the butcher's aprons which she washed for a living.
>
> Louis, she explained was "bad." He did not "cure his head," and what would become of him, for they would not take him into the school because of it? Louis, hanging the offending head, said he had been to the dispensary a good many times. . . . But "every time I go to school Teacher tells me to go home".
>
> It needed only intelligent application of the dispensary ointments to the affected area, and in September I had the joy of securing the boy's admittance to school for the first time in his life (Woodfill and Beyrer, 1991).

Public health efforts in those days concentrated on the control of communicable disease. Thousands of immigrants were crowding into the tenement areas of large cities such as New York and Boston. With the tenements came the diseases that resulted from poverty and overcrowding. Having identified this child and many more like him, Lillian Wald and her staff carefully compiled a data-based report that soon convinced city officials to introduce physicians into schools to examine students and exclude those with contagious diseases. As an isolated event, these daily inspections created more problems than they solved. Follow-up of treatment and counseling was definitely needed be-

cause students and their families were frequently unable to understand the instructions on the exclusion card:

> In many cases the excluded children, not fully understanding the instructions, played on the street with their companions as they came out of school and lost or destroyed the cards. In other instances the cards were taken home, but the parents, often ignorant of the English language, did not understand what the child tried to explain and the Latin names were uncomprehended. . . . In many instances the cards were never looked at but remained in their sealed envelopes while the child played on the street (Rogers, 1908).

After 5 years of medical inspections in schools, thousands of children were excluded because of trachoma, and classrooms were empty. "In a single school three hundred children were out at one time" (Rogers, 1905). Lillian Wald proposed to the boards of health and education that a nurse be sent into the schools. As a demonstration project, Lena Rogers visited four schools daily, spending an hour in each:

> Here she dresses or cleanses all such cases as the physician directs, mild cases of conjunctivitis, minor skin infections, such as ring-worm, etc., and the children need not then miss their class-work, as otherwise they would have to do as a matter of protection to the rest. She then visits those who have been sent home, and keeps records of them (Dock, 1902).

Between 1903 and 1904, 39 nurses were recruited by the New York City Health Department, and they were remarkably successful. According to health department records, 98% of students previously excluded from school were retained in classrooms. Improvised dispensaries were set up to treat students on-site. Nurses provided the counseling and instruction necessary to overcome parental fear and indifference. During home visits, nurses found that many students were out of school for social reasons rather than because of disease, and many were "victims of the temptations of the streets" (Struthers, 1917). Others, however, needed clothing and food before they could come to school, and some were caring for younger children while their mothers worked. In a few instances, these children were providing nursing care to family members who were ill. Steps were taken by the nurses to relieve a number of these social problems, and the children returned to school.

By 1909, municipalities throughout the United States were employing school nurses. Initially, the visiting nurse association provided the nursing service on a demonstration basis. If the project was effective, the tax-supported boards of education or health would assume administrative control (Waters, 1909). In 1912 the American Red Cross created a nursing service to meet the school health needs in rural areas (Woodfill, 1991).

The need for school nurses to provide treatment in schools and to focus their efforts almost exclusively on the control of contagious diseases began to diminish around 1916. Different priorities arose with the onset of World War I. In a time when able-bodied men were needed to defend their country, literally thousands of recruits were found to be physically unfit to serve because of poor eyesight, hearing loss, advanced dental disease, or orthopedic defects. Consequently, the importance of early case finding and corrective follow-up during childhood became clear to public health officials. School nurses soon shifted their attention from communicable disease control to primary prevention efforts such as vision and hearing screening. It was the first organized large scale attempt to proactively improve the long-term health status of American children.

By the 1920s, the role of the school nurse had expanded to include the functions of health educator and counselor. The dual role of school nurse-teacher evolved in 1937. Subsequently, a school nurse-teacher group became a section of the newly formed Department of School Health and Physical Education of the National Education Association (NEA). Later a separate department of school nurses was formed, which eventually evolved into the National Association of School Nurses (NASN). This organization is now constitutionally separate from the NEA, but a close alliance still exists.

Over the past 40 years, school nurses have been recognized for their humanitarian, preventive, and educational contributions to child and adolescent health. However, the role of school nurse-teacher has been the subject of almost continual debate, and significant clinical roles for school nurses are only now emerging. Fortunately, the duties and functions of school nurses are less ambiguous today, largely because of numerous attempts at standardization of the role and state certification.

During World War II, the nursing shortage became acute, and the school health program became the responsibility of school personnel other than the school nurse and the few physicians who still worked in the field. Consequently, most school nurses gave up their more labor intensive roles as health teachers and counselors to take on the role of health consultant/coordinator/liaison between school, home, and community. Ironically their school assignments doubled and tripled under this arrangement and no extra personnel (e.g., health assistants) were added at the building level to carry out the various screenings, simple health instructions, and follow-up activities. Consequently, the quality of school health programs deteriorated.

By the end of the 1960s, many working mothers and worried school administrators recognized the educational and economic advantages of offering more diagnostic services and treatment services at school. Thus, the clinical role of the school nurse practitioner appeared. Over the last two decades, the importance of the health consultant role and school nurse-teacher roles has diminished, and the school nurse practitioner role has become more prominent. In turn, all school nurses have gradually become more clinically competent and are providing more case management services.

Various studies have shown that success with the school nurse clinician role requires administrative support, clerical and paraprofessional assistance, available medical consultation, and the presence of others to participate in the planning, coordination, operation, and management of the overall school health program (Goodwin, 1981; Meeker, 1986). In the past, the only dollars allocated for school health were salaries for school nurses. Consequently, the strategy today for finding the resources necessary to develop a comprehensive school health program, in which the school nurse clinician is a member of an interdisciplinary team, requires reorganization of schools and community health agencies to consolidate child and adolescent health efforts. Therefore, to be truly effective, school health programs need to include an array of health, social service, and education personnel, in addition to the nurse, who are prepared to deal with the health-related problems of students. These new developments in school health also present new opportunities for nurses to become school health managers or health coordinators.

With one foot in nursing and the other in education, school nurses often have balanced precariously on the periphery of both fields. Unfortunately, there has been little power or recognition in either field. However, major changes are underway, and these frustrations have become tolerable as the public and policymakers now recognize the value of improving health programs in schools. Here it is possible to enhance the health status of all boys and girls and to provide special attention to those who have no other regular source of health care or whose health condition requires special nursing care for them to attend school. The history of school nursing clearly reflects the evolving nature of this role. A chronology of other health, education, and social events that have contributed to its development and to the school health movement is in Table 40-1.

COMPONENTS OF THE SCHOOL HEALTH PROGRAM

The three core components of school health are health services, health education, and a healthy environment. Figure 40-1 illustrates the services and the personnel involved. The rough estimate for 1987 expenditures for basic school health services, not including primary health care and the services of nurse practitioners, was $13/student/year (Walker, Butler, and Bender, 1990). This figure is exclusive of the costs involved in providing classroom health education and maintaining a healthy environment. No national estimates for these components of school health are currently available.

Health Services

School health services generally include health screenings, basic care for minor complaints, administration of medications, surveillance of immunization status, case-finding for the early identification of problems, case management, health counseling, nursing care of students with special health needs, and in some districts, primary health care. All of these activities are family-centered and intended to prevent disease and promote health. School nurses are generally the persons responsible for this component of school health. These nurses may or may not have medical and psychological consultation available to them, depending on the size of their school health program and its level of development.

Recent advances in nursing research have substantially increased the knowledge base for the design and delivery of school health services of high quality. The University of Colorado School Health Programs in Denver, Colorado, manages a resource center, clearinghouse, reference collection, and newsletter. School nurses and others interested in school health have access to this information. The system also provides referrals to nurses working in model school health programs throughout the country.

Text continued on p. 716.

TABLE 40-1

Chronology; a listing of events significant in the history of school health services

Developments in school health services	Developments in education
1800 First school physicians and nurses hired in Europe (1834-1892)	1800 Child labor reform and emergence of a public education system
1894 First medical inspections began in Boston schools to identify and exclude students with communicable disease. No follow-up.	1890 Responsibility for school health assigned to local school boards as health departments not in existence in every town Minimal school health instruction
Communicable disease control	
1900 Classroom inspections expand to include screening for ringworm, scabies, impetigo, malnutrition Proper hygiene practices demonstrated in school and home Minor cases of contagion treated at school (e.g., dressing changes)	1910 School health instruction is combined with medical inspection. Teachers rarely participate and health professionals do the health teaching.
1902 Home visits for sanitary inspection, follow-up on excluded students, truancy, social problems. As a result, school attendance escalates.	
1910 Emergency services now available in schools School inspections expand to individualized medical examinations to identify and correct defects	
1920 Red Cross provides school nursing services to rural America	1930 Federal school lunch program starts. Department of Agriculture
1924 Employee health services incorporated into school health. Roger's report recommends teachers have health exams and tuberculin tests.	
1930 Mass screenings for early casefinding (i.e., vision, hearing, dental caries, orthopedic defects) increasingly widespread Counseling, health education and consultation offered in conjunction with health services	
1934 School nurses/physicians services are overextended and quality of services deteriorates (National Organization of Public Health Nursing [NOPHN] Study)	
Health guidance & consultation	
1940 Nonstatutory ban on school-based diagnosis and treatment widely enforced First aid/emergency services closely identified with school nurses despite their "no more bandaides" campaign to delegate more responsibilities for nonnursing tasks to other school personnel Service more public health oriented (e.g., coordinating community services for students)	1940 First coordinated integrated health education curriculum developed
1945 School health councils advocated as a means for organizing school health programs	
1950 School health services under review by American Public Health Association (APHA), American Nurses Association (ANA), American School Health Association (ASHA)	

From Office of School Health, University of Colorado Health Sciences Center 1991.   *Continued.*

TABLE 40-1

Chronology; a listing of events significant in the history of school health services—cont'd

Developments in school health services	Developments in education

Primary care

1960   Comprehensive health histories recommended in lieu of cursory school examinations; record-keeping excessive and not effective for planning purposes

1969   Introduction of the first pilot for school based primary health care using school nurse practitioners (Denver Public Schools)

1974   Special services available for students with disabilities, handicaps, chronic illness (i.e., medication administration, catheterization)

New school health personnel (clerks, occupational therapist, physical therapist, psychologist, speech pathologist, substance abuse counselors)

1979   Private agencies (including hospitals) assume the management of some school health programs on an experimental basis in New York.

1960   Title I-Elementary and secondary education act authorized provisions for health and nutrition services OED

1970   Child Find Screenings begin to identify students eligible for special services under PL 94-142 Handicapped Children's Act

White House Conference on Children and Youth recommendations for early childhood education and day care

Immigration of Vietnamese/Indo-Chinese refugees with third world health problems; complex cultural and language barriers must be overcome

1978   School Health Education Study produces comprehensive curriculum models for health education (grades K-12)

1979   Growing Healthy curriculum adopted nationwide. Well-validated program reported to produce health behavior changes in elementary school students.

Teenage Health Modules will develop later and will also be disseminated nationally.

Health promotion/special needs

1980   National School Health Services Program, Robert Wood Johnson Foundation (1980-1985). Demonstrates the effectiveness of school-based diagnosis and treatment by school nurse practitioners. Emphasis on elementary schools.

1986   The School Based Adolescent Health Care Program (SBAHC), Robert Wood Johnson Foundation. Increased the number of school-based health centers with diagnostic and treatment services (1986-1992). School based clinics now concentrate on adolescent services. Main obstacles: conservative public opinion, financing, integration with the rest of school health program.

Disease prevention, health promotion services flourish: health hazard appraisals; fitness/endurance/cardio-vascular risk screening; student health fairs.

1990   Clinical services, health education, health promotion, environmental measures increasingly overlap. Growing emphasis on environmental health.

1980   School Reform movement underway. Parent participation increases.

Carnegie Foundation Report *Turning Points* recommends numerous changes in middle school including the establishment of family resource centers and a new role for a health coordinator

Student assistance programs to prevent drug and alcohol abuse proliferate under the leadership of guidance counselors

1987   Youth 2000 campaign launched by the business community to combat the school dropout problem

Division of Adolescent and School Health, Center for Chronic Disease Prevention and Health Promotion, Centers for Disease Control established.

Continued.

TABLE 40-1

Chronology; a listing of events significant in the history of school health services—cont'd

Developments in pediatrics, nursing, public health	Social and legislative developments
1800 Fundamental discoveries in bacteriology	1897 First appropriation by states for care of handicapped children, Minnesota
1908 First Bureau of Child Hygiene established in N.Y.C. 1909 School nursing services provided from visiting nurse associations First White House Conference recommends Federal Children's Bureau 1912 Discovery of numerous serious health defects among army recruits 1913 School Nursing Committee created within the National Organization for Public Health Nursing (NOPHN) Lina Rogers Struthers, chairman. 1918 Schools of Public Health open	1904 Child labor legislation 1912 Act of 1912, Children's Bureau established 1915 Rockefeller Foundation well child clinics and clean milk stations
1920 All cities with population of 100,000+ have maternal and child health services in most state health departments Second White House Conference advocates standards of MCH; consumer education is stressed School nurse established as faculty member in New York State and referred to as School Nurse-Teacher 1926 National Organization for Public Health Nursing published its first statement on the objectives, scope of work, and methods in school nursing 1927 American School Health Association (ASHA) is formed 1930 American Academy of Pediatrics is formed 1937 School nurses became a section of the new Department of School Health and Physical Education of the National Education Association; eventually this section evolved into the National Association of School Nurses 1939 Crippled Children's Services from State Health Department expand	1921 Maternity and Infancy Act (Sheppard-Towner) federal grant-in-aid to the states 1924 An alliance develops between the National Education Association and the American Medical Association. "Health education, not health services is the proper role for the schools." 1935 Title V; Social Security Act enacted; Maternal and Child Health Care Services authorized
1940 Delegation of school nurse tasks to teachers, health clerks, volunteers 50% of all public health nurses are employed in school health 1941 First edition of *The Nurse in the School* published by the Joint Committee of the National Education Association and the American Medical Association. (Second edition released in 1955) 1944 Selective service reports Army recruits have numerous health defects. Committee on School Nursing Policies and Practices of the American School Health Association established. (Name changed in 1958 to School Nursing Committee and since the late 1960s referred to as the Study Committee on School Nursing) 1949 Significant increases in number of school nurses employed by health departments 1950 White House Conference demands a ban on racial public school segregation. Concept of school health team develops	1954 Brown v. Board of Education; a civil rights case that overturned the "separate but equal" doctrine in public schools

Continued.

TABLE 40-1

Chronology; a listing of events significant in the history of school health services—cont'd

Developments in pediatrics, nursing, public health	Social and legislative developments
1960 White House Conference on Children and Youth has youth participation for the first time. Profound concern about drug abuse, increases in the incidence of venereal diseases, illegitimate births, inadequate opportunities for youth employment and concern for the environment	1960 "New Frontier", "Great Society", "War on Poverty" Partnership for Health act—comprehensive neighborhood health centers
1961 National Institute of Child Health and Human Development established, a national center for basic research in child development	1963 MCH funds authorized for children and youth projects
	1965 Headstart Title V; Social Security Act; provides preschoolhealth, education
1962 Two-thirds of school nurses are employed by Boards of Education; number of nurses swell to 30,000	Medicaid, medical services for low income families (Title XIX)
1969 School Nurse Practitioner program developed at the University of Colorado in conjunction with Denver Public Schools	National Health Promotion/Disease Prevention Campaign underway with release of the Surgeon General's report on smoking
1970 Position Statement "Role of the School Nurse Practitioner" developed by various public health, school health and medical associations	1970 Family Planning Services and Population Research Act (PL 94:142); Education of the Handicapped legislation Rehabilitation Act of 1973
1975 National Association of State School Nurse Consultants organized	Early Periodic Screening, Diagnosis and Treatment (EPSDT); (Title XIX, Social Security Act); comprehensive and preventive health services for diagnosis and treatment of physical and mental defects
1976 23 of 50 states have mandatory school nurse certification requirements; 10 states have permissive legislation	1973 Child Abuse ACT (PL 934-247)
	1974 The Education of All Handicapped Children Act (PL 94:142) helps states provide a free and appropriate public education
	1975 School-based initiative developed, states improve on child abuse reporting laws and include school personnel
1980 AIDS epidemic fully recognized	1980 Refugee Education Assistance Act
1983 *Standards for School Nursing Practice,* a set of guidelines for nursing practice in the schools developed jointly by five professional health and nursing organizations, published by the American Nurses' Association	1981 Select Panel for the Promotion of Child Health
	1986 Education of the Handicapped Act Amendments (PL 99-457) (Part H); program for infants and toddlers with handicaps
1989 Position statement *Role of the School Nurse in Disease Prevention, Health Promotion and Health Protection* receives American School Health Association endorsement	
1990 Bureau of Maternal and Child Health re-established National Health Agenda and Objectives for the Year 2000 launched	

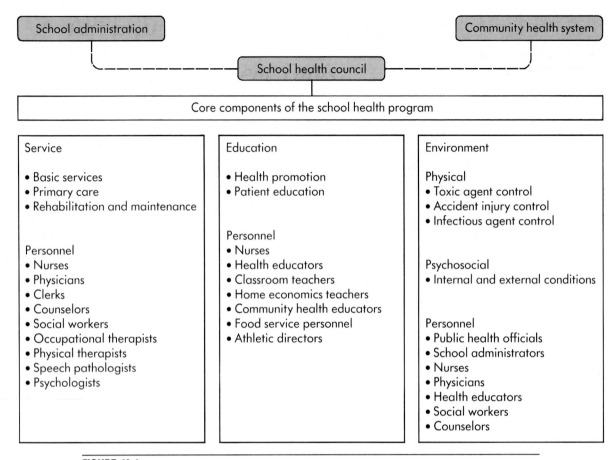

FIGURE 40-1

The organization of the school health program. *(From School Health Programs, University of Colorado Health Science Center, 1989.)*

Screening

The school nurse's responsibility in the screening process is to work with families and other team members to (1) establish what screening will be done, (2) develop a plan for the screening and a data management system, (3) teach paraprofessionals and others (including students and volunteers) how to conduct the screenings, (4) determine the appropriate resources for additional diagnostic work-up for children with signs and symptoms, (5) refer students in need of further evaluation to other school and community resources, and (6) collaborate with others in implementing and evaluating treatment plans.

Preventive health screenings may include vision, hearing, scoliosis, dental, cardiovascular risk factor analysis, and more comprehensive surveys of personal health habits known as behavioral risk surveys. These screenings usually take place as close to the beginning of the school year as possible to uncover problems that may interfere with learning. The box lists recommended screenings for school-age youth.

Special screening packages for preschool children are also available in school. One such program is the Early and Periodic Screening Diagnosis and Treatment (EPSDT) Program. This program is a part of the Medicaid program (Title XIX of the Social Security Act), a means-tested entitlement program for medical assistance to needy families with de-

pendent children. All states have an EPSDT program that offers early screening, diagnosis, treatment, and periodic follow-up services to children and youth who meet the financial eligibility requirements and who are under the age of 21 years.

There are two other preschool programs that include a number of health screenings. Head Start is an early childhood education program for children who are at risk for academic problems because of poverty and lack of sufficient social stimulation. Child Find is the other screening program and is part of the IDEA legislation (PL 101-476). Its purpose is early identification of preschool children who are at risk for school failure because of mental retardation, other disabilities, chronic health conditions, or special health needs. Currently, school administrators including school health personnel face the challenge of combining all of these preschool programs into a more consolidated screening package to control costs and avoid unnecessary duplication. Although the EPSDT, Head Start, and Child Find programs offer services only to selected children, there is a national trend underway to offer early childhood education and health screenings to all students.

Controversy surrounds some screenings. What should be provided, who should do the screening, and who will finance the service are questions that are raised frequently. Persons skilled in epidemiology (most often health department personnel) need to work with schools and school nurses in identifying which screenings are sufficiently valid, reliable, cost effective, simple, safe, and acceptable to be worthwhile. Many states mandate certain screenings through either statutes or regulations. Currently there are serious questions about the high priority assigned to scoliosis screening (Mann, 1990).

In addition to the traditional school health screenings, various circumstances have developed that now necessitate the delivery of more complex clinical services at school. Consequently, selective screening has become available for pregnancy, emotional disorders, and sexually transmitted diseases. In conjunction with this type of screening, students need psychosocial and behavioral counseling and other disease prevention and health promotion services as well as traditional medical treatments.

Case-Finding

Case-finding is a form of selective screening, which involves a search for certain students whose behavior, family circumstances, or health status place them at particular risk for ill health, absenteeism, and poor school performance. Instead of mass screening in which all students in various grades are involved, case-finding efforts begin by identifying risk factors and then locating students whose behavior suggests they are at risk for certain problems and in need of further assessment and possible referral. Therefore case-finding techniques are more intensive efforts and usually require the clinical judgment of school nurses to determine whether further assessment and diagnosis is necessary.

Case-finding is carried out by practicing careful, systematic observation of all children with whom nurses come in contact, looking for anomalies or suspect symptoms. Case-finding efforts should concentrate on identifying students who have these kinds of risk factors:

1. Students who are absent more than 10% of school days.
2. Students frequently sent to the principal's office for illness.
3. Students frequently sent to the principal's office for "acting out in the classroom."
4. Students who appear chronically ill to the teacher.
5. Students with subtle, as well as obvious, physical defects who are experiencing problems in functioning at school.
6. Students with subtle, as well as obvious, emotional problems.
7. Students who frequently seek out the nurse with vague, nonspecific complaints.
8. Students who have been seriously injured or who have a history of repeated injuries.
9. Students who are genetically predisposed to certain conditions such as sickle cell disease.

Because the frequency rates for absenteeism, visits to the school nurse's office, injuries, referrals to the principal's office, as well as the practice of various personal health habits vary a great deal from school to school, the first step in case-finding is to establish these rates for each school building and for the district as a whole. This is done by keeping track of the students seen by the nurse, reviewing screening results and absenteeism records, collecting information from teachers and school administrators, and having students complete personal lifestyle inventories. Once the overall frequency rates for student behavior in these instances have been established, it becomes possible to determine whether the responses of certain students are the same or different from the rest of their classmates. Within most schools there are school administrators with experience in setting up surveillance systems that can help the school nurse in gathering this type of information and learning how to interpret it if a school health supervisor is not available. In 29 states, there are school nurse consultants located in the state departments of health and education who are also available to help.

The most likely place to begin case-finding efforts is with observation of children who are obviously physically or mentally different; children who are part of a desegregation program or who have moved from rural, mountain, urban, or suburban settings into a totally different social environment; and children from stressful situations where parental expectations may sometimes seem unreasonable for the child's stage of cognitive, physical, and psychosocial development. School nurses are especially concerned with detecting children who are victims of social illness (e.g., neglect or abuse). The nurse's responsibility in working with children suspected of being abused is to provide them with a nonthreatening environment, providing comfort, a safe place, support, encouragement, and compassion. It is also the nurse's responsibility to report the problem to appropriate authorities such as the Children's Protective Services.

Surveillance of Immunization Status

Legally, entry into school requires that students be currently immunized unless exempted for religious or medical reasons. Consequently, up-to-date Certificates of Immunization Status must be presented to school personnel for admission. This usually applies to preschool students as well as to boys and girls who are older. Each of the following vaccines are required: polio, measles, mumps, rubella, and diphtheria/tetanus, and in the instance of preschoolers, pertussis. Because of recent measles outbreaks, an additional booster during adolescence is now recommended and, in many instances, is required by state law.

The school should have a procedure for dealing with immunizations. First, an administrator (or designee, often a secretary or a teacher) who has received the necessary instruction from the school nurse conducts a primary review of the child's health record to determine the immunization status. Next, the information collected from the school is shared with the local county health department. Those children not in compliance with the immunization law are cited with an exclusion order by the health department. This information is then routed back to the school, where administrators exclude the unimmunized students. If students do not return to school in a reasonable length of time (i.e., 3 to 4 days), follow-up measures are taken to investigate the truancy. Often families have no access to immunization services because of poverty. Consequently, some schools have reintroduced school-based immunization clinics to alleviate the problem. Previously, Goodwin found that this alternative was by far the most efficient and economical approach (Goodwin, 1978).

Managing Minor Complaints

Each school building should have first-aid supplies and equipment in accordance with accepted first-aid guidelines. Local district policies, as well as state and federal occupational health regulations, need to be followed. A health room or area should be available in which to deliver first aid and emergency care as well as care for such common complaints as abdominal pain, headaches, earaches, fatigue, nonspecific complaints, and nuisance diseases such as pediculosis.

Increasingly, nurses have begun to involve teachers and students in the responsibilities associated with first aid. Often first-aid kits are located in the classrooms, and nurses work with school personnel and students to enable them to deal directly with minor injuries. American Red Cross classes are often an excellent means of preparation. This approach is especially important if the nurse is not in the building on a full-time basis.

All school nurses need physical assessment skills and equipment to diagnose, treat, or refer students with common health complaints. This type of information also needs to be recorded on the student's health record at school and, to ensure continuity of care, on written referrals prepared and sent with the student if another health care provider becomes involved. It is also important for the nurse to receive feedback from the community health care provider. Frequently, a regular system of communication has to be worked out to establish this kind of collaboration. Although this is more complicated in larger communities, the place to begin is to identify the students' health care providers. This is handled by having parents complete emergency cards that not only specify where the parent may be located during the day but also the name of their health care provider and the health facility or managed care system they use.

Some creative school nurses have established an ongoing link to community health professionals in various ways, including inviting them to visit and tour the school with the nurse, inviting them to join the school health council, and placing them on the mailing list for the school health newsletter.

Administration of Medications

One type of drug problem that occurs in children is improper use of medication. Based on a recent study by the National Council on Patient Information and Education, "In any two-week period, about 13 million people in the United States under the age of 18 take medicines prescribed or recommended by a physician. Of those, 46% either stop treatment too soon, do not take enough medication, take too much, or refuse to take any at all. When children use medicines improperly, lives are lost, treatable chronic diseases remain uncontrolled, and acute illnesses needlessly continue or recur" (National Council on Patient Information and Education, 1989). Many of these medications are administered in school.

Medication policies are essential in schools today. However, these policies should not serve as a barrier to gaining access to the classroom and learning. Some students with chronic disease (i.e., asthma) are in special self-management programs to help them learn how to function independently. School nurses need to support this approach by

individualizing overall medication policies as appropriate. The five basic requirements for administration of medications in schools are the following:

1. Medications are given only with parents' written permission.
2. Medications requiring a prescription are given only on the written authorization of a physician.
3. For medications requiring a prescription there must be an individual, pharmacy-labeled bottle for each student.
4. Medications must be recorded by the school personnel who administer them. This record states the student's name, medication, dosage, time, and the person administering the medication.
5. Medications must be stored in a secure, locked, clean container or cabinet.

The administration of medications in schools is so prevalent today that in many instances nonnursing personnel have this responsibility. In these cases instruction is needed, and manuals do exist for this purpose (Iowa Department of Education, 1991). States vary in their interpretation of the school nurse role, relationship, and responsibility to the persons dispensing the medications. The state board of nursing is the agency responsible for establishing this policy.

Counseling

The ability to counsel students or others skillfully is an art. The counselor's responsibility is to provide information; to listen objectively; and to be supportive, caring, and trustworthy. Counselors do not make decisions; they help clients arrive at the decisions that best suit them. Counseling therefore differs from teaching and interviewing. For example, teaching is giving information; interviewing is obtaining information from someone; counseling is helping people arrive at workable solutions to their problems or conflicts. The box at right lists recommended counseling topics for school-age youth.

Students usually require counseling when they are unable to make decisions about personal concerns that affect their lives, for example, taking medication and changing lifestyle habits. If the nurse lacks the ability to counsel or to recognize that counseling is needed, the student may be unable to fully comprehend the extent of the problem or to find alternatives to resolve the problem. Students' peers can be used as counselors. However, students who act as counselors must be trained for the role. After providing students who are acting as peer counselors with technical advice, school nurses should encourage them to also use their personal experiences, to role-play, and to be available and accessible to other students.

Students with vague, nonspecific complaints who visit the health room frequently should be of special concern to school nurses. This may be the first warning sign of a student who is not doing well in school and who is at risk for eventually dropping out. Lewis and others have previously identified that children at risk of becoming school dropouts develop this type of maladaptive response to stress (vague health complaints) in early school years. This behavior continues into adulthood, thereby jeopardizing work as well as school performance (Lewis and Lewis 1990). However, with the right assistance and counseling from the school nurse,

SCREENING AND COUNSELING FOR SCHOOL-AGE YOUTH

AGES 7-12

Leading causes of death:

Motor vehicle crashes
Injuries (nonmotor vehicle)
Congenital anomalies
Leukemia
Homicide
Heart disease

Recommended screening

Height and weight
Blood pressure
HIGH-RISK GROUPS
Tuberculin skin test (PPD)

Patient and parent counseling

Diet and Exercise
Fat (especially saturated fat), cholesterol, sweets and be-
    tween-meal snacks, sodium
Caloric balance
Selection of exercise program
Injury Prevention
Safety belts
Smoke detector
Storage of firearms, drugs, toxic chemicals, matches
Bicycle safety helmets
Dental Health
Regular tooth brushing and dental visits
Other Primary
Preventive Measures
HIGH-RISK GROUPS
Skin protection from ultraviolet light

Remain alert for:

Vision disorders
Diminished hearing
Dental decay, malalignment, mouth breathing
Signs of child abuse or neglect
Abnormal bereavement

AGES 13-18

Leading causes of death:

Motor vehicle crashes	Injuries (nonmotor vehicle)
Homicide	Heart disease
Suicide	

Recommended screening

History

| Dietary intake | Tobacco/alcohol/drug use |
| Physical activity | Sexual practices |

Physical Exam

Height and weight	
HIGH-RISK GROUPS	Blood pressure
Complete skin exam	Clinical testicular exam

Laboratory/Diagnostic Procedures

HIGH-RISK GROUPS

Rubella antibodies	Counseling and testing for HIV
VDRL/RPR	Tuberculin skin test (PPD)
Chlamydial testing	Hearing
Gonorrhea culture	Papanicolaou smear

Patient and parent counseling

Diet and Exercise
Fat (especially saturated fat), cholesterol, sodium, iron, cal-
    cium
Caloric balance
Selection of exercise program
Substance Use
Tobacco: cessation/primary prevention
Alcohol and other drugs: cessation/primary prevention
Driving/other dangerous activities while under the influence
Treatment for abuse
HIGH-RISK GROUPS
Sharing/using unsterilized needles and syringes
Sexual Practices
Sexual development and behavior
Sexually transmitted diseases: partner selection, condoms
Unintended pregnancy and contraceptive options
Injury Prevention
Safety belts
Smoke detector
Storage of firearms, drugs, toxic chemicals, matches
Bicycle safety helmets
Dental Health
Regular tooth brushing and dental visits
Other Primary Preventive Measures
HIGH-RISK GROUPS
Discussion of hemoglobin testing
Skin protection from ultraviolet light

Remain alert for:

Depressive symptoms	Tooth decay, malalignment,
Suicide risk factors	gingivitis
Abnormal bereavement	Signs of child abuse or neglect

From American School Health Association: School health in America, Kent, Ohio, 1989, The Association.

which involves making sure the child is not physically ill and developing plans to enhance the student's self-concept, improve their problem-solving skills, and reduce stress levels, these students can be helped to manage their problems more effectively.

Case Management

As a case manager, there are a number of general activities performed by the school nurse. Parents need to be contacted to seek permission to discuss their child's health problem with the family physician. The nurse will also need to inform teachers and administrators accurately about the nature and prognosis of the health problem and the specific therapies required during the school day. Situations occurring at school that either interfere with the treatment plan or exacerbate the health condition need to be identified, communicated to the parties involved, and managed. Problems that arise from the student's health condition that deter learning also need to be recognized and handled. This usually involves obtaining and conveying information between health and school personnel. The school nurse is usually the person who bridges this gap through the process of case management.

Primary Health Care

School-wide campaigns to improve diet and physical exercise habits, contraceptive advice, individual and small group counseling to reduce stress and improve self-image, and social skills training and cognitive therapies to prevent substance abuse and delay the onset of sexual activity are just a few examples of the kind of generalized primary care health services and health promotion activities now available in schools. The American School Health Association also recommends fitness screening, school breakfast and lunch programs, physical education, and mental health programs (Healthy People 2000, 1990). Detailed handbooks are available to assist school nurses and other school health personnel in developing these programs (Allensworth and Wolford, 1988). If school nurse practitioners are available, students also will be able to receive comprehensive health evaluations in schools.

An increasing number of boys and girls today need to obtain additional primary health care services in their schools. This type of care includes a health history, physical examination, simple laboratory tests, and diagnosis and treatment of minor health problems. A 24-hour a day, 7-day a week, year-round referral system also must be in place in case students' problems require additional medical attention or they become ill when school is closed. The 1984 National Health Interview Survey found that 4.5 million (14%) students aged 10 to 18 years are from poor and minority households. These students are the ones who are least likely to have health insurance and access to primary health care.

Increasingly, school nurse practitioners are also becoming involved in more specialized forms of primary care. For example, some nurses serve as sports trainers, offering evaluations and special interventions to reduce the likelihood of sports injuries. Other nurses who are primary care providers work exclusively with students experiencing emotional disorders or with students who are medically fragile

and technology-dependent. Still other school nurse practitioners deliver primary care in special settings such as the diagnostic center for a school system.

Health Services for Students with Special Needs

According to the IDEA bill (PL 101-476), students eligible for service must have a comprehensive interdisciplinary evaluation followed by the preparation of an individualized education plan (IEP). This plan is reviewed and modified at regular intervals during the school year and throughout the student's school experience. Parent conferences always occur in conjunction with the evaluation and preparation of the IEP. Students frequently join their parents and school staff for these meetings. For students whose health status significantly interferes with their ability to learn, a health care plan is a component of the IEP.

The health component of the IEP includes the following types of information: specific notations of any special preparation and supervision that may be required in caring for the student, health counseling that is necessary for the student to function in the class, and any changes in the school environment that are necessary, such as the removal of architectural barriers. Also included in the health component of the IEP would be safety measures, measures required to relieve pain and discomfort (i.e., suctioning, skin care), special diet, medications, and special assistance with activities of daily living. Finally, any special adaptations of school health activities (i.e., screenings, health education, case-finding) are described so that the student is able to have full access to this program.

School staff members often need preparation and supervision by the school nurse to competently manage health care plans and the special health needs of students. Fortunately, the professional organizations for teachers and school nurses have developed policies to delineate their roles and responsibilities (Guidelines, 1990). Unfortunately, often it is difficult to enforce policies and guidelines that are issued from professional organizations because they have no statutory authority over local school systems.

In 1986, PL 94-142 was amended by PL 99-457, which changed the limit for mandated health and education services to include disabled children 3 to 5 years of age. Moreover, in section H of the amendment, called infants and toddlers, the states also were given the option to extend these early intervention services to children from birth to age 3 years to include those infants and toddlers who are disabled or who have special health needs that could eventually interfere with their ability to learn. In these instances, individualized family service plans (IFSP) are developed by an interdisciplinary team in partnership with parents, setting in place an early intervention program to prepare the infant/toddler/preschooler for school. Those states involved in section H also designate one community agency to coordinate these efforts. The school has been the designated agency in some states, however, other agencies also have been selected, including departments of health and social services.

Health Education

During the past decade, health education has been closely identified with the health promotion movement. Basically, health promotion is a social concept or campaign as well as a set of health education activities intended to develop healthy lifestyles among Americans (Green, 1984). Although not all health educators agree, many believe that the two areas are practically synonymous or that health promotion is the more encompassing activity and health education is a technique for its achievement. Health education efforts must therefore relate to the values and beliefs of students and their families. Because the potential exists for health education to infringe on the constitutional rights of individuals, health education at school is best developed locally, by committee, and should be open for public inspection and parental approval.

The health education component should include instructional efforts that foster wellness, such as health classes and courses to prevent the spread of infectious diseases like acquired immune deficiency syndrome (AIDS). Health education also includes education for students with chronic health problems who need to learn more about their diseases, self-care, and how to effectively use the health care system. Three general goals for the health education component of school health are: (1) to teach all children about their bodies and how to keep them healthy, (2) to instill in boys and girls lifelong healthy habits and the knowledge to make responsible decisions concerning their own health, the health of their families when they become adults, and the health of their communities (Wold, 1981), and (3) to teach students how to use the health care system wisely and effectively.

There are a number of validated health education curricula available today. Five programs are particularly well known. The Growing Healthy curriculum for elementary grades is a generalized program aimed at improving students' personal lifestyles (Kolbe, 1984). At the high school level, the Teenage Health Teaching Modules (THTM) have been widely used (Kolbe and Iverson, 1984). A more targeted type of health instruction is the Know Your Body course, which focuses on making students aware of their own cardiovascular risk factors through screening activities followed by special instruction related to risk reduction (Kolbe and Iverson, 1984). The Quest and Dare programs are often used in schools for drug and alcohol prevention (Kolbe and Iverson, 1984).

The HealthPACT course is a different type of health instruction. Designed as consumer health affairs lessons, it is intended to prepare children to communicate effectively with health professionals during visits for health care. HealthPACT teaches children to communicate effectively by using five basic communication skills: (1) Talk with the health care provider; (2) Listen and learn; (3) Ask questions; (4) Decide what to do, with help from the provider; (5) Do follow through. The letters (TLADD) are used as an acronym to help children learn and remember their health consumer responsibilities.

This program may be used as a supplement to an established health education curriculum, or it may be taught to children in a wide range of locations, including school classrooms, clinics, youth organizations, and at home. Since 1971, it has been implemented in varying degrees and at various times by school nurses, general health educators, dentists, teachers, physicians, clinic and hospital staff, par-

ents, nurses, and physicians' assistants. A variety of program evaluations have been done over the years, with successful outcomes (Stember, 1988).

A 3-year national investigation of the HealthPACT program demonstrated that the program was successful in teaching students in elementary grades how to actively participate during visits for health care. Fourth grade is apparently the best age for this type of instruction (Stember, 1988).

The implications from the HealthPACT program and its evaluation are threefold: (1) the role of the patient/consumer is changing; (2) the concept of the patient as partner even during childhood is acceptable; (3) children can learn consumer behaviors for use in health settings if they have support. The HealthPACT program also demonstrates that a new kind of health education is needed and is acceptable. Starting with instruction about active participation in a health facility, children and youth and their parents also need to learn self-help health measures (e.g., how to do their own vision screening, how to use an otoscope), and they also need to know more about the overall health care system and how it operates so that they can successfully negotiate their way around this system and can change its nature and operation if, as citizens, they see the need for change (Igoe, 1990).

Environmental Health

The third component of the school health program is environmental health, which involves physical and psychosocial factors such as infectious agent control and the physical and social environment of children. This component has received little attention until recently. Evaluating the need to improve the social environment in schools today is complex and involves instilling a sense of pride in students and measuring the morale of teachers and parents as well as evaluating the attitudes of the rest of the school team for signs of apathy, powerlessness, and hostility (Comer, 1988).

The physical environment in schools also needs to be evaluated. School nurses should work closely with local public health officials to ensure that this area of school health is not overlooked. Safety programs are most important. Often nurses enlist the active involvement of students in identifying areas in the school in which injuries are most frequent and in planning intervention strategies to reduce the risk. Incident reports need to be completed by school personnel when injuries occur, and school health personnel should review this information regularly to improve conditions. Asbestos, lead poisoning, and toxic substances in the chemistry and art classrooms are areas of concern to school administrators. Nurses must be well informed and have a close working relationship with the environmental health personnel at the local health department to be a useful resource for school officials. Often the nurse will be involved in surveying areas for risks, collecting information from parents, and providing school administrators, parents, and students with the most current approach to these problems to avoid unnecessary scares and instances of consumer fraud.

ROLES, FUNCTIONS, AND CREDENTIALS FOR SCHOOL NURSES

The majority of the 26,000 professional registered professional nurses now employed in school health are generalists prepared at the baccalaureate level who function in the consultant/coordinator role. The newer role for school nurses is as school health manager or coordinator. The functions associated with this role include: (1) policy-making activities to ensure a more comprehensive and integrated school health program, (2) case management functions to help families find the help they need, (3) program management duties so that a system of formalized school health activities and protocols develops as an integral part of both the private and public community health system, and (4) health promotion and health protection responsibilities. Because children's health problems are becoming more complex, knowledge of nursing, pediatrics, adolescent health, and public health is essential. These nurses must also be prepared to identify health-related situations that place the student at risk and that other school personnel might fail to recognize. In addition school nurses also must be very familiar with community resources and how to gain access to them. 'People' skills also are necessary because this nurse serves as the key link between the school and community health agencies.

A number of school nurses have dual degrees. Although health education has been a popular second degree, the guidance and counseling degree is a new goal for many school nurses. Efforts are underway now to inform school nurses that this content is integrated into graduate nursing programs, which should alleviate the need for school nurses to seek degrees outside of nursing.

Specialists

For nurses wishing to pursue a specialty in school nursing, a graduate degree in nursing is highly recommended. Two types of degree plans are designed specifically for them: the clinician role and the administrative/managerial role. The most common clinical role now seen in schools is as a school nurse practitioner (SNP) or as a specialist in such areas as child psychiatry, mental health, rehabilitation, and developmental disabilities. Only 400 certified SNPs are available and employed in schools. Thousands are needed. The number of other nurse specialists working in schools is unknown. The number of nurses in this group is probably much smaller than the number of SNPs but is just as much in demand.

School nurse practitioners are registered professional nurses whose advanced practice area is primary health care. They can serve as primary care providers for students who have no access to health care or whose parents prefer that their child receive this care at school. In addition to working with this group of students, SNPs also evaluate any students coming to their health office with complaints of illness and injuries. Earlier studies have demonstrated that (1) SNPs send home from school 50% fewer students than regular school nurses, (2) parents are more likely to act on the advice of SNPs, (3) SNPs handle 87% of the health complaints referred to them, and (4) SNPs resolve 96% of the health problems they see. In addition the difference in cost in relation to other community health facilities is substantial (Igoe, 1990; Meeker, et al., 1986).

In addition to working in a clinical setting, evaluating students in need of primary health care and those who are sick and injured, SNPs are also part of the interdisciplinary team involved in screening students with special health needs who may be eligible for services under the IDEA

legislation PL 101-476. One of their unique functions is the performance of neurodevelopmental evaluations. These evaluations contribute greatly to the overall assessment of a child by helping primary care providers identify the student's strengths and deficits in processing information.

The community health nurse specialist for school-aged children is the newest role proposed for school nurses. This role encompasses the functions of the school health manager previously described. These nurses function in nontraditional health facilities (alternative health care delivery systems), using various community settings such as schools, juvenile corrections facilities, group homes for the disabled and chronically ill, day care centers, and shelters for the homeless. Special organizational skills and management expertise are needed to provide more accessible public/community health programs in these settings, especially if the nurse is to have a leadership role. These settings frequently lack the necessary policies and procedures, data management systems, coordinated networks with other community health systems, and effective financing mechanisms to function effectively. Nurses functioning in this role have the organizational and political skills to design and implement health programs in these settings that cut across systems and produce results (Igoe, 1991).

Credentials

In addition to their nurses' license, school nurses often elect to become certified as a school nurse, school nurse practitioner, community health nurse, or other type of clinical nurse specialist through one or more of their national professional nursing associations. In some states the State Department of Education offers an additional state certification program for school nurses. In fact, depending on the state, it may not be possible to be employed in some school systems (or for school administrators to receive any federal reimbursement for school nursing care for students with handicaps) without a state certificate. Currently, many school nurses are striving to establish this type of credentialing to upgrade the quality of school nursing.

MANAGEMENT OF THE SCHOOL HEALTH PROGRAM

A school health program requires good management to operate smoothly and effectively. Four essential steps are involved in reaching this goal: planning, organizing, directing, and controlling the quality of the program through proper evaluation. Planning for school health should be a joint endeavor involving members of a school health council. To ensure broad-based representation, this council should be composed of teachers, school nurses, parents, students, administrators, and community leaders. Members of this team need to set the direction for the program, ensuring that the mission of the school health program is consistent with the goals of the school district and the rest of the community health system. The council plans and sets goals for the school health program and develops and then implements strategies to meet these goals. The council also evaluates the program in view of these goals and makes changes as necessary. A school health council is a valuable support mechanism for the proper development, revision, implementation, and evaluation of the school health program. Although technically school health councils are advisory bodies, the current emphasis in schools on community participation and parental involvement conveys a special sense of authority to the school health council. This influence, if used properly, provides the school health program the support it needs to operate successfully.

The Relationship Between Education Reform and School Health

In 1990 the National Governor's Association established the following goals for education by the year 2000.

1. All children will start school ready to learn.
2. The high school graduation rate will increase to at least 90% for all groups.
3. All students will leave grades 4, 8, and 12 having demonstrated competency over challenging subject matter in English, mathematics, science, history, and geography.
4. U.S. students will be first in the world in mathematics and science achievement.
5. Every adult will be literate and possess the knowledge and skills necessary to compete in a global economy and to exercise the rights and responsibilities of citizenship.
6. Every school in America will be free of drugs and violence and will offer a disciplined environment conducive to learning (U.S. Department of Education, 1990).

The impetus for this action and the need for major reform movements within education in recent years is the result of the growing public awareness that academic achievement scores of American youth are slipping; school dropout rates are rising; violence and drug abuse is threatening the integrity of many school communities; and minority youth as well as those who are disabled or who have special health needs still do not have equal opportunities for learning. All of these factors threaten the ability of students to become productive adults.

The educational goals for the year 2000 along with *Healthy People 2000: National Disease Prevention and Health Promotion Objectives* (U.S. Office of Disease Prevention and Health Promotion 1990) are the guidelines that set the direction for school health planning. In June 1990 the National Commission on the Role of the School and Community in Improving Adolescent Health issued a designated planning document for school health in secondary schools, *Code Blue: Uniting for Healthier Youth* (Code Blue, 1990). The commission that authored this report was composed of community leaders from health, education, and religious organizations, business, and government. The Commission was cosponsored by the National Association of State Boards of Education (NASBE) and the American Medical Association (AMA), with funding from the Centers for Disease Control.

Planning

Many school nurses are themselves the managers or coordinators of school health programs. School health requires a unique type of management known as pivot management. Under this plan, nurses organize a school health team using the personnel already in the school system or closely associated with it: teachers, students, parents, administrators, psychologists, health educators, social workers, speech pathologists, counselors, secretarial staff, and maintenance

---

SCHOOL HEALTH NEEDS ASSESSMENT

STUDENT HEALTH

Absenteeism: frequency and nature
Health problems presented at school (for example: illness and the nature, frequency, and location of injuries)
Resolution of health problems: frequency
Chronic health conditions, handicapping conditions
Health status of students
  Immunization level
  Dental
  Vision
  Hearing
  Emotional disorders
  Physical/sexual abuse
  Prevalence of positive health behavior (for example: nutrition, exercise, safety, and avoidance of substance abuse)
Change in health status of students

RESOURCES

Community resources available
Use of community resources (overuse as well as underuse)
Health care/education available in regular curriculum (for example: physical education, home economics, special education, science, and health education)
Health services available through current school health programs

EMPLOYEE HEALTH

Health state of school personnel: absenteeism and nature of disability claims

---

personnel. With the help of a school health council, this team develops a comprehensive school health plan, and a budget is developed and proposed to school administrators. Program goals, strategies, and activities are designed and organized so that health services, health education, and environmental components of the program are coordinated with one another. If the health program for students with disabilities is separated from the general school health program, special care must be taken to link these two efforts to avoid unnecessary duplication and fragmentation.

A needs assessment is the starting point for program development. It is used to determine the problems requiring attention and the way to best meet these needs. The box provides an outline of some areas covered in needs assessments for school health.

All three areas of school health must be considered when planning is done, and decisions must reflect innovative and economical ways of combining health services with health education and environmental health measures. Unfortunately, school health programming often is handled haphazardly, with decisions about the health education curriculum made in one department, health services planned and implemented from another office, and the environmental health component attended to in yet another department.

Traditionally, health services have been limited to screening and first aid. However, with the advent of school-based health centers, the increased numbers of uninsured students, and the admission of students with complex health care needs, care now being delivered in schools closely resembles the activities of traditional health facilities, including on-site diagnostic and treatment services and sophisticated nursing care for students with complex health problems. Rehabilitative services also must be available. Consequently, public health codes governing primary health care facilities often apply to school-based health centers. By maintaining a close working relationship with the local public health authorities, the school nurse is aware of local health regulations.

Health education requirements are especially important today because the public health agenda increasingly emphasizes disease prevention and health promotion. By obtaining an aggregated lifestyle profile for individual schools and for the total school district, school health planners will be more aware of the level of need for health education in their district. Health appraisal questionnaires that ask students about their knowledge, attitudes, and lifestyle behaviors in relation to diet, nutrition, exercise, dental health, human sexuality, infectious disease, and substance abuse can provide the needed information. Also, an audit of student health and school records to determine injury rates and illness-related absences provides administrators and the community with data about the overall health status of the student body. This approach often is effective in gaining school board support for a health education curriculum.

Plans also must be made in terms of who will provide the health instruction. Ideally, sufficient numbers of school-employed health educators will teach the classes. More realistically, health educators who are in very short supply develop the health education curriculum and work with classroom teachers, school nurses, and other community health professionals to implement the program.

Clear and appropriate written policies and procedures must exist for a well organized school health program. To be effective, these regulations must address the problems of poor students, students with chronic illnesses or disabilities, and sick and disabled infants and toddlers. The "new morbidities" affecting school-aged children cannot necessarily be managed completely by the health care system alone because many problems have psychosocial, political, and physical features. External environmental and sociopolitical forces that lead to these problems must be considered to implement school health programs effectively. Tools for planning, implementing, and evaluating the school health program should describe a general plan as well as provide regulations for emergencies such as allergic shock, breathing disorders, drug overdose, and head and spinal injuries. Policies and procedures should address these areas as well as others, including disaster plans, communicable diseases, reportable diseases required by the state, child abuse, and the warning signs and incidence of suicide. If state school nurse consultants are available, they should be consulted during the planning stage.

Organizing

There are 15,577 public school systems in this country, which is considerably less than the 100,000 districts that existed at the end of World War II around 1945. School nurses are unevenly distributed from one district to the next and from state to state. While professional organizations recommend a ratio of 1 nurse for every 750 students, a ratio of 1 nurse to 1500 students is more realistic in terms of the supply of prepared nurses that are available and the costs involved. For students with special health needs, the requirements for care are much different and hence ratios must be adjusted accordingly. However, as yet there are insufficient data about the nursing care required to make any reliable recommendations.

More problematic than the number of students per nurse is the number of school buildings the nurse must visit to come in contact with students. For example, 47% of school districts have a total school enrollment of only 2500 students (Digest of Educational Statistics, 1989). This means that one or two school nurses often make up the total school health team in these districts, with an assignment of 3 to 5 schools each. In large urban "inner city" school districts, the ratio of nurses to students and nurses to buildings is far worse (Igoe, 1991). This organizational dilemma adds to the credibility of a recommendation that came from a President's Commission on School Health in the early 1970s, which advised that health assistants be placed in schools to handle basic care (first aid, minor complaints), with nurses assuming managerial positions.

The intermediate education district is another network for organizing school health. Known as area education agencies (AEAs) or boards of cooperative educational services (BOCES), these systems frequently provide related services for special education students in school districts of limited size. School nursing, speech, audiology, occupational and physical therapy, and psychological services are some of the services often provided regionally. Nurses working in regional agencies often help local school district personnel develop and implement health care plans for certain students, such as those who are disabled or at high risk for academic difficulty. These specialized school nurses also work with the school nurse in the local district, if there is one, who is responsible for the overall school health program.

School nurses face a tremendous challenge daily in managing their time effectively. Therefore it is important to have a written plan that sets the direction, priorities, and schedule for the school health program. Within this context, the nurse also must organize the day in such a way that low-priority tasks are not crowding out time to work on high-priority activities. For example, many school nurses have discovered that an open-door policy fosters continual interruptions throughout the day. Consequently, school nurses in many school systems have now initiated an appointment system for seeing students and for parent–teacher conferences. Specified sick-call times are often established as another way of cutting down on the number of unnecessary interruptions.

It is also important for school nurses to organize an epidemiological data base that profiles the health status of the student body both individually and collectively. This is accomplished by using a systematic recording system for the problems that nurses see and the care they provide. Well organized school health programs have policy and procedure manuals that explain the recording system to be used in a

particular school system. Software packages for computerized school health records recently have been introduced,
and school nurses have begun to include personal computers
in their budget requests (Kaplan, 1991). Currently, some
effort is underway to coordinate school and community
health data systems by having school health personnel use
the International Classification of Disease (ICD-9) codes in
recording student health problems. Another approach undertaken in the Multnomah County Educational Service District in Portland, Oregon, has been to use the nursing diagnosis classification system (NANDA). This is in keeping
with the Oregon nurse practice act, which requires nurses
to document their practice in this manner.

Individuals developing new school health programs or
revising old ones must also now consider organizing school
health under a single department, office or division so that
needs are met, services do not overlap, and costs are contained. The ideal organizing process would involve and
consolidate all health personnel responsible for the care of
students in general, for students with special health needs,
and for other students at high risk for school failure (i.e.,
school nurses, speech pathologists, occupational therapists,
physical therapists, social workers, clinical psychologists,
and counselors including student assistant personnel). Although most related service personnel are employed by
school districts to carry out the provisions of the IDEA bill,
this does not mean that school administrators cannot integrate these professionals with other school employees such
as school nurses to achieve a more comprehensive approach
to school health.

There are three barriers to reorganization and consolidation of school health. First, many of the related service
personnel do not identify themselves with school health.
Second, school nurses may be unaccustomed to a team
approach in which the other members of the team are not
nurses. Third, bureaucratic turf battles often interfere with
interdisciplinary and transdisciplinary efforts in which the
students' needs are first identified and then the team decides
who is the person best suited to provide the care.

One way of overcoming the natural resistance to change
would be to organize related service personnel, including
the school nurse, into interdisciplinary teams that service a
cluster of schools. This organizational arrangement allows
various persons with backgrounds in fields other than education to become members of their own team and to gain
a sense of identity. Team development work will be needed
to build trust and a sense of how to operate in this kind of
an interdisciplinary environment. Nevertheless, this personnel arrangement offers the support system school nurses and
other personnel often miss when they function separately.

Once the health service component of school health has
been unified, the next step in restructuring school health is
to strengthen the link between the health service, health
education, and environmental health divisions. Regular
meetings of the persons responsible for these programs is
essential as is the need for them to develop a comprehensive
coordinated strategic management plan for school health.
The school health council is their advisory body.

Although schools traditionally have employed their own
school health personnel or contracted with the public health
agency for these services, new partnerships and organiza-

tional arrangements are emerging. School nurses in California and New York are forming their own school health
companies and contracting directly with schools. Hospitals,
both profit and nonprofit, also have begun to contract with
schools to administer school health programs.

Directing

Leadership for school health programs needs strengthening
at all levels. States currently have school nurse consultants,
with approximately 50% of them employed by state health
departments and the rest responsible to the state department
of education instruction. These individuals frequently provide technical assistance to local school districts, known as
local education agencies (LEA), in the form of inservice
education and on-site evaluation of the program while performing statewide planning for school health.

At the local level, a school nurse supervisor/coordinator
usually oversees the health services program and provides
supervision for other school nurses. In a 1986 national survey of school nurse supervisors, 60% were registered
professional nurses. Other supervisors for school nurses
were school administrators (10%), educators (health and
physical educators) (15%), psychologists and counselors
(12%), and physicians (3%) (Igoe, 1991). As the health
needs of students become increasingly complex and the level
of care delivered in school rises, there is an obvious need
for the school health program (especially the health service
component) to be managed by a health professional who is
knowledgeable about the clinical aspects of care.

School health managers/coordinators require certain
skills to be effective. Among the most frequently cited skills
of effective managers are the following: (1) verbal communication (including listening); (2) managing time and
stress; (3) managing individual decisions; (4) recognizing,
defining, solving problems; (5) motivating and influencing
others; (6) delegating; (7) setting goals and articulating a
vision; (8) self-awareness; (9) team building; and (10) managing conflict (Whetten, Cameron, 1991). Individuals seeking to manage school health programs would definitely need
these abilities in light of the major changes that most school
health programs are undergoing.

Controlling

Efforts to evaluate school health programs are underway,
but this area of program management is still in its infancy.
Fortunately, practice standards for the school nurse and
school nurse practitioner exist, and these serve as useful
guides in determining nurses' effectiveness (Guidelines,
1991). Program evaluations also occur (Igoe, 1991). School
nurses are beginning to include outcome measures as well
as process variables in these evaluations. For example, the
number of referred students who now wear glasses should
be noted in an evaluation (outcome measures) as well as the
number of students screened (process variables). Outcome
measures of the effectiveness of a particular school health
activity also must reflect what impact the activity had on
the child's academic performance.

Another way to improve the quality of school health is
to mandate or require that certain services, health education,
and environmental measures be provided for students. A

OVERVIEW OF STATE REGULATIONS THAT AFFECT ENVIRONMENTAL HEALTH CONDITIONS IN SCHOOLS

RESPONSIBLE AGENCY

◊ 11 states (21%) responsible party employed by State Education Agency

◊ 15 states (30%) responsible party employed by State Health Department

◊ 18 states (35%) both Department of Education/health agencies

◊ 7 states (14%) Department of Education, State Department of Health, plus other agencies

TRADITIONAL

◊ Ventilation—32 states (63%)

◊ Kitchen—45 states (88%)

◊ Illumination—27 states (53%)

◊ Safety glass—31 states (61%)

INSPECTION REQUIREMENTS

◊ Most frequent—Kitchen (46 states, 61%), restrooms (29 states, 57%)

◊ Less than one-third of states required mandatory inspection of the chemical laboratory, classroom, gymnasium, playground, athletic field

OTHER POLICIES/STANDARDS

◊ New Standards (EPA/Office of Water)—Lead in school drinking water

◊ Asbestos—Containing Materials in Schools Rule EPA (40 CFR Part 763 Subpart E)—25 states (49%) developed plan to meet 1989 federal regulations

Source: American School Health Association. *School Health in America,* 1989.

---

regulated approach, however, is not always the best way to proceed. This can turn out to be a highly political process and once things are mandated it is often difficult to change them if there is evidence that a practice is no longer necessary. Finally, the area of school health that is probably most in need of quality control is the environment. Generally, environmental health standards are not always relevant, available, or enforced. The box provides an overview of the environmental health regulations that are currently in effect (Lovato, 1990).

INNOVATIONS IN SCHOOL HEALTH
School-Based Health Centers

School-based health centers (SBHC) were established as a result of several demonstration projects conducted during the past two decades (Meeker et al., 1986). These projects demonstrated that the school can be an effective site for primary health care services because most children and youth attend school and have access to this facility. The projects also demonstrated that nurse practitioners with appropriate physician consultation provide excellent health care, reduce unnecessary referrals, and cut down on the time away from school if a student's only other access to care is a public clinic where the waiting time is extensive

(Kornguth, 1990). Presently, there are an estimated 300 school-based health centers in the United States located in secondary schools. No accurate estimates exist of the number that are established in elementary schools, preschools, or in school-based after-school day care centers.

Schools encounter financial problems with even the most basic school health program. Therefore if a community's school-age population is to benefit from the advantages of using the school setting as the student health center, the responsibility for organizing, financing, and delivery of school health services in these sites must be shared with other community health systems, including state and local health departments. School-based health centers are cost effective in comparison to other community health facilities, with estimates ranging from $90/student/year to $150/student/year (Model School Health Programs, 1991). Consequently, financing mechanisms must be found to support SBHCs such as third party reimbursement for services rendered to students who have Medicaid benefits or other health insurance plans as is done in the Hartford, Connecticut school district (Model School Health Programs, 1991).

School-based health centers change the school nurse responsibilities in several ways. In some instances the school nurse takes on the responsibility for providing the care as a school nurse practitioner. In other settings the school nurse acts as the manager for the center and designs the programs and activities necessary for its operation. In other settings, nurses serve as team members for the center and their responsibility is triage and case management. However, it should be pointed out that the delivery of individualized personal health services is but one aspect of the total school health program. Therefore policy makers would be ill advised to trade away all the rest of their school health program (generalized health services for the entire student body, health education, and a healthy environment) for a school-based health center.

Family Resource/Service Centers

In Florida, Kentucky, and New Jersey the idea of family resource/service centers is attracting attention. Within this organizational structure, a number of school and community resources for families are consolidated into one agency for the sake of efficiency and cost containment. Various public agencies, including the school, pool their child and adolescent health and child care resources and reduce their overhead and management expenses by offering a one-stop shopping arrangement. An extension of the school health program logically belongs within these centers.

Family resource centers may be either geographically located in the school or linked to the school in some other way. In addition to student services, education and employment opportunities for parents are also offered.

Employee Health

Another key aspect of some school health programs is that the program should meet some of the health needs of the teaching staff and other employees of the school system. Currently, a number of school districts have wellness programs for employees as well as medical services (i.e., physical examinations, counseling for drug and alcohol abuse) and in-house evaluations for workmen's compensation claims. These services are often highly valued by the school board and school administrators because of the potential for health care cost containment and reduction in absences. School nurses also have offered various consumer health education programs (such as an adult version of the HealthPACT course) in an effort to enhance teacher satisfaction with the health care system and to improve their use of their health care benefits.

CLINICAL APPLICATION

A referral was made to the school nurse by Monique's sixth grade teacher. Mr. Mather had noticed that Monique was having increasing problems in the classroom—with attention, behavior problems, and poor work, for about the last 2 weeks. Could the nurse see whether any of these problems might be health-related?

Conversation with the teachers revealed that Monique was new to the school, having moved into the district only 2 months ago. Monique was the daughter of an immigrant; the family had been in the United States for 10 years. Her mother spoke limited English, but Monique appeared to have a good command of the language. When the teacher spoke with the mother, Monique would assist with interpretation. The teacher stated that Monique did respond to questions appropriately "when she paid attention." He noted that Monique appeared to have few friends in the class. So far as her behavior was concerned, she would talk or 'day dream' in class instead of listening and was disruptive with her irrelevant remarks.

The nurse agreed that it was appropriate to investigate the possible causes of Moniques' classroom difficulties. Parental permission was sought and granted. Plans were made to meet Monique in the school clinic. The findings would be discussed with Monique, her parents, and the teacher.

When seen in the clinic, Monique was a quiet, shy girl, neatly but plainly dressed. At first, she responded only when questioned. Little information was volunteered. However, as the interview progressed she soon relaxed enough to talk more spontaneously with the nurse. Monique was feeling left out of activities with the other students—they had their own friends to sit with at lunch and she did not really see any of them after school. Sometimes Monique would try to get their attention in class or ask questions about what the teacher said because she could not always understand him. She was "feeling ok" now, but was tired and sometimes her neck and jaw would ache, usually on one side only. Yes, she would get colds every year and her mama would buy "medicine for her ears," but she had not had any for a long time. The nurse noticed that Monique would turn her head to the right side when she was spoken to. Her partial physical examination revealed a low-grade temperature of 99.2° F, caries in a right molar, and a dull right tympanic membrane (tm) with decreased mobility and mild erythema. The left tm showed evidence of scarring from previous infection. The lymph nodes in her neck were enlarged, the right more than the left. She also had nasal congestion with clear nasal drainage. She denied any pain. Her speech was clear.

A quick review of Monique's health records from her previous school indicated that several referrals had been made for earaches and dental care. There were few notations regarding behavior.

Assessment of the information indicated that Monique had acute otitis media (om) and chronic dental caries. The recent onset of classroom difficulties indicated that there was a possible association between these conditions and her behavior in the classroom. A more long-term problem was her sense of isolation from her classmates and acting out behaviors to get their attention.

A call was placed to Monique's mother regarding the nurse's findings. Although Monique's mother spoke limited English, the nurse was bilingual and was able to convey the information that Monique needed treatment for an ear infection and would need to see a dentist because she had cavities. With Monique's additional help with interpretation, the nurse learned that the family was uninsured and had no regular source of medical and dental care. The family would be interested in low cost medical care because they had limited financial resources and no insurance. Transportation to receive medical care would also be a problem because Monique's father would be at work and unable to take her for medical care.

The nurse had the address and phone number of the local community health clinic. She helped call and arranged an appointment time for Monique and her mother to go to the clinic. Monique could be seen the same day that her mother applied for clinic services. No interpreter would be available at the clinic to help with the details of the financial qualifying interview or with the health history. It was apparent that additional assistance was needed since the nurse's schedule prevented her from accompanying the family, and Monique's mother agreed.

The community resource book listed a local agency responsible for assistance to immigrant groups within the community. A call to the agency yielded the name of a representative who could serve as an interpreter. The agent agreed to contact Monique's mother and arrange assistance with transportation for medical care and an interpreter for the visit.

Follow-up with Monique and her mother was made by the nurse. Monique was seen in the local health clinic and treated for acute otitis media. Future appointments were made for follow-up visits to assess the response to medication, for a complete physical examination, and for dental care. The mother was pleased with the clinic and planned to use the clinic services for regular health care needs for the entire family. Because she had a contact with an agency that would assist with language difficulties, the mother felt more comfortable seeking care for herself and her family.

The nurse also maintained contact with Monique's teacher. He was made aware of the ear infection and in the following weeks reported an improvement in her attention to school work. Behavior problems lessened as Monique's ear infection resolved and she was able to understand what was being said. There were still attempts by Monique to get the attention of other students, so it was agreed that the teacher would use class activities to encourage student interaction and offer opportunities for students to know each other better. The nurse counseled Monique and her mother, encouraging Monique's involvement in activities (both in and out of school) that would foster friendships with her classmates.

As a final step, the nurse and teacher agreed that Monique would be encouraged to develop friendships, and the nurse would be notified if other problems were noted. The previously identified physical problems would be followed through the routine screenings alone in each school and special attention would be given to any indications of recurring physical problems.

The preceding case study illustrates the role of the school nurse in providing care to school-age youth. Use of available school and community resources is not only wise but necessary if the nurse is to function effectively. Care of a student requires collaboration between teachers, students and their families, and community resources if needs are to be properly identified and met. The school nurse is a key resource for assessment and preventive health maintenance and coordination of services.

SUMMARY

School health is a component of the community health system. Traditionally, school health programs have been limited in scope. However, societal changes have produced a need to restructure school health and to offer more complex health care services and more effective health education approaches. The school environment also requires more attention than it previously was given.

School nurses, by virtue of their ability to offer clinical services, provide health instruction, and recognize environmental health hazards, are well prepared to organize, coordinate, and manage the school health program. In addition, school nurses frequently are case managers for students with special health needs, chronic disease, and other disabilities.

New models for school health are emerging. School and community health systems are becoming more closely integrated. This arrangement offers a variety of new possibilities for school health programming and school nursing.

KEY CONCEPTS

The health problems of school-age youth vary substantially between the younger years and the adolescent years.

Health problems are major risk factors for absenteeism and academic failure.

Children and adolescents who are poor are at high risk for absenteeism and school failure.

The three core components of school health are health services, health education, and promotion of a healthy environment.

School health services generally include health screenings, basic care for minor complaints, administration of medications, surveillance of immunization status, case-finding for the early identification of problems, and nursing care of students with special needs.

Historically, reducing absenteeism has been the single most important reason for school nursing services. With the current emphasis on education reform and academic performance, reducing absenteeism continues to be a top priority for school nurses.

The role of the school nurse includes the functions of health education and counseling as well as the delivery of clinical care to students with disabilities. Coordination of the overall school health program and case management of individual student health problems are other responsibilities of the nurse.

School health activities are family-centered and are intended to promote health as well as reduce the incidence of disease.

Although health screenings are an integral component of school health services, nurses must prepare other school personnel, students, and volunteers for this work.

Administration of medications and clinical care of students with disabilities in schools is increasing in frequency. Nevertheless the risks associated with these practices can be managed successfully provided there are well developed policies and procedures.

School health education involves health promotion instruction for all students to develop their positive personal health habits; self-help classes for students with special health needs; and consumer education for all so that the next generation will be prepared to use the health care system effectively.

The school environment requires attention, and certain measures are necessary if the climate at school is to be both physically and psychologically healthy.

Schools are nontraditional health care settings. Consequently, it is important to establish health policies, procedures, and plans to provide direction for the school health program.

Planning and operation of the school health program involves parents and community health professionals as well as school personnel.

LEARNING ACTIVITIES

1. Visit a school. Observe the activities and interactions of students as a group both inside and outside the classroom. What are the advantages and disadvantages of learning collectively as opposed to being tutored? What are the implications for health teaching and counseling?

2. Interview a school nurse, school nurse practitioner, or community health nurse specialist for school-aged youth working in schools. How do they explain their roles in the school? What are the rewards? What are the frustrations?

3. Visit a school with a school nurse. Observe how the nurse works with individual children with disabilities and with boys and girls who are at high risk for academic failure because of chronic illness, poverty, and family problems. Inquire about any special procedures and precautions they observe in caring for these students. Look at the record keeping system. Ask to review an individual education plan (IEP) and an individualized family service plan (IFSP). Find out whether the school nurse is involved with the school district's preschool program. Does the school also have a program for those infants and toddlers 0 to 3 years of age who have disabilities? How is the nurse involved with this effort?

4. Find a journal or textbook for school teachers. Review the table of contents to determine the areas of interest and importance to them. Select and read one of these articles/chapters. Compare and contrast the school teacher's approach to problem solving with the way nurses solve problems. What benefits and constraints could these differences present when nurses and teachers try to work together?

5. Attend a school board meeting. In preparation for this activity find out whether the board members are appointed or elected. Also find out something about the board members: their names, occupations, special concerns about education. At the time of the meeting, review the agenda, notice the amount of preparatory work the board members must do before meetings, observe the interactions between the board, school administrators, and members of the audience. What are the chief concerns expressed at this meeting? How will this affect the school health program and school nurses?

6. Find a group of children or adolescents. Ask them to draw you a picture (or explain) the nature of the health program at their school. What services are provided? What health classes are taught? What activities go on at school to keep it a safe and healthy environment for students? Ask the students to identify one change in the school health program that they would like to make.

7. Contact a parent who is a member of the Parent Teachers Organization (PTO). Discover the purpose and functions of this organization. Find out whether the PTO is involved in school health locally or nationally. Also discover whether the PTO represents all parents. Are parents who are poor or from minority groups involved?

8. Is there a state school nurse consultant in your state? Find out by contacting the State Department of Health and the State Department of Education/Instruction. If there is a nurse consultant available, find out the answers to these questions: (a) How many school nurses are there in your state? (b) Is there a current statewide policy/procedure manual for school health that is available to guide the practice of all school health personnel, especially those people working in districts too small to develop their own? How is this manual developed? (c) What is the major school health concern right now in your state and the nurse consultant's strategy for addressing this issue? (d) Where are the school health programs in your state that work well? What are the ingredients in these school systems that make these programs successful?

9. Review the Chronology of School Health Events in Table 40-1 and predict what type of school health program will be needed in the year 2015.

BIBLIOGRAPHY

A children's defense budget FY 1989. An analysis of our nation's investment in children, Washington, DC, 1988, Children's Defense Fund.

Allensworth D and Wolford C: Achieving the 1990 health objectives for the nation, Kent, Ohio, 1988, American School Health Association.

Califano Jr J: America's health care revolution, who lives? who dies? who pays?, New York, 1986, Random House.

Children and America's other drug problem: guidelines for improving prescription medicine use among children and teenagers, Washington, DC, 1989, National Council on Patient Information.

Code blue: uniting for healthier youth a call to action, The National Commission on the Role of the School and Community in Improving Adolescents Health, Alexandria VA, 1990, NASBE.

Comer J: Educating poor minority children, Scientific American, 259:42-48, 1988.

Committee on vision: Myopia: prevalence and progression. Commission on Behavioral and Social Sciences and Education. National Research Council. Washington, DC, 1989, National Academy Press.

Council. Washington, DC, 1989, National Academy Press.

Current Population Reports, Series P-60, No. 161, U.S. Department of Commerce, Washington, DC, 1988, Bureau of the Census.

Digest of educational statistics (NCES86-643), Washington, DC, 1989, U.S. Department of Education Office of Educational Research and Improvement.

Department of Health and Human Services: Child Health USA 89, DHHS Pub. No (PHS) Bureau of Maternal and Child Health and Resource Development, Office of Maternal and Child Health HRS-M-CH8915, Washington, DC, 1989, Department of Health and Human Services.

Dever A: Epidemiology of health service management, Rockville, Md, 1984, Aspen Systems Corp.

Dock LL: School-nurse experiment in New York, Am J Nurs 3:108-110, 1902.

Family health in an era of stress. General Mills American Family Report, 1979, General Mills, Inc.

Flinn foundation special report. The health of Arizona's school children. Key findings of two

surveys by Louis Harris and Associates, Inc and the UCLA School of Medicine, Phoenix, Ariz 1989, Flinn Foundation.

Goodwin L: The effectiveness of school nurse practitioners: a review of the literature, J Sch Health, 51:623-624, 1981.

Goodwin L: Immunizations in schools: pros and cons. Unpublished report, 1978.

Green LW: Health education models. In Matarazzo JD, Weiss SM, Herd JA, Miller N, and Weiss SM, editors: Behavioral health: a handbook of health enhancement and disease prevention, New York, 1984, John Wiley and Sons.

Guide to Clinical Preventive Services. Report of the US preventive services task force: 305-313, Baltimore, 1989, Williams and Wilkins Co.

Guidelines for a model school nursing services program, Scarborough Maine, 1990, National Association of School Nurses, Inc.

Guidelines for the Delineation of Roles and Responsibilities for the Safe Delivery of Specialized Health Care in the Educational Setting. Developed by the joint task force for the management of children with special health needs of the American Federation of Teachers (AFT), The Council for Exceptional Children (CEC), National Association of School Nurses, Inc. (NASN), National Education Association (NEA), Scarborough, Maine, 1990, National Association of School Nurses.

Health: United States, 1989, DHHS Pub. No (PHS) 90-1232, Washington, DC, 1990, Department of Health and Human Services.

Igoe J: Healthy long-term attitudes on personal health can be developed in school-age children, Pediatrician, 15:127-136, 1988.

Igoe J: Empowering the health care consumer, Pediatric nursing forum on the future: looking toward the 21st century, New Jersey, 1989, Anthony Jannetti, Inc.

Igoe J: School nursing and school health. In Natapoff J and Wieczarek R, editors: Maternal child health policy: a nursing perspective, New York, 1990, Springer.

Igoe J and Campos EL: Report of a national survey of school nurse supervisors, School Nurse 6:8-20, 1991.

Igoe J: Is health a school issue? School-based health services. In Aiken L and Fagin C, editors: Nursing and health policy: issues of the 1990's, Philadelphia, 1991, J.B. Lippincott.

Iowa Department of Education: Administering medications to students in Iowa schools. A training guide, Unpublished report, 1991.

Kaplan D: School health care ONLINE!!!! School-based clinic management information system, Denver, Colo, 1991, Medical and Educational Software, Inc.

Kids count data book. State profiles of child well-being. Washington, DC, 1991, The Center for the Study of Social Policy.

Klerman L: School absence—a health perspective, Pediatr Clin North Am 35:1253-1269, 1988.

Kolbe L and Iverson D: Comprehensive school health education programs. In Matarazzo J, Weiss S, Herd J, Miller N, and Weiss S, editors: Behavioral health: a handbook of health enhancement and disease prevention, New York, 1984, John Wiley and Sons.

Kornguth M: School absences for illness: who's absent and why, Pediatric Nursing, 16:95-99, 1990.

Kovar M: The health status of preschool and school-age children. In Wallace H, Ryan G, Oglesby A, editors: Maternal and child health practices, Oakland, Calif, 1988, Third Party Publishing Company.

Lewis C and Lewis MA: Consequences of empowering children to care for themselves, Pediatrician 17:63-67, 1990.

Lovato C, editor: School health in America, Kent, Ohio, 1990, American School Health Association.

Mann K: Screening for scoliosis: a review of the evidence. In Goldbloom RB and Lawrence R, editors: Preventing disease beyond the rhetoric, New York, 1990, Springer-Verlag.

Meeker R, De Angelis C, Berman B, et al: A comprehensive school health initiative. Image 18:86-91, 1986.

Model school health programs. Unpublished report, 1991.

National Council on Patient Information and Education: Guidelines for improving prescription medicine use among children and teenagers. A report of the national council on patient information and education, Washington, DC, 1989, The Council.

Northern J and Downs M: Hearing in children, Baltimore, 1989, Williams & Wilkins.

US Office of Disease Prevention and Health Promotion: Healthy People 2000, DHHS Publication No. 90-502-12, Washington, DC, 1990, US Government Printing Office.

Rogers L: Some phases of school nursing, Am J Nurs 8:966-974, 1908.

Rogers L: The nurse in the public school, Am J Nurs 5:763-769, 1905.

School Health in America Kent, Ohio, 1989, American School Health Association.

School nurses working with handicapped children: a statement of the American Nurses Association Divisions on Nursing Practice, The American School Health Association and the National Association of School Nurses, Kansas City, Mo, 1980, American Nurses Association.

Starfield B: Family income, ill health and medical care of U.S. children. J Public Health Policy, 3:244-259, 1982.

Stember M: Kids as consumers: effectiveness of HealthPACT, final report of "a study of school nurses' use of project HealthPACT" Division of Nursing, Bureau of Health Professions, Health Resources and Services Administration, U.S. Public Health Service R01NU0093, 1988.

Stoto M, Behrens R, and Rosemont C, editors: Healthy People 2000: citizens chart the course. Institute of Medicine, Washington, DC, 1990, National Academy Press.

Struthers LR: The school nurse, New York, 1917, G.P. Putnam's Sons.

US Department of Education: National Goals for Education, 1990, Washington, DC.

Walker D, Butler J, and Bender A: Children's health care and the schools. In Schlesinger M and Eisenberg L, editors: Children in a changing health system. Assessments and proposals for reform, Baltimore, 1990, John Hopkins University Press.

Waters Y: Visiting nursing in the United States, New York, 1909, Charities Publications Committee.

Whetten D and Cameron K: Developing management skills, New York, 1991, Harper Collins.

Wold SJ: School nursing: a framework for practice, North Branch, Minn, 1981, Sunrise River Press.

Woodfill M and Beyrer M: The role of the nurse in the school setting: an historical view as reflected in the literature. Kent, Ohio, 1991, American School Health Association.

41

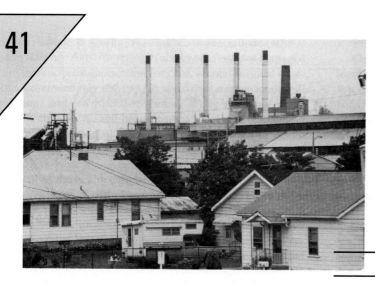

The Community Health Nurse in Occupational Health

Charlene C. Ossler

OBJECTIVES

After reading this chapter, the student should be able to:

Describe the nursing role in occupational health.

Describe at least three characteristics of the American work force.

Describe the extent of work-related illnesses and injuries.

Use the epidemiological model to explain work-health interactions.

Cite at least three host factors associated with increased risk from an adverse response to hazardous workplace exposure.

Define hypersusceptible workers.

Explain one example each of biological, chemical, ergonomic, physical, and psychosocial workplace hazards.

Differentiate between health promotion programs and employee assistance programs.

Describe the functions of OSHA and NIOSH.

Describe an effective disaster plan.

Complete an occupational health history.

KEY TERMS

agents
biological agents
chemical agents
cumulative trauma
disaster planning
employee assistance programs
environment
epidemiological triad
ergonomists
ergonomic agents
first aiders

Hazard Communication Standard
host
hypersusceptible
National Institute for Occupational Safety and Health
occupational health history
Occupational Safety and Health Act

Occupational Safety and Health Administration
physical agents
plant survey
psychosocial agents
workers' compensation act
work health interactions
worksite survey

he past two decades have witnessed revolutionary changes in the nature of work and the workplace, the global economy, and the health care system. These complex changes are shaping future health priorities. An analysis of these trends suggests that work-health interactions will continue to grow in importance, especially as the demand for healthy workers exceeds the supply. As a result of these changes, impressive developments in occupational health and safety programs have occurred that are designed to control and prevent work-related illness and injury. Nurses, particularly occupational health nurses, have performed critical roles in the planning and delivery of work-site health and safety services, which must continue to grow in comprehensiveness and cost effectiveness. The continuing escalation of the cost of health care and concern about the quality of care have prompted American businesses to add management of nonwork-related health problems to their health services programs.

The health impact of work is an important aspect of most clients for whom the community health nurse provides care. At least one-third of the average adult's life is spent at work; therefore, the workplace has a significant potential influence on individuals' health and is a primary site for the delivery of preventive health care. According to Bezold, Carlson, and Peck (1986, p. 168), "The dominant institutions of health—the hospital, the clinic, the laboratory, the nursing home—will steadily shrink in influence and scope in the decades ahead. They will yield to the home, the community center, and the workplace as the dominant settings in which health is pursued."

The prevalence and significance of the interactions between health and work underscore the importance of incorporating principles of occupational health and safety into general nursing practice. The types of interactions and the frequent use of the general health care system for the identification, treatment, and prevention of occupational illnesses and injuries require nurses to use this knowledge in all practice settings.

This chapter describes the community health nurse's role with the working population. It provides an introduction to work-related health and safety concerns and the principles for the prevention and control of adverse work-health interactions. The focus is on the knowledge and skills needed to promote the health and safety of workers through work-site occupational health programs, as well as through off-site interventions from agencies other than the employing business organizations. The epidemiological triad is used as the model for understanding these interactions as well as risk factors and effective nursing care for promoting health and safety among employed populations. The assessment, prevention, and management of occupational health problems are skills that can be applied in all types of nursing care settings.

NURSING ROLES IN OCCUPATIONAL SETTINGS

Nurses perform a variety of roles and functions in occupational settings. The specialty of occupational health nursing in the United States began in 1898 with the employment of Ida Mayo Stewart, the first occupational health nurse

(OHN), at the Vermont Marble Company (Babbitz, 1984). Although occupational health nursing has been a major force in promoting worker health since that time, rapid technological transformations, changes in the health care system, and societal expectations have demanded an increasingly complex and expanded role for occupational health nursing in the twentieth century. The primary focus of occupational health nurses' practices is the health and safety of workers, with an emphasis on the prevention of illness and injury.

As American industry has shifted from agrarian to industrial to highly technological processes, the role of the occupational health nurse has continued to evolve. The focus on work-related health problems now includes the spectrum of human responses to multiple, complex interactions of biopsychosocial factors that occur in the community, home, and work environments. The customary role of the occupational health nurse has extended beyond emergency treatment and prevention of illness and injury to include the promotion and maintenance of health, overall risk management, and efforts to reduce health-related costs in businesses.

The occupational health nurse offers direct care to employees, as well as managerial functions such as program evaluation and analysis of work-related injuries and illnesses. The role changes with the goals of an organization's occupational health and safety program and is therefore diversified. The interdisciplinary nature of occupational health nursing has become more critical as occupational health and safety problems require more complex solutions. The OHN frequently collaborates closely with multiple disciplines and management as well as representatives of labor.

Occupational health nurses constitute the largest group of occupational health professionals. The most recent national survey of registered nurses indicates that there are approximately 21,000 licensed occupational health nurses (U.S. Department of Health and Human Services, 1988). In the most recent survey conducted on OHNs, nearly 70% report that they are employed as staff nurses; the majority of these manage one-nurse units in a variety of businesses. Other occupational health nurses hold positions as nurse practitioners, clinical nurse specialists, managers, supervisors, consultants, and educators (Cox, 1985). The occupational health nursing role is unique in that it adapts to an organization's needs as well as to the needs of specific groups of workers.

The professional organization for this specialty, the American Association of Occupational Health Nurses, Inc. (AAOHN), describes five job titles for OHNs: solo practitioner, manager, educator, consultant, and corporate director (AAOHN, 1987). The majority of OHNs work as solo practitioners, but an increasing number of positions have developed in the other categories. New roles in case management and in environmental assessment and control have developed in larger firms. In many companies, management positions have been pared, and the OHN has assumed expanded responsibilities in job analysis, safety, and benefits management. Specialization in the field is often a requirement for the other positions. Graduate education in occupational health nursing is currently available through 14 universities (see box at right).

CURRENT COLLEGIATE PROGRAMS IN OCCUPATIONAL HEALTH NURSING AND NIOSH FUNDED EDUCATIONAL RESOURCE CENTERS (ERC)

University of Alabama (ERC)
School of Nursing
University Station
Birmingham, AL 35294

University of California
School of Nursing
10833 Le Conte
Los Angeles, CA 90024-1702

University of California (ERC)
School of Nursing
San Francisco, CA 94143-0608

Harvard University (ERC)
School of Public Health
633 Commonwealth Ave.
Boston, MA 02115

University of Cincinnati (ERC)
College of Nursing
3110 Vine St.
Cincinnati, OH 45221

Emory University
School of Nursing
Atlanta, GA 30322

University of Illinois (ERC)
College of Nursing
845 S. Damen St.
Chicago, IL 60612

Johns Hopkins University (ERC)
School of Hygiene & Public Health
615 North Wolfe Street
Baltimore, MD 21205

University of Michigan (ERC)
School of Nursing
Ann Arbor, MI 48109

University of Minnesota (ERC)
School of Public Health
420 Delaware St., S.W.
Minneapolis, MN 55455

University of North Carolina (ERC)
School of Public Health
Rosenau Hall cb 7400
Chapel Hill, NC 27599

University of Texas Health Science Center
School of Public Health
P.O. Box 20186
Houston, TX 77025

University of Washington (ERC)
SM-24 Community Health Care Systems
Seattle, WA 98195

Texas Women's University
College of Nursing
1130 M.D. Anderson Blvd.
Houston, TX 77030

University of Wisconsin-Milwaukee
School of Nursing
P.O. Box 413
Milwaukee, WI 53201

Simmons College
Department of Nursing
300 Fenway
Boston, MA 02115

University of Pennsylvania
School of Nursing
420 Service Dr.
Philadelphia, PA 19104

Certification in the specialty is provided by the American Board for Occupational Health Nurses, Inc. (ABOHN). OHNs must meet requirements for experience, continuing education, and professional activities before they are eligible to take the ABOHN certification examination. Approximately 10% of the OHNs practicing in the specialty are certified occupational health nurses (COHN). The AAOHN is listed as a resource in Appendix H2.

WORKERS AS A POPULATION AGGREGATE

There are approximately 108 million workers over the age of 16 in the United States, employed in over 6.5 million different work sites (Bureau of Labor Statistics, 1989). This number represents 64% of the total workforce and does not indicate the full number of individuals who have potentially been exposed to work-related health hazards. More than

91% of those who are able to work outside of the home do so for some portion of their lives (Bureau of Labor Statistics, 1989). Although some individuals may currently be unemployed or retired, they continue to bear the increased health risks of past occupational hazards. For the community health nurse, the number of affected individuals may be even larger, as work-related illnesses are found among the spouses, children, and neighbors of exposed workers.

Americans are employed in diverse industries that range in size from one to tens of thousands of employees. Types of industries include traditional manufacturing (e.g., automotive and appliances), service industries (e.g., banking, health care, and restaurants), agriculture, and the newer high-technology firms, such as computer chip manufacturers. Approximately 85% of business organizations are considered small; they employ fewer than 500 people (Bureau of Labor Statistics, 1989). Although some industries are noted for the high degree of hazards associated with their work (e.g., foundries, mines, construction, and agriculture), no work site is free of occupational health and safety hazards. The larger the company, the more likely it is that there will be health and safety programs for employees. Smaller companies are more likely to rely on the external community to meet their needs for health and safety services.

Characteristics of the Workforce

The demographic trends in the American work force describe a changing population aggregate, and this has implications for the preventive services targeted to that group. Major changes in the working population are reflected in the increasing numbers of women, older individuals, and those with chronic illnesses that are part of the workforce. Because of changes in the economy, extension of life-span, legislative initiatives, and societal acceptance of working women, the proportion of the employed population that these three groups represent will probably continue to grow.

In an era in which the demand for workers is expected to outstrip the available supply (Naisbitt and Aburdene, 1990, p. 230), businesses must be concerned about strategies to optimize the health, employment longevity, and satisfaction of workers. For example, nearly 60% of women are now employed, and it is predicted that women will account for 67% of the increase in the labor force over the next decade (Rix, 1988). These workers tend to be married with children and aging parents for whom they are responsible. This aggregate of workers poses new issues for individual and family health promotion (such as child care and elder care) that can be addressed in the work environment. Other trends shaping the profile of the workforce include more education and mobility as well as increasing mismatches in the 1990s between skills of workers and types of employment.

Characteristics of Work

There has been a dramatic shift in the types of jobs held by workers. Following the evolution from an agrarian economy to a manufacturing society and then to a highly technological workplace, the greatest proportion of paid employment is now in the occupations of service (e.g., health care, information processing, banking, and insurance), professional and technical positions (e.g., managers and computer specialists), and clerical work (e.g., word processors and secretaries). Of the new jobs created from 1984 to 1989, 73% were in the categories of professional administrative, sales and technical, and precision crafts (Bureau of Labor Statistics, 1989). In the traditional manufacturing setting, modernization with robots and other mechanization of work processes have altered job requirements. This change in the nature of work has been accompanied by many new occupational hazards such as complex chemicals, non-ergonomic workstation design (the adaptation of the workplace or equipment used to do work to meet the employee's health and safety needs), and job stress. In addition, the emergence of a global economy with free trade and multinational corporations presents new challenges for health and safety programs that are culturally relevant.

Work-Health Interactions

The influence of work on health is shown by statistics on illnesses, injuries, and deaths associated with employment. In 1988, 6.4 million reported work-related illnesses and injuries resulted in lost time from work. Of these, one-third were severe enough to result in temporary or permanent disability that prevented the worker from returning to a usual job. Over the past few years, the incidence and severity of work-related injury have increased (Bureau of Labor Statistics, 1989). During 1988, 3270 deaths were attributed to the work environment, and there were 100,000 deaths resulting from primary illnesses in which work was a contributing or exacerbating factor. More than 300,000 cases of occupationally induced illness are diagnosed annually (Office of Technology Assessment, 1986). These figures are often described as "the tip of the iceberg" because many work-related health problems go unreported; but even the recorded statistics are significant in depicting the amount of human suffering, economic loss, and decreased productivity associated with workplace hazards.

APPLICATION OF THE EPIDEMIOLOGICAL MODEL

The epidemiological model can be used to understand the relationship between work and health (Figure 41-1). With a focus on the health and safety of the employed population, the *host* is described as any susceptible human being. Because of the ubiquitous nature of work-related hazards, nurses must assume that all employed individuals and groups are potentially at risk of being exposed to occupational hazards. The *agents*, factors associated with illness and injury, are occupational hazards that are classified as biological, chemical, ergonomic, physical, or psychosocial. The third

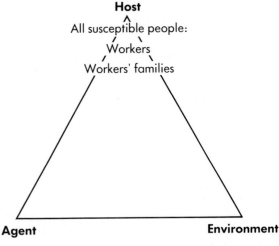

Host
All susceptible people:
Workers
Workers' families

Agent

Workplace hazards:
  Biological
  Chemical
  Ergonomic
  Physical
  Psychosocial

Environment

All other external factors that influence host-agent interactions: physical and social

FIGURE 41-1

Elements of the epidemiologic triad applied to occupational health.

element, the *environment*, includes all external conditions that influence the interaction of the host and agents. These may be workplace conditions such as temperature extremes, crowding, shiftwork, and inflexible management styles. The basic principle of epidemiology is that health status interventions for restoring and promoting health are the result of complex interactions among these three elements. To understand these interactions and to design effective nursing strategies for dealing with them in a proactive manner, nurses must look at each element and how it influences the others.

Host

Each worker represents a host within the worker population-group. Certain host factors correlate with increased risk of adverse response to the hazards of the workplace. These include age, gender, chronic illness, work practices, immunological status, ethnicity, and lifestyle habits. For example, the population group at greatest risk for experiencing a work-related accident with subsequent injury are young males (18 to 30 years old) with less than 6 months experience in their current job. The host factors of age, gender, and work experience combine to increase this group's risk of injury because of characteristics such as risk-taking, lack of knowledge, and low dexterity on the new job. This population aggregate of workers is also more likely to be impaired by chronic use and abuse of drugs and alcohol.

Older workers may be at increased risk in the workplace because of diminished sensory abilities, the effects of chronic illnesses, and delayed reaction times (Poore, 1986). A third population group that may be very susceptible to workplace exposures is women in their childbearing years. The hormonal changes during these years along with the increased stress of new roles and additional responsibilities are host factors that may influence this group's response to potentially toxic exposures.

In addition to these host factors, there may be other, less well-understood individual differences in responses to occupational hazard exposures. Even if employers maintain exposure levels below the level recommended by occupational health and safety standards, 15% to 20% of the population may have health reactions to the "safe" low-level exposures. This group has been termed *hypersusceptible*. A number of host factors appear to be associated with this hypersusceptibility: light skin, malnutrition, compromised immune system, glucose 6-phosphate dehydrogenase deficiency, serum alpha 1-antitrypsin deficiency, chronic obstructive pulmonary disease, sickle cell trait, and hypertension (Stokinger, 1977). Individuals who have known hypersusceptibility to chemicals that are respiratory irritants, hemolytic chemicals, organic isocyanates, and carbon disulfide may also be hypersusceptible to other agents in the work environment (Zenz, 1988, p. 109). Although this has prompted some industries to consider preplacement screening for such risk factors, the associations between these individual health markers and hypersusceptible response are speculative and require further research.

Agents

Work-related hazards, or agents, present potential and actual risks to the health and safety of workers in the 6 million business establishments in the United States. These agents are classified in five categories: *biological, chemical, ergonomic, physical,* and *psychosocial*. Any worksite commonly presents multiple and interacting exposures from all five categories of agents. Table 41-1 lists some of the more common workplace exposures, their known health effects, and the types of jobs associated with these hazards.

Biological Agents

Biological agents are living organisms whose excretions or parts are capable of causing human disease, usually by

---

TABLE 41-1
Common workplace exposures by job with known health effects

Workplace hazard	Health effects	Jobs with potential exposure
Carbon monoxide	Headache, angina	Firefighters, auto mechanics, drive-in bank tellers
Solvents	Dermatitis, cancer	Foundry workers, wood finishers, dry cleaners, textile workers, microelectronics
Lead	Abdominal pain, hypertension, behavioral changes	Battery makers, smelter workers, painters, shoemakers, gasoline station attendants
Asbestos, silica, coal dust	Chronic bronchitis, emphysema, lung cancer	Insulators, pipe fitters, miners, shipyard workers
Benzene	Aplastic anemia, leukemia	Furniture finishers, chemists
Hepatitis B virus	Hepatitis	Health services workers
Sunlight	Melanoma	Farmers, fishermen, highway workers
Heat	Burns, hyperthermia	Foundry and smelter workers, food services workers, firefighters
Lifting heavy loads	Back pain, muscle strain, sprains	Health services workers, truckers who load and unload vehicles
Vibration	Kidney disease, bladder disease, carpal tunnel	Semi-trailer truck drivers, jack hammer operators
Postural strain	Headaches, blurred vision, neck pain	VDT operator

an infectious process (Cheremisinoff, 1984). Biological hazards are common in workplaces such as hospitals and clinical laboratories. In these worksites, employees are potentially exposed to a variety of infectious agents including viruses, fungi, and bacteria. Health services workers are at increased risk of contracting disease from these exposures. For example, hepatitis B and tuberculosis rates are generally higher than expected among hospital personnel; a hospital employee is 41% more likely than the average worker to lose work time because of a serious occupational injury or illness (National Safety Council, 1989). Many workers in these settings are employed as maintenance workers, security guards, aides, or cleaning people, who tend not to be well-protected from inadvertent exposures which include contaminated bed linen in the laundry, soiled equipment, and trash containing contaminated dressings or specimens.

Other occupations with exposures to biological agents include agriculture (farmer's lung) and commercial baking (baker's asthma) (McCunney, 1988; Kusnetz and Hutchison, 1979). In addition, new biological agents (such as AIDS, *Legionella* infection, and herpes) have developed.

Chemical Agents

Over 300 billion pounds of chemicals are produced annually in the United States. Of the approximately 2 million known chemicals in existence, only several hundred have been adequately studied for their effects on humans. Of those chemicals that have been assayed for carcinogenicity, approximately one-half test positive as animal carcinogens. Most chemicals have not been studied epidemiologically to determine the effects of exposure on humans (Huff, McConnell, and Haseman, 1985; Levy and Wegman, 1988, p. 221-223). As a consequence of general environmental contamination with chemicals from work, home, and community activities, a variety of chemicals are found in the body tissues of the general population. These tissue loads may result in part from the accidental release of chemicals into the environment, such as that which occurred in Love Canal when chemicals leached out from buried industrial wastes. In many workplaces, significant exposure to a daily, low-level dose of workplace chemicals may be below the exposure standards but still may constitute a potentially chronic and perhaps cumulative assault on workers' health. Predicting human responses to such exposures is further complicated because several chemicals are often combined to create a new chemical agent; human effects may be associated with the interaction of these agents rather than with a single chemical.

An evolving concern about occupational exposure to chemicals is reproductive health effects. Workplace reproductive hazards have become important legal and scientific issues. Toxicity to male and female reproductive systems has been demonstrated in common agents such as lead, mercury, cadmium, nickel, and zinc, as well as in antineoplastic drug administration (Mattison, 1983). These concerns are addressed in a recent governmental report that calls for additional legislative intervention with occupational reproductive hazards (Office of Technology Assessment, 1985).

On March 20, 1991, the US Supreme Court issued a decision, *Auto Workers vs. Johnson Controls, Inc.*, that will have far-reaching health effects. The Court ruled that women of childbearing age cannot be excluded from jobs that could result in reproductive hazards. Parents are to be informed about the potential work-related hazards, but they must make the decision about whether the women continue to work in a potentially dangerous environment. The Court based its decision in part, on the aim of being non-discriminatory in allowing women to work in better-paying jobs even though these jobs may pose hazards to the fetus. In this case, the women working in a battery manufacturing plant were exposed to lead, which can cause anomalies in a developing fetus.

Since data for predicting human responses to many chemical agents are inadequate, workers should be assessed for all potential exposures and cautioned to work preventively with these agents. High-risk or vulnerable workers should be carefully screened and monitored for optimal health protection.

Ergonomic Agents

Ergonomic agents are those that involve the transfer of mechanical energy from the work processes or pose postural or other strains that can produce adverse health effects when certain tasks are performed repetitively. Examples are vibration, repetitive motion, poor workstation-worker fit, and the lifting of heavy loads. Vibration, which accompanies the use of power tools and vehicles such as trucks, affects internal organs, supportive ligaments, the upper torso, and the shoulder-girdle structure. Localized effects are seen with handheld power tools; the most common is Raynaud's phenomenon (Cheremisinoff, 1984). Carpal tunnel syndrome, tendonitis, and tendosynovitis are the most frequently seen occupational diseases observed in workers who are chronically exposed to repetitive motion (Putz-Anderson, 1988). The research on these hazards, related human responses, and prevention is evolving. Injuries and illnesses related to this category of agents have been termed *cumulative trauma*, and this comprises the largest category of work-related illness and disability claims in the United States. The most productive strategy in preventing these exposures appears to be redesigning the workplace and the work machinery or processes.

Physical Agents

Physical agents are those that produce adverse health effects by the transfer of physical energy. Commonly encountered physical agents in the workplace include extremes of temperature, noise, radiation, and lighting. The control of worker exposure to these agents frequently depends on the worker's compliance with preventive actions such as safe work habits and wearing personal protective equipment. Examples of safe work habits include taking appropriate breaks from environments with temperature extremes and not eating or smoking in radiation-contaminated areas. Personal protective equipment includes hearing protection, eye guards, protective clothing, and devices for monitoring exposures to agents such as radiation. This class of agents is considered one of the most easily controlled. Frost bite, heat stroke, hearing loss, radiation sickness, and headaches from improper lighting can be prevented through engineering controls and appropriate education of the worker in preventive work practices.

Psychosocial Agents

Psychosocial hazards are conditions that pose a threat to the psychological and/or social well being of individuals and groups. A psychosocial response to the work environment occurs as an employee acts selectively toward his environment in an attempt to achieve a harmonious relationship. When such a human attempt at adaptation to the environment fails, an adverse psychosocial response may occur. Work-related "burnout" is a response to excessive and continuous occupationally induced stress. Responses to negative interpersonal relationships, particularly those with authority figures in the workplace, are often the cause of vague health symptoms and increased absenteeism. Epidemiological work in mental health has pointed to environmental variables such as these in the incidence of mental illness and emotional disorder (Baker, 1985; Cooper and Payne, 1978).

Environment

Environmental factors influence the occurrence of host-agent interactions and may mediate the course and outcome of those interactions. While there may be aspects of the physical environment (e.g., heat, odor, or ventilation) that influence the host-agent interaction, the psychological environment can be of equal importance. Consider an employee who is working with a potentially toxic liquid. Providing education about safe work practices and fitting the employee with protective clothing may not be adequate if the work must occur in a very hot and humid environment. As the worker becomes uncomfortable in the hot clothing, his protection may be compromised by rolling up a sleeve, taking off a glove, or wiping his face with a contaminated piece of clothing. If the psychosocial norms in the workplace condone such work practices, i.e., "Everyone does it when it's too hot," the interventions that address only the host and agent will be ineffective.

The psychosocial environment includes characteristics of the work itself, as well as the interpersonal relationships required in the work setting. Job characteristics such as low autonomy, poor job satisfaction, and limited control over the pace of work have been associated with an increased risk of heart disease among clerical and blue collar workers (Haynes, 1980). Interpersonal relationships among employees and co-workers or bosses and managers are often sources of conflict and stress. Another environmental aspect is organizational culture. This refers to the norms and patterns of behavior that are sanctioned within a particular organization (Deal and Kennedy, 1982). Such norms and patterns set guidelines for the types of work behaviors that will enable employees to succeed within a particular firm. Examples include following organizational norms for working overtime, expressing dissatisfaction with management, and making work the first priority. These factors and the employee's response to them must be assessed if strategies for influencing the health and safety of workers are to be effective.

The epidemiologic model can be used as the basis for planning interventions to restore and promote the health of workers. These efforts are influenced by societal and organizational activities related to occupational health and safety.

ORGANIZATIONAL AND SOCIETAL EFFORTS TO PROMOTE WORKER HEALTH AND SAFETY

Promotion of worker health and safety is the goal of occupational health and safety programs. These programs are offered primarily by the employer at the workplace, but the range of services and the models for delivering them have been changing dramatically over the past few years. In addition to specific services, legislation at the federal and state levels has had a significant impact on efforts to provide a healthy and safe environment for all workers. Although the initial response to this legislation was an increased use of occupational health and safety professionals, the 1980s were a time of decreased enforcement of these laws. This effect, along with economic compression and cost cutting, resulted in "down-sizing": occupational health and safety services decreased in scope in some firms and were provided by paraprofessionals such as medical technicians, licensed practical nurses, or first aiders employed as production workers in the company. Under new administration of the Occupational Safety and Health Act, and increased public concern about worker health and safety, there have recently been citations of companies that do not meet minimal occupational health and safety standards. Criminal charges have been filed against business owners when preventable work-related deaths occurred. These events have redirected an emphasis on preventive occupational health and safety programming.

Unless a company has OSHA-regulated exposures, business firms are not required to provide occupational health and safety services that meet any specified standards. With few exceptions, there is no legal mandate for specific services or level of personnel provided by employers to protect worker health and safety. Therefore, the range of services offered and the qualifications of the providers of occupational health and safety vary widely across industries. An important stimulus for health and safety programs is cost avoidance that can be attributed to the effectiveness of preventive services.

On-site Occupational Health and Safety Programs

Optimally, on-site occupational health and safety services are provided by a team of occupational health and safety professionals. The core members of this team are the occupational health nurse, occupational physician, industrial hygienist, and safety professional. The largest group of health care professionals in business settings is occupational health nurses; therefore, the most frequently seen model is that of the one—nurse unit or solo practicing occupational health nurse. This nurse collaborates with a community physician who provides consultation and accepts referrals for specific employee medical problems. The collaboration may occur primarily through telephone contact, or the physician may be under contract with the company to spend a certain amount of time on-site each week. As companies

---

SCOPE OF SERVICES PROVIDED THROUGH AN OCCUPATIONAL HEALTH AND SAFETY PROGRAM

Health assessments
  Preplacement
  Periodic: mandatory, voluntary
  Transfer
  Retirement/termination
  Executive
  Health risk appraisal
Preventive health screening with education
Employee assistance programs
Lifestyle classes: smoking cessation, weight control, stress
  management, physical fitness and conditioning
Rehabilitation
Treatment of illness and injury
Primary health care for workers and dependents
Fitting of protective equipment
Worker safety and health education related to occupational
  hazards
Job analysis and design
Prenatal and postnatal care and support groups
Medical self-help and consumerism classes
Safety audits and accident investigation
Plant surveys and environmental monitoring
Workers' compensation and processing of OSHA claims and
  reports
Health-related cost-containment strategies such as medical
  care utilization review, case management, and advice on
  benefit use
Risk management, loss control
Emergency preparedness
Preretirement counseling

FUNCTIONS OF FEDERAL AGENCIES INVOLVED IN OCCUPATIONAL HEALTH AND SAFETY

OSHA

Determine and set standards for hazardous exposures in the
  workplace
Enforce the occupational and health standards (includes the
  right of entry for inspection)
Educate employers about occupational health and safety
Develop and maintain a database of work-related injuries,
  illnesses, and deaths
Monitor compliance with occupational health and safety
  standards

NIOSH

Conduct research and review of research findings to recommend permissible exposure levels for occupational
  hazards to OSHA
Identify and research occupational health and safety hazards
Educate occupational health and safety professionals
Distribute research findings relevant to occupational health
  and safety

---

become larger, they are likely to hire additional nurses, part-time or full-time physicians, safety professionals, and industrial hygienists. An increasingly popular option is to contract some health, safety, and industrial hygiene work to external providers. The largest firms often have corporate occupational health and safety professionals who set policy and participate in company decision making at the corporate level. These professionals work with the nurses employed at the individual sites within the company.

Depending on the needs of the company and the workers, additional professionals may be on the occupational health and safety team. These may include employee assistance counselors or social workers, health educators, physical fitness specialists, toxicologists, and human factors engineers (ergonomists). The personnel and services in an organization's occupational health and safety program differ across companies and result from decisions made by management.

The services provided by on-site occupational health programs range from those focused only on work-related health and safety problems to a wide scope of services that includes primary health care (see box). In industries that have exposures regulated by law, certain programs are mandated. The ability of a company to offer additional programs depends on management's attitudes and understanding about health and safety, acceptance by the workers, and the eco-

nomic status of the firm. A significant increase in the number of health promotion and employee assistance programs offered in industry has occurred over the past few years. Health promotion programs focus on lifestyle habits that pose risks to health (e.g., obesity, smoking, stress responses, and lack of exercise). Employee assistance programs are designed to address personal problems (e.g., marital discord, substance abuse, and financial difficulties) that affect the employee's productivity. Since such efforts are cost-effective for businesses, they should continue to increase (Girdano, 1986).

A similar array of occupational health and safety programs is available on a contractual basis from community-based providers. These may be offered by free-standing industrial clinics, health maintenance organizations, hospitals, emergency clinics, and other health care organizations. In addition, consultants in each discipline work in the private sector (self-employed, in group practice, or in insurance companies) and in the public sector (in local and state health departments or departments of labor and industry). These services may be brought on-site, delivered elsewhere in the community, or offered through a mobile van that visits companies. These multiple resources have increased the options for companies that need occupational health and safety services and have also broadened the employment opportunities for health and safety professionals.

Legislation

The occupational health and safety services provided by an employer are influenced by specific legislation at federal and state levels. Although the relationship between work and health has been known since the second century (Ramazzini, 1713), public policy that effectively controlled occupational hazards was not enacted until the 1960s. The Mine Safety and Health Act of 1968 was the first legislation that specifically mandated certain preventive programs for workers. This was followed by the Occupational Safety and Health Act of 1970. The Occupational Safety and Health Act established two agencies to carry out the act's purpose of ensuring "safe and healthful working conditions for working men and women" (Public Law 91-596, 1970). The functions of these agencies are described in the box.

The Occupational Safety and Health Administration (OSHA) is a federal agency within the U.S. Department of Labor. The other agency, the National Institute for Occupational Safety and Health (NIOSH), is part of the Centers for Disease Control, which is within the U.S. Public Health Service. The standards that regulate workers' exposure to potentially toxic substances are OSHA standards and regulations that OSHA enforces at the federal, regional, and state levels. Specific standards and information about compliance can be obtained from federal, regional, and state OSHA offices. NIOSH maintains a computerized database that can be accessed for the most recent international research and recommendations for occupational hazards.

One of the most far-reaching OSHA standards is the *Hazard Communication Standard*. Also known as the federal *"right-to-know"* law, this standard is based on the premise that working environments cannot eliminate **all** potentially toxic agents; therefore, an important line of defense is an educated work force. The Hazard Communication Standard, which took effect in May 1986, required that all manufacturing firms inventory their toxic agents, label them, and develop information sheets, called *Material Safety Data Sheets* (MSDSs), for each agent. In addition, the employer must have in place a Hazard Communication Program that provides workers with education about these agents. This education must include identification, toxic effects, and protective measures. In 1988, this standard was extended to all employers covered by the Occupational Safety and Health Act. Noncompliance with the standard has been one of the most frequently cited OSHA violations. Similar right-to-know legislation exists at many state and local levels. The next legislative approach will focus on the right to act: standards and guidelines that protect workers' rights to use the information from right-to-know efforts to change unsafe or unhealthy working conditions.

In addition to standards, which are prescriptive laws, OSHA recently has been publishing non-binding *guidelines* that may be used by OSHA compliance officers to determine conformity with general health and safety recommendations. An example is the "Guidelines for Worker Protection Against Hepatitis, AIDS, and Other Bloodborne Diseases," which requires specific employer and employee actions to safeguard employees in human services jobs.

Workers' compensation acts are important state laws that govern financial compensation of employees who suffer work-related health problems. These acts vary by state; each sets rules for the reimbursement of employees with occupational health problems for medical expenses and lost work time associated with the illness or injury. Workers' Compensation also pays death benefits. The increased costs and frequency of workers' compensation claims and the experience-based insurance premiums paid by industry have been important motivations for increasing the health and safety of the workplace.

DISASTER PLANNING AND MANAGEMENT

Although disaster planning and management have been functions of occupational health and safety programs (Lee, 1978), this is an area of new legislation that affects businesses and health professionals. The legislation of the Superfund Amendment and Reauthorization Act (SARA) requires written disaster plans shared with key resources in the community, such as fire departments and emergency rooms (McCunney, 1988). Public concern about disasters such as the methyl isocyanate leak in Bhopal, India or the community exposure to chemicals at Times Beach, Missouri has mandated more attention to disaster planning.

The goals of a disaster plan are to prevent or minimize injuries and deaths of workers and residents, minimize property damage, effectively triage, and facilitate the resumption of necessary business activities. A disaster plan requires the cooperation of different personnel within the company and community. The nurse is often a key person on the disaster planning team, along with safety professionals, physicians, industrial hygienists, the fire chief, and company management. The potential for disaster (e.g., explosions, fires, and leaks) must be identified, and this is best achieved by completing an exhaustive chemical and hazard inventory of the workplace. The material safety data sheets and plant blueprint are critical for correctly identifying substances and work areas that may be hazardous. Workplace surveys are the first step to completing this inventory.

Effective disaster plans are designed by those with knowledge of the work processes and materials, the workers and workplace, and the resources in the community. Specific steps must be detailed for actions to be put in place by specific individuals in the event of a disaster. The written plan must be shared with all who will be involved in its execution. Employees should be prepared in first aid, CPR, and fire brigade procedures. Plans must be clear, specific, and comprehensive (i.e., covering all shifts and all work areas). Plans must include activities to be conducted within the worksite and those that require community resources. Transportation plans, fire response, and emergency services response should be coordinated with the agencies that would be involved in an actual disaster. The disaster plan, emergency and safety equipment, and the first response team's capabilities should be tested annually with a drill. Practice results should be carefully evaluated with changes incorporated as needed.

Hospital and other emergency services, such as the fire department, should be involved in developing the disaster plan and should receive a copy of the disaster plan and a current hazard inventory. It is imperative that the disaster plan and hazard inventory are periodically updated. The occupational health nurse or another company representative should provide emergency health care providers with updated clinical information on exposures and appropriate treatment. It should never be assumed that local services will have current information on substances used in industry. Representatives of these agencies should visit the worksite and accompany the nurse on a worksite walk-through so that they are familiar with the operations.

In disaster planning, the nurse is often assigned or assumes the responsibility for coordinating the planning and implementation efforts. The nurse works with appropriate key people within the company and in the community to develop a workable, comprehensive plan. Other tasks include providing ongoing communication to keep the plan current; planning the drills; educating the employees, management, and community providers; and assessing the equipment and services that may be used in a disaster.

In the event of a disaster, the nurse should play a key role in coordinating the response. Principles of triage may be employed as the response team determines the extent of the disaster and the ability of the company and community to respond. Postdisaster nursing interventions are also critical. Examples include identification of ongoing disaster-related health needs of workers and community residents, collection of epidemiological data, and assessment of the cause and the necessary steps to prevent a recurrence.

NURSING INTERVENTIONS WITH WORKING POPULATIONS

The nurse is often the first health care provider seen by an individual with a work-related health problem. Consequently, nurses are in key positions to intervene with working populations at all three levels of prevention.

Assessment of Individuals and Families

The initial step of assessment involves the traditional history and physical assessment, emphasizing exposure to occupational hazards and individual characteristics that may predispose the client to increased health risk at certain jobs.

The occupational health history is an indispensable component of the health assessment of individuals. Since work is a part of life for most people, incorporating an occupational health history into all routine nursing assessments is important. Many workers in the United States do not have access to health care services in their workplaces. Yet it is not unusual to encounter health care providers in the community who have little or no knowledge about workplaces or expertise in occupationally related illnesses and injuries. Because of the large number of small businesses that do not have the resources for maintaining on-site health care, injured and ill workers are seen first in the public and private health care sector: in clinics, emergency rooms, physicians' offices, hospitals, HMOs, and ambulatory care centers. Nurses are often the first-line assessors of these individuals and perhaps the only contact for education about self-protection from workplace hazards. The identification of workplace exposures as sources of adverse health effects may influence the client's course of illness and rehabilitation and also prevent similar illnesses among others with potential for exposure.

Incorporating occupational health data into client assessments begins with recognizing the possible relationship between health and occupational factors. The next step is to integrate into the history-taking procedure some routine assessment questions that will provide the data necessary to confirm or rule out occupationally induced symptoms. Symptoms of hazardous workplace exposures may be indicated by vague complaints involving any bodily system and often mimicking common medical problems. Goldman and Peters (1982) suggest three points that occupational

health histories should include: a list of current and past jobs the client has held; questions about exposures to specific agents and relationships between the symptoms and activities at work, job titles, or history of exposures; and other factors that may enhance the client's susceptibility to occupational agents (e.g., smoking history, underlying illness, previous injury, or handicapping condition).

Questions about the client's occupational history can be woven into existing assessment tools. The more complete the data collected, the more likely the nurse is to notice the influence of work-health interactions. All clients should be queried about their employment history. To describe only a current status of "retired" or "housewife" may lead to the omission of relevant data. The nurse should be aware that not all workers are well-informed about the materials with which they work or about potential hazards. For this reason the nurse must develop basic knowledge about the types of jobs held by clients and the possible hazards associated with them. Since there is an increased likelihood of multiple exposures from other environments that may interact with workplace exposures, the nurse should extend the questioning to include this information.

Identification of work-related health problems does not require an extensive knowledge of occupational agents and their effects. A systematic approach for evaluating the potential for workplace exposures is the most effective intervention for detection and prevention of occupational health risks. Figure 41-2 shows one short assessment tool that can be incorporated into routine history-taking. Similar questions can be included in the assessment of workers' spouses and dependents, who may receive secondhand or indirect exposure to occupational hazards.

During these health assessments the nurse has the opportunity to teach about workplace hazards and preventive measures the worker can use. At the same time, the nurse is obtaining information that will be valuable in optimizing worker-job fit. Such assessments may be done as preplacement exams before the client begins a job, on a periodic basis during employment, or with the onset of a work-related health problem or exposure. Work-related health assessments can also be conducted when an employee is being transferred to another job with different requirements and exposures, at termination, and at retirement. The goal of these assessments is to identify agent and host factors that could place the employee at risk and to determine preventive steps that can be taken to eliminate or minimize the exposure and potential health effect.

When the health data from such assessments are considered collectively, the nurse may determine some patterns in risk factors associated with the occurrence of work-related injuries and illnesses (Ossler, 1986). For example, a nurse practitioner in a clinic noted a dramatic increase in the number of bladder cancer cases among her clients. When she looked at factors in common among these individuals, she determined that they all worked at a firm that used benzidine dyes, which are known bladder carcinogens. She worked with the union and the company to assess the environmental exposures to the employees. This nursing intervention led to a safer work environment and a subsequent decrease in bladder cancer among this population group.

I. Present Job
    A. What do you do for a living? _____
    B. How long have you had this job? _____
    C. Describe the specific tasks this job involves: _____
        _____

    D. What product or service is produced by the company where you work?

    E. Are you exposed to any of the following on your present job?
        Chemicals   Vapors. gases   Radiation
        Loud noise   Vibration   Extreme heat or cold
        Infectious   Dusts   Stress
            agent   Others:

    F. Do you feel you have any health problems related to your work?

        If yes, describe:

    G. How would you describe your satisfaction with your job?
        Very satisfied   Satisfied   Somewhat satisfied
        Dissatisfied   Very dissatisfied

    H. Have there been any recent changes in your job or the hours you work?

        Comments:

    I. Do you use protective clothing and/or equipment on your job?

        If yes, describe:

    J. Have any of your co-workers been complaining of illnesses or injuries that they associate with their jobs?

        If yes, describe:

II. All Past Work
     Starting with your first job, please provide the following information:

Job Title	Years Held from to	Description of work	Exposures	Injuries/ Illnesses

III. Other Exposures
      A. Do you have any hobbies which involve exposure to chemicals, metals or any of the other agents mentioned before? If yes, describe:

      B. Are any other members of your household exposed to any of the substances listed above? If yes, describe:

      C. Do you live near any factories, dump sites, or other sources of pollution? If yes, describe:

FIGURE 41-2

Occupational health history.

Name of company _____ Date _____

   Address _____

                _____

Parent company (if any) _____

   Location of corporate offices _____

SIC code _____ Major products _____

Major processes and operations:

Raw materials used/created:

Potential health hazards:

Organizational chart that includes the occupational health professionals:

Employees

   Total number: _____ Number in production: _____ Others: _____

   % Fulltime _____ % Men _____ % Women _____

   First shift _____ Second shift _____ Third shift _____

   Age distribution _____

   % Unionized _____ Names of unions _____

Health Data

   Work related illnesses, injuries, deaths per annum: _____

   OSHA recordable _____ Workers' Compensation _____

      Other _____ Most frequent complaints: _____

   Average number of monthly calls to the health unit: _____

   Absenteeism rate: _____

Description of health and safety services:

   Providers:

   Examinations offered:

   Employee assistance programs:

   Treatment if illness/injury:

   Health education: Preventive screening:

   Physical fitness, health promotion activities:

   Mandatory programs:

   Health and safety committee;

   Safety audits:

   Environmental monitoring:

Comments:

FIGURE 41-3

Guide for worksite survey.

Such an approach can be used at the company, industry, and community levels; the initial collection of data and the questioning about workplace exposures are vital steps for any intervention.

Assessment of the Workplace

The nurse may conduct a similar assessment of the workplace itself. The purpose of this assessment, known as a *worksite survey* or *walk-through*, is to become knowledgeable about the work processes and materials, the requirements of various jobs, the presence of actual or potential hazards, and the work practices of employees (AAOHN, 1988). Figure 41-3 shows a brief outline that can be used to guide a walk-through. More complex surveys are performed by industrial hygienists and safety professionals when the purpose of the walk-through is environmental monitoring or a safety audit (Lee, 1983). Some occupational health nurses have developed expertise in these areas and include such tasks as part of their functions. For any health care provider who assesses workers, this information makes up an important data base. For the on-site health care provider, worksite walk-throughs assist the professional in establishing rapport with and credibility among the employees.

A worksite survey begins with an understanding of the type of work that occurs in the workplace. All business organizations are classified by the U.S. Department of Commerce with a numerical code, the Standard Industrial Classification (SIC) Code. This code, usually a two- to four-digit number, indicates a firm's product and therefore the possible types of occupational health hazards that may be associated with the processes and materials used by its employees. SIC codes are used to collect and report data on businesses. For example, illness and injury rates of one company are compared to the rates of other companies of similar size with the same SIC code to determine whether the company is experiencing an excess of illness or injury. All OSHA and workers' compensation data are reported by SIC code. In addition, by knowing the SIC code of a company, a health care professional can access reference books that describe the usual processes, materials, and by-products of that kind of firm. A simple drawing of the work processes and work areas categorizes information by jobs or locations in the workplace. These preliminary data provide clues about what hazards may be present and an understanding of the types of jobs and health requirements that may be

involved in a particular industry.

Characteristics of the employee group comprise the second area of important information. The nature, availability, and utilization of health and safety services are also assessed. The structure of the organization, the chain of command for occupational health professionals, and the incidence rates for work-related illnesses and injuries complete the survey data. The more information that can be collected before the walk-through, the more efficient will be the process of the survey. After the survey is conducted, the nurse can use this information with the aggregate health data to evaluate the effectiveness of the occupational health and safety program and to plan future programs.

CLINICAL APPLICATION: INTERACTIONS OF THE HOST, AGENT, AND ENVIRONMENT IN THE WORKPLACE

An example of how the epidemiological model can be used to assess clients and plan nursing care illustrates the usefulness of approaching occupational health problems with an epidemiological perspective. An insurance company recently renovated their claims-processing office area. All typewriters were replaced with video display terminals (VDTs) and associated hardware for handling all future work by computer. The company's occupational health nurse noticed an increase in visits to the health unit for complaints of headache, stiff neck muscles, and visual disturbances. These health problems have been associated with VDT operation (McKay-Rossignol, 1987). To conduct a complete investigation of this problem, the nurse assessed the workers, the new agent (the VDTs), previously existing potential agents, and the work environment (Ossler, 1985). Table 41-2 depicts the factors that the nurse assessed for each of these areas. By collecting data for each of the three elements of the epidemiological triad, the nurse could respond most effectively to the aggregate health problem suggested by the increased use of the health unit.

This information led to the conclusions that certain workers may be at increased risk of adverse responses to this new agent; workstation design contributes to these unhealthy responses; and the work environment influences the host-agent interaction. Interventions should always focus on designing the health hazard out of the work, if possible; for example, with hazardous chemicals the strategy may include substituting a safer chemical, isolating the chemical in the work process, or isolating the worker from the chemical. In the present example, the first level of intervention was

---

TABLE 41-2
Areas to be assessed in applying the epidemiological model to the use of VDTs in an office setting

Host: workers	Agent: VDTs	Work environment: office
Previous musculoskeletal injury	Height of work station	Pacing of work
Age	Adjustable keyboard	Worker control of work
Other use of VDT outside of employment	Lighting	Noise, other distractions
Underlying chronic illness	Wrist supports	Employee-supervisor relationships
Eyeglasses or other sign of visual impairment	Tiltable screen	Policies about rest breaks
Work habits	Chair with lumbar support and stability	Adequate space for rest breaks
	CRT shield	

design of the workstation, the component used by the VDT operators in doing their work. Minimizing the possible hazards of the agent involved recommendations for desk, chair, and lighting design that would accommodate the individual worker and allow shielding of the VDT (Grandjean, 1987). The nurse's recommendations about designing these components to minimize strain on the worker's comfort and health were based on principles of ergonomics—the study of adapting work and workplaces to fit humans.

The nursing interventions could include strengthening the resistance of the host by prescribing appropriate rest breaks, eye exercises, and relaxation strategies. Recognizing that previous cervical neck injury or impaired vision may increase the risk of adverse effects from VDT work, the nurse would include assessment for these factors in employees' preplacement and periodic health examinations.

For the environmental concerns, the nurse could educate the manager about the health risks of paced, externally controlled work expectations and recommend alternatives. Such an approach is likely to address most factors involved in this example of work-related illness and to result in interventions that are effective in promoting worker health and safety while increasing the productivity and morale of the work group.

SUMMARY

Although nurses can specialize in occupational health nursing, the principles of occupational health and safety are important to the practice of all nurses. Multiple risks to workers' health and safety in workplace settings include biological, chemical, ergonomic, physical, and psychosocial agents. Basic nursing education prepares generalists who are capable of providing nursing care to individuals, families, and groups across the lifespan and along the health-illness continuum. This includes all workers, their families, and those who live in industrial areas. Incorporation of work-related exposures and health risks is a critical part of any nursing assessment. The preventive interventions for clients with workplace health and safety risks are often in the realm of nurses in occupational and other settings.

This chapter has introduced the epidemiological approach to assessing and intervening with occupational health and safety problems. The key to minimizing or eliminating many of these hazards lies in the identification of the potential or actual exposures and effective education about protective measures. Two tools to assist in meeting this goal were described: the occupational health history and the worksite survey. The nurse's role in this preventive approach is to incorporate occupational health data into each client assessment and to use this information to identify workplace exposures and to implement appropriate worker education.

The bibliography includes basic texts for health care providers who wish to increase their familiarity with occupational hazards and their effects on health. Appendix H2 provides information for contacting agencies involved in worker health and safety protection.

KEY CONCEPTS

The health impact of work is an important aspect for most clients for whom the community health nurse provides care.

Two major changes in the working population are the increasing number of women and older individuals in the workplace.

Host factors known to be associated with increased risk of adverse response to exposures in the workplace are age, gender, underlying chronic illness, work practices, immunological status, ethnicity, and lifestyle.

Work-related hazards, or agents, are classified as biological, chemical, ergonomic, physical, and psychosocial.

Promotion of worker health and safety is the goal of occupational health and safety programs. Effective programs are proactive. The work should be redesigned to eliminate or minimize health hazards. Using personal protective equipment is an important strategy, but it should not substitute for redesigning.

Services provided by on-site occupational health programs range from those focused only on work-related health and safety problems to a wide scope of services that may include primary care.

The ability of a company to offer health and safety programs depends on the management's attitudes and understanding about health and safety, acceptance of the program by workers, and the economic status of the company.

Although the relationship between work and health has been known since the second century, public policy that effectively controlled occupational health hazards was not enacted in the United States until the 1960s.

Nurses are often the first health care providers seen by individuals with work-related health problems. Consequently, nurses are in key positions to intervene with working populations at all three levels of prevention.

The occupational health history is an indispensable component of the health assessment of individuals, and it should include all prior potential occupational health exposures.

A worksite survey, or walk-through, is important in assessing the workplace for actual and potential hazards. It enables the nurse to gain knowledge of the requirements of various jobs, the presence of actual or potential hazards, and work practices of employees.

KEY CONCEPTS

The primary focus of occupational health nurses' practice is the health and safety of workers, with an emphasis on the prevention of illness and injury.

As American industry has shifted from agrarian to industrial to highly technological processes, the occupational health nurse's role has evolved and expanded.

Although nurses can specialize and become certified in occupational health, the principles of occupational health and safety are important to the practice of all nurses.

LEARNING ACTIVITIES

1. Visit a worksite and describe the workers. What are their ages? What percentage are women? What type of work are the employees doing? Can you detect anything about the workers' or management's attitudes about health and safety? Ask to see a Material Safety Data Sheet and the company's disaster plan.

2. After your worksite visit, describe at least two real or potential occupational health hazards that you observed.

3. Describe at least one preventive strategy that could be used or that you observed being used for each hazard.

4. Select an individual with an injury or illness that could be work-related and ask to trace the work history. Look for risk factors that may have precipitated these symptoms or health problems.

5. Interview a worker to evaluate the psychosocial environment of the work setting. Identify hazards and possible interventions. Ask what the worker has done to minimize work stress.

6. Review your own work history and identify the potential hazards to which you have been exposed. What controls existed or could have been put in place?

7. Complete a thorough assessment of a workplace and develop a model occupational health and safety plan. Include hazards, goals, resources, and deficits.

8. Identify at least one community resource for workers and employers that provides occupational health and safety-related services. What programs are available? How are they accessed? How can potential users contact them most effectively?

BIBLIOGRAPHY

Alderson M: Occupational cancer, London, 1986, Butterworths.

American Association of Occupational Health Nurses: A comprehensive guide for establishing an occupational health service, Atlanta, 1988, AAOHN.

American Nurses Association: Division of Governmental Affairs, Capital Update 9(6):1, March 29, 1991.

Babbitz MA: The practice of occupational health nursing in the United States, Occupational Health Nursing 31(6):23-25, 1984.

Baker DB: The study of stress at work, Annu Rev Public Health 6:367, 1985.

Bellingham R and Cohen B editors: The corporate wellness sourcebook, Amherst, Mass, 1987, Human Resource Development Press.

Bezold C, Carlson RJ, and Peck JC: The future of work and health, Dover, Mass, 1986, Auburn.

Bureau of Labor Statistics: Handbook of labor statistics, Washington, DC, 1984, US Department of Labor.

Bureau of Labor Statistics: Handbook of labor statistics, Washington, DC, 1989, US Department of Labor.

Centers for Disease Control: Legionnaire's disease, Morbidity and Mortality Weekly Report 26:439-441, 1978.

Cheremisinoff PN: Management of hazardous occupational environments, Lancaster, PA, 1984, Technomic Publishing.

Cooper CL and Payne R, editors: Stress at work, New York, 1978, John Wiley & Sons.

Cooper CL and Payne R editors: Current concerns in occupational stress, New York, 1980, Wiley.

Cox AR: Profile of the occupational health nurse, Occupational Health Nursing 33(12):591-593, 1988.

Cralley LJ and Cralley LV: Patty's industrial hygiene and toxicology, New York, 1985, John Wiley & Sons, Inc.

Deal TE and Kennedy AA: Corporate cultures: The rites and rituals of corporate life, Reading, Mass, 1982, Addison-Wesley.

Dyal LE: Plant profile: A contemporary interpretation of the nursing process, Occupational Health Nursing 29(3):17-21, 1982.

Girdano DA: Occupational health promotion: a practical guide to program development, New York, 1986, MacMillan.

Goldman R and Peters JW: The occupational and environmental health history, JAMA 246:2831-2836, 1982.

Grandjean E: Ergonomics in computerized offices, London, 1987, Taylor & Francis.

Haynes S and Feinleib M: Women, work, and coronary heart disease, Am J Public Health 70(2):133-141, 1980.

Huff JE, McConnell EE, Haseman JK: On the proportion of positive results in carcinogenicity studies in animals, Environ Mutagen 7:427-428, 1985.

Isernhagen SI: Work injury prevention and management, Rockville, Md, 1988, Aspen.

Jacobs K and Ogden-Niemeyer L: Work-hardening: state of the art, Thorofare, NJ, 1985, Slack.

Karvonen M and Mikheev MI, editors: Epidemiology of occupational health, Geneva, 1986, World Health Organization Publication No 20.

Key MM: Occupational diseases—a guide to their recognition, Cincinnati, 1977, National Institute for Occupational Safety and Health.

Klarreich SH: Health and fitness in the workplace, New York, 1987, Praeger.

Klaassen CD, Amdur MO, and Doull J: Casarett and Doull's toxicology, New York, 1986, MacMillan.

Kustnetz A and Hutchison M: A guide to the work-relatedness of disease, Cincinnati, 1979, National Institute for Occupational Safety and Health.

LaDou J, editor: Occupational medicine, Norwalk, Conn, 1990, Appleton & Lange.

Lee JA: New nurse in industry, Cincinnati, 1978, Washington, DC, USDHEW, NIOSH, Pub. No. 78-143, US Government Printing Office.

Lee JS: Environmental evaluation of the work place, Family and Community Health, 16-23, 1983.

Levy BS and Wegman DH: Occupational health: recognizing and preventing occupational disease, Boston, 1988, Little, Brown & Co, Inc.

Matheson LN: Work capacity evaluation, Anaheim, Calif, 1986, Employment and Rehabilitation Institute of California.

Mattison DR: Reproductive toxicology, New York, 1983, Alan R. Liss.

McCunney R: Handbook of occupational medicine, Boston, 1988, Little, Brown & Co, Inc.

McKay-Rossignol A, Morse E, Summers V, and Pagnotto L: Video display terminal use: reported health symptoms among Massachusetts workers, J Occup Med 29(2):112-118, 1987.

National Safety Council: National Safety News, July, 1984.

National Safety Council: Accident facts, Chicago, 1989.

Office of Technology Assessment, U.S. Congress: Preventing illness and injury in the workplace, Pub No OTA-H-256, Washington, DC, 1985, US Government Printing Office.

Ossler CC: Work environments and men's health risks, Nurs Clin North Am 21(1):25-36, 1986.

Ossler CC: Distributive nursing practice in occupational health and safety. In JE Hall and BR Weaver, editors: Distributive nursing practice: a systems approach to community health, ed 2, pp. 483-505, Philadelphia, 1985, JB Lippincott.

Poore M: Older workers, Occup Health Saf 55(8):12-15, 1986.

Proctor NH, Hughes JP, and Fischman ML: Chemical hazards of the workplace, ed 2, Philadelphia, 1988, JB Lippincott.

Putz-Anderson V: Cumulative trauma disorders: a manual for musculoskeletal diseases of the upper limbs, London, 1988, Taylor & Francis.

Ramazzini B: Diseases of workers. Translated by Wright WC. From DeMorbis Artificum. Diatriba, 1713. New York, 1964, Hafner.

ReVelle P and ReVelle C: The environment: issues and choices for society, New York, 1981, D Van Nostrand.

Rix S: The American woman, 1988-1989, New York, 1988, WW Norton.

Rom WN: Occupational and environmental medicine, Boston, 1983, Little, Brown & Co, Inc.

Rosenstock L and Cullen M: Clinical occupational medicine, Philadelphia, 1986, Saunders.

Sax NI: Dangerous properties of industrial materials, ed 5, New York, 1986, Van Nostrand.

Schwartz RM: Injured on the job, Boston, 1979, Mass Coalition for Occupational Safety and Health.

Stellman JM and Daum SM: Work is dangerous to your health, New York, 1973, Random House.

US Department of Health and Human Services: Unpublished data from the national sample survey of registered nurses, Rockville, Md, Bureau of Health Professions, 1988.

US Department of Labor, Bureau of Labor Statistics: Handbook of labor statistics, Washington, DC, 1989, US Government Printing Office.

US Department of Labor, Bureau of Labor Statistics: Occupational injuries and illnesses in the United States by industry, Washington, DC, 1988, US DoL.

Wicker AW: An introduction to ecological psychology, Belmont, CA, 1979, Wadsworth.

Williams PL and Burson JL editors: Industrial toxicology: Safety and health implications in the workplace, New York, 1985, Van Nostrand Reinhold.

Zenz C: Occupational medicine: Principles and practical applications, ed 2, Chicago, 1988, Year Book Medical Publishers.

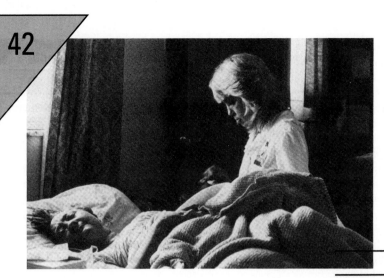

42

The Community Health Nurse In Home Health and Hospice Care

Mary N. Albrecht

OBJECTIVES

After reading this chapter, the student should be able to:

Review the history of home health care nursing.
Formulate a definition of home health care.
Discuss the importance of contracting.
Describe the roles of the various disciplines involved in providing home health care.
Discuss the impact of high-technology on the client and family in the home.
Discuss the impact of chronic illness on the client and family in the home.
Describe payment mechanisms for home health care.
Describe ways to measure quality of care in home health care agencies.
Discuss a nursing model for home health care.
Apply concepts from the nursing model to a clinical situation in the home.

KEY TERMS

ANA standards	high technology	NLN standards
benefits of home care	model for home care	payment
chronic illness	nursing role	quality of care
discharge		

Note: Excerpts from this chapter may reflect contributions by Eileen Wiles and Jacqueline Logue from the second edition of this text.

T his chapter deals with community health nurses' roles in home health care. The history of home health care and definitions related to home care are discussed. The focus is on care of clients and families with chronic illnesses, as well as those with high-technology needs.

The purpose of this chapter is to present client and family concerns in the home and assessment and intervention strategies. A nursing model to facilitate assessment, planning, and interventions for clients with various needs in the home setting is included.

HISTORY OF HOME HEALTH CARE

Home health care began in the United States around the 1800s. The Boston Dispensary served as one of the initial providers of home care, dating back to 1796. During this era, few hospitals were available, and people did not always go to the hospital when they became ill.

Public health nursing began in the United States when philanthropic organizations sponsored visiting nurses, who gave care to individuals in their homes and taught families how to take care of the sick. In 1877 the New York City Mission and the New York Society for Ethical Culture began to use visiting nurses. The idea grew slowly, with nurses being paid by clients or by philanthropic societies. Eventually the community became more involved and developed projects and funds to support the cause of home care. In 1890 there were 21 visiting nurses associations in the United States, most of them employing only one nurse. After 1894, the use of visiting nurses grew more rapidly.

In 1842 a nurse society was established in Philadelphia to supply nurses to the independent sick and to those individuals who could pay. American communities established similar organizations primarily because visiting nursing in England had developed into a viable social service. The Waltham (Massachusetts) Training School was established in 1885 by Dr. Alfred Worcester after he conferred with Florence Nightingale and designed a course to train nurses for private duty. The course included experience in the home. Later, public health nursing with field experience was added to the program. The school was criticized for sending students into homes to earn money for the hospital and for overworking and not supervising the students (Dolan, 1958).

In the 1940s, hospitals began to take a more serious interest in home care because of the increased number of chronically ill clients being hospitalized. The Montefiore Hospital Home Care Program in New York began in 1947 and offered comprehensive home care services such as medical nursing and social services. Before enactment of Medicare in 1966, most agencies relied on charity and public contributions for survival.

Home care reached a turning point with the arrival of Medicare, which regulated reimbursement mechanisms for home care practice. In 1967, one year after Medicare was enacted, there were 1753 Medicare-participating home health agencies in the United States. The majority of these were visiting nursing associations or programs in public health departments. By 1974, there were 2237 home health agencies, an increase of about 48% (Callender and Lavor, 1975). The Health Care Financing Agency (HCFA) reported 5949 Medicare-certified home health agencies as of October 1986, a 62% growth in 11 years (NAHC Report, 1986). This dramatic growth was due largely to the implementation of diagnostic-related groups (DRGs), which resulted in earlier discharge from hospitals and an increased demand for home care.

As the end of the 20th century approaches, the United States is experiencing a great increase in the elderly population. Many of these elderly people will be living at home, suffering chronic health problems, and requiring intermittent home health care services. To meet this growing need, the number of types of home health agencies has increased rapidly (Green, 1989). The nature of home health care can be more fully understood by reviewing the definitions of home health care.

DEFINITION OF HOME HEALTH CARE

Home health care cannot be defined simply as "care at home." It includes an arrangement of health-related services provided to people in their place of residence. A more comprehensive definition of home health care was prepared by a Department of Health and Human Services interdepartmental work group (Warhola, 1980).

> *Home health care* is that component of a continuum of comprehensive health care whereby health services are provided to individuals and families in their places of residence for the purpose of promoting, maintaining or restoring health, or of maximizing the level of independence, while minimizing illness. Services appropriate to the needs of the individual patient and family are planned, coordinated, and made available by providers organized for the delivery of home care through the use of employed staff, contractual arrangements, or a combination of the two patterns.

Another definition, prepared by the American Medical Association (1979), described home health care as follows:

> The provision of nursing care, social work, therapies (such as diet, occupational, physical, psychological, and speech), vocational and social services, and homemaker-home health aide services may be included as basic components of home health care. The provision of these needed services to the patient at home constitutes a logical extension of the physician's therapeutic responsibility. At the physician's request and under his medical direction, personnel who provide these home health care services operate as a team in assessing and developing the home care plan.

Home health care, as defined by Medicare, includes the following items and services (HCSA, 1989):
1. Part-time or intermittent nursing care provided by or under the supervision of a registered professional nurse.
2. Physical, occupational, or speech therapy.
3. Medical social services under the direction of a physician.
4. Part-time or intermittent services of a home health aide as permitted by the regulations.
5. Medical supplies (other than drugs and biological materials such as serum and vaccinations) and the use of medical applications.
6. Medical services provided by an intern or resident enrolled in a teaching program in hospitals affiliated or under contract with a home health agency.

CONCEPTS AND DEFINITIONS OF HOME HEALTH CARE

Client: rational, biologic, emotional, social being desiring the use of home care services

Family, loved one(s): any other individuals present in the home and willing to participate in care as needed by the client to maintain self-care at home.

Provider agency: any official, voluntary, private, hospital-based, nonprofit, or proprietary agency providing health care services at home

Professional nurse: individual with license to practice professional nursing in state

Health team: members coordinated by the professional nurse; any LPN, ADN, or professional in speech, social work home health aide, physical therapy, occupational therapy, nutrition, dental hygiene, and respiratory therapy; physician; durable medical equipment; home meals, homemaker, transportation, or volunteers available to provide care or service at home

Client classification: complexity or difficulty of nursing care required

Costs: charges or fees per visit or for agency operation

Demand: number of client or families requesting home care services

Availability: number of home care agencies available for client/family use, or availability of health team and nurse to accept new cases

Productivity: number of clients nurses can visit in one day or number staff can visit in a month or year

Accountability: health teams and nurse responsibility for actions, agency to standards, and consumer to participation in care

Accessibility: ease at which one can enter home health care system

Efficiency: high ratio of output to input in system, minimum wasted effort

Type of care: focus and intensity of care given by nurse/others in the home

Coordination of care: case management by professional nurse for continuity and comprehensive services in the home according to professional, agency, and federal guidelines, and use of other community resources

Intervention: actions taken by professional nurse, health team members, client, or family to promote or enhance self-care capabilities

Satisfaction: verbal or written expression of positive statements toward care given and/or received

Quality of care: care meets ANA standards for home health care practice/certification/NLN accreditation standards

Cost effective: costs of delivering a set of services while maintaining ANA/NLN quality standards

Health status: cured, self-care, self-care with assistance, dependent on others, alternative care (nursing home, hospital, clinic, hospice); deceased

Self-care capability: ability to perform activities of daily living that permit the individual to live independently at home

Modified from Albrecht M: The Albrecht nursing model for home health care: implications for research, practice, and education, Public Health Nurs 7(11), 122, 1990.

Trager (1972) describes *home health care* as ". . . an array of services which may be brought into the home singly or in combination in order to achieve and sustain the optimum state of health, activity, and independence for individuals of all ages who require such services because of acute illness, exacerbations of chronic illness, or long-term permanent limitations due to chronic illness and disability."

The definitions integrate the components of home health care: client, family, health care professionals (multidisciplinary), and goals to assist the client to return to an optimum level of health and independence. The definitions differ because interpretation and actual delivery of home health care can vary according to the client, provider, and reimburser of these services.

Family, which includes any caretaker or significant person who takes the responsibility to assist the client in need of care at home, is an integral part of home health care. Roles of the caretaker include supervising clients by ensuring that their basic needs are being met and providing direct care such as personal hygiene, meal preparation, and medication administration. This person is valuable in providing the needed maintenance care between the skilled visits of the professional provider. The *place of residence* is unique in terms of the location for providing care, depending on what a client calls home.

Client goals are always related to the principles of health promotion, maintenance, and restoration, regardless of the primary health care provider. By maximizing the level of independence, home health care nurses can help clients function at the best possible level for preventing dependency. This assistance can include teaching or linking clients with community services providing limited assistance that enables them to stay at home. Also, preventing complications of chronically ill persons can help to minimize the effects of disability and illness. Many complications of long-term illness that result in disability are preventable with adequate home health care intervention. Terminal illness can be handled at home instead of in the hospital if the client and family accept hospice home care programs. Alleviating pain and suffering is also possible in the home care setting. Pain control using medications is closely supervised by nurses in the home. They assess the client's response to the medication and report these findings to the client's physician, who then modifies the medication as needed.

Services can be tailored to any client need or problem. When a client's level of independence increases, the need for services decreases. The services are coordinated so that quality care and continuity of care are maintained.

The box provides a summary of the concepts and definitions relevant to home health care nursing.

CONTRACTING WITH CLIENTS AND FAMILIES

Contracting is a vital component of all nurse/client relationships. Constantly evolving legislative guidelines, third-party payer dictates, the high risk of liability, and the intense level of nurse autonomy, require that contracting be reviewed in the home care context.

The process of contracting in home care involves not only the client and the nurse but also the family. *Contracting* refers to a working (renegotiable) agreement between the nurse, client, and family. The process of contracting can be reflected in the client's care plan and clinical notes. Contracting allows the client and family to set their own goals and alleviates the problem of nurses who set unrealistic expectations of themselves or of the client and family.

Contracting is directly related to use of the nursing process and can be done at each phase of the nursing process. For example, during an initial home visit, nurses gather data for establishing the client-home health care nurse-family contract. They determine the components of the agreement and plan for subsequent actions by establishing the contract with the client and family. During that visit, if appropriate, portions of the contract may be implemented. If not, subsequent visits will afford the opportunities.

Contracts can be formal (written) or informal (verbal), depending on the client's needs. In either case, the process is recorded in the client's chart. The most important aspect is not the type of contract, but the client's actual participation in establishing, implementing, and evaluating the process.

The home care nurse must establish both short-term and long-term goals with the client and family. The purpose of this is not only for continuity of care but also for evaluating the client's condition and progress toward an optimum level of self-care. In a study of community health nurses who made home visits, half of the purposes of the visit went unknown to the clients. This was because nurses in the study did not share the purposes for the visits with them. Much of the dialogue failed to show any *development* of the interrelationship between the client and the nurse.

NURSING ROLES

The *roles* of clinician, educator, researcher, administrator, and consultant are seen in home health care. They can be demonstrated by the experienced home health care nurse, the nursing supervisor, the director of nursing, or the administrator.

Home health care nurses in a staff position are clinicians because they provide direct nursing care to clients and families. They are educators because they teach clients and families the "how to's" and "why's" of self-care. Formally, they may teach classes to community groups regarding health education topics. The researcher role in home health care has been relatively dormant, even though home health care nurses often provide the data required for clinical or administrative change within their agency of employment. The home health care setting abounds with potential research areas. This role needs to take priority in the future if quality and cost effectiveness are to be maintained. A home health care administrator can be a nurse who has had advanced education with community health experience; requirements are stipulated by both federal and state rules and regulations. Consultants advise and counsel staff and clients.

RESPONSIBILITIES OF OTHER DISCIPLINES

The responsibilities and functions of the disciplines in home health care are dictated by Medicare regulations, professional organizations, and state licensing boards. The home health care providers' roles discussed in the following sections are different from providers' roles in other health care settings. Other professional services can be provided in the home such as podiatry, pharmacology, follow-up nutrition counseling, respiratory therapy, and psychiatric or mental health nursing when indicated. Much of these contributions can be provided on a consultant basis in the form of in-service training or direct referral information.

Physician

Each client in the home care program must be under the current care of a doctor of medicine or osteopathy to certify that the client does have a medical problem. A nurse can make an *assessment* visit without physician approval but must have the physician's certification if a plan of care with follow-up is developed. The physician must *certify* a plan of treatment for the home health agency before care is provided to the client. This plan must be reviewed at least every 60 days to modify or continue the client's plan of care.

The plan of treatment must include the following information: diagnosis, functional limitations, anticipated length of care, type and frequency of services needed (nursing, physical therapy, occupational therapy, speech therapy, home health aide, medical social services) medications, diet activities permitted, medical supplies and appliances. Additionally, the plan of treatment should be reviewed by the physician in collaboration with home care professionals at least every 60 days but more often if the person's condition warrants more frequent assessment and alteration of care. This process is called *recertification*.

Physicians in the community also serve in an advisory capacity to the home health agency by assisting in the development of home care policies and procedures relative to client care. Physician involvement in and acceptance of home health care are to be recognized. In the early 1960s the American Medical Association urged physicians to "participate in organized home health care programs for any patient who can benefit from the program and to promote such programs in their communities." The Physician Guide to Home Health Care (AMA, 1979, pp. 1-3) explains the important role of home health care and the benefits that clients can receive from this service. Examples cited include a more rapid client recovery, improved client emotional well-being, early discharge from the hospital, reduction in readmissions, and a savings over costs of institutional care.

Physical Therapist

Physical therapists are graduates of a baccalaureate or master's level physical therapy program and must be licensed by the state in which they practice. They provide maintenance, preventive, and restorative treatment for clients in the home. Like home health care nurses, a physical therapist also provides direct and indirect care. Direct care activities include strengthening muscles, restoring mobility, controlling spasticity, gait training, and teaching active-passive resistive exercises. The treatment modalities used include therapeutic exercise, massage, transcutaneous electrical nerve stimulation, heat, water, ultraviolet light, ultrasound, postural drainage, and pulmonary exercises. The therapist is also responsible for teaching the client and family the treatment regimen to promote self-care and responsibility. Indirect care activities of the physical therapist include consulting with the staff and contributing to client care conferences by sharing skills and area of expertise.

Physical therapy assistants provide some therapy under the direction of a registered physical therapist. Assistants are high school graduates who have completed an approved assistants' program and have been licensed.

Occupational Therapist

Occupational therapists (OT) help clients achieve their optimum level of functioning by teaching them to develop and maintain the abilities to perform activities of daily living in their home. Occupational therapists focus most of their treatment on the client's upper extremities by assisting to restore muscle strength and mobility for functional skills. Occupational therapists earn baccalaureate degrees. When OT becomes registered by the National Occupational Therapy Association, he or she is subsequently referred to as an OTR.

Direct functions of the OTR include evaluating the client's level of function and ability by testing muscles and joints. The OTR teaches self-care activities, assesses the client's home for safety with possible modifications for removing barriers, and provides adaptive equipment when needed. Indirect care is similar to the other home care professional's roles of serving as a consultant for special client needs regarding self-care activities and adapting the home for the client. Occupational therapy has not been used to its full potential in the home because other health care providers have been unaware of its potential contributions. This discipline is a valuable resource in assisting the client to become independent in self-care, a mutual goal of all home health care professionals.

Certified occupational therapy assistants (COTAs) are high school graduates with an approved continuing education certificate from an occupational therapy program. The COTA works under the supervision of the OTR.

Speech Pathologist

Speech pathologists are therapists who are certified by the American Speech and Hearing Association and are educated at the master's level. Speech pathologists work with people with a communication problem related to speech, language, or hearing. Most clients receive direct care services, such as evaluation of speech and language ability, with specific plans being taught to the client and family for follow-up. The goal of speech therapy is to assist individuals to develop and maintain optimum speech and language ability. Speech pathologists also work with eating and swallowing problems. By serving as a consultant to other home care staff members, the speech pathologist can teach other providers of care and families how to encourage development of the best method of communication for clients.

Social Worker

The social worker in home health care holds a master's degree in social work (MSW) and helps clients and families deal with social, emotional, and environmental factors that affect their well-being. Social workers assist directly in intervening or referring clients to appropriate community resources. Often after an episode in the hospital the clients return home unable to cope with their present state of functioning and need assistance in getting their lives reorganized. Many indirect care duties are performed by the social worker, since consultation and referral constitute the major focus of their practice. Other functions include resource identification and application, crisis intervention, and equipment procurement when payment is a problem.

Social work assistants are prepared at the baccalaureate level and function similar to the social worker, who directly supervises the activities of the assistant.

Homemaker/Home Health Aide

With the advent of Medicare, the *home health aide,* sometimes referred to as the homemaker, became an important member of the home health care team. The home health aide (HHA) is directly supervised by the home health care nurse or physical therapist. The role of the HHA is to help clients reach their level of independence by temporarily assisting with personal hygiene. Additional duties include light housekeeping and other homemaking skills. The HHA must be experienced as an aide and be trained to provide home care services. The HHA implements the plan of care established by the nurse or other professionals to reinforce teaching. The role of the homemaker, as distinct from the HHA, emphasizes housekeeping chores.

INTERDISCIPLINARY APPROACH TO HOME HEALTH CARE

Interdisciplinary collaboration is required in the home health care setting. Its use is mandated for Medicare-certified home care agencies, and it is also inherent in the definition of home health care (Warhola, 1980). Without effective collaboration there would be no continuity of care and the client's and family's understanding of the home care program would be fragmented. Each client has an individualized care plan even though the client may have problems similar to others in a specific disease category classification.

Generally, the collaborative process for home care begins in the hospital. The discharge planner and hospital nurse identify a client's need for home care and then review their observations and plans with the physician for approval and orders. The discharge planner then calls the referral intake coordinator of the home care agency, specifying the services requested by the physician. If persons from several disciplines, such as registered nurses, home health aides, and physical therapists, will be involved, the clinical services director notifies the appropriate persons and monitors the interdisciplinary collaboration. In terms of legal accountability and compliance with federal regulatory mechanisms, the physician must certify the plan of treatment for the client. Yet in most instances, it is the health care professional (nurse or physical therapist) who reevaluates the client's status, reports the finding to the physician, and then with the physician modifies the plan of treatment for the client.

Medicare requires that interdisciplinary services be documented. This requirement allows for accountability for each professional and fosters continuity of care. Documentation in the client's chart reflects interdisciplinary collaboration as evidenced by case conferences and contracts made between the care givers. Documentation is the evidence or means, not the end product of care. Quality assurance mechanisms (chart audits, peer review, etc.) verify the appropriateness and effectiveness of the collaboration.

Successful interdisciplinary functioning depends on numerous factors of knowledge, skills, and attitudes. The most important requirement is that the team members must be competent practitioners in their own field. It is unrealistic to assume that there is a clear-cut way to avoid role stress, ambiguity, or overlapping. Professionals in home care are in a unique setting in which they can truly work together to accomplish the client's care goals. Again, regulations require that appropriate resources are used with documentation of collaboration with other disciplines. Care plans and treatments by each discipline are to be built on by other health care providers involved. As an example, nurses must reinforce the teaching of exercise regimens and gait training by the physical therapist.

HOME CARE AND HIGH TECHNOLOGY

Once viewed as something that could be done only in the hospital, high-technology home care has now become part of community health nursing (Stiller, 1988). Because of diagnostic-related groups (DRGs), hospitals are sending clients home earlier than usual, and many clients need high-technology treatment such as IV therapy, mechanical ventilator therapy, phototherapy, and apnea monitoring.

The exact number of cases of high-technology care provided in the home is unknown, but it is increasing. A study by Andrews and Neilson in the western United States (1988) showed that a total of 2492 children required home technology. The technology involved 1115 apnea monitors, 436 photo-therapy interventions, 372 oxygen therapies, 357 enteral feeding pumps, 186 tracheostomies, 24 IV antibiotic therapies, 17 ventilator therapies, and 10 renal dialyses.

The increased use of high-technology equipment in the home increases the need for home health care nurses. Nurses working in the hospital setting need to provide proper discharge teaching for clients going home with specific high-technology equipment. Nurses and clients must ensure that all information regarding the correct operation of the equipment is understood before discharge. Home health nurses must also be educated. Some professionals suggest training home health nurses for the specific needs of the high-technology equipment; however, organizing a case load, using community resources, understanding reimbursement, and working closely with the family are as important to a client's well-being as starting an IV correctly (Handy, 1988). Administrative issues must also be addressed (Handy, 1988): Who is going to pay for the care and equipment expenses? Will insurance companies pay? If they do, are there specific circumstances involved? Both clinical and administrative aspects need to be considered when providing high-technology home health care.

Discharge to Home

High technology in the home is becoming more popular in the health care field. Before returning home, the client and the family must be thoroughly assessed by the professional health care team. The client and care giver must be capable of and committed to learning and carrying out the prescribed regimen (Loewenhardt, 1987).

Most information and research about high technology in the home involves stress factors in the families and the nurse's role with the family. Assessment of the family and client is the most important factor in determining whether home care is a good possibility. McCarthy (1986) states that family members must be assessed for their desire and readiness. A good way to assess readiness is by having the client take "field trips" home and evaluating the family members' reactions and how they divide the responsibilities of care.

Regardless of a client's age, someone must assume the role as the care giver although some clients may be able to take responsibility for some of their care. Handy (1989) states that today it is becoming almost mandatory for the spouse to assume this responsibility. Wildblood and Strezo (1987) report similar findings. They also state that when infants or young children receive IV therapy, the parents must assume some responsibility for maintaining the infusions and administering medication.

Assessment for discharge from the hospital to the home is an important priority. The decision about discharge may be made by the agency, family, or the client. Certain conditions must be met for a client to be transferred from the hospital setting to the home setting, including whether the client is stable and whether the family unit is able and willing to accept the technology-dependent family member (Handy, 1989; Donar, 1988). McCarthy (1986) states that family members should be assessed for their willingness, and ability to provide care. Once family members feel comfortable about the situation, they can approach the staff for actual discharge.

Education is an important aspect during the discharge process (Donar, 1988; Handy, 1989; Gorski, 1987; Smith and Marien, 1989). The primary responsibility of staff members is to assist family members by reviewing all available alternatives and to support them in making an informed and responsible decision. Rapid decision for discharge is almost impossible. The emotional needs of family members are often overlooked (Handy, 1989). Family members may be more concerned about the equipment and neglect the client's other needs. This may result in anxiety and resentment about the equipment, leading to negative feelings about having a "sick" person at home. When discussing emotional tension and anxiety, home care nurses realize that these are feelings the entire family shares. They may be very capable of handling the equipment, but they may not be coping with the role changes they are experiencing. Smith and Marien (1989) indicate that family coping skills, role disruption, and the client's prognosis will worsen in families that are unable to deal with emotional tension and anxiety. These families suffer from mental or emotional problems, especially fatigue to the care givers.

Siblings of young clients needing high-technology care must also be considered. Donar (1988) reported on siblings who felt that their parents did not love them or rejected them because of the sick child. Donar (1988) discusses cases in which siblings unplug ventilators for attention. They need education and emotional support as much as their parents (Handy, 1989; Donar, 1988).

Benefits of High-Technology Home Care

How beneficial is going home with high-technology equipment? Although high-technology home care is fairly new, it is often the best alternative for clients, especially young children. Home care can offer a safer and more nurturing environment than the hospital. Children at home with high-technology equipment have fewer infections and socialization occurs more rapidly (Handy, 1989; Donar, 1988). There is less chance of nosocomial infection in the home, and being in the home environment allows for normal growth and development for the child and other family members.

A study of children dependent on high technology in the home found that parents had many concerns, especially regarding support from the health care provider. Some providers are located many miles away. The discharge teaching is often forgotten or poorly comprehended by parents. Many parents had problems trouble-shooting alarms on respiratory monitors or monitoring IV or enteral feeding fluid levels. Home care nurses must therefore provide teaching about the equipment, previous discharge instructions, and available community resources. They need to ensure that the client and care givers feel comfortable and experience minimal stress. An example is the case study by Braun (1987). This was an elderly couple where the wife had Chronic Obstructive Pulmonary Disease (COPD) and was on a ventilator for a long time in the hospital. The husband was taught how to care for the equipment and both were taught to suction and bag the tracheostomy. On the day of discharge she could not suction or bag herself without the nurse being present. The husband admitted he did not feel comfortable suctioning his wife since he had performed the procedure only on a model. Discharge was postponed for a week but they stated that it would be impossible to reteach the husband in that short a period of time. On the actual day of discharge the husband still had not performed the procedures on his wife, but she was still discharged. This is a example of what can cause families and care givers to become very stressed and burned out.

Determining the interventions for high-technology home care depends on the type of home situation and necessary equipment. Areas that should be assessed include the following: Is the client in a safe environment? Are family members satisfied with their responsibilities? Is the client receiving proper care in the home? Are the client and family experiencing normal socialization and growth and development?

HOME CARE AND CHRONIC ILLNESS

The elderly make up a large part of society. The number of persons aged 65 and over has increased from 4% of the population in 1900 to 12% in 1985. Since 1960, the population under 65 years of age increased by 24%, the proportion of those over 65 years of age rose 55%, and the proportion of those aged 85 years and older rose 174% (Van Ort and Woodtli, 1989). Thus the elderly constitute the most rapidly growing segment of the United States and need increased attention to their health care needs. Home health care nurses will be providing care to this group in greater frequency than in the past.

Factors to Consider

Some areas to evaluate when providing home care to the elderly are the following: Does the care plan consider the overall satisfaction of the elderly person and family? Where will the client be living in the home setting (upstairs or downstairs)? Who will be available as a support person?

Other concerns include family anguish about placing a loved one in a nursing home or continuing support in the home environment; the appropriateness of the home care versus nursing home care; the cost of care and its effect on the decision of the setting for care; and the outside support, resources, and help in the home. Home care nurses should realize that the entire family will be burdened, yet the client may not be involved enough in the decision. If nurses meet client's needs, they will adjust better to the situation thereby increasing adaptation and coping while decreasing stress.

Thus when helping families decide about home care, there are four major considerations: (1) the appropriateness of home care, (2) family resources and preferences of the client and care taker, as well as health, education level, physical ability to provide care, motivation, and availability of outside assistance, (3) the cost of care, and (4) the client's functional status (Powers, 1989).

Important in home health care is family and client satisfaction. Nurses cannot estimate the joy and burdens involved in caring for an elderly loved one with chronic illness. Social and physical environmental characteristics affect morale and the life satisfaction level of older persons (Namazi, Eckert, Kahana et al., 1989). Client and environment must be compatible for successful home health care.

The Richmond/Hopkins Family Coping Index assesses how well a client's family is coping or functioning at home. Nine domains were used when rating family coping: (1) physical independence, (2) therapeutic competence, (3) knowledge of health condition, (4) application of principles of general hygiene, (5) health care attitude, (6) emotional competence, (7) family living patterns, (8) physical environment, and (9) use of community resources (Choi, Josten, and Christensen, 1987).

As with all clients, alternatives for care are important for aging clients. Knowledge of the client's medical status, family and client resources and preferences, cost factors, and the client's functional status provide needed information for the home care nurse, elderly client, and the family when deciding about the appropriateness of home care.

HOSPICE HOME CARE

Historically, the word *hospice* referred to a place of refuge for travelers. The contemporary meaning refers to caring for people nearing the end of their life and faced with dying from a terminal illness. Originating in nineteenth century England, the earliest hospices first provided palliative care to terminally ill patients in hospitals and later extended the services into homes. In 1970 the hospice movement in the United States gained momentum in response to awakened public interest generated by Dr. Elisabeth Kübler-Ross' book, *Death with Dignity*. Public-sponsored hospices, successful in meeting the special needs of the dying patient, attracted congressional attention. After evaluation of a limited trial hospice benefit, Congress enacted legislation in 1985 that provided coverage for hospice services under Medicare. Stringent controls and criteria for quality hospice care are imposed both by the Health Care Financing Agency (HCFA) and the Joint Commission on Accreditation of Healthcare Organizations (JCAHO).

As a result of the hospice movement, people with terminal disease now are offered the opportunity to die at home, if that is their choice, with the supportive services that home care can provide. A variety of hospice care models in the United States use institutional services, home care service, or both. Those that use an existing hospital in conjunction with an established home health agency (hospital-based or contracted services) are probably the most cost-efficient because each organization can contribute a portion of its resources to this concept of care. In addition to prescribed home care services, core services unique to hospice are a medical director who actively participates as a member of the hospice team, volunteers, chaplain support, respite care, financial assistance with medicines and equipment, and bereavement support of the family after the death of the patient.

Hospice care requires a team of professionals and paraprofessionals with experience in caring for the terminally ill. Interdisciplinary coordination is imperative for a smooth transfer of clients to the home care setting from the hospital. In keeping clients at home, the primary goal is to help both the client and family in maintaining the client's integrity and comfort. Palliative rather than curative care is the objective. This goal is met by nursing actions such as alleviating symptoms and meeting the special needs of the dying client and client's family.

Health care providers who work with the dying often experience stress, which must be identified and appropriately addressed to deliver quality client care and to maintain the care provider's integrity. Employee stress factors related to hospice care differ from general job-related stressors. Understanding these differences will enable the hospice nurse to practice self-care while delivering client care. Some stress factors are: (1) difficulty accepting the fact that a patient's problems cannot always be controlled, (2) frustration from investing large amounts of energy for people who then die, (3) anger at being subjected to high performance expectations, (4) difficulty setting limits on involvement with patients and family, and (5) difficulty establishing realistic limitations as to what can be provided by hospice.

The hospice nurse needs a firm foundation in home care skills, knowledge of community resources, the ability to function constructively as a team member, and the mature ability to meet personal emotional needs and the emotional needs of the hospice patient and family.

A major issue in hospice care is the reimbursement structure in the health care delivery system. Initially, many hospices provided free services as a mission of ministering to the dying. Others accepted available payment from third-party payers for billable services. In November 1983, the federal government legislated a Medicare hospice benefit for reimbursement to Medicare hospice-certified agencies.

The hospice reimbursement benefit is optional for the Medicare-eligible patient. Hospices may bill for skilled home care services under regular Medicare part A benefits if the patient does not want to use the hospice benefit. Responding to the perceived cost-containment potential of hospice care and the public demand for caring services during terminal illness, third-party payors are following Medicare's lead in providing hospice service options.

Not all terminally ill patients choose hospice care, and of those that do, not all are eligible for Medicare or covered by private insurance. If reimbursement potential becomes an admission criterion for hospice care, it will no longer be a viable option for all terminally ill patients. The community health nurse choosing hospice as a specialty area must be prepared to deal with this and other potentially ethical issues. Despite the many unresolved issues, (e.g., patient choice, hospice availability, reimbursement status, admission criteria) hospice nursing is a rewarding specialty.

Home health care nurses working with chronic terminal illness in hospice settings must clarify their own values on death. Nurses should prepare for their own death by having life insurance, wills, and funeral plans arranged in advance.

For information about home care and hospice care, nurses can contact The National Association for Home Care, 519 C Street, N.E., Washington, D.C. 20002 (202-547-7424) and the Visiting Nurse Association of America, 3801 East Florida Avenue, Suite 806, Denver, CO 80210, (800-426-2547).

The National League for Nursing (NLN) developed specific standards for home care organizations that offer hospice as a major service. Home care agencies accredited by the NLN must demonstrate that the structure and function of the agency supports the consumer-oriented philosophy, provides high-quality services, has adequate resources, and is positioned for long-term viability (NLN, 1989). The NLN community health accreditation program (CHAP) has been accrediting home care organizations since 1965. CHAP is committed to ensuring that home care agencies adhere to the highest standards of excellence and certifies to the consumer that the accredited agency has voluntarily met the highest standards for home care and community health in the nation (NLN, 1989, p. 1).

In addition to having standards for hospice, CHAP also has specific standards for professional services, paraprofessional services, home infusion therapy, home medical equipment, pharmacy services, public health programs, and community nursing centers (NLN, 1989). The services the agency offers determine the set of standards that will be used for accreditation.

FINANCIAL ASPECTS OF HOME HEALTH CARE
Reimbursement Mechanisms

Before federal intervention, home health care was funded by clients who could pay for the service and by donations, which subsidized the care provided to those who could pay only a portion or not at all. Now, Medicare and Medicaid are the principal funding sources, with private third-party health insurance providing another major source.

Medicare

Reimbursement of home health services is handled through insurance companies under contract to the Social Security Administration to pay home health care agencies for Medicare-covered services rendered to beneficiaries. To qualify for home health services a beneficiary must be over 65 years of age or disabled and (1) under the care of a physician; (2) confined to the home (homebound); or (3) in need of skilled nursing services, physical therapy, occupational therapy, or speech therapy on an intermittent basis.

The person's attending physician establishes the plan of treatment and also certifies the necessity of home health services. The plan must specify (1) types of services required, (2) frequency of visits, (3) anticipated length of care, (4) diagnosis, (5) description of the client's functional limitations, (6) medications, (7) diet, (8) activities permitted, (9) medical supplies and appliances needed, and (10) safety of home environment. This plan must be reviewed at least every 60 days; continuance of care requires recertification of the plan by physician.

A beneficiary is considered eligible for home health services provided that a physician certifies that the client is confined at home. Clients do not have to be bedridden, but they must be unable to leave their residence without assistance because of illness or injury. Feebleness and insecurity brought on by advanced age do not qualify the person to receive home health care.

Skilled services are those required by an individual that are *reasonable* and *necessary* for treatment of an illness or injury. The following factors are evaluated in determining the degree of skill: (1) complexity of service and condition of client, (2) performance or supervision of performance by a registered nurse, (3) teaching of service by skilled professional, and (4) whether the service can be accomplished by nonmedical person.

Services directed toward the prevention of illness or injury are not covered by Medicare. This does not mean, however, that these activities cannot be performed. They must be done in conjunction with a "skilled" service. The following are examples of services that are reimbursable and covered under Medicare because they require skill, knowledge, and judgment on the part of the practitioner: (1) observation and evaluation of physical status; (2) teaching and training activities to client, family, or caregiver; (3) therapeutic exercises (for restoration or loss of function); (4) insertion and irrigation of catheters; (5) administration of medication (intravenous and intramuscular injections and teaching of medication regimen), and (6) skin care (extensive decubitus ulcer).

Because they are elderly, Medicare beneficiaries usually suffer from chronic conditions with multiple disease processes. Medicare beneficiaries rely on federal reimbursement criteria that definitely influence the provision of care. Medicare places an emphasis on episodic care because of its limitation in benefits and requirement for skilled care. One of the shortcomings of Medicare is its limited protection. Medicare usually reimburses 80% of "usual, customary and reasonable charges." The remaining 20% must be "coinsured" for protection against excessive expense. The nurse should encourage the elderly client to acquire supplemental

TABLE 42-1

Comparison of the two major federally supported programs for home health care

Medicare (Title XVIII)	Medicaid (Title XVIX)
Federal *insurance* program administered by Social Security Administration	Federal and state *assistance* program administered by the state
Age 65 and over or disabled	Income-based eligibility
Conditions of participation	Conditions of participation
Homebound status	Not necessarily homebound status
Intermittent service	Intermittent service
Skilled service	Not necessarily skilled service
Restorative program maintenance	Custodial and program
Physician certification	Physician certification
Therapies, medical social service	State option—therapist, medical social service
Pays rental and purchase	Pays purchase
Reimbursement—"reasonable cost"	Reimbursement—maximum allowed at state level

health insurance to cover the cost of charges that Medicare does not pay. The use of home health services under Medicare has increased significantly since the passage of the 1972 amendments and since the implementation of the prospective payment system for hospitals in 1983. New rules and regulations are written for Medicare and intermediaries as needed. These changes are published in bulletins sent to agencies. For example, currently, Medicare does not assume the role of primary insurer in cases of accidents of liability when other insurances are available.

Medicaid

Authorized by Title XIX of the Social Security Act, Medicaid provides health services to low income persons. It is a medical assistance program for eligible people under Title XVI (Aid to Families with Dependent Children) or Title XVI (Supplemental Security Income) of the Social Security Act and also is available for those individuals whose income is insufficient to cover medical services and for disability coverage. Medicaid is administered by the states but is both state and federally subsidized. Providers are directly reimbursed by the state, which is also responsible for monitoring the operations and enforcing the regulations. Medicaid covers home health including skilled and unskilled services such as personal care. Needy children are eligible under Medicaid, whereas the elderly usually receive Medicare as their primary method of payment.

Table 42-1 compares Medicare with Medicaid. If an elderly client has both Medicare and Medicaid or a private insurance plan, Medicare is used as the primary payment source, provided the services being delivered to the client are "skilled." When the client is no longer eligible under Medicare, the Medicaid benefits can be used.

Private Insurance

Third-party payers are represented by private insurance companies to which the person subscribes individually or with a group such as an employer. Some states (e.g., Connecticut) have laws that require home health care to be a provision in health insurance coverage. Individuals under 65 years of age who need home care follow-up after surgery or prolonged hospitalization use this benefit the most. This benefit can decrease a client's length of stay in the hospital, thereby assisting clients to return to their former level of functioning.

Payment by Individual

Some individuals who require home health services but do not have health insurance may pay the home health agency directly. Individuals who do not meet their insurance coverage requirements and still want the services pay the established charge or may be offered the service on a sliding scale or established fee, based on their financial status. For example, clients may no longer require skilled nursing service for assessment of their condition but still need the help of a home health aide to assist with personal hygiene needs. Some persons may pay for home health services the Medicare program offers.

Nursing Visit Charges

Home health care is growing because it is assumed to be more cost-effective than hospital care. It is likely that financiers will closely scrutinize the implementation of home health services and adjustments and restrictions will evolve as needed to maintain cost containment. Several factors influence the cost and charge data: (1) type of service provided, (2) geographical location of the agency, and (3) current community staffing patterns. The term *cost* refers to the dollar amount agencies spend to provide the service. The term *charge* is the dollar amount expected or billed for rendering service.

The Health Care Financing Administration continuously gathers data regarding use of home care services by analyzing factors such as cost, frequency, duration of services, and number of visits. The federal government is interested in cost containment and also in quality of care.

THE PRACTICE OF HOME HEALTH CARE NURSING
Quality of Care and Standards

In 1986 the House Republican Select Committee on Aging questioned the type of services provided by home care agencies. To this point, there had been limited research on quality of care. Because of the extensive media coverage of this report, consumers began questioning health care professionals about the type and effectiveness of home care services (Martin and Scheet, 1988). To provide accountability to consumers, home care providers must document that their care is appropriate and effective (NLN, 1987).

In addition to providing consumer accountability, documenting the quality of care provided by agencies fulfills other purposes. Nurses have accurate data documenting protection of the client's right to appropriate and competent care. This data also assists consumers in making informed decisions about home care. Research and documentation of

---

> ### STANDARDS OF HOME HEALTH NURSING PRACTICE
>
> #### STANDARD I. ORGANIZATION OF HOME HEALTH SERVICES
>
> All home health services are planned, organized, and directed by a master's prepared professional nurse with experience in community health and administration.
>
> #### STANDARD II. THEORY
>
> The nurse applies theoretical concepts as a basis for decisions in practice.
>
> #### STANDARD III. DATA COLLECTION
>
> The nurse continuously collects and records data that are comprehensive, accurate, and systematic.
>
> #### STANDARD IV. DIAGNOSIS
>
> The nurse uses health assessment data to determine nursing diagnoses.
>
> #### STANDARD V. PLANNING
>
> The nurse develops care plans that establish goals. The care plan is based on nursing diagnoses and incorporates therapeutic, preventive, and rehabilitative nursing actions.
>
> #### STANDARD VI. INTERVENTION
>
> The nurse, guided by the care plan, intervenes to provide comfort, to restore, improve, and promote health, to prevent complications and sequelae of illness, and to effect rehabilitation.
>
> #### STANDARD VII. EVALUATION
>
> The nurse continually evaluates the client's and family's responses to interventions in order to determine progress toward goal attainment and to revise the data base, nursing diagnoses, and plan of care.

From American Nurses' Association: Standards of home health nursing practice, Kansas City, Mo, 1986, The Association.

---

quality of home care services advances the welfare of the community by ensuring that individual members receive adequate health care. Both the ANA and NLN have developed professional standards of home care that include requirements for evaluation of quality of care. NLN standard S17.1 states that "Annual program evaluation includes assessment of quality of care . . . and client outcomes" (NLN, 1987, p. 29). ANA standard VII (see box) requires" . . . an ongoing, organized quality assurance program to evaluate care" (ANA, 1986, p. 13). Emphasis on meeting professional standards fosters the development and strengths of home care nursing as a viable alternative to hospital care. Previously, home care providers have primarily met requirements set by Medicare and third-party payers (Hough and Schmele, 1987). Accurate data that documents fulfillment of professional standards is evidence of quality care being provided.

Quality of Care Measurement

Peters and Poe (1988) have proposed a system of monitoring for measuring all aspects of quality of care in the home—

structure, process and outcome. They suggest using a retrospective chart audit or other types of data collection that classify clients by medical or nursing diagnoses. Monitoring is different from an evaluation/audit because monitoring involves identifying opportunities to improve care. Rinke (1988) proposes measuring client outcomes through client outcome program objectives. These are goal statements measuring a client's response to home care on three levels: knowledge, behavior, and health status. Clients are classified by nursing problems such as "wound healing" and "bedbound," and a retrospective chart audit is also used. The standard is that 70% to 80% of patients meet the criteria.

Several public health associations and private home care agencies have published information about implementation of quality assurance programs. The Florida Association of Home Health Agencies (NLN, 1987) describes using clients' medical diagnoses in writing outcome criteria, which are evaluated through a peer review of clients' charts. The Colorado Association of Home Health Agencies (NLN, 1987) also measures client outcomes through a retrospective chart audit, classifying clients by both medical diagnoses and nursing problems, and emphasizing the importance of documenting abnormal outcomes and developing a new plan. The Visiting Nurse Association of Omaha uses a retrospective chart audit in evaluating client outcomes on three levels: knowledge, behavior, and physical status (Martin and Scheet, 1988).

The Visiting Nursing Association of Pennsylvania classifies clients by nursing diagnoses and rehabilitation potential (e.g., recovery, maintenance, and terminal), with patient physiological and self-care knowledge outcome objectives for each category (Harris, Peters, and Yuan 1987). They do not use a retrospective chart audit; nurses document patient outcomes during home visits, using flow sheets listing specific outcome criteria. There is a strong emphasis on relating cost and quality, and the cost of providing care for each client is related to the outcomes achieved. The United Home Health Service of Philadelphia uses standardized nursing care plans for measuring nursing process and patient outcomes (Gould, 1985). Specific nursing interventions and client outcome criteria have been developed for each nursing diagnosis, and nurses document these criteria on flow sheets during home visits. The Minnesota Department of Public Health documents client outcomes in two ways: 1) For clients with acute physical, medical, and nursing problems, outcomes are measured by considering the client's knowledge, self-care management, psychosocial adjustment, and physiological status. 2) For clients with more chronic conditions, outcomes are measured by considering the client's level of functioning, such as degree of independence in bathing, dressing, feeding, transferring, or continence (NLN, 1987).

Each of these agencies has developed its own instruments and criteria because there are few reliable and valid tools for measuring quality of care outcomes. The Slater scale and the Schmele Instrument to Measure the Process of Nursing Care (SIMP) are other tools that can be used to determine the quality of care (Hough and Schmele, 1987; Schmele and Foss, 1989). There are few studies providing actual data on quality of care provided in the home.

As mentioned before, most of these criteria and studies have used either process or outcome measures. Retrospective chart audits have been the primary data source, with data collection done either as a peer review process or by impartial observers. Various client classification systems have been used (Albrecht, 1991), including medical and nursing diagnoses, and nursing problems, with many types of outcome criteria, including client's physiological status, self-care behavior and knowledge, and psychosocial coping.

THE ALBRECHT NURSING MODEL FOR HOME HEALTH CARE

Albrecht (1990) describes a nursing model for home health care (Figure 42-1) that distinguishes three main components of home care services—structure, process, and outcome. Albrecht describes structural elements as including the client, family/loved one, provider agency, professional nurse, and health team. Process elements include type of care, coordination of care, and intervention. Outcome elements are satisfaction with care, quality of care, cost effectiveness, health status, self-care capability, and use of home care. The structural and process elements are modified by client classification, cost, demand, availability, productivity, accountability, accessibility, and efficiency. Albrecht emphasizes the dynamic interaction between the overall structural, process, and outcome elements and between the variables that make up these elements. According to this model, positive outcome elements are determined by adequate structural and process elements. Therefore, quality of care is an especially important variable because it may reflect the elements constituting a home care agency and the care given.

The model gives direction for research, practice, and education in home health care. It can be used for assessing and planning care for a family and for analysis of the agency. It provides the necessary framework for providing quality care to the family and client in their home.

Structure and process consist of the client's use of high-technology equipment in the home. Does the client desire the home care service? Are the family members or significant others willing to participate in the care of the client dependent on high-technology equipment? Is a provider agency available to provide the home care services and give support as needed? Has the care giver been properly taught? The process outcomes relate by identifying the types of care needed in the home. Is the client receiving proper care from the nurse or family member? The outcome is the most important aspect of the model because it will tell whether or not the structural and process elements worked. One way this can be determined is by whether or not the client is satisfied with the care provided.

Quality of care could be measured by client's physical status, self-care knowledge, and psychosocial coping. It is anticipated that nurses are providing good care, and this will be shown by the clients meeting most of the physical criteria. Perhaps clients not meeting physical criteria may not be due to poor quality care, but rather to other structural factors, such as the client demographic and psychological variables listed in Albrecht's model. For example, elderly clients may have difficulty understanding and following all

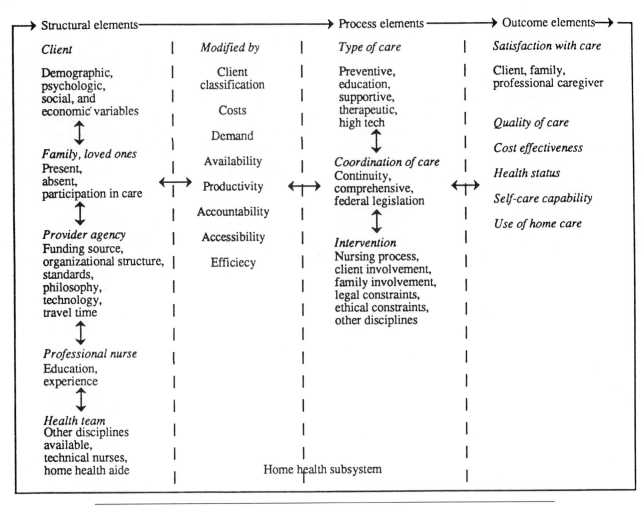

FIGURE 42-1

The Albrecht nursing model for home health care. *(From Albrecht M: The Albrecht nursing model for home health care: implications for research, practice, and education. Public Health Nurs 7(11), 123.)*

the self-care responsibilities posed by such complex chronic diseases as cancer, congestive heart failure, arthritis, diabetes, and chronic obstructive lung disease. Also, clients may demonstrate impaired coping, even though the nurses are meeting the clients' psychosocial needs. Once again this may be due not to poor quality care, but to structural elements such as client's psychological, social, and economic variables and family's presence or absence and participation in care.

CLINICAL APPLICATION

Mrs. S. is a 71-year-old woman admitted to home care with diagnoses of diabetes, renal insufficiency, angina, and COPD. She receives renal dialysis three times per week and insulin injections at home. She lives alone in a poor home environment, with limited financial and family support. Her activity tolerance is limited due to severe dyspnea and poor disease management.

According to the Albrecht Nursing Model, she has limited structural supports (limited client and family support) and will probably need therapeutic high-technology care. Services provided will depend on the costs and availability

from her provider home care agency. Coordination of care will be necessary to promote self-care capability.

Cynthia, community health nursing student, has been assigned to accompany Susan, staff nurse, to Mrs. S.'s home to *assess* the home, family, and client needs. It is obvious that Mrs. S. would have benefitted from a joint discharge planning arrangement between the hospital, the home health agency, the client, and the client's daughter, who lives 50 miles away in a nearby community.

During the assessment it is determined that Mrs. S. will need a live in companion, a respiratory therapist, and the nurse to monitor her renal dialysis and to teach Mrs. S., the companion, and her daughter proper dialysis techniques and proper care of the diabetic client. On return to the agency, Cynthia and Susan arrange a clinical conference with the physician, the companion, the respiratory therapist, and the nurse to *plan* Mrs. S.'s care. The group determines that they will request from Medicare certification for three nurse visits per week plus daily respiratory therapy visits for 1 month, at which time an assessment will be made to determine continued need.

Nursing *intervention* will involve teaching; providing dialysis care and diabetic care until such time as the companion and the daughter can properly demonstrate their ability to perform the client's care; increasing Mrs. S.'s involvement in her care as she is able to with improved management of illness; and checking the community resources available to improve the home environment so that Mrs. S. can live safely in her own home.

The contract arranged with the client and her family included an *evaluation* of the client's progress at the end of each visit, the family's and care giver's knowledge and ability to care for the client, the benefits derived from the community resources.

SUMMARY

Families are a major part of home care, and home care nurses must educate and support all family members. When one person needs home care, the whole family is affected. Whether it is a child or an elderly person in need of home care, the effects on the family will be similar. The Albrecht model (1990) suggests that regardless of the client's status, with the right combination of structural and process variables the client can have an outcome of self-care capability.

KEY CONCEPTS

The use of high technology in the home care setting is increasing.

Home health care nurses must be prepared to respond to various high-technology chronic, and hospice situations in the home.

Home health care nurses need to assist families dealing with stress associated with care in the home.

Home care nurses must provide for the needs of the caregiver in home.

The age of the elderly population is increasing.

Clients with chronic illnesses are being cared for in the home.

The ANA and NLN have developed standards for home health care nursing.

Research on quality of care in the home has to consider the structure, process, and outcome variables.

The Albrecht nursing model provides a framework for home health care nursing practice.

LEARNING ACTIVITIES

1. Interview a home health care nurse and a nursing supervisor in your home health care agency. What percentage of the clients are over 65 years of age? What are the major nursing and medical diagnoses of these clients?

2. In addition to the above questions, determine the percentage of clients using high-technology equipment in the home. What equipment is being used? What types of stress does this equipment cause the nurse and family?

3. Discuss with your instructor in a group setting how the ANA and NLN standards are being met in this agency.

4. Discuss how the Albrecht Nursing Model can be used to assess and plan for nursing care in the home for the following clients.
   a. Mrs. P. is an 84-year-old woman who lives with her son. Her medical diagnoses included decubitus ulcer, pneumonia, and Parkinson's disease. She needs total care, is incontinent of bowel and bladder, is bedbound due to contractures, is mentally lethargic and cries frequently, and is

fed via a gastrostomy tube.
   b. Mr. W. is an 87-year-old man who lives with a companion. He was admitted to home care with degenerative arthritis, s/p fractured right ankle, and terminal cancer. He is receiving morphine drip for pain.
   c. Mrs. F. is a 60-year-old woman who lives at home with her husband. Mrs. F. has a diagnosis of Alzheimer's, and it is clearly unsafe for her to be left unattended at any time. Mrs. F. often awakens in the morning before her husband and wanders outside, without shoes or a coat, regardless of the weather, and is unable to find her way home. She has an inconsistent pattern of attending to basic hygiene, nutrition, and safety needs. She enjoys ironing but has burned her hands on several occasions. Mr. F. is finding it increasingly difficult to help his wife to care for herself. He calls your home care agency and asks for your help. How do you proceed?

BIBLIOGRAPHY

Albrecht M: The Albrecht nursing model for home health care: implications for research, practice, and education, Public Health Nursing, 7(2):118-126, 1990.

Albrecht M: Home health care: reliability and validity testing of patient-classification instrument, Public Nursing, 8(2):124-131, 1991.

American Medical Association: Physician guide to home health care, Monroe, Wis, 1979, The Association.

American Nurses Association: Guidelines for review of nursing care at the local level. In Rinke LT and Wilson AA, editors: Outcome measures in home care, vol 2: service, New York, 1987, National League for Nursing.

American Nurses Association: Standards of home health nursing practice, Kansas City, 1986, The Association.

Anderson K: Long-term oxygen therapy: indications and guidelines for use, Home Health Care Nurse 7(3):40-47, 1989.

Andrews M and Nielson D: Technology dependent children in the home, Pediatr Nursing 14(2): 111-114, 151, 1988.

Braun L: Discharge of a patient with chronic respiratory failure, Home Health Care Nurse, 7(3):17-21, 1987.

Callender M and Lavor J: Home health care: development, problems, and potential, Washington, D C, 1975, Office of the Assistant Secretary

for Planning & Evaluation, Social Services & Human Development, Department of Health, Education, & Welfare.

Christensen ML: Development and use of functional client outcome measures. In Rinke LT and Wilson AA, editors: Outcome measures in home care, vol 2: service, New York, 1987, National League for Nursing.

Choi T, Josten L, and Christensen M: Health-specific family coping index for noninstitutional care. In Rinke LT, editor: Outcome measures in home care, vol 1: research, New York, 1987, National League for Nursing.

Colorado Association of Home Health Agencies: Colorado quality assurance audit criteria, In

Rinke LT and Wilson AA, editors: Outcome measures in home care, vol 2: services, New York, 1987, National League for Nursing.

Decker F, Stevens L, Vancini M, and Wedeking L: Using patient outcomes to evaluate community health nursing. In Rinke LT and Wilson AA, editors: Outcome measures in home care, vol 2: service, New York, 1987, National League for Nursing.

Dolan J: Goodnow's history of nursing, Philadelphia, 1958, WB Saunders Co.

Donabedian A: Some basic issues in evaluating the quality of health care, In Rinke LT, editor: Outcome measures in home care, vol 1: research, New York, 1987, National League of Nursing.

Donar M: Community care: pediatric home, Holistic Nursing Practice, 2(2):68-70, 1988.

Florida Association of Home Health Agencies: Quality assurance program. In Rinke LT and Wilson AA, editors: Outcome measures in home care, vol 2: service, New York, 1987, National League for Nursing.

Gorski L: Effective teaching of home IV therapy, Home Health Care Nurse 7(5):10-17, 1987.

Gould DJ: Standardized home health nursing care plans: a quality assurance tool, QRB 11:334-338, 1985.

Green JH: Long-term home care research. In National League for Nursing, editor: Indices of quality in long-term care research, New York, 1989, National League for Nursing.

Handy C: Home care of patients with technically complex nursing needs—high technology in the home, Nurs Clin North Am 23(2):315-327, 1988.

Handy C: Patient-centered high technology home care, Holistic Nursing Practice, 3(2):46-53, 1989.

Harris MD, Peters DA, and Yuan J: Relating quality and cost in a home care agency, QRB 13:175-181, 1987.

Health Care Financing Administration (HCSA)

HIM-II Medicare Home Health Agency Manual, April 1989, Baltimore, Md, HCFA.

Hegyvary ST, and Haussmann D: The relationship of nursing process and patient outcomes. In Rinke LT, editor: Outcome measures in home care, vol 1: research, New York, 1987, National League for Nursing.

Hough BL and Schmele JA: The Slater scale: a viable method for monitoring nursing care quality in home health. J Nursing Quality Assurance 1(3):28-38, 1987.

Longway L: Hospice care: personal death awareness for hospice nurses, Home Health Care Nurse 7(5):8-9, 45, 1987.

Loewenhardt P: Assuring successful home enteral feedings, Home Health Care Nurse, 7(5):16-21, 1987.

Martin KS and Scheet NJ: The Omaha system: providing a framework for assuring quality of home care, Home Health Care Nurse 6(3):24-28, 1988.

McCarthy M: A home discharging program for ventilator assisted children. Pediatric Nursing 12(5):338-340, 1986.

Minnesota Department of Health: Outcome criteria: public health nursing and home care services. In Rinke LT and Wilson AA, editors: Outcome measures in home care, vol 2: service, New York, 1987, National League for Nursing.

Namazi K, Eckert K, Kahana E, and Lyon S: Psychosocial well-being of elderly board and care home residents, The Gerontologist, 4(29): 511-516, 1989.

National Association for Home Care: Report #152, February 4, 1986.

National League for Nursing: Accreditation criteria, standards, and substantiating evidences for home care and community health, New York, 1987, NLN.

National League for Nursing: Standards of excellence for home care organizations, New York, 1989, NLN.

Oleske DM, Otte DM, and Heinze S: Development and evaluation of a system for monitoring the quality of oncology nursing care in the home setting, Cancer Nursing 10(4):190-198, 1987.

Peters DA and Poe SS: Using monitoring in a home care quality assurance program, J Nursing Quality Assurance 2(2):34-37, 1988.

Powers J: Helping family and patients decide between home care and nursing home care, South Med J 6(82):723-726.

Raulin A and Shannon K: PNP's case managers for technology-dependent children, Pediatric Nursing 12(5):338-340, 1986.

Rinke LT: Outcome standards in home health: state of the art, New York, 1988, National League for Nursing.

Schmele JA, and Foss SJ: A process method for clinical practice evaluation in the home health setting, J Nurs Quality Assurance, 3(3):54-63, 1989.

Smith C and Marien L: Transitional care of adults dependent on technological care at home, The Kansas Nurse 1-2, 1989.

Stiller S: Success and difficulty in high-tech home care, Public Health Nursing 5(2):68-75, 1988.

Trager B: Home health services in the United States: a report to the Special Committee on Aging, 92nd Congress, 2nd session, Washington, D C, 1972, US Government Printing Office.

Van Ort S and Woodtli A: Home health care: providing a missing link, J Gerontological Nursing 15(9):4-9, 1989.

Warhola C: Planning for home health services: a resource handbook, Pub. No. (HRA) 80-14017, Washington, DC: August 1, 1980, Public Health Service, Department of Health & Human Services.

Wildblood A and Stezo P: The how-to's of home IV therapy, Pediatric Nursing 13(1):42-46, 68, 1987.

Wilson J: Filling the family fuel tank, Home Health Care Nurse 5(1):46-48, 1987.

Appendixes

A1—DISCHARGED PATIENTS QUESTIONNAIRE*
(Chapter 13)

We are asking patients and families who have recently received services from the agency to assist us in the evaluation of our programs. As a consumer of the services we offer, your answers to the enclosed questionnaire will help us determine if we are meeting our objectives as a provider of skilled nursing care in the home designed to meet the needs of residents of our county.

We would appreciate it if you could complete the questionnaire and return it to us in the envelope provided. It will not be necessary to sign the questionnaire as we are not interested in identifying a patient or the nurse who gave care.

Instructions: Please circle the *Yes* or *No* following each question below, as you feel it answers the question.

1. When the public health nurse visited your home, did you know why she was there?   Yes   No

2. Did you and the nurse arrange a time for the visits that was convenient for both of you?   Yes   No

3. Did the nurse do any of the following treatments?   Yes   No
   - Change or irrigate catheter   Yes   No
   - Irrigate colostomy or give an enema   Yes   No
   - Change dressings   Yes   No
   - Inject a medication   Yes   No
   - Assist with exercise routine   Yes   No
   - Suction or care for tracheotomy   Yes   No
   - Insert a nasal-gastric tube   Yes   No

   If you answered *Yes* to any of the above, did you understand what the treatment was expected to do for you?   Yes   No

4. Did the nurse teach you or any member of your family to do a treatment?   Yes   No

   Did you or your family learn to do the treatment yourself?   Yes   No

5. Did you take medication by mouth?   Yes   No

   Did you understand how to take the medication (i.e., amount to take; number of times during the day; if taken before, after, or with meals)?   Yes   No

   Did the nurse help you understand what the medication was expected to do?   Yes   No

6. Did the nurse examine you at any time (i.e., take blood pressure, pulse, listen to your chest with a stethoscope, examine your skin)?   Yes   No

   If yes, did you understand why she was making these observations?   Yes   No

7. Did the nurse help you to understand your illness?   Yes   No

8. Did you understand what the nurse was planning to accomplish by visiting you?   Yes   No

9. Did the nurse's visits make it easier for you to remain in your home and care for yourself?   Yes   No

10. Did you have other problems (e.g., financial) that the public health nurse could not assist you with by herself?   Yes   No

    If yes, did the nurse assist you to contact another agency that could help you?   Yes   No

11. Do you feel the nursing visits were (circle one):
    Too few   Too many   Right number

12. Were you aware that the nurse was going to discharge you from her service?   Yes   No

13. Did you feel you could function on your own when the nurse dismissed you from the service?   Yes   No

14. If you need skilled nursing service in your home at some time in the future, will you contact the agency?   Yes   No

15. If you have any comments, please write them in the space below:

---

*From Administrator's handbook for the structure, operation, and expansion of home health agencies, Pub. No. 21-1653, pp. 409-410, New York, 1977, National League for Nursing.

A2—SUMMARY OF A HEALTH HISTORY*
(Chapters 28 and 29)

Information	Comments

IDENTIFYING INFORMATION

1. Name
2. Address
3. Telephone number
4. Age and birthdate
5. Birthplace
6. Race
7. Sex
8. Religion
9. Nationality
10. Date of interview
11. Informant

Additional information appropriate to older adolescent may include occupation, marital status, and temporary and permanent address

Under informant include subjective impression of reliability, general attitude, willingness to communicate, overall accuracy of data, and any special circumstances, such as use of an interpreter

Informants should include parent and child, as well as others who may be primary caregivers, such as grandparent

CHIEF COMPLAINT (CC)

To establish the major specific reason for the individual's seeking professional health attention

Record in patient's own words; include duration of symptoms

If informant has difficulty isolating *one* problem, ask which problem or symptom led person to seek help *now*

In case of routine physical examination, state CC as reason for visit

PRESENT ILLNESS (PI)

To obtain all details related to the chief complaint
1. Onset
   a. Date of onset
   b. Manner of onset (gradual or sudden)
   c. Precipitating and predisposing factors related to onset (emotional disturbance, physical exertion, fatigue, bodily function, pregnancy, environment, injury, infection, toxins and allergens, or therapeutic agents)
2. Characteristics
   a. Character (quality, quantity, consistency, or other)
   b. Location and radiation (i.e., pain)
   c. Intensity or severity
   d. Timing (continuous or intermittent, duration of each, temporal relationship to other events)
   e. Aggravating and relieving factors
   f. Associated symptoms
3. Course since onset
   a. Incidence
      (1) Single acute attack
      (2) Recurrent acute attacks
      (3) Daily occurrences
      (4) Periodic occurrences
      (5) Continuous chronic episode
   b. Progress (better, worse, unchanged)
   c. Effect of therapy

In its broadest sense, *illness* denotes any problem of a physical, emotional, or psychosocial nature

Present information to chronologic order; may be referenced according to one point in time, such as *prior to admission* (PTA)

Concentrate on reason for seeking help now, especially if problem has existed for some time

PAST HISTORY (PH)

To elicit a profile of the individual's previous illnesses, injuries, or operations
1. Pregnancy (maternal)
   a. Number (gravida)
      (1) Dates of delivery
   b. Outcome (parity)
      (1) Gestation (full-term, premature, postmature)
      (2) Stillbirths, abortions
   c. Health during pregnancy
   d. Medications taken

Importance of prenatal history depends on child's age; the younger the child, the more important the perinatal history

Explain relevance of obstetric history in revealing important factors relating to the child's health

Assess parents' emotional attitudes toward the pregnancy and birth

---

*From Wong DL and Whaley LF: Clinical manual of pediatric nursing, ed 3, St. Louis, 1990, Mosby–Year Book, Inc.

A2—SUMMARY OF A HEALTH HISTORY—cont'd
(Chapters 28 and 29)

Information	Comments

2. Labor and delivery
  a. Duration of labor
  b. Type of delivery
  c. Place of delivery
  d. Medications
	Assess parent's feelings regarding delivery; investigate factors affecting bonding, such as if awake and able to hold infant or if asleep and separated from infant

3. Birth
  a. Weight and length
  b. Time of regaining birth weight
  c. Condition of health
  d. Apgar score
  e. Presence of congenital anomalies
  f. Date of discharge from nursery
	If birth problems are reported, inquire about treatment, such as use of oxygen, phototherapy, surgery, and so on, and parents' emotional response to the event

4. Previous illnesses, operations, or injuries
  a. Onset, symptoms, course, termination
  b. Occurrence of complications
  c. Incidence of disease in other family members or in community
  d. Emotional response to previous hospitalization
  e. Circumstances and nature of injuries
	Make positive statement about diphtheria, scarlet fever, measles, chickenpox, mumps, tonsillitis, pertussis, and common illnesses such as colds, earaches, or sore throats
	Elicit a description of disease to verify the diagnosis
	Be alert to areas of injury prevention

5. Allergies
  a. Hay fever, asthma, or eczema
  b. Unusual reactions to foods, drugs, animals, plants, or houshold products
	Have parent describe the type of allergic reaction
	
	Note sensitivity to egg albumin and reactions to certain immunizations

6. Current medications a. Name, dose, schedule, duration, and reason for administration	Assess parents' knowledge of correct dosage of common drugs, such as acetaminophen; note underusage or overusage

7. Immunizations
  a. Name, number of doses, ages when given
  b. Occurrence of reaction
  c. Administration of horse or other foreign serum, gamma globulin, or blood transfusion
	May refer to immunizations as "baby shots"
	Whenever possible, confirm information by checking medical or school records

8. Growth and development
  a. Weight at birth, 6 months, 1 year, and present
  b. Dentition
    (1) Age of eruption/shedding
    (2) Number
    (3) Problems with teething
  c. Age of head control, sitting unsupported, walking, first words
  d. Present grade in school, scholastic achievement
  e. Interaction with peers and adults
  f. Participation in organized activities, such as scouts, sports, and so on
	Compare parents' responses with own observations of child's achievement and results from objective tests, such as DDST or DASE
	
	School and social history can be more thoroughly explored under Family Assessment

9. Habits
  a. Behavior patterns
    (1) Nail biting
    (2) Thumb sucking
    (3) Pica
    (4) Rituals, such as "security blanket"
    (5) Unusual movements (headbanging, rocking)
    (6) Temper tantrums
  b. Activities of daily living
    (1) Hour of sleep and arising
    (2) Duration of nocturnal sleep/naps
    (3) Age of toilet training
    (4) Pattern of stools and urination; occurrence of enuresis
    (5) Type of exercise
  c. Use/abuse of drugs, alcohol, coffee, or cigarettes
  d. Usual disposition; response to frustration
	Assess parents' attitudes toward habits and any remedies used to curtail them, such as punishment for bedwetting
	
	Record child's usual terms for defecation and urination
	
	With adolescents, estimate the quantity of drugs used

Continued.

A2—SUMMARY OF A HEALTH HISTORY—cont'd
(Chapters 28 and 29)

Information	Comments

REVIEW OF SYSTEMS (ROS)

To elicit information concerning any potential health problem
 1. *General*—overall state of health, fatigue, recent and/or unexplained weight gain or loss, period of time for either, contributing factors (change of diet, illness, altered appetite), exercise tolerance, fevers (time of day), chills, night sweats (unrelated to climatic conditions), frequent infections, general ability to carry out activities of daily living
 2. *Integument*—pruritus, pigment or other color changes, acne, eruptions, rashes (location), tendency to bruising, petechiae, excessive dryness, general texture, disorders or deformities of nails, hair growth or loss, hair color change (for adolescent, use of hair dyes or other potentially toxic substances, such as hair straighteners)
 3. *Head*—headaches, dizziness, injury (specific details)
 4. *Eyes*—visual problems (ask about behaviors that indicate blurred vision, such as bumping into objects, clumsiness, sitting very close to television, holding a book close to the face, writing with head near desk, squinting, rubbing the eyes, bending the head in an awkward position), "cross-eye" (strabismus), eye infections, edema of lids, excessive tearing, use of glasses or contact lenses, date of last optic examination
 5. *Nose*—nosebleeds (epistaxis), constant or frequent running or stuffy nose, nasal obstruction (difficulty in breathing), sense of smell
 6. *Ears*—earaches, discharge, evidence of hearing loss (ask about behaviors such as need to repeat requests, loud speech, inattentive behavior), results of any previous auditory testing
 7. *Mouth*—mouth breathing, gum bleeding, toothaches, toothbrushing, use of fluoride, difficulty with teething (symptoms), last visit to dentist (especially if temporary dentition is complete), response to dentist
 8. *Throat*—sore throats, difficulty in swallowing, choking (especially when chewing food, which may be caused by poor chewing habits), hoarseness or other voice irregularities
 9. *Neck*—pain, limitation of movement, stiffness, difficulty in holding head straight (torticollis), thyroid enlargement, enlarged nodes or other masses
10. *Chest*—breast enlargement, discharge, masses, enlarged axillary nodes (for adolescent female, ask about breast self-examination)
11. *Respiratory*—chronic cough, frequent colds (number per year), wheezing, shortness of breath at rest or on exertion, difficulty in breathing, sputum production, infections (pneumonia, tuberculosis), date of last chest x-ray examination; date of last tuberculin test and type of reaction, if any
12. *Cardiovascular*—cyanosis or fatigue on exertion, history of heart murmur or rheumatic fever, anemia, date of last blood count, blood type, recent transfusion
13. *Gastrointestinal*—(much of this in regard to appetite, food tolerance, and elimination habits has been asked elsewhere) concentrate on nausea, vomiting (if not associated with eating, it may indicate brain tumor or increased in-

Explain relevance of questioning to parents (similar to pregnancy section) in comprising total health history of child
Make positive statements about each system, for example, "Mother denies headaches, bumping into objects, squinting, or excessive rubbing of eyes"
Use terms parents are likely to understand, such as "bruises" for ecchymoses

A2—SUMMARY OF A HEALTH HISTORY—cont'd
(Chapters 28 and 29)

Information	Comments

tracranial pressure), jaundice or yellowing skin or sclera, belching, flatulence, recent change in bowel habits (blood in stools, change of color, diarrhea, or constipation)

14. *Genitourinary*—pain on urination, frequency, hesitancy, urgency, hematuria, nocturia, polyuria, unpleasant odor of urine, direction and force of stream, discharge, change in size of scrotum, date of last urinalysis (for adolescent, sexually transmitted disease, type of treatment; for adolescent male, ask about testicular self-examination)

15. *Gynecologic*—menarche, date of last menstrual period, regularity or problems with menstruation, vaginal discharge, pruritus, date and result of last Pap test (include obstetric history as discussed under birth history when applicable), if sexually active, type of contraception

16. *Musculoskeletal*—weakness, clumsiness, lack of coordination, unusual movements, back or joint stiffness, muscle pains or cramps, abnormal gait, deformity, fractures, serious sprains, activity level

17. *Neurologic*—seizures, tremors, dizziness, loss of memory, general affect, fears, nightmares, speech problems, any unusual habits

18. *Endocrine*—intolerance to weather changes, excessive thirst, excessive sweating, salty taste to skin, signs of early puberty

NUTRITION HISTORY

To elicit information about adequacy of child's dietary intake and eating patterns

FAMILY MEDICAL HISTORY

To identify the presence of genetic traits or diseases that have familial tendencies; to assess family habits and exposure to a communicable disease that may affect family members

Choose terms wisely when asking about child's parentage, for example, inquire about paternal history by referring to the child's "father" rather than mother's husband; use term "partner," rather than spouse

1. Family pedigree (Fig. A-1) and guidelines for construction (boxed material)

A pedigree is a pictorial representation or diagram of a family tree to visualize patterns of disease transmission

2. Familial diseases and congenital anomalies, such as heart disease, hypertension, cancer, diabetes mellitus, obesity, congenital anomalies, allergy, asthma, tuberculosis, sickle cell disease, mental retardation, convulsions, insanity or other emotional problems, syphilis, or rheumatic fever; indicate symptoms, treatment, and sequelae

3. Family habits, such as smoking or chemical use

4. Geographic location, such as recent travel or contact with foreign visitors

Important for identification of endemic diseases

FAMILY PERSONAL/SOCIAL HISTORY

To gain an understanding of the family's structure and function

SEXUAL HISTORY

To elicit information concerning young person's concerns and/or activities and any pertinent data regarding adults' sexual activity that influences child
   a. Sexual concerns/activity of youngster
   b. Sexual concerns/activity of adults if warranted

Sexual history is an essential component of preadolescents' and adolescents' health assessment

Degree of investigation into parents' sexual history depends on its relevance to the child's health. It may be limited to family planning concerns or it may be more detailed if overt sexual activity or abuse is suspected

Investigate toward end of history when rapport is greatest

Respect sensitive and complex nature of questioning
   Give parents and youngster option of discussing sexual matters alone with nurse

Continued.

A2—SUMMARY OF A HEALTH HISTORY—cont'd
(Chapters 28 and 29)

Information	Comments
	Assure confidentiality
	Clarify terms such as "sexually active" or "having sex?"
	Refer to sexual contacts a "partners" not "girlfriends" or "boyfriends" to avoid biasing discussion of homosexual activity
	Discussion may flow easily after review of genitourinary tract, such as asking female about menstruation or male about urinary problems
	Suggestions for beginning discussion include:
	"Tell me about your social life."
	"Who are your closest friends?"
	"Is there one very special friend?"
	"Some teenagers have decided to have sex. What do you think about that?"
	Take detailed history of all contacts if sexually transmitted disease is suspected or diagnosed

PATIENT PROFILE (P/P)

To summarize the interviewer's overall impression of the child's and family physical, psychologic, and socioeconomic background

1. Health status
2. Psychologic status
3. Socioeconomic status

A comprehensive summary often identifies nursing diagnoses based on subjective and objective findings

---

GUIDELINES FOR PEDIGREE CONSTRUCTION

1. Begin diagram in the middle of a large sheet of paper.
2. Represent males by a square placed to the left and females by a circle placed to the right.
3. Represent the proband (index case, original patient) with an arrow (if the counselee or patient is different, place a "C" under that person's symbol).
4. Use a horizontal line between a square and a circle for a mating or marriage.
5. Suspend offspring vertically from the mating line and place in order of birth with oldest to the left (regardless of sex).
6. Symbolize generations by Roman numerals with the earliest generation at the top.
7. Include three generations: grandparents, parents, offspring, siblings, aunts, uncles, and first cousins of proband.
8. Include name of each person (maiden names for married women), their date of birth, health problems, and date and cause of death.
9. Date the pedigree.

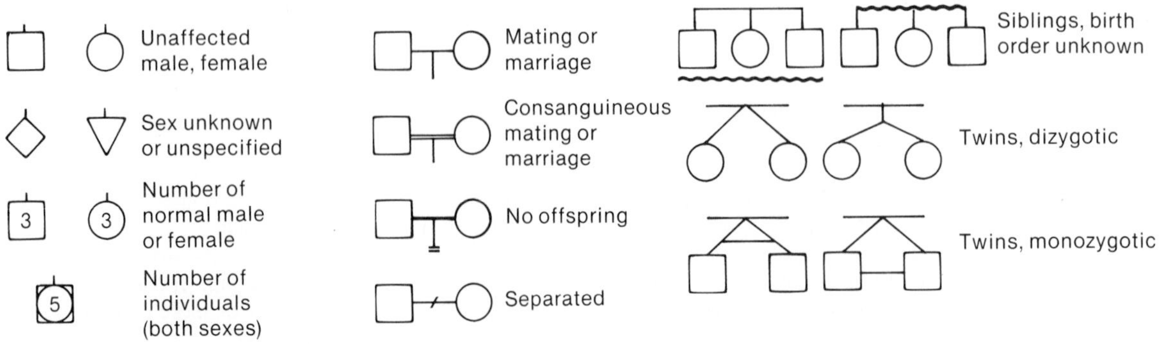

FIGURE A-1

Common pedigree symbols. If symbols other than these are used, add to the pedigree a key to explain their meaning.

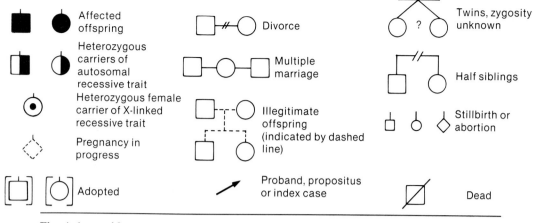

	Affected offspring		Divorce		Twins, zygosity unknown

Heterozygous carriers of autosomal recessive trait

Multiple marriage

Half siblings

Heterozygous female carrier of X-linked recessive trait

Illegitimate offspring (indicated by dashed line)

Stillbirth or abortion

Pregnancy in progress

Adopted

Proband, propositus or index case

Dead

Fig. A-1, cont'd.

A3—HEALTH ASSESSMENT FOR NURSE-FAMILY ENCOUNTERS: SELECTED AGES*
(Chapters 28 and 29)

Health history physical exam	Nutrition	Development	Commonly recommended laboratory procedures and immunizations
FIRST INFANT ENCOUNTER			
Prenatal concerns Prenatal history Birth history Neonatal history History of familial diseases Interval history Family and social history Length, weight, and head circumference Complete physical exam Discussion of normal variants and abnormal physical findings with parents	Assess caloric needs for optimal growth: 100-110 cal/kg/day Discuss need for iron, vitamins, fluoride Discuss current feeding methods	2 weeks: sucking and rooting reflexes, Moro reflex, and tonic neck reflex (TNR) Sensitive to light and noise One month: responds to bell, eyes follow to midline, regards face, lifts head when prone	Urine ferric chloride for PKU Discuss PKU with parents Discuss immunization schedule and its importance
HEALTH ASSESSMENT AT 5 TO 9 WEEKS			
Parental concerns Interval history to include past illnesses, eating, sleeping, elimination, behavior Family and social history Length, weight, and head circumference Complete physical exam Discussion of findings with parents	Assess caloric needs for optimal growth Discuss parental attitudes and expectations re: solids Discuss need for water	5 weeks: rooting and Moro reflexes and TNR May "smile" Fist to mouth Follows light; tracks sound 9 weeks: smiles, vocalizes, hands to midline, listens, follows light past midline, holds head up 90° in prone position	Diphtheria, tetanus, pertussis vaccine (DTP) Trivalent oral polio vaccine (TOPV)
HEALTH ASSESSMENT AT 2½ TO 4 MONTHS			
Parental concerns Interval history Family and social history Length, weight, and head circumference Complete physical exam Discussion of findings with parents	Continued need for iron-enriched formula Digestive system now mature enough to handle solids Introduction of cereal, fruits at 4 months	2½ months: holds head and chest to 90° in prone position Laughs, babbles TNR and moro reflex diminishing	DTP and TOPV No. 2

*Modified from Chow MP, et al.: Handbook of pediatric primary care, New York, 1979, John Wiley & Sons, Inc.

A3—HEALTH ASSESSMENT FOR NURSE-FAMILY ENCOUNTERS: SELECTED AGES—cont'd
(Chapters 28 and 29)

Health history physical exam	Nutrition	Development	Commonly recommended laboratory procedures and immunizations
HEALTH ASSESSMENT AT 2½ TO 4 MONTHS—cont'd	Teething biscuits may be used; avoid wheat products	4 months: holds head erect and steady in sitting position Bears weight on legs May roll over, do not leave unattended	
HEALTH ASSESSMENT AT 6 MONTHS			
Parental concerns Interval history Family and social history Length, weight, and head circumference Complete physical exam, including eye cover test for strabismus Discussion of findings with parents	Limit milk to 24 oz/24 hr Discuss iron-containing foods, finger foods Advise waiting to wean until after 1 year Discuss fluoride, avoidance of sugared foods Discuss cleaning of teeth Avoid all bottle propping	Laughs, babbles Passes object from hand to hand and mouths objects—permit no small objects or toys Tooth eruption Turns to voice Rolls over, may get to sitting position Beginning stranger anxiety Stronger attachment to mother	DTP and TOPV No. 3
HEALTH ASSESSMENT AT 9 MONTHS			
Parental concerns Interval history Family and social history Length, weight, and head circumference Complete physical exam, including hearing assessment (infant should turn head at least 45° to locate sound) Discussion of findings with parents	Advise 3 meals/day May introduce cup if child ready; advise waiting to wean until after 1 year Normal drop in appetite Restriction of sugared foods, milk, and juices in bedtime bottles Advise having ipecac syrup on hand	Jabber, babbles Thumb-finger grasp Imitates speech sounds Plays pat-a-cake May pull to stand and/or crawl—secure furniture, knickknacks; cover outlets	Hematocrit, hemoglobin, and RBC indices Sickle cell and G-6 PD screening No immunizations if up to date
HEALTH ASSESSMENT AT 12 MONTHS			
Parental concerns Interval history Family and social history Length, weight, and head circumference Complete physical exam Discussion of findings with parents	Review basic food groups, table foods, and amounts appropriate for age Lessened appetite Milk limited to 16-20 oz/24 hr Avoidance of sugared foods and drinks Discuss weaning from bottle	Indicates wants Drinks from cup Pincer grasp May use spoon Ma-ma, da-da Crawls, walks holding on or alone—time to childproof home	Urinalysis Hemogram if not obtained sooner Tuberculin test

Continued.

A3—HEALTH ASSESSMENT FOR NURSE-FAMILY ENCOUNTERS: SELECTED AGES—cont'd
(Chapters 28 and 29)

Health history physical exam	Nutrition	Development	Commonly recommended laboratory procedures and immunizations
HEALTH ASSESSMENT AT 15 TO 18 MONTHS			
Parental concerns Interval history Family and social history Height and weight Complete physical exam Discussion of findings with parents	Review basic food groups Stress need for iron and avoidance of sugared foods and drinks May feed self Discuss dental care	More than 5-6 words Uses spoon Scribbles on paper Points to one or more parts of body Climbing, running	PRP-D (Haemophilus b diphtheria toxoid conjugate) vaccine at 15 months Measles, mumps, and rubella (MMR) vaccine at 15 months DTP and TOPV No. 4 at 18 months if No. 3 was given at 6 months
HEALTH ASSESSMENT AT 2 YEARS			
Parental concerns Interval history Family and social history Height, weight, and head circumference Complete physical exam Discussion of findings with parents	Review basic food groups and appropriate amounts for age Reduce milk intake to 16 oz/24 hr Discuss importance of proper snacks (low sugar, high protein) Discuss teaching use of toothbrush	May talk well and follow directions Purposeful markings on paper Balances 4 blocks Performs simple household tasks Later may throw ball overhand	Urinalysis if not done earlier
HEALTH ASSESSMENT AT 3 YEARS			
Parental concerns Interval history Family and social history Height and weight; blood pressure Complete physical exam Vision screening Hearing screening Language screening (Denver Articulation Screening Examination [DASE]) Discussion of findings with parents	Review basic food groups and appropriate amounts for age Discuss proper snack foods Eating patterns are influenced by family members Discuss dental visit	Talks well, uses plurals Jumps, runs Pedals tricycle Washes and dries hands Separates from mother easily	Tuberculin skin test Urinalysis for girls Hemoglobin or hematocrit
HEALTH ASSESSMENT AT 4 YEARS			
Parental concerns Interval history Family and social history Height and weight; blood pressure Complete physical exam Vision screening Hearing screening Discussion of findings with parents Assess preschool readiness (PRESS)	Review basic food groups and appropriate amount for age Continued need for iron-containing foods Avoidance of sugared snacks and drinks	Knows first and last names Copies circles and crosses Understands prepositions and opposites May dress self Separates from mother easily Heel-to-toe walk	Hematocrit and RBC indices Tuberculin skin test, if not done at 3 years
HEALTH ASSESSMENT AT 5 TO 10 YEARS			
Parental and client concerns Interval history: illnesses, injuries, major changes in lifestyle Review of systems Family and social history Weight, height, blood pressure,	Basic food groups: milk, 3 servings; meat (including poultry, fish, eggs, peanut butter, dried beans), 4 servings; fruits, vegetables, 4 servings; breads,	5-6 years: balance on one foot for 10 seconds; backward heel-to-toe-walk; draws person with more than 6 parts; performs self-care activities	DTP and trivalent OPV boosters are given between 4 and 6 years of age Tuberculin testing every 3 years

Continued.

A3—HEALTH ASSESSMENT FOR NURSE-FAMILY ENCOUNTERS: SELECTED AGES—cont'd
(Chapters 28 and 29)

Health history physical exam	Nutrition	Development	Commonly recommended laboratory procedures and immunizations
pulse, and respiration Complete physical exam Discussion of findings with parents and client Screening: visual acuity and audiogram, language (DASE)	cereals, 4 servings Food likes and dislikes Types of food used for snacking Sugar intake Other considerations: milk fortified with vitamin D; iodized salt; whole grain or enriched breads and cereals; evaluate calcium fluoride, iron source Discuss preventive dental care	6-9 years: latency period of physical and psychological growth; questions about sex and conception 9-11 years: concrete thinking continues; judges thoughts only in reference to own experience, learns by trial and error Beginning growth spurt: females at approximately 9½ years and males at approximately 10½ years Females: beginning growth of pubic hair and breast budding; tomboy activities Males: male-dominated social activity	Routine urinalysis and complete blood count if not done within the last 3 years

HEALTH ASSESSMENT AT 11 TO 14 YEARS

Past history: birth, maternal medications during pregnancy, developmental milestones, illnesses, injuries, immunizations, communicable diseases, family history Present history: client and parental concerns, history of current concern, nutrition; social: relationships with peers, school marks, social interests, future goals, sexual information and activity Review of systems Complete physical exam is done including weight, height, blood pressure, pulse, and respiration; pelvic exam if indicated Screening: visual acuity and audiogram	Eating habits: number of regular meals a day, snacking pattern and types of food; use of crash diets, fasting, food fads; source of protein and iron; knowledge of balanced food choices; availability of nutritious snacking foods Discuss need for continued dental care	Hormonal influences: as a defense mechanism against changing body image there are increased somatic complaints Males: beginning growth of pubic hair, enlargement of testicles; wet dreams Females: continued breast development, growth of axillary and pubic hair Thought process: beginning of abstract thinking to manipulate concepts outside of own experience; self-centered (egocentrism); feelings of autonomy, mood swings, antisocial behavior Family: negativism as a manifestation of rejection of parents' values and seeking own identity, testing of parental controls, beginning emancipation from family Peers: importance of peer group for psychologic support and social development	Td and TOPV boosters TB test Routine urinalysis Complete blood count (CBC) Rubella titer (females) VDRL Pap smear and gonorrhea cervical culture if sexually active (females) Sickle cell screening if indicated Vision testing Audiometry Gonorrhea and chlamydia, serologic test for syphillis if sexually active Liver function tests are Hepatitis B surface antigen and antibody if sexually active homosexual male or drug and/or alcohol-using adolescent

Continued.

A3—HEALTH ASSESSMENT FOR NURSE-FAMILY ENCOUNTERS: SELECTED AGES—cont'd
(Chapters 28 and 29)

Health history physical exam	Nutrition	Development	Commonly recommended laboratory procedures and immunizations
HEALTH ASSESSMENT AT 15 TO 18 YEARS Health history Complete physical exam is done including weight, height, blood pressure, pulse, and respiration; pelvic exam if indicated	Basic food groups Eating habits Continued dental care	Hormonal influences: continued development of secondary sexual characteristics Males: increased size of penis, testes, scrotum	Td and TOPV boosters if not given within the last 10 years Routine urinalysis and CBC if not done within the last 3 years
HEALTH ASSESSMENT AT 15 TO 18 YEARS—cont'd Screening: visual acuity and audiogram		growth of body hair; voice and skin changes Females: enlarged breasts, broadened pelvic bones, growth of body hair, menstruation Thought process: use of formal logic in solving problems; feelings and goals directed away from self toward idealistic causes; future goals become more clear Family: movement away from family into own relationships and activities; views family's morals and culture with criticism because of idealism Peers: regular group social activity and/or individual dating	Rubella titer (females) VDRL Pap smear and gonorrhea cervical culture if sexually active (females) Sickle cell screening if indicated Vision testing Audiometry Gonorrhea and chlamydia, serologic testing for syphilis if sexually active. Liver function tests and hepatitis B surface antigen and antibody if sexually active homosexual male or drug and/or alcohol-user.

A4—DIET HISTORY QUESTIONNAIRE FOR INFANTS THROUGH TEENAGERS*
(Chapters 28 and 29)

Questionnaire I—Infants (Birth to 1 Year)

Date _____ Age _____

Name _____ Birth date _____

Please answer the following questions by checking the appropriate box or filling in the blank. Answer only those questions that apply to you or your child. All information is confidential.

1. Is the baby breast fed: Yes __ No __
   If yes does he/she also receive milk or formula?
   Yes __ No __
   If yes, what kind? _____

2. Does the baby receive formula? Yes __ No __
   If yes: Ready-to-feed   __
   Concentrated liquid __
   Powdered   __
   Evaporated milk   __
   Other _____
   How is formula prepared? _____
   Is the formula iron fortified? _____
   Yes __ No __
   Don't know __

3. Does the baby drink milk? Yes __ No __
   If yes: Whole milk __
   2% milk   __
   Skim milk   __
   Other _____

4. Does the baby drink any fluids other than milk or formula?
   Yes __ No __
   If yes, what? _____

*For Bureau of Maternal and Child Health/Nutrition: Diet history questionnaire for infants, Washington, D.C., 1985.

5. How many times does the baby eat each day, including milk or formula feedings? _____

6. Does the baby usually take a bottle to bed?
Yes ___ No ___
If yes, what is usually in the bottle? _____

7. If the baby drinks milk or formula, what is the usual amount in a day?
Less than 16 oz (2 cups)   ___
16 to 32 oz   ___
More than 32 oz (1 quart)   ___

8. Does the baby take vitamin or iron drops?
Yes ___ No ___
If yes, how often? ___ What kind? _____

9. Is the baby on a special diet now?   Yes ___ No___
If yes: Allergy   ___
         Weight reduction   ___
         Other _____
Who recommended the diet? _____

10. Does the baby eat clay, paint chips, dirt, paper, or anything else that is not considered food?
Yes ___ No ___
If yes, what? _____ How often?_____

11. Do you think the child has a feeding problem?
Yes ___ No ___
If yes, describe _____

12. Who usually feeds the baby? _____
Does the person have the use of:
Working stove ___
Refrigerator   ___
Piped water   ___

13. Does the family participate in
Food stamp program   Yes ___ No ___
WIC program   Yes ___ No ___
Day care food program   Yes ___ No ___

14. Please check which, if any, of the following foods the baby eats and how often.

	LESS THAN ONCE A WEEK	NOT DAILY BUT AT LEAST ONCE A WEEK	EVERY DAY OR NEARLY EVERY DAY
Cheese, yogurt, ice cream, pudding	___	___	___
Milk or formula	___	___	___
Eggs	___	___	___
Dried beans, peas, peanut butter, nuts	___	___	___
Meat, fish, poultry, wild game	___	___	___
Bread, rice, grits, cereal, tortillas, noodles, spaghetti	___	___	___
Fruits or fruit juices	___	___	___
Vegetables (including potatoes)	___	___	___
Candy, desserts, sweets	___	___	___

15. If the baby eats fruits or drinks fruit juices every day or nearly every day, which ones does he/she eat or drink most often (not more than three)?
_____   _____   _____

16. If the baby eats vegetables every day or nearly every day, which ones does he/she eat most often (not more than three)?
_____   _____   _____

17. Does the baby eat:
Sticky or sweet foods? Yes ___ No ___
Salty foods?   Yes ___ No ___
If yes, what are the foods? _____
_____

Is salt added to the baby's food?   Yes ___ No ___

18. Below list the foods and beverages the baby has had during the last 24 hours.

Time	Food eaten	Amount	How is this food prepared?

Questionnaire II—Preschool and Young School-Age Child (Guardian Responds)

Date _____ Age _____
Name _____ Birth date _____

Please answer the following questions by checking the appropriate box or filling in the blank. Answer only those questions that apply to you or your child. All information is confidential.

1. Does the child drink milk?   Yes ___ No ___
If yes: Whole milk ___
         2% milk   ___
         Skim milk   ___
         Other _____
If yes: Less than 8 oz (1 cup)   ___
         8-32 oz   ___
         More than 32 oz (1 qt)   ___

2. Does the child drink anything from a bottle?
Yes ___ No ___
If yes: Milk ___
         Other _____
Does the child take a bottle to bed?   Yes ___ No___
If yes, what is usually in the bottle?
_____

3. How many times a day does the child usually eat, including snacks? _____
Does the child eat anything after he/she has gone to bed?
Yes ___ No ___
If yes, what? _____

4. Does the child take vitamins or iron?
   Yes ___ No ___
   If yes, how often? _____
   What kind? _____

5. Is the child on a special diet now?   Yes ___ No ___
   If yes: Allergy   ___
           Weight reduction   ___
           Other _____
   Who recommended the diet? _____

6. Does the child eat clay, paint chips, dirt, paper, or anything else not usually considered food?
   Yes ___ No ___
   If yes, what? _____ How often? _____

7. How would you describe the child's appetite?
       Good ___
       Fair ___
       Poor ___
       Other (specify) _____

8. Who usually feeds the child? _____
   Does this person have use of:
       Working stove ___
       Refrigeration ___
       Piped water ___

9. Does the family participate in:
       Food stamp program   Yes ___ No ___
       WIC program   Yes ___ No ___
   Does the child participate in:
       School breakfast   Yes ___ No ___
       School lunch   Yes ___ No ___
       Day care food program Yes ___ No ___
       Summer food program   Yes ___ No ___

10. Please check which, if any, of the following foods the child eats and how often.

	LESS THAN ONCE A WEEK	NOT DAILY BUT AT LEAST ONCE A WEEK	EVERY DAY OR NEARLY EVERY DAY
Cheese, yogurt, ice cream, pudding	___	___	___
Milk	___	___	___
Eggs	___	___	___
Dried beans, peas, peanut butter, nuts	___	___	___
Meat, fish, poultry, wild game	___	___	___
Bread, rice, grits, cereal, tortillas, noodles, spaghetti	___	___	___
Fruits or fruit juices	___	___	___
Vegetables (including potatoes)	___	___	___
Candy, desserts, sweets	___	___	___

11. If the child eats fruits or drinks fruit juices every day or nearly every day, which ones does he/she eat or drink most often (not more than three)?
    _____ _____ _____

12. If the child eats vegetables every day or nearly every day, which ones does he/she eat most often (not more than three)?
    _____ _____ _____

13. Does the child usually eat between meals?
    Yes ___ No ___
    If yes, name the two or three snacks (including bedtime snacks) that the child has most often.
    _____ _____ _____

14. Does the child eat:
    Sticky or sweet foods? Yes ___ No ___
    Salty foods?   Yes ___ No ___
    If yes, what are the foods? _____
    _____
    Is salt added to the child's food?   Yes ___ No ___

15. Below list the foods and beverages the child has had during the last 24 hours.

Time	Food eaten	Amount	How is this food prepared?

Questionnaire III—School-Age Child and Teenager

Date _____ Age _____
Name _____ Birth date _____

Please answer the following questions by checking the appropriate box or filling in the blank. Answer only those questions that apply to you or your child. All information is confidential.

1. Do you drink milk?   Yes ___ No ___
   If yes: Whole milk ___
           2% milk   ___
           Skim milk ___
           Other _____
   How often? _____
   Are there other beverages you often drink?
   Yes ___ No ___
   If yes, what? _____

2. How many times a day do you eat, including snacks?
   _____

3. Do you take vitamins or iron?
   Yes ___ No ___
   If yes, how often? _____ What kind? _____

4. Are you on a special diet now?   Yes ___ No ___
   If yes: Allergy   ___
           Weight reduction   ___
           Other _____
   Who recommended the diet? _____

5. Do you eat clay, paint chips, dirt, paper, or anything else not usually considered food? Yes ___ No ___
   If yes, what? _____ How often?_____

6. Does anyone in your household participate in:
   Food stamp program   Yes ___ No ___
   WIC program   Yes ___ No ___
   Do you participate in:
   School breakfast   Yes ___ No ___
   School lunch   Yes ___ No ___
   Summer food program   Yes ___ No ___

7. Who usually prepares your meals? _____
   Does this person have use of:
   Working stove ___
   Refrigerator ___
   Piped water   ___

8. Do you eat any:
   Sticky or sweet foods? Yes ___ No ___
   Salty foods?   Yes ___ No ___
   Do you add salt to your food?   Yes ___ No ___

9. Please check which, of the following foods you eat and how often:

	LESS THAN ONCE A WEEK	NOT DAILY BUT AT LEAST ONCE A WEEK	EVERY DAY OR NEARLY EVERY DAY
Cheese, yogurt, ice cream, pudding	—	—	—
Milk	—	—	—
Eggs	—	—	—
Dried beans, peas, peanut butter, nuts	—	—	—
Meat, fish, poultry, wild game	—	—	—
Bread, rice, grits, cereal, tortillas, noodles, spaghetti	—	—	—
Fruits or fruit juices	—	—	—
Vegetables (including potatoes)	—	—	—
Candy, desserts, sweets	—	—	—

10. If you eat fruits or drinks fruit juices every day or nearly every day, which ones does he/she eat or drink most often (not more than three)?

    _____ _____ _____

11. If you eat vegetables every day or nearly every day, which ones does he/she eat most often (not more than three)?

    _____ _____ _____

12. Do you usually eat between meals?
    Yes ___ No ___
    If yes, name the two or three snacks (including bedtime snacks) that the child has most often.

    _____ _____ _____

13. Below list the foods and beverages you have had in the last 24 hours.

Time	Food eaten	Amount	How is this food prepared?

A5—NEEDS SATISFACTION SCALE FOR INDIVIDUALS WITH A DISABILITY
(Chapter 30)

Section A: Demographic Data

Name _____
Address _____
Telephone _____
Social Security no. _____
Age _____ Birth date ____ ____ ____
                                Month Day Year

Sex ___ F ___ M
Date of interview _____
Primary disability _____
Secondary disabilities _____

Marital status
___ Married   ___ Never married
___ Separated   ___ Divorced
___ Widowed   ___ Marriage annulled

Education
___ None
___ 1-5 grade
___ 6-8 grade
___ 9-12
___ High school graduate
___ Vocational-technical without licensure/certification
___ Vocational-technical with licensure/certification
___ Attended college 1-2 years
___ Attended college 3-4 years
___ 4-year college degree
___ Graduate degree (master's)
___ Graduate degree (doctorate)

Number of dependents
___ Self only   ___ 3
___ 1   ___ 4
___ 2   ___ 5 or more

Heritage
___ African American   ___ Pacific Islander
___ Caucasian   ___ Hispanic
___ Native American   ___ Other
___ Asian

Living arrangement
___ Living alone
___ Living with spouse
___ Living with one or both parents (including step-parents)
___ Living with nonrelatives
___ Living with other relatives
___ Other

Names and relationships of household members

_____
_____
_____
_____
_____
_____
_____

Military status
___ Previous military service
___ Currently in the military
___ Never in the military

Income sources
___ Earnings
___ Interest
___ Rent
___ Dividends
___ Private insurance, disability benefits
___ Family
___ Friends

___ Private agency
___ Annuities
___ Public assistance, state
___ Workman's Compensation
___ Social Security
___ Public assistance, federal

Income category
___ $0-3,000
___ $3,100-6,000
___ $6,100-9,000
___ $9,100-12,000
___ $12,100-15,000

___ $15,000-18,000
___ $18,100-21,000
___ $21,100-24,000
___ Above $24,000

Work status
___ Employed outside the home
   ___ Competitive labor market
   ___ Sheltered workshop
___ Employed, home
___ Unemployed

___ Self-employed, home
___ Self-employed, outside home
___ Homemaker
___ Student
___ Retired

Pervious occupation
___ Professional
___ Technical

___ Laborer
___ Semiprofessional
___ Nontechnical

Currently under the services of
___ Vocational Rehabilitation Services
   ___ Regular
   ___ Homebound

___ Medicaid
___ Medicare
___ Crippled Children's Service

Source of transportation
___ Private automobile
___ Private van, specially equipped

___ Public
___ None

Main care giver
___ Self
___ Family member

___ Full-time attendant
___ Part-time attendant

My birth order position is _____
                                         (rank)

in a family of _____
             (total no. of children)

Sexes of children in the family are: M ___   F ___
                                        (no.) (no.)

Functional abilities	Yes	No	N/A
Dress self			
Feed self, unassisted			
Feed self with assistance			
Brush teeth			
Comb hair			
Self-help, bowel elimination			
Self-help, bladder elimination			
Bathe self			
Walk			
Other independent mobility			

Section B: Satisfaction of Needs

Directions: Please choose the response that most nearly describes your answer to the question regarding your present needs.

Basic physiological needs

1. My current state of health is ___ Poor ___ Fair
                                        1   2
   ___ Satisfactory ___ Good ___ Excellent
     3   4   5

2. Rate each of the following health needs on a scale from 1 to 5 (1—extremely problematic, 2—somewhat problematic, 3—controlled problem, 4—inactive problem, 5—no problem).

	1	2	3	4	5
a. Vision					
b. Hearing					
c. Mobility					
d. Respirations					
e. Sleep					
f. Anxiety; depression					
g. Energy level					
h. Nutrition—food intake					
i. Nutrition—fluid intake					
j. Bowel elimination					
k. Bladder elimination					
l. Exercise					
m. Recreation, play					
n. Sexual libido					

Rate the following items on a scale from 1 to 5 (1—never, 2—hardly ever, 3—sometimes, 4—often, 5—almost all the time).

	1	2	3	4	5
3. I drink 2000-3000 cc of fluid per day.					
4. I eat a well-balanced diet.					
5. I take vitamins as prescribed.					
6. I avoid smoking cigarettes, cigars, and pipes.					
7. I drink alcoholic beverages only as prescribed.					
8. I take prescribed medicines.					
9. I take patent medicines only as directed by my physician.					
10. I have ROM or other exercises daily.					
11. I get 6-8 hours sleep minimum daily.					
12. I take rest periods during the day.					
13. I experience a high energy level.					
14. My bowel elimination habits are satisfactory.					
15. My urinary elmination habits are satisfactory.					
16. I keep my immunizations up to date.					
17. I practice regular dental care daily.					
18. I watch myself for signs of cancer.					
19. I have visual examinations as suggested by physician.					
20. I am able to relax.					
21. I take special measures to conserve my health.					
22. I do not object to having to take special measures to conserve my health.					
23. I do not object to giving up things I like for the sake of my health.					
24. I am confident I can meet my future health needs.					

Need for security

	1	2	3	4	5
25. I am secure about my physical safety in my home environment.					
26. I feel secure about special precautions I take regarding physical safety.					
27. I feel secure about my financial position.					
28. I feel secure about meeting the expenses of my routine medicine and supplies.					

	1	2	3	4	5
29. I feel satisfied about my transportation plans.					
30. I am satisfied about long-term plans for my care.					
31. I am satisfied with my present vocational/occupational status.					

Need for love and belongingness

	1	2	3	4	5
32. I am satisfied with the amount of love from family.					
33. I am satisfied with the amount of love from friends.					
34. I cope satisfactorily with stress in the home life.					
35. I cope satisfactorily with stress in other aspects of life.					
36. I am satisfied with my level of social effectiveness.					
37. I am satisfied with my social participation.					
38. I am comfortable asking for help when needed.					
39. I am satisfied with the amount of religion in my life.					
40. I am satisfied with family activities and traditions in which I participate.					
41. I am satisfied with my role in the family.					
42. I am satisfied with my level of sexual fulfillment.					
43. I am satisfied with my level of knowledge about human sexuality.					
44. I am satisfied with the feelings of love and belongingness I receive from others.					
45. I am satisfied with the feelings of love and belongingness I give to others.					
46. I have get-togethers with friends my own age.					

Need for self-esteem

	1	2	3	4	5
47. I am satisfied with the appearance of my body.					
48. I am satisfied with my intellectual functioning.					
49. I am satisfied with the kind of characteristics that could be said to describe me.					
50. I am satisfied with past accomplishments in my life.					
51. I am satisfied with present accomplishments in my life.					
52. My predominant emotional state is happy and content.					
53. I am satisfied with my level of education/occupation.					

	1	2	3	4	5

Need for self-actualization

54. I am satisfied with my state of fulfillment.

55. I am satisfied with the amount of enjoyment in my everyday life.

56. I make plans to increase my level of fulfillment.

57. I am optimistic about my potential to reach higher life.

58. I am satisfied with task accomplishment in my present life.

59. I am satisfied with my own motivational level.

60. I am satisfied with motivational level of family and friends to support my goals.

61. I am satisfied with amount of responsibilities I have in life.

62. I am satisfied with the amount of spontaneity in life.

63. I have a satisfactory level of hope in my life.

64. I have new interests in life.

65. I am satisfied with the amount of meaning and purpose in my life.

66. I am reconciled to the change in my life-style from the disability I have.

67. I am satisfied with my coping reaction to suffering.

68. I am satisfied with amount of strength (courage) I have now.

Needs	Client score	Possible score	Percentage
Basic physiological		185	
Security		35	
Love and belonging ness		75	
Self-esteem		35	
Self-actualization		75	
TOTALS		405	

A6—KATZ INDEX OF INDEPENDENCE IN ACTIVITIES OF DAILY LIVING
(Chapter 22; see Figure 22-5, p. 385)

B1—FAMILY HEALTH CARE PLAN*
(Chapter 26)

Goal: To reduce the risk of hypertension in the family

Objectives

To reduce by ⅓ to ½ the salt (sodium) intake of both family members within 5 weeks

Target activities

a. Will use only ½ as much salt in cooking at once
b. In 1 week will no longer add salt to foods at the table
c. Will increase by 50% the use of herbs, spices, and lemon in cooking in place of salt by the end of 1 week
d. Will avoid snack foods with visible salt by end of 1 week
e. Will avoid all foods prepared in brine (e.g., ham, bacon, pickles) within 2 weeks
f. Will stop drinking carbonated beverages within 3 weeks
g. Will start using salt (sodium)-free vegetables (fresh, frozen, canned) after present canned vegetable supply is depleted

Formative Evaluation

Family and community health nurse together measure progress made toward accomplishing target activities at check points.

At end of week 1 measure the following
Progress toward meeting target activities, a, b, c, and d
Problems encountered meeting target activities
FINDING
Husband having difficulty meeting target activity b
PLAN
Obective b modified from 1 week to 2 weeks
Plan developed for a health counseling visit

At end of week 2 measure the following
Progress made toward meeting activity e
Husband's progress toward meeting activity b
Continuing ability to meet activities a, b (wife), and d

At end of week 3 measure the following
Progress made toward meeting activity f
Continuing ability to meet all other activities except g (because of canned vegetable supply on hand)

At end of week 4 measure the following
Continuing ability to meet activities

---

*Sample of an approach to a health care plan for a family consisting of a middle-aged husband and wife. The family health care plan is completed by adding objectives and target activities regarding stress, weight, and exercise.
Developed by R. Johnson. Ed 1 for Stanhope & Lancaster.

Summative Evaluation

Conducted by family and community health nurse at time when care plan fully implemented and executed. Measures extent to which the objective and target activities were met at end of 5 weeks. Also examine problems encountered in meeting target activities.

B2—FAMILY–COMMUNITY HEALTH NURSE CONTRACT
(Chapter 27)

Family health situation: Family members at high risk for hypertension.
Goal: To increase the family's knowledge about hypertension and low-sodium foods

FAMILY RESPONSIBILITIES (HUSBAND AND WIFE)	NURSE'S RESPONSIBILITIES
1. Demonstrate increased knowledge about hypertension Explain (from a lay perspective) the physiology of hypertension and attending risks Explain the relationship between preventive measures and reducing the risk of hypertension	1. Provide information to family about hypertension Provide reading materials about hypertension and related self-care Counsel with the family regarding the physiology and risks associated with hypertension; describe preventive measures (e.g., life-style changes)
2. Demonstrate increased knowledge about low-sodium foods Able to list common high-sodium and low-sodium foods Modifies food purchasing habits so more low-sodium foods included and more high-sodium foods excluded Uses low-sodium recipes Increasingly uses low-sodium menus	2. Provide information to family about low-sodium foods: Provide lists of high-sodium and low-sodium foods Provide low-sodium recipes and menus congruent with family's resources and life-style

Length of contract _____
Date started _____ Date concluded _____
Evaluation plan _____

We mutually agree to the above goal and responsibilities. This contract may be renegotiated if it becomes necessary to do so.
Signatures:
Family members _____ Date _____
_____ Date _____
Community _____ Date _____
health nurse

B3—FAMILY HEALTH ASSESSMENT GUIDE
(Chapter 26)

General instructions: Content areas of the guide should be modified and adapted as appropriate for individual families and the circumstances of the family and/or community health nurse contact(s). The factors listed for many of the major family assessment areas are examples and should be added to or omitted as necessary.

Family Unit
Family Composition (see accompanying box)

Extended family (e.g., parents, children, and other relative outside of household)
  Relationship
  Place of residency
  Frequency of contact
Residential history
  Length of time at present address
  Frequency of residential and geographical changes
Education of family member (present and/or highest level attained)
  Educational level
  Attending school/college
  Educational goal
Vocational interests of family member
  Interest
  Goal
Avocational interests of family member (hobbies, other creative endeavors)
  Interest
  Goal
Occupation of family member
  Type of work
  Hours of work
  Satisfaction with job
  Goal(s)
Financial resources
  Sources (e.g., salaries, pension, and public assistance)
  Total income
  Distribution of income (e.g., housing, food, clothing, health/illness care, utilities, recreation, and insurance)
  Adequacy of income
Religious practices of family members
  Religious preferences
  Extent of involvement
  Relative importance of religion in everyday life (e.g., influence on activities of daily living and relationships)
Rituals
  Holidays and celebrations related to activities of daily living

Recreational interests of family members
  Interests around home (alone and with family)
  Interests outside home (alone and with family)
  Activities with relatives
  With friends
  With community groups
  What does the family do for "fun" around home? Outside of home?

Family Environment
Residence

Housing
  Type of dwelling
  Number and types of rooms
  General condition
Furnishings
  Condition
  Adequacy
Living space
  Adequate for family size
  Privacy for family members
Sleeping arrangements
  Where members sleep
  Sharing of bed(s)
  Adequacy of sleeping arrangements
Bathroom facilities
  Location
  Adequacy
  Sanitation
Food preparation arrangements
  Cleanliness
  Cooking
  Refrigeration
Eating arrangements and mealtime environment
General state of cleanliness and sanitation
Adequacy of
  Water supply and source
  Waste/garbage disposal
  Lighting
  Heating and cooling
  Ventilation
  Laundry facilities
  Telephone
Condition of yard
Pets
  Number
  Kinds
  Care

Family member	Age	Sex	Ethnicity/race	Family position (e.g., mother, spouse)	Special status (e.g., adopted, single, divorced)
_____	___	___	_____	_____	_____
_____	___	___	_____	_____	_____
_____	___	___	_____	_____	_____

Automobile
  Number
  Conditions
Provisions for emergencies
  Smoke alarm
  Emergency numbers by telephone
Environmental stressors
  Noise
  Lack of individual territory
Environmental hazards
  Storage of medicines and household cleaners/poisons
  Sharp tools
  Fire dangers
  Unsafe toys
  Loose rugs
  Clutter
  Swimming pool
Family attitudes toward home, neighborhood, and community

Goals for Future
Neighborhood

Type
  Residential
  Semicommercial
  Urban/nonmetropolitan
Dwellings
  Single-family house
  Apartment
  Combination
Age of area
  Newly constructed
  Deteriorating
  Foilage (trees, shrubbery)
Sociocultural characteristics
  Age composition
  Ethnic groups
  Employment/unemployment
General condition of structures, yards, streets, alleys, etc.
Traffic patterns
Efficiency of street lighting systems
Availability of fire hydrants
Resources
  Shopping
  Transportation
  Recreational
  Educational
  Religious
  Protective services
  Health/illness
  Emergency
  Human services
  Business
  Garbage/refuse disposal
Environmental stressors
  Noise
  Crime rate
  Substance abuse
  Crowding
  Poverty

Environmental hazards
  Air pollution
  Garbage/debris
  Traffic flow
  Unsafe play areas
In-migration and out-migration of residents
Neighbors' attitude toward the family
Famiy's involvement in the neighborhood

Community

Leadership and government
Resources (essentially the same as those listed for neighborhood)
Occupations, industries, businesses
Family's involvement in the community
  Community memberships
  Interaction with social institutions
  Use of resources

Family Structure

Organization
  As a system
  Subsystems
Roles
  Roles being filled
  Satisfaction/dissatisfaction with role(s)
  Level of role functioning
  Perceptions about roles
  Acceptance of roles
  Flexibility of roles/interchangeable
Socialization processes for roles
Division of labor
  How is delegation of tasks determined?
  Who carries out which tasks?
  What is the flexibility of task responsibilities?
  What is the extent of satisfaction/dissatisfaction with task delegation and performance?
Authority and power
  Degree of autonomy for each family member
  Locus of authority
  Power relationships
  How authority is exercised
  How power is demonstrated
  Satisfaction/dissatisfaction with autonomy, authority, and power in family
Values, attitudes, and beliefs regarding family organization, roles, division of labor, autonomy, authority, and power
Stresses related to family organization, roles, division of labor, autonomy, authority, and power—how handled?

Family Processes
Communication

Patterns
  Ways used to communicate effectively
  Content of communications
  Interpretation of content
  Linguistic characteristics (cultural)
  Frequency of communications
  How do joy, love, anger, sadness, frustration get communicated?

Communication patterns within family subsystems

Effectiveness of communications—understood, clear, consistent, etc.

Satisfaction/dissatisfaction with family communication patterns

Values, attitudes and beliefs regarding family communications

Stresses related to family communications

Decision Making

How are decisions made?

What is the process?

Who makes decisions affecting adults?

Children?

Entire group?

How are decisons implemented?

How are decision-making skills learned in the family?

Satisfaction/dissatisfaction with family decision-making process

Values, attitudes, and beliefs regarding family decision making

Stresses related to family decision making

Problem Solving

How are problems handled?

What is the process?

Who is involved in the problem-solving process?

Who provides leadership in the process?

Extent to which family can deal with problem solving and for what types of problems

Flexibility in approaches to problem solving

Ability to use information from outside family in problem-solving process

Satisfaction/dissatisfaction with family's problem-solving ability and process

Values, attitudes, and beliefs regarding family's problem solving

Stresses related to family problem solving

Family Functions
Physical

How are needs for food, shelter, clothing, etc., met?

Are physical needs being met satisfactorily? If not, what solutions have been tried by the family?

Values, attitudes, and beliefs regarding family's physical needs and functions

Stresses related to meeting family's physical needs

Emotional

Affectional relationships

Between adults

Between adults and children

Between siblings

Ways of obtaining and giving emotional support: distribution of support, when given, how given, acceptance by other family member(s)

Ways in which family members do or do not assist each other in developing self-esteem

In developing autonomy

How do family members show respect for each other?

To what extent and how is intimacy expressed?

Physical affection and companionship?

Satisfaction/dissatisfaction regarding how family's emotional needs are met

Values, attitudes, and beliefs regarding family's emotional needs and functions

Stresses related to family's emotional functions

Social

Goals for family and individual family members

Support for individual creativity, initiative, and leadership

Process for developing and supporting family and individual leadership

Process for strengthening family members' competency regarding adjustment in social organizations (e.g., school)

Competency regarding appropriate use of social organizations

Seeking new experiences—king, etc.

Discipline and limit-setting practices

Individual developmental tasks (physical, affective, intellectual, language, psychosocial, sexual, moral, personality)

Level of knowledge

Seeks information as needed

Provides support

Seeks support resources as needed

Adopts socialization approaches to meet individual needs and tasks

Family developmental tasks

Level of knowledge

Seeks information as needed

Intrafamily support

Uses resources as needed

Satisfaction/dissatisfaction regarding social functions

Values, attitudes, and beliefs regarding social functions

Stresses related to social functions

Coping
Conflict

To what extent and how are conflicts expressed covertly and overtly?

Frequency of conflicts? Kinds? Attributed causes?

How are conflicts avoided? How are conflicts resolved?

Satisfaction/dissatisfaction regarding conflict resolution process

Values, attitudes, and beliefs regarding conflict resolution

Stresses related to conflicts and conflict resolution

Life Changes

Recent, present, and anticipated life changes

Impact of change(s) on family's functioning as a unit

Impact of change(s) on family roles and functions

Ability to cope wtih change(s): practices, behaviors, values, attitudes, beliefs

Stresses associated with change(s)

Support Systems

Resources within family—what, how used, when, effectiveness

External support systems—how used, when, effectiveness
  Significant others (e.g., extended family members and friends)
  Nonprofessional organizations
  Professional systems
  Understand how to use—seek relevant information
  Availability, accessibility, use patterns
Satisfaction/dissatisfaction with support systems
Values, attitudes, and beliefs related to using support systems

Life Satisfaction

How does family feel about its quality of life?
What influences family's quality of life?
What influences the family's feelings about life?
Would the family like to change anything about its life? What? What impedes change?
What can family do? Others do?

Health Behavior
Health History

Genetic or familial diseases (e.g., diabetes, heart disease)
Family history of emotional problems, suicide, etc.
Past illnesses, operations, accidents, injuries
Present illnesses and/or physical discomforts
Use of prescribed and/or over-the-counter medications
Present symptoms such as anxiety, depression, etc.
Concerns about hearing, vision, speech
Recent history regarding physical and dental examinations, immunizations, Pap smear, etc.

Health Status

Family's assessment of present health status
Concerns about present health status and/or potential health problems
Family's perceptions of vulnerability to disease/illness
What does the family perceive as a health problem?
What present and potential health problems are identified by the family? Priorities for health problems?
What is family's belief about cause of problem(s)?
What is family's belief(s) about cure/treatment for problem(s)?

Activities of Daily Living

Eating patterns and foods
Personal hygiene and daily grooming
Physical activity
Sleeping behavior
Dental practices
What are family members' daily rhythms (e.g., morning person, night person)?
How does family describe a typical weekday? A weekend?

Risk Behaviors

Inadequate nutritional behavior (overeating; undereating; irregular meals; diet high in sugar, sodium; beverages high in caffeine)
Physical inactivity
Limited sleep or irregular sleeping patterns
Smoking
Use of alcohol

Nonuse of seat belts
Excessive exposure to stress situations (family, work, social)

Health Beliefs

How does family define health? Illness?
How does family define health and illness for each family member?
What value does family assign health? Health promotion? Prevention?
What are family's perceptions about cause(s) of illness?
What are family's perceptions about control over health and illness?
What are family's perceptions about how illness/disease are cured?
What are family's health goals?
How are values, attitudes, and beliefs regarding health promotion communicated to children? What is the socialization process? How does family members' involvement in the community influence family's health values, attitudes, and beliefs?

Self-care

Knowledge
Level of knowledge regarding health promotion, preventive measures, emergency care, causes and treatment of illnesses/diseases
How is health knowledge transmitted to family members?
What are sources of health information?
How does family assess its level of health knowledge?
What would family like to know about health promotion? Prevention? Illness care?
Practices
What does family do to protect its health (physical, emotional, social, spiritual)?
What does family do to improve its health status?
What does family do to prevent illness/disease?
What does family do to generate and support health protective behaviors in family members?
What does family do to care for health problems and illnesses in the home?
How are health and illness care responsibilities distributed in the family? Is there flexibility of family roles and tasks?
What are family's perceptions regarding ability to protect family's health?
How does family care for health problems and illnesses in the home?
What are the family's values, attitudes, and beliefs regarding self-care?
Family planning
Family's values, attitudes, and beliefs regarding family planning (e.g., methods, child spacing, childlessness, and appropriateness for which family members)
Decision-making process
Practices

Health Care Resources

Utilization practices regarding formal informal health and illness care systems (e.g., what systems and frequency of use)

Availability of emergency care resources

Availability, accessibility, and attractiveness of health and illness care resources

Effectiveness and efficiency with which family uses resources

How is health/illness care financed? What are other costs for family such as transportation and work time lost?

Family's knowledge about health and illness care resources

Family's perceptions of and attitudes about experiences with health/illness care resources and health care providers (e.g., nurses and physicians)

What are the family's feelings about the kinds of health services available to them in the community?

What kinds of health services would they like to receive?

What suggestions do they have about making any necessary changes in the delivery of services?

What are the family's feelings about health care providers?

What kind of relationship would the family like to have with health care providers?

What suggestions do they have about helping the health care providers to better meet the needs of the family?

Family's values and beliefs related to health/illness care resources and health care providers

Stresses related to use of health/illness care resources and interactions with health care providers

Community Health Nursing Services

Knowledge about community health nursing

Attitudes toward community health nursing services

Expectations of community health nursing services

Family Health Assessment Summary

Family's sociodemographic profile

Family's environment—strengths and problems regarding home, neighborhood, and community

Family structure, processes, functions—strengths and limitations; existing and/or potential problems

Family's coping profile

Conflict management—strengths and limitations

Life changes—strengths and limitations regarding coping with changes

Support systems—strengths and limitations

Life satisfaction profile

Family's health behavior profile

Health history—existing and/or potential problems

Health status—existing and/or potential problems

Activities of daily living—strengths and limitations/problems

Risk profile—for family unit and family members

Health beliefs—profile of values, attitudes, and beliefs regarding health and illness

Self-care—strengths and limitations

Health care resources—adequacy of availability, accessibility, attractiveness, and use; general practices

Community health nursing services—attitudes and expectations

B4—FAMILY PROBLEM-SOLVING GUIDE*
(Chapter 25)

I. Types of family problems
   A. Problems that can be resolved by the family without the community health nurse
   B. Problems that can be resolved by the family with the community health nurse's assistance
   C. Problems that should be referred to another health care professional or other human services worker

II. Problem-solving process (family and community health nurse)
   A. Assessment of the problem
      1. Who identified problem—family, community health nurse, others?
      2. Extent of problem—is the problem a threat to the health and well-being of the family? An individual family member? Others? The community?
      3. Family's assessment of the problem—seriousness? Implications of the problem for the family? If family did not identify the problem, does the family view the situation as a problem?
      4. Community health nurse's assessment of the problem (using criteria regarding extent of problem)—if the problem is of a threatening nature but not recognized as a problem by the family, the nurse will need to assist the family ro recognize and understand the implications of the problem
   B. Problem solving
      1. What is the history of the problem—when started, how started, why existing, effect on family?
      2. Is family attempting ro resolve or handle problem?
         If yes
         How? How successful is approach? If approach is succeeding, support should be given to the family to continue its efforts.
         If approach is not successful, assist family to explore possible reasons for limited or lack of resolution.
         What other possible approaches has family considered?
         Have any of these approaches been tried with the present situation or similar situations in the past? If so, how effective was the approach? If approach was successful, why? If approach was unsuccessful, why?
         Would an approach used in the past be appropriate for the present situation? Would it meet with some degree of success? Explore possibilities regarding implementation and outcomes.
         If family has considered alternate approaches but has not tried them, family should be assisted to (1) think how approach could be imple-

---

*Developed by R Johnson for Stanhope M and Lancaster J: Community Health Nursing, ed 1.

mented and (2) consider effectiveness of outcomes.

If family perceives that implementation and outcomes will be successful, explore why—is the reasoning realistic? If not, explore other possibilities regarding implementation and outcomes which might be more realistic and workable.

If family perceives that implementation and/or outcomes will be unsuccessful, use same exploratory process as preceding example.

The family should be assisted to explore the implications for each possible approach to decide on the one most effective for the problem situation and the family.

If it becomes necessary for the community health nurse to supplement the family's ideas with other suggested approaches, the same exploratory approach as in the previous example should be used by the family—and the final decision regarding a problem-solving approach resides with the family.

If no (family not attempting to resolve problem)

Must the family do something because of the nature of the problem?

What are the family's reasons for not working on the problem? For example, is there some other family situation that must be resolved first? The problem-solving process may need to refocus unless both problems can be approached simultaneously.

The family is provided with information about the resolution of the problem as well as the risks associated with neglecting the problem to make an informed decision about a course of action.

The family is assisted in its problem solving in the same manner as discussed previously.

C. Evaluation (jointly by family and community health nurse)

1. Evaluation of problem-solving process and experience.

2. Evaluation of the implementation and outcomes of the family's selected approach to the problem.

B5—FAMILY ASSESSMENT RECORDING
(Chapter 8)

FAMILY RECORD

AREAS TO ASSESS		FINDINGS AND INTERVENTIONS
		COMMENTS "S" =
PHYSIOLOGICAL FACTORS	—Family Medical History —Genogram	
PSYCHOLOGICAL FACTORS	—Communication Patterns —Coping Patterns —Decision Making Patterns —Management of Change —Privacy	
SOCIOCULTURAL FACTORS	—Economic Situation —Ethnicity —Ecomap —Support Systems —Family Role Patterns —Community Involvement —Agency and/or Professional Involvement	
DEVELOPMENTAL FACTORS	—Family Stage	
SPIRITUAL FACTORS	—Value Systems —Religious Affiliation	

ANALYSIS	FAMILY'S PERCEPTION	P.H.N.'S PERCEPTION
INTRAFAMILIAL FACTORS		
INTERFAMILIAL FACTORS		
EXTRAFAMILIAL FACTORS		
NURSING DIAGNOSIS		

DATE OF ASSESSMENT	PUBLIC HEALTH NURSE'S SIGNATURE

K.C.H.U. - PH1 - 1988

From Allison EM: Family assessment recording, Kent-Chatham Health Unit, Chatham, Ontario, Canada.

KEY TO GENOGRAM SYMBOLS

| Male | Female | Twins (Girls) | Twins (Boys) | Adopted Child | Pregnancy | Miscarriage or Abortion | Unknown Sex | Death | Separation | Divorce |

| Relationship | Marriage Relationship | Parent-Child Relationship | D Distant Relationship | Overclose Relationship | Conflictual Relationship | Overclose Conflictual Relationship |

SUMMARY — ANALYSIS	FAMILY'S PERCEPTION	P.H.N.'s PERCEPTION
INTRAFAMILIAL FACTORS		
INTERFAMILIAL FACTORS		
EXTRAFAMILIAL FACTORS		
NURSING DIAGNOSIS		

DATE OF ASSESSMENT   PUBLIC HEALTH NURSE'S SIGNATURE

ECOMAP

SURNAME   ADDRESS

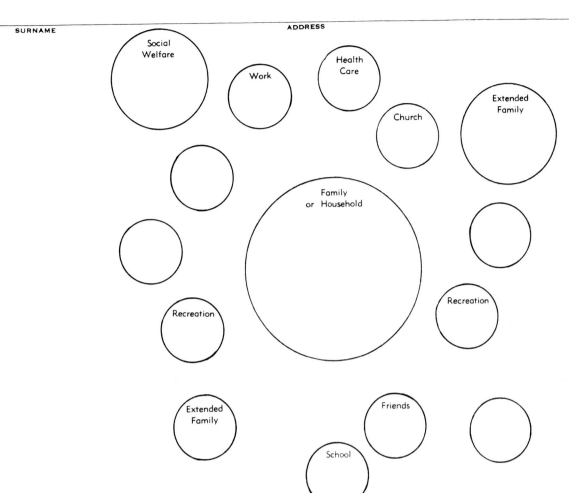

Fill in connections where they exist.

Indicate nature of connections with a descriptive word or by drawing different kinds of lines, ——————— for **strong**, – – – – – – – for **tenuous**, /////////////// for **stressful**.

Draw arrows along lines to signify flow of energy, resources, etc.

Identify significant people and fill in empty circles as needed.

SUMMARY — ANALYSIS	FAMILY'S PERCEPTION	P.H.N.'s PERCEPTION
INTRAFAMILIAL FACTORS		
INTERFAMILIAL FACTORS		
EXTRAFAMILIAL FACTORS		
NURSING DIAGNOSIS		

DATE OF ASSESSMENT   PUBLIC HEALTH NURSE'S SIGNATURE

K.C.H.U. - PH - E/G - 1988

B6—HOME OBSERVATION FOR MEASUREMENT OF THE ENVIRONMENT
(Chapters 28 and 29)

Birth to Three

Date of interview _____

Child designee _____
             Name

Age   Sex   Ethnicity

Child's birthday _____   Birth order _____
Mother's name _____   Father's name _____
Address _____

_____

Categories

	Raw scores	Percentile scores
I. Emotional and verbal responsivity of mother	_____	_____
II. Avoidance of restriction and punishment	_____	_____
III. Organization of physical and temporal environment	_____	_____
IV. Provision of appropriate play materials	_____	_____
V. Maternal involvement with child	_____	_____
VI. Opportunities for variety in daily stimulation	_____	_____
TOTALS	_____	

I. Emotional and verbal responsivitiy of mother

	Yes	No
1. Mother spontaneously vocalizes to child at least twice during visit (excluding scolding).	_____	_____
2. Mother responds to child's vocalizations with a verbal response.	_____	_____
3. Mother tells child the name of some object during visit or says name of person or object in a "teaching" style.	_____	_____
4. Mother's speech is distinct, clear, and audible.	_____	_____
5. Mother initiates verbal interchanges with observer—asks questions and makes spontaneous comments.	_____	_____
6. Mother expresses ideas freely and easily and uses statements of appropriate length for conversation (e.g., give more than brief answers).	_____	_____
* 7. Mother permits child occasionally to engage in "messy" type of play.	_____	_____
8. Mother spontaneously praises child's qualities or behavior twice during visit.	_____	_____
9. When speaking of or to child, mother's voice conveys positive feeling.	_____	_____
10. Mother caresses or kisses child at least once during visit.	_____	_____
11. Mother shows some positive emotional responses to praise of child offered by visitor.	_____	_____
SUBSCORE	_____	_____

II. Avoidance of restriction and punishment

12. Mother does not shout at child during visit.	_____	_____
13. Mother does not express overt annoyance with or hostility toward child.	_____	_____
14. Mother neither slaps nor spanks child during visit.	_____	_____
*15. Mother reports that no more than one instance of physical punishment occurred during the past week.	_____	_____
16. Mother does not scold or derogate child during visit.	_____	_____
17. Mother does not interfere with child's actions or restrict child's movements more than three times during visit.	_____	_____
18. At least 10 books are present and visible.	_____	_____
*19. Family has a pet.	_____	_____
SUBSCORE	_____	_____

III. Organization of physical and temporal environment

20. When mother is away, care is provided by one of three regular substitutes.	_____	_____
21. Someone takes child into grocery store at least once a week.	_____	_____
22. Child gets out of house at least four times a week.	_____	_____
23. Child is taken regularly to doctor's office or clinic.	_____	_____
*24. Child has a special place in which to keep his toys and "treasures."	_____	_____
25. Child's play environment appears safe and free of hazards.	_____	_____
SUBSCORE	_____	_____

IV. Provision of appropiate play materials

	Yes	No
26. Child has some muscle activity toys or equipment.	_____	_____
27. Child has push or pull toy.	_____	_____

*Items that may require direct questions.

28. Child has stroller or walker, kiddie car, scooter or tricycle. _____ _____
29. Mother provides toys or interesting activities for child during interview. _____ _____
30. Provides learning equipment appropriate to age—cuddly toy or role-playing toys. _____ _____
31. Provides learning equipment appropriate to age—mobile, table and chairs, high chair, play pen. _____ _____
32. Provides eye-hand coordination toys—times to go in and out of receptacle, fit-together toys, beads. _____ _____
33. Provides eye-hand coordination toys that permit combinations—stacking or nesting toys, blocks or building toys. _____ _____
34. Provides toys for literature and music. _____ _____

SUBSCORE _____ _____

V. Maternal involvement with child
35. Mother tends to keep child within visual range and to look at him often. _____ _____
36. Mother talks to child while doing her work. _____ _____
37. Mother consciously encourages developmental advance. _____ _____
38. Mother invests "maturing" toys with value via her attention. _____ _____
39. Mother structures child's play periods. _____ _____
40. Mother provides toys that challenge child to develop new skills. _____ _____

SUBSCORE _____ _____

VI. Opportunities for variety in daily stimulation
41. Father provides some caregiving every day. _____ _____
42. Mother reads stories at least three times weekly. _____ _____
43. Child eats at least one meal per day with mother and father. _____ _____
44. Family visits or receives visits from relatives. _____ _____
45. Child has three or more books of his own. _____ _____

SUBSCORE _____ _____

Three to Six

Date of interview _____

Child designee _____
                          Name   Age   Sex   Ethnicity

Child's birthday _____   Birth order _____

Mother's name _____   Father's name _____

Address _____

Categories

	Raw scores	Percentile scores
I. Provision of stimulation through equipment, toys, and experiences	_____	_____
II. Stimulation of mature behavior	_____	_____
III. Provision of stimulating physical and language environment	_____	_____
IV. Avoidance of restriction and punishment	_____	_____
V. Pride, affection, and thoughtfulness	_____	_____
VI. Masculine stimulation	_____	_____
VII. Independence from parental control	_____	_____
TOTALS	_____	_____

I. Provision of stimulation through equipment, toys, and experiences

1-12 The following are present in home and either belong to child subject or he is allowed to play with them:

	Yes	No
1. Toys to learn colors, sizes, shapes (e.g., typewriter, pressouts, play school, and peg boards).	_____	_____
2. Toy or game facilitating learning letters (e.g., blocks with letters, toy typewriter, letter sticks, and books about letters).	_____	_____
3. Three or more puzzles.	_____	_____
4. Two toys necessitating some finger and whole hand movements (e.g., crayons and coloring books, paper dolls).	_____	_____
5. Record player and at least five children's records.	_____	_____
6. Real or toy musical instrument (e.g, piano, drum, toy xylophone, or guitar).	_____	_____
7. Toy or game permitting free expression (e.g., finger paints, play dough, and crayons or paint and paper).	_____	_____
8. Toys or game necessitating refined movements (paint by number, dot book, paper dolls, crayons and coloring books).	_____	_____

9. Toys to learn animals (e.g., books about animals, circus games, and animal puzzles).

10. Toy or game facilitating learning numbers (e.g., blocks with numbers, books about numbers, games with numbers).

11. Building toys (e.g., block, Tinker Toys, and Lincoln Logs).

12. Ten children's books.

13. At least 10 books are present and visible in the apartment.

14. Family buys a newspaper daily and reads it.

15. Family subscribes to at least one magazine.

16. Family member has taken child on one outing (picnic, shopping excursion) at least every other week.

17. Child has been taken out to eat in some kind of restaurant three or four times in the past year.

18-20 Child has been taken by a family member to the following within the past year:

18. Airport

19. A trip more than 50 miles from his home (50 miles radial distance, not total distance).

20. A scientific, historical, or art museum.

21. Child is taken to grocery store at least once a week.

SUBSCORE

II. Stimulation of mature behavior

	Yes	No

22-29 Child is encouraged to learn the following:

22. Colors

23. Shapes

24. Patterned speech (e.g., nursery rhymes, prayers, songs, and TV commercials)

25. The alphabet

26. To tell time

27. Spatial relationships (e.g., up, down, under, big, and little)

28. Numbers

29. To read a few words

30. Tries to get child to pick up and put away toys after play session—without help.

31. Child is taught rules of social behavior that involve recognition of rights of others.

32. Parent teaches child some simple manners—to say, "Please," "Thank you," and "I'm sorry."

33. Some delay of food gratification is demanded of the child, e.g., not to whine or demand food unless within ½ hour of meal time.

SUBSCORE

III. Provision of a stimulating physical and language environment
(Observation items, except *45*)

	Yes	No

34. Building has no potentially dangerous structural or health defect (e.g., plaster coming down from ceiling, stairway with boards missing, or rodents).

35. Child's outside play environment appears safe and free of hazards (no outside play area requires an automatic "No").

36. The interior of the apartment is not dark or perceptibly monotonous.

37. House is not overly noisy—television, shouts of children, radio, etc.

38. Neighborhood has trees, grass, birds—is esthetically pleasing.

39. There is at least 100 square feet of living space per person in the house.

40. In terms of available floor space, the rooms are not overcrowded with furniture.

41. All visible rooms of the house are reasonably clean and minimally cluttered.

*42. Mother uses complex sentence structure and some long words in conversing.

43. Mother uses correct grammar and pronunciation.

44. Mother's speech is distinct, clear, and audible.

45. Family has TV and it is used judiciously, not left on continuously (no TV requires an automatic "No"—any scheduling scores "Yes").

SUBSCORE

IV. Avoidance of restriction and punishment
(Observation items, except *51* and *52*)

	Yes	No

46. Mother does not scold or derogate child more than once during visit.

47. Mother does not use physical restraint, shake, grab, or pinch child during visit.

---

*Throughout interview this refers to mother *or* other care giver who is present for interview.
From Caldwell B: Home observation measurement of the environment, Little Rock, Ark., 1976, University of Arkansas Center for Child Development and Education.

48. Mother neither slaps nor spanks child during visit. _____ _____
49. Mother does not express over-annoyance with or hostility toward child—complain, say child is _____ _____
"bad" or won't mind.
50. Child is not punished or ridiculed for speech. _____ _____
51. No more than one instance of physical punishment occurred during the past week (accept parental _____ _____
report).
52. Child does not get slapped or spanked for spilling food or drink. _____ _____

SUBSCORE _____ _____

V. Pride, affection, and thoughtfulness | **Yes** | **No**
(Observation items, except *53* through *59*)

53. Parent turns on special TV progam regarded as "good" for children (e.g., *Captain Kangaroo,* _____ _____
Walt Disney, Flipper, Lassie, or educational TV).
54. Someone reads stories to child or shows and comments on pictures in magazines five times weekly. _____ _____
55. Parent encourages child to relate experiences or takes time to listen to him relate experiences. _____ _____
56. Parent holds child close 10 to 15 minutes per day (e.g., during TV, story time, or visiting). _____ _____
57. Parent occasionally sings to child, or sings in presence of child.
58. Child has a special place in which to keep his toys and "treasures." _____ _____
59. Child's art work is displayed some place in house (anything that child makes).
60. Mother introduces interviewer to child.
61. Mother converses with child at least twice during visit (scolding and suspicious comments not _____ _____
counted).
62. Mother answers child's questions or requests verbally.
63. Mother usually responds verbally to child's talking. _____ _____
64. Mother provides toys or interesting activities or in other ways structures situation for child during _____ _____
visit when her attention will be elsewhere. (To score "Yes" mother must make an active guiding
gesture or suggestion to structure child's play.)
65. Mother spontaneously praises child's qualities or behavior twice during visit. _____ _____
66. When speaking of or to child, mother's voice conveys positive feeling. _____ _____
67. Mother caresses, kisses, or cuddles child at least once during visit. _____ _____
68. Mother sets up situation that allows child to show off during visit. _____ _____

SUBSCORE _____ _____

VI. Masculine stimulation | **Yes** | **No**
69. Child sees and spends some time with father four days a week. _____ _____
70. Child eats at least one meal per day, on most days, with mother (or mother figure) and father (or _____ _____
father figure). (One-parent families get an automatic "No.")

B7—SUMMARY CHARACTERISTICS OF NINE FAMILY ASSESSMENT TOOLS
(Chapters 28 and 29)

Tools	Dimensions measured	Understandable	Ease of administration and scoring	Appropriate for all types of families	Clinical relevance
FFI*	Communication Togetherness Closeness Decision making Child orientation	Yes	15 items Quickly administered Complicated scoring	Not for families without children or those with adult children	Not sensitive to short-term change
FAD†	Problem solving Communication Roles Affective responsive-ness Affective involve-ment Behavior control General functioning	Yes	53 items Easy to administer	Requires individual to "speak for fam-ily"	Measures areas that nurses could change through care plans

From Speer, JJ and Sachs B: Selecting the appropriate family assessment tool, Pediatr Nurs 11:349-355, 1985. Reprinted with permission: A.J. Jannetti, Inc.
*Family Functioning Index
†The Family Assessment Device

B7—SUMMARY CHARACTERISTICS OF NINE FAMILY ASSESSMENT TOOLS—cont'd

(Chapters 28 and 29)

Tools	Dimensions measured	Understandable	Ease of administration and scoring	Appropriate for all types of families	Clinical relevance
FES*	Relationships Personal growth System maintenance and change	Yes	90 items, true/false Length for clinical use (short form available) Scoring is complex Standardized scores, two categories	Universally appropriate	Useful to measure change after interventions
SFIS†	Enmeshment/disengagement Neglect/overprotection Rigidity/flexibility Conflict/avoidance Client management Triangulation of parent/child coalition Detouring	Easier to understand for those familiar with Minuchin's family functioning theory	85 items on 4-point agreement scale Easy to administer	Unknown at this time	Further testing required Useful for family counseling assessment
FFS‡	Parent's perception of relationship and family functions	Somewhat difficult	Somewhat complicated scoring	Useful with middle-class families	Measures factors that nurses could help change through care plans
CICI:PQ§	Perceptions of stressors Coping strategies	Yes	48 items Scoring unknown	Only for families with chronically ill children	Identifies nursing intervention areas for families with chronically ill children
Family APGAR‖	Adaptability Partnership Growth Affection Resolve	Requires global assessment of five areas	Five items Quick to administer	No data reported	Measures relevant factors
IFF[a]	Positive/negative feelings toward each member	Yes Complicated for large families	38 items, 3-point Likertlike scale Easily scored	Unknown at this time	Limited clinical usefulness because of lack of dimension
FACES II[b]	Cohesion Adaptability Social desirability	Easily understood	30 items on 4-point Likertlike scale Easy to administer	Universally useful Family members may be unwilling to assess themselves	Measures relevant factors for nursing Can use as real and ideal

*Family Environment Scale
†Structural Family Interaction Scale
‡Feetham Family Functioning Survey
§Chronicity Impact and Coping Instrument: Parent Questionnaire
‖Family Adaptability, Partnership, Growth, Affection, and Resolve Test
[a]The Inventory of Family Feelings
[b]Family Adaptability and Cohesion Evaluation Scale

C1 LIFESTYLE ASSESSMENT QUESTIONNAIRE (5TH EDITION)

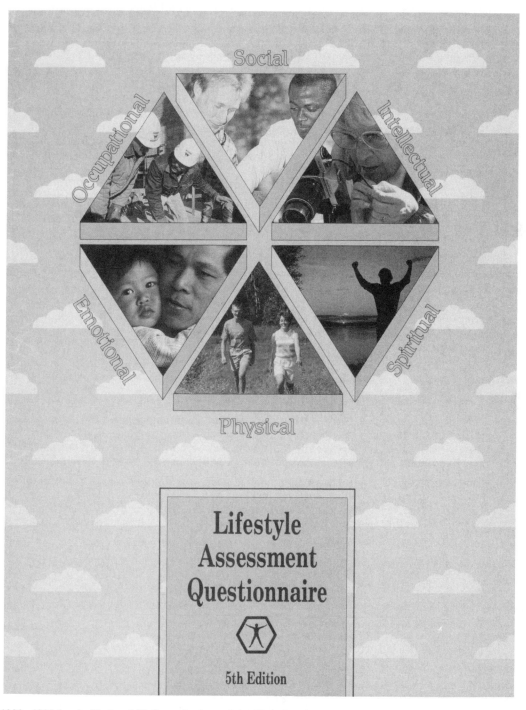

Purpose

This assessment tool and the analysis it provides are designed to help you discover how the choices you make each day affect your overall health.

By participating in this assessment process, you will also learn how you can make positive changes in your lifestyle, enabling you to reach a higher level of wellness.

Some of the questions are personal. While you may leave them blank, the more information you provide about your current lifestyle, the more accurately the LAQ can assess your current level of wellness and risk areas.

Confidentiality

The National Wellness Institute, Inc. subscribes to the guidelines established by the Society of Prospective Medicine concerning confidentiality in the use of health risk appraisals and risk reduction systems. These guidelines specifically state that only the participant and health professionals authorized by the participant should receive copies of his/her own health risk appraisal results.

The National Wellness Institute, Inc. strongly encourages all users of the LAQ to strictly follow these guidelines and maintain the confidentiality of all answers.

What is Wellness?

Wellness is an active process of becoming aware of and making choices toward a higher level of well-being. **Remember,** leading a wellness lifestyle requires your **active involvement.** As you gain more knowledge about what enhances your well-being, you are encouraged to use this information to make informed choices which lead to a healthier life.

General Instructions

The enclosed answer sheet is for you to record your answers to the Lifestyle Assessment Questionnaire. Please make certain that you complete all of the information at the top of the answer sheet including your zip code, group code, and social security number. If a group code has not been provided for you, leave this item blank.

Your questionnaire will be scored by an optical mark reading instrument; therefore, please use only a No. 2 (soft) pencil for marking your responses. To assure the most accurate results, follow the instructions shown on the answer sheet. Only your answer sheet needs to be returned for scoring. You may keep this questionnaire.

The Lifestyle Assessment Questionnaire was written by the National Wellness Institute, Inc.'s Board of Directors and Cofounders; Dennis Elsenrath, Ed.D., Bill Hettler, M.D., and Fred Leafgren, Ph.D.

⬡ Lifestyle Assessment Questionnaire™ Results

Making Wellness Work for You

Do you want to know how you can increase your level of wellness?

If you answered "yes" to this question, a plan is outlined below that you can use to increase your level of well-being and potentially reduce your risk of premature death.

STEP 1: Choose a behavior you would like to change:
Target Behavior _____

STEP 2: Take the Target Behavior Test:

TARGET BEHAVIOR TEST

		Yes	No
1.	I really want to change this behavior.	☐	☐
2.	I am likely to be healthier by changing this behavior.	☐	☐
3.	If necessary, I am willing to spend some money as part of changing this behavior.	☐	☐
4.	I am willing to devote the necessary time to changing this behavior.	☐	☐
5.	I have chosen a target behavior that I am able to count or measure.	☐	☐
6.	I have selected a goal which I can achieve. (e.g., "I will lose one pound per week by eliminating all between-meal snacks and walking one mile per day" is probably a realistic goal. "I will lose twenty pounds this month" is probably too large of a goal and may be unsafe.)	☐	☐

If you answered "no" to any of these questions, this behavior may not be the best place to start. You may want to choose another behavior which appeals to you and allows you to answer "yes" to all the questions on the **Target Behavior Test**. When you're ready, go on to the next step.

STEP 3: Create a place to begin.

To measure your success, you will want to know where you started. You can measure your starting point by recording a current behavior which you plan to change. You may create a measure of this starting point by writing down answers to questions like: How much? How little? How often? How long? Where and in what situations does it occur? The following chart will assist you.

Lifestyle Assessment Questionnaire™ Results

Name: _____   Date: _____

Target Behavior: _____

	WHERE	HOW OFTEN OR HOW MUCH	WHEN			BEHAVIOR DESCRIPTION What I did & with whom
			Start	Stop	Date	
Day 1						
Day 2						
Day 3						
Day 4						
Day 5						
Day 6						
Day 7						

BEHAVIOR TOTAL   TIME TOTAL

STEP 4: Design your surroundings to make changes easier.
Create a work and/or home space where it is harder to use the old negative pattern.

Examples:

A. If you want to stop smoking and you usually smoke and talk on the phone, both at home and at work, don't have cigarettes, matches, or an ashtray anywhere near the telephone or in the room.

B. If you are losing weight and often snack and watch television, write letters or read a book rather than watch television. Remember, don't bring snacks into the room, house or office.

C. Put a saying or picture which pleases and/or motivates you in a place where you will often see it.

STEP 5: Reward yourself when you act in the wellness way.
Pick a reward which is positive and which you enjoy. You may list your own in the first blanks or pick from the list of suggested rewards.

My rewards or what I like or want:

1) _____

2) _____

3) _____

HINT: Use only one reward each time and use the largest reward for the biggest accomplishment.

Lifestyle Assessment Questionnaire™ Results

SUGGESTED REWARDS:

1. Time with friends.
2. Go to a movie or concert.
3. Buy a new piece of clothing.
4. Enjoy a special food or beverage.
5. Tell yourself how well you are doing.
6. Take a walk or bicycle ride.

MORE HINTS ABOUT REWARDS:

1. Do not demand too much work or success for too little reward.
2. Reward yourself as quickly as possible when you are successful.
3. Change your rewards as necessary.
4. After you are doing well, don't reward yourself as often.

STEP 6: Get help from friends and family.
Use the *Contract for Behavior Change* or ask for their help.

Contract for Behavior Change

I, _____, have pledged to meet the following

goal(s). 1) _____   2) _____

3) _____. The goal I will begin with is _____

_____ .

The friends of_____who have signed below have

agreed to provide the following: (Please write them down.)

_____

_____

We will meet on _____ _____, _____, to discuss progress
                    Month   Day   Year
and provide support.

Signed:

_____ _____ _____
Signature   Date   Signature   Date   Signature   Date

STEP 7: Measure and record your progress.

	Week 1	Week 2	Week 3	Week 4
Behavior Total:				
Time Total:				
What I Learned From Behavior Descriptions:				

FINAL HELPFUL HINTS:

1. Don't criticize yourself; don't expect perfection.
2. Focus on the positive. Develop an optimistic attitude.
3. Learn by watching others who are doing a good job with the behaviors you are changing.
4. Don't stop if the goal is not accomplished quickly. Practice! Practice! Practice!
5. If you have doubts or it seems much too hard, consult with knowledgeable others and/or a professional counselor.

LIFESTYLE ASSESSMENT QUESTIONNAIRE ANSWER SHEET

Please Do Not Mark In This Box

38326

NAME

LAST   FIRST

RETURN ADDRESS

INSTRUCTIONS

- USE #2 PENCIL ONLY
- MARK BUBBLE COMPLETELY
- DO NOT MAKE ANY STRAY MARKS
- ERASE ONLY MARKS YOU WISH TO CHANGE

SAMPLE

ZIP CODE

GROUP CODE

SOCIAL SECURITY #

Printed in U.S.A.   NCS Trans-Optic® MP30-78818-3   A2202

SECTION 1-PERSONAL DATA

1 Ⓐ Ⓑ

2 Ⓐ Ⓑ Ⓒ Ⓓ Ⓔ Ⓕ

3 [Ⓞ①②③④⑤⑥⑦⑧⑨ / Ⓞ①②③④⑤⑥⑦⑧⑨]

4 [Ⓞ①②③④⑤⑥⑦⑧⑨ / Ⓞ①②③④⑤⑥⑦⑧⑨⑩⑪]

5 [Ⓞ①②③④⑤⑥⑦⑧⑨ / Ⓞ①②③④⑤⑥⑦⑧⑨ / Ⓞ①②③④⑤⑥⑦⑧⑨]

6 Ⓐ Ⓑ Ⓒ

7 Ⓐ Ⓑ Ⓒ Ⓓ Ⓔ Ⓕ

8 Ⓐ Ⓑ Ⓒ Ⓓ Ⓔ Ⓕ Ⓖ

9 Ⓐ Ⓑ Ⓒ Ⓓ Ⓔ Ⓕ

10 Ⓐ Ⓑ Ⓒ Ⓓ

11 Ⓐ Ⓑ Ⓒ Ⓓ

12 Ⓐ Ⓑ Ⓒ Ⓓ Ⓔ

SECTION 2-LIFESTYLE

A. Physical Exercise

1 Ⓐ Ⓑ Ⓒ Ⓓ Ⓔ
2 Ⓐ Ⓑ Ⓒ Ⓓ Ⓔ
3 Ⓐ Ⓑ Ⓒ Ⓓ Ⓔ
4 Ⓐ Ⓑ Ⓒ Ⓓ Ⓔ
5 Ⓐ Ⓑ Ⓒ Ⓓ Ⓔ
6 Ⓐ Ⓑ Ⓒ Ⓓ Ⓔ
7 Ⓐ Ⓑ Ⓒ Ⓓ Ⓔ
8 Ⓐ Ⓑ Ⓒ Ⓓ Ⓔ
9 Ⓐ Ⓑ Ⓒ Ⓓ Ⓔ
10 Ⓐ Ⓑ Ⓒ Ⓓ Ⓔ

B. Nutrition

11 Ⓐ Ⓑ Ⓒ Ⓓ Ⓔ
12 Ⓐ Ⓑ Ⓒ Ⓓ Ⓔ
13 Ⓐ Ⓑ Ⓒ Ⓓ Ⓔ

14 Ⓐ Ⓑ Ⓒ Ⓓ Ⓔ
15 Ⓐ Ⓑ Ⓒ Ⓓ Ⓔ
16 Ⓐ Ⓑ Ⓒ Ⓓ Ⓔ
17 Ⓐ Ⓑ Ⓒ Ⓓ Ⓔ
18 Ⓐ Ⓑ Ⓒ Ⓓ Ⓔ
19 Ⓐ Ⓑ Ⓒ Ⓓ Ⓔ
20 Ⓐ Ⓑ Ⓒ Ⓓ Ⓔ
21 Ⓐ Ⓑ Ⓒ Ⓓ Ⓔ
22 Ⓐ Ⓑ Ⓒ Ⓓ Ⓔ
23 Ⓐ Ⓑ Ⓒ Ⓓ Ⓔ

C. Self-Care

24 Ⓐ Ⓑ Ⓒ Ⓓ Ⓔ
25 Ⓐ Ⓑ Ⓒ Ⓓ Ⓔ
26 Ⓐ Ⓑ Ⓒ Ⓓ Ⓔ
27 Ⓐ Ⓑ Ⓒ Ⓓ Ⓔ
28 Ⓐ Ⓑ Ⓒ Ⓓ Ⓔ
29 Ⓐ Ⓑ Ⓒ Ⓓ Ⓔ
30 Ⓐ Ⓑ Ⓒ Ⓓ Ⓔ
31 Ⓐ Ⓑ Ⓒ Ⓓ Ⓔ
32 Ⓐ Ⓑ Ⓒ Ⓓ Ⓔ
33 Ⓐ Ⓑ Ⓒ Ⓓ Ⓔ
34 Ⓐ Ⓑ Ⓒ Ⓓ Ⓔ
35 Ⓐ Ⓑ Ⓒ Ⓓ Ⓔ
36 Ⓐ Ⓑ Ⓒ Ⓓ Ⓔ
37 Ⓐ Ⓑ Ⓒ Ⓓ Ⓔ

D. Vehicle Safety

38 Ⓐ Ⓑ Ⓒ Ⓓ Ⓔ
39 Ⓐ Ⓑ Ⓒ Ⓓ Ⓔ
40 Ⓐ Ⓑ Ⓒ Ⓓ Ⓔ
41 Ⓐ Ⓑ Ⓒ Ⓓ Ⓔ
42 Ⓐ Ⓑ Ⓒ Ⓓ Ⓔ

43 Ⓐ Ⓑ Ⓒ Ⓓ Ⓔ
44 Ⓐ Ⓑ Ⓒ Ⓓ Ⓔ
45 Ⓐ Ⓑ Ⓒ Ⓓ Ⓔ
46 Ⓐ Ⓑ Ⓒ Ⓓ Ⓔ
47 Ⓐ Ⓑ Ⓒ Ⓓ Ⓔ
48 Ⓐ Ⓑ Ⓒ Ⓓ Ⓔ

E. Drug Usage Awareness

49 Ⓐ Ⓑ Ⓒ Ⓓ Ⓔ
50 Ⓐ Ⓑ Ⓒ Ⓓ Ⓔ
51 Ⓐ Ⓑ Ⓒ Ⓓ Ⓔ
52 Ⓐ Ⓑ Ⓒ Ⓓ Ⓔ
53 Ⓐ Ⓑ Ⓒ Ⓓ Ⓔ
54 Ⓐ Ⓑ Ⓒ Ⓓ Ⓔ
55 Ⓐ Ⓑ Ⓒ Ⓓ Ⓔ
56 Ⓐ Ⓑ Ⓒ Ⓓ Ⓔ
57 Ⓐ Ⓑ Ⓒ Ⓓ Ⓔ
58 Ⓐ Ⓑ Ⓒ Ⓓ Ⓔ
59 Ⓐ Ⓑ Ⓒ Ⓓ Ⓔ
60 Ⓐ Ⓑ Ⓒ Ⓓ Ⓔ
61 Ⓐ Ⓑ Ⓒ Ⓓ Ⓔ
62 Ⓐ Ⓑ Ⓒ Ⓓ Ⓔ
63 Ⓐ Ⓑ Ⓒ Ⓓ Ⓔ

F. Social/Environmental

64 Ⓐ Ⓑ Ⓒ Ⓓ Ⓔ
65 Ⓐ Ⓑ Ⓒ Ⓓ Ⓔ
66 Ⓐ Ⓑ Ⓒ Ⓓ Ⓔ
67 Ⓐ Ⓑ Ⓒ Ⓓ Ⓔ
68 Ⓐ Ⓑ Ⓒ Ⓓ Ⓔ
69 Ⓐ Ⓑ Ⓒ Ⓓ Ⓔ
70 Ⓐ Ⓑ Ⓒ Ⓓ Ⓔ
71 Ⓐ Ⓑ Ⓒ Ⓓ Ⓔ

72 Ⓐ Ⓑ Ⓒ Ⓓ Ⓔ
73 Ⓐ Ⓑ Ⓒ Ⓓ Ⓔ
74 Ⓐ Ⓑ Ⓒ Ⓓ Ⓔ
75 Ⓐ Ⓑ Ⓒ Ⓓ Ⓔ
76 Ⓐ Ⓑ Ⓒ Ⓓ Ⓔ
77 Ⓐ Ⓑ Ⓒ Ⓓ Ⓔ
78 Ⓐ Ⓑ Ⓒ Ⓓ Ⓔ
79 Ⓐ Ⓑ Ⓒ Ⓓ Ⓔ
80 Ⓐ Ⓑ Ⓒ Ⓓ Ⓔ
81 Ⓐ Ⓑ Ⓒ Ⓓ Ⓔ
82 Ⓐ Ⓑ Ⓒ Ⓓ Ⓔ
83 Ⓐ Ⓑ Ⓒ Ⓓ Ⓔ
84 Ⓐ Ⓑ Ⓒ Ⓓ Ⓔ

G. Emotional Awareness & Acceptance

85 Ⓐ Ⓑ Ⓒ Ⓓ Ⓔ

H. Emotional Management

86 Ⓐ Ⓑ Ⓒ Ⓓ Ⓔ
87 Ⓐ Ⓑ Ⓒ Ⓓ Ⓔ
88 Ⓐ Ⓑ Ⓒ Ⓓ Ⓔ
89 Ⓐ Ⓑ Ⓒ Ⓓ Ⓔ
90 Ⓐ Ⓑ Ⓒ Ⓓ Ⓔ
91 Ⓐ Ⓑ Ⓒ Ⓓ Ⓔ
92 Ⓐ Ⓑ Ⓒ Ⓓ Ⓔ
93 Ⓐ Ⓑ Ⓒ Ⓓ Ⓔ
94 Ⓐ Ⓑ Ⓒ Ⓓ Ⓔ
95 Ⓐ Ⓑ Ⓒ Ⓓ Ⓔ
96 Ⓐ Ⓑ Ⓒ Ⓓ Ⓔ
97 Ⓐ Ⓑ Ⓒ Ⓓ Ⓔ
98 Ⓐ Ⓑ Ⓒ Ⓓ Ⓔ
99 Ⓐ Ⓑ Ⓒ Ⓓ Ⓔ
100 Ⓐ Ⓑ Ⓒ Ⓓ Ⓔ
101 Ⓐ Ⓑ Ⓒ Ⓓ Ⓔ

102 Ⓐ Ⓑ Ⓒ Ⓓ Ⓔ
103 Ⓐ Ⓑ Ⓒ Ⓓ Ⓔ
104 Ⓐ Ⓑ Ⓒ Ⓓ Ⓔ
105 Ⓐ Ⓑ Ⓒ Ⓓ Ⓔ
106 Ⓐ Ⓑ Ⓒ Ⓓ Ⓔ
107 Ⓐ Ⓑ Ⓒ Ⓓ Ⓔ
108 Ⓐ Ⓑ Ⓒ Ⓓ Ⓔ
109 Ⓐ Ⓑ Ⓒ Ⓓ Ⓔ
110 Ⓐ Ⓑ Ⓒ Ⓓ Ⓔ
111 Ⓐ Ⓑ Ⓒ Ⓓ Ⓔ
112 Ⓐ Ⓑ Ⓒ Ⓓ Ⓔ
113 Ⓐ Ⓑ Ⓒ Ⓓ Ⓔ
114 Ⓐ Ⓑ Ⓒ Ⓓ Ⓔ
115 Ⓐ Ⓑ Ⓒ Ⓓ Ⓔ
116 Ⓐ Ⓑ Ⓒ Ⓓ Ⓔ
117 Ⓐ Ⓑ Ⓒ Ⓓ Ⓔ
118 Ⓐ Ⓑ Ⓒ Ⓓ Ⓔ
119 Ⓐ Ⓑ Ⓒ Ⓓ Ⓔ
120 Ⓐ Ⓑ Ⓒ Ⓓ Ⓔ
121 Ⓐ Ⓑ Ⓒ Ⓓ Ⓔ
122 Ⓐ Ⓑ Ⓒ Ⓓ Ⓔ
123 Ⓐ Ⓑ Ⓒ Ⓓ Ⓔ
124 Ⓐ Ⓑ Ⓒ Ⓓ Ⓔ
125 Ⓐ Ⓑ Ⓒ Ⓓ Ⓔ
126 Ⓐ Ⓑ Ⓒ Ⓓ Ⓔ
127 Ⓐ Ⓑ Ⓒ Ⓓ Ⓔ
128 Ⓐ Ⓑ Ⓒ Ⓓ Ⓔ
129 Ⓐ Ⓑ Ⓒ Ⓓ Ⓔ
130 Ⓐ Ⓑ Ⓒ Ⓓ Ⓔ
131 Ⓐ Ⓑ Ⓒ Ⓓ Ⓔ

132 Ⓐ Ⓑ Ⓒ Ⓓ Ⓔ
133 Ⓐ Ⓑ Ⓒ Ⓓ Ⓔ
134 Ⓐ Ⓑ Ⓒ Ⓓ Ⓔ
135 Ⓐ Ⓑ Ⓒ Ⓓ Ⓔ
136 Ⓐ Ⓑ Ⓒ Ⓓ Ⓔ
137 Ⓐ Ⓑ Ⓒ Ⓓ Ⓔ
138 Ⓐ Ⓑ Ⓒ Ⓓ Ⓔ
139 Ⓐ Ⓑ Ⓒ Ⓓ Ⓔ
140 Ⓐ Ⓑ Ⓒ Ⓓ Ⓔ

I. Intellectual

141 Ⓐ Ⓑ Ⓒ Ⓓ Ⓔ
142 Ⓐ Ⓑ Ⓒ Ⓓ Ⓔ
143 Ⓐ Ⓑ Ⓒ Ⓓ Ⓔ
144 Ⓐ Ⓑ Ⓒ Ⓓ Ⓔ
145 Ⓐ Ⓑ Ⓒ Ⓓ Ⓔ
146 Ⓐ Ⓑ Ⓒ Ⓓ Ⓔ
147 Ⓐ Ⓑ Ⓒ Ⓓ Ⓔ
148 Ⓐ Ⓑ Ⓒ Ⓓ Ⓔ
149 Ⓐ Ⓑ Ⓒ Ⓓ Ⓔ
150 Ⓐ Ⓑ Ⓒ Ⓓ Ⓔ
151 Ⓐ Ⓑ Ⓒ Ⓓ Ⓔ
152 Ⓐ Ⓑ Ⓒ Ⓓ Ⓔ
153 Ⓐ Ⓑ Ⓒ Ⓓ Ⓔ
154 Ⓐ Ⓑ Ⓒ Ⓓ Ⓔ
155 Ⓐ Ⓑ Ⓒ Ⓓ Ⓔ

J. Occupational

156 Ⓐ Ⓑ Ⓒ Ⓓ Ⓔ
157 Ⓐ Ⓑ Ⓒ Ⓓ Ⓔ
158 Ⓐ Ⓑ Ⓒ Ⓓ Ⓔ
159 Ⓐ Ⓑ Ⓒ Ⓓ Ⓔ
160 Ⓐ Ⓑ Ⓒ Ⓓ Ⓔ

Lifestyle Assessment Questionnaire™

Answer Sheet

SIDE 2

J. Occupational (Cont.)

161 Ⓐ Ⓑ Ⓒ Ⓓ Ⓔ
162 Ⓐ Ⓑ Ⓒ Ⓓ Ⓔ
163 Ⓐ Ⓑ Ⓒ Ⓓ Ⓔ
164 Ⓐ Ⓑ Ⓒ Ⓓ Ⓔ
165 Ⓐ Ⓑ Ⓒ Ⓓ Ⓔ
166 Ⓐ Ⓑ Ⓒ Ⓓ Ⓔ
167 Ⓐ Ⓑ Ⓒ Ⓓ Ⓔ
168 Ⓐ Ⓑ Ⓒ Ⓓ Ⓔ
169 Ⓐ Ⓑ Ⓒ Ⓓ Ⓔ
170 Ⓐ Ⓑ Ⓒ Ⓓ Ⓔ
171 Ⓐ Ⓑ Ⓒ Ⓓ Ⓔ

K. Spiritual

172 Ⓐ Ⓑ Ⓒ Ⓓ Ⓔ
173 Ⓐ Ⓑ Ⓒ Ⓓ Ⓔ
174 Ⓐ Ⓑ Ⓒ Ⓓ Ⓔ
175 Ⓐ Ⓑ Ⓒ Ⓓ Ⓔ
176 Ⓐ Ⓑ Ⓒ Ⓓ Ⓔ
177 Ⓐ Ⓑ Ⓒ Ⓓ Ⓔ
178 Ⓐ Ⓑ Ⓒ Ⓓ Ⓔ
179 Ⓐ Ⓑ Ⓒ Ⓓ Ⓔ
180 Ⓐ Ⓑ Ⓒ Ⓓ Ⓔ
181 Ⓐ Ⓑ Ⓒ Ⓓ Ⓔ
182 Ⓐ Ⓑ Ⓒ Ⓓ Ⓔ
183 Ⓐ Ⓑ Ⓒ Ⓓ Ⓔ
184 Ⓐ Ⓑ Ⓒ Ⓓ Ⓔ
185 Ⓐ Ⓑ Ⓒ Ⓓ Ⓔ

SECTION 3-HEALTH RISK APPRAISAL

1 Ⓐ Ⓑ
2 Ⓐ Ⓑ Ⓒ
3 Ⓐ Ⓑ Ⓒ Ⓓ
4 Ⓐ Ⓑ
5a ⓪①②③④⑤⑥⑦⑧⑨ / ⓪①②③④⑤⑥⑦⑧⑨ / ⓪①②③④⑤⑥⑦⑧⑨
5b ⓪①②③④⑤⑥⑦⑧⑨ / ⓪①②③④⑤⑥⑦⑧⑨ / ⓪①②③④⑤⑥⑦⑧⑨
6 Ⓐ Ⓑ Ⓒ
7 ⓪①②③④⑤⑥⑦⑧⑨ / ⓪①②③④⑤⑥⑦⑧⑨ / ⓪①②③④⑤⑥⑦⑧⑨
8 ⓪①②③④⑤⑥⑦⑧⑨ / ⓪①②③④⑤⑥⑦⑧⑨ / ⓪①②③④⑤⑥⑦⑧⑨
9 ⓪①②③④⑤⑥⑦⑧⑨ / ⓪①②③④⑤⑥⑦⑧⑨
10 ⓪①②③④⑤⑥⑦⑧⑨ / ⓪①②③④⑤⑥⑦⑧⑨
11 ⓪①②③④⑤⑥⑦⑧⑨ / ⓪①②③④⑤⑥⑦⑧⑨
12 Ⓐ Ⓑ Ⓒ
13 ⓪①②③④⑤⑥⑦⑧⑨ / ⓪①②③④⑤⑥⑦⑧⑨
14a ⓪①②③④⑤⑥⑦⑧⑨ / ⓪①②③④⑤⑥⑦⑧⑨
14b ⓪①②③④⑤⑥⑦⑧⑨ / ⓪①②③④⑤⑥⑦⑧⑨

15a ⓪①②③④⑤⑥⑦⑧⑨ / ⓪①②③④⑤⑥⑦⑧⑨ / ⓪①②③④⑤⑥⑦⑧⑨
15b ⓪①②③④⑤⑥⑦⑧⑨ / ⓪①②③④⑤⑥⑦⑧⑨ / ⓪①②③④⑤⑥⑦⑧⑨
16 Ⓐ Ⓑ Ⓒ Ⓓ Ⓔ Ⓕ Ⓖ Ⓗ
17 ⓪①②③④⑤⑥⑦⑧⑨ / ⓪①②③④⑤⑥⑦⑧⑨
18 Ⓐ Ⓑ Ⓒ Ⓓ
19 ⓪①②③④⑤⑥⑦⑧⑨ / ⓪①②③④⑤⑥⑦⑧⑨
20 ⓪①②③④⑤⑥⑦⑧⑨ / ⓪①②③④⑤⑥⑦⑧⑨
21 ⓪①②③④⑤⑥⑦
22 ⓪①②③④⑤⑥⑦⑧⑨ / ⓪①②③④⑤⑥⑦⑧⑨
23 ⓪①②③④⑤⑥⑦⑧⑨ / ⓪①②③④⑤⑥⑦⑧⑨
24 Ⓐ Ⓑ Ⓒ Ⓓ Ⓔ
25 ⓪①②③④⑤⑥⑦⑧⑨ / ⓪①②③④⑤⑥⑦⑧⑨
26 Ⓐ Ⓑ Ⓒ
27 Ⓐ Ⓑ Ⓒ Ⓓ Ⓔ
28 Ⓐ Ⓑ Ⓒ
29 Ⓐ Ⓑ Ⓒ Ⓓ Ⓔ
30 Ⓐ Ⓑ Ⓒ Ⓓ Ⓔ
31 Ⓐ Ⓑ Ⓒ Ⓓ Ⓔ
32 Ⓐ Ⓑ Ⓒ

33 Ⓐ Ⓑ Ⓒ
34 Ⓐ Ⓑ Ⓒ Ⓓ Ⓔ
35 Ⓐ Ⓑ Ⓒ Ⓓ
36 Ⓐ Ⓑ Ⓒ Ⓓ
37 Ⓐ Ⓑ Ⓒ
38 Ⓐ Ⓑ Ⓒ Ⓓ

39 Ⓐ Ⓑ
40 Ⓐ Ⓑ
41 Ⓐ Ⓑ Ⓒ
42 Ⓐ Ⓑ Ⓒ

SECTION 4-TOPICS FOR PERSONAL GROWTH

1 ○   23 ○
2 ○   24 ○
3 ○   25 ○
4 ○   26 ○
5 ○   27 ○
6 ○   28 ○
7 ○   29 ○
8 ○   30 ○
9 ○   31 ○
10 ○   32 ○
11 ○   33 ○
12 ○   34 ○
13 ○   35 ○
14 ○   36 ○
15 ○   37 ○
16 ○   38 ○
17 ○   39 ○
18 ○   40 ○
19 ○   41 ○
20 ○   42 ○
21 ○   43 ○
22 ○

Section 1: PERSONAL DATA

INSTRUCTIONS:

Please complete the following general information about yourself by marking your answers in the appropriate places on the LAQ answer sheet. Please take your time and read each question carefully.

1. Sex
   a) male
   b) female
2. Race
   a) White
   b) Black
   c) Hispanic
   d) Asian
   e) American Indian
   f) other
3. Age
4. Height (feet and inches)
5. Weight (pounds)
6. Body frame size
   a) small
   b) medium
   c) large
7. Marital Status
   a) married
   b) widowed
   c) separated
   d) divorced
   e) single
   f) cohabiting
8. What was the total gross income of your household last year?
   a) under $12,000
   b) $12,000-$20,000
   c) $20,001-$30,000
   d) $30,001-$40,000
   e) $40,001-$50,000
   f) $50,001-$60,000
   g) over $60,000
9. What is the highest level of education you have completed?
   a) grade school or less
   b) some high school
   c) high school graduate
   d) some college or technical school
   e) college graduate
   f) postgraduate or professional degree
10. On the average day, how many hours do you watch television?
   a) 0 hours
   b) 1-3 hours
   c) 4-7 hours
   d) more than 8 hours
11. Where do you live?
   a) in the country
   b) in a city
   c) suburb
   d) small town
12. If you live in a city, suburb, or small town, what is the population?
   a) under 20,000
   b) 20,000-50,000
   c) 50,001-100,000
   d) 100,001-500,000
   e) over 500,000

Section 2: LIFESTYLE

INSTRUCTIONS:

This section will help determine your level of wellness. It will also give you ideas for areas in which you might improve. Some questions touch on very personal subjects. Therefore, if you prefer to skip certain questions, you may. However, the more questions you answer, the more you will learn about your health and how to improve it.

Please respond to these statements using the following responses. If an item does not apply to you, do not mark it.

A *Almost always (90% or more of the time)*
B *Very often (approximately 75% of the time)*
C *Often (approximately 50% of the time)*
D *Occasionally (approximately 25% of the time)*
E *Almost never (less than 10% of the time)*

PHYSICAL EXERCISE

Measures one's commitment to maintaining physical fitness.

1. I exercise vigorously for at least 20 minutes three or more times per week.
2. I determine my activity level by monitoring my heart rate.
3. I stop exercising before I feel exhausted.
4. I exercise in a relaxed, calm, and joyful manner.
5. I stretch before exercising.
6. I stretch after exercising.
7. I walk or bike whenever possible.
8. I participate in a strenuous activity (tennis, running, brisk walking, water exercise, swimming, handball, basketball, etc.).
9. If I am not in shape, I avoid sporadic (once a week or less often), strenuous exercise.
10. After vigorous exercise, I "cool down" (very light exercise such as walking) for at least five minutes before sitting or lying down.

NUTRITION

Measures the degree to which one chooses foods that are consistent with the dietary goals of the United States as published by the Senate Select Committee on Nutrition and Human Needs.

11. When choosing non-vegetable protein, I select lean cuts of meat, poultry, fish, and low-fat dairy products.
12. I maintain an appropriate weight for my height and frame.
13. I minimize salt intake.
14. I eat fruits and vegetables, fresh and uncooked.
15. I eat breakfast.
16. I intentionally include fiber in my diet on a daily basis.
17. I drink enough fluid to keep my urine light yellow.
18. I plan my diet to insure an adequate amount of vitamins and minerals.
19. I minimize foods in my diet that contain large amounts of refined flour (bleached white flour, typical store bread, cakes, etc.).
20. I minimize my intake of fats and oils including margarine and animal fats.

1

21. I include items from all four basic food groups in my diet each day (fruits and vegetables; milk group; breads and cereals; meat, fowl, fish or vegetable proteins).
22. To avoid unnecessary calories, I choose water as one of the beverages I drink.
23. I avoid adding sugar to my foods. I minimize my intake of pre-sweetened foods (sugarcoated cereals, syrups, chocolate milk, and most processed and fast foods).

SELF-CARE

Measures the behaviors which help one prevent or detect early illnesses.

24. I use footgear of good quality designed for the activity or the job in which I participate.
25. I record immunizations to maintain up-to-date immunization records.
26. I examine my breasts or testes on a monthly basis.
27. I have my breasts or testes examined yearly by a physician.
28. I balance the type and amount of food I eat with exercise to maintain a healthy percent body fat.
29. I take action to minimize my exposure to tobacco smoke.
30. When I experience illness or injury, I take necessary steps to correct the problem.
31. I engage in activities which keep my blood pressure in a range which minimizes my chances of disease (e.g., stroke, heart attack, and kidney disease).
32. I brush my teeth after eating.
33. I floss my teeth after eating.
34. My resting pulse is 60 or less.
35. I get an adequate amount of sleep.
36. If I were to have sex, I would take action to prevent unplanned pregnancy.
37. If I were to have sex, I would take action to prevent giving and/or getting sexually transmitted disease.

VEHICLE SAFETY

Measures one's ability to minimize chances of injury or death in a vehicle accident.

38. I do not operate vehicles while I am under the influence of alcohol or other drugs.
39. I do not ride with drivers who are under the influence of alcohol or other drugs.
40. I stay within the speed limit.
41. I practice defensive driving techniques.
42. When traffic lights change from green to yellow, I prepare to stop.
43. I maintain a safe driving distance between cars based on speed and road conditions.
44. Vehicles which I drive are maintained to assure safety.
45. Because they are safer, I use radial tires on cars that I drive.
46. When I ride a bicycle or motorcycle, I wear a helmet and have adequate lights/reflectors.
47. Children riding in my car are secured in an approved car seat or seat belt.
48. I use my seat belt while driving or riding in a vehicle.

DRUG USAGE AND AWARENESS

Measures the degree to which one functions without the unnecessary use of chemicals.

49. I use prescription drugs and over-the-counter medications only when necessary.
50. If I consume alcohol, I limit my consumption to not more than one drink per hour and no more than two drinks per day.
51. I avoid the use of tobacco.
52. Because of the potentially harmful effects of caffeine (e.g., coffee, tea, cola, etc.), I limit my consumption.
53. I avoid the use of marijuana.
54. I avoid the use of hallucinogens (LSD, PCP, MDA, etc.).
55. I avoid the use of stimulants ("uppers"—e.g., cocaine, amphetamines, "pep pills," etc.).
56. I avoid the use of nonmedically prescribed depressants ("downers"—e.g., barbituates, quaaludes, minor tranquilizers, etc.).
57. I avoid using a combination of drugs unless under medical supervision.
58. I follow the instructions provided with any drug I take.
59. I avoid using drugs obtained from illegal sources.
60. I understand the expected effect of drugs I take.
61. I consider alternatives to drugs.
62. If I experience discomfort from stress or tension, I use relaxation techniques, exercise, and meditation instead of taking drugs.
63. I get clear directions for taking my medicine from my doctor or pharmacist.

SOCIAL/ENVIRONMENTAL

Measures the degree to which one contributes to the common welfare of the community. This emphasizes interdependence with others and nature.

64. I conserve energy at home.
65. I consider energy conservation when choosing a mode of transportation.
66. My social ties with family are strong.
67. I contribute to the feeling of acceptance within my family.
68. I develop and maintain strong friendships.
69. I do my part to promote a clean environment (i.e., air, water, noise, etc.).
70. When I see a safety hazard, I take action (warn others or correct the problem).
71. I avoid unnecessary radiation.
72. I report criminal acts I observe.
73. I contribute time and/or money to community projects.
74. I actively seek to become acquainted with individuals in my community.
75. I use my creativity in constructive ways.
76. My behavior reflects fairness and justice.
77. When possible, I choose an environment which is free of **noise** pollution.
78. When possible, I choose an environment which is free of **air** pollution.
79. I participate in volunteer activities benefiting others.
80. I help others in need.
81. I beautify those parts of my environment under my control.

2

82. Because of limited resources, I do my part to conserve.
83. I recycle aluminum, glass, and paper products.
84. I involve myself with people who support a positive lifestyle.

EMOTIONAL AWARENESS AND ACCEPTANCE

Measures the degree to which one has an awareness and acceptance of one's feelings. This includes the degree to which one feels positive and enthusiastic about oneself and life.

85. I have a good sense of humor.
86. I feel positive about myself.
87. I feel there is a satisfying amount of excitement in my life.
88. My emotional life is stable.
89. I am aware of my needs.
90. I trust and value my own judgment.
91. When I make mistakes, I learn from them.
92. I feel comfortable when complimented for jobs well done.
93. It is okay for me to cry.
94. I have feelings of sensitivity for others.
95. I feel enthusiastic about life.
96. I find it easy to laugh.
97. I am able to give love.
98. I am able to receive love.
99. I enjoy my life.
100. I have plenty of energy.
101. My sleep is restful.
102. I trust others.
103. I feel others trust me.
104. I accept my sexual desires.
105. I understand how I create my feelings.
106. At times, I can be both strong and sensitive.
107. I am aware when I feel angry.
108. I accept my anger.
109. I am aware when I feel sad.
110. I accept my sadness.
111. I am aware when I feel happy.
112. I accept my happiness.
113. I am aware when I feel frightened.
114. I accept my feelings of fear.
115. I am aware of my feelings about death.
116. I accept my feelings about death.

EMOTIONAL MANAGEMENT

Measures the degree to which one controls and expresses feelings, and engages in effective, related behaviors.

117. I share my feelings with those with whom I am close.
118. I express my feelings of anger in appropriate ways.
119. I express my feelings of sadness in healthy ways.
120. I express my feelings of happiness in desirable ways.
121. I express my feelings of fear in appropriate ways.
122. I compliment myself for a job well done.
123. I accept constructive criticism without reacting defensively.
124. I set appropriate limits for myself.

125. I stay within the limits that I have set.
126. I recognize that I can have wide variations of feelings about the same person (such as loving someone even though you are angry with her/him at the moment).
127. I am able to develop close, intimate relationships.
128. I say "no" without feeling guilty.
129. I would feel comfortable seeking professional help to better understand and cope with my feelings.
130. I reduce feelings of failure by setting achievable goals.
131. I relax my body and mind without using drugs.
132. I can be alone without feeling lonely.
133. I am able to be spontaneous in expressing my feelings.
134. I accept responsibility for my actions.
135. I am willing to take the risks that come with making change.
136. I manage my feelings to avoid unnecessary suffering.
137. I make decisions with a minimum of stress and worry.
138. I accept the responsibility for creating my own feelings.
139. I can express my feelings about death.
140. I recognize grieving as a healthy response to loss.

INTELLECTUAL

Measures the degree to which one engages her/his mind in creative, stimulating mental activities, expanding knowledge, and improving skills.

141. I read a newspaper daily.
142. I read twelve or more books yearly.
143. On the average, I read one or more national magazines per week.
144. When I watch TV, I choose programs with informational/educational value.
145. I visit a museum or art show at least three times yearly.
146. I attend lectures, workshops, and demonstrations at least three times yearly.
147. I regularly use some of my time participating in hobbies such as photography, gardening, woodworking, sewing, painting, baking, art, music, writing, pottery, etc.
148. I read about local, state, national, and international political/public issues.
149. I learn the meaning of new words.
150. I engage in some type of writing activity such as a regular journal, letter writing, preparation of papers or manuscripts, etc.
151. I am interested in understanding the views of others.
152. I share ideas, concepts, thoughts, or procedures with others.
153. I gather information to enable me to make decisions.
154. I listen to radio and/or TV news.
155. I think about ideas different than my own.

OCCUPATIONAL

Measures the satisfaction gained from one's work and the degree to which one is enriched by that work. Please answer these items from your primary frame of reference, (e.g., your job, student, homemaker, etc.).

156. I enjoy my work.

78818 - 3/3

3

157. My work contributes to my personal needs.

158. I feel that my job in some way contributes to my well-being.

159. I cooperate with others in my work.

160. I take advantage of opportunities to learn new work-related skills.

161. My work is challenging.

162. I feel my job responsibilities are consistent with my values.

163. I find satisfaction from the work I do.

164. I find healthy ways of reducing excessive job-related stress.

165. I use recommended health and safety precautions.

166. I make recommendations for improving worksite health and safety.

167. I am satisfied with the degree of freedom I have in my job to exercise independent judgments.

168. I am satisfied with the amount of variety in my work.

169. I believe I am competent in my job.

170. My co-workers and supervisors respect me as a competent individual.

171. My communication with others in my work place is enriching for me.

SPIRITUAL

Measures one's ongoing involvement in seeking meaning and purpose in human existence. It includes an appreciation for the depth and expanse of life and natural forces that exist in the universe.

172. I feel good about my spiritual life.

173. Prayer, meditation, and/or quiet personal reflection is/are important part(s) of my life.

174. I contemplate my purpose in life.

175. I reflect on the meaning of events in my life.

176. My values guide my daily life.

177. My values and beliefs help me to meet daily challenges.

178. I recognize that my spiritual growth is a lifelong process.

179. I am concerned about humanitarian issues.

180. I enjoy participating in discussions about spiritual values.

181. I feel a sense of compassion for others in need.

182. I seek spiritual knowledge.

183. My spiritual awareness occurs other than at times of crisis.

184. I believe in something greater or that I am part of something greater than myself.

185. I share my spiritual values.

Section 3: HEALTH RISK APPRAISAL

INSTRUCTIONS:

This section is intended to help you identify the problems most likely to interfere with the quality of your life. It will also show you choices you can make to stay healthy and avoid the most common causes of death for a person your age and sex.

This Health Risk Appraisal is not a substitute for a checkup or physical exam that you get from a doctor or nurse. It only gives you some ideas for lowering your risk of getting sick or injured in the future. It is NOT designed for people who already have HEART DISEASE, CANCER, KIDNEY DISEASE, OR OTHER SERIOUS CONDITIONS. If you have any of these problems and you want a Health Risk Appraisal anyway, ask your doctor or nurse to read this section of the printout with you.

If you don't know or are unsure of an answer, please leave that item blank.

1. Have you ever been told that you have diabetes (or sugar diabetes)?
   a. yes
   b. no

2. Does your natural mother, father, sister or brother have diabetes?
   a. yes
   b. no
   c. not sure

3. Did either of your natural parents die of a heart attack before age 60? (If your parents are younger than 60, mark no.)
   a. yes, one of them
   b. yes, both of them
   c. no
   d. not sure

4. Are you now taking medicine for high blood pressure?
   a. yes
   b. no

5. What is your blood pressure now?
   a. _____ systolic (high number)
   b. _____ diastolic (low number)

6. If you *do not* know the number, select the answer that describes your blood pressure.
   a. high
   b. normal or low
   c. don't know

7. What is your TOTAL cholesterol level (based on a blood test)?
   _____ (mg/dl)

8. What is your High Density Lipoprotein (HDL) cholesterol level (based on a blood test)?
   _____ (mg/dl)

9. How many cigars do you usually smoke per day?
   _____

10. How many pipes of tobacco do you usually smoke per day? _____

11. How many times per day do you usually use smokeless tobacco (chewing tobacco, snuff, pouches, etc.)? _____

12. How would you describe your cigarette smoking habits?
    a. never smoked **Go to 15**
    b. used to smoke **Go to 14**
    c. still smoke **Go to 13**

4

13. How many cigarettes a day do you smoke?
_____ cigarettes per day **Go to 15**

14. a. How many years has it been since you smoked cigarettes regularly?
_____ years
b. What was the average number of cigarettes per day that you smoked in the 2 years before you quit?
_____ cigarettes per day

15. In the next 12 months, how many thousands of miles will you probably travel by each of the following? (NOTE: U.S. average = 10,000 miles)
a. car, truck, or van: _____,000 miles
b. motorcycle: _____,000 miles

16. On a typical day how do you USUALLY travel? (Check one only)
a. walk
b. bicycle
c. motorcycle
d. sub-compact or compact car
e. mid-size or full-size car
f. truck or van
g. bus, subway, or train
h. mostly stay home

17. What percent of the time do you usually buckle your safety belt when driving or riding?
_____%

18. On the average, how close to the speed limit do you usually drive?
a. within 5 mph of limit
b. 6-10 mph over limit
c. 11-15 mph over limit
d. more than 15 mph over limit

19. How many times in the last month did you drive or ride when the driver had perhaps too much alcohol to drink?
_____ times last month

20. When you drink alcoholic beverages, how many drinks do you consume in an average day? (If you *never* drink alcoholic beverages, write 0.)
_____ alcoholic beverages/average day

21. On the average, how many days per week do you consume alcohol?
_____ days/week

(MEN GO TO QUESTION 31)

WOMEN ONLY (QUESTIONS 22-30)

22. At what age did you have your first menstrual period?
_____ years old

23. How old were you when your first child was born (if no children, write 0)?
_____ years old

24. How long has it been since your last breast x-ray (mammogram)?
a. less than 1 year ago
b. 1 year ago
c. 2 years ago
d. 3 or more years ago
e. never

25. How many women in your natural family (mother and sisters only) have had breast cancer?
_____ women

26. Have you had a hysterectomy?
a. yes
b. no
c. not sure

27. How long has it been since you had a pap smear test?
a. less than 1 year ago
b. 1 year ago
c. 2 years ago
d. 3 or more years ago
e. never

28. How often do you examine your breasts for lumps?
a. monthly
b. once every few months
c. rarely or never

29. About how long has it been since you had your breasts examined by a physician or nurse?
a. less than 1 year ago
b. 1 year ago
c. 2 years ago
d. 3 or more years ago
e. never

30. About how long has it been since you had a rectal exam?
a. less than 1 year ago
b. 1 year ago
c. 2 years ago
d. 3 or more years ago
e. never

WOMEN GO TO QUESTION 35

MEN ONLY (QUESTIONS 31-34)

31. About how long has it been since you had a rectal or prostate exam?
a. less than 1 year ago
b. 1 year ago
c. 2 years ago
d. 3 or more years ago
e. never

32. Do you know how to properly examine your testes for lumps?
a. yes
b. no
c. not sure

33. How often do you examine your testes for lumps?
a. monthly
b. once every few months
c. rarely or never

34. About how long has it been since you had your testes examined by a physician or nurse?
a. less than one year ago
b. 1 year ago
c. 2 years ago
d. 3 or more years ago
e. never

35. How many times in the last year did you witness or become involved in a violent fight or attack where there was a good chance of a serious injury to someone?
a. 4 or more times
b. 2 or 3 times
c. 1 time or never
d. not sure

5

36. Considering your age, how would you describe your overall physical health?
    a. excellent
    b. good
    c. fair
    d. poor

37. In an average week, how many times do you engage in physical activity (exercise or work which lasts at least 20 minutes without stopping and which is hard enough to make you breathe heavier and your heart beat faster)?
    a. less than 1 time per week
    b. 1 or 2 times per week
    c. at least 3 times per week

38. If you ride a motorcycle or all-terrain vehicle (ATV), what percent of the time do you wear a helmet?
    a. 75% to 100%
    b. 25% to 74%
    c. less than 25%
    d. does not apply to me

39. Do you eat some food every day that is high in fiber, such as whole grain bread, cereal, fresh fruits, or vegetables?
    a. yes
    b. no

40. Do you eat foods every day that are high in cholesterol or fat, such as fatty meat, cheese, fried foods, or eggs?
    a. yes
    b. no

41. In general, how satisfied are you with your life?
    a. mostly satisfied
    b. partly satisfied
    c. not satisfied

42. Have you suffered a personal loss or misfortune in the past year that had a serious impact on your life? (For example, a job loss, disability, separation, jail term, or the death of someone close to you.)
    a. yes, 1 serious loss or misfortune
    b. yes, 2 or more
    c. no

Section 4: TOPICS FOR PERSONAL GROWTH

This section will help you identify areas in which you would like more information. In response to your selection from the following topics, we will provide you with resources or services to meet your requests.

Select topics on which you would like information. (Maximum of 4 topics.)

1. Responsible alcohol use
2. Stop-smoking programs
3. Sexuality
4. Gay issues
5. Depression
6. Loneliness
7. Exercise programs
8. Weight reduction
9. Self-breast exam
10. Medical emergencies
11. Nutrition
12. Relaxation
13. Stress reduction
14. Parenting skills
15. Marital or couples problems
16. Assertiveness training (how to say "no" without feeling guilty)
17. Biofeedback for tension headache and pain
18. Overcoming fears (i.e., high places, crowded rooms, etc.)
19. Educational career goal setting/planning
20. Spiritual or philosophical values
21. Communication skills
22. Automobile safety
23. Suicide thoughts or attempts
24. Substance abuse
25. Anxiety associated with public speaking, tests, writing, etc.
26. Enhancing relationships
27. Time-management skills
28. Death and dying
29. Learning skills (i.e., speed-reading, comprehension, etc.)
30. Financial management
31. Divorce
32. Alcoholism
33. Men's issues
34. Women's issues
35. Medical self-care
36. Dental self-care
37. Self-testes exam
38. Aging
39. Self-esteem
40. Premenstrual syndrome (PMS)
41. Osteoporosis
42. Recreation and leisure
43. Environmental issues

> **IMPORTANT— If you have finished completing all sections of the LAQ, please make sure you have answered the questions in Section 1 requesting your sex, race, age, height and weight. Results cannot be generated for the Health Risk Appraisal section without this information.**

6

You and Your Lifestyle Are the Major Determinants for Joyful Living

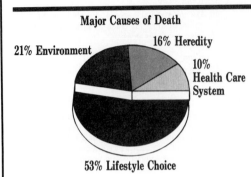

Major Causes of Death

21% Environment

16% Heredity

10% Health Care System

53% Lifestyle Choice

The circle graph to the left indicates the factors which contribute to your enjoyment and quality of life. While medical professionals contribute to the quality of your life, this graph clearly shows that the majority of those factors which contribute to your well-being are controlled by you. As you make responsible, informed choices, your chances of improving your health and well-being increase.

The LAQ's Role...

We believe this instrument is useful in helping individuals identify the most likely causes of death and disability. More importantly, it identifies those areas of self-improvement which will lead to higher levels of health and well-being.

The areas assessed in the LAQ emphasize the importance of creating a balance among the many different aspects of your lifestyle. Each of these areas affects one another and determines your overall wellness status. Also, each provides an opportunity for learning, making responsible decisions, and personal growth.

We invite you to use the information provided by the LAQ to your best advantage to increase your level of wellness.

Words from the Past

Wellness is a term that has enjoyed growing popularity during the past several decades. Although the term was introduced relatively recently, the concept of prevention has been present for centuries. The following passages provide a brief glimpse of the wellness philosophy through the years. Wellness is a movement which has become a major part of modern culture and is the most important weapon available to combat lifestyle illnesses.

"For many years, while engaged in the practice of medicine, the author of this volume has been more and more impressed with the idea that the causes of suffering, diseases, and premature deaths, which we witness around us on every hand, lie near our own doors ... and that the men and women of today, are, at least, equally as responsible for existing suffering, as those who have gone before them, and often much more so. In fact, he feels satisfied that by far the greatest portion of all the suffering, disease, deformity, and premature deaths which occur are the direct result of either the violation of, or the want of compliance with the laws of our being; calamities, which, were the requisite knowledge possessed by the community, can and should be avoided."

—JOHN ELLIS, M.D., 1859

"It is universally admitted at the present time that preventive medicine is of far greater importance than curative medication, and many of the most eminent members of the profession are devoting themselves exclusively to this branch."

—J. H. KELLOGG, M.D., 1902

"To ward off disease or recover health, men as a rule find it easier to depend on the healers than to attempt the more difficult task of living wisely."

—RENE DUBOS, Ph.D., 1959

"It's what you do hour by hour, day by day, that largely determines the state of your health; whether you get sick, what you get sick with, and perhaps when you die."

—LESTER BRESLOW, M.D., 1969

A National Wellness Institute, Inc.
Publication

National Wellness Institute, Inc.
South Hall, 1319 Fremont Street
Stevens Point, Wisconsin 54481
(715) 346-2172

PHOTO CREDITS: Occupational, Social, Intellectual — Educational Media Service (UW-Stevens Point; Emotional, Spiritual — Becker Communications, Inc.; Physical — Tan Yorks, NWI, Inc.

C2 HEALTHIER PEOPLE HEALTH RISK APPRAISAL
(CHAPTER 33)

THE
CARTER CENTER
OF EMORY UNIVERSITY

Healthier People
Health Risk Appraisal

No. _____

Detach this coupon and put it in a safe place.
You will need it to claim your appraisal results.

✂ —

Healthier People
Health Risk Appraisal
The Carter Center of Emory University

No. _____

_____

Health Risk Appraisal is an educational tool. It shows you choices you can make to keep good health and avoid the most common causes of death for a person your age and sex. This Health Risk Appraisal is not a substitute for a check-up or physical exam that you get from a doctor or nurse. It only gives you some ideas for lowering your risk of getting sick or injured in the future. It is NOT designed for people who already have HEART DISEASE, CANCER, KIDNEY DISEASE, OR OTHER SERIOUS CONDITIONS. If you have any of these problems and you want a Health Risk Appraisal anyway, ask your doctor or nurse to read the report with you.

DIRECTIONS: To keep your answers confidential DO NOT write your name or any identification on this form. Please keep the coupon with your participant number on it. You will need it to claim your computer report. To get the most accurate results answer as many questions as you can and as best you can. If you do not know the answer leave it blank. Questions with a ★ (star symbol) are important to your health, but are not used by the computer to calculate your risks. However, your answers may be helpful in planning your health and fitness program.

Please put your answers in the empty boxes. (Examples: ⬚x⬚ or ⬚125⬚)

1. SEX	1 ☐ Male 2 ☐ Female
2. AGE	☐ Years
3. HEIGHT (Without shoes) (No fractions)	☐ Feet ☐ Inches
4. WEIGHT (Without shoes) (No fractions)	☐ Pounds
5. Body frame size	1 ☐ Small 2 ☐ Medium 3 ☐ Large
6. Have you ever been told that you have diabetes (or sugar diabetes)?	1 ☐ Yes 2 ☐ No
7. Are you now taking medicine for high blood pressure?	1 ☐ Yes 2 ☐ No
8. What is your blood pressure now?	☐ / ☐ Systolic (High number) / Diastolic (Low number)
9. If you *do not* know the numbers, check the box that describes your blood pressure.	1 ☐ High 2 ☐ Normal or Low 3 ☐ Don't Know
10. What is your TOTAL cholesterol level (based on a blood test)?	☐ mg/dl
11. What is your HDL cholesterol (based on a blood test)?	☐ mg/dl
12. How many cigars do you usually smoke per day?	☐ cigars per day
13. How many pipes of tobacco do you usually smoke per day?	☐ pipes per day
14. How many times per day do you usually use smokeless tobacco? (Chewing tobacco, snuff, pouches, etc.)	☐ times per day

From The Carter Center of Emory University, Decatur, Ga.

Health Risk Appraisal is an educational tool. It shows you choices you can make to keep good health and avoid the most common causes of death for a person your age and sex. This Health Risk Appraisal is not a substitute for a check-up or physical exam that you get from a doctor or nurse. It only gives you some ideas for lowering your risk of getting sick or injured in the future. It is NOT designed for people who already have HEART DISEASE, CANCER, KIDNEY DISEASE, OR OTHER SERIOUS CONDITIONS. If you have any of these problems and you want a Health Risk Appraisal anyway, ask your doctor or nurse to read the report with you.

Your report may be picked up at _____ on _____.

15. CIGARETTE SMOKING

How would you describe your cigarette smoking habits?

1 ☐ Never smoked   ☞ Go to 18
2 ☐ Used to smoke   ☞ Go to 17
3 ☐ Still smoke   ☞ Go to 16

16. STILL SMOKE

How many cigarettes a day do you smoke?

☞ GO TO QUESTION 18

[   ] cigarettes per day ☞ Go to 18

17. USED TO SMOKE

a. How many years has it been since you smoked cigarettes fairly regularly?

[   ] years

b. What was the average number of cigarettes per day that you smoked in the 2 years before you quit?

[   ] cigarettes per day

18. In the next 12 months how many thousands of miles will you probably travel by each of the following? (NOTE: U.S. average = 10,000 miles)

a. Car, truck, or van: [   ],000 miles
b. Motorcycle: [   ],000 miles

19. On a typical day how do you USUALLY travel?

(Check one only)

1 ☐ Walk
2 ☐ Bicycle
3 ☐ Motorcycle
4 ☐ Sub-compact or compact car
5 ☐ Mid-size or full-size car
6 ☐ Truck or van
7 ☐ Bus, subway, or train
8 ☐ Mostly stay home

20. What percent of the time do you usually buckle your safety belt when driving or riding?

[   ] %

21. On the average, how close to the speed limit do you usually drive?

1 ☐ Within 5 mph of limit
2 ☐ 6-10 mph over limit
3 ☐ 11-15 mph over limit
4 ☐ More than 15 mph over limit

22. How many times in the last month did you drive or ride when the driver had perhaps too much alcohol to drink?

[   ] times last month

23. How many drinks of alcoholic beverages do you have in a typical week?

☞ (*MEN GO TO QUESTION 33*)

(Write the number of each type of drink)

[   ] Bottles or cans of beer
[   ] Glasses of wine
[   ] Wine coolers
[   ] Mixed drinks or shots of liquor

WOMEN

24. At what age did you have your first menstrual period?

[   ] years old

25. How old were you when your first child was born?

[   ] years old
(If no children write 0)

26. How long has it been since your last breast x-ray (mammogram)?

1 ☐ Less than 1 year ago
2 ☐ 1 year ago
3 ☐ 2 years ago
4 ☐ 3 or more years ago
5 ☐ Never

27. How many women in your natural family (mother and sisters only) have had breast cancer?

☐ women

28. Have you had a hysterectomy operation?

1 ☐ Yes
2 ☐ No
3 ☐ Not sure

29. How long has it been since you had a pap smear test?

1 ☐ Less than 1 year ago
2 ☐ 1 year ago
3 ☐ 2 years ago
4 ☐ 3 or more years ago
5 ☐ Never

★ 30. How often do you examine your breasts for lumps?

1 ☐ Monthly
2 ☐ Once every few months
3 ☐ Rarely or never

★ 31. About how long has it been since you had your breasts examined by a physician or nurse?

1 ☐ Less than 1 year ago
2 ☐ 1 year ago
3 ☐ 2 years ago
4 ☐ 3 or more years ago
5 ☐ Never

★ 32. About how long has it been since you had a rectal exam?

1 ☐ Less than 1 year ago
2 ☐ 1 year ago
3 ☐ 2 years ago
4 ☐ 3 or more years ago
5 ☐ Never

☞ (WOMEN GO TO QUESTION 34)

MEN
★ 33. About how long has it been since you had a rectal or prostate exam?

1 ☐ Less than 1 year ago
2 ☐ 1 year ago
3 ☐ 2 years ago
4 ☐ 3 or more years ago
5 ☐ Never

★ 34. How many times in the last year did you witness or become involved in a violent fight or attack where there was a good chance of a serious injury to someone?

1 ☐ 4 or more times
2 ☐ 2 or 3 times
3 ☐ 1 time or never
4 ☐ Not sure

★ 35. Considering your age, how would you describe your overall physical health?

1 ☐ Excellent
2 ☐ Good
3 ☐ Fair
4 ☐ Poor

★ 36. In an average week, how many times do you engage in physical activity (exercise or work which lasts at least 20 minutes without stopping and which is hard enough to make you breathe heavier and your heart beat faster)?

1 ☐ Less than 1 time per week
2 ☐ 1 or 2 times per week
3 ☐ At least 3 times per week

★ 37. If you ride a motorcycle or all-terrain vehicle (ATV) what percent of the time do you wear a helmet?

1 ☐ 75% to 100%
2 ☐ 25% to 74%
3 ☐ Less than 25%
4 ☐ Does not apply to me

★ 38. Do you eat some food every day that is high in fiber, such as whole grain bread, cereal, fresh fruits or vegetables?

1 ☐ Yes   2 ☐ No

★ 39. Do you eat foods every day that are high in cholesterol or fat, such as fatty meat, cheese, fried foods, or eggs?

1 ☐ Yes   2 ☐ No

★ 40. In general, how satisfied are you with your life?

1 ☐ Mostly satisfied
2 ☐ Partly satisfied
3 ☐ Not satisfied

★ 41. Have you suffered a personal loss or misfortune in the past year that had a serious impact on your life? (For example, a job loss, disability, separation, jail term, or the death of someone close to you.)

1 ☐ Yes, 1 serious loss or misfortune
2 ☐ Yes, 2 or more
3 ☐ No

★ 42a. Race

1 ☐ Aleutian, Alaska native, Eskimo or American Indian
2 ☐ Asian
3 ☐ Black
4 ☐ Pacific Islander
5 ☐ White
6 ☐ Other
7 ☐ Don't know

★ 42b. Are you of Hispanic origin such as Mexican-American, Puerto Rican, or Cuban?

1 ☐ Yes   2 ☐ No

★ 43. What is the highest grade you completed in school?

1 ☐ Grade school or less
2 ☐ Some high school
3 ☐ High school graduate
4 ☐ Some college
5 ☐ College graduate
6 ☐ Post graduate or professional degree

★ 44. What is your job or occupation?

(Check only one)

1 ☐ Health professional
2 ☐ Manager, educator, professional
3 ☐ Technical, sales or administrative support
4 ☐ Operator, fabricator, laborer
5 ☐ Student
6 ☐ Retired
7 ☐ Homemaker
8 ☐ Service
9 ☐ Skilled crafts
10 ☐ Unemployed
11 ☐ Other

★ 45. In what industry do you work (or did you last work)?

(Check only one)

1 ☐ Electric, gas, sanitation
2 ☐ Transportation, communication
3 ☐ Agriculture, forestry, fishing
4 ☐ Wholesale or retail trade
5 ☐ Financial and service industries
6 ☐ Mining
7 ☐ Government
8 ☐ Manufacturing
9 ☐ Construction
10 ☐ Other

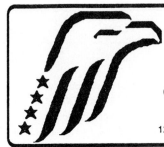

THE CARTER CENTER OF EMORY UNIVERSITY

1276 McConnell Drive, Suite D. Decatur, Ga. 30033

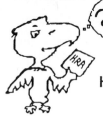

User's Guide to Interpreting the
HEALTH RISK APPRAISAL REPORT FORM

Unhealthy habits lead to early death or chronic illness. Every year 1.3 million people die prematurely in the United States from conditions which could be prevented or delayed. This Health Risk Appraisal (HRA) may help you avoid becoming one of these statistics by giving you a prediction of your health risks related to your particular characteristics and habits.

WHAT IS A HEALTH RISK APPRAISAL ?

The health risk appraisal is an estimation of your risk of dying in the next ten years from each of forty-two causes of death. The twelve most important of these are printed individually on your Report Form; the others are grouped together and printed as "All Other" on the form. These risks are calculated by a computer which compares your characteristics to national mortality statistics using equations developed by epidemiologists. The Health Risk Appraisal does not tell you how long you will live, nor does it diagnose or treat disease; it gives you a way to compare yourself to large groups of people on which medical data have been collected.

RISK FACTORS

Most chronic diseases develop slowly in the presence of certain risk factors. Risk factors are either controllable or uncontrollable. Uncontrollable risk factors include factors such as your age, sex, and the health history of your family. Controllable risk factors include lifestyle habits that you can change such as blood pressure, exercise, smoking, weight, cholesterol, and stress.

The Health Risk Appraisal uses both uncontrollable and controllable risk factors in calculating health risks, however, you should focus on controllable risk factors. To help you decide which controllable risk factors you should concentrate on, the Health Risk Appraisal identifies the controllable factors for each cause of death. The report gives you an idea of their relative importance by indicating the number of risk years you could gain by controling each factor.

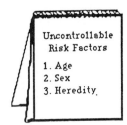

To see what the numbers on your Report Form mean, where to find your relative risks, and which risk factors you need to control, turn the page.

User's Guide to Interpreting the Health Risk Appraisal Report Form

An example using a 48 year old woman: 5'7", 175 lbs, 250mg/dl cholesterol, 160/95 B.P., 30 cigarettes/day, 7 drinks/week, seat belt use 15%, drives 4,000 mi/yr, menarche 13 yrs, 1st child at 32.

Your **RISK AGE** compares your total risk from 42 causes of death to the total risk of those who are your age and sex. It merely gives you an idea of your risks compared with the population average in terms of an age. Your **TARGET** risk age indicates how much you could improve.

If your **TARGET** risk age seems too high, and you have medical factors you can not change, such as diabetes and a family history of breast cancer, it may be helpful for you to see how you compare with others who are more like you than just the same sex and age.

Your actual age is here

12345
Female Age 48

	YOUR	NOW	TARGET
RISK AGE		55.57	47.68

THIS REPORT CONTAINS ESTIMATES DUE TO MISSING ITEMS, INCLUDING THE FOLLOWING

HDL Cholesterol

If you did not answer items on the questionnaire which are used for calculations, these missing items will be listed here. The computer substitutes national average values for the items you left blank and calculates your risks with these numbers.

Many serious injuries and health problems can be prevented. Your Health Risk Appraisal lists factors you can change to lower your risk. For causes of death that are not directly computable, the report uses the average risk for persons of your age and sex. More technical detail about the report is on page 2.

Beside each cause of death are listed the modifiable risk factors which your questionnaire responses indicate you need to work on. The list is specific for you unless you have none of the risk factors or if there are no known risk factors for a cause of death. In this case, a short statement of general advice related to risk reduction is printed.

MOST COMMON CAUSES OF DEATH	NUMBER OF DEATHS IN NEXT 10 YEARS FOR 1000 WOMEN AGE 48			MODIFIABLE RISK FACTORS
	YOUR GROUP	TARGET	POPULATION AVERAGE	
Heart attack	33	7	7	Avoid Tobacco Use, Blood Pressure, Cholesterol Level, HDL Level, Weight
Lung cancer	11	6	4	Avoid Tobacco Use
Stroke	7	2	3	Avoid Tobacco Use, Blood Pressure
Breast cancer	7	2*	6	A Low-Fat Diet and Regular Exams Might Reduce Risk
Colon Cancer	2*	2*	2	A High-Fiber and Low-Fat Diet Might Reduce Risk
Ovary Cancer	2	2	<2	Continue to Avoid Heavy Drinking
Emphysema/Bronchitis	2*	1	2	Get Regular Exams
Esophagus Cancer	1	1	1	Avoid Tobacco Use
Diabetes mellitus	1	<1	1	Avoid Tobacco Use
Pancreas Cancer	1	<1	<1	Control Your Weight and Follow Your Doctor's Advice
				Avoid Tobacco Use
All Other	22	21	22	* = Average Value Used
TOTAL:	91	49	51	Deaths in Next 10 Years Per 1,000 WOMEN, Age 48

The numbers in the **YOUR GROUP** column refer to the number of predicted deaths for each cause of death in the next 10 years from among 1,000 people who have habits and characteristics just like you.

The numbers in the **TARGET** column refer to those predicted to die in the next 10 years from among 1,000 people who have characteristics just like you, but who have adopted the habits recommended below in the **TO IMPROVE YOUR RISK PROFILE** box.

The numbers in the **POPULATION AVERAGE** column refer to the national average of deaths in 10 years for people of your same sex and age.

For Height 5'7" and Large Frame, 175 pounds is about 20% Overweight.   Desirable Weight Range: 139-153

Your **DESIRABLE WEIGHT RANGE** is based on your height and frame size.

```
******************
* HERE'S THE IMPORTANT PART! *
******************
```

In this box is our prescription to lengthen your life and a prediction of how much life you may be expected to gain by adopting these health habits. The **TOTAL RISK YEARS** you could gain by making these habit changes are printed here. This is also the difference between your present Risk Age and your Target Risk Age. Also important are the recommendations on page 2.

TO IMPROVE YOUR RISK PROFILE:	RISK YEARS GAINED
- Quit smoking	4.07
- Lower your blood pressure	1.58
- Lower your cholesterol	1.27
- Improve your HDL Level	.76
- Bring your weight to desirable range	.11
- Always wear your safety belt.	.10

GOOD HABITS
+ Regular pap tests
+ Safe driving speed
+ You don't use smokeless tobacco

This box lists your **GOOD HABITS**. Congratulations!

Total Risk Years you could gain = 7.89

Page two of your Report Form lists some **ROUTINE PREVENTATIVE SERVICES**. These services are specific for people of your age and sex. The Report Form also lists some **GENERAL RECOMMENDATIONS FOR EVERYONE**. For the particular woman used in this example, the Report Form printed the following messages:

ROUTINE PREVENTIVE SERVICES FOR WOMEN YOUR AGE
Blood Pressure and Cholesterol test
Pap Smear test
Breast cancer screening (check with your doctor or clinic)
Rectal exam (or Sigmoidoscopy)
Eye exam for glaucoma
Dental Exam
Tetanus-Diptheria booster shot (every 10 years)

GENERAL RECOMMENDATIONS FOR EVERYONE
* Exercise briskly for 15-30 minutes
  at least three times a week
* Use good eating habits by choosing a
  variety of foods that are low in fat
  and cholesterol and high in fiber
* Learn to recognize and handle stress -
  get help if you need it.

The Standard Report Form also prints a message about AIDS and some additional information about the Report.

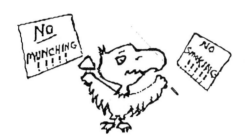

CHOOSING A HABIT TO WORK ON

Your Health Risk Appraisal is intended to encourage you to work on the habits you can change - to be the best that you can be. You don't have to change your entire lifestyle overnight - in fact, trying to change too many habits at once is probably the quickest way to discouragement and failure. The Health Risk Appraisal, therefore, may help you by showing you which behaviors should have priority. If you can not change the behavior that is top on the list (the one that would give the greatest amount of **RISK YEARS GAINED**), try to concentrate on changing the next highest on the list.

HRA LIMITS

Your Health Risk Appraisal does have limits. It is not a predictor, but rather an educational tool. It does not take into consideration whether or not you already have a medical condition and it does not consider more rare diseases and other health problems which are not fatal but can limit your enjoyment of life (such as arthritis).

What it does consider are the lifestyle factors over which you have a great degree of control and which account for a large number of premature deaths. Now that you are familiar with your particular health risks, it's time to do something about them!

MAKE A PLAN

Make a plan of how to change the habit you chose to work on. Write the plan down and keep it in sight. Be prepared for temptation! Observe the time, situation, or place that most often triggers your unhealthy habit and be ready to combat the urge when it appears. Let family and friends know of your goals, and ask for their encouragement.

REWARD YOURSELF

Rewards are an important part of changing behavior. Give yourself a reasonable reward when you accomplish your goal. Don't eat half a gallon of ice cream after losing 10 pounds! Choose a healthy and enjoyable reward. You've worked hard and are on the road to good health!

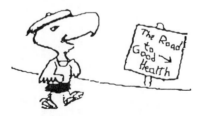

APPENDIX

Drug and Immunization Information

D1—RECOMMENDATIONS FOR PROPHYLAXIS OF HEPATITIS A
(Chapter 19)

1. *Close personal contact.* IG is recommended for all household and sexual contacts of persons with hepatitis A.

2. *Day-care centers.* Day-care facilities with children in diapers can be important settings for HAV transmission. IG should be administered to all staff and attendees of day-care centers or homes of (1) one or more hepatitis A cases are recognized among children or employees; or (2) cases are recognized in two or more households of center attendees. When an outbreak (hepatitis cases in three or more families) occurs, IG should also be considered for members of households whose diapered children attend. In centers not enrolling children in diapers, IG need only be given to classroom contacts of an index case.

3. *Schools.* Contact at elementary and secondary schools is usually not an important means of transmitting hepatitis A. Routine administration of IG is not indicated for pupils and teachers in contact with a patient. However, when epidemiological study clearly shows the existence of a school- or classroom-centered outbreak, IG may be given to those who have close personal contact with patients.

4. *Institutions for custodial care.* Living conditions in some institutions, such as prisons and facilities for the developmentally disabled, favor transmission of hepatitis A. When outbreaks occur, giving IG to residents and staff who have close contact with patients with hepatitis A may reduce spread of disease. Depending on the epidemiologic circumstances, prophylaxis can be limited or can involve the entire institution.

5. *Hospitals.* Routine IG administration is not indicated. Rather, sound hygienic practices should be emphasized. Staff education should point out the risk of exposure to hepatitis A and emphasize precautions regarding direct contact with potentially infective materials. Outbreaks of hepatitis A among hospital staff occur occasionally, usually in association with an unsuspected index patient who is fecally incontinent. Large outbreaks have occurred among staff and family contacts of infected infants in neonatal intensive-care units. In outbreaks, prophylaxis of persons exposed to feces of infected patients may be indicated.

6. *Offices and factories.* Routine IG administration is not indicated under the usual office or factory conditions for persons exposed to a fellow worker with hepatitis A. Experience shows that casual contact in the work setting does not result in virus transmission.

7. *Common-source exposure.* IG might be effective in preventing food-borne or waterborne hepatitis A if exposure is recognized in time. However, IG is not recommended for persons exposed to a common source of hepatitis infection after cases have begun to occur in those exposed, because the 2-week period during which IG is effective will have been exceeded.

If a foodhandler is diagnosed as having hepatitis A, common-source transmission is possible but uncommon. IG should be administered to other foodhandlers but is usually not recommended for patrons. However, IG administration to patrons may be considered if (1) the infected person is directly involved in handling, without gloves, foods that will not be cooked before they are eaten; (2) the hygienic practices of the foodhandler are deficient; and (3) patrons can be identified and treated within 2 weeks of exposure. Situations in which repeated exposures may have occurred, such as in institutional cafeterias, may warrant stronger consideration of IG use.

For postexposure IG prophylaxis, a single intramuscular dose of 0.02 ml/kg is recommended.

Drug	Dosage	Route	Onset	Duration
STIMULANTS				
Caffeine	50-100 mg	Oral	15-30 minutes	3-5 hours
Amphetamines				
Amphetamine (Benzedrine)	5-30 mg	Oral	15-30 minutes	4-14 hours
Dextramphetamine (Dexedrine)	5-60 mg	Injection		Up to 24 hours
Methamphetamine (Methedrine)	2.5-15 mg	Inhalation (Ice)		6-12 hours and up to 24 hours
Cocaine	25 mg per "line"	Intranasal	3-5 minutes	15-30 minutes
		IV	<10 seconds	
		Inhalation	<5 seconds	10-15 minutes
Nicotine	1-2 mg delivered per cigarette	Inhalation Sublingual	Within seconds	30 minutes
DEPRESSANTS				
Alcohol		Oral		Depends on amount consumed
Barbiturates				
Phenobarbital	30-200 mg	Oral	15-30 minutes	12-24 hours (phenobarbital and barbital)
Amobarbital (Amytal)	15-120 mg bid to qid	Injection		
Pentobarbital (Nembutal)	20-40 mg bid to qid	Suppository		6-7 hours
Secobarbital (Seconal)	200-300 mg			
Chloral hydrate	500 mg-1 gm	Oral	15-30 minutes	5 hours
Methaqualone (Quaaludes)	75-300 mg			
Glutethamide (Doriden)	250-500 mg			
Methyprylon (Noludar)	200-400 mg		30-45 minutes	7 hours
Ethchlorvynol (Placidyl)	500 mg			
Minor tranquilizers				
Benzodiazepines				
Diazepam (Valium)	2-10 mg tid to qid	Oral		
Chlordiazepam (Librium)	5-10 mg qid	IV (Valium, Librium, Ativan)	15-30 minutes	
Lorazepam (Ativan)	2-6 mg	IM (Ativan)		

Desired effects	Side effects/adverse reactions	Tolerance	physical dependency	psychological dependency	Overdose
Increased mental activity, elevates mood, increased alertness	Cardiac muscle stimulant, insomnia, irritability, tremulousness, diuresis, anxiety, stomach irritant, bladder irritant, headache, muscle twitching	Y	Y	Y	Vomiting, dehydration, mild delirium, fever, cardiac arrhythmias, convulsions, possibly death
Increased alertness, weight loss, increased energy, elation, increased confidence (medicinal: obesity, fatigue, depression, narcolepsy) IV: amphetamin psychosis—hallucinations, paranoia, aggressiveness, panic	Insomnia, irritability, jitteriness, decreased sex drive, dry mouth, anorexia, dilated pupils, tachycardia, hypertension, fever	Y	Some	Strong	Agitation, fever, hallucinations, cardiac arrhythmias, panic, convulsions, possibly death
Euphoria, elation, increased energy, increased confidence (medicinal: local anesthetic)	Tachycardia, hypertension, anorexia, weight loss, dilated pupils, runny nose, anxiety, insomnia, dry mouth, paranoia, psychosis, "cocaine bugs"	Y	Y	High	Agitation, hyperthermia, hallucinations, cardiac arrhythmias, convulsions, possibly death
Relaxation, increased alertness	Dizziness, nausea	Rapid	Y	Y	
Relaxation, decreased inhibitions, euphoria	Decreased alertness, impaired judgement, impaired coordination and reflexes, constricted pupils	Y	Y	Y	Respiratory depression, dilated pupils, coma, death
Decrease anxiety, sedative, hypnotic	Same	Y	Y	Y	Same
Relaxation, increased self-confidence, decrease anxiety, muscle relaxant (medicinal: anxiety disorders, insomnia, muscle spasms, seizures)	Inferferes with spatial judgement, vision, and sense of time: hypotension, slurred speech, drowsiness, headache	Some	Y	Y	Drowsiness, confusion, hypotension

D2—Commonly Abused Substances—cont'd
(Chapter 23)

Drug	Dosage	Route	Onset	Duration
Alprazolam (Xanax)	0.25-0.5 mg tid			
Oxazepam (Serax)	15-30 mg tid to qid			
Flurazepam (Dalmane)	15-30 mg at HS			
Temazepam (Restoril)				
Triazolam (Halcion)	0.125-0.5 mg at HS			
Meprobamate (Miltown)	1.2-1.6 gm			
Opiates				
Morphine sulfate	4-15 mg q4h	Oral	20 minutes	4 hours
Heroin		IM IV		
Opium				
Codeine	15-60 mg q4h	Inhalation	Within seconds	1 hour
Meperedine (Demerol)	50-150 mg q4h	Suppository		
Methadone	2.5-10 mg q4-12h			22-48 hours
Propoxyphene (Darvon)	65 mg q4h			
Hydromorphone (Dilaudid)	1-6 mg q4-6h			
Oxycodone (Percodan)	1-2 tabs q4h			
MARIJUANA				
Sinsemilla	5-20 mg THC per joint	Inhalation	Within minutes	2-4 hours
Hash				
Nabilone (oral THC)	1-2 mg bid	Oral	½ to 1½ hours	3-10 hours
PHENCYCLIDINE (PCP)	2-15 mg	Oral	15-30 minutes	14 hours
		Inhalation	30-60 seconds	4-6 hours
		Intranasal		
HALLUCINOGENS				
LSD	100-200 mcg	Oral	15-80 minutes	6-12 hours
Psilocybin	20-60 mg			4-6 hours
Mescaline	1-50 gm			
Peyote	6-12 buttons			12 hours

Desired effects	Side effects/adverse reactions	Tolerance	physical dependency	psychological dependency	Overdose
Analgesia, euphoria, relaxation, detachment from reality (medicinal: analgesia, cough suppressant, combat diarrhea)	Drowsiness, constricted pupils, anorexia, nausea, slurred speech, constipation, impaired judgement, disorientation, clammy skin, respiratory depression	Y	Strong	Strong	Unconsciousness, hypothermia, respiratory depression, circulatory depression, coma, cardiac or respiratory arrest, death
Relaxation, increase perception, euphoria (medicinal: increase appetite, anti-emetic, decrease intraocular pressure, decrease muscle spasticity)	Dry mouth, increased appetite, tachycardia, reddens eyes, disorientation, anxiety	Some	Some	Some	Fatigue, anxiety, paranoia
Distortion of senses, feeling of disconnection from the body	Tachycardia, hypertension, flushing, diaphoresis, dizziness, numbness in extremities, agitation, blank stare, muscle rigidity, confusion, amnesia, horizontal/vertical nystagmus, psychosis	Y	N	Some	Catatonia, convulsions, coma, respiratory failure, death
Heightened sense of awareness, distorted perceptions, syesthesia	Nausea, depersonalization, dilated pupils, hypertension, increased salivation, panic, psychosis	N / Y / Y	N / N / N	N / N / N	Panic, psychosis

D3—IMMUNIZATION INFORMATION

Routine immunizing agents

Agent	Age to administer	Administration	Reaction and treatment
DTP diphtheria toxoid, tetanus toxoid, and pertussis vaccine	2, 4, 6 months; 1½ years; 4-6 years (may be given through the sixth year)	a. Primary course: three 0.5 cc doses at 8-week intervals followed by fourth 0.5 cc dose 1 year after third dose. b. Booster course: one 0.5 cc dose at 4-6 years of age; thereafter Td 0.5 cc every 10 years. *Contraindications:* (1) any acute febrile illness; (2) exposure to disease (diphtheria and pertussis): booster dose given of appropriate single antigen, unless fourth dose has been given within past year; (3) tetanus prophylaxis in wound management; (4) any severe allergic reaction; (5) encephalopathy or residual seizure disorder; (6) specific contraindications include: encephalopathy within 7 days of DTP administration; a convulsion with or without fever occurring within 3 days of immunization; persistent unconsolable screaming or crying for 3 or more hours or unusual high-pitched cry within 48 hours; shocklike state within 48 hours; temperature 40.5 C (104.9 F) or greater, unexplained by another cause within 48 hours; an immediate allergic reaction.	a. Local reaction: induration, redness, or nodule at injection site. Treatment: warm compress to site; rotation of injection sites. b. Systemic reaction: temperature elevation and irritability not lasting more than 24-48 hours. Treatment: acetaminophen for fever. If febrile or local reactions are severe, fractional doses should be considered.
DT: pediatric—diphtheria toxoid and tetanus toxoid	May be given through the sixth year	Same as DTP; indicated for use in infants and young children under 6 when pertussis vaccine is contraindicated. *Contraindications:* same as for DTP	Same as DTP.
Td: adult type—diphtheria toxoid and tetanus toxoid	Children over 6 years; 14-16 years and every 10 years thereafter	a. Primary course: two 0.5 cc doses at 8-week interval followed by third 0.5 cc dose 6-12 months after second dose. b. Booster course: one 0.5 cc dose at 14-16 years and every 10 years thereafter. *Contraindications:* same as for DTP.	Same as DTP.
OPV: live, oral poliovirus vaccine; vaccine must be kept frozen	2, 4, 6 months; 1½ years, 4-6 years (do not give to persons over 18 years) Population at risk: children not vaccinated, especially a large number in 0 to 4 age group	a. Primary course: two doses at 8-week intervals in first 6 months of life with third dose at 18 months of age. b Booster course: one dose at 4-6 years. c. Course for children or adolescents under 18 years: two doses at 8-week intervals followed by third dose in 8-14 months. *Contraindications:* same as for DTP. See Chapter 26.	Risk of vaccine: live virus persists in GI tract for 4-6 weeks after vaccination and paralytic disease can occur. Populations with immune deficiency disorders are particularly at risk, as are those over 18 years who have had no previous polio immunization and have been exposed. Use of inactivated vaccine (Salk) is recommended for these populations.

Adapted from American Academy of Pediatrics: Report of Committee on Infectious Diseases, ed 22, Elk Grove Village, Ill, 1991; and Phillips CF: Keeping up with the changing immunization schedule, Contemporary Pediatrics 8:20-46, 1991.   *Continued.*

D3—IMMUNIZATION INFORMATION
Routine immunizing agents—cont'd

Agent	Age to administer	Administration	Reaction and treatment
Measles: live attenuated virus vaccine; also available in combination as (a) measles-rubella or (b) measles-mumps-rubella	15 months of age Booster at 5 years or 10-12 years of age	One subcutaneous injection of total volume of reconstituted vaccine. *Contraindications:* hypersensitivity to eggs (See Chapter 23). Vaccine should be given anytime after 6 months of age if exposed to measles and repeated at 15 months. *Indications* for revaccination include children vaccinated before 13 months of age, children vaccinated with simultaneous administration of gamma globulin at any age, and children for whom doubt exists about immunization status. Tuberculin testing should be done prior to, simultaneously, or 4-6 weeks after measles vaccine administration.	Reaction: mild noncommunicable infection with symptoms of fever, faint rash, and minor toxicity in 15% of vaccinated population. May occur 5-12 days after vaccination. Treatment: symptomatic.
Rubella: live attentuated virus; in combination as (a) measles-rubella, (b) mumps-rubella, or (c) measles-mumps-rubella	15 months of age Booster at 5 years or 10-12 years of age.	Same as for measles *Contraindications:* pregnant women. In susceptible nonpregnent females, administration if Hl titer is less than 1:10 and pregnancy is not planned for 2 months.	Reaction: rarely fever and rash. Treatment: symptomatic. In older age populations transient arthritis and arrthralgia may occur 2-4 weeks after vaccination. Treatment: symptomatic.
Mumps: live attenuated virus. In combination as (a) mumps-rubella or (b) measles-mumps-rubella	15 months of age Booster at 5 years or 10-12 years of age.	Same as measles. *Contraindications:* see Chapter 26. Indicated for use in susceptible children approaching puberty, in adolescents, and in males who have no history of mumps.	Reaction: no serious side effects. Occasionally mild fever treated symptomatically.
Haemophilus influenzae Type b Conjugate Vaccines 1. HbOC: oligosaccharide of capsular antigen of Hib conjugated to diphtheria	2, 4, 6 months with booster at 15 months	3 0.5 ml intramuscular injections at 8 week intervals with one 0.5 intramuscular booster	For all conjugate vaccines: Reaction: fever, erythema swelling and tenderness at injection site in first 24 hours.
2. PRP-OMP: outer membrane protein complex of *Neisseria* meningitis	2, 4 months with booster at 12 months	2 0.5 ml intramuscular injections at 8-week intervals with one 0.5 ml booster	
3. PRP-D: diptheria toxoid conjugate	Appropriate for 15 month booster or for one-time immunization of children 15-60 months who did not receive initial series.	1 0.5 ml intramuscular booster or one-time immunization All Hib conjugates may be given concurrently with DTP, OPV and MMR at different sites. *Contraindications:* delay in presence of any febrile illness or acute infection.	Treatment: warm compresses to site: acetaminophen for fever.

Contracts and Forms: Samples

E1—COMMUNITY ORIENTED HEALTH RECORD (COHR)
(Chapter 16)
Community Health Assessment Model

Definition of *community:* A locality-based entity—composed of systems of formal organizations reflecting societal institutions, informal groups, and aggregates, which are interdependent—whose function (expressed intent) is to meet a wide range of collective needs.

Definition of *community health:* The meeting of collective needs, through identifying problems and managing interactions within the community and between the community and the larger society. This requires commitment, self-other awareness and clarity of situational definitions, articulateness, effective communication, conflict containment and accommodation, participation, management of relations with the larger society, and machinery for facilitating participant interaction and decision making.

Community Health Assessment Guide Categories

A. Community
   1. Place
      a. Geopolitical boundaries of community
      b. Local or folk name for community
      c. Size in square miles/areas/blocks/census tracts
      d. Transportation avenues
      e. Physical environment
   2. People
      a. Number and density of population
      b. Demographic structure of population
      c. Informal groups
      d. Formal groups
      e. Linking structures
   3. Function
      a. Production—distribution—consumption of goods and services
      b. Socialization of new members
      c. Maintenance of social control
      d. Adapting to ongoing and unexpected change
      e. Provision of mutual aid
B. Community health
   1. Status
      a. Vital statistics
      b. Disease incidence and prevalence for leading causes of mortality and morbidity
      c. Health risk profiles
      d. Functional ability levels
   2. Structure
      a. Health facilities
      b. Health related planning groups
      c. Health manpower
      d. Health resource utilization patterns
   3. Process
      a. Commitment
      b. Self-other awareness and clarity of situational definitions
      c. Articulateness
      d. Effective communication
      e. Conflict containment and accommodation
      f. Participation
      g. Management of relations with the larger society
      h. Machinery for facilitating participant interaction and decision making

Database

This form provides a structured method for recording data. The name of the community and the assessment category and/or subcategory are noted at the top of the page. These categories correspond to those of the assessment guide. The data are collected and the source of the information and the data are recorded. Data are often entered using the SOAP format. An example of the COHR Database form is depicted on the next page.

Community Problem List

Headings of columns for the Community Problem List are Date, Number, Problem/Concern, and Supportive Data (title of appropriate section of Data Base and capsule summary of relevant data).

Community Capability List

Headings of columns for this list are Date, Number, Capability, Supportive Data (title of appropriate section of Data Base and capsule summary of relevant data).

Problem Analysis

A line labeled Problem/Statement is included at the top of the form below Name of Community. Headings of columns are Problem Correlates, Relationship of Correlates to Problem, and Data Supportive to Relationships (refer to appropriate sections of Data Base *and* relevant research findings in current literature). An example of a completed Problem Analysis is depicted on p. 262.

Problem Prioritization

Headings of columns are Criteria, Criteria Weights (1-10). Problem, Problem Rating (1-10), Rationale for Rating, Problem Significance/(Weight × Rate).

DATABASE

Name of community _____

Assessment category _____ Subcategory _____

Date	Data source	Data*

*Note with an asterisk the themes identified and meanings given.

Goals and Objectives

This form includes a line labeled Problem/Concern as well as lines for Goal Statement at the top under Name of Community. Column headings are Date, Objectives (number and statement), and By Date. An example of a completed goals and objectives statement is depicted on p. 264.

Plan

A line labeled Objective Number and Statement is included under Name of Community. Column headings are Date, Intervener Activities/Means, Value (1-10)/Probability (1-10), and Activity/Means Selected for Implementation. Sample plan sheets from the interventions related to infant malnutrition are presented on pp. 265 and 266.

Progress Notes

A line labeled Goal is included under Name of Community. Column headings are Date, Narrative, Assessment, Plan (NAP), and Budget and Time. A footnote to the second column explains the NAP procedure: Record both objective and subjective data. Interpret these data in terms of (1) whether the objectives were achieved and (2) whether the intervener activities utilized were effective. The plan is dependent on the assessment and may include both new (or revised) objectives and activities. Progress Notes reflecting evaluation of interventions aimed at decreasing the incidence of malnutrition are presented on p. 268.

E2—AUDIT FORM
(Chapter 13)

SCHMELE INSTRUMENT TO MEASURE THE PROCESS OF NURSING PRACTICE IN HOME HEALTH

INSTRUCTIONS: On the scale provided for each item, please *circle the number* that best describes the nursing care observed during the home visit. If not observed or not applicable, indicate the reason under the item.

NOTE: Whenever "family" occurs in an item, consider it to mean "family or significant other." Whenever "nursing diagnoses" occurs in an item, consider it to mean "nursing diagnosis or nursing problem."

I. Assessing

Objective: To measure the quality of nursing care observed for the *assessment* component of the nursing process.

	Best care		Average care		Worst care	Not applicable	Not observed
	5	4	3	2	1	0	0
1. The nurse collects data about the client's response to his/her medical illness.	5	4	3	2	1	0	0
2. The nurse collects data about the client's ability to care for self in the home.	5	4	3	2	1	0	0
3. The nurse collects data about client and/or family strengths that maintain or promote health.	5	4	3	2	1	0	0
4. During the visit, the nurse obtains pertinent data by questioning the client and/or family.	5	4	3	2	1	0	0
5. During the visit, the nurse's objective examination (auditory visual, palpable) of the client if either indicated* and made or *not* indicated and *not* made.	5	4	3	2	1	0	0
6. During the visit, the client is given an opportunity (time and encouragement) to initiate discussion or questions.	5	4	3	2	1	0	0
7. The nurse inquires about financial conditions of the client that affect his/her health.	5	4	3	2	1	0	0
8. Environmental data is collected (home, neighborhood, community).	5	4	3	2	1	0	0
9. The nurse collects data about cultural beliefs that affect his/her health.	5	4	3	2	1	0	0
10. The nursing diagnoses are validated with the client and/or family during the visit.	5	4	3	2	1	0	0
11. The nurse collects data about client use and/or ability to use community health care resources.	5	4	3	2	1	0	0
12. The nurse asks questions about health history.	5	4	3	2	1	0	0
13. The data gathered supports the nursing diagnosis, which is noted in the record.	5	4	3	2	1	0	0
14. Nursing diagnoses are prioritized with the client during the visit.	5	4	3	2	1	0	0
15. The nursing diagnosis can be treated by nursing interventions.	5	4	3	2	1	0	0

II. Planning

Objective: To measure the quality of nursing care observed for the *planning* component of the nursing process.

16. The client and family participate in goal setting.	5	4	3	2	1	0	0
17. A long-term goal (hoped for outcome) is established.	5	4	3	2	1	0	0
18. Short-term goals (steps to meet long-term goal) are established.	5	4	3	2	1	0	0
19. Action plans (steps to achieve goals) are established.	5	4	3	2	1	0	0
20. The client participates in action planning.	5	4	3	2	1	0	0
21. The nurse and client discuss the resources (community, agency, family, personal, etc.) needed to fulfill the plan.	5	4	3	2	1	0	0
22. The nurse and client mutually decide upon an expected date of goal accomplishment.	5	4	3	2	1	0	0
23. The nurse discusses costs and benefits of the nursing plan.	5	4	3	2	1	0	0
24. The plan includes community resources.	5	4	3	2	1	0	0
25. The plan is revised as goals are achieved or changed.	5	4	3	2	1	0	0
26. Goals are measurable.	5	4	3	2	1	0	0
27. Goals are achievable.	5	4	3	2	1	0	0
28. Goals are based on the nursing diagnosis.	5	4	3	2	1	0	0
29. The nursing plan indicates what the nurse will do.	5	4	3	2	1	0	0
30. The nursing plan indicates what the client will do.	5	4	3	2	1	0	0

III. Intervention

Objective: To measure the quality of nursing care observed for the *intervention* component of the nursing process.

31. The nurse periodically reinforces client and family strengths.	5	4	3	2	1	0	0
32. Nursing actions provide for client participation in health promotion, maintenance, or restoration.	5	4	3	2	1	0	0

*"Indicated" means that the nature of the client's problem requires examination.

Continued.

	Best care		Average care		Worst care	Not applicable	Not observed

33. During the visit, one of the following takes place regarding a referral to another agency or discipline: referral indicated* and made or referral *not* indicated and *not* made. 5 4 3 2 1 0 0

34. The communication pattern that illustrates the decision-making process during this visit is:

----->

Nurse <----- Client

----->

<----- 5 4 3 2 1 0 0

35. Teaching regarding the client's problems or need is done during the visit. 5 4 3 2 1 0 0

36. The client participates in the intervention(s) if capable. 5 4 3 2 1 0 0

37. The intervention is performed to reach the nursing care goal. 5 4 3 2 1 0 0

38. The nurse explains the rationale for the intervention. 5 4 3 2 1 0 0

39. The nursing action reflects currently accepted standards of practice. 5 4 3 2 1 0 0

40. The nurse coordinates health care services when more than one discipline is involved. 5 4 3 2 1 0 0

41. The nurse advocates for the client. 5 4 3 2 1 0 0

42. The nurse informs the client about nursing interventions being carried out. 5 4 3 2 1 0 0

43. The nurse assists the client to modify the environment according to need. 5 4 3 2 1 0 0

44. The nurse explores the use of health care resources with the client and/or family. 5 4 3 2 1 0 0

45. The nurse adapts or uses alternative interventions based on the client's response. 5 4 3 2 1 0 0

IV. Evaluating

Objective: To measure the quality of nursing care observed for the *evaluation* component of the nursing process.

46. The nurse refers to the nursing care goal set at the previous visit. 5 4 3 2 1 0 0

47. The communication pattern used to illustrate the evaluation of the client's progress to goal achievement is:

----->

Nurse <----- Client

----->

<----- 5 4 3 2 1 0 0

48. The family and nurse discuss the accomplishment of the nursing care goal(s). 5 4 3 2 1 0 0

49. The nurse informs the client about his/her health status. 5 4 3 2 1 0 0

50. There is mutual consideration of the short-term goals. 5 4 3 2 1 0 0

51. There is mutual consideration of the long-term goals. 5 4 3 2 1 0 0

52. New data is validated with the client and family. 5 4 3 2 1 0 0

53. The nurse and the client discuss how actions will be evaluated. 5 4 3 2 1 0 0

54. Changes in the care plan are discussed with the client and family. 5 4 3 2 1 0 0

55. During the visit, there is evidence of ongoing assessment. 5 4 3 2 1 0 0

56. During the visit, there is consideration of priorities. 5 4 3 2 1 0 0

57. Revision of the nursing care plan is based on progress toward the goal. 5 4 3 2 1 0 0

58. The nurse and the client and/or family discuss progress toward goal achievement. 5 4 3 2 1 0 0

59. The client's ongoing response to the medical illness is discussed. 5 4 3 2 1 0 0

60. The client and/or family demonstrates the ability to follow the nursing care plan. 5 4 3 2 1 0 0

*"Indicated" means that there was evidence of a problem requiring assistance of someone other than the nurse.

APPENDIX

Criteria and Standards for Community Health Nursing Practice

F1—ANA STANDARDS OF COMMUNITY HEALTH NURSING PRACTICE*
(Chapter 8)

Standard I. Theory: The nurse applies theoretical concepts as a basis for decisions in practice.

Standard II. Data collection: The nurse systematically collects data that are comprehensive and accurate.

Standard III. Diagnosis: The nurse analyzes data collected about the community, family, and individual to determine diagnoses.

Standard IV. Planning: At each level of prevention, the nurse develops plans that specify nursing actions unique to client needs.

Standard V. Intervention: The nurse, guided by the plan, intervenes to promote, maintain, or restore health, to prevent illness, and to effect rehabilitation.

Standard VI. Evaluation: The nurse evaluates responses of the community, family, and individual to interventions in order to determine progress toward goal achievement and to revise the data base, diagnoses, and plan.

Standard VII. Quality assurance and professional development: The nurse participates in peer review and other means of evaluation to assure quality of nursing practice; the nurse assumes responsibility for professional development and contributes to the professional growth of others.

Standard VIII. Interdisciplinary collaboration: The nurse collaborates with other health care providers, professionals, and community representatives in assessing, planning, implementing, and evaluating programs for community health.

Standard IX. Research: The nurse contributes to theory and practice in community health nursing through research.

F2—CRITERIA FOR DOCUMENTATION TO MEASURE THE QUALITY OF CARE IN THE HOME HEALTH AGENCY†
(Chapters 13 and 42)

1. The agency assesses the community served.
2. The agency is responsive to community health needs.
3. The agency has a legally constituted body that is responsible for the effective governing of the agency. It involves consumers in broad agency affairs.
4. Administrative responsibilities and relationships are established and clearly defined.
5. The governing body delegates to a qualified individual the authority and responsibility for overall agency administration.
6. If the agency has a person (or persons) other than the chief executive officer responsible for the administration and direction of the agency's programs, this individual (or individuals) is delegated the authority and responsibility for program administration.
7. If the agency has a person other than the chief executive officer responsible for the fiscal and business affairs of the agency, this individual is delegated the authority and responsibility for fiscal and business practices.
8. Fiscal policies and practices assure effective and efficient implementation of the program(s) of the agency.
9. The agency has agreements with organizations, agencies, and/or individuals for securing or providing services.
10. Program and fiscal management activities are coordinated to promote effective planning and implementation of programs within the agency.
11. The agency coordinates its services with other health and social agencies; consumers are kept informed of services available.
12. The agency has established programs in response to community health needs.
13. For each program and service, the agency has priorities that are responsive to agency purpose and community need.
14. The agency has policies and procedures governing programs, services, and professional practices.
15. Service records are maintained for each client.
16. All agency services are coordinated.
17. The agency has the responsibility for participation, if feasible, in the education of student health personnel.
18. The staff includes professional and nonprofessional personnel commensurate with the needs of the programs of the agency. There are written job descriptions for all classifications of personnel.
19. The agency provides consultation as needed for the administrative, supervisory, and direct-service personnel.
20. The agency has written personnel policies for all personnel.

---

*From American Nurses' Association: Standards of community health nursing practice, Kansas City, MO, 1986, The Association. Reprinted with the permission of ANA.

†From National League for Nursing: Criteria and standards manual for National League for Nursing/American Public Health Association Accreditation of Home Health Agencies and Community Nursing Services. New York, 1980, Publ. No. 21-1306. Used with permission.

21. The agency provides ongoing professional and/or technical supervision for all personnel.
22. The agency provides for staff development.
23. The agency has a structure and plan for evaluation.
24. The agency evaluates its organizational structure and administrative policies and practices.
25. The agency evaluates its programs.
26. The agency evaluates its staffing patterns, policies, and practices.
27. The agency establishes goals as a result of its overall evaluation. It communicates its status to the public.
28. Long-range planning is conducted by the agency to provide for future direction and viability.

Governmental Influences on Health Care Delivery

G1—SELECT MAJOR HISTORICAL EVENTS DEPICTING FINANCIAL INVOLVEMENT OF FEDERAL GOVERNMENT IN HEALTH CARE DELIVERY
(Chapter 4)

1798   Marine Hospital Service Act was passed to provide medical care to Merchant Marines.

1878   Port Quarantine Act was passed to prevent epidemic diseases from entering the country through seaports.

1879   National Health Department was established by Congress with a budget of $500,000.

1887   Laboratory of Hygiene at Staten Island Marine Hospital marked the beginning of Public Health Service research activities. This bacteriologic research laboratory later evolved into the National Institute of Health.

1890   Marine Hospital Service was given authority to inspect all immigrants to bar "lunatics and others unable to care for self" from entering the country.

1902   National Health Department was renamed the Public Health and Marine Hospital Service.

1912   National Institute of Health functions were expanded to study and investigate diseases of persons and the conditions influencing the origin and spread of disease.

1912   The Public Health and Marine Hospital Service was renamed the United States Public Health Service.

1912   The Child Health Bureau was established within the USPHS.

1917   National leprosarium was established at Carville, Louisiana under the aegis of the USPHS.

1917   USPHS became responsible for the physical and mental examination of all aliens.

1917   Congress appropriated $25,000 to USPHS to study and provide demonstration projects sharing state and federal cooperative rural health services.

1918   Because of increased veneral disease incidence during World War I, the Division of Venereal Disease was established in USPHS providing for cooperative federal and state control and prevention programs.

Sources for this listing were Hanlon J and Picker G: Public health administration and practice, ed 2, St. Louis, 1984, The CV Mosby Co.; Congressional Research Service: Summary of health legislation. 1959-1981. Library of Congress Pub No 82-127 EPW, Washington, DC, May 7, 1981, US Government Printing Office; Congressional Research Service: Major legislation of the 97th Congress, Library of Congress Pub No 9, Washington, DC, Oct 6, 1982 U.S. Government Printing Office; Congressional Research Service: Major Legislation of the 98th Congress, Library of Congress Pub No 9, Wash, DC, Oct, 1986 U.S. Government Printing Office.

1921   Shepherd-Towner Maternity Infancy Act was passed to provide for the establishment of state maternal and infant programs. The Act provided for mother-child health conferences, home delivery supplies, improved prenatal care, improved infant and child care, more public health nurses, and health education.

1929   USPHS Narcotics Division was developed to provide facilities for the confinement and treatment of drug addicts (renamed Division of Mental Hygiene in 1939).

1935   Congress passed the Social Security Act. Title VI of the Act was written for the purpose of assisting states, counties, health districts, and other political subdivisions in establishing and maintaining adequate public health service, including the training of personnel for state and local health work.

1935   The Social Security Act provided for grants-in-aid to states to finance the public's health. *Grants-in-aid* resulted in increased numbers of new health departments and the strengthening and expansion of existing health departments.

1937   National Cancer Act called for the establishment of the National Cancer Institute for research into the causes, diagnosis, and treatment of cancer; for assistance to public and private agencies; and for the promotion of the most effective prevention and treatment.

1938   The second Federal Veneral Disease Control Act was passed to promote investigation and control and to provide funds for the development and maintenance of state and local programs.

1939   The Federal Security Agency was established to bring health, welfare, and education services of the federal government together.

1940   Communicable Disease Center (National Center for Disease Control) was established in Atlanta for the purpose of conducting epidemiological studies, providing health personnel training, and establishing methods of communication and education.

1940   National Office of Vital Statistics (National Center for Health Statistics) was authorized to provide data about health, illness, injuries, and death.

1941   Nurse training appropriations provided monies to nursing programs to increase enrollment and improve programs.

1943   Nurse Training Act established the U.S. Nurse Cadet Corps in USPHS to support nurse training.

1946   National Mental Health Act was passed for constructing and equipping hospitals and laboratories to stimulate research and training in mental health.

1946   Hill-Burton Act provided for hospital services and construction.

1947   National Institute of Health Division of Research Grants were established to administer and award grants for research projects and training.

1947   A permanent Nursing Corps in the Army and Navy was established.

1948   National Heart Institute was established (renamed Heart, Lung, and Blood Institute in 1976).

1948   Microbiological, Experimental Biology, and Medicine Institutes were established (renamed National Institute of Allergy and Infectious Diseases in 1955).

1948   National Institute of Dental Research was authorized.

1948   National Institute of Health became National Institutes of Health (NIH).

1949   National Institute of Mental Health was established (renamed Alcoholism, Drug Abuse, and Mental Health Administration in 1974).

1950   National Institute of Neurological Diseases and Blindness was established (renamed National Eye Institute in 1968 and the National Institute of Neurological and Communicative Disorders and Strokes in 1975).

1950   Health Manpower Training Acts evolved to provide for training of Health Personnel.

1953   National Clinical Center was founded to accelerate research and to confirm and apply research findings. A 600-bed research hospital evolved.

1954   Congress extended Hill-Burton Act to allow monies for construction of other types of health facilities, such as general, mental, tuberculosis, and chronic disease hospitals; public health centers; diagnostic and treatment centers; rehabilitation facilities; nursing homes; state health laboratories; and nurse training facilities.

1954   Taft Sanitary Engineering Center was founded in Cincinnati for research and training in environmental health.

1955   National Institutes of Health Division of Biological Standards was established to oversee the growth of the pharmaceutical industry and market.

1955   Polio Vaccination Assistance Act was passed to aid state vaccination programs.

1956   U.S. Army Medical Library was transferred to USPHS, which became the Library of Medicine at the National Institutes of Health. The library provides MEDLARS, the Medical Literature Analysis and Retrieval System.

1956   CHAMPUS program was established for dependents of military personnel.

1956   National Health Survey was established for continuous monitoring of sickness and disability in the United States.

1959   National Institute of Arthritis and Metabolic Diseases was established (renamed National Institute of Arthritis, Metabolic, and Digestive Diseases in 1981).

1960   Social Security Amendments provided grants to states for medical assistance to the aged.

1962   National Institute of Child Health and Human Development was founded.

1962   Program for state assistance in preschool vaccination programs was authorized.

1963   Aid program was established for the construction of mental retardation and community mental health facilities and the development of programs to combat health problems, e.g., maternal health, crippled children, and the mentally retarded.

1965   Heart disease, cancer, and stroke legislation was provided for the establishment of Regional Medical Programs to coordinate existing services for these three health problems.

1965   Appalachian Regional Development Act was passed to provide for construction of health services facilities in economically depressed area.

1965   Social Security Act was amended to provide for Medicare and Medicaid programs.

1966   Division of Environmental Health Services was established in Public Health Service.

1966   Partnership for health legislation consolidated preexisting projects and *formula grants* to states through a new system of grants for comprehensive health planning. The legislation allowed health planning but did not give authority to control program development, spending, or construction of health facilities.

1968   Fogarty International Center for Advanced Study in Health Sciences was founded at NIH for international collaboration, study, and research by world scholars.

1970   Occupational Health and Safety Act was passed to assure safe and health working conditions.

1971   Environmental Protection Agency was founded to establish an umbrella agency for all environmental programs.

1971   National Center for Toxicological Research was established at Pine Bluff, Arkansas under the aegis of the Food and Drug Administration of USPHS.

1972   National programs were established for research, screening, counseling, and treatment of sickle cell anemia and Cooley's anemia.

1972   Social Security Act amended to encourage Professional Standards Review Organizations (PSRO). PSROs were designed to review hospital services ordered by physicians to determine overuse and underuse of services for patient care.

1972   National commission was established to study and investigate causes, cures, and treatment of multiple sclerosis.

1973   Social Security Act was amended to provide for the development of health maintenance organizations (HMOs)—prepaid comprehensive health care delivery systems designed to introduce competition into the health care arena.

1973   Program of grants (contracts for establishing and operating emergency medical services systems) was authorized.

1974   National Health Planning and Resources Development Act was passed to provide a triad health planning system. The system was designed as a comprehensive planning structure to review health services and facilities and to control and limit the expenditure of federal monies by discouraging the development and continuation of unnecessary new and existing programs.

1974   National Diabetes Mellitus Research and Education Act was passed to authorize NIH to establish a National Commission on Diabetes to formulate long-range plans to combat the disease.

1974   Sudden Infant Death Syndrome Act was passed to provide a program of dissemination of research and information to the public.

1976   National Swine Flu Immunization Program was established and implemented.

1976   Toxic Substances Control Act was passed to require testing of certain chemical substances to protect human health and environment.

1977   Rural Health Clinics Services Act was passed to provide for the establishment of health clinics in rural underserved communities. The clinics were to be staffed by nurse practitioners or physician assistants. The bill marked the first national legislation passed for reimbursement of nurse practitioner and physician assistant services under Medicare and Medicaid.

1980   Civil Rights of Institutionalized Persons Act was passed to protect mentally ill, disabled, retarded, chronically ill, or handicapped persons from flagrant conditions in state-affiliated institutions.

1980   Infant Formula Act was passed to require that such formulas meet certain standards of nutrition, quality, and safety in manufacturing.

1980   Department of Health, Education, and Welfare reorganized. Department of Health and Human Services oversees the regulation of health programs.

1981   Omnibus Budget Reconciliation Act (OBRA) provided for maternal and child health block grants to states under Title V of the Social Security Act to assist the states in advancing the health of mothers and children. Legislation allows states to make decisions on how to spend monies for nine maternal-child health programs.

1981   Omnibus Budget Reconciliation Act provided preventive health services block grants to allow states to make decisions about monies spent for 10 preventive health programs like hypertensive screening, rape crisis centers, etc.

1981   Omnibus Budget Reconciliation Act provided alcohol, drug abuse, and mental health block grants for states to provide direct service through community health centers and alcohol and drug abuse programs.

1981   Omnibus Budget Reconciliation Act provided primary care block grants to states for community health center funding.

1982   Defense appropriations amendments allowed for direct, independent nurse practitioner reimbursement under CHAMPUS.

1982   The Tax Equity and Fiscal Responsibility Act established reductions in Medicare and Medicaid spending, called for the development of a prospective reimbursement system, authorized Medicare payments for hospice service, and replaced PSRO with a new utilization and quality control peer review program.

1983   Public Health Emergency Act provided for a permanent revolving fund for use by the Secretary of DHHS in responding to public health emergencies.

1983   Social Security Amendments of 1983 contained provisions providing for the establishment of a prospective payment system under Medicare.

1983   Amendments to the Public Health Act authorized grants, contracts, and loans for the development of home health agencies and training of home health personnel.

1985   Health Research Extension Act establishes a new National Center for Nursing Research.

1986   Supplemental appropriations bill passed to allow hospitals to include capital building costs in payment requests under PPS beginning in 1987.

1987   Omnibus Budget Reconciliation Act provided increased quality control measures for the nursing home industry, and required nurse aide training for nursing home and home health.

1989   Medicare/Medicaid regulations established a PPS for ambulatory surgery; provided Medicaid coverage for children 6 years and under and pregnant women with incomes of 133% of poverty level; and provided reimbursement of certified pediatric nurse practitioners and family nurse parctitioners for Medicaid services; and provided for nurse practitioners and clinical nurse specialists to certify patients needs for nursing home care.

Community Resources

H1—PARTIAL LIST OF HEALTH ORGANIZATIONS USED BY COMMUNITY HEALTH NURSES

AL-ANON Family Group Headquarters, Inc.

1372 Broadway, New York, NY 10018

Founded in 1951. Al-Anon, including Alateen for teenagers, offers a self-help recovery program for relatives and friends who have been adversely affected by someone else's drinking problem. Members share experiences, strength, and hope in an effort to make their own lives manageable. Membership: 15,600 groups worldwide.

Alcohol and Drug Problems Association of North America, Inc.

444 North Capitol Street, NW, Suite 181, Washington, DC 20001

Founded in 1949, the association serves as a focal point for action and a medium of exchange for professionals in the alcohol and drug problems field at the national, state, and local governmental levels and in the private sector.

Alcoholics Anonymous World Services

PO Box 459, Grand Central Station, New York, NY 10163

Founded in 1935. AA is a program of recovery from alcoholism.

American Burn Association

c/o Shriners Burns Institute, 202 Goodman Street, Cincinnati, OH 45219

Founded in 1967.

American Cancer Society

261 Madison Avenue, New York, NY 10016

Founded in 1913. ACS conducts research on cause, prevention, treatment of cancer; public education programs alert Americans to protective and preventive measures; informs physicians on developments in diagnosis and treatment of cancer; provides service and rehabilitation program for patients.

American Dental Association

211 East Chicago Avenue, Chicago, IL 60611

Founded in 1859. The ADA is the national voluntary organization for the U.S. dental profession and is the second largest health profession in the country.

American Diabetes Association National Service Center

PO Box 25757, 1660 Duke Street, Alexandria, VA 22313

Founded in 1940. ADA funds research and conducts education programs in the field of diabetes. Publishes patient magazine and two medical journals.

American Epilepsy Society

c/o Priscilla S. Bourgeois, 179 Allyn Street, #304, Hartford, CT 06103

Founded in 1946. AES works to foster research and treatment of epilepsy in all of its phases—biological, clinical, and social—and the promotion of better care and treatment of persons subject to seizures.

American Fertility Society

2140 11th Avenue, S, Suite 200, Birmingham, AL 35205

Founded in 1944. The primary objective of the Society is to disseminate that body of knowledge which encompasses all aspects of infertility, related endocrinology, conception control, and reproductive biology. The greater emphasis is on those matters that are clinical in nature.

American Foundation for Maternal and Child Health

439 East 51st Street, New York, NY 10022

Founded in 1925.

American Foundation for the Blind

15 West 16th Street, New York, NY 10011

Founded in 1921. The objective of the foundation is to stimulate, facilitate, and coordinate a national effort for improving services to blind and psychological, technological/social research, gathering, preparation, publishing information to professional and general public, sponsoring workshops, seminars, conferences.

American Geriatrics Society

770 Lexington Avenue, Suite 400, New York, NY 10021

Founded in 1942. AGS provides dissemination of information relating to the etiology, prevention, diagnosis, and treatment of diseases of the aging and aged, rehabilitation of patients and problems relating to the health care of the older patient.

American Health Care Association

1201 L Street, NW, Washington, DC 20005

American Health Foundation

320 East 43rd Street, New York, NY 10018

Founded in 1969. AHF is a unique, non-profit institution, totally committed to disease prevention and health promotion. Today, on national and community levels, AHF is achieving its goals through laboratory and clinical research, preventive health care services and public education.

American Heart Association

7320 Greenville Avenue, Dallas, TX 75231

Founded in 1948. The AHA mission is to reduce death and disability from cardiovascular diseases.

American Hepatitis Association

30 East 40th Street, Rm 305, New York, NY 10016

American Laryngological Association

c/o Eugene N. Meyers, MD, Eye and Ear Hospital,

230 Lothrop Street, Rm 1115, Pittsburgh, PA 15213

Founded in 1878. ALA conducts annual meetings, publishes transactions in field of laryngology, rhinology, head, and neck surgery.

American Liver Foundation

998 Pomptom Avenue, Cedar Grove, NJ 07009

Founded in 1976. The ALF seeks to improve the understanding, prevention, and cure of liver diseases through professional and public education and by supporting vitally needed research training of young scientific investigators.

American Lung Association

1740 Broadway, New York, NY 10019

Founded in 1904. ALA is primarily an educational organization to fight lung disease and work for lung health. It also works against cigarette smoking and air pollution.

American Mental Health Foundation

2 East 86th Street, New York, NY 10028

Founded in 1924. The AMHF is dedicated to extensive and intensive research in the theories of psychotherapy and to the implementation of needed reforms.

American Optometric Association

243 Lindbergh Boulevard, St. Louis, MO 63141

Founded in 1898. The objectives of the AOA as stated in its constitution are: To improve the vision care and health of the public and to promote the art and science of the profession of optometry.

American Parkinson Disease Association

116 John Street, Suite 417, New York, NY 10038

American Pediatric Society

c/o Audrey Brown, MD, Department of Pediatrics,

Box 49, SUNY Health Sciences Center, 450 Clarkson Avenue, Brooklyn, NY 11207

Founded in 1888. APS provides an annual scientific meeting during which short papers are presented in all the pediatric subspecialties. The subspecialty sessions are preceded by a plenary session as well as a symposium on important research achievements in pediatrics.

American Physical Fitness Research Institute

654 N Sepulveda Boulevard, Los Angeles, CA 90049

Founded in 1958. APFRI provides research and development of motivational and educational information on all aspects of health, fitness, and well-being directed toward personal responsibility toward one's health.

American Psychosomatic Society

6728 Old McLean Village Drive, McLean, VA 22101

Founded in 1943. APS works to advance the research of psychosomatic medicine.

American Red Cross

17th and D Streets, NW, Washington, DC 20006

Founded in 1881. The aims of the Red Cross are to improve the quality of human life and enhance individual self-reliance and concern for others. It works toward these aims through national and chapter services governed and directed by volunteers.

American Rescue Workers

716 Ritchie Road, Capitol Heights, MD 20743

Founded 1880. American Rescue Workers is an international religious and charitable organization providing health and welfare services throughout the world. In the United States a wide range of services is based upon needs of community and available local resources.

American School Health Association

7263 State Route 43, PO Box 708, Kent, OH 44240

American Venereal Disease Association

c/o Edward W. Hook III, MD, Blalock 111, 600 N. Wolfe Street, Baltimore, MD 21205

AVDA is an association of physicians, nurses, and other public health professionals concerned with research, professional education, and control of sexually transmitted diseases. Publishes a quarterly journal, *Sexually Transmitted Diseases*.

Arthritis Foundation

1314 Spring Street, NW, Atlanta, GA 30309

Founded in 1948.

Arthritis Society

920 Yonge Street, Suite 420, Toronto, Ontario, M4W 3J7, Canada

Founded in 1948. The AS is organized for the development of rheumatological manpower through associateships and fellowships; the support of research projects deemed relevant to the rheumatic diseases; and the communication about arthritis with general public and medical profession.

Association for the Care of Asthma

c/o Herbert C. Mansmann, Jr, MD, Jefferson Medical College, 1025 Walnut Street, Rm 727, Philadelphia, PA 19107

Founded in 1963. ACA conducts an annual postgraduate course in allergy and clinical immunology for the advancement of the knowledge and practice of the care and treatment of asthma, by discussion at such meetings, promoting and encouraging research and study.

Association for the Care of Children's Health

3615 Wisconsin Avenue, NW, Washington, DC 20016. Founded in 1965. ACCH seeks to foster and promote the health and well-being of children and families in health care settings by education, interdisciplinary interaction and planning, and research.

Association for Children and Adults with Learning Disabilities

4156 Library Road, Pittsburgh, PA 15234

Founded in 1963.

Association for Children with Retarded Mental Development

162 Fifth Avenue, 11th Fl, New York, NY 10010

Founded in 1951. ACRMD is a non-profit membership corporation offering services to mentally retarded adults throughout New York City. Services include rehabilitation and sheltered workshops; day training and activities centers; day treatment centers; job placement; evening and weekend social centers; various community services.

Association for Education and Rehabilitation of the Blind and Visually Impaired

206 N. Washington Street, Suite 320, Alexandria, VA 22314

Founded 1984. Works to expand the opportunities for the visually handicapped in society.

Association for Retarded Citizens

PO Box 6109, Arlington, TX 76005

Founded in 1950.

Association for Vital Records and Health Statistics

c/o George Van Amburg, Michigan Department of Public Health, 3423 Logan Street, North, PO Box 30195, Lansing, MI 48909

Founded in 1933, the AVRHS provides the only national forum for the study, discussion, and solution of the problems related to programs of vital and health statistics by state and local representatives without undue influence of Federal government officials.

Asthma and Allergy Foundation of America

1717 Massachusetts Avenue, Suite 305, Washington, DC 20036

Founded in 1953. The AAFA provides public education booklets and newletters; answers inquiries on asthma and allergy; arranges for professional speakers and audio-visual materials and encourages community activities through its local chapters.

Autism Society for America

1234 Massachusetts Avenue, NW, Suite C-1017, Washington, DC 20005

Founded in 1965. The ASA is a nonprofit organization of parents, professionals and other concerned citizens working for better education, research, treatment, and legislation on behalf of autistic persons.

Biofeedback Society of America

c/o Francine Butler, PhD, 10200 West 44th Ave, #304, Wheat Ridge, CO 80033

Founded in 1969. The BSA is an interdisciplinary organization dedicated to the applied, research, and educational aspects of biofeedback.

Braille Institute

741 North Vermont Avenue, Los Angeles, CA 90029

Founded in 1919. The institute provides training, education, and special services for the blind of all ages.

Child Abuse Listening Mediation

PO Box 718, Santa Barbara, CA 93102

Founded in 1971. CALM is organized for the prevention of child abuse and neglect, and provides a hotline listener, child care to reduce stress, a speakers bureau, and parent support groups.

Child Health Associate Program

4200 East Ninth Avenue, Box C219, Denver, CO 80262

Founded in 1969. The CHAP is a training program to prepare health care professionals capable of providing a wide range of diagnostic, preventive and therapeutic services to children. Working principally in ambulatory settings as colleagues and associates of physicians, child health associates have the knowledge and skill to care for a large percentage of the patients seen in a typical pediatric practice. The training program is 3 years in length. Prerequisites include 2 years of college preparation.

Children's Foundation

815 15th Street, NW, Suite 928, Washington, DC 20005

The foundation was established in 1969 as a national, non-profit advocacy organization focusing upon the quality and availability of the federal food assistance programs for children and their families.

Council on Arteriosclerosis of the American Heart Association

7320 Greenville Avenue, Dallas, TX 75231

Founded in 1946.

Council on Education for Public Health

1015 15th Street, NW, Washington, DC 20005

Founded in 1974. CEPH is the independent agency officially recognized by the U.S. Office of Education and the Council on Postsecondary Accreditation to accredit graduate schools of public health and certain graduate programs outside of schools of public health.

Council of World Organizations Interested in the Handicapped

432 Park Avenue, South, New York, NY 10016

Founded in 1953. The council provides a coordinating mechanism for international organizations and the UN agencies to avoid duplication of programs for disabled people.

Drug Information Association

PO Box 113, Maple Glen, PA 19002

Founded in 1965. The DIA is an international multidisciplinary professional association of specialists engaged in furthering modern technology of communication in medical, pharmaceutical, and allied human/animal fields. Publishes quarterly *Drug Information Journal* as proceedings of meetings and for submitted relevant papers.

Gerontological Society of America

1411 K Street, NW, Suite 300, Washington, DC 20005

Founded in 1945. The society is a national multidisciplinary organization of researchers, educators, and professionals in aging devoted to stimulating and promoting research and its application to practice. Publishes two bimonthly journals: *Journal of Gerontology* and *The Gerontologist*.

Goodwill Industries of America

9200 Wisconsin Avenue, Bethesda, MD 20814

Founded in 1902. Goodwill Industries provides services, materials, and information to assist member Goodwill Industries in their programs of service to handicapped people.

Gray Panthers

311 S. Juniper Street, Suite 601, Philadelphia, PA 19107

Founded in 1970. The Gray Panthers are people of all ages, working for social change. It tries to develop creative alternatives to the injustices in society which confront people at every phase of life.

Guide Dog Users, Inc.

c/o Kim Charlson, 12 Riverside Street, Apt 1-2, Watertown, MA 02172

Founded in 1969. The goals of GDU are to improve the quality of the educational, cultural, employment, and rehabilitation services of all blind persons, to promote the acceptance of guide dog users by federal and state agencies, employers, educational institutions, business establishments, and places of entertainment. National basis members at large; publication *Pawtracks* quarterly.

Health and Education Resources

4733 Bethesda Avenue, Suite 735, Bethesda, MD 20814

Founded in 1969. HER is a non-profit organization developing programs and communications in health, education, and social services including continuing education for clinical laboratory personnel, technical assistance for implementation of a skill-and-knowledge-based task analysis method; production of audio-visual instructional materials.

Health Sciences Communications Association

6105 Lindell Blvd, St Louis, MO 63112

Founded in 1959. HSCA is a non-profit organization devoted to advancement of education in health sciences by means of varied contemporary educational technology.

Healthy America

315 West 105th St, #1F, New York, NY 10025

Founded in 1977 the coalition is a national, non-profit organization emphasizing health advocacy, disease prevention and promotion of good health habits as means to attain lasting good health. It encourages health promotion policies and programs at all levels of government and within private sectors, sponsors seminars, conferences, etc, and serves as congressional liaison for membership.

Huntington's Disease Society of America

140 West 22nd Street, 6th Floor, New York, NY 10011-2420

Founded 1986.

International Association Cancer Victims and Friends

7740 W. Manchester Avenue, Suite 110, Playa del Rey, CA 90293

Founded in 1963. IACVF is a non-profit (tax exempt) corporation organized under the laws of the state of California. Its purpose is the dissemination of educational materials concerning the prevention and control of cancer through the use of non-toxic therapies. Chapters have symposiums and seminars in their respective areas throughout the year.

International Childbirth Education Association

PO Box 20048, Minneapolis, MN 55420

Founded in 1960. The ICEA promotes family centered maternity care and helps groups and individuals promote same through classes in prepared childbirth, teacher training, publications, conferences, and conventions.

International Commission for Prevention of Alcoholism and Drug Dependency

6830 Laurel Street, NW, Washington, DC 20012

Founded in 1952. The commission is a non-government organization of the UN, focusing on prevention programming through organizing of congresses, seminars, personal contacts, educational material and other community endeavors.

International Council on Health, Physical Education and Recreation

1900 Association Drive, Reston, VA 22091

Founded in 1958. The council represents and brings together teachers, administrators, leaders, national departments of physical education, and related associations in health, physical education, sports, dance and recreation into one organization at the international level. It fosters international understanding, goodwill, and encourages development and expansion of educationally sound programs.

Juvenile Diabetes Foundation International

432 Park Avenue, South, New York, NY 10016

Founded in 1970. JDFI is a non-profit voluntary agency whose prime objective is to support and fund research aimed at preventing the complications and curing the disease itself. JDF chapters provide educational and counseling services in addition to fund raising.

W.K. Kellogg Foundation

400 North Avenue, Battle Creek, MI 49017

Founded in 1930. The foundation is committed to the application of existing knowledge to problems of people in the areas of health, education, and agriculture. It currently assists programs of four continents, including the United States and Canada, Latin America, Europe, and Australia. A grant-making organization, the foundation does not operate programs.

La Leche League International

9616 Minneapolis Avenue, PO Box 1209, Franklin Park, IL 60131

Founded in 1956. The league is a non-profit organization that provides help for breastfeeding mothers in a series of four meetings, annual seminar for physicians, biennial international conferences for parents and professionals, and a 24 hour telephone hotline.

Leukemia Society of America

733 Third Avenue, New York, NY 10017

Founded in 1949. The LSA promotes and provides support into the causes, treatment, and cure or control of the leukemias and related lymphomas. Allied programs are patient service, public and professional education, and community services.

Living Bank

PO Box 6725, Houston, TX 77625

Founded in 1968. The LB is an organ and body donor registry, educating the public about the importance of organ and body donations, registration, and referral of donations, at the time of death, to the appropriate medical facility closest to the point of death.

Lupus Foundation of America

1717 Massachusetts Ave, NW, Suite 203, Washington, DC 20036

Founded in 1977. The corporation is organized exclusively for charitable, educational, and scientific purposes to encourage development of research programs designed to discover the causes of, and to improve the methods of treating, diagnosing, curing and preventing Lupus Erythematosus.

March of Dimes Birth Defects Foundation

1275 Mamaroneck Avenue, White Plains, NY 10605
Founded in 1938. The goal of the foundation is the prevention of birth defects, our most serious child health problem, through support of research, medical services, and education.

Maternity Center Association

48 East 92nd Street, New York, NY 10128
Founded in 1918. The MCA provides complete maternity service for low-risk families; childbirth education and information service; support of nurse-midwifery education; institutes on parent education and literature on childbearing and maternity care.

Medic Alert Foundation International

2323 Colorado, Turlock, CA 95381
Founded in 1956. Medic Alert provides emergency medical identification in either necklace or bracelet style, which includes hidden medical condition, membership number, and emergency telephone number that can be called collect. A wallet card is provided with additional emergency information. $10 membership fee includes stainless steel emblem.

Mended Hearts

c/o American Heart Association, 7320 Greenville Ave, Dallas, TX 75231
Founded in 1951.

Muscular Dystrophy Association

810 Seventh Avenue, New York, NY 10019
The MDA is a voluntary national health agency—a dedicated partnership between scientists and concerned citizens aimed at conquering nueromuscular diseases that affect thousands of Americans.

Myasthenia Gravis Foundation

53 W Jackson Blvd, Suite 909, Chicago, IL 60604
Founded in 1952. The foundation fosters, coordinates, and supports research into the cause, prevention, alleviation, and cure of myasthenia gravis, and gives research grants to MG clinics, hospitals, medical schools throughout the United States, and awards at least 10 medical student fellowships each year and a $20,000 post-doctoral fellowship.

National Association for Down's Syndrome

PO Box 4542, Oak Park, IL 60522
Founded in 1960. NADS is a not-for-profit organization comprised of parents and professionals involved with the individual with Down's Syndrome.

National Association on Drug Abuse Problems

355 Lexington Avenue, New York, NY 10017
Founded in 1971. NADAP provides a placement service for rehabilitated drug abusers and a workshop for drug treatment counselors and corporate management.

National Association of the Physically Handicapped

76 Elm Street, London, OH 43140
Founded in 1958. The NAPH advances the social, economic, and physical welfare of physically handicapped. It is not a resource center for information. We give no type services; nor give financial aid. We support legislation to benefit handicapped; trying to make public aware of needs of handicapped.

National Association of School Nurses

PO Box 1300, Scarborough, ME 04074

National Association for Visually Handicapped

22 West 21st Street, New York, NY 10010
Founded in 1954. The NAVH offers guidance and counsel for all partially-seeing people and professionals and paraprofessionals working with them, informational literature. It publishes and distributes large print books, textbooks, and testing material. Serves as referral agency for all services for partially seeing. Only national health agency serving only the partially-seeing (not the totally blind).

National Ataxia Foundation

600 Twelve Oaks Center, 15500 Wayzata Blvd, Wayzata, MN 55391
Founded in 1957. NAF works to combat all types of hereditary ataxia and related disorders through four major objectives: education, service, prevention and research.

National Committee for the Prevention of Alcoholism and Drug Dependency

RR 1, Box 635, Appomattox, VA 24522
Founded in 1950. The committee periodically holds institutes and seminar-workshops throughout the U.S. It gathers and distributes information and materials concerning the effects of alcohol and other drugs on the physical, mental and moral powers of the individual citizen and promotes an educational program for prevention with visual and teaching aids throughout the country. Willing to cooperate with other organizations in holding seminar-workshops in their area.

National Council on Alcoholism

12 West 21st Street, New York, NY 10010
Founded in 1944. The council is the only national voluntary agency founded to combat the disease of alcoholism.

National Council on Stuttering

PO Box 8171, Grand Rapids, MI 49518
Founded in 1965. Promotes and encourages programs and studies on the problems of stuttering.

National Genetics Foundation

PO Box 1374, New York, NY 10101
Founded in 1903.

National Health Council

622 Third Avenue, 34th Floor, New York, NY 10017
Founded in 1920. NHC is a membership organization of national voluntary, professional, and related organizations interested in improving the health of all Americans in the areas of planning, coordination, and delivery of health services.

National Health Federation

PO Box 688, Monrovia, CA 91016
Founded in 1955.

National Hearing Aid Society

20361 Middlebelt Road, Livonia, MI 48152
Founded in 1951. NHAS is the professional association for those engaged in fitting and selling of hearing aids.

National Hemophilia Foundation

110 Green Street, Rm 406, New York, NY 10012
Founded in 1948. The foundation provides information for those interested in the field, and promotes research.

National Indian Council on Aging

PO Box 2088, Albuquerque, NM 87103

Founded in 1976. The council is a national advocacy organization to bring about improved services to American Indian and Alaskan Native elders, including health-related services.

National Indian Health Board

PO Box 6940, Denver, CO 80206

Founded in 1969. The board provides review and comment on federal legislation that affects Indian tribes and serves as an advisory board to HEW on Indian health concerns.

National Kidney Foundation

2 Park Avenue, New York, NY 10003

Founded in 1958. NKF is a national voluntary health organization supporting research and public information on the diagnosis and treatment of diseases of the kidney.

National Lupus Erythematosus Foundation

5430 Van Nuys Boulevard, Suite 206, Van Nuys, CA 91401

Founded in 1950. NLEF is a non-profit organization for the distribution of Lupus literature; compiling of information gathered from Lupus patients; funding of Lupus research, and establishing Lupus City of Hope Chapters throughout the country.

National Mental Health Association

1021 Prince Street, Alexandria, VA 22314

Founded in 1909. The MHA is a lay, volunteer organization that provides social action and public education in the area of mental health.

National Spinal Cord Injury Association

600 West Cummings Park, Suite 2000, Woburn, MA 01801

Founded in 1948. The foundation addresses the needs of persons with spinal cord injuries through programs in the areas of care, cure, and coping.

National Sudden Infant Death Syndrome Foundation

8200 Professional Plaza, Suite 104, Landover, MD 20785

Founded in 1962. NSIDSF provides support for SIDS research, services to families of victims of SIDS and SIDS-related disorders, and educational programs for health and emergency personnel. It also fulfills a consumer advocacy role for SIDS families.

National Tay-Sachs and Allied Diseases Association

385 Elliot Street, Newton, MA 02164

Founded in 1957. The association conducts programs in support of research, family counseling, and public and professional education into the genetic disease Tay-Sachs and many other diseases due to inborn errors of metabolism.

Pediatric Pulmonary and Cystic Fibrosis Center

St Christopher's Hospital for Children, 2600 North Lawrence Street, Philadelphia, PA 19133

Focuses upon research on cystic fibrosis and other chronic respiratory diseases in infants and children; examines new therapeutic modalities.

Planned Parenthood Federation of America

810 Seventh Avenue, New York, NY 10019

PPF works to make effective means of birth control available for all.

School Health Programs

University of Colorado Health Sciences Center School of Nursing, 4200 East 9th Avenue, C-287, Denver, CO 80262

Synanon Foundation, Inc.

6055 Marshall Petalvma Road, Marshall CA 94940

Founded in 1958. Synanon was the first community designed for the re-education of drug addicts and other character disorders, and it continues to do that work. Since 1974 Synanon has been providing re-education for children as young as 10 years of age. Facilities in Marshall, San Francisco, Los Angeles, and Badger, Calif.; Kerhonkson and New York, N.Y.; Chicago, Ill., and Detroit, Mich.

United Cerebral Palsy Association

66 East 34th Street, New York, NY 10016

Founded in 1948. UCP is the only nationwide voluntary organization targeting its services on the specific and multiple needs of persons with cerebral palsy and their families. UCP's more than 240 affiliates provide a variety of community services, support research, and conduct programs of public education pertaining to cerebral palsy.

H2—RESOURCES FOR OCCUPATIONAL HEALTH (CHAPTER 41)

American Association of Occupational Health Nurses (AAOHN)

50 Lenox Pointe, Atlanta, GA 30324

Founded in 1942. Members: 12,000. The AAOHN is the professional association for registered nurses involved in occupational health. Its mission is to promote occupational health nursing, maintain professional integrity, and enhance its professional status.

American Foundation for Maternal and Child Health (AFMC)

439 East 51st Street, New York, NY 10022, Doris Haire, Pres

Founded in 1972. Serves as a clearinghouse for interdisciplinary research on maternal and child health; focuses on the perinatal or birth period and its effect on infant development. Sponsors medical research designed to improve application of technology in maternal and child health; conducts educational programs; compiles statistics. Operates extensive reference library.

American Foundation for the Blind

15 West 16th Street, New York, NY 10011

Founded in 1921. The objective of the foundation is to stimulate, facilitate, and coordinate a national effort for improving services to blind and psychological, technological/social research, gathering, preparation, publishing information to professional and general public, sponsoring workshops, seminars, conferences.

American Geriatrics Society

770 Lexington Avenue, Suite 400, New York, NY 10021

Founded in 1942. AGS provides dissemination of information relating to the etiology, prevention, diagnosis, and treatment of the aging and aged, rehabilitation of patients and problems relating to the health care of the older patient.

American Health Care Association (AHCA)

1200 15th Street, NW, Washington, DC 20005, Dr. Paul R. Willging, Exec Vice Pres

Founded in 1949. Members: 9000. Federation of state associations of long-term health-care facilities. Promotes standards for professionals in long-term health care delivery, and quality care for patients and residents in a safe environment. Focuses on issues of availability, quality, affordability, and fair payment. Conducts seminars and conferences that provide continuing education for nursing home personnel. Maintains liaison with governmental agencies, Congress, and professional associations. Presents awards; compiles statistics. Publications: (1) Notes, biweekly; (2) Provider, monthly; also publishes Health Career Opportunities; Thinking About a Nursing Home; Welcome to Our Nursing Home; and training manuals and audiovisual aids.

American Health Foundation

320 East 43rd Street, New York, NY 10018

Founded in 1969. AHF is a unique, non-profit institution, totally committed to disease prevention and health promotion. Today, on national and community levels, AHF is achieving its goals through laboratory and clinical research, preventive health care services, and public education.

American Heart Association

7320 Greenville Avenue, Dallas, TX 75231

Founded in 1948. The AHA mission is to reduce death and disability from cardiovascular diseases.

American Hepatitis Association (AHA)

30 East 40th Street, Room 305, New York, NY 10016, Gerald Meltzer, Pres.

Founded in 1983. Persons having hepatitis in any form; persons who have a high risk of contracting hepatitis; interested individuals. Conducts educational and prevention programs concerning hepatitis; provides low-cost blood screening and vaccines. Offers support groups for individuals with hepatitis. Sponsors talks for high risk groups including health care workers, medical personnel, homosexual men, IV drug abusers, and those who work with infants with hepatitis. Facilitates research on the treatment and prevention of hepatitis. Sponsors Hepatitis Awareness Week; offers blood screenings and vaccinations. Maintains speakers' bureau; operates children's services. Publications: AHA Newsletter, periodic; also publishes dietary guidelines, pamphlets, and brochures.

American Laryngological Association

c/o Eugene N. Myers, MD, Eye & Ear Hospital, 230 Lothrop Street, Room 1115, Pittsburgh, PA 15213

Founded in 1878. ALA conducts annual meetings, publishes transactions in field of laryngology, rhinology, head, and neck surgery.

American Liver Foundation

998 Pompton Avenue, Cedar Grove, NJ 07009

Founded in 1976. The ALF seeks to improve the understanding, prevention, and cure of liver disease through professional and public education and by supporting vitally needed research training of young scientific investigators.

American Lung Association

1740 Broadway, New York, NY 10019

Founded in 1904. ALA is primarily an educational organization to fight lung disease and work for lung health. It also works against cigarette smoking and air pollution.

American Mental Health Foundation

2 East 86th Street, New York, NY 10028

Founded in 1924. The AMHF is dedicated to extensive and intensive research in the theories of psychotherapy and to the implementation of needed reforms.

American Optometric Association

243 Lindbergh Boulevard, St. Louis, MO 63141

Founded in 1898. The objectives of the AOA as stated in its constitution are: to improve the vision care and health of the public and to promote the art and science of the profession of optometry.

American Parkinson Disease Association

116 John Street, Suite 417, New York, NY 10038

American Pediatric Society

c/o Audrey Brown, MD, Dept of Pediatrics, Box 49, SUNY Health Sciences Center, 450 Clarkson Avenue, Brooklyn, NY 11207

Founded in 1888. APS provides an annual scientific meeting during which short papers are presented in all the pediatric subspecialties. The subspecialty sessions are preceded by a plenary session as well as a symposium on important research achievements in pediatrics.

American Physical Fitness Research Institute

654 N Sepulveda Boulevard, Los Angeles, CA 90049

Founded in 1958. APFRI provides research and development of motivational and educational information on all aspects of health, fitness, and well-being directed toward personal responsibility toward one's health.

American Psychosomatic Society

6728 Old McLean Village Drive, McLean, VA 22101

Founded in 1943. APS works to advance the research of psychosomatic medicine.

American Red Cross

17th and D Streets, NW, Washington, DC 20006

Founded in 1881. The aims of the Red Cross are to improve the quality of human life and enhance individual self-reliance and concern for others. It works toward these aims through national and chapter services governed and directed by volunteers.

American Rescue Workers

716 Ritchie Road, Capitol Heights, MD 20743

Founded in 1884. American Rescue Workers is an international religious and charitable organization providing health and welfare services throughout the world. In the United States a wide range of services is based upon needs of community and available local resources.

American School Health Association

1521 South Water Street, PO Box 708, Kent, OH 44240, Dana A. Davis, Exec Dir

Founded in 1927. Members: 8000. School physicians, dentists, nurses, nutritionists, health educators, dental hygienists, and public health workers. To promote comprehensive and constructive school health programs including the teaching of health, health services, and promotion of a healthful school environment. Offers a professional referral service, classroom teaching aids, and professional reference materials. Conducts research programs; maintains placement service; compiles statistics. Sponsors annual foreign travel study tour. Presents William A. Howe Award annually for distinguished service in school health. Maintains numerous committees including: College Health and Professional Preparation; Mental Health; Special Health Problems of Children. Publications: (1) Journal of School Health, 10/year, (2) Topical Index of Articles From the Journal, annual; also publishes School Health in America (survey), A Pocketguide to Health and Health Problems in School Physical Activities, and other books.

Association for Vital Records and Health Statistics

c/o George Van Amburg, Michigan Department of Public Health, 3423 Logan Street, N, PO Box 30295, Lansing, MI 48909

Founded in 1933. The AVRHS provides the only national forum for the study, discussion, and solution of the problems related to programs of vital and health statistics by state and local representatives without undue influence of federal government officials.

Asthma and Allergy Foundation of America

1717 Massachusetts Avenue, Suite 305, Washington, DC 20036

Founded in 1953. The AAFA provides public education booklets and newsletters; answers inquiries on asthma and allergy; arranges for professional speakers and audiovisual materials, and encourages community activities through its local chapters.

Autism Society for America

1234 Massachusetts Avenue, NW, Suite C-10, Washington, DC 20005

Founded in 1965. The NSAC is a non-profit organization of parents, professionals, and other concerned citizens working for better education, research, treatment, and legislation on behalf of autistic persons.

Biofeedback Society of America

c/o Francine Butler, PhD, 10200 West 44th Avenue, #304, Wheat Ridge, CO 80033

Founded in 1969. The BSA is an interdisciplinary organization dedicated to the applied, research, and educational aspects of biofeedback.

Braille Institute

741 North Vermont Avenue, Los Angeles, CA 90029

Founded in 1919. The institute provides training, education, and special services for the blind of all ages.

Child Abuse Listening Mediation

PO Box 718, Santa Barbara, CA 93102

Founded in 1971. CALM is organized for the prevention of child abuse and neglect, and provides a hotline listener, child care to reduce stress, a speakers bureau, and parent support groups.

Children's Foundation

815 15th Street, NW, Suite 928, Washington, DC 20005

The foundation was established in 1969 as a national, non-profit advocacy organization focusing upon the quality and availability of the federal food assistance programs for children and their families.

Health and Education Resources

4733 Bethesda Avenue, Suite 735, Bethesda, MD 20814

Founded in 1969. HER is a non-profit organization developing programs and communications in health, education, and social services including continuing education for clinical laboratory personnel; technical assistance for implementation of a skill-and-knowledge based task analysis method; production of audiovisual instructional materials.

Health Sciences Communications Association

6105 Lindell Boulevard, St. Louis, MO 63112

Founded in 1959. HSCA is a non-profit organization devoted to advancement of education in health sciences by means of varied contemporary educational technology.

Healthy America

315 West 105th Street, #1F, New York, NY 10025

Founded in 1977 the coalition is a national, non-profit organization emphasizing health advocacy, disease prevention, and promotion of good health habits as means to attain lasting good health. It encourages health promotion policies and programs at all levels of government and within private sector, sponsors seminars, conferences, etc., and services as congressional liaison for membership.

Huntington's Disease Society of America

140 West 22nd Street, 6th Floor, New York, NY 10011-2420

Founded in 1986. Members: 12,000. Individuals and groups of volunteers concerned with Huntington's disease, an inherited and terminal neurological disease causing progressive brain and nerve deterioration. Goals are to: identify HR families; educate the public and professionals, with emphasis on increasing consumer awareness of HR; promote and support basic and clinical research into the causes and cure of HR; maintain patient services program, coordinated with various community services, to assist families in meeting the social, economic, and emotional problems resulting from HR. HDSA is working to change the attitude of the working community toward the HR patient, and in doing so, enhance the lifestyle of the individual and promote better health care and treatment, both in the community and in facilities. Has launched nationwide legislative campaign in support of enacting federal and state legislation for the establishment of clinics, genetic counseling and screening centers, and diagnostic and treatment centers for the HR patient as well as those suffering from chronic, debilitating disease. Actively cooperates with researchers in ongoing studies; co-sponsors and support services are available. Maintains lending library of audiovisual materials and general and scientific displays. Publications: (1) The Marker (newsletter), 3/year; (2) Annual Report; also publishes booklets and pamphlets.

International Association Cancer Victims and Friends

7740 W. Manchester Avenue, Suite 110, Playa del Rey, CA 90293

Founded in 1963. IAC is a non-profit (tax exempt) corporation organized under the laws of the state of California. Its purpose is the dissemination of educational materials concerning the prevention and control of cancer through the use of non-toxic therapies. Chapters have symposiums and seminars in their respective areas throughout the year.

International Childbirth Education Association

PO Box 20048, Minneapolis, MN 55420

Founded in 1960. The ICEA promotes family centered maternity care and helps groups and individuals promote same through classes in prepared childbirth, teacher training, publications, conferences, and conventions.

National Association of the Physically Handicapped

76 Elm Street, London, OH 43140

Founded in 1958. The NAPH advances the social, economic, and physical welfare of physically handicapped. It is not a resource center for information. We give no type services; nor give financial aid. We support legislation to benefit handicapped; trying to make public aware of needs of handicapped.

National Association of School Nurses

PO Box 1300, Scarborough, ME 04074

Founded in 1969. Members: 4500. School nurses who conduct comprehensive school health programs in public and private schools. Objectives are: to provide national leadership in the promotion of health services for school children; to promote school health interests to the nursing and health community and the public; to monitor legislation pertaining to school nursing. Provides continuing education programs at the national level and assistance to states for program implementation. Offers certification for school nurses. Has established numerous workshops and grants for study of child and drug abuse, the female body, and skin care. Bestows the Lillian Wald Research Award and an annual recognition award for contributions to school nursing. Publications: (1) Newsletter, quarterly; (2) School Nurse Journal, quarterly; also published Guide Lines for a Model School Nurse Services Program and Hearing Screening Guidelines for School Nurses and vision guidelines.

National Association for Visually Handicapped

22 West 21st Street, New York, NY 10010

Founded in 1954. The NAVH offers guidance and counsel for all partially-seeing people and professionals and paraprofessionals working with them, informational literature. It publishes and distributes large print books, textbooks, and testing material. Serves as referral agency for all services for partially seeing. Only national health agency serving only the partially-seeing (not the totally blind).

National Ataxia Foundation

600 Twelve Oaks Center, 15500 Wayzata Boulevard, Wayzata, MN 55391

Founded in 1957. NAF works to combat all types of hereditary ataxia and related disorders through four major objectives: education, service, prevention, and research.

National Committee for the Prevention of Alcoholism and Drug Dependency

RR 1, Box 635, Appomattox, VA 24522

Founded in 1950. The committee holds institutes and seminar-workshops throughout the US periodically. It gathers and distributes information and materials concerning the effects of alcohol and other drugs on the physical, mental, and moral powers of the individual citizen and promotes an educational program for prevention with visual and teaching aids throughout the country. Willing to cooperate with other organizations in holding seminar-workshops in their area.

National Council on Alcoholism

12 West 21st Street, New York, NY 10010

Founded in 1944. The council is the only national voluntary agency founded to combat the disease of alcoholism.

National Council of Stuttering

PO Box 8171, Grand Rapids, MI 49518

Founded in 1965. Promotes and encourages programs and studies on the problems of stuttering.

National Genetics Foundation

PO Box 1374, New York, NY 10101

Founded in 1903.

National Sudden Infant Death Syndrome Foundation

8200 Professional Plaza, Suite 104, Landover, MD 20785

Founded in 1962. NSIDSF provides support for SIDS research, services to families of victims of SIDS and SIDS-related disorders, and educational programs for health and emergency personnel. It also fulfills a consumer advocacy role of SIDS families.

National Tay-Sachs and Allied Diseases Association

385 Elliot Street, Newton, MA 02164

Founded in 1957. The association conducts programs in support of research, family counseling, and public and professional education into the genetic disease Tay-Sachs and many other diseases due to inborn errors of metabolism.

Pediatric Pulmonary and Cystic Fibrosis Center

St. Christopher's Hospital for Children, 2600 North Lawrence Street, Philadelphia, PA 19133

Focuses upon research on cystic fibrosis and other chronic respiratory diseases in infants and children. Examines new therapeutic modalities.

Planned Parenthood Federation of America

810 Seventh Avenue, New York, NY 10019

PPF works to make effective means of birth control available for all.

School Health Programs

University of Colorado Health Sciences Center School of Nursing, 4200 East 9th Avenue, C-287, Denver, CO 80262

Founded in 1969. The SHP is a training program to prepare health care professionals capable of providing a wide range of diagnostic, preventive, and therapeutic services to children. Working principally in ambulatory settings as colleagues and associates of physicians, child health associates have the knowledge and skill to care for a large percentage of the patients seen in a typical pediatric practice. The training program is 3 years in length. Prerequisites include 2 years of college preparation.

Synanon Foundation, Inc.

6055 Marshall Petalvma Road, Marshall, CA 84840

Founded in 1958. Synanon was the first community designed for the re-education of drug addicts and other character disorders, and it continues to do that work. Since 1974 Synanon has been providing re-education for children as young as 10. Facilities in Marshall, San Francisco, Los Angeles, and Badger, CA; Kerhonkson and New York, NY; Chicago, IL; and Detroit, MI.

United Cerebral Palsy Association

66 East 34th Street, New York, NY 10016

Founded in 1948. UCP is the only nationwide voluntary organization targeting its services on the specific and multiple needs of persons with cerebral palsy and their families. UCP's more than 240 affiliates provide a variety of community services, support research and conduct programs of public education pertaining to cerebral palsy.

APPENDIX

Sample Guides

I1—INFECTION CONTROL GUIDELINES FOR HOME CARE (CHAPTER 20)

The practice of universal precautions means that all blood and body fluids are treated as potentially infectious. Universal precautions is implemented to prevent exposure and infection of caregivers. It is an important practice because many infections are subclinical.

Use extreme care when handling needles, scalpels, and razors to prevent injuries. Do not recap, bend, break, or remove the needle from a syringe before disposal. Discard needles and syringes in puncture-resistant containers made of plastic or metal and dispose them in a local landfill.

Barrier precautions such as gloves, masks, eye covering, and gowns should be worn when contact with blood and body fluids is expected. Gloves must be worn when in contact with body fluids, mucous membranes, non-intact skin, and when drawing blood. Masks and eye cover are recommended when droplets or splashes of blood or other body fluids is expected. Wear gowns, aprons, or smocks to protect regular clothing from splashes of blood or body fluids.

Handwashing is the single most important practice in preventing infections. Handwashing should be done before and after providing client care and before and after preparing food, eating, feeding, or using the bathroom.

Soiled dressings and perineal pads should be placed inside polyethylene garbage bags by using two bags and double lining them.

HIV is easily decontaminated by common disinfectants such as lysol and is rapidly killed by household bleach. Surfaces can be disinfected with a solution of 1 part bleach to 10 parts water. This solution must be mixed daily to retain its disinfectant properties. Bathrooms and kitchens can be safely shared with persons infected with HIV, but towels, razors and toothbrushes should not be shared. Household cleaning can be done in a regular manner unless there are spills of blood or body fluids. If a spill occurs, wear gloves and decontaminate the area by flooding the spill with a disinfectant, then use paper towels to remove visible debris, and reapply disinfectant.

Kitchen counters, dishes, and laundry should be cleaned in warm water and detergent after use. Bathrooms may be cleaned with a household disinfectant.

I2—SAFER SEX GUIDELINES (CHAPTER 20)

The following information is intended to be given to clients during risk reduction counseling.

Discuss injectable drug use, sexual history, and safer sex practices with potential partners before sexual activity. If you are infected with any sexually transmitted disease such as genital herpes, HIV, or genital warts, let sexual partners know. Drugs and alcohol may impair judgement and reduce your ability to make wise decisions.

Recommendations for Use of Condoms

Use latex condoms to prevent exchange of body fluids because they offer greater protection against STD than natural membrane condoms. The use of condoms that contain spermicides, such as nonoxynol-9, can be effective in rendering HIV inactive. Nonoxynol-9 can also be put in the condom before putting it on. Oil-based lubricants, such as petroleum jelly (Vaseline), are unsafe because they weaken condoms and diminish protection. Only water-based lubricants such as K-Y jelly should be used. Condoms should be put on before any genital contact. Hold the tip of the condom and unroll it onto the erect penis. Leave a space at the tip for collection of semen but make sure that no air is trapped in the tip of the condom. Withdrawal should occur before loss of erection. The base of the condom should be held throughout withdrawal and the condom should be removed slowly to avoid tearing the condom or spilling body fluids. If the penis relaxes before withdrawal, the condom may fall off and body fluids may spill, thus causing potential exposure. Avoid mouth contact with the penis, vagina, or anus. Wear condoms during oral sex. Condoms should never be reused and should be stored in a cool, dry place.

I3—GUIDE FOR EVALUATION OF GROUP EFFECTIVENESS (CHAPTER 17)

The following questions focus evaluation on group task accomplishment, member satisfaction, conflict management, and group purpose. Answer each question for the group, then write a descriptive summary of group effectiveness.

1. Describe the group's task goal. List the steps proposed or acted on by members relative to the goal. How well do members achieve these steps?
2. Describe leadership behavior for the group. How well do members carry out other group roles?
3. Describe comfort level for group members. Do members support each other? Is the level of tension conducive to productive behavior?
4. Is disagreement expressed clearly and openly? How do members manage and resolve conflict?
5. By what bonds are members attracted to each other and to the group?
6. Are there implicit goals for the group, and do these goals interfere with the group's work toward the explicit goal?

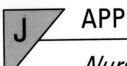

APPENDIX

Nursing Intervention Tools

J1—NORMAL VARIATIONS AND MINOR ABNORMALITIES IN NEWBORN PHYSICAL CHARACTERISTICS
(CHAPTERS 28 and 29)

Variant	Cause	Course	Nursing anticipatory guidance
HEAD			
Cephalhematoma	Usually caused by trauma of birth.	Soft, fluctuant, well-outlined mass of blood trapped beneath the pericranium and confined to one bone. This is a subperiosteal hematoma with no extension across suture lines.	Observe for any changes in the size or shape of the hematoma. Reassure parents.
Caput succedaneum	Caused by head pressing on the pelvic outlet in the last period of labor.	Clear fluid trapped between the scalp and bone. It is ill-defined, pits on pressure, not fluctuant. Fluid usually disappears in 1 to 2 weeks.	Explain the cause to parents and reassure them it will disappear.
Facial asymmetry	Overriding of the cranial sutures at birth caused by intrauterine molding or molding from delivery. Bones are soft and pliable.	Flattening of part of head or face. Generally disappears a few days after birth.	If the occipital area is flat because of labor and delivery, reassure parents about its disappearance in a few days. If it is caused by the "same" positioning of the child in the crib, instruct the parents to alternate the positioning of the child in the crib daily.
Asymmetry of the scalp	Usually occurs from molding during delivery or the use of forceps during delivery. Also can be caused by positioning the infant repeatedly on the same side without rotating.	Flattening of part of head.	Same as facial asymmetry.
Craniotabes	Unknown.	Softening of localized areas in the cranial bone. Sometimes found in the parietal bones at the vertex near the sagittal suture. The areas are spongelike and can be indented by the pressure of a fingertip. They resume their shape when the pressure is removed.	Usually inconsequential, but if they persist, could be indicative of a pathological cause. There is no specific treatment. It is normal for these craniotabes to persist for months. They should eventually disappear.

Continued.

Normal variations and minor abnormalities in newborn physical characteristics—cont'd

Variant	Cause	Course	Nursing anticipatory guidance
Fontanelle	An irregular-shaped area enclosed by a membrane which occurs where the sutures of the bone of the skull meet. These areas are called anterior fontanelle, posterior fontanelle, and temporal fontanelles.	The anterior fontanelle should be open; the posterior fontanelle may be closed.	Explain to the parents that the open fontanelle helped to protect the baby's head during the birth process. The fontanelle allows the brain to grow and will continue to do so for the next 18 months. Reassure parents that fontanelle can be touched and scalp scrubbed without ill effect.
MOUTH			
Bednar's aphthae (ulcers)	Unknown. May be caused by vigorous sucking.	Usually located on hard palate posteriorly; generally bilateral	Reassure and support parents. Explain to the parents that there is no specific treatment, and condition will disappear without any treatment.
Epstein's epithelial pearls	Small epithelial cysts.	Located along both sides of the middle of the hard palate or along the alveolar ridge.	Reassure parents that cysts will disappear. There is no specific treatment.
Bohn's pearls (nodules)	Small white papules.	Located on each side of the midline of the hard palate. They disappear spontaneously in several weeks.	Reassure and support parents. Parents sometimes think that these lesions look like thrush. Reassure that these lesions are not thrush and will go away without treatment.
High palatal arch		Of no significance if there are no other findings present.	Reassure, support, and explain the lack of significance.
EYES			
Chemical conjunctivitis	Irritation from silver nitrate solution instilled after birth.	Eyes red with purulent exudate. Lids swollen. Onset occurs within first 24 hours and lasts about 2 to 4 days.	Cleanse eyelids with cotton balls soaked in warm saline solution. Wipe the eyes from the inner canthus out toward the outer canthus. Reassure parents that the infant's eyesight will not be affected.
Subconjunctival hemorrhage	Caused from pressure in the birth process.	Occurs at the limbus. It may be crescent shaped or may form a red halo around the iris. The hemorrhage resolves itself without any specific treatment in a few days.	Reassure parents that no residual defects occur from the hemorrhage. The blood will reabsorb itself in a few days.
Pseudostrabismus	Poor muscle coordination of the eye.	Movements of the newborn's eyes are poorly coordinated. The eyes do not necessarily move together. Very common and usually disappears spontaneously.	Reassure parents that this generally disappears spontaneously as the eye muscles strengthen and the infant's eyes continue to develop and grow.
SKIN			
Vernix caseosa	Cheeselike material that sticks to the skin. Protective covering for infant in utero.	Skin of newborn covered with varying amounts of this substance.	Will dry and disappear within a few days. Discourage mother from trying to vigorously rub it off. Encourage good skin care.

Continued.

Normal variations and minor abnormalities in newborn physical characteristics—cont'd

Variant	Cause	Course	Nursing anticipatory guidance
SKIN—cont'd			
Lanugo	Fine downy type of hair.	Usually found on the back, shoulders, and ear lobes.	Usually disappears in time as a result of the friction of the skin rubbing on the bassinet linens. Reassure parents.
Desquamation	Skin in the newborn is very tender and soft. Following birth, the skin reacts to the changed environment by becoming very red. When the redness subsides, desquamation of the skin tends to occur.	Shedding, flaking, or peeling of the skin. Usually occurs during the first week of life. Can vary from extensive to so slight it almost goes unnoticed.	Reassure, support, and explain the cause to parents. Encourage good skin care, which avoids overuse of lotions, oils, and powders.
Ecchymosis	Blood under the skin caused by superficial trauma to the skin.	Bruise—disappears as the blood is reabsorbed.	Provide reassurance.
Acrocyanosis	Venous stasis.	Blue hands and feet.	No specific treatment. Make sure the baby is warm and that the cause of the acrocyanosis is not from being cold.
Erythema toxicum	Unknown.	A rash consisting of small, red, flat or raised lesions. Looks splotchy and sometimes resembles chicken pox or flea bites. Usually occurs during the first 2 weeks.	No specific treatment. Reassure, support, and explain.
Nevi, pigmented Nevus spilus (hairless mole)	Increased pigmentation.	Range from smooth, flat, hairless pigmented areas to those with hair; some can look like warts.	No treatment unless for cosmetic reasons. Provide reassurance.
Nevi, telangiectatic	Widening of surface capillaries.	Small red areas due to widening of surface capillaries; disappear momentarily with blanching of skin, but usually do not disappear completely.	Provide reassurance.
Capillary hemangiomata (sometimes called Balmar patches)	Capillary lesions of the skin.	Irregular blotchy pink spots at the nape of the neck, eyelids, globella, or lumbosacral areas. Gradually fade; usually disappear by 2 years.	Reassurance and support. No specific treatment.
Mongolian spots	Large aggregations of melanin–rich dark cells, which give the affected area a purple or blue/black color. Occur most frequently in black children but may occur in white children.	Generally found over the sacrum and coccygeal area of a large percentage of infants of black, Chicano, and Asiatic Indian origin. They do not have any significance and most disappear with time.	Explain cause and reassure parents. The spots usually disappear within the first year of life.
Mottling	Vasoconstriction—general circulatory instability.	Overall red and white coloration of the skin. Generally occurs in fair children who become chilled. Disappears when child becomes warm.	Explain causes and reassure parents; use a blanket to warm the infant.

Normal variations and minor abnormalities in newborn physical characteristics—cont'd

Normal variations and minor abnormalities in newborn physical characteristics—cont'd

Variant	Cause	Course	Nursing anticipatory guidance
SKIN—cont'd			
Milia	Retained sebum in the skin.	Yellow-white, pinpoint-size lesions located on the bridge of the nose, the chin, or the cheeks. Disappear after first few weeks of life.	No specific treatment necessary. Explain to parents that lesions will disappear.
Café au lait	Variations in pigment.	Light to dark brown pigmented spots. One or two patches considered normal. If infant has several patches, may indicate fibromas or neurofibromatosis.	Assess nature of spots. If number of spots exceeds two, refer to physician or neurologist. Reassurance and support.
Accessory nipples (supernumerary nipples)	Not adequately explained (sometimes referred to as developmental cutaneous defect).	Occurs in a unilateral or bilateral distribution along the ''mammary lines'' from midaxilla to the inguinal area.	Reassure parents that the nipples may be excised for cosmetic reasons.
Harlequin coloring	Thought to be caused by poorly developed vasomotor reflexes.	Half of the infant's body appears red/white, the other half is pale. Transitory condition, which usually occurs when the infant cries forcefully.	Explain to parents that this is not significant. It is apparently harmless and the cause is not adequately explained.
Cyanosis (localized)	Inadequate oxygenation of tissues; localized cyanosis because of immature peripheral circulation and venous stasis.	Usually involves lips, hand and feet or cyanosis of the presenting parts. Usually present at birth and for variable number or days afterwards.	Keep child warm; cyanosis will decrease as peripheral circulation improves. Reassure and support parents. Explain cause.
Cyanosis (general)	Numerous causes of general cyanosis (e.g., atelectasis, congenital heart disease, central nervous system damage, obstructed airway).	Depends on the cause.	Reassurance and support. Try to determine the relationship of cyanosis to crying, (i.e., if cyanosis is relieved or improved when the child cries, then the cause may be atelectasis). Crying tends to make infants with cardiac malformations worse. Refer to physician.
ABDOMEN			
Umbilical cord variations	Natural process for sloughing tissues.	Blue/white at birth. Dull and yellow/brown within 24 hours, then black/brown and dry. Usually drops off at the end of the second week.	Keep cord area clean and dry. Reassure parents. Instruct parents in cord care.
Umbilical hernia	Occurs at the defect in the musculature of the abdominal wall near the umbilicus.	Skin-covered protuberance at the umbilicus. Very common in black infants and some Italian infants. Usually disappears spontaneously at the end of one year.	Reassure parents that it will probably disappear spontaneously. If it does not, it can be treated surgically when the child is older. Discourage home remedies (e.g., coin taped to hernia, binding, etc.)
OTHER			
Vaginal discharge	Physiological manifestation of increased maternal hormonal influences.	Milky white discharge, sometimes blood–tinged or whole blood. Usually disappears in 2 weeks.	Reassure mother that this is nothing to worry about. It occurs quite frequently and is considered normal. Explain that it will disappear in a few weeks.

Continued.

Normal variations and minor abnormalities in newborn physical characteristics—cont'd

Variant	Cause	Course	Nursing anticipatory guidance
Brachial palsy	Sometimes caused when lateral traction is exerted on the head and neck during delivery of the shoulder in a vertex presentation, or in a breech presentation when the arms are extended over the head, or when there is excessive traction on the shoulders.	Should be suspected when there is asymmetric response of the upper extremities during a Moro response. The asymmetric response occurs because there is paralysis of the muscles of the upper arm or paralysis of the entire arm. Prognosis depends on the extent of damage to the nerves.	Treatment usually consists of partial immobilization and appropriate positioning. Problem needs to be evaluated and the appropriate treatment initiated. Depending on the severity of damage, there could be complete return of function within a few months or there may be permanent damage. Teach parents the importance of carrying out the immobilization-positioning treatment on a daily basis. Reassure and support parents. Observe for any changes in the movement of the upper extremities.

J2—INTERVENTIONS FOR THE ALLERGIC CHILD
(CHAPTERS 28 and 29)
Home allergy-proofing techniques

Potential antigen	Proofing actions
House dust (leading cause of respiratory allergy)	1. Restrict use of bedroom to sleeping. 2. Use shades instead of blinds or curtains. 3. Place washable plastic over mattresses. 4. Use no carpeting or wool scatter rugs. 5. Damp dust daily with child out of room. 6. Allow no stuffed animals or knickknacks. 7. Have minimum furniture; if stuffed, it should be with foam rubber. 8. Either close off heat ducts or cover with cheesecloth. (Wash often.) 9. Keep doors and windows closed. 10. Avoid storing wool in closets and avoid use of wool blankets. 11. Heating system: forced-air heat that circulates dust should not be used unless vents or ducts are covered with cheesecloth, which must be washed frequently. 12. Use electric heaters instead of forced air heat wherever possible, but beware of fire potential. 13. Use clean-air machines or purifiers to cleanse air of dust. 14. Use washable paint or wallpaper on ceiling and walls.
Mold, mildew	1. Eliminate plants and aquariums from child's bedroom and play area; keep to a minimum throughout the home. 2. Avoid use of cellars as play or living area. 3. Clean bathroom and tile areas with anti-mold agent (e.g., Lysol) regularly. 4. Cleanse vaporizers or humidifiers frequently. 5. Use dehumidifier in humid or damp areas.
Danders, feathers	1. Use Dacron or foam rubber pillows and mattresses. 2. Get rid of pets or keep them outdoors. 3. Allow no stuffed animals or furniture and no clothing stuffed or insulated with feathers (down).
Contactants	1. Buy no wool clothing. 2. Wash all new clothing and linens before using. 3. Double-rinse infant's clothing and diapers. 4. Wash baby articles in mild soap. 5. Use mild soap to bathe baby and rinse well. 6. Avoid use of perfumed lotions, powders, oils.

PROCEDURE FOR AN ELIMINATION DIET

The procedure is as follows:

1. A diary of each food, beverage, or medication that is ingested at meals or between meals without alteration in customary patterns is to be recorded for 7 to 10 days.
2. Constituents of all home-prepared foods must be listed as well as ingredients of all packaged foods. Concealed foods may be included in prepared products.
3. Symptoms are also recorded for 7 to 10 days. By correlating symptoms with the information in the diary, the nurse frequently can determine the elimination diet suitable for the particular case; e.g., milk-free, salicylate-free, or others.
4. The elimination diet is initiated.
5. Two weeks following the start of an elimination diet, the client is interviewed, and the diet is reviewed. Improvement can be expected within 2 to 3 weeks if the correct food has been eliminated.
6. Two weeks later another interview and review are conducted.
7. If symptoms have not subsided, the program is abandoned, and another diet regimen is implemented.
8. If the diet is successful in eliminating symptoms it should be continued for at least 2 months before attempting additions of new foods to the diet.
9. New foods can then be added individually every 5 to 7 days.
10. If symptoms return, the food should be discontinued.
11. If the second attempt at introducing the food is not successful, the food should be permanently excluded from the diet.
12. This procedure is repeated with other foods, each one taken individually, until a well-balanced and varied diet is provided for the client.
13. The diet diary should be continued for a few months, if possible, in the event of a recurrence of symptoms.
14. All labels, especially of prepared foods, must be read carefully.
15. Home-prepared foods are preferable because the ingredients can be controlled.
16. Absolute adherence to the diet is imperative. If undesirable weight loss occurs, more of the prescribed carbohydrates, sugar, fats, and oils must be taken. This may require eating four to five meals a day.
17. Caution should be taken not to place a child on a nutritionally deficient diet for long periods of time when no specific results have been obtained.

From Chow MP, et al.: Handbook of pediatric primary care, ed 2, New York, 1984, John Wiley & Sons, Inc.

J3—INFANT STIMULATION
(CHAPTERS 28 & 29)

BIRTH TO 1 MONTH

Babies like to
  Suck
  Listen to repeated soft sounds
  Stare at movement and light
  Be *held* and *rocked*
Give your baby
  Your *talking* and *singing*
  Lamps throwing light patterns
  Your *arms*
  Rocking

1 MONTH

Babies like to
  Listen to your voice
  Look up and to the side
  Hold things placed in their hands
Give your baby
  A lullaby *record*
  A *mobile* overhead
  Pictures on the walls
  Your *face* near his
  A *change in scenery* and *position*

2 MONTHS

Babies like to
  Listen to musical sounds
  Focus, especially on their hands
  Reach and *bat* nearby objects
  Smile

Give your baby
  A *music box* or a soft *musical toy*
  A soft security *cuddle toy* tied to crib
  Your *smile*
  Play time with you

3 MONTHS

Babies like to
  Reach and *feel* with open hands
  Grasp crudely with two hands
  Wave their fists and *watch* them
Give your baby
  Musical records
  Rattles
  Dangling toys
  Textured toys

4 MONTHS

Babies like to
  Grasp things and *let go*
  Kick
  Laugh at unexpected sights and sounds
  Make *consonant sounds*
Give your baby
  Bells
  A *crib gym*
  More *dangling toys*
  Space to kick and move

5 MONTHS

Babies like to
  Shake, feel, and *bang* things

  Sit with support
  Play peek-a-boo
  Roll over
Give your baby
  A *high chair* with a rubber *suction toy*
  A *play pen*
  A *kicking toy*
  Toys that make noise

6 MONTHS

Babies like to
  Shake, bang and throw things down
  Gum objects
  Recognize familiar *faces*
Give your baby
  Many *household objects*
  Tin *cups, spoons,* and pot *lids*
  Wire *whisks*
  A *clutch ball* and *squeaky toys*
  A *teether* and *gumming toys*
  Bouncing, swinging seat

7 MONTHS

Babies like to
  Sit alone
  Use their *fingers* and *thumb*
  Notice *cause* and *effect*
  Bite on their *first tooth*

Continued.

Give your baby
- *Bath tub toys*
- More *'things'*
- *String*
- More *squeaky toys*
- *Finger foods*

8 MONTHS

Babies like to
- *Pivot* on their stomachs
- *Throw, wave,* and *bang* toys together
- *Look* for toys they have
- Make *vowel sounds*

Give your baby
- *Space* to pivot and creep
- 2 *toys* at once to *bang* together
- Big *soft blocks*
- A *Jack-in-the-box*
- *Nested* plastic *cups*
- Your *conversation*

9 MONTHS

Babies like to
- *Pull themselves up*
- *Creep*
- *Place* things generally where they're wanted
- *Say "da-da"*
- *Play pat-a-cake*

Give your baby
- A *safe corner* of the room to *explore*
- *Toys* tied to the *high chair*
- A metal *mirror*
- *Jack-in-the-box*

10 MONTHS

Babies like to
- *Poke* and *prod* with their forefingers
- *Put things in* other things
- *Imitate sounds*

Give your baby
- A big *pegboard*
- Some *cloth books*
- *Motion toys*
- *Textured toys*

11 MONTHS TO 1 YEAR

Babies like to
- *Use* their *fingers*
- *Lower themselves from standing*
- *Drink* from a cup
- *Mark* on paper

Give your baby
- *Pyramid disks*
- A large *crayon*
- A baking *tin* with *clothespins*
- Personal *drinking cup*
- More *picture books*

J4—FEEDING AND NUTRITION GUIDELINES FOR INFANTS AND CHILDREN
(CHAPTERS 28 and 29)

Age	Type of feeding	Specific recommendations
Birth-6 months	Breast-feeding	Most desirable complete diet for first half of year
		Requires supplements of flouride (0.25 mg) regardless of the fluoride content of the local water supply, and iron by 6 months of age
		Requires supplements of vitamin D (400 units) if mother's diet is inadequate or if infant is not exposed to sufficient sunlight
		Average number of feedings 6-8 in first 2 weeks, decreasing to 4-5 by 6 months
	Formula	Iron-fortified commercial formula is a complete food for the first half of the year
		Requires fluoride supplements (0.25 mg) when the concentration of fluoride in the drinking water is below 0.3 parts per million (ppm)
		Evaporated milk formula requires supplements of vitamin C, iron, and fluoride (in accordance with the fluoride content of the local water supply)
		Average total of 22 oz at 2 weeks; 28-30 oz at 2 months; 32-34-oz at 3 months; 32-38-oz at 6 months
		Frequency and amount ranges from 2-3 oz 6-8 times a day at 2 weeks to 5-oz, 5-6 times a day at 2 months to 7-8-oz, 4-5 times a day at 5 months
6-12 months	Solid foods	May begin to add solids by 4-6 months of age; earlier introduction tends to contribute to overfeeding
		First foods are strained, pureed, or finely mashed
		"Finger foods" such as teething crackers, raw fruit, or vegetables can be introduced by 6 to 7 months
		Chopped table food or commercially prepared junior foods can be started by 9 to 12 months
		With the exception of cereal, the order of introducing foods is variable; a recommended sequence is weekly introduction of other foods, beginning with fruit, followed by vegetables and then meat
		Breast-fed infants require more high-protein foods than formula-fed children
		As the quantity of solids increases, the amount of formula should be limited to 28-30 oz daily

Continued.

J4—FEEDING AND NUTRITION GUIDELINES FOR INFANTS AND CHILDREN
(CHAPTERS 28 and 29)/cont'd

Age	Type of feeding	Specific recommendations
	Cereal	Introduce commercially prepared iron-fortified infant cereals, and offer daily until 18 months of age Rice cereal is usually introduced first because of its low allergenic potential Can discontinue supplemental iron once cereal is given
	Fruits and vegetables	Applesauce, bananas, and pears are usually well-tolerated Avoid fruits and vegetables marketed in cans that are not specifically designed for infants, because of variable and sometimes high lead content and addition of salt, sugar, or preservatives Offer fruit juice only from a cup, not a bottle, to reduce the development of "nursing bottle carries"
	Meat, fish, and poultry	Avoid fatty meats Prepare by baking, broiling, steaming, or poaching Include organ meats such as liver, which has a high content of iron, vitamin A, and vitamin B complex If soup is given, be sure all ingredients are familiar in child's diet
	Eggs and cheese	Serve egg yolk hard–boiled and mashed, soft cooked, or poached Introduce egg white in small quantities (1 tsp) toward end of first year to detect any allergic manifestation Use cheese as a substitute for meat and as "finger food"
	Progession of starting solids	Start enriched baby cereal 2-2½ tb at breakfast and supper at 4-5 months; progress to 3 tb at breakfast and supper by months. Continue to progress not to exceed ½ cup by 9 months. Add 1½ to 3 tb strained fruits for breakfast and supper at 5 months; progress to 3 tb at breakfast and supper by 6 months. Continue to progress, not to exceed 2-3 tb two times a day at 8 months. Add 1-2 tb strained vegetables at lunch at 5 months; progress to 2-3 tb at lunch by 6 months. Continue to progress, not to exceed 3 tb two times a day by 8-9 months. Add strained meats, 1-2 tb at lunch at 6 months; progress to 1-2 tb at lunch and supper by 7-8 months. Continue to progress to 2 to 2½ tb two times a day at 9-10 months. Add egg yolk, 1 yolk or 2 tb at 7 months. Add bread and starch at 8-9 months. Progress to mashed table food at 8-9 months and finger foods at approximately same time.
	Food texture	Liquids, birth to 4 months. Baby-soft, 4-6 months. Thickened soft, 6-7 months. Mashed table food, 8-9 months. Finger foods, 9 months. Finely cut, 11-12 months.

Adapted from Whaley, LF and Wong D: Nursing care of infants and children, ed 4, St. Louis, 1991, Mosby–Year Book, Inc.

Older children and adolescents

Food group	Servings per day	Average size of servings					
		1 year	2-3 years	4-5 years	6-9 years	10-12 years	13-15 years
MILK AND CHEESE 1.5 oz cheese = 1 cup milk (1 cup = 8 oz or 240 gm)	4	½ cup	½-¾ cup	¾ cup	¾-1 cup	1 cup	1 cup
MEAT GROUP (PROTEIN FOODS)	3 or more						
Egg		1	1	1	1	1	1 or more
Lean meat, fish, poultry (liver once a week)		2 tb	2 tb	4 tb	2-3 oz (4-6 tb)	3-4 oz	4 oz or more
Peanut butter			1 tb	2 tb	2-3 tb	3 tb	3 tb
FRUITS AND VEGETABLES	At least 4, including:						
Vitamin C source (citrus fruits, berries, tomato, cabbage, cantaloupe)	1 or more (twice as much tomato as citrus)	⅓ cup citrus	½ cup	½ cup	1 medium orange	1 medium orange	1 medium orange
Vitamin A source (green or yellow fruits and vegetables)	1 or more	2 tb	3 tb	4 tb (¼ cup)	¼ cup	⅓ cup	½ cup
Other vegetables (potato and legumes, etc.) *or*	2	2 tb	3 tb	4 tb (¼ cup)	⅓ cup	½ cup	¾ cup
Other fruits (apple, banana, etc.)		¼ cup	⅓ cup	½ cup	1 medium	1 medium	1 medium
CEREALS (WHOLE-GRAIN OR ENRICHED)	At least 4						
Bread		½ slice	1 slice	1½ slices	1-2 slices	2 slices	2 slices
Ready-to-eat cereal		½ oz	¾ oz	1 oz	1 oz	1 oz	1 oz
Cooked cereal (including macaroni, spaghetti, rice, etc.)		¼ cup	⅓ cup	½ cup	½ cup	¾ cup	1 cup or more
FATS AND CARBOHYDRATES	To meet caloric needs						
Butter, margarine, mayonnaise, oils: 1 tb = 100 calories (kcal)		1 tb	1 tb	1 tb	2 tb	2 tb	2-4 tb
Desserts and sweets: 100-calorie portions as follows: ⅓ cup pudding or ice cream, 2 3-inch cookies, 1 oz cake, 1⅓ oz pie, 2 tb jelly, jam, honey, sugar		1 portion	1½ portions	1½ portions	3 portions	3 portions	3-6 portions

From Behrman RE, and Vaughan VC: Nelson textbook of pediatrics, ed 13, 1987, WB Saunders Co., p. 123.
*Based on food groups and the average size of servings at different age levels.

J5—COMMON CONCERNS AND PROBLEMS OF FIRST YEAR (NEONATE AND INFANT)

Problem or concern	Assessment	Nursing intervention
Burping	Swallowed air bubbles trapped in stomach; occurs more frequently in bottle-fed infants who cry during feeding.	Burp frequently during feeding (i.e., before, during, and after, or after every 1 ounce of formula or after every 4-5 minutes at breast). Use upright position to burp (gently rub infant's back while baby sits on parent's knee and rests forward against parent's arm). Try to burp every 10-15 minutes while awake if not successful burping during and after feeding. Sit upright in infant seat for 30-45 minutes after feeding if awake or position with head elevated and on right side if sleeping.
Colic	Unexplained bouts of crying frequently occurring at same time of day (usually busiest) and often accompanied by abdominal distention, spasms, drawing up legs to stomach and/or passing gas. May be caused by feeding problems, maternal anxiety, allergy, and is aggravated by tension in household. Can last 3 months. Also see Crying.	Review basic infant needs with parents (i.e., is infant hungry, wet, have air bubble, in uncomfortable position)? Review feeding method, technique and burping, review maternal diet for offending foods if breastfed. Record time when colic episodes occur. Soothe and comfort before "attack." Swaddle infant, i.e., wrap warmly and in an encompassing manner. Walk, rock, and hold infant over shoulder. Try a monotonous soothing noise (music, ticking clock) or activity (ride in a car). Change infant position from stomach to side to back to sitting position. Rest infant on abdomen on warm hard surface (i.e., parent knee, warmed crib surface). Change household routine if indicated, create a quiet environment. Try pacifier or sugar water; if bottle fed, try soy formula. Reassure parents that infant is not ill, that they are providing good care, and that colic will definitely go away. Provide support to parents, giving opportunity to discuss feelings. Explain theories about origin and cycle of colic.
Crying	Periodic crying for unexplained reason; ascertain if a pattern exists for crying spells; may be related to colic; obtain a detailed history of time and length of spell; feeding frequency, method, technique and burping; stool patterns; meeting contact and sucking needs; parental handling of crying and feelings about crying; other household factors, (i.e., siblings, relative advice, parental support of each other, presence of other symptoms and/or allergies).	See previous section on colic. Reinforce that babies crying for a reason. Best to respond to crying versus letting baby cry it out. Crying is a release and/or exercise for infant. One or two periods a day of 5-10 minutes is normal for most infants. Assist parents to develop positive, relaxed approach. Reassure and support parents in this time of stress. Suggest parents alternate infant care and alternate meeting infant demands.
Constipation	Consistency of stool which is hard, pebbly, rocklike. Not related to frequency, straining, grunting or number of days between stools. Ascertain color, consistency and frequency as well as presence of blood or mucus. Review infant diet and verify parent perception of constipation and expectation of normal stool patterns.	Discuss normal elimination/stool patterns for type of feeding method (i.e., breast fed stools versus bottle fed stools). Reassure that straining, grunting, infrequent number are normal. Reinforce that each infant has individual stool pattern and educate parents about *what* constipation actually is (i.e., consistency). Discuss parents' attitude regarding toilet habits and expectations about stool patterns.

Continued.

Common concerns and problems of first year (neonate and infant)—cont'd

Problem or concern	Assessment	Nursing intervention
		If constipated, increase liquids in diet; may offer water between meals.
		If introduced to solids too early or in too large a quantity, discontinue use until constipation clears, then begin again with smaller amounts.
		Karo syrup, 1 tsp/3 oz of water may be given several times a day.
		If appropriate for feeding stage, add prunes (up to 3 tb.) or prune juice to diet.
Flatus	Air in stomach or intestines causing abdominal distress, distension, and discomfort, frequently expelled through anus. May be caused by excess swallowing of air, overfeeding, underfeeding, or allergy. Ascertain details about feeding, (i.e., frequency and size of nipple, type bottle used, breast feeding technique, maternal diet, use of pacifier, propping of bottle, burping, etc.).	Burp frequently during and after feedings. See first section. Calm infant when crying and burp after crying. Place on left side to ease expelling of gas. If suspect allergies, try soy formula or elimination diet (Appendix J2, p. 849). Reassure parents.
Hiccoughs	Sudden sharp involuntary spasms of diaphragm, usually occur following a meal.	Reassure patient that infant will cry if truly distressed. Offer infant something to suck (pacifier, breast, bottle with warm water).
Pacifier	Infants demonstrate a need for non-nutritional sucking.	Assist parents to understand aspects of positive and negative use of pacifier. Positive use: indicated immediately after birth before newborn can manipulate thumb into mouth; assists in developing sucking function; contributes to establishment of breast feeding; good means of satisfying sucking need, especially for bottle fed infants who need extra sucking time; does not usually become a habit unless child sucks beyond infancy; most infants substitute thumb for pacifier around 3 to 4 months. Parents should look for clues to eliminate pacifier use at this time and provide stimulation suitable for the age. Negative use: pacifiers do not replace holding; stimulation, or needs satisfaction; pacifiers should not be used constantly, especially before tending to infant's needs; parents should be encouraged to discontinue use by 5 months since continued use may become a hard habit to overcome. If thumb is substituted, generally it is used less frequently than pacifier.
Spoiling	Ascertain parent definition of spoiling. Generally it is the result of basic needs not being met in early infancy leading to a demanding, undisciplined child because need for gratification continues beyond normal time. Overgratification usually occurs then. Generally it is believed that infants cannot be spoiled under 6 months of age.	Parents require counseling and education that reinforces the following: Early infant needs must be gratified. A child cannot handle frustrations well until 8-9 months and is unable to delay gratification of needs until this age. A gradual and gentle approach to limits and delaying gratification is best. A relaxed, positive approach is helpful. Parents often find support groups helpful in dealing with this problem.
Biting	In first year, frequently related to teething. Particularly a problem for breast-feeding mothers. In toddlerhood related to normal aggressive impulses.	If related to teething, see later section on teething for alleviation of discomfort. Breast-feeding mothers should remove infant from breast at every occurrence and may accompany with a "no," should also allow time to lapse before finishing feeding. If related to impulsivity of toddlerhood, see first section of table on p. 865.

Continued.

Common concerns and problems of first year (neonate and infant)—cont'd

Problem or concern	Assessment	Nursing intervention
Separation anxiety	Occurs at 9-10 months as infant is learning to differentiate self from mother. Can occur again in toddlerhood as child is learning to distance and separate self from mother in attempt to establish autonomy.	Reassure mother that this is normal developmental process. Advise parents, especially mother, to do the following: Play "peek-a-boo" games. Allow sufficient time (30-45 minutes for child to acquaint him/herself with new person (i.e., visitor, babysitter). Avoid "sneaking out." Tell child firmly that "mommy leaves, mommy comes back." Reinforce this with "peek-a-boo" or "hide and seek" games. Avoid making major changes in child's or household routines during this period (i.e., mother returning to work; changing child's room; changing regular babysitter or day care situation, etc.).
Stranger anxiety	Begins at 6-8 months, gradually diminishing by 18 months. Process of child development.	See preceding section on separation anxiety. Advise parents, particularly mother, to hold infant in presence of strangers. If infant is to be left, mother should spend a short time with stranger.
Infant sleep patterns	Some infants have difficulty releasing into sleep or awaken easily. Separation anxiety, teething, illness are among the common causes. Ascertain history of problem to include how long infant sleeps, what feeding schedule is, bedtime and household routines, presence of illness or teething, and how problem is handled.	Counseling should be directed toward education of parents; infants need gratification and normal sleep patterns, emphasizing the following: Differences in temperament and incidence of sleep problems can be related. Infants generally sleep through the night by 3 months. Infant may need help getting to sleep by rocking, holding, pacifier, walking, etc. Environment and atmosphere conducive to sleep, (e.g., quiet, dim) should be provided. If sleep problem is related to a physical problem, measures to remedy should be implemented.
Teething	Eruption of primary or deciduous teeth starting at about 6 months usually with lower incisors. Will continue every 2 months for first 2 years. Signs may include, but are not always present: red, swollen gums; irritable; crying and rubbing gums. Since other events in infant development are occurring simultaneously, nursing must assist parents to distinguish between these and teething as follows: Drooling, which normally occurs at 3-4 months and has little to do with teething, although it may persist throughout teething. Fevers do not usually accompany teething. Must be assessed separately because maternal antibody protection is diminishing and presence of fever is suspect for infectious process. Separation anxiety, sleep disturbances, or fussiness from other causes are all common developmental symptoms associated with infant age group, as is reaching for and mouthing objects.	Recommend to parents hard, clean objects for baby to chew on, such as rubber teething rings, or beads, hard rubber toys, cool spoon, teething biscuits or pretzels, etc. Parents should avoid use of teething toys or rings filled with liquid because plastic covers are easily broken and liquid can be ingested.

Continued.

Common concerns and problems of first year (neonate and infant)—cont'd

Problem or concern	Assessment	Nursing intervention
Diaper rashes	Rashes of varying types occurring in diaper area. Persistent rashes which do not respond to home management or continue to occur in spite of preventive measures should be referred for medical evaluation.	Preventive measures to keep area clean, dry, and aerated: Frequent diaper changing. Cleansing with water (and mild soap after bowel movement) at each changing, dry area well. Thick diapers and/or absorbent pads are recommended; plastic or rubber pants are not suggested. A *thin* film of lubrication may be used, such as A and D ointment, petroleum jelly. Remove diapers for short periods every day. Wash diapers well as follows: 1. Soak soiled diapers in Borateen or borax solution (½ cup to 1 gallon of water). 2. Prerinse before washing. 3. Wash in full cycle with mild soap such as Ivory, Dreft, or Lux. 4. Avoid softeners and strong detergents. 5. Rinse diapers 2-3 times, and may be added ¼ to ½ cup vinegar to final rinse. 6. Dry in sun if possible.
	Home management of diaper rash:	Follow preventive measures with emphasis on leaving diaper off more frequently, changing when wet, and cleaning area thoroughly during changes. Zinc oxide ointment often is helpful in checking early nonfungal rashes. Cornstarch is never recommended for rashes or their prevention. Seek medical help if rash worsens or does not improve.
Cradle cap	Form of seborrheic dermatitis in neonate characterized by scalping, flaking of scalp skin especially over anterior fontanelle. May persist beyond neonate into infancy period.	Preventive measures: Teach parents how to shampoo infant head and recommend shampooing every other day. Reassure that vigorous scrubbing will not injure fontanelle or skull. Home management for mild cases: Shampoo head daily with warm water and soap, using firm pressure on scalp. Loosen cap by applying mineral or baby oil to scalp 15-20 minutes before shampooing. Remove with shampoo. Comb scalp with fine comb to loosen and dislodge scaly cap. Severe cases will require medical attention and are generally managed with antiseborrheic shampoos.
PROBLEMS RELATED TO FEEDING		
Parental concerns about overfeeding or underfeeding	Some parents find it difficult to determine appropriate amount of milk and/or solid food to give infant. Ascertain parent understanding, knowledge, and perceptions through the following: Diet history Height and weight measurement and charting on growth curve. Elimination habits and description.	Assist parents to construct a workable feeding schedule. Discuss normal feeding pattern for breast and bottle fed infants (see discussion in this chapter). Discuss infant need for nonnutrient sucking. Convey that infants will eat more than they need or require if food is offered at each cry. Offer water between feedings to postpone next feeding to reasonable time. Suggest schedule of solid food introduction (Appendix J4, p. 850).

Continued.

Common concerns and problems of first year (neonate and infant)—cont'd

Problem or concern	Assessment	Nursing intervention

Refusal of solids	Infant may refuse new foods for a number of reasons, e.g., temperature, texture, manner presented by person feeding, or too early introduction. Ascertain through diet history which foods accepted, and likes and dislikes, and parental feelings and perception regarding solid foods.	Reassure parents that if infant is gaining weight he is not underfed.
		Explain growth and appetite spurts.
		Discuss normal feeding patterns for age.
		Review indications for starting or not starting solid foods;
		  No need before 4-6 months.
		  Digestion begins with salivation around 4 months.
		  Feeding of solid foods is not necessarily related to sleeping through the night.
		  Tongue thrusting of solid food is normal and not a refusal.
		Discuss ways to encourage solid food acceptance:
		  Allow infant to feed self.
		  Avoid forcing infant to eat since this will only increase resistance.
		  Solids may be stopped for a while, offering only ones that infant likes.
		  Offer solid foods before milk when infant is hungriest.
		  Offer food in calm positive manner.

Refusal of food and variations in appetite	Once solid foods have been introduced and established, infants and especially toddlers will go through periods of refusal, pickiness, and preference. Obtain diet history as reviewed in preceding section (Refusal of solids).	See preceding section (Refusal of solids).
		Discuss following with parents:
		  Refusal may be due to loss of interest in food when more active or due to form of negativism and means to control.
		  Avoid use of food as substitute for attention or stimulation.
		  Some degree of refusal and variation in appetite is normal for age.
		Try following approaches:
		  Offer small amounts of food frequently.
		  Emphasize favorite foods as much as possible.
		  Use as few nonnutritive foods as possible.
		  Allow child to feed self if child desires to, and provide finger foods.
		  Be patient as child tries to master use of utensils.
		  Eating should be an enjoyable and sociable time. If hunger does not permit infant to wait until family dinner time, feed before and offer nibbles during family meal.
		  Give older infant and toddler place, chair, utensils, plate at the table.

Spitting up	Regurgitation commonly following a feeding. Usually related to air swallowed with food, inability to relax esophageal sphincter, possible overfeeding, or allergy to milk. Ascertain nature of regurgitation (frequency, amount, color, consistency, etc.) as well as diet history and data regarding weight gain. Frequently outgrown by time infant is sitting well in upright position.	Reinforce the following with parents:
		  Correct preparation of formula.
		  Use of appropriate size nipple and nipple hole.
		  Regular and frequent burping is needed.
		  Place infant in an upright position for 30 minutes after feeding.
		  Correct position of infant during feeding.
		Determine need to change method of feeding or formula.

Continued.

Common concerns and problems of first year (neonate and infant)—cont'd

Problem or concern	Assessment	Nursing intervention
Weaning	A transition of feeding methods. May be from bottle to cup or from breast to bottle and/or cup. Weaning from breast is difficult if parents (especially mother) have ambivalent feelings or if infant refuses alternative methods. Ascertain who wants baby weaned and why as well as schedule of feedings. Weaning from bottle should be attempted gradually, when child is ready, usually around 1 year. Ascertain who wants child weaned, what has been tried, feeding schedule and number of bottles, and ability to use cup.	Assist parents to make decision to wean: Should be discussed and decided by both parents. If breast feeding, it is helpful to mother to assess every 3 months whether or not to continue nursing. Positive attitude toward weaning is essential, especially for breast-feeding mothers. Weaning at times of separation anxiety is not advised, especially in breast-fed infants. If possible, an infant should be weaned from breast to cup. This avoids having to wean from bottle later on. Active weaning for breast feeding mothers: Start by substituting bottle or cup for breast at one feeding and allow 5-6 days before substituting second breast feeding. If resistance is encountered try giving water or juice in bottle or cup before weaning starts, using nipple similar to breast or pacifier if one is used, heating milk before offering, and having someone other than mother offer bottle or cup. Keep to a schedule and be firm, positive, and patient. Active weaning to cup: continue preceding steps with following additions: Reinforce idea of accomplishment in using a cup to child. May give one bottle a day but should contain only water to avoid incidence of dental caries. Avoid forcing child to wean; forcing use of cup may increase need to suck. Calm, relaxed, positive approach is essential.

J6—ACCIDENT PREVENTION IN CHILDREN
(CHAPTERS 28 and 29)

Age	Development	Major accidents	Anticipatory guidance
Neonate to 1 month	Is unable to protect self; when on abdomen can lift and turn head; dependent, requires protection; little control over body and movements	Motor vehicles	Use approved car seat Do not hold infant in lap Never leave infant in car unattended For long trips, firmly secure car bed with seat belts in back seat
		Strangulation	Spacing between crib bars should be no more than 2⅜ inches apart Avoid tying anything, including pacifiers, around neck Fasten mobiles securely
		Suffocation and injuries	Crib mattress should fit firmly to sides Do not use pillows; use bumper pads Support infant's head when lifting, holding, or bathing
		Burns including sunburn	Avoid bathing near hot water faucets Test water temperature before bath Avoid handling hot liquids and do not smoke while handling infant Keep out of direct sunlight and use sun screen Use flame-resistant clothing and furniture

Continued.

Accident prevention—cont'd

Age	Development	Major accidents	Anticipatory guidance
2-3 months	Begins gross motor movements of wiggling, squirming, thrashing, rolling	Falls	Never leave infant unattended (at any age) for any reason Keep one hand on infant while giving care Keep crib sides up Use infant seat on floor or playpen
4-5 months	Mouths objects; brings hands to mouth	Aspiration and choking	Do not prop bottles (at any age) Burp well before putting infant in crib and place on stomach with head to side or propped on side Toys should be too large for infant to swallow, nonbreakable, and free of sharp edges, strings, and detachable parts Keep diaper pins closed during changing Keep small objects (e.g., buttons, coins) out of reach Use only pacifiers with a large shield
		Suffocation	Keep all plastic bags out of reach Keep stuffed animals out of crib
		Lead poisoning	Check toys and other objects for lead-free paint
6-7 months	Sits without support; has a firm grasp; rolls and creeps	Falls and falling objects	Use safety strap in stroller or high chair Use sturdy high chair or feeding table Keep doors to stairs and outside locked; use safety gates Avoid use of hanging table-cloths Remove knickknacks and breakables
		Ingestion	Keep small objects, medicine, and plants out of reach Keep ipecac on hand and understand use Have poison control number posted Lock up medicine, cleaning agents, insecticides, etc. Keep trashcans out of reach or use locklids
		Injuries and electric shock	Cover wall outlets Place furniture so cords are inaccessible Check furniture for sharp corners—remove or pad Inspect toys for breakage Keep sharp objects out of reach
8-12 months	Pulls to stand; crawls, grabs; beginning to walk; enjoys exploring	Burns	Crawl around on floor and investigate what child could reach or get into Keep all hot food and drinks away from table edge; turn pot handles inward on stove Keep matches and lighters out of reach Keep kitchen closed up or gated Never leave child unattended near fireplace or stove Place guards around open hearths, registers, stoves, and fans Do not iron when child is crawling nearby
		Choking	Do not give child small hard foods, such as peanuts, raw vegetables, popcorn Inspect toys for broken parts Keep floors, counters, tables free of small objects
		Motor vehicle accidents	Continue use of car seat Keep doors locked
		Poisoning	See previous discussion
1-2 years	Walks up and down stairs; stoops and recovers; climbs; likes to take things apart	Falls and injuries	Supervise children in most activities, especially up and down stairs, out of doors, and at playgrounds Lock all windows; when opening, do so from top only Remove any objects or furniture in front of window that child could use as a ladder Permit climbing within child's capabilities

Continued.

Accident prevention—cont'd

Age	Development	Major accidents	Anticipatory guidance
			Remove bumper pads or toys in crib which child could use to climb on
			Check toys, especially riding ones, for damage
			Keep small, pointed, or sharp objects out of reach
			Keep out of way of swings
		Burns	Teach child meaning of *hot*
			Avoid use of flowing clothing
		Drowning	Continue to supervise bath
			Supervise all water sport activity (e.g., swimming, boating); use floats and/or life jackets
			Teach child to respect water and seek swimming lessons
		Automobile-related accidents	Continue to use appropriate car seat
			Keep doors and windows locked
			Do not permit child to hang out of windows
			Hold onto child when crossing street or in parking lots
			Do not permit child to ride toys near street
		Poisoning and ingestion	Have ipecac in any household child frequents (babysitter, grandparents)
			Use childproof caps on medications
			Do not regard medicine as candy
			Do not give one child another's prescription
2-4 years	More adventuresome and curious; explores body orifices; more independent, with limited cognition; imitates	Falls and injuries	Teach child to be cautious around strange animals
			Supervise play at playground
			Keep out of reach small objects and foods (peanuts, beans) that can be inserted into orifices; check buttons on clothes and toys
			Discontinue use of crib when height of crib rail is ¾ of toddler's height
			Keep stairs well lighted and free of clutter
			Give toys a safety check
			Discourage running in house and limit outdoor running to safe places
			Teach child to respect street and cars
			Teach child to stay away from and out of old appliances
		Drowning	Continue to teach water safety
			Supervise all water activities
			Continue with swimming lessons
		Automobile-related accidents	See previous discussion
	Play increases to include rougher games and bike riding	Burns	Teach child what to do if fire breaks out; hold household drills
			Teach child to roll and smother clothes if they catch on fire
	Cognition improving and can identify good and bad	Drowning	Continue swimming lessons
			Use floats or lifejacket if child cannot swim
			Swim only where supervision is available (parent or lifeguard)
		Automobile-related accidents	Teach pedestrian safety, providing example for child
			Do not permit playing in street
			Use adult seat belt, if child is over 40 pounds
			If over 55 inches tall, use shoulder restraints
			If under 55 inches tall, only lap belt is used
		Falls, injuries	Make periodic checks on playground or play area used frequently
			Check on child when out playing

Continued.

Accident prevention—cont'd

Age	Development	Major accidents	Anticipatory guidance
			Instruct child in safe use of toys; keep in good condition
			Keep away from driveways and streets
			If possible, provide fenced-in play area
			Set a good example by using seat belt, looking before crossing street, etc.
		Burns	Teach child about danger of matches, lighters, stove
			Recheck radiators, space heaters, fireplaces, and protective guards
		Poisoning and ingestions	Do not become lax about keeping medication, etc., locked up
			Teach child to respect harmful objects and use a symbol to indicate "danger or harmful" to child
			Routinely check house, basement, and garage for harmful substances within reach
4-6 years	Continues to be curious, daring, and imitative; frequently plays out of sight		Involve child in safety discussions
			Continue previously described activities when using household tools and equipment
School age	Increased motor coordination and cognitive ability; increased peer and group activity and involvement in sports; assumes more responsibility for self and well-being.	Motor vehicle and bicycle accidents	Involve child in safety discussion and planning
			Assign safety responsibilities, such as checking bike
			Teach child not to ride with strangers
			Teach child how to contact police and fire department and physician
			Be certain child knows address and phone number
			Discuss bicycle and pedestrian safety
			Discuss bicycle riding rules:
			Do not hitch ride on moving vehicles
			Do not ride on dark street
			Use headlight or reflector light at night; wear bright clothes
			Do not dart from behind parked cars
			Do not carry passengers on bicycle
			Keep bike in good repair
			Do not use street as a playground
			Use seat belts
		Injuries	Teach child to participate in sports safely using appropriate gear
			Permit only supervised sport activities
			Teach child proper use of household gadgets and equipment; supervise as necessary
		Drowning	Teach the following swimming rules:
			Swim only where a lifeguard is present
			Use buddy system
			Know water depth before diving
			Wear life jacket while boating or skiing or if nonswimmer
			No horseplay or call for help jokingly
		Falls	See bicycle rules
			Discuss climbing trees:
			Avoid slippery shoes
			Avoid weak or dead branches
			Keep a secure handhold
		Burns	Continue household drills
			Camp with supervision
			Teach proper campfire and barbecue care
			Use safe camping gear, including flame-retardant clothes

Age	Development	Major accidents	Anticipatory guidance
Adolescence	Seeking identity and establishment of independence; subject to strong peer pressure; rejects unsought advice; has a need for physical activity; spends most of free time away from home	Drowning	Most important to have cooperation of adolescent when discussing and implementing safety measures See previous sections Never too late to learn to swim Enroll in lifesaving classes
		Firearms accidents	Avoid having loaded guns in household Learn safety handling if involved in sport hunting Keep guns in locked closet and ammunition in separate locked area Never assume gun is not loaded Never point gun at another
		Automobile–related accidents	Take drivers education Use seat belts for self and passengers Practice pedestrian safety Do not drive under influence of drugs or alcohol Do not hitchhike or pick up hitchhikers
		Alcohol, drugs, and tobacco	Discuss effects of substance use and abuse Assist teen to identify other ways to achieve self-esteem, independence, and peer acceptance

J7—INFECTIOUS DISEASES
(CHAPTERS 28 and 29)

Disease	Presentation	Management
VIRAL INFECTIONS		
Conjunctivitis	Bacterial: purulent drainage, accompained by crusting of eyelids; conjunctiva is inflamed; lids are swollen; frequently affects both eyes. Viral: swollen eyes, inflamed conjuctiva with watery discharge; can be accompanied by subconjunctival hemorrhage and photophobia.	Medical: both bacterial and viral forms are self limiting; however, bacterial is treated with topical antibiotics. Supportive: removal of accumulated discharge by cleansing from inner canthus down and outward; warm, moist compresses are useful in removing crusts; use of disposable materials for cleansing; avoid rubbing eyes; wash hands after handling infected area.
Diptheria	Fever, sore throat, serosanguineous to mucopurlent nasal discharge occurs; progresses to hoarseness; cough with smooth, white, adherent gray membrane in pharyngeal area.	Treatment: administration of antitoxin and antibiotics; readiness for tracheostomy; treatment of contacts and carriers. Supportive: maintain strict bedrest and isolation; suction as needed; regulate humidity; tracheostomy care; observe for signs of respiratory obstruction.
Erythema infectionsum (Fifth disease)	Rash appearing in three stages. First on face; "slapped cheek" appearance; progressing to upper and lower extremities; further progression from proximal to distal surface and lasting a week or more. Third stage is rash subsiding with reappearance if skin is irritated.	Medical: none indicated. Supportive: reassurance that condition is benign; fever and URI management if occur coincidentally.

Continued.

Disease	Presentation	Management
Gastroenteritis	Usually abrupt in onset, frequently accompanied by vomiting and abdominal discomfort; loss of appetite, fever, and diarrhea.	Medical: antimicrobial medication if bacterial in origin. Supportive: isolation varying from strict to stool precautions if bacterial in origin; frequent handwashing; assess hydration status; prevent skin break down; maintain hydration and reinstitute diet as appropriate.
Hepatitis	See Chapters 19 and 28	Home care and supportive treatment, including rest and well-balanced diet with sufficient calories and vitamin B complex supplements Isolation: enteric precautions Prophylaxis: Gamma globulin or hepatitis B immune globulin
Herpes simplex	Seen as gingivostomatitis in young children with reinfections being localized as "cold sores" or "fever blisters"; abrupt onset with fever, irritability, anorexia, and sore mouth; red swollen gums with small vesicles appearing on palate, tongue, and mucosa	Supportive treatment, particularly mouth care of petroleum jelly for cracking and mouth washes, rinses, and analgesics for pain; secretion precautions should be observed Diet: soft, bland foods; cool liquids—avoidance of citrus juices General measures as for influenza
Herpes zoster (shingles)	Uncommon under age 10; characterized by pain and crops of vesicles confined to an area of distribution of one of spinal or cranial sensory nerves; malaise and fever may accompany vesicles	Symptomatic treatment of wet compresses, calamine lotion (for lesions), and aspirin (for pain)
Influenza	Rapid onset of chills, fever, headache, generalized aches and malaise, anorexia, and prostration; frequently young children experience vomiting and diarrhea; hacking cough and rhinitis frequently develop	Symptomatic treatment including these general measures: A. Fever 　1. Antipyretic medication 　2. Tepid sponge bath 　3. Liberal fluid intake 　4. Rest and limited activity B. Upper respiratory infections 　1. Liberal fluid intake 　2. Cool mist vaporizer 　3. Decongestants 　4. Warm gargle, saline mouth/throat irrigations 　5. Cool liquids and soft foods for throat and mouth irritations 　6. Petroleum jelly to protect nares and lips C. Aches and malaise 　1. Rest and limited activity 　2. Warm bath 　3. Body massage 　4. Cold compresses for headache 　5. Analgesics D. Anorexia 　1. Small, frequent feedings of favorite foods and liquids 　2. Relaxed approach to oral intake E. Rash 　1. Proper hygiene and bathing 　2. Cool baths, calamine lotion, mild anesthetic ointment, or systemic antihistamines 　3. Short, clean fingernails; gloves or mittens for young children

Continued.

Disease	Presentation	Management
		4. Saline mouthwashes if mucous membranes are involved
Measles (rubeola)	Malaise, fever, conjunctivitis, cough 3-4 days before appearance of red-brown or purple-red macropapular rash, first on face, hairline, and neck, proceeding to trunk and extremities; Koplek's spots appear about 12 hours before rash on buccal mucosa; rash lasts 5-7 days	General measures as for influenza; emphasis on avoiding bright lights if photophobic and using warm water to cleanse eyes. Respiratory and discharge precautions. Prevention: active immunization
Mononucleosis (infectious)	Mild symptoms of headache, malaise, and fatigue; fever and sore throat, tonsils enlarged, red and covered with membrane; lymph adenopathy and splenomegaly are common	General measures as for influenza; emphasis on bed rest with gradual increase in activity; no strenuous activity while spleen is enlarged; no social contact until acute phase is over
Mumps (parotitis)	Prodrome of fever, headache, anorexia, malaise, and muscle pain. Local pain around ear and jaw within 24-48 hours, followed by swelling of parotid gland.	General measures as for influenza; emphasis on avoidance of citrus foods and fluids; alleviation of pain with aspirin and warm or cold compresses; respiratory precautions.
Pertussis (whooping cough)	Begins with URI symptoms and low grade fever, continuing for 1-2 weeks and progressing to dry hacking cough; progress to paroxysmal cough with a high pitched crowing or "whoop" sound; cough usually produces a thick mucous plug; vomiting frequently follows coughing episode; may persist 4-6 weeks.	Medical: antimicrobial therapy and administration of pertussis immune globulin. Supportive: bedrest; increased oxygen and humidity; increased fluids and readiness for intubation; respiratory isolation is indicated; assess for airway obstruction; reduce environmental factors that produce paroxysms (dust, smoke, temperature changes, excitement).
Roseola (exanthem subitum)	High fever and irritability for 3-4 days followed by rose-pink, maculopapular rash, beginning on chest and spreading to trunk and face; rash lasts several hours to 2 days; fever falls to normal as rash appears	General measures as for influenza; support for parents as fever may not respond or subside for 3-5 days
Rubella (german measles)	No prodrome. Pink-red maculopapular rash first on face, progressing to neck, trunk, extremities; lasts 3-5 days	General measures as for influenza; exposure of first-trimester pregnant women to be avoided. Prevention: active immunization
Varicella (chickenpox)	May have 1-2 days of fever and malaise followed by macular rash that evolves to papular to vesicles to crusts; rash appears on trunk and in crops and may progress to hairline and face; all lesions eventually dry and crust	General measures as for influenza; emphasis on skin care, alleviation of itching by cornstarch baths, systemic antipruritic medication (Benadryl) and topical lotions (calamine); general skin hygiene of bathing, changing bed linen and clothes frequently, keeping nails short and clean; isolate until vesicles dried and observe respiratory and secretion precautions

BACTERIAL INFECTIONS

Disease	Presentation	Management
Cellulitis	See Appendix J10	Employ general measures as described under influenza; systemic antibiotic therapy; warm compresses and immobilization of affected part
Meningitis	Varies with age and causative organism. *Neonates.* Escherichia coli and group B streptococci common causative agents; onset is insidious; poor tone, sucking feeding difficulties, poor cry, vomiting, irritability, drowsy or irritable, jittery; tense, full, bulging fontanelle. *Infants.* Most common causative agents: hemophelus influenza, neisseria meningitides. Unexplained febrile illness preceded by respiratory or gastrointestinal infection; accompanied by irritability, fever, anorexia, vomiting, drowsiness, and high pitch cry; fontanelle may be bulging, nuchal rigidity signs may be difficult to elicit	Requires medical referral and antibiotic therapy that will be determined by weight of child and depends on causative agent. Parent counseling regarding diagnosis and disease process is indicated as well as convalescent care and follow-up care

Continued.

Age	Development	Major accidents	Anticipatory guidance
	Older children. Causative agent as for infants; fever, chills, vomiting, severe headache, stiff neck; nuchal rigidity and positive Kernig's and Brudzinski's signs *Meningococcemia.* A medical emergency with rapidly developing petechial and purpuric rash, preceded by 24-hour period of fever, vomiting, irritability, and nuchal rigidity		
Scarlet fever (scarlatini)	Abrupt onset of fever, sore throat, vomiting, headache, and chills followed by bright red rash that blanches on pressure; rash has rough sandpaper texture and appears first on flexor surfaces, rapidly becoming more generalized; lasts 7 days, followed by desquamation of hands and feet.		General measures as for influenza; Penicillin is antibiotic of choice, unless allergy is present and erythromycin is indicated; prepare parents for skin desquamation; follow-up care and throat culture is advisable as well as examination for signs of rheumatic fever and glomerulonephritis; advisable to obtain throat cultures on household contacts
Tuberculosis	See Appendix J10		Active tuberculosis: antimicrobial therapy and general supportive measures Prevention: if positive skin test and no clinical demonstrated disease, prophylactic treatment with INH is recommended if child is under 4 years Child has recently converted from negative to positive skin reaction Child with positive skin test has known exposure to active TB Child with inactive primary TB has never been treated All contacts with person with active tuberculosis should be skin tested, positive reactions treated and negative skin tests retested in 6 weeks and at least every 3 months for duration of contact; infants should be removed from contact with infected person until at least 6 months after all cultures are reported as negative Prevention: tuberculin testing

J8—COMMON CONCERNS AND PROBLEMS OF TODDLER AND PRESCHOOL YEARS
(Chapters 28 and 29)

Problem and assessment	Nursing intervention

AGGRESSIVE AND NEGATIVE BEHAVIORS
Biting and hitting

Temporary behaviors occurring as a result of normal aggressive impulses and most frequently happening in new or difficult situations, when tired or hungry or frustrated or when expectations are too high in terms of social behaviors (ability to play with peers); used as a means of asserting control or power	Reassure parents that behaviors are normal; discuss development and tasks child is trying to accomplish
	Advise parents to:
	  Avoid retaliation by hitting or biting back
	  Cup chin or hold hand giving reminder that biting and/or hitting is unacceptable
	  Anticipate circumstances in which behaviors occur and circumvent them
	  Use limits such as isolation if helpful
	  Limit playmates and playtime to what is reasonable for child and his age
	  Allow child and playmate to work out difficulties as much as possible, redirecting their play when necessary

Continued.

Common concerns and problems of toddler and preschool years—cont'd

Problem and assessment	Nursing intervention

Verbal negativism

Use of the word "no" as means of control in striving for independence; often used indiscriminately and inappropriately

Advise parents to:
  Offer child a choice when possible, making alternatives simple
  Avoid bargaining and arguments
  If no choice is available, do not offer one—approach with a matter-of-fact attitude
  Develop strategy for times when child will choose and then change his mind

Temper tantrums

Developmental behavior directed at gaining control; Frequently triggered by unmet needs (tired, hungry), frustration and/or overgratification and need for limits; ascertain when tantrums occur and how they are handled

Management by parents should be directed at finding cause and prevention; counseling is directed toward approaches to discipline and limit setting (see section on discipline) and the following:
  Discussion of child's needs for limits at this age
  Diary can be kept to identify pattern when tantrums occur
  Intervention is made before tantrum begins
Should tantrum occur, possible approaches include the following:
  Calm, matter-of-fact approach by parents
  Isolation of child by removal to neutral room until control is achieved
  Hold and comfort child until control is achieved, possibly offering substitue for desired object or activity that triggered tantrum
  Use of corporal punishment (spanking) to achieve control

DISCIPLINE

Discipline is guidance offered by parents to assist child in demonstrating correct, acceptable safe behaviors; discipline is based on the parent's concepts, feelings, and attitudes regarding desirable behaviors and rules of conduct for them; mechanisms of discipline will set limits and control undesirable behaviors

Advise parents regarding different approaches to discipline:
  Permissiveness
  Overpermissiveness
  Authoritarianism
Advise parents that setting limits should permit self-respect and protection of parent and child integrity; parents should be aware that discipline is essential to healthy growth
Parent techniques include the following:
  Set examples of desirable behaviors (honesty, unselfishness, good manners)
  Be fair, clear, and consistent
  Agree on methods of discipline
  Give simple clear directions; bend a little by giving warnings
  Allow child to express feelings
  Respect your child; be sure to praise, show approval, and encourage
  Be realistic in behaviors expected
  Avoid arguing, threatening, promising, sermonizing, overpermissiveness, and an overauthoritarian manner
  Discipline (punishing the act)

PUNISHMENT

A method of controlling behaviors when limits are exceeded and based on child being made to feel guilty for misdeed; guilt will eventually inhibit impulse to commit act; punishment may be verbal, restrictive, or physical and should always be appropriate to the act; most punishment is the result of parent loss of temper

Advise parents to:
Allow a cooling-off period
Direct anger at situation or act, not child
Avoid retaliation by hitting, belittling, sarcasm, ridicule, humiliation, or shame
Avoid sending to bed or going without food
Avoid depriving child of love to examine their feelings and experiences regarding punishment. Remind them that it can be an effective method of discipline with appropriate motivation and intent
Review points discussed in discipline section

Continued.

Common concerns and problems of toddler and preschool years—cont'd

Problem and assessment	Nursing intervention

BREATHHOLDING

A high indicator of a disturbed parent-child relationship, this symptom may be caused by overprotection, a tense rigid daily schedule, or prematurely enforced toilet training regime; it has a high familial incidence and is characterized by a preceding temper tantrum, with child holding breath and turning blue

Ascertain circumstances that trigger episodes and how handled by parents

Counseling directed toward guidance and education regarding parent-child relationship; parents will need reassurance and support as they attempt to

Ignore breathholding in an attempt to prevent child satisfaction in gaining control

Redirect relationship with child emphasizing meeting of his needs in a positive way, reinforcing desirable behaviors

See section on discipline

ROCKING, HEAD BANGING, BED SHAKING

Forms of self-stimulation as a result of undergratification; frequently occurs at bedtime; ascertain how child's needs are met

Counseling directed toward advising parents regarding
Gratification of needs
Avoidance of letting child "cry it out"
Provision of comfort and extra stimulation time
Provision of relaxed, calm atmosphere through holding, singing, music

MASTURBATION

A normal reaction, which is an exploration of body that results in stimulation of pleasurable sexual feelings; generally occurs at bedtime and starts accidentally becoming more purposeful and frequent around 4 years
Ascertain frequency, how parents handle, and their attitude and feelings

Advise parents that masturbation is normal and that censoring of open masturbation is appropriate; otherwise parents should convey to child that they are aware of and understand the behavior
Avoidance of placing excessive importance on masturbation which may only encourage it; it is best to ignore it and/or set limits as appropriate to situation
A punitive attitude should be avoided

PERSISTENT THUMB SUCKING

A form of self-comfort occurring in times of stress and persisting beyond 3-4 years; generally sporadic sucking is harmless and regular sucking until 2 or 3 is considered normal

Assist parents to identify source of stress and ways to alleviate it.
Reassure and support parents when thumb sucking is within normal range
Suggest parents remove fingers or thumb from mouth after asleep
Suggest parents avoid constant nagging and reminding; pulling thumb from mouth; use of restraints, foul-tasting medications, or bandages

FEEDING-RELATED PROBLEMS
Loss of variations of appetite; refusal of food

Common problems related to: "too busy to eat," development of food preferences; a normal decrease in amount of food required and/or an attempt to control and assert independence

See Chapter 22 for anticipatory guidance and Appendix J5, pp. 853-858

SLEEP-RELATED PROBLEMS
Nightmares

Problems may follow a tiring busy day, be associated with illness, or be the result of working things out in dreams
Nightmares are frightening dreams that awaken child who feels fear and helplessness; they generally occur as a result of increased aggressive urges

Review normal sleep patterns with parents (see Chapter 28)
Reassure parents that dreams and terrors are normal and tend to disappear spontaneously
Parents should comfort child when awakened by dream—may attempt to explain they are not "real"
Parents should avoid making a fuss over these sleep problems

Night terrors

These are dreams, generally frightening in nature, from which a child does not awaken; after acting out dream and/or a period of disorientation, child returns to sleep

•

Problem and assessment	Nursing intervention

TOILET TRAINING

Achievement of control over bodily elimination; development of habits that make child self-sufficient in toileting; parents need to understand child's development and readiness before instituting a toilet training regime (see following); parent must ascertain attitude and expectations regarding toilet training as well as measures previously used

Indicators of readiness to toilet train	Approximate age (yr)
1. Manipulates sphincter muscles	1½-2
2. Manual dexterity needed to manipulate clothing	2-2½
3. Can hold urine for up to 4 to 5 hours	2-2½
4. Can understand simple directions	1½-2
5. Can communicate needs using words or gestures	1½-2
6. Developed a sense of self	1-2
7. Demonstrates trust in mother and desire to please	1½-2
8. Demonstrates sense of independence and a desire to do for self	2-2½
9. Is proud of own accomplishments	2-2½
10. Demonstrates behavioral control	2-2½

Direct counseling toward parental understanding of realistic expectations, readiness of child, types of toilet training and frequent problems encountered

Types of toilet training:

A. Early training from ages 10-15 months; points to emphasize:
   1. Child is not physiologically able to use toilet at this age
   2. Parents may be ready to train child, but they will be the ones who will have to pick up signals, put child on toilet, undress and dress, etc.; therefore, they should be highly motivated
   3. Bowel training may be accomplished but accidents will happen and will be due to trainer (parent), not trainee (child)
   4. Training should not be stressful for parent or child

B. Training at 18-30 months; points to emphasize:
   1. Review readiness signs and check off which ones child has accomplished. If the majority have been achieved, probably appropriate to start training
   2. Select a good time such as when
      There are no major changes in household and child has shown some interest after observing others
      Nursery school friends are trained
      Child is aware of wet and dirty versus dry and clean
   3. Select a method and stick to it
   4. Training should not be stressful; if child resists it is best to forget for awhile then try again
   5. Accomplishment of training is variable; it may be a few days or several weeks or months
   6. Parents need to develop a relaxed, positive attitude
   7. Alternative methods include
      Place child on own potty chair at given intervals during the day
      Place child on potty before elimination is expected
      Place child on potty when parent goes
      Always positively reinforce a successful attempt

C. "Natural" toilet training (children training themselves), points to emphasize:
   1. Toileting is brought to child's attention when readiness is indicated
   2. Child handles situation by himself
   3. Child needs to know parents are willing to help
   4. Although enjoying a sense of independence and accomplishment, child also needs limits set at this age

Problems are frequently encountered; reassure parents about naturalness, normalcy and transient nature of these problems:

1. Problem with sitting or standing for boys; suggest starting training with sitting progressing to standing
2. Problem using large toilet; suggest potty chair with portable seat which can be taken on excursions
3. Regression; suggest reinforcing as little as possible; depending on severity may require going back to diapers for a while
4. Need help with wiping; suggest allowing child to try if wants to clean self
5. Being able to communicate toilet needs to others; suggest parents make sure other caretakers are aware of child's progress in training, how he communicates need, what words and what degree of independence have been achieved
6. Child does not wish to flush bowel movements; suggest this point not be emphasized; flush toilet later
7. Playing with feces; suggest play with clay or fingerpaints; parent should matter-of-factly state displeasure when this occurs

OBSERVATIONS OF PARENTS-TO-BE

1. Are the parents overconcerned with the baby's sex?
2. Are they overconcerned with the baby's performance? Do they worry that he will not meet the standard?
3. Is there an attempt to deny that there is a pregnancy (mother not willing to gain weight, no plans whatsoever, refusal to talk about the situation)?
4. Is this child going to be one child too many? Could he be the "last straw"?
5. Is there great depression over this pregnancy?
6. Is the mother alone and frightened, especially by the physical changes caused by the pregnancy? Do careful explanations fail to dissipate these fears?
7. Is support lacking from husband and/or family?
8. Where is the family living? Do they have a listed telephone number? Are there relatives and friends nearby?
9. Did the mother and/or father formerly want an abortion but not go through with it or waited until it was too late?
10. Have the parents considered relinquishment of their child? Why did they change their minds?

Adapted from Kempe CH: Approaches to preventing child abuse, Am J Dis Child 130:941-947, 1976.

OBSERVATIONS TO BE MADE AT POSTPARTUM CHECKUPS AND PEDIATRIC CHECKUPS

1. Does the mother have fun with the baby?
2. Does the mother establish eye contact (direct en face position) with the baby?
3. How does the mother talk to her baby? Is everything she expresses a demand?
4. Are most of her verbalizations about the child negative?
5. Does she remain disappointed over the child's sex?
6. What is the child's name? Where did it come from? When did they name the child?
7. Are the mother's expectations for the child's development far beyond the child's capabilities?
8. Is the mother very bothered by the baby's crying? How does she feel about the crying?
9. Does the mother see the baby as too demanding during feedings? Is she repulsed by the messiness? Does she ignore the baby's demands to be fed?
10. What is the mother's reaction to the task of changing diapers?
11. When the baby cries, does she or can she comfort him?
12. What was/is the husband's and/or family's reaction to the baby?
13. What kind of support is the mother receiving?
14. Are there sibling rivalry problems?
15. Is the husband jealous of the baby's drain on the mother's time and affection?
16. When the mother brings the child for check-ups does she get involved and take control over the baby's needs and what's going to happen (during the examination and while in the waiting room) or does she relinquish control to the physician or nurse (undressing the child, holding him, allowing him to express his fears, etc.)?
17. Can attention be focused on the child in the mother's presence? Can the mother see something positive for her in that?
18. Does the mother make nonexistent complaints about the baby? Does she describe to you a child that you don't see there at all? Does she call with strange stories that the child has, for example, stopped breathing, turned color, or is doing something "on purpose" to aggravate the parent?
19. Does the mother make emergency calls for very small things, not major things?

Adapted from Kempe CH: Approaches to preventing child abuse, Am J Dis Child 130:941-947, 1976.

SPECIAL WELL-CHILD CARE FOR HIGH-RISK FAMILIES

1. Promote maternal attachment to the newborn.
2. Phone the mother during the first 2 days at home.
3. Provide more frequent clinic visits.
4. Give more attention to the mother.
5. Emphasize nutrition.
6. Counsel discipline only for accident prevention.
7. Emphasize accident prevention.
8. Use compliments rather than criticism.
9. Be available during nonworking hours to provide support.
10. Arrange for regular home visits.

Adapted from Kempe CH: Approaches to preventing child abuse, Am J Dis Child 130:941-947, 1976.

J10—HEALTH PROBLEMS OF SCHOOL AGE CHILD AND ADOLESCENT
(CHAPTERS 28 and 29)

Health problem	Etiology	Incidence	Assessment	Management	Prevention
Acne	Sebaceous glands over produce sebum which inflames skin pores	70% of adolescents experience acne	Noninflamed comedones or inflamed papules, pustules and nodulocystic lesions on face, neck, upper chest, back and shoulders; hair and skin are often oily	Use of benzoyl peroxide agent; more severe cases may require retinoic acid and/or antibiotics; thorough cleansing of the skin two or three times a day using warm water and a mild soap; drying and peeling lotions may be used overnight; avoid exposure to sun and wind; frequent shampooing of the scalp; proper diet with added liquids; no diet restrictions are indicated, but should the adolescent feel a certain food aggravates the acne, it should be avoided; avoid greasy make-up, powder is better.	No known prevention but severity of symptoms can reduced with appropriate management.
Impetigo	Superficial skin lesion invaded by staphylococci or streptococci, spread by direct contact with incubation of 2-10 days	Potential risk for glomerulonephrites	Appearance of discolored spots that form vesicles or bullae; these vesicles break and form yellow, honey-colored seropurulent lesions Most frequently on hands, face, or perineum and accompanied by regional lymphadenopathy Culture fluid from lesion or at base of lesion	Topical treatment with Bacitracin or neomycin ointment after soaking with warm compresses Systemic antibiotic if numerous lesions are present Follow-up if not improved with 3 days	Teach child not to pick or scratch insect bites, healing lesions, etc. Keep nails short and clean Frequent handwashing Isolate child's washing and bed linen, drinking glass, and clothes Inspect other family members Adequate rest and nutrition

Continued.

Health problems of school age child and adolescent—cont'd

Health problem	Etiology	Incidence	Assessment	Management	Prevention
Cellulitis	Bacterial invasion of skin (both dermis and subcutaneous tissue) caused by Staphylococcus aureus, group A beta-hemolytic streptococci, or Hemophilus influenza Less communicable than impetigo but suspect throughout infection; more apt to lead to septicemia	Frequently a secondary infection to impetigo or other skin lesions	Warm tender, erythematous, swollen, and indurated area on skin Lymphangitis seen on extremities Fever, malaise, lymphadenapathy often present	Warm compresses Immobilization of affected part Rest and symptomatic measures Systemic antibiotic therapy	Prevention as for impetigo All family members should be cultured and those with positive cultures treated
Streptococcal pharyngitis	Group A-Beta hemolytic streptococcus	Increased incidence in winter and spring 30%-50% of cases appear in school-age children	Must differentiate from viral pharyngitis Obtain throat culture	10-day course of penicillin when strep confirmed by culture Repeat culture at end of medication course	Culture all symptomatic exposed family contacts Avoid contact with infected child and his eating/drinking utensils
Reye Syndrome	Masking of symptoms linked to aspirin use; frequent sequelae of influenzae	Stablilized over past decade but continues to affect 10-19-year-olds, primarily due to self-treatment.	Characterized by encephalopathy, severe brain edema, increased intracranial pressure, hypoglycemia and fatty infiltration of liver.	Immediate hospitalization and medical treatment of neurologic symptoms	Educate parents and particularly school-age and adolescent children to eliminate use of aspirin for self-treatment of viral illnesses; develop school and/or community program about Reye syndrome, its prevention and early recognition
Streptococcal pharyngitis— cont'd		At risk for complications of cervical adenitis, otitis media, peritonsillar abscess, sinusitis, acute glomerulonephritis, acute rheumatic fever		Symptomatic treatment for fever reduction; normal saline gargles, hard sour candy for sore throat; hot or cold compresses for tender cervical nodes	Education regarding illness and necessity of full treatment course of medication
Toxic shock syndrome	*Staphylococcus aureus* is causative agent with use of super absorbant tampons a significant contributing factor	42% of cases are adolescents	Sudden onset of fever, headache, sore throat, nausea, vomiting, and diarrhea, abdominal pain, hypotension, rash, arthralgia and desquamation of soles and palms	Immediate hospitalization antibiotics and monitoring and treatment of shock	Counseling to avoid use of tampons; if must use tampons, use regular not superabsorbant and change every 3-4 hours; use sanitary pads at night; Employ general genitourinary hygiene measures

Continued.

Health problems of school age child and adolescent—cont'd

Health problem	Etiology	Incidence	Assessment	Management	Prevention
Tuberculosis	Communicated through sputum and cough spray of infected person Causative organism are Mycobacterium tuberculosis and M. bovis Incubation range is 2-10 weeks	Most at risk in first 3 years and the second year preceding puberty For children of all ages, an average of 4000 new cases are reported annually Predisposing factors include state of health and nutrition; age; environmental and socioeconomic circumstances (crowding, poor sanitation); virulence and number of bacilli	Development of overt symptoms occurs in small percentage Demonstrated systemic hypersensitivity as evidenced by positive skin test Chest x-ray to determine presence and extent of active lesions Sputum smears	Rest, adequate diet, and gradual return to normal activity; prevention of other infection Drug therapy Counseling and support	Screening tests particularly for at risk population Identify, screen, and treat contacts Hygiene and sputum precautions/measures
Urinary tract infections	Bacteria enter urinary tract through urethra	5%-10% of girls and 1% of boys experience a UTI before 18 years	History of signs and symptoms: urgency, frequency, burning, dribbling, foul-smelling urine, fever, irritability, GI symptoms; *may be asymptomatic*	2-week medication course based on causative organism, age, weight of child, sensitivity of organism to drug and previous occurrences	Routine urine screening, particularly for girls early in life (1-2 years)
	Predisposing factors include Short female urethra Obstruction Foreign body Poor hygiene and/or fecal contamination Incomplete bladder emptying resulting in urine stasis Chemical irritants Pinworms Indwelling catheter or catheterization Sexual intercourse Pregnancy	More frequent in girls than boys	Laboratory signs: bacteria on urine culture of greater than 100,000 colonies of a single bacteria per ml of urine confirms infection in symptomatic child	Medication frequently used: Sulfisoxazole (Gantrisin) Ampicillin Nitrofurantoin (Furadantin) Cephalexin (Keflex)	Hygiene education: Wipe front to back Frequent voiding (3-4 hours) with complete bladder emptying Avoid bubble baths and harsh detergents Use cotton versus nylon panties Avoid tight clothing Adequate fluid intake

Continued.

Health problems of school age child and adolescent—cont'd

Health problem	Etiology	Incidence	Assessment	Management	Prevention
	Causative organisms: *Escherichia coli* accounts for 80% to 85% of cases Gram-positive organisms *(Staphylococcus aureus)* *Klebsiella, enterobacteria, Pseudomonas,* and *Proteus* sp.			Increased fluid and rest	Prompt attention for recurrent symptoms
				Symptomatic measures for generalized signs Follow-up is essential: Urine culture 48-72 hours after medication is instituted Urine culture on completion of medication Further follow-up at 1 month (U/A culture); 3 months; 6 months; 12 months (physical exam); 18 months; 24 months (physical exam); annually	
Osteomyelitis	Causative organisms are *Staphylococcus aureus* in older children and Haemophilus in younger children; organisms may enter directly to bone or through a preexisting infection	Occurs most frequently between the ages of 5 and 14 years and more commonly in boys than girls	Frequently a history of trauma usually localized tenderness, warmth and redness with pain on movement. Laboratory signs: marked leukocytes, elevated erythrocyte sedimentation rate and positive blood culture	Antibiotic therapy for 3-4 weeks; complete bedrest and immobilization	Prompt attention to penetrating injuries or suspect skin lesions Proper treatment and hygiene of injuries and skin lesions.

Continued.

Health problems of school age child and adolescent—cont'd

Health problem	Etiology	Incidence	Assessment	Management	Prevention
PARASITIC INFECTIONS					
Scabies	Caused by parasite, female mite that burrows into stratum corneum of skin and lays eggs in the tunnel. Transmitted by direct contact with infected person; can be contracted from infected bedding and clothing	Pandemic in U.S. since 1974	Vesicular or papulo-vesicular rash occurring typically on genitals, buttocks, between fingers and in folds of wrist, elbows, armpits, and at beltline. Appear as fine wavy line; gray to pink in color. Pruritus is worse at night. Skin scrapings from over lesion reveal mite presence under microscope	Scabicide (Kwell) applied to affected areas; one application is generally sufficient—may be repeated. Clothing and bedding should be washed	Avoid contact with infected person's bedding and clothing. Family members should do self-skin inspection
Tinea capitis (scalp), corporis (body), pedis (foot)	Fungal infection frequently transmitted by dogs and cats; caused by Microsporum canis or by Trichophyton transmitted by humans	Increased incidence in puberty. Permanent baldness may occur with severe capitis	Capitis: bald patches with erythema, gray scaling, and crusting. Corporis: macule that enlarges peripherally, healing in center to present as scaly, circular lesions found on face, upper extremities, and trunk; may have mild pruritus. Pedis: vesicular eruptions with skin maceration between toes. Laboratory procedures: (1) microscopic exam with KOH; (2) ultraviolet light fluoresces Microsporum infections; (3) microscopic culture	Capitis: griseofulvin—follow-up cultures should be done. Corporis: tolnaftate (Tinactin) 1% solution or cream. Pedis: tolnaftate (Tinactin) solution or cream and Desenex or Tinactin powder prophylactically	Capitis: avoid exchange of head gear; avoid/treat infected animal; wash scalp after haircuts; avoid use of infected person's personal care articles. Corporis: preceding plus avoiding exchange of clothing and community showers or bathing places. Pedis: preceding plus thoroughly dry between toes; use cotton socks and change frequently; wear well ventilated shoes; air feet; wear rubber sandals in community showers

Continued.

Health problems of school age child and adolescent—cont'd

Health problem	Etiology	Incidence	Assessment	Management	Prevention
Pediculosis Capitis (head lice)	Causative agent is parasite and lice infestations are communicable	Very common among school children	Itching of occipital area, behind ears and nape of neck; Diagnosis made by observation of eggs attached to hair shafts, which fluoresce white under wood light	Application of pediculocidal shampoo, with manual removal of nits	Wash clothing and bed linen of infected person in hot water; vacuum furniture; wash hair care items with louse shampoo; advise child against sharing hair care items or head coverings.
Insect bites	A variety of stinging and biting insects	Very common in children of all ages	Localized erythema, itching and a local wheal are common	Cool compresses, antipruritic agents and antihistamines are recommended; removal of stinger	Wear shoes outside, avoid wooded, overgrown areas; use insect repellants; avoid scratching to prevent secondary infections.
Lyme disease	Causative agents is a spirochete, *Borrelia burdorferi.* Transmitted by tick bite	High in Northeastern, coastal, Great Lakes, and western states.	Maculopapular rash at tick bite site progressing to an expanded area of erythema; progresses to neurologic and cardiac symptoms if not treated	Careful removal of tick, pulling out with tweezers close to its mouth. Antibiotic therapy Monitoring of progressive symptoms	Avoid wooded, grassy areas; wear light colored clothing for easier visualization of ticks; wear hats, long sleeve shirts tucked inside pants and white socks; check thoroughly for ticks if in woods; inspect children everyday if playing outside especially checking head, neck, ears, axilla, naval, buttocks and groin; and use DEET-containing insect repellants

DENTAL

Health problem	Etiology	Incidence	Assessment	Management	Prevention
Caries	Progressive lesions of calcified dental tissue characterized by tooth structure loss Bacteria, carbohydrates, and plaque are definite factors producing tooth decay	50%-97% of children have 1 or more cavities by 6 years of age Greatest incidence occurs between 4 to 8 years and 12 to 18 years	Characterized as discolored areas or actual lesion in fissures of chewing surfaces of teeth May be visible on inspection Dental equipment and x-rays most reliable in detecting caries	Dental referral Prevention	Preventive measures: Early institution of dental care and visits Brushing and flossing after every meal Water fluoridation; oral supplemental fluoride if indicated; fluoride rinses Topical fluoride application and use of toothpaste containing fluoride Limit carbohydrate content of diet

Continued.

Health problems of school age child and adolescent—cont'd

Health problem	Etiology	Incidence	Assessment	Management	Prevention
Malocclusion	Irregularities of tooth alignment and improper fitting of teeth Causative factors: abnormal jaw alignment; abnormal muscle function; incompatibility of tooth and jaw size creating abnormal spacing, crowding or teeth irregularities; delayed permanent teeth eruption; prolonged retention of primary teeth; neglected teeth; prolonged occurrence of lip biting, mouth breathing, tongue twisting, teeth grinding, thumb sucking	Most frequently recognized in early school age years Not common in deciduous teeth	Variation of normal occlusion of top molars meeting firmly on opposing bottom posterior teeth with upper incisors barely overlapping and touching bottom anterior incisors	Dental referral Prevention	Preventive measures: Meeting early sucking needs Avoidance of prolonged use of bottle over 2 years Weaning to cup at 1 year to promote jaw and mouth development after sucking Gentle reminder about finger/thumb sucking, lip biting, etc. Remove finger, thumb from mouth when child is sleeping

PSYCHOSOCIAL

Health problem	Etiology	Incidence	Assessment	Management	Prevention
Enuresis	Exact cause is not known but potential factors include: delayed development of neuromuscular control, organic causes, deep sleep and high threshold for nocturnal arousal; psychologic/emotional factors	Up to 15% of 6- to 7-year-olds and 3% of 13- to 14-year olds Males affected more than females	Primary: in children who have never achieved bladder control Secondary: in children who have achieved bladder control for 3-6 months then lose it Complete history to include: Amount and times of fluid intake Number of enuretic episodes per week/month Sleeping patterns Voiding patterns Any recent stressful events Occurrence at home and/or away from home or both	INITIAL MEASURES Fluids are restricted after supper Child voids before bedtime Before retiring for night, parents should wake child to void A night light is provided CONDITIONING Enuretone, a moisture-sensitive device that rings an alarm bell upon initiation of wetting, can be used Imipramine (Tofranil), which exerts an anticholinergic effect on bladder muscle and/or an antidepressant effect on central nervous system, can be used	Preventive measures: Avoid too early toilet training Avoid negative reinforcement if accidents happen Empty bladder before bedtime Get up at night to void Decrease fluid intake from dinner time on Be supportive if accidents happen Identify stresses child may have and help resolve

Continued.

Health problem	Etiology	Incidence	Assessment	Management	Prevention
			Child's response to enuresis Emotional atmosphere of home Details of toilet training Family history of enuresis Past medical history Laboratory tests Routine urinalysis		
Enuresis—cont'd				**BLADDER TRAINING (A BEHAVIOR MODIFICATION PROCEDURE)** Child drinks large fluid amount during day and retains urine as long as possible When child must void, urine is measured and recorded in a daily log Dry nights are recorded Wall charts are maintained Positive reinforcers such as stars or points are maintained for advances (e.g., two dry nights, dry all day, breaking record of previous voiding volume) **COUNSELING** Family and child should be encouraged to express feelings about enuresis Parents and child should be informed that enuresis is not intentional and is no one's fault Punitive or shaming techniques should be avoided Explanation of the many variables involved in enuresis is essential for parents and child	

Continued.

Health problems of school age child and adolescent—cont'd

Health problem	Etiology	Incidence	Assessment	Management	Prevention
				Nurse should assist parents and child to accept problem Nurse should help provide support for child Nurse should maintain a positive attitude and assist parents and child to do the same	
Encopresis	Commonly caused by chronic constipation or psychogenic problems Fecal incontinence with constipated movements; frequently impactions occur	Occurs in children over 5 years Boys affected more frequently than girls	*Primary:* children have never been toilet trained. *Secondary:* children had established bowel control. Children state they are unaware of having bowel movement. Complete history focusing on patterns of occurrence, bowel habits and toilet training. Explore psychosocial development for significant factors (i.e., illness, loss, stress)	Removal of fecal impactions by use of enemas Use of stool softeners High residue diet Counseling and support to child and parents Establishment of regular bowel routine Assist parents to help child deal with anxiety Identify practical solutions (i.e., wear extra underwear) Skin care measures	Preventive measures: Avoid too early toilet training Avoid punitive techniques in toilet training Avoid negative feedback when incontinent Increase fluid intake High residue diet

EATING DISORDERS

Health problem	Etiology	Incidence	Assessment	Management	Prevention
Anorexia	Psychosomatic disorder which frequently begins with weight reduction diet even though weight is within normal range.	Primarily affects adolescent girls.	Weight loss and refusal of food accompanied by denial of hunger. Definitive diagnostic criteria include (1) loss of at least 25% of original body weight; (2) delay or cessation of menstruation for at least 3 months; and (3) distorted body image.	Frequently requires hospitalization for both anorexic and/or bulimic adolescent.	Promote healthy eating habits and attitudes; early recognition of behavioral indicators such as: obsessive-compulsive traits; setting of perfectionistic standards for self; neat, clean, well-behaved manner; a general immaturity; and difficulty with peer and social relationships; other nursing activities include (1) liaison contracts with the client, family, and teritary care management team; (2) provision

Continued.

Health problems of school age child and adolescent—cont'd

Health problem	Etiology	Incidence	Assessment	Management	Prevention
					of support and reassurance; and (3) faciliation of home management and follow-up care by assisting the discharged client and family to maintain normal eating patterns through use of a food journal and education about balancing caloric intake requirements and exercise.
Bulimia	Psychsomatic disorder of recurrent episodes of binge eating followed by self induced vomiting.	Primarily affects adolescent girls.	Rapid consumption of large amounts of high-calorie, easily digested food in a short time period, sudden weight loss or dramatic weight fluctuations are common, dental erosion, electrolyte imbalance, and menstrual irregularities.		See measures under anorexia.
Latch-key Children	Increased number of single working parent families and inadequacy of child care options.	As many as 10 million children lack adequate adult supervision after school.	Inadequacy of care leaves children vulnerable to injury, deliquent behavior, feeling lonely, isolated and fearful.	Teach self-help skills to children; develop programs that focus on safety, how to handle telephone calls, answering door, calling parent when arrives at home; explore alternative after school activities; discuss feelings of loneliness, isolation and fear with child and explore ways to reduce these feelings; promote employer-based day care and after school care; assist parent and child to plan time alone with activities.	See Management

Continued.

Health problems of school age child and adolescent—cont'd

Health problem	Etiology	Incidence	Assessment	Management	Prevention
Obesity	Causes are related to organic problem and imbalance between caloric intake and energy expenditure Influencing factors: Genetic Activity patterns Metabolic rate Number and size of fat cells Nutritional habits Attitude about feeding Quantity of food ingested	Approximately 10% to 30% of American children are considered obese	Clinically children with weight 20% above the mean for their age and height are obese with those 10% to 20% over mean defined as overweight Organic problems must be ruled out Nutritional status and diet history (see Table 29-5 and Appendix J, p. 853)	Referral if organic problem indicated Weight control or reduction plan that modifies eating habits, reduces caloric intake, increases energy expenditure, and promotes sense of well-being and self-esteem Early prevention	Preventive measures: Encourage breast feeding Avoid overfeeding in infancy/early childhood including milk Teach nutritional needs to parents Encourage healthful eating habits Avoid extra caloric foods (sweetened water, candy as reward) Delay early introduction of solids Encourage home-prepared baby foods and meals for older children Avoid commercially prepared baby dinners and meals for older children Encourage physical activity
Stuttering	Child's advancing mental ability and level of comprehension exceeds vocabulary ability	Common until 6 years, reversal difficult after 7 years.	Hesitancy or dysfluency in speech pattern	Avoid helping child to speak; speak clearly to child, avoid rushing child, look at child when speaking, praise fluent speech	Understand normalcy of dysfluency to age 6, avoid situations where stuttering increases.

J11—COMMON BEHAVIORS OF SCHOOL AGE CHILD AND ADOLESCENT
(CHAPTERS 28 and 29)

Behavior	Development	Guidance
SCHOOL AGE		
Cheating	Testing right and wrong; generally follow parents' rules and authority but may succumb to peer pressure to "break rules"; becoming more aware of their parents' "cheating" in different ways	Assist parents to Reinforce positive "good" behaviors Maintain limits and discipline standards Recognize that most children confess or are caught and that disciplinary action must be immediate Identify what prompted cheating
Lying	Differentiating between fantasies and realities; use of untruth to avoid the unpleasant; becoming more aware of parents not always telling the truth	Confront and assess problem with assistance from teacher and involvement of child Reassure child that a real world of absolute truthfulness does not exist Point out to child untruths that are fantasies, emphasizing the real component Use discipline for act and discuss meaning of untruths Reinforce honest behaviors positively

Continued.

Common behaviors of school age child and adolescent—cont'd

Behavior	Development	Guidance
Stealing	Curiosity about other possessions; continue to learn and internalize concept of "mine" versus "yours"; not easy to resist temptations; limited idea of property	Act as role model; respect child's property and spouse's property; ask before use Reinforce concept of property and ownership verbally as well as behaviorally Discipline for petty acts, e.g., have child return or pay back item; use verbal disapproval Assess, help, and seek referral if problem is persistent
Fighting	More boys than girls fight; siblings usually fight; an attempt to establish position for self; may be result of frustration	Act as role model; parents who verbally and physically fight indicate behavior is acceptable Establish behaviors that are acceptable vents for frustration/and anger Emphasize the need to share, exchange, and interact in positive manner Separate siblings when fighting; then allow them to work out differences once composure is regained Avoid condoning physical assault as a means of retaliation with peers; assist child to find other solutions Discover reason for fighting if it is continual
Scatology	Uses dirty words as means of attention and testing parents; frequently has no understanding of meaning	Set an example; do not use dirty words in front of child Indicate unacceptability of dirty words; remind when child uses Avoid a struggle, argument, or excessive discipline unless profound problem exists Seek help if persistent
Fears	Often learned from parents; indicative of struggle to cope with unknown or unpleasant experience; may be result of learning right from wrong	Deal with each fear separately Avoid overemphasis of own fear Identify what specifically about situation evokes fear Reassure child; reinforce that some fears are healthy and protective in nature Seek help if fears interfere with daily life
ADOLESCENT		
Moodiness/non-communicative	Result of emotional conflicts of establishing an identity, developing sexually, and worries over body image and social relationships	Assist adolescent and parents to: Feel reassured about normalcy of wanting to be alone, mood swings, and fears Recognize and discuss family conflicts and possible solutions Recognize and discuss importance of communication and need to validate feelings
Preoccupation with body image and sexuality	Physical changes are dramatic; need to be the same as peers; sexual fantasies and erotic urges and behaviors are heightened with physiological changes	Recognize normalcy of feelings and preoccupation Understand normal physical growth, physiological changes, and individual patterns Accept self; develop constructive coping behaviors (e.g., sublimate into activity; need to verbalize feelings) Identify other resources of information: courses at school, books, etc. Encourage physical activity as tension release
Rebellion	Need to establish own value and belief system	Alleviate conflicts through open communication and validation of feelings Role-play and offer reflective feedback to each other Focus on individual needs and place value and pressure from others in perspective
Conformity	Need for allegiance and belonging; assists in challenge of authority and developing of self; serves as validation mechanism	Reinforce positive aspects of peer group and what is taught by them Recognize normalcy of need Find solutions when conformity interferes with adolescent's and family's goals

Continued.

Common behaviors of school age child and adolescent—cont'd

Behavior	Development	Guidance
Inferiority feelings	Result of feelings of loneliness and being different when unable to conform to peer group	Relate importance of social involvement to individual goals Explore interest and participation in after-school activities Recognize feelings about self (what he or she likes and dislikes and what are desired changes) Identify solutions to problem behaviors identified
Poor study habits	May result from disinterest, preoccupation, excessive parent expectations	Identify cause of poor habits; may need remedial help or assistance in developing constructive habits Avoid nagging or conflict over issue Identify constructive solutions Identify feelings and attitudes Discuss individual goals, methods of meeting goals as related to ability and consequences
Ambivalence	An attempt to identify dependent versus independent needs; reflects conflict between parental rules and own wishes	Identify conflict and possible solutions Maintain a system of accountability for behavior and compliance with rules of system Deal with feelings constructively (e.g., verbally, physical exercise) Recognize importance and normalcy of behavior

J12—EDUCATIONAL TOOL FOR CONTRACEPTION COUNSELING
(CHAPTERS 28 and 29)

	The pill	Minipills	Intrauterine device (IUD)	Diaphragm with spermicidal jelly or cream	Cervial cap
Description	Pills with two hormones, estrogen and progestin, similar to the hormones a woman makes in her own ovaries.	Pills with just 1 type of hormone: progestin, similar to a hormone a woman makes in her own ovaries.	A small piece of plastic with nylon threads attached. Some have copper wire wrapped around them. One IUD gives off a hormone, progesterone.	A shallow rubber cup used with a sperm-killing jelly or cream.	A flexible rubber, dome-shaped cap filled with spermicidal jelly or cream.
Action	Prevents egg's release from woman's ovaries, makes cervical mucus thicker and changes lining of the uterus.	May prevent egg's release from woman's ovaries; makes cervical mucus thicker and changes lining of uterus, making it harder for a fertilized egg to start growing there.	The IUD is inserted into the uterus. It is not known exactly how the IUD prevents pregnancy.	Fits inside the vagina. The rubber cup forms a barrier between the uterus and the sperm. The jelly or cream kills the sperm.	Fits around the cervix by suction seal, forming a barrier between the uterus and the sperm; cream or jelly kills any sperm that may escape the barrier.

Continued.

J12—EDUCATIONAL TOOL FOR CONTRACEPTION COUNSELING
(CHAPTERS 28 and 29)

	The pill	Minipills	Intrauterine device (IUD)	Diaphragm with spermicidal jelly or cream	Cervial cap
Problems	Must be prescribed by a doctor. All women should have a medical exam before taking "the Pill," and some women should not take it.	Must be prescribed by a practitioner. All women should have a medical exam first.	Must be inserted by a practitioner after a pelvic examination. Cannot be used by all women. Sometimes the uterus "pushes" it out.	Must be fitted by a practitioner after a pelvic exam. Some women find it difficult to insert, inconvenient, or messy.	Cap insertion and removal can be difficult; must be fitted by a practitioner after a pelvic exam; some cervixes are unsuitable for fitting.
Advantages	Convenient, extremely effective, does not interfere with sex, and may diminish menstrual cramps.	Convenient, effective, does not interefere with sex, and less serious side–effects than with regular birth control pills.	Effective, always there when needed, but usually not felt by either partner.	Effective and safe.	Can leave in for up to 3 days and retain safety and effectiveness.
Procedure	Either of two ways: 1. A pill a day for 3 weeks, stop for 1 week, then start a new pack. 2. A pill every single day with no stopping between packs.	Take 1 pill every single day as long as you want to avoid pregnancy.	Check string at least once a month right after the period ends to make sure your IUD is still properly in place.	Insert the diaphragm and jelly (or cream) before intercourse. Can be inserted up to 6 hours before intercourse. Must stay in at least 6 hours after intercourse.	Insert the cap filled with cream or jelly before intercourse. May stay inserted for 3 days. Suction seal over cervix must be obtained and checked by running finger around cap rim to detect any gaps.

Spermicidal foam, jelly, or cream	Condom (rubber)	Condom and foam	Periodic abstinence (natural family planning)	Sterilization
Cream and jelly come in tubes; foam comes in aerosol cans or individual applicators and is placed into the vagina.	A sheath of rubber shaped to fit snugly over the erect penis.	Condom and foam used together.	Method to find out days each month when you are most likely to get pregnant. Intercourse is avoided at that time.	Vasectomy (male) or tubal ligation (female). Ducts carrying sperm or the egg are tied and cut surgically.
Foam, jelly, and cream contain a chemical that kills sperm and acts as a physical barrier between sperm and the uterus.	Prevents sperm from getting inside a woman's vagina during intercourse.	Prevents sperm from getting inside the uterus by killing the sperm and by preventing sperm from getting out into the vagina.	Techniques include maintaining chart of basal body temperature, checking vaginal secretions, and keeping calendar of menstrual periods, all of which can help predict when an egg is most likely to be released.	Closing of tubes in male prevents sperm from reaching egg; closing tubes in female prevents egg from reaching sperm.
Must be inserted just before intercourse. Some find it inconvenient or messy.	Objectionable to some men and women. Interrupts intercourse. May be messy. Condom may break.	Requires more effort than some couples like. May be messy or inconvenient. Interrupts intercourse.	Difficult to use method if menstrual cycle is irregular. Sexual intercourse must be avoided for a significant part of each cycle.	Surgical operation has some risk but serious complications are rare. Sterilizations should not be done unless no more children are desired.
Effective, safe, a good lubricant, and can be purchased at a drugstore.	Effective, safe, and can be purchased at a drugstore; excellent protection against sexually transmitted infections.	Extremely effective, safe; both may be purchased at a drugstore without a doctor's prescription. Excellent protection against sexually transmitted infections.	Safe, effective if followed carefully; little if any religious objection to method. Teaches women about their menstrual cycles.	The most effective method; low rate of complications; many feel that removing fear of pregnancy improves sexual relations.
Put foam, jelly, or cream into your vagina each time you have intercourse, not more than 30 min beforehand. No douching for at least 8 hours after intercourse.	The condom should be placed on the erect penis before the penis ever comes into contact with the vagina. After ejaculation, the penis should be removed from the vagina immediately.	Foam must be inserted within 30 min before intercourse and condom must be placed onto erect penis before contact with vagina.	Careful records must be maintained of several factors: basal body temperature, vaginal secretions, and onset of menstrual bleeding. Careful study of these methods will dictate when intercourse should be avoided.	After the decision to have no more children has been well thought through, a brief surgical procedure is performed on the man or the woman.

J-13 — SYSTEM ASSESSMENT AND CARE PLAN FOR THE CHILD WITH AIDS
(CHAPTERS 28 and 29)

System	Problem Identification	Primary/Secondary Causative Agents	Interdisciplinary Involvement	Plan of Care
Neurologic	Developmental delays Loss of developmental milestones Loss of reflexes Lack of coordination Loss of memory Ataxia Irritability Visual disturbance	AIDS encephalopathy, CMV, toxoplasmosis, CNS lymphomas	Nursing/PT/OT/child life	Individualize plan for PT, OT, Speech Encourage self-care Establish daily routine Provide developmentally appropriate activities/toys Increase stimulation Increase school attendance/Special Education
ENT	Hearing loss Dental caries	Chronic otitis media, oral candidasis, strep, staph, other flora	Nursing/speech therapy Nursing/dentist	Instruct sign language Instruct lip reading Administer consistent, gentle oral hygiene
Respiratory	Dry, hacking cough (baseline) Oxygen dependency Rhonchi, rales Tachypnea	Chronic pneumonias, lymphoid interstitial pneumonitis (LIP)	Nursing/medicine/RT	Assess baseline respiratory status Encourage ambulation/positioning Avoid over-exertion Continue CPT on regular basis Maintain adequate hydration
Cardiac	Activity tolerance decreases Cardiac output decreases Tachycardia Fluid retention/edema Audible gallop/murmur	Cardiac myopathy secondary to repeated infections and arteriopathy	Nursing/medicine	Assess baseline cardiac status Avoid over-exertion Restrict fluid intake Administer cardiac glycoside and diuretics
GI	Failure to thrive (FTT) less than 5% for height and weight for age Loss of appetite Chronic diarrhea Painful oral/esophageal lesions Nausea, vomiting Intractable pain	Oral/esophageal candidiasis, painful suck/swallow, malabsorption problems, damage to intestinal flora	Nursing/dietary	Monitor daily weights Track progress on growth charts Encourage self-menu planning (creative) Avoid citrus fruits Provide lactose-free formulas, milk products Provide anesthetic agents for oral cavity Administer antiemetics (rectally) Administer pain relievers, narcotics (if necessary)

System assessment and care plan for the child with aids — cont'd

System	Problem Identification	Primary/Secondary Causative Agents	Interdisciplinary Involvement	Plan of Care
Integument	Perianal abscess Oral/lip lesions Generalized body rashes	Herpes simplex, fungal infections, chronic diarrhea, Kaposi's Sarcoma (rare)	Nursing/medicine	Encourage ambulation/positioning Moisturize skin every day Administer consistent, thorough hygiene Use special mattresses
Renal	Urine output decreases BUN, creatine increases Fluid retention	Antigen/antibody phenomenon, nephrotoxic antibiotics	Nursing/medicine	Maintain fluid and electrolyte balance Restrict fluid intake Administer vitamin K supplements
Psychosocial	Depression Regressive/Aggressive behaviors Withdrawal Emotional lability	Social isolation, chaotic family situation, abandonment, medication side effects	Nursing/psychology/social work	Establish daily routine Maintain consistency of care Provide "anger-release" activities Assess for alternate living arrangements Behavior modification activities

From: Williams AD: Nursing management of the child with AIDS, Pediatric Nursing 15:260, 1989.

J14—NATURAL HISTORY, PIH: PREGNANCY INDUCED HYPERTENSION
(CHAPTER 9)

Prepathogenesis events	Primary prevention strategies

1. Susceptibility

The following conditions predispose to PIH: hydatid mole, hydramnios, multiple pregnancy, hypertensive vascular disease, chronic renal disease and diabetes mellitus. "Pure" PIH is almost exclusively found in primigravida. It occurs more frequently in advancing pregnancy. Except for hydatid mole, it does not occur in the first 6 months of pregnancy. Blacks are at increased risk, also residents of the SE United States, the Phillipines, and among women in lower socioeconomic strata. It affects women at extremes of reproductive age (<20 and >35 yrs).

Some studies have shown that 93% of normotensive nulliparous women who later develop PIH showed an elevation of the diastolic BP of at least 20 mm Hg when turned from a lateral to supine position between 28-32 wks gestation. These women showed an increased sensitivity to the infusion of angiotension II. (Rollover test)

PIH is a very common complication of pregnancy; it is seen in 6-7% of all gravidas.

2. Adaptation

The etiology of PIH is unclear; however, the theory of "uterine ischemia" is the most widely accepted. Relative ischemia of the uterus and its contents alters the maternal-placental-fetal mechanisms controlling sodium and water balance, and fluid retention results. After a variable period of time, if there is further alteration of the utero-placental complex, the release of vasoconstrictor agents into the maternal circulation is triggered.

(1) Direct strategies to socioeconomically deprived groups.

Educate clients on the need for a 1 gm/kg protein diet with vitamins and minerals.

Develop programs to help women increase their economic status and alleviate the physical and social stresses associated with poverty.

Educate public on the need for early and frequent prenatal care.

Support funding for prenatal services for indigent women.

Target populations with predisposing medical problems. Educate these groups on the need for careful, planned pregnancies and achievement of optimal physical/mental condition *before* becoming pregnant.

Target adolescent population. Educate regarding responsible sexuality and risks associated with pregnancy during the teen years.

Natural history, PIH: pregnancy induced hypertension—cont'd

Pathogenesis events	Secondary interventions/tertiary interventions

1. Early pathogenesis.

The vasoconstrictive agents cause the kidneys to release inordinate amounts of renin from the kidneys. From a reaction with renin, angiotensin is produced and the vasoconstriction process is perpetuated. Disturbances in the metabolic, electrolyte and fluid compartments begin.

2. Discernible early lesions.

Laboratory findings are usually of little assistance in predicting the development of PIH. As the disease progresses the hematocrit and hemoglobin levels rise and Na^+ may decrease. Fibrinogen increases. Urine volume may decrease, along with 24 hour clearance of Na^+, K^+, and Ct. Weight gain is a most important parameter in recognizing developing PIH, with or without demonstrable edema. Increments of >1 kg/ week in the third trimester are frequently seen. Swelling in excess of hands and ankles may start to develop.

(1)
1. Accurate prenatal history for assessment of risk factors
2. Monitor edema, BP, and proteinuria on each prenatal visit
3. Teach importance of high protein diet and vitamins

(2) Early recognition of sodium and H_2O retention. Prevention of progression of the disease

1. High protein diet
2. Bed rest (12 hrs per day) in lateral recumbent position
3. Phenobarbitol 30-60 mg tid
4. More frequent monitoring of fetal status

Continued.

Natural history, PIH: pregnancy induced hypertension—cont'd

Pathogenesis events	Secondary interventions/tertiary interventions

3. Clinical disease

PIH is usually diagnosed when the patient develops hypertension, proteinuria and usually edema. Both elevated blood pressure and proteinuria are considered late manifestations of the disease. Proteinuria (3+ protein or 5 grams in 25 hour sample) usually is indicative of an advanced and probably irreversible phase of the syndrome. Symptoms/signs indicative of severity include: hyperreflexia, epigastric pain, visual disturbances, oliguria, and drowsiness, severe headache, convulsions, and coma. Pathophysical alterations seen in severe cases include cerebral edema, cerebral hemorrhage. There is marked glomeruli edema. The liver may be damaged as evidenced by necrosis in patients who have died from PIH, but in many cases there is no hepatic involvement. Severe retinal constriction may result in retinal detachment. Acute pulmonary edema is often prominent in the lungs of PIH patients. The placenta develops infarcts. The fetus may be malnourished and underweight and in 2%-10% of cases will die. Abruptio placenta is a frequent occurrence in severe PIH. The necrosis in the tissues mentioned above may often be explained by the development of disseminated intravascular coagulation (DIC). PIH is one of the leading causes of maternal death and accounts for some 250 maternal deaths each year. Prognosis varies. "Pure" PIH is completely reversible and does not produce chronic hypertension. PIH will not occur in subsequent pregnancies unless one or more of the major predisposing factors are present. Perinatal mortality rates range from 2%-30%. The infant may also have residual ECG abnormalities, seizures, and/or developmental delays.

(3) If B/P >140/90 or >30 mm Hg systolic and 15 mm Hg diastolic and proteinuria, hospitalize

1. Bedrest with BRP
2. Daily weighing
3. Monitor FHT, fetal stress tests
4. Phenobarbitol qid
5. High protein diet
6. 24 hour urine estriols
7. Delivery at 37 weeks gestation. Delivery before 37 weeks if disease progresses

(4) Severe cases

1. Bedrest absolute
2. Close observation, decrease stimulation
3. Magnesium sulfate to hyperreflexia
4. Monitor I and O
5. Fetal monitoring
6. Seizure precautions
7. Delivery after adequate sedation

After delivery monitor for vasomotor collapse and hypovolemia. In severe cases assess residual organ damage. Supportive therapy and follow-up for infant.

Bobak I, Jensen M, and Zalar M, editors: Maternity and gynecologic care: the nurse and the family, ed 4, St. Louis, 1989, Mosby–Year Book, Inc.

J15 — SUMMARY OF NUTRIENTS FOR HEALTH
(CHAPTER 34)

Nutrient	Sources	Examples of major functions	Deficiency symptoms	Toxicity symptoms	RDA Men	RDA Women
Protein	Milk products, fish, poultry, eggs, meat, beans, peas, nuts	Supplies 4 calories per gram; constitutes part of structure of all cells; supports growth and maintains healthy body cells; constitutes part of enzymes, hormones, antibodies that regulate body processes	Protein calorie malnutrition	Elevated uric acid and urea in serum, calcium loss, fluid imbalance	56 g 15%-20% of total calories	44 g
Carbohydrate Fiber Starch Sugar	Cereals, breads, potatoes, beans, corn, sugar, honey	Supplies 4 calories per gram; major source of energy for CNS; supplies energy so protein can be used for growth and maintenance of cells; unrefined products supply fiber important for regular elimination	Poor GI function	Flatulence, trace mineral deficiencies	No RDA 50%-55% of total calories	
Fat Saturated	Meats, dairy products, tropical oils	Supplies 9 calories per gram; constitutes part of all cells; carries fat-soluble vitamins	Essential fatty acid deficiency	Obesity	No RDA 25%-30% of total calories	
Monounsaturated	Olive and peanut oils					
Polyunsaturated	Fish, liquid vegetable oils					
Cholesterol	Animal meats, egg yolks					

Continued.

Summary of nutrients for health – cont'd

Nutrient	Sources	Examples of major functions	Deficiency symptoms	Toxicity symptoms	RDA Men	RDA Women
Fat Soluble Vitamins						
Vitamin A (Retinol)	Milk fat, cod liver oil, liver; yellow, orange, leafy green vegetables	Assists formation and maintenance of skin and mucous membranes, thus increasing resistence to infection; promotes bone growth; promotes health of eye tissue and eye adaptation in dim light	Eye, skin, bone, blood, immune system disorders	Headaches, skin, blood, bone disorders	1000	800 IU
Vitamin D	Exposure to sunlight, fortified milk, fish	Required for body use of calcium and phosphorus in mineralization of bones and teeth	Rickets, other bone and tooth disorders	Calcium deposits in kidney and soft tissues, GI symptoms, headaches, weakness	5 mcg	5 mcg
Vitamin E	Vegetable oils, nuts	Antioxidant; protects Vitamin A and unsaturated fatty acids, integrity of normal cell membranes; important for wound healing, immune system health	Anemia	Possbily blood coagulation disorders	10 mg	8 mg
Vitamin K	Lettuce, cabbage, egg yolk, soybean oil, liver	Coagulation of blood; bone maintenance	Prolonged blood clotting time	Kernicterus	80 mcg	65 mcg
Water Soluble Vitamins						
Vitamin C (ascorbic acid)	Citrus fruits, strawberries, cabbage, potatoes, broccoli, greens	Aids utilization of iron, forms cement that holds cells together, strengthens blood vessels promotes healing, increases resistance to infection	Scurvy, skin, blood, GI, neurologic disorders	Rare	60 mg	60 mg

Continued.

Summary of nutrients for health — cont'd

Nutrient	Sources	Examples of major functions	Deficiency symptoms	Toxicity symptoms	RDA Men	RDA Women
Thiamin (B₁)	Meats, whole grains, nuts, lentils, potatoes	Coenzyme in carbohydrate metabolism, promotes normal appetite, function of heart, nerves, muscles	Beriberi, deep muscle pain, nerve, GI, heart disorders, depression, irritability, fatigue, Wernicke-Korsakoff syndrome (alcoholics)	Rare	1.5 mg	1.1 mg
Riboflavin (B₂)	Liver, fish, eggs, cereals, green leafy vegetables	Coenzyme in protein and energy metabolism; promotes healthy skin, eyes	Eye symptoms, frontal headaches, sore dry skin	Rare	1.7 mg	1.3 mg
Niacin (tryptophan, nicotinic acid, niacinamide)	Liver, meat, fish, eggs, whole grains, legumes	Coenzyme in energy production; promotes healthy skin, GI, and nervous system function	Pellagra, dermatitis, diarrhea, depression	Liver damage, flushing, itching, nausea, fainting	19 mg	15 mg
Vitamin B₆ (pyridoxine)	Meats, seeds, grains, potatoes, bananas, green vegetables	Important in protein metabolism, hemoglobin synthesis, integrity of CNS	Anemia, CNS disturbances	Rare	2.0 mg	1.6 mg
Vitamin B₁₂	Animal foods	Important for function of all body cells; essential for red blood cell maturation	Pernicious anemia	Rare	2 mcg	2 mcg
Minerals Calcium	Milk products, fish with bones, vegetable greens	Combines with other minerals (phosphorus) within protein framework to give strength and structure to bones and teeth, functions in blood clotting, muscle contraction, nerve action	Tooth and bone loss, hypertension, muscular cramps and tremors	Hypercalcemia	800 mg	
Iron	Liver, red meat, dried beans and peas, egg yolk, dark green vegetables, enriched breads and cereals	Combines with protein to form hemoglobin, which carries oxygen in blood, increases resistence to infection, functions as part of enzymes involved in tissue respiration	Lowered resistance to infection, anemia, fatigue	Hemosiderosis, hemochromotosis (bronze coloration), liver damage	10 mg	15 mg

APPENDIX

Screening Tools

K1—GROWTH MEASUREMENTS: BIRTH TO 18 YEARS
(CHAPTERS 28 and 29)
Height and weight measurements for boys

	Height by percentiles						Weight by percentiles					
	5		50		95		5		50		95	
Age*	cm	inches	cm	inches	cm	inches	kg	lb	kg	lb	kg	lb
Birth	46.4	18¼	50.5	20	54.4	21½	2.54	5½	3.27	7¼	4.15	9¼
3 months	56.7	22¼	61.1	24	65.4	25¾	4.43	9¾	5.98	13¼	7.37	16¼
6 months	63.4	25	67.8	26¾	72.3	28½	6.20	13¾	7.85	17¼	9.46	20¾
9 months	68.0	26¾	72.3	28½	77.1	30¼	7.52	16½	9.18	20¼	10.93	24
1	71.7	28¼	76.1	30	81.2	32	8.43	18½	10.15	22½	11.99	26½
1½	77.5	30½	82.4	32½	88.1	34¾	9.59	21¼	11.47	25¼	13.44	29½
2†	82.5	32½	86.8	34¼	94.4	37¼	10.49	23¼	12.34	27¼	15.50	34¼
2½†	85.4	33½	90.4	35½	97.8	38½	11.27	24¾	13.52	29¾	16.61	36½
3	89.0	35	94.9	37¼	102.0	40¼	12.05	26½	14.62	32¼	17.77	39¼
3½	92.5	36½	99.1	39	106.1	41¾	12.84	28¼	15.68	34½	18.98	41¾
4	95.8	37¾	102.9	40½	109.9	43¼	13.64	30	16.69	36¾	20.27	44¾
4½	98.9	39	106.6	42	113.5	44¾	14.45	31¾	17.69	39	21.63	47¾
5	102.0	40¼	109.9	43¼	117.0	46	15.27	33¾	18.67	41¼	23.09	51
6	107.7	42½	116.1	45¾	123.5	48½	16.93	37¼	20.69	45½	26.34	58
7	113.0	44½	121.7	48	129.7	51	18.64	41	22.85	50¼	30.12	66½
8	118.1	46½	127.0	50	135.7	53½	20.40	45	25.30	55¾	34.51	76
9	122.9	48½	132.2	52	141.8	55¾	22.25	49	28.13	62	39.58	87¼
10	127.7	50¼	137.5	54¼	148.1	58¼	24.33	53¾	31.44	69¼	45.27	99¾
11	132.6	52¼	143.3	56½	154.9	61	26.80	59	35.30	77¾	51.47	113½
12	137.6	54¼	149.7	59	162.3	64	29.85	65¾	39.78	87¾	58.09	128
13	142.9	56¼	156.5	61½	169.8	66¾	33.64	74¼	44.95	99	65.02	143¼
14	148.8	58½	163.1	64¼	176.7	69½	38.22	84¼	50.77	112	72.13	159
15	155.2	61	169.0	66½	181.9	71½	43.11	95	56.71	125	79.12	174½
16	161.1	63½	173.5	68¼	185.4	73	47.74	105¼	62.10	137	85.62	188¾
17	164.9	65	176.2	69¼	187.3	73¾	51.50	113½	66.31	146¼	91.31	201¼
18	165.7	65¼	176.8	69½	187.6	73¾	53.97	119	68.88	151¾	95.76	211

From: Whaley LF, and Wong DL: Nursing care of infants and children, ed. 4, St. Louis, 1991, Mosby–Year Book, Inc., pp. 1962-1963 as adapted from National Center for Health Statistics, Health Resources Administration, Department of Health, Education and Welfare, Hyattsville, Md. Values correspond with NCHS percentile curves (see Figs. D-1 to D-4). Conversion of metric data to approximate inches and pounds by Ross Laboratories.

*Years unless otherwise indicated.

†Height data include some recumbent length measurements, which make values slightly higher than if all measurements had been of stature (standing height).

Height and weight measurements for girls

| | Height by percentiles | | | | | | Weight by percentiles | | | | | |
| | 5 | | 50 | | 95 | | 5 | | 50 | | 95 | |
Age*	cm	inches	cm	inches	cm	inches	kg	lb	kg	lb	kg	lb
Birth	45.4	17¾	49.9	19¾	52.9	20¾	2.36	5¼	3.23	7	3.81	8½
3 months	55.4	21¾	59.5	23½	63.4	25	4.18	9¼	5.4	12	6.74	14¾
6 months	61.8	24¼	65.9	26	70.2	27¾	5.79	12¾	7.21	16	8.73	19¼
9 months	66.1	26	70.4	27¾	75.0	29½	7.0	15½	8.56	18¾	10.17	22½
1	69.8	27½	74.3	29¼	79.1	31¼	7.84	17¼	9.53	21	11.24	24¾
1½	76.0	30	80.9	31¾	86.1	34	8.92	19¾	10.82	23¾	12.76	28¼
2†	81.6	32¼	86.8	34¼	93.6	36¾	9.95	22	11.8	26	14.15	31¼
2½†	84.6	33¼	90.0	35½	96.6	38	10.8	23¾	13.03	28¾	15.76	34¾
3	88.3	34¾	94.1	37	100.6	39½	11.61	25½	14.1	31	17.22	38
3½	91.7	36	97.9	38½	104.5	41¼	12.37	27¼	15.07	33¼	18.59	41
4	95.0	37½	101.6	40	108.3	42¾	13.11	29	15.96	35¼	19.91	44
4½	98.1	38½	105.0	41¼	112.0	44	13.83	30½	16.81	37	21.24	46¾
5	101.1	39¾	108.4	42¾	115.6	45½	14.55	32	17.66	39	22.62	49¾
6	106.6	42	114.6	45	122.7	48¼	16.05	35½	19.52	43	25.75	56¾
7	111.8	44	120.6	47½	129.5	51	17.71	39	21.84	48¼	29.68	65½
8	116.9	46	126.4	49¾	136.2	53½	19.62	43¼	24.84	54¾	34.71	76½
9	122.1	48	132.2	52	142.9	56¼	21.82	48	28.46	62¾	40.64	89½
10	127.5	50¼	138.3	54½	149.5	58¾	24.36	53¾	32.55	71¾	47.17	104
11	133.5	52½	144.8	57	156.2	61½	27.24	60	36.95	81½	54.0	119
12	139.8	55	151.5	59¾	162.7	64	30.52	67¼	41.53	91½	60.81	134
13	145.2	57¼	157.1	61¾	168.1	66¼	34.14	75¼	46.1	101¾	67.3	148¼
14	148.7	58½	160.4	63¼	171.3	67½	37.76	83¼	50.28	110¾	73.08	161
15	150.5	59¼	161.8	63¾	172.8	68	40.99	90¼	53.68	118¼	77.78	171½
16	151.6	59¾	162.4	64	173.3	68¼	43.41	95¾	55.89	123¼	80.99	178½
17	152.7	60	163.1	64¼	173.5	68¼	44.74	98¾	56.69	125	82.46	181¾
18	153.6	60½	163.7	64½	173.6	68¼	45.26	99¾	56.62	124¾	82.47	181¾

Adapted from National Center for Health Statistics, Health Resources Administration, Department of Health, Education and Welfare, Hyattsville, Md. Values correspond with NCHS percentile curves (see Figs. D-5 to D-8). Conversion of metric data to approximate inches and pounds by Ross Laboratories.

*Years unless otherwise indicated.

†Height data include some recumbent length measurements, which make values slightly higher than if all measurements had been of stature (standing height).

Continued.

K2—DENVER DEVELOPMENTAL SCREENING TEST

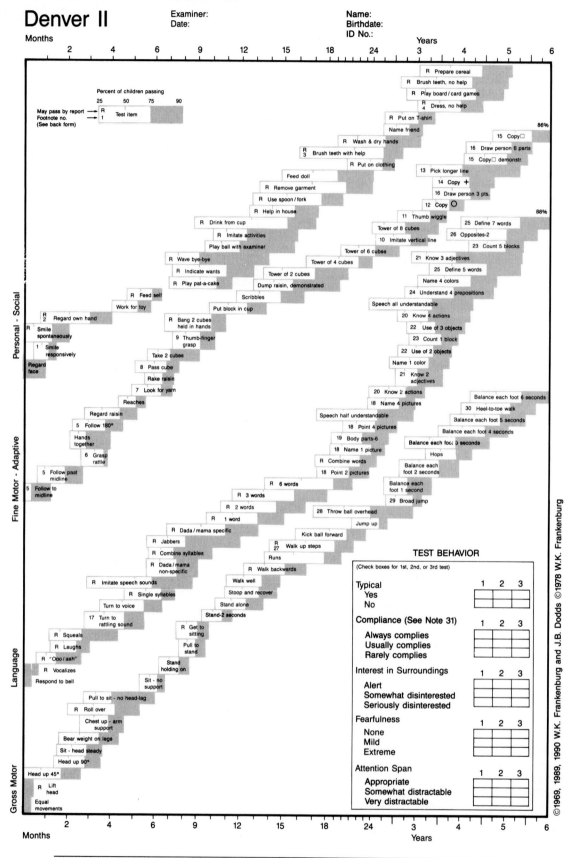

FIGURE K-1

A, Denver II. *From W.K. Frankenburg and J.B. Doss, 1990.*

DIRECTIONS FOR ADMINISTRATION

1. Try to get child to smile by smiling, talking or waving. Do not touch him/her.
2. Child must stare at hand several seconds.
3. Parent may help guide toothbrush and put toothpaste on brush.
4. Child does not have to be able to tie shoes or button/zip in the back.
5. Move yarn slowly in an arc from one side to the other, about 8" above child's face.
6. Pass if child grasps rattle when it is touched to the backs or tips of fingers.
7. Pass if child tries to see where yarn went. Yarn should be dropped quickly from sight from tester's hand without arm movement.
8. Child must transfer cube from hand to hand without help of body, mouth, or table.
9. Pass if child picks up raisin with any part of thumb and finger.
10. Line can vary only 30 degrees or less from tester's line. /
11. Make a fist with thumb pointing upward and wiggle only the thumb. Pass if child imitates and does not move any fingers other than the thumb.

     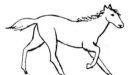   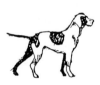

12. Pass any enclosed form. Fail continuous round motions.
13. Which line is longer? (Not bigger.) Turn paper upside down and repeat. (pass 3 of 3 or 5 of 6)
14. Pass any lines crossing near midpoint.
15. Have child copy first. If failed, demonstrate.

When giving items 12, 14, and 15, do not name the forms. Do not demonstrate 12 and 14.

16. When scoring, each pair (2 arms, 2 legs, etc.) counts as one part.
17. Place one cube in cup and shake gently near child's ear, but out of sight. Repeat for other ear.

B 18. Point to picture and have child name it. (No credit is given for sounds only.)
   If less than 4 pictures are named correctly, have child point to picture as each is named by tester.

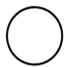   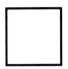   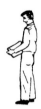

19. Using doll, tell child: Show me the nose, eyes, ears, mouth, hands, feet, tummy, hair. Pass 6 of 8.
20. Using pictures, ask child: Which one flies?... says meow?... talks?... barks?... gallops? Pass 2 of 5, 4 of 5.
21. Ask child: What do you do when you are cold?... tired?... hungry? Pass 2 of 3, 3 of 3.
22. Ask child: What do you do with a cup? What is a chair used for? What is a pencil used for? Action words must be included in answers.
23. Pass if child correctly places <u>and</u> says how many blocks are on paper. (1, 5).
24. Tell child: Put block **on** table; **under** table; **in front of** me, **behind** me. Pass 4 of 4. (Do not help child by pointing, moving head or eyes.)
25. Ask child: What is a ball?... lake?... desk?... house?... banana?... curtain?... fence?... ceiling? Pass if defined in terms of use, shape, what it is made of, or general category (such as banana is fruit, not just yellow). Pass 5 of 8, 7 of 8.
26. Ask child: If a horse is big, a mouse is __? If fire is hot, ice is __? If the sun shines during the day, the moon shines during the __? Pass 2 of 3.
27. Child may use wall or rail only, not person. May not crawl.
28. Child must throw ball overhand 3 feet to within arm's reach of tester.
29. Child must perform standing broad jump over width of test sheet (8 1/2 inches).
30. Tell child to walk forward, ⌒⌒⌒⌒➤ heel within 1 inch of toe. Tester may demonstrate. Child must walk 4 consecutive steps.
31. In the second year, half of normal children are non-compliant.

OBSERVATIONS:

B, Directions for administration of numbered items on Denver II. *From W.K. Frankenburg and J.B. Dodds, 1990.*

K3—INFANT REFLEXES
(CHAPTERS 28 and 29)

Reflex	How to elicit	Response of infant	Clinical implications
Acoustic blink	Produce a sharp loud noise (a clap of the hands) about 30 cm from the head.	By second or third day of life infant blinks both eyes. Disappearance of reflex is variable.	Absence may indicate decreased hearing.
Ankle clonus	Flex the leg at the hip and knee, sharply dorsiflex the foot, and maintain pressure.	Rhythmic flexions and extensions of the foot at the ankle.	Abnormal if more than 10 beats during the first 3 months or more than 3 beats after 3 months. Sustained clonus indicates upper motor neuron disease.
Babinski	Stroke lateral aspect of the plantar surface of foot from heel to toes. Use a blunt object.	Hyperextension or fanning of toes occurs. As myelinization is completed, the normal response becomes flexion (downward curling) of all toes; the positive (pathological) sign is hyperextension (dorsiflexion) of the great toe with or without fanning of the remaining toes.	After 2 years of age, a positive sign is the most significant clinical symptom of the presence of an upper motor neuron (pyramidal tract) lesion.
Blinking	Shine a light suddenly at the infant's open eyes.	Eyelids close in response to light. Disappears after first year.	Absence may indicate poor light perception or blindness.
Landau	Suspend infant carefully in prone position by supporting infant's abdomen with examiner's hand.	By 3 months of age the expected response consists of extension of head, trunk, and hips. Head is slightly above horizontal plane. Disappears by 2 years of age.	If newborn collapses into a limp concave position, it is abnormal.
Moro	With infant in supine position gently support head and lift it a few centimeters off the surface. As soon as neck relaxes, suddenly release the head and let it drop back to the surface. *or* Produce sudden loud noise, or jar the table or crib suddenly.	Normal response is present at birth and is one in which the arms extend outward, the hands open, and then are brought together in midline. The legs flex slightly. Usually disappears by 3 to 4 months. Infant may cry.	Asymmetry indicates possible paralysis. Absence suggests severe neurological problem. Persistence beyond 4 months may indicate neurological disease. If it lasts longer than 6 months, it is definitely abnormal.
Neck righting	With infant in supine position turn head to one side.	Infant's trunk rotates in direction in which head is turned. Appears at 4 to 6 months. Disappears at 24 months.	Absent or decreased reflex may indicate spasticity.
Palmar grasp	With infant's head positioned in midline place examiner's index fingers from ulnar side into infant's palm and press against palm.	Normal response is flexion of all fingers around examiner's fingers. Present at birth and disappears by 4 months when infant is ready to reach.	Note symmetry and strength. Persistence of grasp beyond 4 months suggests cerebral dysfunction.
Parachute	Infant is held in a prone position and is quickly lowered toward the surface of the examining table or floor.	Normal response is extension of arms, hands, and fingers, as if to break a fall. Appears by 9 months and persists.	Asymmetry or absence of response is abnormal.

Continued.

Infant reflexes—cont'd

Reflex	How to elicit	Response of infant	Clinical implications
Perez	Infant is held in a suspended prone position in one of the examiner's hands. The thumb of the other hand is moved firmly from sacrum along entire spine.	Normal response is extension of head and spine, flexion of knees on the chest, a cry, and emptying of the bladder. Present at birth and disappears by 3 months.	Absence indicates severe neurological disease.
Placing	Infant is held erect and the dorsum of one foot touches the undersurface of the examining table top.	Infant flexes hip and knee and places stimulated foot on top of the table. Present at birth and disappears by 6 weeks or variable.	Absent in paralysis or in infants born by breech delivery.
Plantar grasp	Examiner's finger is placed firmly across base of infant's toes.	Toes curl downward. Present at birth and disappears by 10 to 12 months.	Absent in defects of lower spinal column. Infant cannot walk until this reflex disappears.
Rooting	Infant is held in supine position with head in midline and hands against chest. Examiner strokes perioral skin at corner of mouth or cheek.	Infant opens mouth and turns head toward stimulated side. Present at birth and disappears by 3 to 4 months (awake); by 7 months (asleep).	Absence indicates severe central nervous system disease or depressed infant.
Rotation test	Infant is held upright facing examiner and rotated in one direction and then the other.	Infant's head turns in the direction in which the body is being turned. If head is restrained the eyes will turn in the direction in which the infant is turned.	If head and eyes do not move, it indicates a vestibular problem.
Spontaneous crawling (Bauer's response)	Infant is lying prone and examiner presses soles of feet.	Infant makes crawling movements. Present at birth.	Crawling is absent in weak or depressed infants.
Stepping	Infant is held upright and soles of feet are put in touch with solid surface.	Infant "walks" along surface. Present at birth and disappears at 6 weeks.	Absence indicates depressed infant, breech delivery, or paralysis.
Sucking	With infant in supine position place nipple or finger 3 to 4 cm into mouth.	Vigorous sucking of finger or nipple. Present at birth and disappears by 3 to 4 months (awake) and 7 months (asleep). Tongue action should push finger up and back. Note rate of suck, amount of suction, and patterns or groupings of sucks.	Absence in term infants indicates central nervous system depression. Weak reflex may lead to feeding problems.
Tonic neck	With infant in supine position passively rotate head to one side.	Arm and leg on side to which head is turned extend, and opposite arm and leg flex (fencer's position). Present sometimes at birth but usually by 2 to 3 months. Disappears by 6 months.	Obligatory response is always abnormal. Persistence beyond 6 months is abnormal and indicates central motor lesions (e.g., cerebral palsy).
Trunk incurvation (Galant's)	Infant is held prone in examiner's hand. With the other hand the examiner moves a finger down the paravertebral portion of the spine, first on one side, then on the other.	Infant's trunk should curve to the side being stimulated. Present at birth and disappears by 2 months.	Presence of spinal cord lesions interrupts this reflex.
Vertical suspension positioning	Infant is held upright, head is maintained in midline.	Legs are flexed at the hips and knees. Present at birth and disappears after 4 months.	Scissoring or fixed extension indicates spasticity.

K4—VISION, HEARING, AND LANGUAGE SCREENING PROCEDURES
(CHAPTERS 28 and 29)

Method	Age	Procedure	Normal response
VISION			
Following	Infancy	Shine light or hold bright object directly in front of infant's line of vision; move slowly from side to side.	Follow light or bright object up to 180 degrees
Turn to light response	Infancy	Hold back of head to bright light source.	Eyes turn toward source of light
Optokinetic drum	Infancy	Twirl drum with stripes slowly in front of infant's eyes.	Nystagmus occurs.
Herschberg reflex (corneal light reflex)	Infancy through adolescence	Shine penlight into child's eyes; note where light reflex falls. For older children: have child focus and stare at point 14 inches and then 20 inches away before shining light into eyes.	Light reflex falls in same position in eye
Cover test	Toddler through adolescence	Have child focus on specified spot first 14 inches, then 20 inches away. While child is focusing, one eye is completely covered for 5 to 10 seconds. Cover is then removed and eye observed for movement. Procedure repeated for other eye.	No wandering or sharp jerky movement of eyes noted, indicating ability to focus
Snellen E	Preschool	Child is instructed to point finger in direction that the E or table legs are pointing from a distance of 20 feet. Test each eye separately, then together. Test as far down on chart as child can go.	Visual acuity of 20/30
Snellen alphabet	School age through adolescence	Child stands 20 feet from chart and reads letters. Each eye is tested separately and then together. Testing usually started at 20/30 or 20/40 line and child allowed to test as far down chart as possible. Passing score consists of reading majority of letters (or Es) on each line.	Visual acuity of 20/20
HEARING			
Startle reflex	Newborn	Loud noise or bang made near infant's ears.	Jumps at noise, blinks, cries or widen eyes
Tracks sound	3-6 months	Make noise, call name or sing.	Eyes shift toward sound; responds to mother's voice; coos to verbalization
Recognizes sound	6-8 months	As preceding, from out of line of vision.	Turns head toward sound; responds to name, babbles to verbalization
Localization of sound	8-12 months	Call name, or use tuning fork or say words.	Localizes source of sound; turns head (and body at times) toward sound, repeats words
Pure tone screening—play	Toddler to preschool	Demonstrate to child by putting headphones on and making believe you hear sound. As you say "I hear it," put a block in box or ring on holder. Put headphones on child and give block or ring to use. Sound a 50 dB tone at 1000 Hz and guide child's hand with block to box. When child can do this alone, begin screening. Set at 25 dB at 1000 Hz. If child responds, go to 2000, 4000, and 6000 Hz. Praise child and place new block in hand. Switch to other ear and test.	Should respond at 25 dB at any frequency

Continued.

Vision, hearing, and language screening procedures—cont'd

Method	Age	Procedure	Normal response
HEARING—cont'd			
Pure tone audiometry	School age through adolescence	Explain procedure to child. Place headphones on ears. Test 1 ear at a time in sequence as preceding (i.e., 25 dB at 1000, 2000, 4000 and 6000 Hz). Have child raise hand to indicate sound is heard.	Should respond at 25 dB at any frequency
Tuning fork test	Some pre-schoolers; school age through adolescence		
A. Weber test		Strike tuning fork to make it vibrate and place the stem in midline of scalp. Ask child if sound is same in both ears or louder in either ear.	Sound heard equally well in both ears
B. Rinne test		Strike tuning fork until it vibrates, place stem on child's mastoid until he no longer hears it. Then place vibrating fingers of fork 1 to 2 inches in front of concha. Ask child if he can still hear sound.	Sound from fingers of fork vibrating in air should be heard when child can no longer hear sound with stem against mastoid, i.e., air conduction is greater than bone conduction
LANGUAGE			
Assessment of child's language comprehension	3-6 years	Child points to picture named by examiner. Assesses single word vocabulary and two-word, three-word, and four-word phrases.	Child able to name picture understandably
Peabody Picture Vocabulary Test-Revised	2½-18 years	Child looks at picture and points to one named by examiner.	Child able to respond correctly by following directions
Preschool Language Scale	Birth to 3 years	Observation of child's performance.	Depending on age level, child should be able to point to picture, follow direction, or manipulate objects
Expressive One Word Picture Vocabulary	2-12 years	Child looks at picture and names what is seen.	Child able to follow directions and articulate response at age level
Denver Articulation Screening Examination (DASE) (See Appendix K7)	2½-6 yrs	Child repeats words spoken to him.	Child of 2½ years is understandable half of time. Child 3 years and older is understandable all the time.

K5—SCREENING FOR COMMON ORTHOPEDIC PROBLEMS IN INFANCY AND CHILDHOOD
(CHAPTERS 28 and 29)

Deformity	Screening

CONGENITAL HIP DISLOCATION (CHD)

Complete or partial displacement of femoral head out of the acetabulum

Barlow's maneuver (for dislocation of femoral head): flex hip to 90 degrees; grasp symphysis in front and sacrum in back with one hand; with other hand, apply lateral pressure to medial thigh with thumb and longitudinal pressure to knee with palm; abduct flexed hip. A positive sign is sensation of abnormal movement. Reverse hands for examining other hip. See Figure K-1.

Ortolani's maneuver (for reduction of femur): abduct hip to 80 degrees, lifting proximal femur anteriorly with fingers placed on lateral thigh. A positive sign is sensation of a jerk or snap with reduction into socket. See Figure K-2.

Limited full abduction of hips: with child flat on back, abduct hips one at a time, then together. See Figure K-3 for degrees of hip abduction.

Apparent shortening of femur:

1. Allis sign: with child lying on back, pelvis flat, knees flexed and feet planted firmly, observe knees. If the knee projects further anteriorly, femur is longer; if one knee is higher, the tibia is longer.
2. With child on back, both legs are extended out with pressure on knees. Heels are matched and observed for equal or unequal length.
3. Trendelenburg sign: with child standing on one leg, observe pelvis. When child stands on abnormal leg, the pelvis drops on normal side. See Figure K-4.

METATARSUS ADDUCTUS (VARUS)

Adduction or turning in of forefoot with high longitudinal arch and wide space between first and second toes. Commonly associated with tibial torsion

Test foot for flexibility and elicit tonic foot reflexes. Rigidity is indicated by eversion or inversion when foot does not move beyond neutral position or does not respond to toe grasping or by dorsiflexing. Signs of metatarsus adductus are illustrated in Figure K-5.

PES PLANUS (FLAT FEET)

When child is weight bearing, longitudinal arch of foot appears flat on floor

(1) Pseudo flat feet: very common until ages 2 to 3; created by plantar fat pad. Feet are flexible, exhibit hypermobility of joint, and have a low arch

1. Observe feet in weighted and unweighted position
2. Stand child on toes. Arch disappears with weight bearing in flexible flat foot and reappears when on toes. See Figure K-6.
3. Elicit dorsal and plantar flexion to rule out tight heel cord.
4. Elicit eversion and inversion flexion to rule out tarsal coalition.

(2) Rigid flat feet: Uncommon; created by tightness of heel cord or tarsal coalition (a cartilaginous fibrous or bony connection between bones)

Same as for preceding No. 1 (pseudo flat feet)

GENU VALGUM (KNOCK-KNEES)

A deviant axis of thighs and calves of more than 10 to 15 degrees; (normal from ages 2-6)

1. Observe axis of thighs and calves with child standing. Normally axis are parallel with 10 to 15 degrees deviance. See Figure K-7.
2. Observe space between the knees from front to back. Normal spacing is 1½ inches.
3. Observe space between ankles from front and back. Normal spacing between medial malleoli at heel is 2 inches.

GENU VARUM (BOWLEGS)

Deviant axis of thighs and calves which is

(1) Physiological: normal until ages 2 to 3; occurs with internal tibial torsion and genu valgum

(2) Pathological

Same for genu valgum

Continued.

Screening for common orthopedic problems in infancy and childhood—cont'd

Deformity	Screening

INTERNAL TIBIAL TORSION

Twisting or torsion of tibia usually accompanied by metatarsus adductus

1. Examine legs for range of motion, flexibility of ankle and elicit tonic foot reflexes.
2. Holding knee firmly with foot in neutral position, observe medial and lateral
   mallioli. The normal angle between them is approximately 15 to 20 degrees.
   See Figure K-8.
3. Have child sit on examining table and draw a circle over patellar and external
   mallioli. With patella facing forward only anterior edge of malleolar circle
   should be seen. See Figure K-9.

SCOLIOSIS

S-shaped lateral curvature of spine with
rotation of vertical bodies.

Screening is implemented as follows:
1. Ask the child to bend forward in a 50% flexing position with shoulders droop-
   ing forward, arms and head dangling. Observe the spine from above the head
   and inspect for any lateral curvature or prominent projection of the rib cage on
   one side (Figure K-10).
2. While the child is standing erect with weight equal on both feet, observe for
   Difference in levels of shoulders, scapula, and hips
   Differences in the size of the spaces between the arms and the trunk
   Prominence of either scapula or hip
   A curve in the vertebral spinous process alignment
3. Ask the child to walk and make observations discussed in No. 2 and observe
   for the presence of a waddle, limp, or tilt.

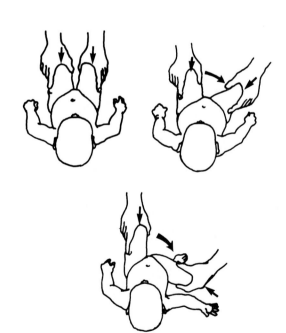

FIGURE K-2.

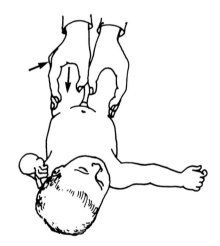

FIGURE K-1.

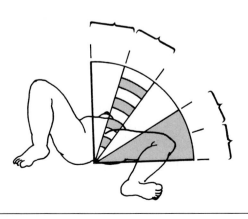

FIGURE K-3.

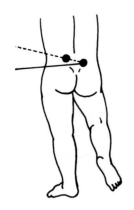

FIGURE K-4.

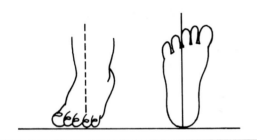

FIGURE K-5.

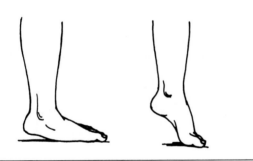

FIGURE K-6.

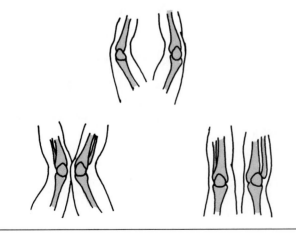

FIGURE K-7.

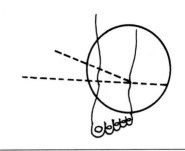

FIGURE K-8.

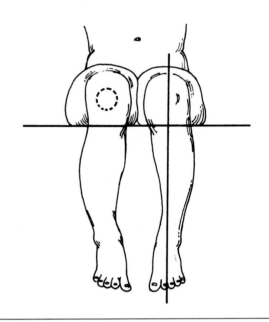

FIGURE K-9.

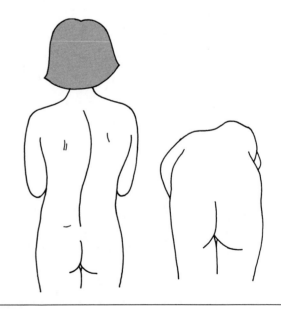

FIGURE K-10.

K6—DENVER ARTICULATION SCREENING EXAMINATION
(CHAPTER 28)

```
        DENVER ARTICULATION SCREENING EXAM          NAME
        for children 2 1/2 to 6 years of age
                                                    HOSP. NO.
   Instructions:  Have child repeat each word after
   you.  Circle the underlined sounds that he pro-  ADDRESS
   nounces correctly.  Total correct sounds is the
   Raw Score.  Use charts on reverse side to score
   results.
```

Date: _____ Child's Age: _____ Examiner: _____ Raw Score: _____
Percentile: _____ Intelligibility: _____ Result: _____

1. table	6. zipper	11. sock	16. wagon	21. leaf
2. shirt	7. grapes	12. vacuum	17. gum	22. carrot
3. door	8. flag	13. yarn	18. house	
4. trunk	9. thumb	14. mother	19. pencil	
5. jumping	10. toothbrush	15. twinkle	20. fish	

Intelligibility: (circle one)   1. Easy to understand   3. Not understandable
                                2. Understandable 1/2   4. Can't evaluate
                                   the time.

Comments:

Date: _____ Child's Age: _____ Examiner: _____ Raw Score _____
Percentile: _____ Intelligibility: _____ Result: _____

1. table	6. zipper	11. sock	16. wagon	21. leaf
2. shirt	7. grapes	12. vacuum	17. gum	22. carrot
3. door	8. flag	13. yarn	18. house	
4. trunk	9. thumb	14. mother	19. pencil	
5. jumping	10. toothbrush	15. twinkle	20. fish	

Intelligibility: (circle one)   1. Easy to understand   3. Not understandable
                                2. Understandable 1/2   4. Can't evaluate
                                   the time.

Comments:

Date: _____ Child's Age: _____ Examiner: _____ Raw Score _____
Percentile: _____ Intelligibility: _____ Result: _____

1. table	6. zipper	11. sock	16. wagon	21. leaf
2. shirt	7. grapes	12. vacuum	17. gum	22. carrot
3. door	8. flag	13. yarn	18. house	
4. trunk	9. thumb	14. mother	19. pencil	
5. jumping	10. toothbrush	15. twinkle	20. fish	

Intelligibility: (circle one)   1. Easy to understand   3. Not understandable
                                2. Understandable 1/2   4. Can't evaluate
                                   the time.

Comments:

To score DASE words: Note Raw Score for child's performance. Match raw score line (extreme left of chart) with column representing child's age (to the closest previous age group). Where raw score line and age column meet number in that square denotes percentile rank of child's performance when compared to other children that age. Percentiles above heavy line are ABNORMAL percentiles, below heavy line are NORMAL.

PERCENTILE RANK

Raw Score	2.5 yr.	3.0	3.5	4.0	4.5	5.0	5.5	6 years
2	1							
3	2							
4	5							
5	9							
6	16							
7	23							
8	31	2						
9	37	4	1					
10	42	6	2					
11	48	7	4					
12	54	9	6	1	1			
13	58	12	9	2	3	1	1	
14	62	17	11	5	4	2	2	
15	68	23	15	9	5	3	2	
16	75	31	19	12	5	4	3	
17	79	38	25	15	6	6	4	
18	83	46	31	19	8	7	4	
19	86	51	38	24	10	9	5	1
20	89	58	45	30	12	11	7	3
21	92	65	52	36	15	15	9	4
22	94	72	58	43	18	19	12	5
23	96	77	63	50	22	24	15	7
24	97	82	70	58	29	29	20	15
25	99	87	78	66	36	34	26	17
26	99	91	84	75	46	43	34	24
27		94	89	82	57	54	44	34
28		96	94	88	70	68	59	47
29		98	98	94	84	84	77	68
30		100	100	100	100	100	100	100

To Score intelligibility:

	NORMAL	ABNORMAL
2 1/2 years	Understandable 1/2 the time, or, "easy"	Not Understandable
3 years and older	Easy to understand	Understandable 1/2 time Not understandable

Test Result: 1. NORMAL on Dase and Intelligibility = NORMAL

2. ABNORMAL on Dase and/or Intelligibility = ABNORMAL

* If abnormal on initial screening rescreen within 2 weeks. If abnormal again child should be referred for complete speech evaluation.

K7—DEVELOPMENT CHARACTERISTICS: SUMMARY FOR CHILDREN
(CHAPTERS 28 and 29)

Waechter developmental guide: the first year

Age	Physical and motor development	Intellectual development	Socialization and vocalization	Emotional development
1 month	Physiologically more stable than in newborn period Wave hands as clenched fists Objects placed in hands are dropped immediately Momentary visual fixation on objects and human face Tonic neck reflex position frequent and Moro reflex brisk Able to turn head when prone, but unable to support head Responds to sounds of bell, rattle, etc. Makes crawling motions when prone Sucking and rooting reflex present Coordinates sucking, swallowing, and breathing	Reflexive No attempt to interact with environment External stimuli do not have meaning	Cries, mews, and makes throaty noises Responds in terms of internal need states Interested in the human face	Response limited generally to tension states Panic reactions, with arching of back and extension and flexion of extremities Derives satisfaction from the feeding situation when held and pleasure from rocking, cuddling, and tactile stimulation Maximum need for sucking pleasures Quiets when picked up
2 months	Moro reflex still brisk Posture still toward tonic neck reflex position Has visual response to patterns Eye coordination to light and objects Follows objects vertically and horizontally Responds to objects placed on face Listens actively to sounds Able to lift head momentarily from prone position Turns from side to back Able to swallow pureed foods	Recognition of familiar face Indicates inspection of the environment Begins to show anticipation before feeding	Begins to vocalize; coos Beginning of social smile Actively follows movement of familiar person or object with eyes Crying becomes differentiated Vocalizes to mother's voice Visually searches to locate sounds of mother's voice	Maximum need for sucking pleasures Indicates more active satisfaction when fed, held, rocked

From Waechter EH and Blake FG: Nursing care of children, ed 9, Philadelphia, 1976, JB Lippincott Co.

Continued.

Waechter developmental guide: the first year—cont'd

Age	Physical and motor development	Intellectual development	Socialization and vocalization	Emotional development
3 months	Frequency of tonic neck reflex position and vigor of Moro response rapidly diminishing Uses arms and legs simultaneously but not separately Able to raise head from prone position; may get chest off bed Holds head in fairly good control Begins differentiation of motor responses Hands are beginning to open, and objects placed in hands are retained for brief inspection; able to carry objects to mouth Indicates preference for prone or supine position "Stepping" reflex disappears Landau reflex appears Eyes converge as objects approach face Has necessary muscular control to accept cereal and fruit	Shows active interest in environment Can recognize familiar faces and objects such as bottle; however, objects do not have permanence Recognition is indicative of recording of memory traces Begins playing with parts of body Follows objects visually Begins to be able to coordinate stimuli from various sense organs Shows awareness of a strange situation	More ready and responsive smile Facial and generalized body response to faces Preferential response to adult voices Has longer periods of wakefulness without crying Begins to use prelanguage vocalizations, babbling and cooing Laughs aloud and shows pleasure in vocalization Shows anticipatory preparation to being lifted Turns head to follow familiar person Ceases crying when mother enters the room	Maximum need for sucking pleasure Wishes to avoid unpleasant situations Not yet able to act independently to evoke response in others
4 months	Ability to carry objects to mouth Inspects and plays with hands Grasps objects with both hands Turns head to sound of bell or bottle Reaches for offered objects Eyes focus on small objects Begins to demonstrate eye-hand coordination Ability to pick up objects Rooting reflex disappears; tonic neck reflex disappearing Sits with minimum support with stable head and back Turns from back to side	Recognizes bottle on sight Becomes bored when left alone for long periods of time Actively interested in environment Indicates beginnings of intentionality and interest in affecting the environment Indicates beginning anticipation of consequences of action	Vocalizes frequently and vocalizations change according to mood Begins to respond to "no, no" Enjoys being propped in a sitting position Turns head to familiar noise Chuckles socially Demands attention by fussing; enjoys attention	Interest in mother heightens Is affable and lovable Shows signs of increasing trust and security

Continued.

Waechter developmental guide: the first year—cont'd

Age	Physical and motor development	Intellectual development	Socialization and vocalization	Emotional development
	Breathing and mouth activity coordination in relation to vocal cords Holds head up when pulled to sitting position Begins to drool			
5 months	Ability to recover near objects Reaches persistently Grasps with whole hand Ability to lift objects Begins to use thumb and finger in "pincer" movement Able to sustain visual inspection Able to sit for longer periods of time when well supported Begins to show signs of tooth eruption Ability to sleep through night without feeding Moro reflex and tonic neck reflex finally disappear	Able to discriminate strangers from family Turns head after fallen object Shows active interest in novelty Attempts to regain interesting action in environment Ability to coordinate visual impressions of an object Begins differentiation of self from environment	Enjoys play with people and objects Smiles at mirror image More exuberantly playful but also more touchy and discriminating	Other members of the family become important as the baby's emotional world expands Begins to be able to postpone gratification Awaits anticipated routines with happy expectation Begins to explore mother's body
6 months	Ability to pick up small objects directly and deftly Ability to lift cup by handle Grasps, holds, and manipulates objects Ability to pull self to sitting position Begins to "hitch" in locomotion Momentary sitting and hand support When lying in prone position, supports weight with hands Weight gain begins to decline Ability to turn completely over	Increasing awareness of self Responds with attentiveness to novel stimuli Begins to be able to recognize mother when she is dressed differently Objects begin to acquire permanence; searches for lost object for brief period	Very interested in sound production Playful response to mirror Laughs aloud when stimulated Great interest in babbling, which is self-reinforcing Begins to recognize strangers	Begins to have sense of "self" Increased growth of ego
7 months	Ability to transfer objects from one hand to another Holds object in one hand Gums or mouths solid foods; exploratory behavior with food	Ability to secure objects by pulling on string Repeats activities that are enjoyed Discovers and plays with own feet Drops and picks up objects in exploration	Vocalizes four different syllables Produces vowel sounds and chained syllables Makes "talking sounds" in response to the talking of others Crows and squeals	Begins to show signs of fretfulness when mother leaves or in presence of strangers Shows beginning fear of strangers Orally aggressive in biting and mouthing

Continued.

Waechter developmental guide: the first year—cont'd

Age	Physical and motor development	Intellectual development	Socialization and vocalization	Emotional development
	Ability to bang objects together Palmar grasp disappears Bears weight when held in standing position Sits alone for brief periods Rolls over adeptly	Searches for lost objects outside perceptual field Has consciousness of desires Growing differentiation of self from environment Rudimentary sense of depth and space		
8 months	Ability to ring bell purposively Ability to feed self with finger foods Begins to experience tooth eruption Sits well alone Ability to release objects at will	Uncovers hidden toy Increased interest in feeding self Differentiation of means from end in intentionality Has lively curiosity about the world	Listens selectively to familiar words Says "da da" or equivalent Babbles to produce consonant sounds Vocalizes to toys Stretches out arms to be picked up	Plays for sheer pleasure of the activity Anxiety when confronted by strangers indicates recognition and need of mother; attachment behavior begins to be obvious and strong
9 months	Rises to sitting position Creeps and/or crawls; maybe backward at first Tries out newly developing motor capacities Ability to hold own bottle Drinks from cup or glass with assistance Begins to show regular patterns in bladder and bowel elimination Good ability to use thumb and finger in pincer grasp Pulls self to feet with help	Ability to put objects in container Examines object held in hand; explores objects by sucking, chewing, and biting	Responds to simple verbal requests Plays interactive games, such as peek-a-boo and patty cake	Mother is increasingly important for her own sake; reacts violently to threat of her loss Begins to show fears of going to bed and being left alone Increasing interest in pleasing mother Active search in play for solutions to separation anxiety
10 months	Ability to unwrap objects Pulls to standing position Uses index finger to poke and finger and thumb to hold objects Finger feeds self; controls lips around cup Plantar reflex disappears Neck-righting reflex disappears Sits without support; recovers balance easily Pulls self upright with use of furniture	Begins to imitate Looks at and follows pictures in book	Extends toy to another person without releasing Responds to own name Inhibits behavior to "no, no" or own name Begins to test reactions to parental responses during feeding and at bedtime Imitates facial expressions and sounds	Has powerful urge toward independence in locomotion, feeding; beginning to help in dressing Experiences joy when achieving a goal and mastering fear

Continued.

Waechter developmental guide: the first year—cont'd

Age	Physical and motor development	Intellectual development	Socialization and vocalization	Emotional developmental
11 months	Ability to hold crayon adaptively Ability to push toys Ability to put several objects in container; releases objects at will Stands with assistance; may be beginning attempts to walk with assistance Begins to be able to hold spoon "Cruises" around furniture	Works to get toy out of reach Growing interest in novelty Heightened curiosity and drive to explore environment	Repeats performance laughed at by others Imitates definite speech sounds Uses jargon Communicates by pointing to objects wanted	Reacts to restrictions with frustration, but has ability to master new situations with mother's help (weaning)
12 months	Turns pages in book; can make marks on paper Babinski sign disappears Begins standing alone and toddling "Cruises" around furniture Lumbar curve develops Hand dominance becomes evident Ability to use spoon in feeding	Dogged determination to remove barriers to action Further separation of means from ends Experiments to reach goals not attained previously Concepts of space, time, and causality begin to have more objectivity	Jabbers expressively Has words that are specific to parents Few, simple words Experimentation with "pseudo-words" of great interest and pleasure	Ability to show emotions of fear, anger, affection, jealousy, anxiety Is in love with the world
15-18 months	Uses spoon and cup with little spilling; builds 2-cube tower; can undress; has refined pincer grasp	Stoops and recovers; walks well; pushes furniture to climb; walks up stairs one at a time with assistance	Rolls ball back and forth with 1 other person; imitates household chores; indicates desires without crying; drinks from a cup	Vocabulary of 10 to 20 words; understands simple questions; forms 2-word phrases; beginning to name pictures
2 years	Builds a 6-cube tower; turns pages of a book one at a time; begins to dress self; washes and dries hands	Runs; walks up and down stairs alone; walks backwards; jumps in place; throws ball overhand	Removes clothes; awareness of ownership; helps out; eats with family but cannot sit through entire meal	Points to body parts; has 300-400 word vocabulary; uses "my" pronouns and prepositions; forms 3- to 4-word phrases
3 years	Opens and closes doors using knob by self; uses fingers to hold pencil; builds 8- to 10-block tower; zips zippers; does simple buttoning	Walks up and down stairs alternating feet; rides tricycle; broad jumps; dresses with assistance	May have imaginary playmates; can put on simple garment; washes and dries hands; likes to have a choice	Uses plurals; forms 3- to 4-word sentences, using correct grammatical structures
4 years	Draws a 3-part man; buttons easily; can cut out pictures	Catches ball with hands; broad jumps; climbs up and down stairs, alternating feet; balances on one foot momentarily	Separates easily from mother; can button clothing; plays interactive and associative games, demonstrating some control; able to share	Comprehends and uses opposites; has increased vocabulary and about 90% comprehensibility; speaks in full sentences, using prepositions, pronouns, adverbs, and adjectives
5 years	Copies a square accurately; draws a 5-part man; begins to tie shoelaces	Runs with speed and agility; dresses without supervision; skips crudely	Developing attachment outside of family; engages in cooperative play; strives for independence	Vocabulary expanding to 3-syllable words; composition increasing to spoken paragraphs

K8 — DEVELOPMENTAL BEHAVIORS: SCHOOL AGE CHILD
(CHAPTERS 28 and 29)

Age (years)	Physical competency	Intellectual competency	Emotional-social competency	Play	Safety
6–12 (General)	Gains an average of 2.5–3.2 kg/year (5½–7 lb/yr). Overall height gains of 5.5 cm (2 in) per year; growth occurs in spurts and is mainly in trunk and extremities. Loses deciduous teeth; most of permanent teeth erupt. Progressively more coordinated in both gross and fine motor skills. Caloric needs increase with growth spurts.	Masters concrete operations. Moves from egocentrism; learns he is not always right. Learns grammar and expression of emotions and thoughts. Vocabulary increases to 3000 words or more; handles complex sentences.	Central crisis: industry vs. inferiority; wants to do and make things. Progressive sex education needed. Wants to be like friends; competition important. Fears body mutilation, alterations in body image; earlier phobias may recur; nightmares; fears death. Nervous habits common.	Plays in groups, mostly of same sex; "gang" activities predominate. Books for all ages. Bicycles a must. Sports equipment. Cards, board, and table games. Most of play is active games requiring little or no equipment.	Enforce continued use of safety belts during car travel. Bicycle safety must be taught and enforced. Teach safety related to hobbies, handicrafts, mechanical equipment.
6–7	Depth perception developed. Vision reaches adult level of 20/20. Gross motor skill exceeds fine motor coordination. Balance and rhythm are good — runs, skips, jumps, climbs, gallops. Throws and catches ball. Dresses self with little or no help.	Vocabulary of 2500 words. Learning to read and print; beginning concrete concepts of numbers, general classification of items. Knows concepts of right and left; morning, afternoon, and evening; coinage. Intuitive thought process. Verbally aggressive, bossy, opinionated, argumentative. Likes simple games with basic rules.	Boisterous, outgoing, and know-it-all, whiney; parents should sidestep power struggles; offer choices. Becomes quiet and reflective during 7th year; very sensitive. Can use telephone. Likes to make things: starts many, finishes few. Give some responsibility for household duties.	Still enjoys dolls, cars, and trucks. Plays well alone but enjoys small groups of both sexes; begins to prefer same sex peer during seventh year. Ready to learn how to ride a bicycle. Prefers imaginary, dramatic play with real costumes. Begins collecting for quantity, not quality. Enjoys active games such as hide-and-seek, tag, jump rope, roller skating, kickball. Ready for lessons in dancing, gymnastics, music. Restrict TV time to 1-2 hours/day.	Teach and reinforce traffic safety. Still needs adult supervision of play. Teach to avoid strangers, never take anything from strangers. Teach cold prevention and reinforce continued practice of other health habits. Restrict bicycle use to home ground; no traffic areas; teach bicycle safety. Teach and set examples regarding harmful use of drugs, alcohol, smoking.

Age	Physical	Intellectual/Language	Social	Activities	Safety
8-10	Myopia may appear. Secondary sex characteristics begin in girls. Hand-eye coordination and fine motor skills well established. Movements are graceful, coordinated. Cares for own physical needs completely. Constantly on move; plays and works hard; enforce balance in rest and activity. Vision and hearing fully developed.	Learning correct grammar and to express feelings in words. Likes books he can read by himself; will read funny papers, scan newspaper. Enjoys making detailed drawings. Mastering classification, seriation, spatial and temporal, numerical concepts. Uses language as a tool; likes riddles, jokes, chants, word games. Rules guiding force in life now. Very interested in how things work, what and how weather, seasons, etc., are made.	Strong preference for same-sex peers; antagonizes opposite-sex peers. Self-assured and pragmatic at home; questions parental values and ideas. Has a strong sense of humor. Enjoys clubs, group projects, outings, large groups, camp. Modesty about own body increases over time; sex conscious. Works diligently to perfect skills he does best. Happy, cooperative, relaxed and casual in relationships. Increasingly courteous and well-mannered with adults. Gang stage at a peak; secret codes and rituals prevail. Responds better to suggestion than dictatorial approach.	Likes hiking, sports. Enjoys cooking, woodworking, crafts. Enjoys cards and table games. Likes radio and records. Begins qualitative collecting now. Continue restriction on TV time.	Stress safety with firearms. Keep them out of reach and allow use only with adult supervision. Know who the child's friends are; parents should still have some control over friend selection. Teach water safety; swimming should be supervised by an adult.
11-12	Vital signs approximate adult norms. Growth spurt for girls; inequalities between sexes increasingly noticeable; boys attain greater physical strength. Eruption of permanent teeth complete except for third molars. Secondary sex characteristics begin in boys. Menstruation may begin.	Able to think about social problems and prejudices; sees others' points of view. Enjoys reading mysteries, love stories. Begins playing with abstract ideas. Interested in whys of health measures and understands human reproduction. Very moralistic; religious commitment often made during this time.	Intense team loyalty; boys begin teasing girls and girls flirt with boys for attention; best friend period. Wants unreasonable independence. Rebellious about routines; wide mood swings; needs some times daily for privacy. Very critical of own work. Hero worship prevails. "Facts of life" chats with friends prevail; masturbation increases. Appears under constant tension.	Enjoys projects and working with hands. Likes to do errands and jobs to earn money. Very involved in sports, dancing, talking on phone. Enjoys all aspects of acting and drama.	Continue monitoring friends; Stress bicycle safety on streets and in traffic.

Adapted from Smith EC: Growth and developement of school age child: maintaining wellness. In Foster R, Hunsberger M, and Anderson J: Family centered care of children and adolescents, Philadelphia, ed. 2. 1989, WB Saunders Co.

K9—SOURCES OF SCREENING AND ASSESSMENT TOOLS/RESOURCES
(CHAPTERS 28, 29, and 32)

AAMD Adaptive Behavior Scale for Children and Adults, 1974 Revision
AAMD Adaptive Behavior Scale Public School Version
Source: American Association for Mental Deficiencies
5101 Wisconsin Avenue, NW
Washington, DC 30016

The Denver Articulation Screening Examination (DASE) by AF Drumwright (2½-6 years)
Source: LADOCA Project and Publishing Foundation
East 51st Avenue and Lincoln Street
Denver, CO 80216

The Denver Developmental Screening Test (DDST) by WK Frankenberg, JB Dodds, A Fandal, E Kazuk, and M Cohrs (birth to 6 years)
Source: LADOCA Project and Publishing Foundation
East 51st Avenue and Lincoln Street
Denver, CO 80216

The Developmental Profile II by GD Alpern, TJ Boll, and M.S. Shearer (birth to 9 years)
Source: Psychological Development Publications
PO Box 3198
Aspen, CO 81612

Education for Multi-handicapped Infants (EMI)
Source: Department of Pediatrics
University of Virginia
Box 232
Charlottesville, VA 22908

The Goodenough Draw-A-Person Test by R Goodenough (3-10 years)
Source: Psychological Corporation
7500 Old Oak Boulevard
Cleveland, OH 44130

Hawaii Early Learning Profile Activity Guide
Source: Vort Corporation
PO Box 60132
Palo Alto, CA 94306

Home Observation for Measurement of the Environment (HOME), B. Caldwell (birth to 3 years, 3-6 years)
Source: Center for Early Development and Education
University of Arkansas
814 Sherman Street
Little Rock, AR 72202

Meeting Street School Screening Test—Early Identification of Children with Learning Disabilities, PK Hainsworth and ML Siqueland (5-7 years, 6 months)
Source: Crippled Children and Adults of Rhode Island, Inc.
Meeting Street School
333 Grotto School
Providence, RI 02906

Sibling Information Network School of Education
Resources: Association for the Care of Children's Health
3615 Wisconsin Avenue, NW
Washington, DC 20016

Recreation Ranch, Inc.
PO Box 292
Signal Mountain, TN 37377

Nursing Child Assessment Satellite Training Developed by K. Barnard
Source: Georgina Sumner
NCAST
WJ-10
University of Washington
Seattle, WA 98195

Peabody Individual Achievement Test (PIAT), LM Dunn and F.C. Markwardt, (2 years, 6 months-18 years)
Source: American Guidance Service, Inc.
Circle Pines, MN 55014

The Portage Guide to Early Education, S Blumar The Portage Project; Cooperative Educational Service—Agency Twelve
Source: The Portage Project
412 East Slifer Street
Portage, WI 53901

Slosson Intelligence Test (SIT), RL Slosson (birth to adult)
Source: Western Psychological Services
Publishers and Distributors
12031 Wilshire Boulevard
Los Angeles, CA 90025

Vineland Social Maturity Scale, EA Doll (birth to adult)
Source: American Guidance Services, Inc.
Circle Pines, MN 55014

Washington Guide to Child Development
Source: Utah Department of Health
Family Health Services Division
Bureau of Maternal and Child Health
44 Medical Drive
Salt Lake City, UT 84113

APPENDIX

L1—PLANNING METHODS AND EVALUATION MODELS
(Chapter 12)

After the need and demand for a program have been determined through the needs assessment process, the next in the development of the program is to choose a procedural method that will assist the community health nurse in planning the program to be offered. The following is offered for students who are more advanced in their career and need to consider several methods of program planning plus more extensive evaluation models for program management.

Five planning methods are discussed in this appendix: (1) the Planning, Programming, and Budgeting System, (2) the Program Planning Method, (3) the Program Evaluation Review Technique, (4) the Critical Path Method, and (5) the Multi-Attribute Utility Method.

PPM and PPBS are more general approaches to program planning, whereas PERT, CPM, and MAUT offer guidelines for identifying and tracking specific program activities essential to program success. All of these approaches establish the basis for program evaluation.

Planning, Programming, and Budgeting System

Planning, Programming, and Budgeting System (PPBS) is a procedural tool initially developed for use by the Department of Defense and other governmental agencies. PPBS is an outcome-oriented accounting system, the effect of which is to determine the most efficient method of resource allocation to attain measurable objectives.

The steps involved in PPBS are (1) setting program goals, (2) defining measurable program objectives, (3) identifying and evaluating alternatives to accomplish program objectives (4) choosing the method for accomplishing the objectives, and (5) developing a program budget with justification for minimizing costs while maximizing program benefits (Figure L-1).

PPBS is an economic method of describing a program plan. In PPBS, *planning* represents formulation of objectives and conceptualization or identification of alternatives and methods for accomplishing objectives; *programming* represents detailing of resources (personnel, facilities, equipment, and financing) for each identified alternative; and *budgeting* represents the assignment of dollar values to resources required for the program implementation, or the evaluation of program costs and benefits.

PPBS is widely used for planning broad-scale governmental programs. It is a system that can also be used to plan programs for an agency or for client groups. For ex-

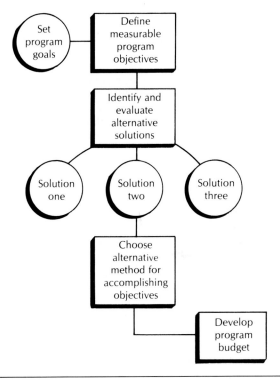

FIGURE L-1

Planning, programming, and budgeting system.

ample, PPBS could be used to develop the annual program plan for the health department or a prenatal program for the local community. A community health nurse could also use this method to develop a health education program for the school population on sexually transmitted diseases. PPBS's use of objectives that are operationally defined by nursing standards or performance criteria is a system that lends itself to effective program evaluation.

Program Planning Method

PPM, or Program Planning Method, is a technique employing the nominal group technique of Delbecq and Van de Van (1971). It can be used by the community health nurse to involve clients more directly in the planning process. This is a five-stage process to identify program needs and focuses on three levels of planning groups comprised of clients, providers, and administrators. The client or consumer group relays a list of problems to the provider group, who in turn aids the client group in presenting the solution to the problem to the administrative group (Nutt, 1984).

The stages of PPM are compared with Nutt's planning process in Table L-1. The *PPM stage one* involves problem

TABLE L-1
Planning methods compared with basic planning process

Basic planning	PPBS	PPM	PERT/CPM	MAUT
1. Formulation	Identify goals and define in measurable terms	Problems identified by client	Identify program activities	Identify target population and program objectives
2. Conceptualization	Identify alternatives	Provider group identifies solution	Explore time and events required to meet program activities	Identify alternative problem solutions
3. Detailing	Evaluate alternatives for use of resources	Analyze available solutions	Determine sequencing of events and resources to meet activities	Identify criteria for choice; rank, rate, and weight; calculate value
4. Evaluation	Choose method for accomplishing objectives and develop budget to evaluate costs vs. benefits	Clients, providers, administrators select best plan	Select appropriate events	Choose best alternatives
5. Implementation		Best plan presented to administrators for funding		

diagnosis. Each client in the group works with all other members of the group to develop a written problem list, one problem at a time. After all problems have been shared and recorded, they are discussed by the total client group. Following the discussion, clients select the problems with the highest priority by voting on the ranking of each problem.

In the *second stage* of PPM the expert provider group identifies solutions for each of the problems identified by the clients. In the *third stage* the client and provider groups present their problems and suggested solutions to the administrative group to determine the possibilities of developing a program to meet one or more of the problems, using one or more of the solutions. In this phase, clients and providers are seeking acceptance from the administrators who control the program resources. *Phase four* of PPM involves identifying the alternative solutions to the problem and analyzing the pros and cons of each. *Phase five* involves the client, providers, and administrators in selecting the best plan for program implementation. In this phase the link between the planned solutions and the problem are evaluated, pointing out strengths and limitations of the proposed program plan.

The community health nurse may use this technique for developing school health services within the total community or in one school. This method may also be used by the nurse working with a senior citizens group to identify their priority needs for nursing or physician clinic services at the health department. It is important to note that this method is used to get consensus among all persons involved in the program—clients, providers, and administrators. Consensus is most helpful in having a successful program.

Program Evaluation Review Technique

The *Program Evaluation Review Technique (PERT)* is a network programming method developed in the 1950s through a joint effort of the United States Navy, Lockheed Aircraft Corporation, and Booz-Allen and Hamilton, Inc. The method was developed for planning and controlling the program activities involved in developing the Polaris missile.

The PERT method is primarily useful for large-scale projects that require planning, scheduling, and controlling a large number of activities. PERT is mentioned here to introduce the reader to the concept of network planning. PERT as a planning method has been used successfully in hospitals to plan for the development of nursing services such as primary care services, and for designing projects such as the installation and use of computers for organizing and providing nursing services.

The major objectives of PERT are to (1) focus attention on the key developmental parts of a program; (2) identify potential program problems that could interfere with movement toward program goals; (3) evaluate program progress toward goal attainment; (4) provide a prompt reporting method; and (5) facilitate decision-making (Nutt, 1984).

PERT involves the concepts of time and events. The basic tool used in the technique is the network or flow plan, which is a series of circles, ovals, or squares representing the program events, or goals, and their interrelationships with the activities of the program. The program activities are the time-consuming events of the program and are represented by arrows that connect the program accomplishments or goals (Figure L-2). Note in the flow plan that it may take several activities to attain a program event (goal) and that some events (goals) must be accomplished before other events may be attained. The interrelationship of several program events (subgoals) may be essential to attain the ultimate program event (goal).

Another element in PERT is the estimate of the time it will take to implement activities leading to program goals.

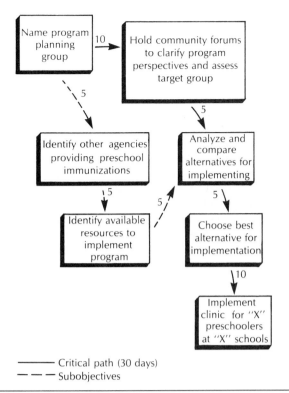

Name program planning group → 10 → Hold community forums to clarify program perspectives and assess target group

Name program planning group ⤏ 5 ⤏ Identify other agencies providing preschool immunizations

Hold community forums to clarify program perspectives and assess target group → 5 → Analyze and compare alternatives for implementing

Identify other agencies providing preschool immunizations → 5 → Identify available resources to implement program

Identify available resources to implement program ⤏ 5 ⤏ Analyze and compare alternatives for implementing

Analyze and compare alternatives for implementing → 5 → Choose best alternative for implementation

Choose best alternative for implementation → 10 → Implement clinic for "X" preschoolers at "X" schools

——— Critical path (30 days)
– – – Subobjectives

FIGURE L-2

Simplified PERT network for planning a preschool immunization program. Numbers represent days required for completion of activities.

In PERT, three estimates of activity time are given: the optimistic time it will take to complete activities, given minimal difficulties; the most likely time it will take to complete activities, given past experiences with normal development of such activities; and the pessimistic time it will take to complete activities, given maximum difficulties. From the time estimates, a simple formula can be applied to indicate the probability of completing a project in a given time period (Barentson, 1970; Roman, 1969; Wiest and Levy, 1969). The numbers appearing along the arrows in Figure L-2 are the estimated numbers of days required for completion of activities leading to a particular event.

PERT embodies three major steps: (1) identification of specific program activities, (2) identification of resources to accomplish the activities, and (3) determination of sequencing activities for the accomplishment of program events.

Critical Path Method

Critical Path Method (CPM) is a network programming planning method that is described by some authors as a technique in itself and by others as an element of PERT.

CPM is a technique that focuses the program planner's attention on the program activities, the sequencing of activities for the best use of time and resources, and the estimated time it will take to complete the project from beginning to end. Using this method the planner can determine the amount of time it will take to accomplish each activity and can identify those activities that may take longer. The planner can then determine the amounts of resources needed

(personnel, money, facilities, and supplies) to accomplish tasks at given points in time along the program's "critical path."

CPM allows for frequent review of progress by program planners. Problems can be identified early in the program implementation, and corrective action can be taken or alternative activities can be substituted for activities that are not meeting program requirements. The amount of time and resources being used during program implementation can be assessed, and time and resources can be increased or decreased as necessary and can be compared to initial estimates of program need.

Hospital nursing services are beginning to use CPM to develop protocols for caring for clients with specific health problems, (e.g., breast cancer or hypertension). The CPM protocols identify the estimated number of days the client will be in the hospital and nursing care activities for each day the client is hospitalized, from admission to discharge. Nurses must document reasons why activities may not have been accomplished. These notes are used to change nursing care plans and set new goals for clients.

PERT and CPM embody the five generic stages of planning described by Nutt. However, these two methods focus on specific activities, times, and events essential to program success. The emphasis in these two models is on detailing and evaluation (Table L-1).

The Multi-Attribute Technique

The *Multi-Attribute Utility Technique (MAUT)* is a planning method based on decision theory (Edwards, Guttentag, and Snapper, 1975). This method can be adapted for making decisions about the care of a single client or about national health care programs. The purpose of MAUT is to separate all elements of a decision and to evaluate each element separately for its impact on the overall decision.

Ten basic steps to MAUT method are described by Edwards, Guttentag, and Snapper (1975):

1. *Identify the person or aggregate whose utilities are to be maximized.* In other words, who is the client for whom the program is being planned?
2. *Identify the issue(s) or decision(s) to which the utilities are relevant.* This step involves the identification of the program objectives.
3. *Identify the entities to be evaluated.* The program planner identifies the available options or action alternatives to accomplish the program goals.
4. *Identify the relevant dimensions of value.* The program planner places a value on competing options or alternatives or identifies criteria to be considered to make a choice between them.
5. *Rank the value dimensions in order of importance.* The program planner will decide which of the criteria are most important and which are least important for meeting program goals.
6. *Rate dimensions in importance.* In this step the program planner assigns an arbitrary rating of 10 to the least important criteria. In considering the next least important criteria, the planner decides how many times more important it is than the least important criteria. If it is considered twice as important, the

dimension will be assigned a 20. If it is only considered half again as important, it will be assigned a 15. If it is considered four times as important, it will be assigned a 40. The process is continued until all dimensions have been rated.

7. *Add the importance rate, divide each by the sum, and multiply by 100.* Edwards refers to this process as "normalizing" the weights. This is considered a purely mechanical step that provides the program planner with a clearer picture of the relative values of the criteria. However, if too many criteria are identified in Step 4, the computational process underestimates the value of some actions and overestimates the value of others. To avoid this problem, it is recommended that the number of criteria be kept between 6 and 15. Therefore, in this initial process the planner can be concerned with only general criteria for choosing action alternatives.

8. *Measure the location of the entity being evaluated on each dimension.* The planner may ask a colleague or expert to estimate on a scale of 0 to 100 the probability that a given option from Step 3 will maximize the value of the criteria from Step 4. An option thought to have a low probability of meeting the criteria may be assigned a value of 20, whereas an option thought to have a high probability may be assigned a value of 80.

9. *Calculate utilities for entities.* The program planner will obtain the usefulness of each identified action alternative by multiplying the weight for each criterion (Step 7) by the rating of an option for each criterion (Step 8) and adding the products. The sum of the products for each action is termed the aggregate utility.

10. *Decide on best alternative to meet program objective.* The action alternative with the highest aggregate utility is considered the best decision for meeting the program objectives. If cost was not considered as one of the criteria on which to evaluate the action alternatives, then the usefulness of each option may need to be considered in relation to cost.

If money is no object, then the option with the highest utility is the best decision. However, if the highest utility option exceeds the budget, the next highest utility option may be the alternative to choose. An example of the application of MAUT to a program decision in community health nursing is given at the end of this discussion. The steps of MAUT relate closely to the basic planning process described by Nutt (1984) as shown in Table L-1.

Steps 1 and 2 of MAUT relate to problem formulation. Step 3 involves conceptualization of the program alternatives, and Steps 4 through 9 focus on detailing and the implications of each option. Step 10 involves the evaluation phase of planning or the choice of the best solution as identified in Steps 4 through 9. Placing quantitative values on solutions to meet program needs is most helpful in the implementation phase of planning (e.g., convincing administrators of the need for such a program). However, caution must be taken in using all planning methods since the best solution reflects the bias of the planner.

Evaluation Models and Techniques
Structure-Process-Outcome Evaluation

The method for evaluation of programs by Donabedian (1982) was initially directed primarily toward medical care but is applicable to the broader area of health care. He described three approaches to assessment of health care: structure, process, and outcome.

Structure refers to settings in which care occurs and includes materials, equipment, qualification of the staff, and organizational structure (Donabedian, 1982). This approach to evaluation is based on the assumption that, given a proper setting with good equipment, good care will follow; but this assumption is not strongly supported.

Process refers to whether the care that was given was "good" (Donabedian, 1982), competent, or preferential. Use of process in program evaluation may consist of observation of practice but more likely consists of review of records. The review may focus on pathology reports to ascertain whether the number of surgeries was strongly indicated or questionable. The review could focus on whether documentation of preventive teaching was on the clinical record. Audits using specific criteria are examples of the use of process.

Outcome refers to client recovery and restoration of function and survival (Donabedian, 1982) but is also used in the sense of changes in health status or changes in health-related knowledge, attitude, and behavior. Thus program outcomes may be expressed in terms of mortality, morbidity, and disability for given populations, such as infants, but could be expressed in a broader sense through health promotion behaviors such as weight control, exercise, and abstinence from tobacco and alcohol.

Donabedian (1982) supports the use of the process approach when possible, followed by outcome, and then by structure. Process and outcome are used more than structure in the evaluation of care. Donabedian's model of evaluating program quality is a popular model and is widely used for evaluation in the health care field. It can be useful in evaluating program effectiveness. Health Care Financing Administration and other third party payers are currently placing more emphasis on outcome evaluation. It is essential that nurses begin to develop outcome criteria for client interventions.

Tracer Method

The board on Medicine of the National Academy of Sciences developed a program to evaluate health service delivery called the tracer method (Kessner and Kalk, 1973). The *tracer method* of evaluation of programs is based on the premise that health status and care can be evaluated by viewing specific health problems called "tracers." Just as radioactive tracers are used to study the thyroid gland, specific health problems are selected to evaluate the delivery of health and nursing services. Examples of conditions selected as tracers are middle ear infection and associated hearing loss, vision disorders, iron deficiency anemia, hypertension, urinary tract infections, and cervical cancer. This program can be used to (1) compare health status among different population groups, (2) compare health status in relation to social, economic, medical care, nursing care, and behavioral variables, and (3) compare various arrangements for health care delivery. The application of this method to the study of health care for children has been reported by Kessner and Kalk (1973) and is discussed by Veney and Kaluzny (1984).

The tracer method is a useful technique for looking at efficiency, effectiveness, and impact of a program. Stevens (1975) has developed a method for evaluating nursing care that is similar to the tracer method (see Chapter 12).

Systems Model

The systems model of evaluation focuses on the process as a working model or social unit capable of achieving the goal (Schulberg, et al., 1969; Shortell, 1978; Liturack, 1985). This *systems model* is concerned with objectives being achieved, subunits functioning in coordination, resources being maintained, and adaptation to the environment. The systems model examines aspects other than the goal; it recognizes that organizations have multiple goals and considers single goal attainment in relation to its effects on other goals in the system.

Three variables are described and evaluated in the systems model: input, throughput, and output. *Input* consists of characters and conditions of people and the resources. *Throughput* refers to the human and nonhuman resources and process. *Output* refers to the products of the system. The systems model is more comprehensive, since it takes more elements into consideration for the evaluation.

Case Register

Systematic registration of contagious disease has been a practice for many years. Denmark began a national register of tuberculosis in 1921 (Horwitz, 1979). Its contribution to the reduction in the incidence of contagious diseases has been widely recognized (Clemesen, 1979). *Case registers* are also used for acute and chronic disease (e.g., cancer and myocardial infarction).

Registers collate information from defined groups, and the information may be used for evaluation and planning of services, disease prevention, provision of care, and monitoring changes in patterns and care of diseases (Holland and Karhausen, 1979). The method is described here because of its use in evaluation of services. Information obtained by the community registers in Europe on myocardial infarction is a good example of the way a case register is used (Keil, 1979). The following are questions that were asked about cases of myocardial infarction for the community registers:

1. What is the incidence of disease? What differences in incidence are there between one community and another?
2. What percentage of clients recover? What percentage die?
3. Where does death occur?
4. How long do clients wait before calling a doctor?
5. How long is it before they see a doctor?
6. How many cases are associated with other major risk factors?
7. How many cases are associated with environmental factors such as water hardness or air pollution?
8. What happens after clients leave the hospital and when they return to work? Are there rehabilitation programs?
9. How many had been seen by a physician shortly before the problem occurred?
10. What prevention measures are taken for persons considered susceptible?

The answers to these questions before and after implementation of a given program would give information about the impact of the program. A tuberculosis register indicates the degree to which infection is being controlled. Cancer registers make state, regional, national, and international comparisons possible, and they provide clues to causes of disease.

Goal Attainment

Goal attainment refers to a process of assessing the efficacy of a program by examination or measurement of the predetermined goals (Kiresuk and Sander, 1979). LaPatra (1975) described the components of the *goal attainment* model as setting objectives, setting measures of the objectives, collecting data, assessing the effect, and modifying the initial objective on the basis of the data analysis and interpretation. Rossi and Freeman refer to this model as goal attainment scaling (1984). The following model by Shields is an example of a goal attainment model. Shields (1974) applied a process to each goal. For each goal the evaluator examines the categories of wherewithal, structure, operations, and outcomes.

Wherewithal refers to resources, materials, equipment, and physical facilities.

Structure consists of the organizational framework (i.e., administrative structure, lines of authority, committee linkages, and patterns of communication).

Operations pertains to the processes and procedures for carrying out the program goals whether they are teaching, treating, or preventing, as well as the performance of the workers doing the processes.

Outcomes refers to whether the goal was attained, to what degree it was attained, and to other significant events related to the outcome.

The criteria applied to outcomes are: (1) effectiveness— whether the immediate purpose was attained; (2) efficiency—how cost efficient the program was; and (3) impact—whether unexpected and potentially harmful events were associated with the program. If the program has more than one goal, the evaluation process is applied to each goal.

Year 2000: National Health Objectives

1. Physical Activity and Fitness
Health Status Objectives

1.1 Reduce coronary heart disease deaths to no more than 100 per 100,000 people.

1.2 Reduce overweight to a prevalence of no more than 20% among people aged 20 and older and no more than 15% among adolescents aged 12 through 19.

Risk Reduction Objectives

1.3 Increase to at least 30% the proportion of people aged 6 and older who engage regularly, preferably daily, in light to moderate physical activity for at least 30 minutes per day.

1.4 Increase to at least 20% the proportion of people aged 18 and older and to at least 75% the proportion of children and adolescents aged 6 through 17 who engage in vigorous physical activity that promotes the development and maintenance of cardiorespiratory fitness 3 or more days per week for 20 or more minutes per occasion.

1.5 Reduce to no more than 15% the proportion of people aged 6 and older who engage in no leisure-time physical activity.

1.6 Increase to at least 40% the proportion of people aged 6 and older who regularly perform physical activities that enhance and maintain muscular strength, muscular endurance, and flexibility.

1.7 Increase to at least 50% the proportion of overweight people aged 12 and older who have adopted sound dietary practices combined with regular physical activity to attain appropriate body weight.

Services and Protection Objectives

1.8 Increase to at least 50% the proportion of children and adolescents in first through twelfth grade who participate in daily school physical education.

1.9 Increase to at least 50% the portion of school physical education class time that students spend being physically active, preferably in lifetime physical activities.

1.10 Increase the proportion of worksites offering employer-sponsored activity and fitness programs.

1.11 Increase community availability and accessibility of physical activity and fitness facilities.

1.12 Increase to at least 50% the proportion of primary care providers who routinely assess and counsel their pa-

tients regarding the frequency, duration, type, and intensity of each patient's physical activity practices.

2. Nutrition
Health Status Objectives

2.1 Reduce coronary heart disease deaths to no more than 100 per 100,000 people.

2.2 Reverse the rise in cancer deaths to achieve a rate of no more than 130 per 100,000 people.

2.3 Reduce overweight to a prevalence of no more than 20% among people aged 20 and older and no more than 15% among adolescents aged 12 through 19.

2.4 Reduce growth retardation among low-income children aged 5 and younger to less than 10%.

Risk Reduction Objectives

2.5 Reduce dietary fat intake to an average of 30% of calories or less and average saturated fat intake to less than 10% of calories among people aged 2 and older.

2.6 Increase complex carbohydrate and fiber-containing foods in the diets of adults to five or more daily servings for vegetables (including legumes) and fruits, and to six or more daily servings for grain products.

2.7 Increase to at least 50% the proportion of overweight people aged 12 and older who have adopted sound dietary practices combined with regular physical activity to attain appropriate body weight.

2.8 Increase calcium intake so at least 50% of youth aged 12 through 24 and 50% of pregnant and lactating women consume 3 or more servings daily of foods rich in calcium, and at least 50% of people aged 25 and older consume two or more servings daily.

2.9 Decrease salt and sodium intake so at least 65% of home meal preparers prepare foods without adding salt, at least 80% of people avoid using salt at the table, and at least 40% of adults regularly purchase foods modified or lower in sodium.

2.10 Reduce iron deficiency to less than 3% among children aged 1 through 4 and among women of childbearing age.

2.11 Increase to at least 75% the proportion of mothers who breastfeed their babies in the early postpartum period and to at least 50% the proportion who continue breastfeeding until their babies are 5 to 6 months old.

2.12 Increase to at least 75% the proportion of parents and caregivers who use feeding practices that prevent baby tooth decay.

2.13 Increase to at least 85% the proportion of people aged 18 and older who use food labels to make nutritious food selections.

From USDHHS: Healthy People 2000: National Health Promotion and Disease Prevention Objectives, Pub No. (PHS)91-50213, 1990. US Government Printing Office, Washington, DC.

Services and Protection Objectives

2.14 Achieve useful and informative nutrition labeling for virtually all processed foods and at least 40% of fresh meats, poultry, fish, fruits, vegetables, baked goods, and ready-to-eat carry-away foods.

2.15 Increase to at least 5000 brand items the availability of processed food products that are reduced in fat and saturated fat.

2.16 Increase to at least 90% the proportion of restaurants and institutional food service operations that offer identifiable low-fat, low-calorie food choices, consistent with the *Dietary Guidelines for Americans*.

2.17 Increase to at least 90% the proportion of school lunch and breakfast services and child care food services with menus that are consistent with the nutrition principles in the *Dietary Guidelines for Americans*.

2.18 Increase to at least 80% the receipt of home food services by people aged 65 and older who have difficulty in preparing their own meals or are otherwise in need of home-delivered meals.

2.19 Increase to at least 75% the proportion of the nation's schools that provide nutrition education from preschool through 12th grade, preferably as part of quality school health education.

2.20 Increase to at least 50% the proportion of worksites with 50% or more employees that offer nutrition education and/or weight management programs for employees.

2.21 Increase to at least 75% the proportion of primary care providers who provide nutrition assessment and counseling and/or referral to qualified nutritionists or dietitians.

3. Tobacco
Health Status Objectives

3.1 Reduce coronary heart disease deaths to no more than 100 per 100,000 people.

3.2 Slow the rise in lung cancer deaths to achieve a rate of no more than 42 per 100,000 people.

3.3 Slow the rise in deaths from chronic obstructive pulmonary disease to achieve a rate of no more than 25 per 100,000 people.

Risk Reduction Objectives

3.4 Reduce cigarette smoking to a prevalence of no more than 15% among people aged 20 and older.

3.5 Reduce the initiation of cigarette smoking by children and youth so that no more than 15% have become regular smokers by age 20.

3.6 Increase to at least 50% the proportion of cigarette smokers aged 18 and older who stopped smoking cigarettes for at least one day during the preceding year.

3.7 Increase smoking cessation during pregnancy so that at least 60% of women who are cigarette smokers at the time they become pregnant quit smoking early in pregnancy and maintain abstinence for the remainder of their pregnancy.

3.8 Reduce to no more than 20% the proportion of children aged 6 and younger who are regularly exposed to tobacco smoke at home.

3.9 Reduce smokeless tobacco use by males aged 12 through 24 to a prevalence of no more than 4%.

Services and Protection Objectives

3.10 Establish tobacco-free environments and include tobacco-use prevention in the curricula of all elementary, middle, and secondary schools, preferably as part of quality school health education.

3.11 Increase to at least 75% the proportion of worksites with a formal smoking policy that prohibits or severely restricts smoking in the workplace.

3.12 Enact in all 50 states comprehensive laws on clean indoor air that prohibit or strictly limit smoking in the workplace and enclosed public places (including health care facilities, schools, and public transportation).

3.13 Enact and enforce in all 50 states laws prohibiting the sale and distribution of tobacco products to youths under age 19.

3.14 Increase to 50 the number of states with plans to reduce tobacco use, especially among youth.

3.15 Eliminate or severely restrict all forms of tobacco product advertising and promotion to which youths under age 18 are likely to be exposed.

3.16 Increase to at least 75% the proportion of primary care and oral health care providers who routinely advise cessation and provide assistance and follow-up for all of their tobacco-using patients.

4. Alcohol and Other Drugs
Health Status Objectives

4.1 Reduce deaths caused by alcohol-related motor vehicle crashes to no more than 8.5 per 100,00 people.

4.2 Reduce cirrhosis deaths to no more than 6 per 100,000 people.

4.3 Reduce drug-related deaths to nso more than 3 per 100,000 people.

4.4 Reduce hospital emergency department visits related to drug abuse by at least 20%.

Risk Reduction Objectives

4.5 Increase by at least 1 year the average age of first use of cigarettes, alcohol, and marijuana by adolescents ages 12 through 17.

4.6 Reduce the proportion of young people who have used alcohol, marijuana, and cocaine in the past month.

4.7 Reduce the proportion of high school seniors and college students engaging in recent occasions of heavy drinking of alcoholic beverages to no more than 28% of high school seniors and 32% of college students.

4.8 Reduce alcohol consumption by people aged 14 and older to an annual average of no more than 2 gallons of ethanol per person.

4.9 Increase the proportion of high school seniors who perceive social disapproval associated with heavy use of alcohol, occasional use of marijuana, and experimentation with cocaine.

4.10 Increase the proportion of high school seniors who associate risk of physical and psychological harm with the heavy use of alcohol, regular use of marijuana, and experimentation with cocaine.

4.11 Reduce to no more than 3% the proportion of male high school seniors who use anabolic steroids.

Services and Protection Objectives

4.12 Establish and monitor in all 50 states comprehensive plans to ensure access to alcohol and drug treatment programs for traditionally underserved people.

4.13 Provide to children in all school districts and private schools primary and secondary school educational programs on alcohol and other drugs, preferably as a part of quality school health education.

4.14 Extend adoption of alcohol and drug policies for the work environment to at least 60% of worksites with 50 or more employees.

4.15 Extend to all 50 states administrative driver's license suspension/revocation laws or programs of equal effectiveness for people determined to have been driving under the influence of intoxicants.

4.16 Increase to 50 the number of states that have enacted and enforce policies to reduce access to alcoholic beverages by minors.

4.17 Increase to at least 20 the number of states that have enacted statutes to restrict promotion of alcoholic beverages that is focused principally on young audiences.

4.18 Extend to all 50 states legal blood alcohol concentration tolerance levels of .04% for motor vehicle drivers aged 21 and older and .00% for those younger than age 21.

4.19 Increase to at least 75% the proportion of primary care providers who screen for alcohol and other drug use problems and provide counseling and referral as needed.

5. Family Planning
Health Status Objectives

5.1 Reduce pregnancies among girls aged 17 and younger to no more than 50 per 1000 adolescents.

5.2 Reduce to no more than 30% the proportion of all pregnancies that are unintended.

5.3 Reduce the prevalence of infertility to no more than 6.5%

Risk Reduction Objectives

5.4 Reduce the proportion of adolescents who have engaged in sexual intercourse by age 15 to no more than 15% and by age 17 to no more than 40%.

5.5 Increase to at least 40% the proportion of adolescents aged 17 and younger who have ever been sexually active that have abstained from sexual activity for the previous 3 months.

5.6 Increase to at least 90% the proportion of sexually active unmarried people aged 19 and younger who use contraception, especially combined-method contraception that both effectively prevents pregnancy and provides barrier protection against disease.

5.7 Increase the effectiveness with which family planning methods are used, as measured by a decrease to no more than 5% in the proportion of couples experiencing pregnancy despite use of a contraceptive method.

Services and Protection Objectives

5.8 Increase to at least 85% the proportion of people aged 10 through 18 who have discussed human sexuality, including values surrounding sexuality, with their parents and/or have received information through other parentally endorsed sources, such as school, religious, or youth programs.

5.9 Increase to at least 90% the proportion of pregnancy counselors who offer positive, accurate information about adoption to their unmarried patients with unintended pregnancies.

5.10 Increase to at least 60% the proportion of primary care providers who provide age-appropriate preconception care and counseling.

5.11 Increase to at least 50% the proportion of the following kinds of clinics that screen, diagnose, treat, counsel, and provide (or refer for) partner notification services for HIV infection and bacterial sexually transmitted diseases (gonorrhea, syphilis, and Chlamydia): family planning clinics, maternal and child health clinics, sexually transmitted disease clinics, tuberculosis clinics, drug treatment centers, and primary care clinics.

6. Mental Health and Mental Disorders
Health Status Objectives

6.1 Reduce suicides to no more than 10.5 per 100,000 people.

6.2 Reduce by 15% the incidence of injurious suicide attempts among adolescents aged 14 through 19.

6.3 Reduce to less than 10% the prevalence of mental disorders among children and adolescents.

6.4 Reduce the prevalence of mental disorders (exclusive of substance abuse) among adults living in the community to less than 10.7%.

6.5 Reduce to less than 35% the proportion of people aged 18 and older who within the past year have experienced adverse health effects from stress.

Risk Reduction Objectives

6.6 Increase to at least 30% the proportion of people aged 18 and older with severe, persistent mental disorders who use community support programs.

6.7 Increase to at least 45% the proportion of people with major depressive disorders who obtain treatment.

6.8 Increase to at least 20% the proportion of people aged 18 and older who seek help in coping with personal and emotional problems.

6.9 Decrease to no more than 5% the proportion of people aged 18 and older who report experiencing significant levels of stress who do not take steps to reduce or control their stress.

Services and Protection Objectives

6.10 In order to facilitate identification and appropriate intervention to prevent suicide by jail inmates, increase to 50 the number of states with officially established protocols that engage mental health, alcohol, drug, and public health authorities with corrections authorities.

6.11 Increase to at least 40% the proportion of worksites employing 50 or more people that provide programs to reduce employee stress.

6.12 Establish mutual-help clearinghouses in at least 25 states.

6.13 Increase to at least 50% the proportion of primary care providers who routinely review with patients their patients' cognitive, emotional, and behavioral functioning and the resources available to deal with any problems that are identified.

6.14 Increase to at least 75% the proportion of providers of primary care for children who include assessment of cognitive, emotional, and parent-child functioning, with appropriate counseling, referral, and follow-up, in their clinical practices.

7. Violent and Abusive Behavior
Health Status Objectives

7.1 Reduce homicides to no more than 7.2 per 100,000 people.

7.2 Reduce suicides to no more than 10.5 per 100,000 people.

7.3 Reduce weapon-related violent deaths to no more than 12.6 per 100,000 people.

7.4 Reverse to less than 25.2 per 1000 children the rising incidence of maltreatment of children younger than age 18.

7.5 Reduce physical abuse directed at women by male partners to no more than 27 per 1000 couples.

7.6 Reduce assault injuries among people aged 12 and older to no more than 10 per 1,000 people.

7.7 Reduce rape and attempted rape of women aged 12 and older to no more than 107 per 100,000 women.

7.8 Reduce by 15% the incidence of injurious suicide attempts among adolescents aged 14 to 19.

Risk Reduction Objectives

7.9 Reduce by 20% the incidence of physical fighting among adolescents aged 14 through 17.

7.10 Reduce by 20% the incidence of weapon-carrying by adolescents aged 14 through 17.

7.11 Reduce by 20% the proportion of weapons that are inappropriately stored and therefore available and dangerous.

Services and Protection Objectives

7.12 Extend protocols to at least 90% of hospital emergency departments for routinely identifying, treating, and properly referring victims of sexual assault, victims of spouse, elder, and child abuse, and those who have attempted suicide.

7.13 Extend to at least 45 states implementation of unexplained child death review systems.

7.14 Increase to at least 30 the number of states in which at least 50% of children identified as physically or sexually abused receive physical and mental evaluation with appropriate follow-up as a means of breaking the intergenerational cycle of abuse.

7.15 Reduce to less than 10% the proportion of battered women and their children turned away from emergency housing because of lack of space.

7.16 Increase to at least 50% the proportion of elementary and secondary schools that teach nonviolent conflict resolution skills, preferably part of quality school health education.

7.17 Extend coordinated, comprehensive violence prevention programs to at least 80% of local jurisdictions with populations over 100,000.

7.18 In order to facilitate identification and appropriate intervention to prevent suicide by jail inmates, increase to 50 the number of states with officially established protocols that engage mental health, alcohol, drug, and public health authorities with corrections authorities.

8. Educational and Community-Based Programs
Health Status Objective

8.1 Increase years of healthy life to at least 65 years.

Risk Reduction Objective

8.2 Increase the high school graduation rate to at least 90%, thereby reducing risks for multiple problem behaviors and poor mental and physical health.

Services and Protection Objectives

8.3 Achieve for all disadvantaged children and children with disabilities access to high quality and developmentally appropriate preschool programs that help prepare children for school, thereby improving their prospects with regard to school performance, behavior, and mental and physical health.

8.4 Increase to at least 75% the proportion of the nation's elementary and secondary schools that provide planned and sequential quality school health education from kindergarten through 12th grade.

8.5 Increase to at least 50% the proportion of postsecondary institutions with institution-wide health promotion programs for students, faculty, and staff.

8.6 Increase to at least 85% the proportion of workplaces with 50 or more employees that offer health promotion activities for their employees, preferably as part of a comprehensive employee health promotion program.

8.7 Increase to at least 20% the proportion of hourly workers who participate regularly in employer-sponsored health promotion activities.

8.8 Increase to at least 90% the proportion of people aged 65 and older who during the preceding year had the opportunity to participate in at least one organized health promotion program through a senior center, lifecare facility, or other community-based setting serving older adults.

8.9 Increase to at least 75% the proportion of people aged 10 and older who have discussed issues related to nutrition, physical activity, sexual behavior, tobacco, alcohol, other drugs, or safety with family members on at least one occasion during the preceding month.

8.10 Establish community health promotion programs that separately or together address at least three of the Healthy People 2000 priorities and reach at least 40% of each state's population.

8.11 Increase to at least 50% the proportion of counties that have established culturally and linguistically appropriate community health promotion programs for racial and ethnic minority populations.

8.12 Increase to at least 90% the proportion of hospitals, health maintenance organizations, and large group practices that provide patient education programs, and to at least 90% the proportion of community hospitals that offer community health programs addressing the priority health needs of their communities.

8.13 Increase to at least 75% the proportion of local television network affiliates in the top 20 television markets that have become partners with one or more community organizations in working toward one of the health problems addressed by the Healthy People 2000 objectives.

8.14 Increase to at least 90% the proportion of people who are served by a local health department that is effectively carrying out the core functions of public health.

9. Unintentional Injuries
Health Status Objectives

9.1 Reduce deaths caused by unintentional injuries to no more than 29.3 per 100,000 people.

9.2 Reduce nonfatal unintentional injuries so that hospitalizations for this condition are no more than 754 per 100,000 people.

9.3 Reduce deaths caused by motor vehicle crashes to no more than 1.9 per 100 million vehicle miles traveled and 17 per 100,000 people.

9.4 Reduce deaths from falls and from fall-related injuries to no more than 2.3 per 100,000.

9.5 Reduce deaths by drowning to no more than 1.3 per 100,000 people.

9.6 Reduce deaths resulting from residential fire to no more than 1.2 per 100,000 people.

9.7 Reduce hip fractures among people aged 65 and older so that hospitalizations for this condition are no more than 620 per 100,000 people.

9.8 Reduce nonfatal head injuries so that hospitalizations for this condition are no more than 106 per 100,000 people.

9.9 Reduce nonfatal head injuries so that hospitalizations for this condition are no more than 106 per 100,000 people.

9.10 Reduce nonfatal spinal cord injuries so that hospitalizations for this condition are no more than 4.5 per 100,000 people.

9.11 Reduce the incidence of secondary disabilities associated with injuries of the head to no more than 16 per 100,000 people, and the incidence of secondary disabilities, associated with injuries of the spinal cord to no more than 2.6 per 100,000 people.

Risk Reduction Objectives

9.12 Increase use of occupant protection systems, such as safety belts, inflatable safety restraints, and child safety seats, to at least 85% of motor vehicle occupants.

9.13 Increase use of helmets to at least 80% of motorcyclists and at least 50% of bicyclists.

Services and Protection Objectives

9.14 Extend to all 50 states laws requiring safety belt and motorcycle helmet use for all ages.

9.15 Enact in all 50 states laws requiring that new handguns be designed to minimize the likelihood of discharge by children.

9.16 Extend to 2000 the number of jurisdictions whose codes address the installation of fire suppression sprinkler systems in those residences at highest risk for fires.

9.17 Increase the presence of functional smoke detectors to at least one on each habitable floor of all inhabited residential dwellings.

9.18 Provide academic instruction on injury prevention and control, preferably as part of quality school health education, in at least 50% of public school systems (grades K through 12).

9.19 Extend requirement of the use of effective head, face, eye, and mouth protection to all organizations, agencies, and institutions sponsoring sporting and recreation events that pose risks of injury.

9.20 Increase to at least 30 the number of states that have design standards for signs, signals, markings, lighting, and other characteristics of the roadway environment to improve the visual stimuli and protect the safety of older drivers and pedestrians.

9.21 Increase to at least 50% the proportion of primary care providers who routinely provide age-appropriate counseling on safety precautions to prevent unintentional injury.

9.22 Increase to 50 the number of states having emergency medical services and trauma systems that link prehospital, hospital, and rehabilitation services in order to prevent trauma deaths and long-term disability.

10. Occupational Safety and Health

10.1 Reduce deaths from work-related injuries to no more than 4 per 100,000 full-time workers.

10.2 Reduce work-related injuries resulting in medical treatment, lost time from work, or restricted work activity to no more than 6 cases per 100 full-time workers.

10.3 Reduce cumulative trauma disorders to an incidence of no more than 60 cases per 100,000 full-time workers.

10.4 Reduce occupational skin disorders or diseases to an incidence of no more than 55 per 100,000 full-time workers.

10.5 Reduce hepatitis B infections among occupationally exposed workers to an incidence of no more than 1250 cases.

Risk Reduction Objectives

10.6 Increase to at least 75% the proportion of worksites with 50 or more employees that mandate employee use of occupant protection systems, such as seat belts, during all work-related motor vehicle travel.

10.7 Reduce to no more than 15% the proportion of workers exposed to average daily noise levels that exceed 85 decibels.

10.8 Eliminate exposures which result in workers having blood lead concentrations greater than 25 $\mu g/dL$ of whole blood.

10.9   Increase hepatitis B immunization levels to 90% among occupationally exposed workers.

Services and Protection Objectives

10.10   Implement occupational safety and health plans in all 50 states for the identification, management, and prevention of leading work-related diseases and injuries within each state.

10.11   Establish in all 50 states exposure standards adequate to prevent the major occupational lung diseases to which their worker populations are exposed (byssinosis, asbestosis, coal workers' pneumoconiosis, and silicosis).

10.12   Increase to at least 70% the proportion of worksites with 50 or more employees that have implemented programs on worker health and safety.

10.13   Increase to at least 50% the proportion of worksites with 50 or more employees that offer back injury prevention and rehabilitation programs.

10.14   Establish in all 50 states either public health or labor department programs that provide consultation and assistance to small businesses to implement safety and health programs for their employees.

10.15   Increase to 75% the proportion of primary care providers who routinely elicit occupational health exposures as part of patient history and provide relevant counseling.

11. Environmental Health
Health Status Objectives

11.1   Reduce asthma morbidity, as measured by a reduction in asthma hospitalizations to no more than 160 per 100,000 people.

11.2   Reduce the prevalence of serious mental retardation among school-aged children to no more than 2 per 1000 children.

11.3   Reduce outbreaks of waterborne disease from infectious agents and chemical poisoning to no more that 11 per year.

11.4   Reduce among children aged 6 months through 5 years the prevalence of blood lead levels exceeding 15 μg/dL and 25 μg/dL to no more than 500,000 and zero, respectively.

Risk Reduction Objectives

11.5   Reduce human exposure to criteria air pollutants, as measured by an increase to at least 85% in the proportion of people who live in counties that have not exceeded any Environmental Protection Agency standard for air quality in the previous 12 months.

11.6   Increase to at least 40 percent the proportion of homes in which homeowners/occupants have tested for radon concentrations and that have either been found to pose minimal risk or have been modified to reduce risk to health.

11.7   Reduce human exposure to toxic agents by confining total pounds of toxic agents released into the air, water, and soil each year to no more than:
—0.24 billion pounds of those toxic agents included on the Department of Health and Human Services list of carcinogens.
—2.6 billion pounds of those toxic agents included

on the Agency for Toxic Substances and Disease Registry list of the most toxic chemicals.

11.8   Reduce human exposure to solid waste-related water, air, and soil contamination, as measured by a reduction in the average amount of municipal solid waste produced per person each day to no more than 3.6 pounds.

11.9   Increase to at least 85% the proportion of people who receive a supply of drinking water that meets the safe drinking water standards established by the Environmental Protection Agency.

11.10   Reduce potential risks to human health from surface water, as measured by a decrease to no more than 15% in the proportion of assessed rivers, lakes, and estuaries that do not support beneficial uses, such as fishing and swimming.

Services and Protection Objectives

11.11   Perform testing for lead-based paint in at least 50% of homes built before 1950.

11.12   Expand to at least 35 the number of states in which at least 75% of local jurisdictions have adopted construction standards and techniques that minimize elevated indoor radon levels in those new building areas locally determined to have elevated radon levels.

11.13   Increase to at least 30 the number of states requiring that prospective buyers be informed of the presence of lead-based paint and radon concentrations in all buildings offered for sale.

11.14   Eliminate significant health risks from National Priority List hazardous waste sites, as measured by performance of clean-up at these sites sufficient to eliminate immediate and significant health threats as specified in health assessments completed at all sites.

11.15   Establish programs for recyclable materials and household hazardous waste in at least 75% of counties.

11.16   Establish and monitor in at least 35 states plans to define and track sentinel environmental diseases.

12. Food and Drug Safety
Health Status Objectives

12.1   Reduce infections caused by key foodborne pathogens (e.g., *Salmonella, Campylobacter jejuni, Escherichia coli* 0157:H7, and *Listeria monocytogenes*).

12.2   Reduce outbreaks of infections due to *Salmonella enteritidis* to fewer than 25 outbreaks yearly.

Risk Reduction Objective

12.3   Increase to at least 75% the proportion of households in which principal food preparers routinely refrain from leaving perishable food out of the refrigerator for over 2 hours and wash cutting boards and utensils with soap after contact with raw meat and poultry.

Services and Protection Objectives

12.4   Extend to at least 70% the proportion of states and territories that have implemented model food codes for institutional food operations and to at least 70% the proportion that have adopted the new uniform food protection code ("Unicode") that sets recommended standards for regulation of all food operations.

12.5 Increase to at least 75% the proportion of pharmacies and other dispensers of prescription medications that use linked systems to provide alerts to potential adverse drug reactions among medications dispensed by different sources to individual patients.

12.6 Increase to at least 75% the proportion of primary care providers who routinely review with their patients aged 65 and older all prescribed and over-the-counter medicines taken by their patients each time a new medication is prescribed.

13. Oral Health
Health Status Objectives

13.1 Reduce dental caries (cavities) so that the proportion of children with one or more caries in permanent or primary teeth is no more than 35% among children aged 6 through 8 and no more than 60% among adolescents aged 15.

13.2 Reduce untreated dental caries so that the proportion of children with untreated caries in permanent or primary teeth is no more than 20% among children aged 6 through 8 and no more than 15% among adolescents aged 15.

13.3 Increase to at least 45% the proportion of people aged 35 through 44 who have never lost a permanent tooth due to dental caries or periodontal disease.

13.4 Reduce to no more than 20% the proportion of people aged 65 and older who have lost all of their natural teeth.

13.5 Reduce the prevalence of gingivitis among people aged 35 through 44 to no more than 30%.

13.6 Reduce destructive periodontal diseases to a prevalence of no more than 15% among people aged 35 through 44.

13.7 Reduce deaths due to cancer of the oral cavity and pharynx to no more than 10.5 per 100,000 men aged 45 through 74 and to 4.1 per 100,000 women aged 45 through 74.

Risk Reduction Objectives

13.8 Increase to at least 50% the proportion of children who have received protective sealants on the occlusal (chewing) surfaces of permanent molar teeth.

13.9 Increase to at least 75% the proportion of people served by community water systems providing optimal levels of fluoride.

13.10 Increase use of professionally or self-administered topical or systemic (dietary) fluorides to at least 85% of people not receiving optimally fluoridated public water.

13.11 Increase to at least 75% the proportion of parents and caregivers who use feeding practices that prevent baby bottle tooth decay.

Services and Protection Objectives

13.12 Increase to at least 90% the proportion of all children entering school programs for the first time who have received an oral health screening, referral, and follow-up for necessary diagnostic, preventive, and treatment services.

13.13 Extend to all long-term institutional facilities the requirement that oral examinations and services be provided no later than 90 days after entry into these facilities.

13.14 Increase to at least 70% the proportion of people aged 35 and older using the oral health care system during each year.

13.15 Increase to at least 40 the number of states that have an effective system for recording and referring infants with cleft lips and/or palates to craniofacial anomaly teams.

13.16 Extend requirement of the use of effective head, face, eye, and mouth protection to all organizations, agencies, and institutions sponsoring sporting and recreation events that pose risks of injury.

14. Maternal and Infant Health
Health Status Objectives

14.1 Reduce the infant mortality rate to no more than 7 per 1000 live births.

14.2 Reduce the fetal death rate (20 or more weeks of gestation) to no more than 5 per 1000 cases of live births and fetal deaths combined.

14.3 Reduce the maternal mortality rate to no more than 3.3 per 100,000 live births.

14.4 Reduce the incidence of fetal alcohol syndrome to no more than 0.12 per 1000 live births.

Risk Reduction Objectives

14.5 Reduce low birth weight to an incidence of no more than 5% of live births and very low birth weight to no more than 1% of live births.

14.6 Increase to at least 85% the proportion of mothers who achieve the minimum recommended weight gain during their pregnancies.

14.7 Reduce severe complications of pregnancy to no more than 15 per 100 deliveries.

14.8 Reduce the Caesarean delivery rate to no more than 15 per 100 deliveries.

14.9 Increase to at least 75% the proportion of mothers who breastfeed their babies in the early postpartum period and to at least 50% the proportion who continue breastfeeding until their babies are 5 to 6 months old.

14.10 Increase abstinence from tobacco use by pregnant women to at least 90% and increase abstinence from alcohol, cocaine, and marijuana by pregnant women by at least 20%.

Services and Protection Objectives

14.11 Increase to at least 90% the proportion of all pregnant women who receive prenatal care in the first trimester of pregnancy.

14.12 Increase to at least 60% the proportion of primary care providers who provide age-appropriate preconception care and counseling.

14.13 Increase to at least 90% the proportion of women enrolled in prenatal care who are offered screening and counseling on prenatal detection of fetal abnormalities.

14.14 Increase to at least 90% the proportion of pregnant

women and infants who receive risk-appropriate care.

14.15 Increase to at least 95% the proportion of newborns screened by state-sponsored programs for genetic disorders and other disabling conditions and to 90% the proportion of newborns testing positive for disease who receive appropriate treatment.

14.16 Increase to at least 90% the proportion of babies aged 18 months and younger who receive recommended primary care services at the appropriate intervals.

15. Heart Disease and Stroke
Health Status Objectives

15.1 Reduce coronary heart disease deaths to no more than 100 per 100,000 people.

15.2 Reduce stroke deaths to no more than 20 per 100,000 people.

15.3 Reverse the increase in end-stage renal disease (requiring maintenance dialysis or transplantation) to attain an incidence of no more than 13 per 100,000.

Risk Reduction Objectives

15.4 Increase to at least 50% the proportion of people with high blood pressure whose blood pressure is under control.

15.5 Increase to at least 90% the proportion of people with high blood pressure who are taking action to help control their blood pressure.

15.6 Reduce the mean serum cholesterol level among adults to no more than 200 mg/dL.

15.7 Reduce the prevalence of blood cholesterol levels of 240 mg/dL or greater to no more than 20% of the adults population.

15.8 Increase to at least 60% the proportion of adults with high blood cholesterol who are aware of their condition and are taking action to reduce their blood cholesterol to recommended levels.

15.9 Reduce dietary fat intake to an average of 30% of calories or less and average saturated fat intake to less than 10% of calories among people aged 2 and older.

15.10 Reduce overweight to a prevalence of no more than 20% among people aged 20 and older and no more than 15% among adolescents aged 12 through 19.

15.11 Increase to at least 30% the proportion of people aged 6 and older who engage regularly, preferably daily, in light to moderate physical activity for at least 30 minutes per day.

15.12 Reduce cigarette smoking to a prevalence of no more than 15% among people aged 20 and older.

Services and Protection Objectives

15.13 Increase to at least 90% the proportion of adults who have had their blood pressure measured within the preceding 2 years and can state whether their blood pressure was normal, high, or low.

15.14 Increase to at least 75% the proportion of adults who have had their blood cholesterol checked within the preceding 5 years.

15.15 Increase to at least 75% the proportion of primary care providers who initiate diet for patients with high blood cholesterol and, if necessary, drug therapy at levels of blood cholesterol consistent with current management guidelines.

15.16 Increase to at least 50% the proportion of worksites with 50 or more employees that offer high blood pressure and/or cholesterol education and control activities to their employees.

15.17 Increase to at least 90% the proportion of clinical laboratories that meet the recommended accuracy standard for cholesterol measurement.

15. Cancer
Health Status Objectives

16.1 Reverse the rise in cancer deaths to achieve a rate of no more than 130 per 100,000 people.

16.2 Slow the rise in lung cancer deaths to achieve a rate of no more than 42 per 100,000 people.

16.3 Reduce breast cancer deaths to no more than 20.6 per 100,000 women.

16.4 Reduce deaths from cancer of the uterine cervix to no more than 1.3 per 100,000 women.

16.5 Reduce colorectal cancer deaths to no more than 13.2 per 100,000 people.

Risk Reduction Objectives

16.6 Reduce cigarette smoking to a prevalence of no more than 15% among people aged 20 and older.

16.7 Reduce dietary fat intake to an average of 30% of calories or less and average saturated fat intake to less than 10% of calories among people aged 2 and older.

16.8 Increase complex carbohydrate and fiber-containing foods in the diets of adults to five or more daily servings for vegetables (including legumes) and fruits, and to six or more daily servings for grain products.

16.9 Increase to at least 60% the proportion of people of all ages who limit sun exposure, use sunscreens and protective clothing when exposed to sunlight, and avoid artificial sources of ultraviolet light (e.g., sun lamps, tanning booths).

Services and Protection Objectives

16.10 Increase to at least 75% the proportion of primary care providers who routinely counsel patients about tobacco use cessation, diet modification, and cancer screening recommendations.

16.11 Increase to at least 80% the proportion of women aged 40 and older who have ever received a clinical breast examination and a mammogram, and to at least 60% those aged 50 and older who have received them within the preceding 1 to 2 years.

16.12 Increase to at least 95% the proportion of women aged 18 and older with uterine cervix who have ever received a Pap test, and to at least 85 percent those who received a Pap test within the preceding 1 to 3 years.

16.13 Increase to at least 50% the proportion of people aged 50 and older who have received fecal occult blood testing within the preceding 1 to 2 years, and to at least 40% those who have ever received proctosigmoidoscopy.

16.14 Increase to at least 40% the proportion of people aged 50 and older visiting a primary care provider who have received oral, skin, and digital rectal examinations during a visit within the preceding year.

16.15 Ensure that Pap tests meet quality standards by monitoring and certifying all cytology laboratories.

16.16 Ensure that mammograms meet quality standards by monitoring and certifying at least 80% of mammography facilities.

17. Diabetes and Chronic Disabling Conditions
Health Status Objectives (Chronic Disabling Conditions)

17.1   Increase years of healthy life to at least 65 years.

17.2   Reduce to no more than 8% the proportion of people who experience a limitation in major activity due to chronic conditions.

17.3   Reduce to no more than 90 per 1000 people the proportion of all people aged 65 and older who have difficulty in performing two or more personal activities, thereby preserving independence.

17.4   Reduce to no more than 10% the proportion of people with asthma who experience activity limitation.

17.5   Reduce activity limitation due to chronic back conditions to a prevalence of no more than 19 per 1000 people.

17.6   Reduce significant hearing impairment to a prevalence of no more than 82 per 1000 people.

17.7   Reduce significant visual impairment to a prevalence of no more than 30 per 1000 people.

17.8   Reduce the prevalence of serious mental retardation in school-aged children to no more than 2 per 1000 children.

Diabetes

17.9   Reduce diabetes-related deaths to no more than 34 per 100,000.

17.10 Reduce the most severe complications of diabetes (i.e., end-stage renal disease, blindness, lower extremity amputation, perinatal mortality, and major congenital malformations).

17.11 Reduce diabetes to an incidence of no more than 2.5 per 1000 people and a prevalence of no more than 25 per 1000 people.

Risk Reduction Objectives

17.12 Reduce overweight to a prevalence of no more than 20% among people aged 20 and older and no more than 15% among adolescents aged 12 through 19.

17.13 Increase to at least 30% the proportion of people aged 6 and older who engage regularly, preferably daily, in light to moderate physical activity for at least 30 minutes per day.

Services and Protection Objectives

17.14 Increase to at least 40% the proportion of people with chronic and disabling conditions who receive formal patient education including information about community and self-help resources as an integral part of the management of their conditions.

17.15 Increase to at least 80% the proportion of providers of primary care for children who routinely refer or screen infants and children for impairments of vision, hearing, speech, and language, and assess other developmental milestones as part of well-child care.

17.16 Reduce the average age at which children with significant hearing impairment are identified to no more than 12 months.

17.17 Increase to at least 60% the proportion of providers of primary care for older adults who routinely evaluate people aged 65 and older for urinary incontinence and impairments of vision, hearing, cognition, and functional status.

17.18 Increase to at least 90% the proportion of perimenopausal women who have been counseled about the benefits and risks of estrogen replacement therapy (combined with progestin, when appropriate) for prevention of osteoporosis.

17.19 Increase to at least 75% the proportion of worksites with 50 or more employees that have a voluntary established policy or program for hiring people with disabilities.

17.20 Increase to 50 the number of states that have service systems for children at risk of or having chronic and disabling conditions, as required by Public Law 101-239.

18. HIV Infection
Health Status Objectives

18.1   Confine annual incidence of diagnosed AIDS cases to no more than 98,000 cases.

18.2   Confine the prevalence of HIV infection to no more than 800 per 100,000.

Risk Reduction Objectives

18.3   Reduce the proportion of adolescents who have engaged in sexual intercourse by age 15 to no more than 15% and by age 17 to no more than 40%.

18.4   Increase to at least 50% the proportion of sexually active unmarried people who used a condom during last sexual intercourse.

18.5   Increase to at least 50% the estimated proportion of all intravenous drug users who are in drug abuse treatment programs.

18.6   Increase to at least 50% the estimated proportion of intravenous drug users not in treatment who use only uncontaminated drug paraphernalia ("works").

18.7   Reduce to no more than 1 per 250,000 units of blood and blood components the risk of transfusion-transmitted HIV infection.

Services and Protection Objectives

18.8   Increase to at least 80% the proportion of HIV-infected people who have been tested for HIV infection.

18.9   Increase to at least 75% the proportion of primary care and mental health care providers who provide age-appropriate counseling on the prevention of HIV and other sexually transmitted diseases.

18.10 Increase to at least 95% the proportion of schools

that have age-appropriate HIV education curricula for students in fourth through twelfth grade, preferably as part of quality school health education.

18.11 Provide HIV education for students and staff in at least 90% of colleges and universities.

18.12 Increase to at least 90% the proportion of cities with populations over 100,000 that have outreach programs to contact drug users (particularly intravenous drug users) to deliver HIV risk reduction messages.

18.13 Increase to at least 50% the proportion of the following kinds of clinics that screen, diagnose, treat, counsel, and provide (or refer for) partner notification services for HIV infection and bacterial sexually transmitted diseases (gonorrhea, syphilis, and *Chlamydia*): family planning clinics, maternal and child health clinics, sexually transmitted disease clinics, tuberculosis clinics, drug treatment centers, and primary care clinics.

18.14 Extend to all facilities where workers are at risk for occupational transmission of HIV regulations to protect workers from exposure to blood-borne infections, including HIV infection.

19. Sexually Transmitted Diseases
Health Status Objectives

19.1 Reduce gonorrhea to an incidence of no more than 225 cases per 100,000 people.

19.2 Reduce *Chlamydia trachomatis* infections, as measured by a decrease in the incidence of nongonococcal urethritis, to no more than 170 cases per 100,000 people.

19.3 Reduce primary and secondary syphilis to an incidence of no more than 10 cases per 100,000 people.

19.4 Reduce congenital syphilis to an incidence of no more than 50 cases per 100,000 live births.

19.5 Reduce genital herpes and genital warts, as measured by reductions to 142,000 and 385,000, respectively, in the annual number of first-time consultations with a physician for the conditions.

19.6 Reduce the incidence of pelvic inflammatory disease, as measured by a reduction in hospitalizations for the condition to no more than 250 per 100,000 women aged 15 through 44.

19.7 Reduce sexually transmitted hepatitis B infection to no more than 30,500 cases.

19.8 Reduce the rate of repeat gonorrhea infection to no more than 15% within the previous year.

Risk Reduction Objectives

19.9 Reduce the proportion of adolescents who have engaged in sexual intercourse by age 15 to no more than 15% and by age 17 to no more than 40%.

19.10 Increase to at least 50% the proportion of sexually active unmarried people who used a condom during last sexual intercourse.

Services and Protection Objectives

19.11 Increase to at least 50% the proportion of the following kinds of clinics that screen, diagnose, treat, counsel, and provide (or refer for) partner notification services for HIV infection and bacterial sexually

transmitted disease (gonorrhea, syphilis, and *Chlamydia*): family planning clinics, maternal and child health clinics, sexually transmitted disease clinics, tuberculosis clinics, drug treatment centers, and primary care clinics.

19.12 Include instruction in preventing transmission of sexually transmitted diseases in the curricula of all middle and secondary schools, preferably as part of quality school health education.

19.13 Increase to at least 90% the proportion of primary care providers treating patients with sexually transmitted diseases who correctly manage cases, as measured by their use of appropriate types and amounts of therapy.

19.14 Increase to at least 75% the proportion of primary care and mental health care providers who provide age-appropriate counseling on the prevention of HIV and other sexually transmitted diseases.

19.15 Increase to at least 50% the proportion of all patients with bacterial sexually transmitted diseases (gonorrhea, syphilis, and *Chlamydia*) who are offered provider referral services.

20. Immunization and Infectious Diseases
Health Status Objectives

20.1 Reduce indigenous cases of vaccine-preventable diseases (i.e., diphtheria, tetanus, polio [wild-type virus], measles, rubella, congenital rubella syndrome, mumps, and pertussis).

20.2 Reduce epidemic-related pneumonia and influenza deaths among people aged 65 and older to no more than 7.3 per 100,000 people.

20.3 Reduce viral hepatitis.

20.4 Reduce tuberculosis to an incidence of no more than 3.5 cases per 100,000 people.

20.5 Reduce by at least 10% the incidence of surgical wound infections and nosocomial infections in intensive care patients.

20.6 Reduce incidence among international travelers of typhoid fever, hepatitis A, and malaria.

20.7 Reduce bacterial meningitis to no more than 4.7 cases per 100,000 people.

20.8 Reduce infectious diarrhea by at least 25% among children in licensed child care centers and children in programs that provide an Individualized Education Program (IEP) or Individualized Health Plan (IHP).

20.9 Reduce acute middle ear infections among children aged 4 and younger, as measured by days of restricted activity or school absenteeism, to no more than 105 days per 100 children.

20.10 Reduce pneumonia-related days of restricted activity.

Risk Reduction Objectives

20.11 Increase immunization levels as follows:
— Basic immunization series among children under age 2: at least 90%.
— Basic immunization series among children in licensed child care facilities and kindergarten through post-secondary education institutions: at least 95%.
— Pneumococcal pneumonia and influenza immu-

nization among institutionalized chronically ill or older people: at least 80%.

— Pneumococcal pneumonia and influenza immunization among noninstitutionalized, high-risk populations, as defined by the Immunization Practices Advisory Committee: at least 60%.

— Hepatitis B immunization among high-risk populations, including infants of surface antigen-positive mothers to at least 90%; occupationally exposed workers to at least 90%; IV-drug users in drug treatment programs to at least 50%; and homosexual men to at least 50%.

20.12 Reduce postexposure rabies treatments to no more than 9000 per year.

Services and Protection Objectives

20.13 Expand immunization laws for schools, preschools, and day care settings to all states for all antigens.

20.14 Increase to at least 90% the proportion of primary care providers who provide information and counseling about immunizations and offer immunizations as appropriate for their patients.

20.15 Improve the financing and delivery of immunizations for children and adults so that virtually no American has a financial barrier to receiving recommended immunizations.

20.16 Increase to at least 90% the proportion of public health departments that provide adult immunization for influenza, pneumococcal disease, hepatitis B, tetanus, and diphtheria.

20.17 Increase to at least 90% the proportion of local health departments that have ongoing programs for actively identifying cases of tuberculosis and latent infection in populations at high risk for tuberculosis.

20.18 Increase to at least 85% the proportion of people found to have tuberculosis infection who completed courses of preventive therapy.

20.19 Increase to at least 85% the proportion of tertiary care hospital laboratories and to at least 50% the proportion of secondary care hospital and health maintenance organization laboratories possessing technologies for rapid viral diagnosis of influenza.

21. Clinical Preventive Services
Health Status Objective

21.1 Increase years of healthy life to at least 65 years.

Risk Reduction Objective

21.2 Increase to at least 50% the proportion of people who have received, as a minimum within the appropriate interval, all of the screening and immunization services and at least one of the counseling services appropriate for their age and sex as recommended by the U.S. Preventive Services Task Force.

Services and Protection Objectives

21.3 Increase to at least 95% the proportion of people who have a specific source of ongoing primary care for

coordination of their preventive and episodic health care.

21.4 Improve financing and delivery of clinical preventive services so that virtually no American has a financial barrier to receiving, at a minimum, the screening, counseling, and immunization services recommended by the U.S. Preventive Services Task Force.

21.5 Assure that at least 90% of people for whom primary care services are provided directly by publicly funded programs are offered, at a minimum, the screening, counseling, and immunization services recommended by the U.S. Preventive Services Task Force.

21.6 Increase to at least 50% the proportion of primary care providers who provide their patients with the screening, counseling, and immunization services recommended by the U.S. Preventive Services Task Force.

21.7 Increase to at least 90% the proportion of people who are served by a local health department that assesses and assures access to essential clinical preventive services.

21.8 Increase the proportion of all degrees in the health professions and allied/associated health profession fields awarded to members of underrepresented racial/ethnic minority groups.

22. Surveillance and Data Systems
Objectives

22.1 Develop a set of health status indicators appropriate for federal, state, and local health agencies and establish use of the set in at least 40 states.

22.2 Identify, and create where necessary, national data sources to measure progress toward each of the Year 2000: National Health Objectives.

22.3 Develop and disseminate among federal, state, and local agencies procedures for collecting comparable data for each of the Year 2000: National Health Objectives and incorporate these into Public Health Service data collection systems.

22.4 Develop and implement a national process to identify significant gaps in the nation's disease prevention and health promotion data, including data for racial and ethnic minorities, people with low incomes, and people with disabilities, and establish mechanisms to meet these needs.

22.5 Implement in all states periodic analysis and publication of data needed to measure progress toward objectives for at least 10 of the priority areas of the National Health Objectives.

22.6 Expand in all states systems for the transfer of health information related to the National Health Objectives among federal, state, and local agencies.

22.7 Achieve timely release of national surveillance and survey data needed by health professionals and agencies to measure progress toward the National Health Objectives.

GLOSSARY

abandonment Forsaking a client in need of service. Determined through the judicial system.

absolute standard Standard Used by the federal government to define a basic set of resources necessary for adequate (not proverty level) existence.

acceptant intervention Consultative mode of client intervention which is a process of catharsis intended to clear emotional blocks in order to engage in objective problem solving.

accommodation Ways in which children modify their view of the world as they have new experiences that influence their responses.

accountability Being answerable to someone for something one has done.
  moral Being answerable to someone for how moral requirements of nursing practice have been carried out.
  legal Being answerable to someone for how legal requirements of nursing practice have been carried out.

accreditation A credentialing process used to recognize agencies for provision of quality services.

accreditation Mechanism for assessing the quality of educational programs.

acculturation Adaptation and incorporation of ideas, values, behaviors, customs, and certain aspects of the majority culture concurrent with maintaining aspects of the traditional or primary culture. Learning one's culture through a process of acquiring knowledge and internalizing values.

achievable age Risk age, expressed in years, which individuals can attain if they comply with suggested medical therapies and life-style changes. Synonymous with survival advantage and compliance age.

acid rain The precipitation of moisture as rain with high acidity caused by release of pollutants into the atmosphere.

acquired immune deficiency syndrome (AIDS) Disease involving a defect in cell-mediated immunity that has a long incubation period, follows a protracted and debilitating course, and has a poor prognosis; transmitted through sexual contact, exposure to contaminated blood, or possibly close personal contact.

active immunization Administration of all or part of a microorganism to stimulate active response by the host's immunological system, resulting in complete protection against a specific disease.

active listening Listening carefully and letting the speaker know that the message was received.

activity theory Theory stating that continuing activities during middle age is required for successful aging.

adaptation Change or response to stress of any kind; may be normal, self-protective, or developmental.

adaptive model of health View of health as individual and family ability to effectively integrate with internal and external environments.

addiction Compulsive, uncontrolled psychological or physical dependence on a substance or a habit.

adolescence A time of discovery of self, of feelings, and of the complexities of society, usually occurring between the ages of 13 and 18 years; the period of psychological maturation.

administrator One who manipulates the resources within an organization to meet the organizational goals.

administrative law Branch of law dealing with organs of government power; precribes the manner of their activity (e.g., state board of nurse examiners).

adult day care center Congregate facility for activities such as socialization, eating, and supervised care of older adults during specified day hours, with the person returning home for the evening hours.

adult nurse practitioner Registered nurse with additional education through a master's degree program in nursing or through a nondegree or certificate continuing education program preparing the nurse to deliver primary health care to adults.

advanced disease A stage in the natural history of a disease in which sufficient anatomical functional changes have occurred to produce recognizable signs and symptoms.

advocacy Engaging in activities for the purpose of protecting the rights of others while supporting the client's responsibility for self-determination; involves informing, supporting, and affirming a client's self-determination in health care decisions. A process to enhance continuity of care.

aerobic exercise Activities involving large muscle groups to produce heart rates which will sustain an individual's endurance and condition the body.

affective domain The learning domain that deals with feelings, attitudes, values, and interests.

affirming Ratifying, asserting, or giving strength to the declarations of self or others.

aftermath The consequences or outcome of a conflict situation.

agent Causative factor invading a susceptible host through an environment favorable to produce disease.

aggregates Populations or defined groups.

aggressive Inclined to move in a hostile manner.

aging The process of growing older as well as related physical and emotional components.

aging network Organizations concerned with advocacy, special populations, and volunteer services relating to older people.

air pollution The presence of foreign materials in the air, either natural or manmade.

akathisia Inability to sit down due to severe anxiety. A feeling of restlessness and an urgent need for movement, with complaints of feelings of muscular quivering.

Alanon Organization of relatives of alcoholic individuals, operated in many communities within the structure of Alcoholics Anonymous.

Alateen Self-help program for children of alcoholics; provides a forum for discussing family stressors, learning coping skills, and gaining support and encouragement from knowledgeable peers.

Alcoholics Anonymous Lay, self-help group that practices a 12-step approach to recovery.

alcoholism Addiction to alcohol.

alternative delivery system Organizations such as HMOs and PPOs that are non-hospital sites for the delivery of health care.

Alzheimer's disease Presenile dementia, characterized by confusion, memory failure, disorientation, restlessness, agnosia, and/or speech disturbances.

ambulatory care centers Hospital or community-based facilities that offer a wide range of outpatient services to treat mental and physical health problems.

amplification Expanding a statement or idea; an objective of comunication.

analytic epidemiology Second stage of epidemiological investigation; focuses on testing etiological hypotheses using observational studies.

anaphylaxis Exaggerated hypersensitivity to a previously encountered antigen; reaction ranges from generalized itching to severe vascular collapse.

andragogy Helping people learn.

anorexia nervosa Syndrome marked by severe and prolonged inability to eat, marked weight loss, amenorrhea, and other symptoms resulting from emotional conflict and biological changes.

Antabuse Drug used as a deterrent to alcohol consumption. When alcohol and Antabuse are mixed, the person experiences a variety of unpleasant physiological reactions.

anthrax Illness with varying symptoms caused by a spore-forming organism; may be endemic to many agricultural areas.

antibody An organism formed in the body that identifies and destroys initial and subsequent invasions of an identified disease-producing organism.

anticipatory guidance Providing advice to clients before an event and discussing potential problems or risks so clients will be aware and may be able to prevent the occurrence of the problem.

antitoxin Solution of antibodies derived from the serum of animals immunized with specific antigens (e.g., diphtheria, tetanus); used to achieve passive immunity.

Apgar scoring A tool used to score neonatal physiological functioning at birth. The newborn characteristics of appearance, pulse, grimace, activity, and respiration are observed and scored.

appraised age Total health risk of an individual, expressed in years. Determined by adjusting the average risk of death from selected causes for the individual's age, sex, and racial group to his own risk.

artificial acquired immunity Immune state that results from immunization or vaccination for a specific disease.

ascariasis (roundworm infection) Infection caused by a parasitic worm, *Ascario lumbriacoides,* that migrates through the lungs in its larval stage; symptoms are coughing, wheezing, and fever.

assertiveness Communicating or expressing one's rights.

assertiveness training Teaching people how to express themselves honestly and directly by identifying what is blocking such behavior and by setting goals for increasing personal assertive behavior.

assessment Systematic calculation of data to assist in identifying needs, questions to be addressed, or abilities and available resources.

assessment of community resources Procedure similar to the process used on behalf of individual clients. The scope of the investigation is more detailed and includes examination of data from health planning groups, including the number of public health facilities, availability of health personnel, availability of funds, and a multitude of other statistics, such as those on mortality and morbidity.

assessment of need Verifying and mapping out the extent and location of a problem and its attendant target population.

assimilation Process of a minority group becoming absorbed into the dominant or majority culture by adopting its behaviors. Also the process of a child's responding to the environment in accordance with his cognitive structures so that elements in the environment are incorporated into his cognitive structures.

attack rates Special rates expressing incidence of a disease.

attentive Fully listening to another.

attributable risk Statistical measure that estimates the reduction in the occurrence of a particular disease which could be affected by elimination of a specific causal agent.

attribute Any physical, psychological, or social characteristic describing an individual.

audit process A six-step process used concurrently or retrospectively for nursing peer review.

authorization The process of placing a ceiling on money to be requested for a program.

autoimmunity Abnormal condition in which the body reacts against parts of its own tissues.

autonomy Freedom of action as chosen by an individual.

autonomic nervous system The part of the nervous system that regulates involuntary functioning, including cardiac muscle, smooth muscle, and the glands.

battered child syndrome Term coined by Kempe to describe the pattern of abuse against children.

battered women Women who are physically and/or emotionally abused by their spouses.

battery Committing bodily harm.

BCG vaccines Several vaccines that vary in their ability to induce active immunity and therefore prevent tuberculosis.

beliefs Statements that a person holds that may or may not correspond with objective facts.

belief statements Statements of beliefs persons hold as true, but which may or may not be based on empirical evidence.

beneficence Ethical principle stating that one should do good and prevent or avoid doing harm.

benefit schedule A list of services with monetary values specifiying the amounts an insurer will pay for the services.

bicultural The straddling of two cultures, lifestyles, and sets of values.

biofeedback Process in which sensitive physiological monitoring instruments serve as teaching tools by helping people become aware of and learn to consciously control many physiological variables previously thought to be automatic.

biological hazards Disease-producing agents primarily consisting of bacteria, viruses, and other microorganisms and parasites.

biological plausibility A reasonable physiological mechanism to explain how a causal factor could operate to bring about a particular disease.

biosphere The world of living things, consisting of numerous ecosystems.

"black lung" Disease common among coal miners, characterized by a large solid black lung mass; caused by deposits of black mining dust in the lungs.

blackouts Intervals of temporary memory loss during which a person remains conscious and active and may even appear sober, but after which there is no memory of what was said or done.

blaming A behavior of accusing another for one's mistakes, stemming from a serious threat to self-esteem.

block nursing A contemporary term for district nursing.

bonding The synchronization of maternal and infant responses resulting in a unique emotional relationship.

botulism Often fatal form of blood poisoning caused by an endotoxin produced by the bacillus *Clostridium botulinum.*

boundary In systems theory the line or border that defines the elements comprising the system.

brainstorming An activity in which spontaneous, free-floating expression of ideas is encouraged. Brainstorming is often a prelude to problem-solving.

breach of contract Unjustified failure to perform the terms of a contract or to meet the contract schedule.

broken record Repeating a word or phrase used by another person to acknowledge that the person has been heard.

brucellosis Infectious disease of nonhuman mammals, which is contagious to humans.

budget A plan stated in financial terms that identifies the costs associated with implementing a program.

bulimia Insatiable craving for food, often resulting in episodes of continuous eating followed by periods of depression and self-denial.

burnout The result of excessive internal and/or external stressors; a physical and behavioral response to stress.

byssinosis Type of lung disease common among cotton mill workers; similar to nonoccupational bronchitis.

capitation A payment system whereby one fee is charged the client to pay for all services received or needed.

carbon monoxide Colorless, odorless, poisonous gas produced by the combustion of carbon or organic fuels in a limited oxygen supply.

carcinogenic agent Single cancer-inducing substance that triggers the change in behavior of cells resulting in uncontrolled growth.

care coordination Linking clients with services.

caregivers Those persons, professional and non-professional, who provide for the social and health needs of others.

case finding Careful, systematic observations of people to identify present or potential problems.

case law Decisions by the courts; judicial opinions.

case management/care management Interchangeable terms used to describe a service given to clients that contain the following activities: screening, assessment, care planning, arranging for service delivery, monitoring, reassessment, evaluation, and discharge. Case management is a process that enhances continuity of care.

case register Systematic registration of acute, chronic, and contagious diseases.

case study A written analysis of program development and implementation throughout the life of the program. An historical depiction of the program.

catalyst A person who promotes activities of others by assisting clients in becoming involved.

catalytic intervention mode A situation whereby a consultant assists a client to broaden his view of an existing situation by gaining additional information or by unifying existing data.

catchment area Designated service area for a community mental health center, consisting of between 75,000 and 200,000 people.

causality Relating of causes to the effects they produce.

census data Composite data, provided by the federal government on the population of states, local and political jurisdictions, and census tracts in organized areas.

Centers for Disease Control Branch of the U.S. Public Health Service whose primary responsibility is to propose, coordinate, and evaluate changes in the surveillance of disease in the United States.

centralization Control or organization by one part of an institution.

cerebral palsy Chronic nonprogressive disorders of the brain occurring in infants and young children and producing abnormalities of posture and significant developmental motor disability.

certificate of need Determination in any given community of the need for new health care facilities on the basis of currently available resources and anticipated demands for use.

certification A mechanism, usually by means of written examination, that provides an indication of professional competence in a specialized area of practice.

chancroid A sexually transmitted disease caused by a bacteria, Hemophilus ducreyi, that results in a highly infectious ulcer on the penis, urethra, vulva, or anus.

charter A mechanism by which a state government agency under state laws grants corporate status to institutions with or without rights to award degrees.

chemical additive contamination Contamination of food, either deliberately or incidentally, by chemical additives.

chemical dependency Addiction to alcohol or other drugs.

child abuse Active forms of maltreatment of children.

child neglect Physical or emotional. Physical neglect refers to failure to provide adequate food, clothing, shelter, hygiene, or necessary medical care; emotional neglect refers to the omission of basic nurturing, acceptance, and caring essential for healthy development.

childbirth center Health facility where prenatal care and delivery services are provided to low-risk pregnant women by a team of nurse-midwives, obstetricians, pediatricians, and ancillary health personnel.

Chlamydia A sexually transmitted disease caused by the organism Chlamydia trachomatis, known to cause infection and/or inflammation of the genitals in males and females.

chlorine Toxic gas used in the chemical and paper industries.

chronic illness diagnosis A system of organizing and naming client problems related to chronicity.

cirrhosis Chronic degenerative liver disease; often caused by chronic alcohol abuse, but can also result from nutritional deprivation, hepatitis, or other infections.

civil law Area of law concerned with the legal rights and duties of individuals.

clarification The process of attempting to make communication or expression clear or easier to understand.

Clean Water Act Legislation passed in 1963 to protect air quality. The goal of the 1990 Act is to reduce acid rain, urban smog, and toxic chemical emissions from industry.

client-centered learning A nondirective, warm, passive, and accepting environment that encourages students to be self-directed and guide their own learning.

client population Individuals, groups, families, organizations, or communities that are the targets of the consultant's interventions.

client problem A current, historic, or potential matter of difficulty or concern that adversely affects any aspect of a client's well-being.

clients' rights Those services, programs, goods, and provider behaviors to which consumers are entitled in order to maintain or achieve health, or to exist.

clinical disease A stage in the natural history of a disease beginning when sufficient anatomical or functional changes have occurred to produce recognizable signs and symptoms of a disease.

clinical horizon Imaginary line demarcating the manifestation signs and symptoms of disease.

clinical judgement Decision-making that results in naming a client problem.

clinical model of health A model in which health is viewed as the absence of disease in individuals and families or as the absence of dysfunction in families.

clinical record A system of collecting information about a client, indicating the extent and quality of services being rendered; commonly referred to as "the chart."

chlorofluorocarbons A family of chemicals containing chlorine and fluorine that damages the ozone layer of the air; found in furniture and bedding foam, carpet padding, foam egg cartons and coffee cups, and insulation.

code of ethics Set of statements encompassing rules that apply to people in professional roles.

Code for Nurses The American Nurses Association professional statement prescribing moral behavior and actions of nurses based on moral principles.

codependency A companion illness in drug addiction in which the codependent is addicted to the addict. Strict rules typically develop in the family to maintain their relationship.

coercive health measures Health care treatment and services required regardless of the client's wishes, choices, or life plans. Such care is usually regulated by law and is instituted to protect the public's health.

cognitive-discovery theory Learning associated with the development of thought, language, and intelligence in infants and children.

cognitive domain Area dealing with the recall or recognition of knowledge and the development of intellectual skills.

cognitive learning Acquisition of facts dealing with recall and recognition of information.

cohesion Attraction of group members to one another and to the group.

cohort Group of people born during the same era who are influenced by some of the same biological, psychological, and social factors.

collaboration Mutual sharing and working together to achieve common goals in such a way that all persons or groups are recognized and growth is enhanced.

collaborative practice Professionals working together in a collegial relationship to provide primary health care to a given population.

common fate, principle of Tendency to see objects moving in the same direction as a perceptual unit.

common law Law based on the opinion of the courts; comes from past court decisions or opinions based on fairness, respect for individuals, autonomy, and self-determination.

communicable disease Disease that is primarily infectious in nature; requires interaction between the host and agent, direct or indirect transmission from the agent reservoir in the environment, and a host that can provide adequate living conditions for the infectious agent.

communication The giving and receiving of verbal or nonverbal messages or information.

communication structure Descriptive framework that identifies message pathways and member participation in sending and receiving messages utilized for a group or groups.

community A locality-based entity, composed of interdependent systems of formal organizations reflecting societal institutions, informal groups, and aggregates, and whose function or expressed intent is to meet a wide variety of collective needs. The target of community-oriented practice.

community attitudes Information gathered from professionals and lay people who work with health-related services in the community.

community client Target of service; i.e., the population group for whom healthful change is sought.

community forum An open meeting for members of a particular community or group to address an issue of interest.

community health Meeting collective needs by identifying problems and managing interactions within the community and larger society. The goal of community-oriented practice.

community health nursing Synthesis of nursing and public health practice applied to promoting and preserving the health of populations. The practice is general and comprehensive, with the dominant responsibility to the population as a whole.

community health problem Actual or potential difficulties within a target population with identifiable causes and consequences in the environment.

community health services Services directed to meet the needs of groups; tend to reflect a public health orientation of health promotion and maintenance of capabilities.

community health strength or capabilities Resources available to meet a community health need.

community mental health Orientation toward health care that seeks to provide a program of continuing and comprehensive mental health care to a specific population.

community oriented practice A clinical approach in which the nurse and community join in partnership and work together for healthful change.

community resident survey A direct assessment of the population of a community to identify the need for a service, the acceptability of the service to the population, and the willingness of the people to use and pay for the service.

community support system (CSS) An organized network of caring and responsible people committed to assisting individuals having long-term mental illness to meet their needs without their exclusion from the community.

compensatory damages Money awarded for proven losses.

competitive medical plans Organization of services within a community for the purpose of bidding on delivery of health care to groups of individuals.

compost Aerobic process whereby bacteria, and especially fungi, feed on organic material; uses a 30:1 carbon-to-nitrogen ratio.

Comprehensive Health Planning and Public Health Services Amendments of 1966 (CHP) Landmark legislation that emphasized regional planning; the first time each person's "right to health care" was acknowledged.

compromise An agreement between two or more people or groups with goals that cannot be met without modification of the positions of each person or group; implies "give and take" in the negotiating process.

computing A fear-based coping mechanism to control self-responses during time of stress. Lack of emotion, aloofness, rigidity, and tenseness are characteristics.

concept Category or class of objects or phenomena that represents either an abstract version of the real world (such as an ideal) or a concrete idea (such as a chair or bench).

conceptual framework A group of concepts and a set of propositions that spells out the relationships between them.

conceptual model A set of concepts and the assumptions that integrate them into a meaningful configuration.

concrete operation A level of cognitive development characterized by non-abstract functioning; e.g., children can think about those things they can see.

concurrent audit A method of evaluating quality of ongoing care through appraisal of the nursing process.

conditioning Strategy for behavior modification that depends on shaping a client's behavior by rewarding changes in the direction of the goal.

confidentiality Controlling the disclosure of personal information and limiting the access of others to sensitive information.

conflict Difference in perception, opinion, or priorities between people; can be spoken or unspoken.

conflict sources Factors that may interfere with the relationship or communication between client and nurse.

confounding variables Factors that interact in some unknown way with other factors thought to cause disease.

confrontation intervention Consultant intervention mode that provides for presentation of ideas and facts to the client and reveals the client's values and assumptions that cannot be disputed.

congenital anomaly Any deviant organ or part existing before or at birth in an abnormal form, structure, or location, but not necessarily detected at birth.

congregate housing An alternative living arrangement that provides shelter and support services to assist the elderly to manage community living.

congruence A condition of agreement between persons or consistency within a person's expressions.

connectionism in stimulus-response theories The idea that the connection is the neural joining between a stimulus and the response.

constituents Clients; individuals represented by other person(s).

constitutional law Branch of law dealing with organization and function of government.

constructs Conceptual components that are not directly observable; deliberately created ideas of references that cannot be seen but allow for explanation and analysis.

consultant One who gives professional advice, services, or information.

consultation Interactional or communication process between two or more persons; one is a consultant, and the other is the consultee. The consultant seeks to help the consultee solve a problem or improve or broaden skills.

consultative contract See contracting.

consultee Person seeking the help of an outside, usually impartial, person in problem resolution.

consumer The recipient of health care. Primary clients are the current or former recipients of care; secondary consumers are the client's family or significant others.

consumerism Organized movement and commitment to the belief that people have both a right and a responsibility to be knowledgeable about the choices they make for health and illness care.

continuity of care A desirable goal in the delivery of health care services as a client utilizes multiple providers and services.

continuity theory Theory that emphasizes continuing a person's unique traits and habits into the later years without much change.

contract A promissory agreement between two or more persons that creates, modifies, or destroys a legal relation. It is a legally enforceable promise between two or more persons to do or not to do something.

contracting Any working agreement, continuously renegotiable and agreed upon by nurse and client.

cool down The period of up to ten minutes after intensive exercise in which a person engages in exercises of diminishing intensity to allow the body temperature and heart rate to decrease slowly. This period reduces complications of intense exercise.

coordination Conscious activity of assembling and directing the work efforts of a group of health providers so that they can function harmoniously in the attainment of the objective of client care.

correctness of temporality Evidence that exposure to a causal factor occurs before the onset of the disease.

corroboration Strengthening or adding to credibility by adding or confirming facts or evidence.

cost-accounting studies Studies finding the actual budgetary cost of a program, procedure, or technique.

cost-benefit studies Studies assessing the desirability of a program, procedure, or technique by placing a specific quantifiable value—a dollar amount—on all costs and benfits of the variable to be evaluated.

cost-effectiveness studies Studies measuring the quality of a program, procedure, or technique relative to cost.

cost-efficiency studies Studies analyzing the actual costs of performing a number of services at different volumes when the same standards are applied.

cost-plus reimbursement Method of payment whereby an agency receives actual costs of services delivered plus added allowable expenses, such as depreciation of facilities and equipment and administrative costs.

creative imagery A way to help people create an environment for their own helping processes to occur; uses mental images.

credentialing A mechanism that seeks to produce performance of acceptable quality by individuals and programs of education and service. The four fundamental features of credentialing are quality, identity, protection, and control.

crisis An event in which circumstances are suddenly and unexpectedly altered which presents challenges and calls for new responses in order to prevent disequilibrium.

crisis intervention A short-term method of providing assistance to persons in crisis.

critical path (CPM) A program planning technique which focuses on activities, best use of time and resources, and estimated time to complete activities.

crude rates Statistical rates in which the events in the numerator and the denominator refer to the entire population.

cultural relativism The value of the culture as defined by its meaning to its members.

cultural values The prevailing and persistent guides influencing thinking and actions of people within a culture.

culture Standards for decisions on what is, what can be, how to feel about it, and how to do it.

culture-bound illnesses Illnesses specific to a particular culture (e.g., *mal ojo* [evil eye] in the Mexican American culture).

culture change The constant process of adding or deleting elements within a culture, such as language, customs, beliefs, attitudes, values, goals, laws, traditions, and moral codes.

culture of poverty A status not merely of economic deprivation but also entailing personality traits passed from one generation to another.

culture shock Feelings of helplessness, discomfort, and disorientation experienced by a person attempting to understand or effectively adapt to a different cultural group because of dissimilarities in practices, values, and beliefs.

data collection The process of acquiring existing information or developing new information.

data generation The development of data, frequently qualitative rather than numerical, by the data collector.

data interpretation The process of analyzing and synthesizing data, which culminates in the identification of community health problems and strengths.

data management A method of collecting, organizing, and prioritizing information to use in resolving client problems.

decentralization Services, authority, responsibility, etc., shared from the top of the organization throughout all levels.

decibel (dB) Unit of measure of the level of noise.

deductive approach The reasoning process of developing specific predictions or ideas from general principles.

deinstitutionalization Effort to move long-term psychiatric patients out of the hospital and back into their own community.

delirium tremens Severe reaction to alcohol withdrawal; characterized by disorientation, paranoia, and outbursts of irrational behavior; symptoms also may include tachycardia, fever, rapid breathing, sweating, vomiting, and diarrhea.

Delta Hepatitis A new form of hepatitis which results from a virus which must piggy-back with hepatitis B to cause infection.

dementia Progressive, organic mental disorder characterized by chronic personality disintegration, confusion, and deterioration of mental functioning.

democratic leadership Cooperative structure that promotes and supports members' functioning in all aspects of decision making and planning.

demographic trends Population trends related to age at first marriage; fertility patterns; birth rates; numbers of individuals engaging in singlehood, divorce, and remarriage; number of dependent children experiencing divorce or life with a never-married parent; and the number of elderly persons.

denial A primary symptom of addiction. The person may lie about use, play down use, and blame; may also use anger or humor to avoid acknowledging the problem to self and others.

Denver Developmental Screening Test (DDST) A simple test to evaluate childhood development in the areas of personal/social, fine motor/adaptive, language, and gross motor development.

deontology Doctrine that moral duty or obligation is binding. Also, what makes acts right are nonconsequential characteristics such as fidelity, veracity, justice, and honesty.

Department of Health and Human Services A regulatory agency of the executive branch of government charged with overseeing health and welfare needs of U.S. citizens.

depression Mental state characterized by dejection, lack of hope, and absence of cheerfulness.

dereflection Logotherapeutic technique of simply taking a person's mind off the goal by a positive redirection to another goal. A technique to direct focus away from the problems at hand and to focus on assets and abilities.

descriptive epidemiology First stage of epidemiological investigation; focuses on describing disease distribution by characteristics relating to time, place, and person.

detoxification Gradual withdrawal from an abused substance; best achieved in a controlled hospital setting.

developmental crisis Disequilibrium occurring at a predictable transition in life.

Developmental Profile II Instrument to measure child development from birth to preadolescence in the areas of physical/motor, self-help, social, academic, and communication skills.

developmental disability Pathological condition that begins before 18 years of age and leads to disruption in the normal maturational process.

developmental theory A way of thinking about how changes occur in human development; includes characteristics such as stages, phases, levels, direction, and forces.

diagnosis-related groups A patient classification scheme that defines 468 illness categories and the corresponding health care services that are reimbursable under Medicare.

dietary guidelines Simple, practical food guides developed to assist health care providers in providing good nutritional education to clients.

dioxin Ingredient in the defoliant Agent Orange which can kill and cause birth defects, cancer, and problems of the liver, kidney, nervous system, and skin.

direct causal association Relationship in which a factor causes a disease with no other factors intervening in the process.

direct provider reimbursement Method of payment to a provider for services delivered (e.g., fee-for-service).

disability The loss, absence, or impairment of physical or mental fitness that is observable or measurable.

discharge planning The process of activities facilitating the client's movement from one setting to another. Discharge planning is a process that enhances continuity of care.

disengagement theory Aging theory postulated on the premise of older people withdrawing from society.

dissenter One who disagrees or blocks the actions of another.

distracting A behavioral response that seems irrelevant and completely unrelated to the situation.

distributive care Health maintenance and disease prevention.

district nursing Early public health nursing whereby a nurse was assigned to each district in a town to provide home health care to needy people.

Division of Nursing A component of the Public Health Service, part of the Health Resources and Services Administration, which oversees nursing education and special nursing demonstration projects in the U.S.

documentation The process of recording data in client records.

domain First level of organizing client problems identified by a nurse. Domains reflect environmental, physiological, psychosocial, and health-related behavior problems.

dosage Regimen governing the size, frequency, and number of doses of a therapeutic agent to be administered to a person.

Down's Syndrome See Trisomy 21.

drug resistance Microorganisms that are not susceptible to the action of a drug because of mutations in the cells of the microorganism.

dual diagnosis Clinical determination that a client has both a mental illness and a chemical dependency problem.

duty Moral or legal obligation, or obligation relating to one's occupation or position. Moral duty is based on moral principles and may or may not be supported by law; carrying out a moral duty may even be prohibited by law. Legal duty is that which is required by law.

absolute Cannot be overridden by any other duty; intrinsically right or wrong.

advocacy Moral obligation to speak, write, or take action in support of the client or client populations.

veracity Obligation to tell the truth and not lie or deceive people.

dysfunctional family A family unit that inhibits clear communication within family relationships and does not provide psychological support for individual members.

early adopters Individuals and/or groups with cosmopolitan rather than local orientations, with abilities to adopt new ideas from mass media rather than face-to-face information sources, and with specialized rather than global interests.

ecological fallacy A myth that assumes the relationships observed among groups will be the same for individuals.

ecological studies Epidemiological studies which compare large aggregates of people with other similar large populations.

ecology The science of the relationship between living and nonliving things; concerned with both structure and function.

economics Social science concerned with the problems of using or administering scarce resources in the most efficient way to attain maximum fulfillment of society's unlimited wants.

ecosystem All living things and nonliving parts that support a chain of life within a selected area.

effectiveness A measure of an organization's performance as compared to its philosophy, goals, and objectives.

efficiency The process of meeting goals in a way that minimizes costs and maximizes benefits.

elder abuse A form of family violence against older members. May include neglect and failure to provide adequate food, clothing, shelter, and physical and safety needs; can also include roughness in care and actual violent behavior toward the elderly.

emancipated Free from parental care and control.

emergency nurse practitioner Registered nurse with additional education through a master's degree program in nursing or through a nondegree or certificate continuing education program preparing the nurse to deliver primary care within an emergency room setting.

emotional abuse Extreme debasement of a person's feelings so that he feels inept, uncared for, and worthless.

empathy A condition existing in a relationship in which the feelings, thoughts, and motives of one person are readily understood by another. The ability to "enter" into another's perceptual world.

employee assistance programs The range of services offered in the workplace to assist employees to cope with personal and work-related problems.

empowerment Enabling a client to use his own personal resources. Empowerment can occur as a result of education, crisis resolution, or other experiences in which a client understands and uses self-attributes to increase control over his life.

enabling The act of shielding or preventing the addict from experiencing the consequences of the addiction.

enabling legislation A bill or law passed by Congress to support the development of a specific program or service.

enculturation The process of acquiring knowledge and internalizing values, or learning a culture.

eudaimonistic model of health A model in which health is viewed as maximizing individual and family well-being and potential.

endemic Indigenous to an area or group.

enterobiasis Pinworm infestation.

entitlement theory Theory that people have rights to resources as determined by the natural lottery and may increase their possessions in any way possible (by purchase, gift, or legitimate exchange), as long as they do not cheat others or acquire the possessions in an unjust manner.

entropy A concept stating that elements in a closed environment will proceed toward greater randomness or less order.

environment The internal and external factors that affect the health of people.

environmental health Aspect of community health concerned with those forms of life, substances, forces, and conditions in the surroundings of people that may exert an influence on their health and well-being.

Environmental Protection Agency Established in 1970 to be responsible for air, water, and land pollution control; never achieved its full goal.

epidemic Occurrence of any given disease phenomenon in excess of normal expectation.

epidemiologic triad The host, agent, and environment relationship necessary for a disease to occur.

epidemiology The study of the distribution of states of health and of the causes of deviations from health in populations.

epididymitis Inflammation of the epididymis that may be a complication of gonorrhea or syphilis, resulting in fever and chills, pain in inguinal region and swollen epididymis.

episodic care Curative and restorative aspect of nursing practice.

equalitarian theory. Doctrine that takes the needs of all people into account equally.

ergonomics The study of people at work in order to understand the complex relationships associated with work.

erythema Reddened raised area on the skin produced by a tissue response to small doses of antigenic substances.

established group An existing group of persons linked by membership and group purpose.

estimation of risk Assessing the nature of a problem, size of the problem, and need for a program within a community to prevent occurrence of the problem.

ethical priniciples Abstract guides that serve as foundations for moral rules.

    autonomy To respect people and their rights to make choices and act according to individual determinations.

    beneficence To do good and prevent or avoid doing harm.

    justice Equals should be treated the same, and those unequal in similar respects should be treated differently according to their similarities.

ethical theories Collection of principles and rules providing theoretical foundations for deciding what to do when moral principles or rules conflict.

ethics Science or study of moral values; also a code of principles and ideals that guide action.

ethnic collectivity Group with common origins, a sense of identity, and shared standards for behavior.

ethnicity Groups whose members share a common social and cultural heritage passed on to each generation.

ethnocentrism Belief that one's own group or culture is superior to others.

eustress Positive form of stress; occurs when people convert negative stress into a positive form by changing their attitudes.

eutrophication Process in which nutrients in lakes promote the growth of algae, which causes cloudy, odorous water.

evaluation Collection of methods, skills, and sensitivities necessary to determine whether a human service is needed and likely to be used, is conducted as planned, and actually does help people in need. Also, provision of information through formal means, such as criteria, measurement, and statistics, for making rational judgments necessary in decision-making situations.

evaluative research A method of collecting information according to the rigors of scientific inquiry for the purpose of evaluating the long-term effect of a program.

evaluative studies Systematic method for collecting information to assess the relevance, progress, effectiveness, efficiency, and impact of a program.

excess mortality Premature death; i.e., occurring before the average life expectancy for persons of the same sex.

existential vacuum Feeling of emptiness and meaninglessness; apathy toward life; an inner void.

experience insurance rate A premium rate that is based on an estimate of the risk of claims by the subscriber.

experimental epidemiology Third stage of epidemiological investigation, which uses experimental design for studies to confirm the causal nature of relationships identified through observational studies.

failed expectations Beliefs and notions about marriage and family that arise from myths about marriage and lead to disappointment when family life is not healthy, happy, and fair.

family Two or more individuals coming from the same or different kinship groups who are involved in a continuous living arrangement, usually residing in the same household, experiencing common emotional bonds, and sharing certain obligations toward each other and toward others.

family assessment Systematic collection, classification, and analysis of family data for the purpose of identifying the family's health-related strengths and problems.

family-centered care A care arrangement enabling families to assume the role of advocates, decision makers, and caregivers.

family demography The study of the structure of families and households and the family-related events, such as marriage and divorce, that alter the structure through the number, timing, and sequence of the events.

family developmental framework A model which assumes that family development follows orderly, sequential changes throughout the family's life-span.

family developmental task A growth responsibility that arises at a certain stage in the life of a family, the successful achievement of which leads to satisfaction, approval, and success with later tasks.

family development task A growth responsibility that must be accomplished by a family at a specified developmental stage.

family dynamics Interactions and relationships within the family that influence the work of the family and its ability to complete its functions and tasks.

family functions Behaviors or activities performed to maintain the integrity of the family unit and to meet the family's needs, individual members' needs, and society's expectations.

family health A condition including the promotion and maintenance of physical, mental, spiritual, and social health for the family unit and for individual family members.

Family Life Cycle A developmental theory which divides family life into a series of stages or phases over time. The stages are qualitatively and quantitatively different from the preceding and succeeding stages.

family nurse practitioner/clinician Registered nurse with additional education through a master's degree program in nursing or a nondegree or certificate continuing education program preparing the nurse to deliver primary health care to individuals, groups, and communities of all ages.

family planning nurse practitioner (obstetric/gynecological nurse practitioner) Registered nurse with additional education through a master's degree program in nursing or a nondegree or certificate continuing education program preparing the nurse to deliver obstetrical and gynecological primary care to women.

family roles Behaviors assumed by family members to maintain the organizational structure of the family and to define the division of labor and the family processes.

family self-care A decision-making process that involves the family in self-observation, symptom perception and labeling, judgment of severity, and choice and assessment of treatment options.

family strengths Those factors or forces that contribute to family unity and solidarity and foster the development of the potentials inherent within the family.

family structure (configuration) Refers to the characteristics of the individual members (gender, age, number) who constitute the family unit.

fee-for-service benefit schedule List of physician services with monetary or unit values attached that specifies the amounts third parties must pay for specific services.

fee screen system The use of usual, customary, and reasonable charges (based on regional evaluations in all specialties) by physicians to set their own reimbursement levels for units of service.

fetal alcohol syndrome A condition that may occur when a woman has consumed alcohol regularly during pregnancy (about six drinks per day). Infants tend to be of low birth weight, mentally retarded, and may have behavioral, facial, limb, genital, cardiac, or neurological impairments.

field theory Belief that the environment consists of interdependent events.

figure-ground relationship A relationship in which the perceptual field is divided into an object of focus (figure) and a diffuse background (ground).

financial resources planning The identification of costs associated with implementing a program or project based on the persons, facilities, equipment, and supplies needed to complete the project or program.

fiscal year Annual operating year of the government (October 1 to September 30 of the next calendar year).

fitness Attainment of wellness on a continuing basis. See wellness.

fogging Agreeing in principle in response to criticism; generates a "fog bank" barrier to criticism.

Food Exchange System Dietary guidelines that include six food groups where goods are grouped according to their similarity in calories and food values, so measured amounts of foods within the group may be traded off in meals.

formal communication Organization of channels for transmitting and receiving information within a network—social, professional, political, or economic.

formal group Persons having a defined membership and specified purpose. The group may or may not have an official or public place in the community's organization.

formal operations Level of cognitive development in which thoughts are independent of physical experience and allow children to deal with hypothetical questions.

formal structure The established power and communication relationships within an organization.

formative evaluation An evaluation instituted for the purpose of assessing the degree to which objectives are met or planned activities are conducted.

freebasing Homemade refining process that extracts a concentrated form of cocaine from its chemical base and then smokes it in a water pipe usually filled with liquor.

free radical theory Theory of aging based on the premise that an imbalance between the production and elimination of free radicals as contributes to aging.

functional family A family unit which provides autonomy and is responsive to the particular interests and needs of individual family members.

functional health patterns A derivature of NANDA, which reflects an organization and naming of client problems based on client functions.

functional nursing A nursing care delivery model which assigns staff nurses and other personnel to perform functions such as giving medicines, performing treatments, and teaching.

fungicide Chemical agent that kills or retards the growth of fungi.

gatekeeper A function of case/care management in which the nurse ensures that clients have access to appropriate and cost effective care within a service system.

general adaptation syndrome Manifestations of stress in the whole body as they develop in time. This happens in three stages: (1) alarm reaction, (2) resistance, and (3) exhaustion.

generalist A nurse who provides a wide range of nursing services to clients.

general systems theory As defined by von Bertalantfy, a complex of elements in mutual interaction. The elements are wholeness, organization, and order.

genital warts Lesions caused by the human papillomavirus.

geriatric day care facility Ambulatory health care facility for elderly people; uses a broad range of professional and community services to maximize functional independence for this age group in the home and community.

geriatric nurse practitioner Registered nurse with additional education through a master's degree program in nursing or a nondegree or certificate continuing education program preparing the nurse to deliver primary health care to older adults.

gerontology A field of study that explores the biopsychosocial issues of aging.

gestalt German word meaning pattern or configuration.

gestational age The number of weeks spent in utero to the time of birth.

goal attainment A process for assessing the efficacy of a program by examination or measurement of predetermined goals.

goals/objectives A consultative problem that involves the inability of a group or individual to accept new goals, change goals, or meet established goals.

Gonorrhea A gram negative intracellular diplococcus bacteria that infects the mucous membranes of the genitourinary tract, the rectum, and the pharynx. Transmitted through direct contact. The sexually transmitted disease caused by a bacteria, Neisseriae gonorrhea, resulting in inflammation of the genital mucous membrane of either sex, dysuria, or no symptoms.

greenhouse effect Global condition resulting from the burning of fossil fuel, which gives off carbon dioxide and is warming the earth's atmosphere, changing weather conditions throughout the world and decreasing water supplies in some parts of the world.

Gross Domestic Product A statistical measure used to compare health care spending between countries.

gross national product (GNP) The total value of all final goods and services produced in the country in one year.

group A collection of interacting individuals who have a common purpose or purposes.

group cohesion Measurement of degree of attraction between members and toward the group.

group culture A composite of the group norms that comes to dictate perceptions and behaviors.

group norms Unwritten and often unspoken standards for group members that guide their behavior and influence their attitudes and perceptions.

group purpose The reason two or more people come together; may be subtle or obvious and easily stated by members.

group structure The particular arrangement of group parts that comprises the whole.

haemophilius influenza A leading cause of serious systematic bacterial disease in the U.S.

hallucinosis A condition that can result from alcohol withdrawal; the person remains oriented and rational but may be confused about time.

handicap The total adjustment to disability that limits functioning at a usual level.

hardiness The ability to adjust to or benefit from stressors; a motivating factor in resolving stressful situations and in adapting to health problems.

hazards Biological, physical, chemical, or psychosocial threats to the environment.

health Balanced state of well-being resulting from harmonious interaction of body, mind, and spirit.

health belief model What one believes about health based on perceptions of susceptibility, seriousness, and advantages or disadvantages of action. Useful in promoting adherence to treatment regimen.

health care Product of health services delivered through personal or public health services.

health contract An agreement, usually written, between client and health care provider which identifies and assigns priorities for health goals and includes measurable criteria to be met within a designated time-frame.

health economics Branch of economics concerned with the problems of producing and distributing the health care resources of the nation in a way that provides maximum benefit to the most people.

health education Any combination of learning experiences designed to facilitate adaptations of behavior conducive to health.

health index A summary of the health features of a community that enables us to determine health care delivery needs.

Health Maintenance Organization (HMO) Organized system of health care that provides for fixed fee physician services, emergency and preventive treatment, and hospital care for people who pre-selected this form of care.

health paradigm A model of practice in which humans are viewed as organismic beings characterized by wholeness.

health planning A continuous social process by which data about a client are collected and evaluated for the purpose of creating "a plan" to guide change in health care delivery.

health policy Public policy that affects health and health services. Delineates options from which individuals and organizations make their health-related choices. Made within a political context.

health practitioners Members of the primary health care team who as colleagues develop strategies for combining their expertise so that they can be integrated in a complementary way to address the health needs of the clients.

health promotion Behaviors designed to increase the health and well-being of individuals, families, and communities.

health promotion model A model organized like the health belief model and directed toward increasing the level of well-being in a person or group.

health risk appraisal Process of identifying and analyzing an individual's prognostic characteristics of health and comparing them with those of a standard age group, thereby providing a prediction of a person's likelihood of prematurely developing the health problems that have high morbidity and mortality in this country.

health risk/health risk factor Disease precursor whose presence is associated with higher-than-average morbidity and/or mortality. Disease precursors include demographic variables, certain individual behaviors, positive individual and/or family history, and some physiological changes.

health risk reduction Application of selected interventions to control or reduce risk factors and minimize the incidence of associated disease and premature mortality. Risk reduction is reflected in greater congruousness between appraised and achievable ages.

health services Personal and public services performed by individuals or institutions for the purpose of maintaining or restoring health.

health status The state or level of health of an individual, family, or community at a given time.

health systems agency Federally funded agency that plans and approves the development of health care facilities in a community.

helminth Wormlike animal.

hepatitis Inflammatory condition of the liver caused by viral or bacterial infection, parasites, alcohol, drugs, toxins, or transfusions of incompatible blood.

herbicide Chemical agent used to destroy unwanted plants.

herpes Any one of five related viruses that attack skin, genitalia, or cranial, cervical, or spinal nerves; infection is characterized by severe pain and various acute symptoms.

Hill-Burton Act First U.S. legislation to focus on planning as a major area of concern. Its primary purpose was to provide for a more equal distribution of hospitals across the nation by matching federal funds for one-third to two-thirds of the total cost of a facility.

HIV antibody test A test used in screening blood for the antibody to HIV, most commonly the enzyme-linked immunosorbent assay (ELISA). The Western Blot is used as a confirmatory test.

HIV disease A disease involving a defect in cell-mediated immunity that has a spectrum of clinical expressions including a long incubation phase and AIDS.

HIV infection Infection with the human immunodeficiency virus. A phase of this infection is subclinical, but infected individuals remain capable of transmitting the virus through specific behaviors.

HIV Seronegative A screening process resulting in lack of identification of the human immunodeficiency virus in a client's blood.

HIV Seropositive A screening process resulting in identification of the human immunodeficiency virus in a client's blood.

HIV Seroprevalence The number of new and old cases of persons in the U.S. identified with human immunodeficiency virus in their blood.

HMO Act Legislation enacted in 1973 to provide a demonstration program for the development of health maintenance organizations.

holism A concept which requires that human behavior not be isolated from the context in which it occurs and that a culture be viewed and analyzed as a whole.

home health agency An organization that provides skilled nursing and other related skills in the home.

home health care An arrangement of health-related services provided to people in their place of residence.

homelessness A state in which a person's primary residence is a public or private shelter, a park, car, or abandoned building.

homeostasis Relative constancy in the internal environment of the body.

home visiting See home health care.

homicide Any violent death that is neither a suicide nor an accident.

hospice Palliative system of health care for terminally ill people; takes place in the home with family involvement under the direction and supervision of health professionals, especially the visiting nurse. Hospice care takes place in the hospital when severe complications of terminal illness occur, or when there is family exhaustion or loss of commitment.

host Human or animal that provides adequate living conditions for any given infectious agent.

household A single dwelling (apartment or house) occupied by an individual or a group of two or more individuals (related or unrelated).

Human Immune Disease A term used to refer to symptomatic HIV infection.

Human Immunodeficiency virus (HIV) The virus that causes AIDS.

humanistic theory Theory emphasizing the importance of feelings, emotions, and personal relationships in determining behavior.

human papillomavirus infection A sexually transmitted disease that results in genital warts (condyloma acuminata) that grow in the vulva, vagina, cervix, urinary meatus, scrotum, or perianal area. A link exists between HPV infections and cancer.

human resources planning Planning for the use of human knowledge and skills available or identified as essential to implementing the goals of a program or project.

hydrocarbons Family of compounds containing carbon and hydrogen.

hydrocephalus Increased accumulation of cerebrospinal fluid in the ventricles of the brain due to interference with the circulation and absorption of the fluid.

hyperactivity A behavior disorder with characteristic clinical manifestations resulting in inappropriate amounts of non-goal-directed activity.

hyperbilirubinemia Elevated levels of unconjugated bilirubin resulting from deficiency or inactivity of bilirubin glucuronyl transferase.

hypothesis A supposition or question that is raised to explain an event or guide investigation.

iatrogenesis Physician-induced illness. Clinical iatrogenesis, the most familiar, includes illnesses created as by-products of medical intervention (e.g., infections caused by antibiotics that alter the body's normal bacterial flora).

iatrogenic guilt Guilt engendered at the time of illness because of assignment of blame for the illness by the care provider to the patient. For example, a patient with heart disease may be told by his physician, "You could have avoided this by not smoking, exercising regularly, and eating a diet low in animal fats."

imagery Creation of mental pictures; can be spontaneously or deliberately created and used for many purposes.

immune globulin (IG) Sterile solution containing antibodies from human blood. IG is primarily indicated for routine maintenance of certain immunodeficient individuals and for passive immunization.

immunity Natural or acquired ability to ward off disease.

immunization A process of protecting an individual from a disease through introduction of a live, killed, or partial component of the invading organism into the individual's system.

immunological theory Aging theory based on the premise that normal cells are unrecognized as such, thereby setting off an immune reaction.

impairment A disturbance in structure or function resulting from anatomical, physiological, and/or psychological abnormalities.

implementation Carrying out a plan that is based on careful assessment of need.

incest Sexual abuse among family members, typically a parent and a child.

incidence rate The rate of newly occurring cases of a disease in a population over a defined period of time.

incidental additives Food additives resulting from the use of pesticides or herbicides, or from chemical changes brought about by processing methods.

incineration Burning of wastes.

incubation period The length of time from host exposure to an infectious agent until the organism multiplies to sufficient numbers to produce a host reaction and clinical symptoms.

independent practice Private practice of a professional who works independently from other professionals.

indirect provider reimbursement Payment to an agency for services delivered by health providers, such as nurses.

individual developmental task A responsibility originating during a certain period of an individual's life; successful achievement of the task leads to satisfaction and to success with later tasks; failure leads to dissatisfaction within the individual, difficulty with later tasks, and social disapproval.

inductive approach The reasoning process of developing general rules or ideas from specific observations.

infection Complex interaction between a host and a specific agent that entails the replication of organisms in the tissue of the host.

infectivity Organisms's ability to spread rapidly from one host to another.

informal caregiver A voluntary caregiver who may or may not be related to the client. This caregiver usually does not receive payment for the caregiving services rendered but may actually give care more hours of the day than the formal (professional or ancillary) health care worker.

informal communication Interaction channels that arise out of the interpersonal relationships of network parts.

informal group A group of persons having no articulated membership or purpose.

informal structure The communication network established by the employees within an organization.

informant interviewing Directed conversation with selected members of a community about community members or groups and events. A direct method of assessment.

informed consent The situation in which the client agrees to a treatment plan after receiving sufficient information concerning the proposal, its incumbent risks, and the acceptable alternatives.

inherent resistance The ability to resist disease independently of antibodies or of specifically developed tissue response.

injectable drug use Includes intravenous and subcutaneous drug injection; the latter usually over the abdominal area and called "popping." The sharing of paraphernalia to prepare or inject the drug can result in transmission of blood-borne pathogens, such as HIV.

insecticide Chemical pesticide used to control insects.

institutional licensure A mechanism for allowing employing agencies to be responsible for the competence of the people they employ.

instructive district nursing Nursing provision begun in Boston, which included health education the family centered health care provided.

integration The incorporation of development tasks and skills into a repertoire of effective behavior.

intentional additives Substances deliberately added in food processing to enhance or conserve nutritional value or to improve or maintain flavor, color, texture, or consistency.

interacting group A cluster of individuals who are linked by personal relationships. The links may be either primary, such as in a family, or secondary, such as in a voluntary association.

interactional framework Model focusing on the family as a unit of interacting personalities which examines the symbolic communication processes by which family members relate to one another.

interaction models Models that rely on the concepts of communication, role, perception, and self-concept.

interdisciplinary Activities involving the collaboration among personnel representing different disciplines (occupational therapists, nurses, physical therapists, physicians, environmental hygienists, etc.).

intervention activities Means or strategies by which objectives are achieved and change is effected.

introspection Process of an individual's inward examination of traits, habits, and qualities.

invasion of privacy Violation of the right to be left alone to live in seclusion without being subjected to unwarranted or undesired publicity.

invasiveness Agent's ability to spread within the host.

involuntary smoking Inhaling by a nonsmoker of tobacco combustion products in a smoke-filled atmosphere.

joint practice Practice in which professionals work together in a complementary and consultative manner.

judicial law Law based on court or jury decisions.

justice Ethical principle which claims that equals should be treated equally and those who are unequal should be treated differently according to their differences.

Kawasaki disease (mucocutaneous lymph node syndrome) Acute febrile illness that occurs predominately in children under 5 years of age. No causative agent has been identified.

kernicterus Neurological damage that occurs when unconjugated bilirubin is deposited in brain tissue.

key informants Professional experts, community leaders, politicians, and entrepreneurs who are in touch with the needs of the community and who are in positions to support new community programs.

Korsakoff's psychosis Condition resulting from excessive alcohol consumption, characterized by disorientation and a memory defect whereby people fill in the gaps by making up forgotten information.

law The sum total of man-made rules and regulations by which society is governed in a formal and legally binding manner.

law of effect A principle in conditioning theories of learning which states that reward increases the strength of a connection while punishment does nothing to the strength of the connection.

law of exercise A principle in conditioning theories of learning which states that connections between a stimulus and a response are strengthened when they are used.

law witness One who testifies to what he has seen, heard, or otherwise observed.

lay advisors Individuals who are influential in approving or disapproving new ideas and who seek advice and information from others about these things.

leader An individual who is given informal power in an oganization by followers.

leadership A process used to move individuals as a group toward a goal.

learning Gaining of knowledge, understanding, or skill.

learning disability A broad range of problems that may interfere with a person's ability in the areas of memory, language, perception, or motor abilities.

least restrictive alternative A response to institutionalization whereby mentally ill people remain in the community and are maintained with the least restrictions they can handle.

legionnaires' disease (legionellosis) Pneumonia-like communicable disease caused by *Legionella pneumophilia*. Mode of transmission is presumed to be airborne.

legislation Bills introduced by Congress for the purpose of establishing laws which direct policy.

legislative process The process used within governments to make laws.

leveling A healthy communication style in which family members under stress are able to say what they feel and believe.

levels of prevention A three-level model of interventions based on the stages of disease, designed to halt or reverse the process of pathological change as early as possible, thereby preventing damage.

liability An obligation one has incurred or might incur through any act or failure to act, or responsibility for conduct falling below a certain standard which is the causal connection to the plaintiff's injury.

licensure Legal sanction to practice a profession after attaining the minimum degree of competence to ensure protection of public health and safety.

life-style-induced health problems Diseases with natural histories that include conscious exposure to certain health-compromising or risk factors. For example, heart disease is life-style-induced; that is, its onset is generally preceded by smoking, unwise eating, failing to exercise, and sustaining unbuffered stress.

litigation Trial in court to determine legal issues and the rights and duties between the parties.

logotherapy Treatment modality based on a blend of humanistic and existential psychology which assists the client in finding meaning and purpose in life and in unique life experiences.

long-term care facility (nursing home) Typically for the older adult, where individuals can receive minimum to maximum skilled nursing care, depending on the type of facility and the need of the client.

macrolevel interventions Health-generating changes carried out at the societal level.

mainstream smoke Smoke inhaled and exhaled by the smoker.

maintenance functions Behaviors that provide physical and psychological support and therefore hold the group together.

maintenance norms Norms that create group pressures to ensure affirming actions for members and are helpful in maintaining comfort

malpractice Professional misconduct, improper discharge of professional duties, or a failure to meet the standard of care by a professional which results in harm to another.

malpractice litigation A lawsuit resulting from client dissatisfaction with the provider and the content or quality of care received; a quality assurance measure.

managed care A system of health care delivery in which clients are subjected to case management that seeks to control access and utilization activities as part of cost-containment and accepted practice parameters. Examples include Health Maintenance Organizations.

manager One who is given official power by the organization to coordinate the individual efforts of others to achieve organizational goals.

mandatory credentialing Certification requiring statutory law (e.g., state nurse practice acts).

mandatory nurse licensure A law that requires all who practice nursing for compensation to be licensed.

mass media Newspapers, TV, radio, or other modes of communication to large audiences.

maternal-infant bond See bonding.

maturational crisis Crisis resulting from an inability to accomplish tasks necessary to move to next developmental stage.

maximin theory Economic theory of distribution of goods and resources to maximize the minimum position in society while at the same time allowing exercise of liberty on the part of all people.

Meals on Wheels Local programs in which one hot meal and sometimes a cold breakfast and sack lunch are delivered to elderly people in their homes.

mediating structures Institutions standing between the individual in private life and the larger institution of public life, such as one's neighborhood, family, church, on voluntary associations.

mediator A role in which the nurse acts to assist parties to understand each other's concerns and to determine their conclusion of the issues. The mediator has no authority to decide on behalf of another.

Medicaid A jointly sponsored state and federal program which pays for medical services for the aged, poor, blind, disabled, and families with dependent children.

medically indigent A portion of the population who are usually above the recognized poverty level and have money to buy the necessities of life but who cannot afford a catastrophic illness or an acute illness crisis.

medical technology A set of interventions, drugs, equipment, and services used to deliver health care.

Medicare A federally funded health insurance program for the elderly, disabled, and persons with end-stage renal disease.

meditation A form of self-discipline that helps people achieve inner peace by focusing uncritically on one thing at a time.

mental retardation Disorder characterized by subaverage general intelligence with impairments in the ability to learn and to fully adapt socially.

methadone A synthetic narcotic analgesic used for anesthesia or as a substitute for heroin.

microbiological food contamination Results from toxins deposited in food.

microlevel interventions Health-generating changes performed at the individual level. Examples are cognitive restructuring, self-confrontation, modeling, conditioning, and stimulus control.

middle adult Individual who is in a transitional stage between young adulthood and old age; person in the 36 to 64 year-old age group, whose psychosocial task is generativity versus stagnation.

middlescence Intermediate stage of life between young adulthood and old age, marked by physical, psychological, and social changes; the developmental task is generativity.

minimal brain dysfunction A descriptive term of a child of average intelligence who has difficulty learning.

minimum data set A minimum set of items of information concerning an aspect or dimension of the health care system. Nursing's minimum data set reveals the comparability of nursing data across clinical populations, settings, geographic areas, and time.

minority A racial, religious, ethnic, or occupational group that constitutes a small part of the population.

mobile clinics A method of providing ambulatory care in a variety of geographic locations via use of specially equipped vans.

model A representation of reality.

modeling Strategy for self-modification that depends on the client's observing the behavior of others who have realized the goal the client has identified as his own.

modifier A set of two terms used with each client problem to name the client and categorize the problem.

moral accountability A moral obligation that directs the professional nurse to act in a particular way according to moral norms and requires the nurse to be answerable for what has been done.

morale/cohesion problem A situation that occurs when a client has lost confidence in his ability to solve problems and feels powerless to institute corrective action.

moral obligation Duty to act in a particular way in response to moral norms.

moral virtue Ideal standard of human behavior or thinking; excellence in respone to moral norms, such as goodness.

morbidity Relative disease rate; usually expressed as incidence or prevalence of a disease.

mortality Relative death rate; the proportion of deaths at a particular time and place.

mothering The process of caring for an infant.

motherliness The capacity of the mother to be gratified by the exchange between herself and her infant and to use gratification for her own growth.

motivation A conscious or unconscious need or desire to act.

multiattribute utility A planning method based on decision theory.

multiproblem family A family unit that faces a number of events within and without the family environment and does not have the ability to solve its own problems.

multisectional approach An approach to improving the status of a person, group, or community that includes many components (e.g., health, education, environment, industry).

mycotoxin Toxic metabolite that can be produced by food molds.

Narcotics Anonymous Support group for narcotics addicts.

National Center for Nursing Research A component of the National Institutes of health charged with promoting the growth and quality of research in nursing.

National Health Planning and Resources Development Act of 1974 (P.L. 93-641) Legislation set forth to coordinate and direct national health policy via state and regional regulatory agencies; its major goal was to establish a nationwide network of health systems agencies.

National Health Service Corps Program established in 1970 by the Public Health Service to recruit health providers to areas experiencing shortages in health work forces.

National Institute of Occupational Safety and Health (NIOSH) The branch of the USPHS responsible for investigating workplace illnesses, accidents, and hazards.

National Joint Practice Commission Organization established by the American Nurses' Association and the American Medical Association to promote collaborative efforts between medicine and nursing; disbanded in 1981.

National Labor Relations Act Passed in 1935 and known as the Wagner Act; protected employees' rights to organize and join unions and also provided for action against unfair labor practices of employers.

National Labor Relation Act Amendments of 1974 (P.L. 93-8360) Amended the Taft Hartley Act of 1947 and extended the right to organize collectively for matters concerning wages, hours, and working conditions to all employees of nonpublic health care facilities.

National Labor Relations Board Administrative agency for implementing federal policy affecting labor relations.

nationally notifiable conditions Certain communicable diseases defined by the Centers for Disease Control as requiring weekly, monthly, and annual reports of occurrence by all states.

natural history Process of development and progression of a disease without intervention by humans.

natural law Doctrine holding that there is a natural moral order or natural moral law inherent in the structure of the universe which can be known by human reason.

natural radiation Radiation that comes from soil, certain rocks, body potassium, and ultraviolet sun rays.

negintropy Energy in a system that propels toward order or can be used for work.

negligence Failure to act as an ordinary, prudent person; conduct contrary to that of a reasonable person under a specific circumstance.

negotiating A process for resolving a difference using principles of communication, conflict resolution, and assertiveness.

neural tube defect Congenital malformation involving defects in the skull and spinal column; caused primarily by failure of neural tube to close during embryonic development.

"Nightingalism" Ideology emphasizing self-sacrifice on the part of the nurse, when the primary concern of the nurse is the welfare of the client with minimum attention to personal economic and general welfare needs.

nitrogen oxide A toxic gas that comes primarily from automobile exhaust or by-products of industry.

Noise Control Act Legislation passed by Congress in 1972 to identify major sources of noise, establish noise emission standards, and provide a mechanism for people to take civil action on their own behalf when a person or agency violates the Act.

nonassertive behavior Denial of one's own rights by failing to express thoughts, beliefs, and feelings honestly.

noncausal association Relationship in which a factor varies systematically with a causal factor and therefore with the occurrence of the disease, but in which the factor is not a cause of the disease.

Nongonococcal Urethritis (NGU) Inflammation of the urethra from microorganisms other than Neisseriae gonorrhea; Chlamydia thrachomatis has been implicated as the cause in 50 percent of all cases.

Nonoxynol-9 A spermicidal gel found in some sexual lubricants, contraceptive foams, and jellies which has viricidal properties. Nonoxynol-9 may also be found in condoms and can be used as a lubricant to protect against HIV.

nontraditional family Alternative family structures comprised of two or more individuals coming from the same or different kinship groups who are involved in a continuous living arrangement, usually residing in the same household, experiencing common emotional bonds and sharing certain obligations toward each other and toward others.

noogenic neurosis Mental health problem caused by spiritual (not religious) problems or moral conflicts; a type of mental conflict in which values are not clarified.

norms Standards that guide, control, and regulate individuals and communities.

norms/standards A consultative intervention when organizational or professional norms, values, or principles are violated or changed.

North American Nursing Diagnosis A classification system for identification and naming of client problems by nurses.

nosocomial infection In the episodic setting an infection that is not present or incubating at the time of admission. In the distributive setting any infection that is not present or incubating at the time the client is initially admitted for care by a given agency or service.

NREM Sleep A quiet brain within a moveable body. Type of sleep which progresses through four stages from a sensation of floating to deep sleep.

nuclear (traditional) family A unit comprised of mother, father, and young children.

nurse practitioner Nursing role that includes a primary care component that focuses on health maintenance, disease prevention, and client counseling.

nursing care delivery model Framework for organizing the work of nurses and assigning tasks. Examples are primary nursing, functional nursing, and team nursing.

nursing centers Health care facilities in which the primary aim is to offer nursing services, including health assessment, promotion, screening, and health teaching.

nursing diagnosis A clinical judgement about individual, family, or community responses to actual or potential health problems/life processes.

nursing practice Nurse clinical activities and behaviors which are performed on behalf of clients.

nursing process A clinical decision-making method which involves assessing, planning, implementing, and evaluating client care. Assessment of client problems results in formulating a nursing diagnosis.

nutrients Vitamins, minerals, proteins, fats, and carbohydrates essential to sustain health.

obesity Weight of 20 percent more than the recommended normal weight for height, body structure, and sex; caused by heredity, interpersonal, and/or environmental factors.

objective A precise behavioral statement of the achievement that will accomplish partial or total realization of a goal. The date by which the achievement is expected is specified.

obstructor One who impedes or blocks the actions of another.

occupational health The state in which a worker is able to function at an optimum level of well-being (see HEALTH) at the worksite; reflected by higher employee productivity, increase in work attendance, reduction in workers' compensation claims, and increase in longevity in employment status.

occupational medicine Special field of preventive medicine concerned with the medical problems and practices relating to occupation and especially to employees of industry.

Occupational Safety and Health Administration (OSHA) Federal agency charged with improving worker health and safety by establishing standards and regulations and by educating workers.

official agencies Agencies operated by state or local governments to provide home health care.

Older American's Act Legislation enacted in 1965 to mandate and provide funds for services, programs, and activities deemed essential to accomplish certain goals for older American meeting specified criteria.

Omaha Problem Classification Scheme A system of organizing and naming client problems using a framework of domains, problems, modifiers, and signs/symptoms.

Omaha System A system of nursing diagnoses, interventions, and evaluations of outcomes of care developed by the Omaha Visiting Nurses' Association.

ombudsman A role of a community health nurse in which the investigation of complaints about health care services and providers is the predominant activity.

operant behavior Behavior not elicited by a known stimulus but simply emitted by the organism.

operant conditioning Form of learning used in behavior therapy whereby a person is rewarded for correct response and punished for incorrect response.

orchitis Inflammation of one or both of the testes; characterized by pain and swelling and often caused by mumps, syphilis, or tuberculosis.

organizational theory A set of observations, assumptions, and hypotheses concerning employees and managers in an organization, and a framework for understanding their behavior.

osteoporosis Disorder characterized by abnormal rarefaction of bone.

Outcome A change in client health status as a result of care or program implementation.

ozone Unstable colorless gas with an oxidizing power surpassed only by fluorine.

pandemic A epidemic that includes widespread geographical areas of the world.

paradoxical intention Logotherapeutic technique whereby the client is encouraged to do what he fears and in fact to exaggerate it to the point of humor; useful in the treatment of phobias.

parent-child bond The synchronization of the parents and the child as a unit, resulting in a unique emotional relationship.

participant observation Conscious and systematic sharing in the life activities and occasionally in the interests and affects of a group of persons; observational methods of assessment; a direct method of data collection.

partner notification Identifying and locating sexual and injectable drug-use partners of people who have been diagnosed with a sexually transmitted disease in order to notify the partners of exposure and encourage them to seek medical treatment. Also known as contact tracing.

partnership Informed, flexible, and negotiated distribution of power among all participants in the process of change for community health. The means for improved community health.

passive Submissive, accepting without objection or resistance.

passive immunization Administration of a preformed antibody to a susceptible host.

paternal-infant bond The development of a reciprocal relationship between a father and infant, which facilitates the development of the paternal role in the family and provides for the emotional and physical needs of the infant.

pathogenic paradigm A model of community health nursing practice in which health is viewed as freedom from disease.

pathogenicity An agent's relative ability to produce disease.

Patient Bill of Rights A document prepared by the American Hospital Association that defines the provider-client relationship within an organization.

pedagogy Art and science of teaching children; based on belief that the purpose of education is the transmittal of knowledge.

pediatric nurse practitioner Registered nurse with certificate or master's level advanced education in the areas of health assessment, diagnosis, and treatment of children. The program prepares the nurse to deliver primary health care to infants and children.

pediculosis Infestation of various hairy body sites by different subspecies of *Pediculus humanus,* or lice.

pelvic inflammatory disease (PID) Infection of the female reproductive organs, especially the fallopian tubes and endometrium, resulting in infertility and/or ectopic pregnancy. Acute symptoms and signs include lower abdominal pain, increased vaginal discharge, urinary frequency, vomiting, and fever. PID results from untreated gonorrhea and chlamydia.

perception A person's interpretation of an event, action, or situation.

perfectionism Characteristic of people devoted to always striving to complete an assignment as nearly perfect as possible.

performance budget A financial plan that shows clearly and concisely the services to be provided in return for the funds available or income generated.

periodontal disease Disease of gum tissue caused by bacterial plaque, resulting in gingivitis (inflammation of the gums) and periodontitis (destruction of supporting bones and ligaments, resulting in loose or drifting teeth). The leading cause of loss of teeth after age 35.

periodontoclasia Loosening of permanent teeth.

peripheral polyneuropathy Affliction of several nerves which usually results from nutritional deficiencies associated with excessive alcohol consumption; characterized by weakness, numbness, partial paralysis of extremities, pain in the legs, and impaired sensory reactions and motor reflexes.

permissive nurse licensure A law that allows a person to practice nursing without a license as long as the term *registered nurse* is not used and the practitioner does not pretend to be licensed.

personal health profiles An assessment of one's health status and risk for specific diseases based on genetics and lifestyle.

personal health services Services directed toward the maintenance of the health status of individuals.

person-year Statistical measure representing one person at risk of developing a disease for one year.

pesticides Chemical poisons used to eliminate pests and to increase annual crop production by generating healthy crops.

physical abuse One or more episodes of extreme disciplining or displaced aggression or frustration, often resulting in serious physical damage to the internal organs, bones, central nervous system, or sense organs.

physical dependency A state of neuroadaption in which continued use of a drug is necessary to prevent withdrawal symptoms.

physical fitness A set of physiological attributes, some of which are health-related, that people have or achieve, including agility, balance, coordination, speed, power, reaction time, cardiorespiratory endurance, muscular endurance, flexibility, muscular strength, and body composition.

physician assistant Health practitioner role created in the 1960s to free physician's time by completing tasks such as taking medical histories and conducting physical examinations.

physician extender Nonphysician health-care provider who performs medical activities typically performed by physicians.

placating Accepting the blame for situations in which one is not at fault.

planning Selecting and carrying out a series of actions designed to achieve stated goals.

planning A systematic approach to developing a plan of action based on a careful assessment.

planning, programming, and budgeting An outcome–oriented accounting system which helps to determine the most efficient use of resources to meet objectives.

plurality patterns Factors related to family size and the pairs of relationships that are a consequence of the number of members in the family.

pneumoconiosis Lung disease associated with dust.

police power States' power to act to protect the health, safety, and welfare of their citizens.

policies Guidelines within which employees of an institution must operate.

pollution Addition of a substance (e.g., noise or toxic chemicals) to an environment that changes its natural qualities.

polysubstance abuse Use of drugs from different categories used together or at different times to regulate how the person feels.

population demography See demographic trends

position (status) Location in a social structure. Occupants of positions are collective categories of people who differ from the general public in some specified shared attribute or behavior.

position power Formal authority associated with an individual's position in the organization.

positive right Claim to other peoples' positive actions

poverty Lack of resources, defined as either an absolute or relative standard.

power/authority issue Question of who has the right to be in charge and who has the right to make a decision.

Practice Acts State laws that govern the practice of health providers.

practice setting Context and/or environment within which nursing care is given.

PRECEDE model A health education model that is outcome–oriented and asks "why" before it asks "how" and can be used with individuals, families, groups, or the community.

precursor or disease precursor Prognostic characteristic or feature of personal health history, health behavior or habit, physical examination, or laboratory or x-ray film findings associated with a higher or lower risk of death than the average.

Preferred Provider Organization (PPO) An organization of providers who contract on a fee-for-service basis with third-party payers to provide comprehensive medical services to subscribers.

prepathogenesis A stage in the natural history of a disease in which the disease has not yet developed although the groundwork has been laid through the presence of factors that favor its occurrence.

presbycusis Loss of hearing and speech intelligibility related to aging.

preschooler A child between the ages of three and six.

prescriptive intervention mode An intervention requiring less collaboration between consultant and client because the consultant explicitly tells the client how to solve the problem.

PRESS Acronym for preschool readiness experimental screening scale, an assessment of the maturational level of children between ages 4 and 5.

presymptomatic disease Early stages of disease when physiological changes have begun but no signs or symptoms are present.

prevalence The number of existing cases of a disease present in a defined population at a given time.

prevention Behaviors designed to avoid disease.

prevention, level of

primary General health promotion.

secondary Identification and prevention of disease and health problems for those who are likely to develop them.

tertiary Health restoration and maintenance.

price inflation Increases in costs of all goods and services in the U.S.

Primary Care Typically the entry point into the health care system; emphasizes health promotion, disease prevention, and management of community–occurring diseases or chronic disease.

primary health care A strategy for delivering essential, affordable, accessible, and acceptable health care to the community.

primary health care team Health care providers with specialized and complementary skills who function together as a team to provide primary health care services.

primary nursing Modality for delivering nursing care in which the client contributes to and receives care, and the provider is not only available but has authority, autonomy, and accountability.

primary prevention Activities directed toward intervening in the natural history of disease before any pathological changes occur in host; these activities seek to keep the agent away from the host or to increase host resistance.

primary relationship Relationship consisting of at least two persons interacting in contingency fashion (the individuals' subjective states and objective behaviors take account of others, are dependent on others, and are reciprocal) within an immediate context as well as a larger milieu.

principles The foundations for rules.

private practice A clinical setting that is usually a single physician's office in which the nurse practitioner is employed.

private sector An individual or any part of society that is not part of the government.

probability Likelihood that an intervention activity can be implemented.

problem analysis Process of identifying problem correlates and interrelationships and substantiating them with relevant data.

problem prioritization Evaluation of problems and establishment of priorities according to predetermined criteria.

problem-solving A process of seeking to find solutions to situations which present difficulty or uncertainty.

professional negligence An unreasonable act or a failure to act when a duty is owed to another, leading to injuries compensable by law.

Professional Standards Review Organizations/Professional Review Organizations Organizations established by law to monitor delivery of health care to clients of Medicaid, Medicare, and Maternal/Child health programs and to monitor implementation of prospective reimbursement.

program budget A financial plan that shows expenses and income related to a specific service.

program evaluation Collection of methods, skills, and sensitivities necessary to determine whether a human service is needed, likely to be used, conducted as planned, and actually helps people.

Program Evaluation and Review Technique (PERT) A network programming method which focuses on key parts, objectives, and time needed to make decisions and evaluate objectives.

program planning method A program planning technique which uses normal groups to assess client problems and find ways to solve the problems.

progressive relaxation Technique for combating tension and anxiety by systematically tensing and relaxing muscle groups.

proportional mortality A measure that relates the number of deaths from a particular condition to all deaths over the same period of time.

prospective medicine Early identification of pathological or potentially pathological processes and the prescription of intervention to stop the processes at this point.

prospective payment system The diagnosis-related group payment mechanism for reimbursing hospitals for inpatient health care services through Medicare.

prospective reimbursement Method of payment to an agency for services to be delivered based on predictions of what an agency's costs will be for the coming year.

protocol Outline or plan for a procedure, written and signed by a physician.

protocols (algorithms) Written, standing orders that have been mutually agreed on by the nurse practitioner and the physician. The nurse practitioner uses them as a guide to manage certain illnesses or conditions.

provider service records A written summary of the provider's work activities on a daily, weekly, or monthly basis.

proximity, principle of Principle that objects that are close together are seen as a perceptual unit.

psittacosis Acute febrile illness that is transmitted to humans by various species of birds.

Psychiatric Mental Health Nursing Domains A system of identification of client mental health problems organized and named according to eight human response patterns.

psychomotor domain Set of tasks including performance of skills that require some degree of neuromuscular coordination.

psychosis Mental disorder often characterized by delusions and hallucinations.

psychotic Pertaining to or affected by psychosis.

psychotropic Drugs that affect psychic function, behavior, or experience.

puberty The biological stage of development during which physical changes occur that make reproduction possible.

public health Organized community efforts designed to prevent disease and promote health.

public health ethic Principle of providing health care services which will offer the greatest good for the greatest number.

public health nursing The field of nursing that synthesizes the public health sciences and the theory of nursing to improve the health of individuals, families, and communities.

public health service An arm of the Department of Health and Human Services that fulfills the function of overseeing health care services within the U.S.

public health services See community health services

pulmonary irritants Substances that get into the respiratory system and induce lung diseases.

quality assurance Monitoring of the activities of client care to determine the degree of excellence attained in the implementation of the activities.

quasivoluntary A form of accreditation that is linked to governmental regulations and encourages programs to participate in a voluntary accrediting process.

race A biological designation whereby group members share distinguishing features, (e.g., skin color, bone structure, and genetic traits such as a blood grouping).

radiation Energy emitted by natural or synthetic radioactive sources. The natural forms come from the sun, soil, and some rocks; synthetic radiation comes from X-rays and radioisotopes in clinical facilities and industry.

radioactive Containing radiation.

radon A radioactive gas caused by the decaying of uranium that can enter homes through floors, cracks, and walls.

rape Natural or unnatural sexual intercourse forced on an unwilling person by threat of bodily injury or loss of life.

rapid eye movement (REM) Movement of the closed eyes during sleep, occurring while the subject is dreaming.

rapport A condition existing in a relationship in which there is mutual trust or emotional affinity.

rate Statistical measure with the frequency of an event as the numerator and the number of persons among whom the event occurred as the denominator.

ratio Statistical measure in which the numerator is not included in the denominator.

rationing Limits placed on health care which may not be beneficial to a client's well being.

reasonable care Degree of skill and knowledge customarily used by a competent health practitioner or student of similar education and experience in treating and caring for the sick and injured in the community in which the individual is practicing.

reasonably prudent person doctrine Requires a person of ordinary sense to use ordinary care and skill.

receptive skills Language skills that provide the toddler with the ability to follow simple instructions.

recertification In home health care, the review and certification performed at least every 60 days by the physician and health care team which demonstrates that the client continues to need a specified plan of care.

reciprocity The recognition and acceptance of a professional's licensure between certain states.

recognition Process whereby one agency accepts the credentialing status of and the credentials conferred by another.

recommended dietary allowances The levels of intake of essential nutrients considered to be adequate to meet the known nutritional needs of practically all healthy people.

referral Guiding clients toward problem-resolution and assisting them in using available resources.

regulations Specific statements of law that relate to and clarify individual pieces of legislation.

rehabilitation Restoration to a former state of functioning, or limiting of impairment and disability to the lowest possible level.

reinforcement To strengthen through added force, support, or encouragement.

relational studies Analytic studies that relate exposure and disease in the same individuals.

relative risk ratio Statistical measure of how much the risk of acquiring a particular disease increases with exposure to a specific causal agent or risk factor.

relative standard Defines poverty in terms of the society's median standard of living.

rem (roentgen-equivalent-man) Measure of the amount of radiation absorbed in human tissues.

representative group Type of community group whose members are elected, appointed, or selected from various community sectors.

rescue fantasy A well-intentioned intervention by a helping person who unwittingly attempts to take over a person's problems to solve them.

respite Relief time from responsibilities for care of a family member.

responeat superior "Let the master answer." The employer is responsible for the legal consequences of the acts of the employee while he acts within the scope of his employment.

retinopathy Noninflammatory eye disorder caused by changes in the retinal blood vessels.

retrospective audit A method of evaluating quality of care through appraisal of the nursing process after the client's discharge from the health care system.

retrospective cost reimbursement Method of payment to an agency based on units of service delivered.

right That to which a person has a just claim.

    legal Claim recognized as valid by a legal system.

    moral Claim recognized as valid by moral principles that in turn may or may not be recognized by legal rules.

right to health Right to not have one's health affected by others (a negative right).

right to health care Right to goods, resources, and services to maintain and improve one's state of health (a positive right).

risk Probability of an unfavorable event, such as developing a disease.

risk appraisal and reduction A quantitative approach comparing data from epidemiologic studies and vital statistics with information supplied by individuals about their 1) health-related practices, 2) health habits, 3) demographic characteristics, and 4) personal and family medical history; the approach is used to predict their individual risks of dying, to provide recommendations for reducing the risks, and to promote healthful behavior changes. Also called health risk or health hazard appraisal.

risk assessment Assessing the probability of developing a disease.

risk factor Disease precursor, the presence of which is associated with higher than average mortality. Disease precursors include demographic variables, certain everyday health practices, family history of disease, and some physiological changes.

risk management Intervention designed to induce and/or sustain changes in health-compromising behaviors, such as counseling, mass media campaigns, or increased production of low-fat dairy goods.

rodenticide Chemical pesticide to kill rodents.

role Identifiable social position associated with a set of behavioral expectations.

role ambiguity Lack of clarity about what is expected.

role behavior What an actor in a position actually does in response to role expectations.

role conflict Presence of contradictory and often competing role expectations.

role negotiation Two or more persons deciding together which tasks, activities, or responsibilities each will accept in a defined situation.

role overload A situation that occurs when there is insufficient time to carry out all of the expected role functions.

role performance model of health A model in which health is viewed as the individual's ability to effectively perform roles and the family's ability to effectively meet their functions and developmental tasks.

role sequence Positions within the family and related behaviors which change over time.

role sharing Arrangement in which both partners have equal claims to the bread–winning role and equal responsibilities for the care of the home and children, including the obligations to contribute equally or equitably to family expenses.

role strain A situation resulting from conditions requiring complex role demands and the fulfillment of multiple roles.

role structure Arrangement of group-member positions according to the expected functions of members.

rubeola (measles) Acute, highly contagious, viral disease involving the respiratory tract and characterized by a rash.

rule of confidentiality Nondisclosure of personal information about others, such as clients, to those not authorized to have this information; also, a rule grounded in the principle of autonomy.

rule of utility Rule derived from the principle of beneficence. Includes the moral duty to weigh and balance benefits and reduce the occurrence of harms.

rules Guidelines, principles, or regulations that govern conduct.

  legal Established by legal principles.

  moral Established by moral principles.

rules and regulations Clear and concise statements mandating or prohibiting certain activity in an institution.

rural areas Areas in open country with a population less than 2,500.

Rural Health Clinic Legislation enacted in 1978 to provide for the development of rural health clinics staffed by new health professionals in existing medically underserved areas of the United States.

salmonellosis A gastroenteritis caused by ingestion of food contaminated with a species of *Salmonella;* characterized by sudden, colicky, abdominal pain, fever, and bloody, watery diarrhea.

Salpingitis Inflammation of the fallopian tubes which may result from gonorrhea or chlamydia. Also referred to as pelvic inflammatory disease.

sampling Selecting a portion of the population to study; can use random or deliberate sampling techniques.

sanitary landfill Method of solid waste disposal whereby waste is taken to canyons, swamps, and ravines, compacted by heavy machines, and covered with earth before rodent infestation occurs.

satellite clinic Health care facility generally operated under the auspices of a large institution but situated in a location away from the institution.

scapegoat Individual in family who is the focus of all family difficulties.

schizophrenia Large group of disorders, usually of psychotic proportion, manifested by characteristic disturbances of thought, mood, and behavior.

school phobia The persistent and abnormal fear of going to school.

school nurse practitioner Registered nurse with certificate or master's level advanced education in the areas of health assessment, diagnosis, and treatment who is prepared to deliver primary health care to school-age children.

scope of practice The usual and customary practice of a profession taking into account how legislation defines the practice of a profession within a particular jurisdiction.

screening Method of dividing people into categories on the basis of the measurement of some characteristic.

secondary analysis Method of assessment in which existing data are used.

secondary care Actions to treat disease in the early, acute phase.

secondary prevention Activities directed toward early detection and treatment of disease.

selected membership group A group of persons brought together for a specific purpose, such as health assessment or promotion. Some members may be linked to others through previous association, or members may be unacquainted before group formation.

self-care Personal and medical care performed by the patient, usually in collaboration with health care providers.

self care diagnostic approach A system of defining a client problem based on health tasks and activities which reflect a client's functional ability and personal resources to practice self care.

self-concept Beliefs one holds about one's self; private self view.

self-confrontation Strategy for self-modification that depends on clients' recognition of and dissatisfaction with inconsistencies in their own values, beliefs, or behaviors or between their own personal systems and those of admired others.

self-determination The right and responsiblity of one to decide and direct one's choices.

self-diagnosis Lay assessment of individual health illness status.

self-esteem The degree of worth one attributes to oneself.

self-health care Continuous or episodic, volitional or unintentional activities that people can do for themselves, individually or collectively, in a variety of health and illness matters.

self health care Lay diagnosis and self treatment, or the process of teaching people how to work with their health care professionals.

self-management The writing and implementation of rules and regulations that are practiced to protect the health of the community or individuals.

self-regulation An essential characteristic of a profession involving activities that have as their goals the overseeing of the rights, obligations, responsibilities, and relationships of a provider to society, to the profession, and to the client. On the individual level, one's ability to exert self-control.

self-regulation One's ability to exert self-control.

self reliance Depending on one's self for maintaining health and for securing needed assistance and care.

senility Mental deterioration associated with old age.

sensitive screening test Laboratory examinations which correctly classify persons with disease as diseased.

seriously mentally ill A term prompted by the consumer movement to reduce the stigma of mental illness; to distinguish from the chronically mentally ill.

seroconversion The appearance of antibodies in serum.

seroprevalence The overall occurrence of HIV antibodies within a specific population at any point in time.

serum sickness Reaction to various serum substances occurring hours or days after the initial injection. It consists of rash, urticaria, arthritis, adenopathy, and fever.

settlement houses Early agencies for visiting nurses.

sexual abuse Abuse ranging from fondling to rape; robs children of the feeling of being in control of themselves; emphasizes their vulnerability.

sexually transmitted disease (STD) Contagious disease usually acquired by sexual intercourse.

shaping Altering behavior by supplying step-by-step reinforcement of actions consistent with desired behavior.

sibling relationship The interaction among brothers and sisters.

sidestream smoke Smoke generated by a smoldering cigarette.

signs/symptoms A cluster of cues and clues suggesting a specific client problem.

situational crisis Crisis resulting from the inability to cope with an unexpected event.

sleep deprivation Condition resulting from distrubed night-time sleep that leads to day-time drowsiness and interference with effective functioning.

social health Level of interpersonal fitness that involves networks of personal contacts established by an individual for the purposes of communication, influence, support, understanding, and prestige.

socialization Process in which people acquire the skills, knowledge, attitudes, and values necessary for performing their social roles.

somatotropin Hormone responsible for growth released by the hypotholamus.

spastic diplegia Classification of cerebral palsy involving paresis of both legs with little or no involvement of the arms.

Special Supplemental Food Program for Women, Infants, and Children (WIC) Federally funded program to promote nutrition among women and children.

specialist A nurse who provides services that are specific to an area of concentration in nursing (e.g., pediatric care).

specific immune globulin Special preparation obtained from human blood preselected for its high antibody count against a specific disease (e.g., varicella zoster immune globulin).

specific protection Measures aimed at protecting individuals against specific agents, such as immunization or attempts to remove agents from the environment.

specific rates Statistical rates in which the events in both the numerator and the denominator are restricted to a specified subgroup of the population.

specificity of the association Uniqueness of a relationship between a causal factor and occurrence of a disease.

specific screening test Laboratory examinations which correctly classify healthy persons as healthy.

spina bifida (neural tube defects) Disturbance in the development of the neural tube early in gestation causing defects in the formation of the spinal cord and possibly the brain. The severity of the condition varies according to the amount of central nervous system tissue involved and may range from absence of brain tissue (anencephaly) to defects anywhere along the spinal column.

spirituality A way of life centered in a human connection with a higher power.

spouse abuse Physical or emotional mistreatment of one's partner.

staff review committees Committees whose function is to monitor client-specific aspects of care appropriate for certain levels of care.

standard of care Those acts performed or omitted that an ordinary prudent person in the defendant's position would or would not have done; a measure by which the defendant's conduct is compared to ascertain negligence.

standardized rates (adjusted rates) Artificial rates of disease that are calculated to allow comparison of rates in populations with differing distributions of characteristics such as age or race.

standards Criteria for measuring conformity to established practice.

statistical indicators Measures of incidence, prevalance, mortality, and other data to 'estimate' client problems, magnitudes of problems, and needs for programs to resolve the problems.

statutes Legislative enactments declaring, commanding, or prohibiting something.

statutory law Law enacted by a legislative body.

stereotypes Exaggerated beliefs and images that are generally false and serve to obscure important differences among members of a group and exaggerate the differences between groups.

stimulus-generalization Conditioning whereby the reaction to one stimulus is reinforced to allow transfer of the reaction to other occurrences.

stimulus-response theory A theory of learning in which environmental conditions (stimuli) affect an organism's reaction (response).

strategic planning A process in which client needs, specific provider strengths, and agency and community resources are successfully matched to offer a service to the community.

strategy Premeditated approach or method of dealing with a situation.

strengthening In stimulus response, an increase in the probability that a response will be made when the stimulus recurs.

strength of the association Degree of a relationship between a causal factor and disease occurrence, usually measured by the relative risk ratio.

stress Condition experienced when physical or emotional demands are placed on people, usually requiring them to change.

stressor Internal or external factors that cause a physical or emotional coping reaction.

structural-functional framework Framework that views the family as a social system with members who have specific roles and functions.

structure In groups, the particular arrangement of group parts that helps to describe the group as a whole.

substance abuse Use of chemicals having actual or potential undesirable effects.

substantive epidemiology Body of knowledge derived from epidemiological studies; for each disease it includes the natural history of the disease, patterns of occurrence, and factors associated with high risk for developing the disease.

suicide Killing oneself.

sulfur oxide Chemical consisting of bluish-white fumes which reduces visibility; generated by burning wood, coal, and petroleum products.

summative evaluation Instituted to assess program outcomes or as a follow-up of the results of program activities.

supervision Denotes line responsibility with active involvement in decision making and implementation activities in an ongoing relationship. It is the antithesis of consultation.

Supplemental Security Income Money awarded to an individual with insufficient resources for the purpose of increasing the income level to a minimum standard.

surveillance The process of monitoring a given population for the occurrence of disease.

survey Method of assessment in which data from a sample of persons are reported to the data collector.

susceptibility Potential to be affected by an agent.

synergism A condition in which factors reinforce one another.

syphilis An infectious, chronic sexually transmitted disease caused by a bacteria, Treponema Pallidum; characterized by the appearance of lesions or chancres which may involve any tissue. Relapses are frequent, and after the initial chancre, syphilis may exist without symptoms for years.

system Complex of elements in interraction.

tactical plan A short-term, flexible, detailed process of defining goals and directions.

Taft-Hartley Act Passed in 1947, a revision of the Wagner Act of 1935; included in the 1947 law was a provision that professional employees should not be organized in the same bargaining unit with nonprofessionals unless a majority of the professional employees voted for such an inclusion.

tardive dyskinesia Disorder characterized by slow, rhythmical, automatic, sterotyped movements, either generalized or in single muscle groups.

target heart rate A heart rate of up to 60% to 85% of age-predicted maximum heart rate during physical activity.

target of service Population group for whom healthful change is sought.

task Function with work or labor overtones assigned to or demanded of a person.

task functions Behaviors that focus or direct movement toward the main work of the group.

taxonomy A framework that provides order to a set of related terms or concepts.

team nursing A nursing care delivery model designed to provide nursing care to a group of clients by a group of nurses. Staff's work is coordinated by a leader.

temporal patterns Seasonal fluctuations in a disease occurrence.

territorialism The perceived or actual assignment of specific client groups or services to a provider group.

tertiary care Actions taken to limit the progression of disease or disability.

tertiary prevention Activities directed toward limitation of disability or restoration of function.

theories of justice Doctrines that indicate how to distribute goods and resources among the population.

theory A clearly stated, operationally defined set of concepts, statements, and hypotheses. A collection of principles and rules.

theory-principles intervention mode A mode in which the client is required to learn theories and their application to problem solving.

therapeutic touch Method of healing that uses a meditative state to enter another person's energy field and passively visualize or free the flow of energy from practitioner to recipient to promote healing.

third-party payments Reimbursement made to health care providers by an agency other than the client for the care of the client (e.g., insurance companies, governments, or employers).

third party payors Insurance companies, governments, and charitable organizations who pay a client's health care bill.

thought-stopping A behavior therapy technique used to help people control obsessive and phobic thoughts by commanding the thought to stop.

threshold limit value Maximum amount of a hazardous substance to which workers can be exposed for 8 hours per day without developing disease.

titer Measure of the concentration of a substance in a solution.

toddler A child of two or three years of age.

tolerance A state characterized by a need to continually increase the dosage of a drug to achieve the desired effects.

tort Legal or civil wrong committed by one person against the person or property of another.

toxic wastes Poisons, inflammables, infectious contaminants, explosives, and radionuclides.

toxicity Ability of a substance to cause injury to biological tissues.

toxoid Modified bacterial toxin that has been made nontoxic but retains the ability to stimulate the formation of antitoxin; used to produce active immunity.

tracer method A method of evaluating programs based on the premise that health status and care can be evaluated by observing the care and outcomes of specific health problems.

transmission agency An epidemiological concept which describes where an infectious agent lives in the environment and how it is transported to a human for disease production.

trend An event which occurs over time and shows a series of fluctuations in its patterns.

triage Deciding which individuals need the most immediate attention and by whom.

triangulation Use of multiple assessment methods. In relationships, the involvement of a third party or object to avoid communication, closeness, or conflict between two individuals.

triggers Temptations that may lead to a relapse in drug usage.

Trisomy 21 Developmental disorder resulting from the presence of an extra chromosome on the 21st pair of chromosomes, causing obvious physical and mental retardation. Also known as Down's syndrome.

tuberculin skin test Intradermal injection of a substance in minute doses in detect or confirm mycobacterial infection.

typology Classification strategies that systematically organize concepts into dimensions of a whole or a configuration of phenomena.

unit of service An entity—individual, family, aggregate, organization, or community—to whom nursing care is given. The level at which service is delivered. The entity from which healthful changes are sought.

urban areas Areas with a population of more than 50,000.

utilitarian theory Economic theory which holds that the best way to distribute resources among people is to decide how expenditures or the use of resources will bring about the greatest net total of good and serve the largest number of people.

utilization review Review directed toward ensuring that care is actually needed and cost is appropriate for the level of care provided.

vaccine Immunizing agent.

validation Substantiating, verifying, or confirming.

values Beliefs about how one should or should not behave. Values are organized into value systems, and individual value systems reflect culture, reference groups, and personal needs.

variables Key characteristics of the problem under study.

vector Agent that actively carries a germ to a susceptible host.

vegetarian Person who abstains from eating animal products.

vertical coordination Hierarchy whereby community health nurses serve as links between their level in the organization and those above and below them. They also serve as links between the agency and the client.

virulence Ability to produce severe disease.

voluntary agency An agency that relies on staff and volunteers to provide a wide range of services; must seek operating funds from a variety of sources, including gifts, dues, and fees.

voluntary certification Process of education, experience, or examination in which a professional elects to engage to be recognized as a specialist.

warm up The period of 5 to 20 minutes before aerobic exercise in which a person engages in activities designed to increase circulation, respiration, and body temperature and gently stretch ligaments and connective tissue to prepare them for more vigorous activity and decrease the possibility of injury.

warts Sexually transmitted, multiple, textured, cauliflower-like lesions which appear on the genitalia, anus, or mouth, caused by human papilloma virus.

wear and tear theory Programmed process wherein cells are constantly wearing out.

web of causation Interrelationships among multiple factors that contribute to the occurrence of a disease.

wellness Dynamic state of health in which individuals progress toward a higher level of functioning, thus maximizing their potential in the environment.

Wernecke's encepholopathy Neurological disorder caused by excessive alcohol consumption; characterized by ophthalmoplegia, nystagmus atoxia, apathy, drowsiness, confusion, and inability to concentrate.

WIC See Special Supplemental Food Program for Women, Infants, and Children.

withdrawal Physical and psychological symptoms that occur when a drug upon which a person is dependent is removed.

Workmen's Compensation Acts Laws requiring employers to assume financial responsibility for wages lost by employees due to occupational injury or illness.

World Health Organization An arm of the United Nations which provides world–wide services to promote health.

yang An ancient Asian health belief of a "male" force that represents light, heat, rejuvenation, and strength. An imbalance of Ying and Yang causes illness.

yin An ancient Asian health belief of a "female" force representing the negative qualities of darkness, cold, weakness, and death.

young adult Individual in the 20- to 35-year-old age group, whose psychosocial task is intimacy versus isolation.

Index